Therapeutic Exercise
Foundations and Techniques

FOURTH EDITION

Carolyn Kisner, ***MS, PT***
Associate Professor
Physical Therapy Program
College of Mount St. Joseph
Cincinnati, Ohio

Assistant Professor Emeritus
The Ohio State University
School of Allied Medical Professions
Physical Therapy Division
Columbus, Ohio

Lynn Allen Colby, ***MS, PT***
Assistant Professor Emeritus
The Ohio State University
School of Allied Medical Professions
Physical Therapy Division
Columbus, Ohio

Illustrations by Jerry L. Kisner, MS

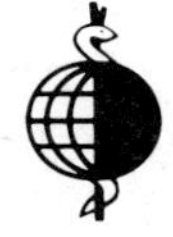

F.A. Davis Company • Philadelphia

F. A. Davis Company
1915 Arch Street
Philadelphia, PA 19103
www.fadavis.com

Printed in the United States of America

Last digit indicates print number: 10 9 8 7 6 5 4 3 2 1

Publisher: Margaret Biblis
Developmental Editor: Peg Waltner
Cover Designer: Louis J. Forgione

As new scientific information becomes available through basic and clinical research, recommended treatments and drug therapies undergo changes. The author(s) and publisher have done everything possible to make this book accurate, up to date, and in accord with accepted standards at the time of publication. The author(s), editors, and publisher are not responsible for errors or omissions or for consequences from application of the book, and make no warranty, expressed or implied, in regard to the contents of the book. Any practice described in this book should be applied by the reader in accordance with professional standards of care used in regard to the unique circumstances that may apply in each situation. The reader is advised always to check product information (package inserts) for changes and new information regarding dose and contraindications before administering any drug. Caution is especially urged when using new or infrequently ordered drugs.

Library of Congress Cataloging-in-Publication Data
Kisner, Carolyn.
Therapeutic exercise: foundations and techniques / Carolyn Kisner, Lynn Allen Colby; illustrations by Jerry L. Kisner.—4th ed.
p. cm.
Includes bibliographical references and index.
ISBN 0-8036-0968-X
1. Exercise therapy—Handbooks, manuals, etc. I. Colby, Lynn Allen. II. Title.

RM725.K53 2002
615.8′2—dc21

2002017442

To Jerry and our growing family—as always, your love and support has sustained me through this project

—CK

To Rick and my extended family—a source of constant support and joy

—LC

To our parents—who have been supportive throughout our lives
To our students—who have taught us so much
To our colleagues—who have been helpful and stimulating in our professional growth

—LC and CK

Contributors

Terri M. Glenn, PhD, PT
Director, Physical Therapy Program
College of Mount St. Joseph
Cincinnati, Ohio

Barbara Settles Huge, PT
Women's Health Specialist/Consultant
Adjunct Faculty, Indiana University Physical Therapy Program
Fishers, Indiana

Janet A. Mulcare, PhD, FASCM
Professor, Physical Therapy Program
Andrews University
Dayton, Ohio

Robert Schrepfer, MS, PT
Former Clinical Director, The Center for Aquatic Rehabilitation
MBA Candidate 2003 Duke University, The Fuqua School of Business
Durham, North Carolina

Preface

Each revision of this textbook is a challenging, demanding, sometimes daunting, and in the final analysis, satisfying task. We believe this edition, as with past editions, is inclusive and up-to-date in light of current research and trends in practice. It continually amazes us how quickly the knowledge base and creative interpretations of basic and applied research including outcome studies influence the delivery of healthcare. Since publication of the Third Edition of *Therapeutic Exercise* in 1996, the American Physical Therapy Association has published and revised the *Guide to Physical Therapist Practice,* many new studies on patient outcomes have been published, technology for communication has expanded, and the healthcare environment has demanded continued high-quality care but more efficient delivery of services. Each of these major factors has influenced the way we think and practice and thus has influenced the presentation of material in this text.

Our original intent when developing the first edition of this textbook over 16 years ago was to provide a foundation of concepts and techniques upon which an individualized program of therapeutic exercise could be built. With each revision we have expanded the content to include new methods of exercise intervention that have been shown to be beneficial in remediating a patient's physical impairments and functional limitations. The foundational material remains an important component of this text. Yet, functional exercise progressions that are built on basic exercise techniques and that prepare patients or clients to return to optimal levels of independence are also integral components of this text. In addition to principles of exercise, background information on various pathologies and musculoskeletal surgeries, descriptions of exercise techniques, and management guidelines are included to assist the reader in the development and progression of comprehensive therapeutic exercise interventions.

What will be most obvious to those who are familiar with previous editions of this text are the changes in format and design of this edition. The double-column format and the use of color were selected to help the reader to locate information more easily and to enhance organization of the material. We have kept the succinct language and straightforward presentation of the content that has been well received in the previous editions; in addition we have expanded the discussion of concepts and techniques to provide the reader with a more comprehensive analysis of the material. Major changes we have made in this Fourth Edition include the following:

- Complete rewriting of Chapter 1 incorporating information on the disablement process and the potential impact of therapeutic exercise on that process, as well as the components of a comprehensive, systematic approach to patient management consistent with the guidelines proposed in the *Guide to Physical Therapist Practice.* A revised outline of a systematic and detailed musculoskeletal examination that used to be in Chapter 1 is now in Appendix A.
- Extensive reorganization of Chapter 3, Resistance Exercise, to include the multi-faceted aspects of muscle performance. In addition, principles and techniques of proprioceptive neuromuscular facilitation for applications of the extremity patterns have been added.
- Addition of material on mobilization with movement (MWM), based on the work of Brian Mulligan, by contributor Jack Miller, an accredited Mulligan concept teacher. The concepts and principles of MWM are presented in Chapter 6, with specific techniques described in each of the respective regional chapters on the extremities (Chapters 9–14).

- Addition of a new chapter on aquatic exercise (Chapter 7) by contributor Robert Schrepfer, MS, PT. Research supporting the use of the aquatic environment in the rehabilitation process of musculoskeletal impairments is integrated with various techniques of exercise interventions.
- Addition of a section at the completion of each chapter entitled *Independent Learning Activities*. This section has several types of activities for students using this text. The subsection called *Critical Thinking and Discussion* has discussion points or a series of questions to stimulate active learning and problem solving or to direct the student to further inquiry. The subsection called *Laboratory Practice* directs the learner toward activities that can be practiced in order to develop specific skills related to the application of therapeutic exercise interventions. The subsection called *Case Studies* presents several case scenarios and questions that reflect the content of the chapter to help the learner integrate the information presented and apply it to real-life situations.
- Reorganization of the spine chapters with the addition of material that reflects current thinking on ways to categorize patient conditions and approaches to intervention (Chapter 15), and the presentation of exercise interventions with emphasis on activation of core stabilizers and stabilization techniques integrated into a comprehensive approach to management of spinal impairments and functional limitations (Chapter 16). Those readers familiar with previous editions will notice that the chapter on spinal traction is not in this edition. Nevertheless we still believe that spinal traction is a useful tool for intervention in the treatment of spinal disorders. Because it can be used to stretch joints and tissues in the spinal region, content specific to this purpose is integrated into the stretching section of the treatment chapter (Chapter 16).
- The chapter on Principles of Exercise for the Obstetric Patient (Chapter 17) has been revised and expanded by contributor Barb Settles Huge, PT, to include basic information and interventions for the management of urinary incontinence.
- A thorough revision of Chapter 18, Management of Vascular Disorders of the Extremities, now includes descriptions and illustrations of exercises for the comprehensive management of lymphedema.
- In previous editions there were two chapters on interventions for and management of pulmonary conditions. The content of those chapters has been reorganized and merged into one chapter (Chapter 19).
- The chapter on Critical Analysis of Exercise Programs, which had been in previous editions, has been deleted from this edition. The idea of using knowledge and skills of kinesiology, examination, and safe application of exercise interventions based on an examination and evaluation of each patient or client is fundamental to all we do as therapists. Therefore it was determined that a separate chapter was no longer needed and the concepts from this chapter were integrated throughout the text.
- Appendices have been added to this edition that include a summary of a systematic musculoskeletal examination and a reprinting of management guideline boxes from multiple chapters for quick reference and for comparison and contrast in Appendix A and B respectively.

As we put the final touches on this revision, we are once again pleased to present our efforts to students and professionals within the healthcare community. It is always our hope that our efforts will contribute to the effective care and services provided to patients and clients. And finally to our families, colleagues and friends who provided encouragement and supported us without hesitation, we extend a resounding THANK YOU!!

Carolyn Kisner
Lynn Allen Colby

Acknowledgments

In addition to all those who helped with the previous editions, we wish to thank and acknowledge the following people for their expertise and contributions to this revision.

Terri Glenn, PhD, PT, and Janet Mulcare, PhD, FASCM—for their revision of Chapter 4, Principles of Aerobic Exercise.

Robert Schrepfer, MS, PT—for writing Chapter 7, Aquatic Exercise.

Barbara Settles Huge, PT—for her revision of Chapter 17, Principles of Exercise for the Obstetric Patient, and inclusion of material on treatment of the client with incontinence.

Jack Miller, BSc(PT), Dip, ManipTher (NZ), FCAMT, Accredited Mulligan Concept Teacher—for writing material on the Mulligan concept of Mobilization with Movement in Chapter 6 and describing techniques for inclusion in each of the extremity chapters.

Marsha Eifert-Mangine, MEd, PT, ATC—for reviewing and contributing material on knee surgeries and rehabilitation and developing tables of intervention for the stages of rehabilitation following various surgical procedures on the knee.

The students and colleagues at the College of Mount St. Joseph in Cincinnati and The Ohio State University in Columbus—who modeled the various exercises and shared ideas in the development of some of the content for this edition.

Peg Waltner, Developmental Editor—who provided insight and direction in the design and development of this edition.

The staff at F.A. Davis—Jean-Francois Vilain, Margaret M. Biblis, Susan Rhyner, Bob Butler, Louis Forgione, Sam Rondinelli, Jack Brandt, and Laura Horowitz.

Contents

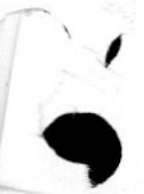

Part I

General Concepts and Techniques

Chapter 1

Therapeutic Exercise: Foundational Concepts

OBJECTIVES

After studying this chapter, the reader will be able to:

1 Define therapeutic exercise in the context of physical therapy care and services.

2 Identify and describe the major areas/aspects of physical function toward which therapeutic exercise interventions are directed.

3 Describe the process of disablement and a model of disablement that serves as a conceptual framework for the use of therapeutic exercise interventions.

4 Describe a comprehensive and systematic approach to patient management that applies critical thinking and sound decision-making throughout the continuum of physical therapy care and services.

5 Develop strategies for effective exercise instruction based on principles of motor learning.

Almost everyone, regardless of age, values the ability to function as independently as possible during everyday life. Healthcare consumers (patients and clients) typically seek out or are referred for physical therapy services because of physical impairments associated with injury, disease, or disorders that interfere with their ability to perform or pursue any number of activities that are necessary or important to them. Physical therapy services may also be sought by those individuals without any impairment who wish to improve their overall level of fitness or reduce the risk of injury or disease. An individually designed therapeutic exercise program is almost always a fundamental component of the physical therapy services provided. This stands to reason because the ultimate goal of a therapeutic exercise program is the achievement of an optimal level of symptom-free movement during basic to complex physical activities.

To develop and implement effective exercise interventions, a therapist must understand how the many forms of exercise affect body systems and how those exercise-induced effects have an impact on key aspects of physical function. A therapist must also integrate and apply knowledge of anatomy, physiology, kinesiology, pathology, and the behavioral sciences across the continuum of patient/client management from the initial examination to discharge planning. To develop therapeutic exercise programs that culminate in positive and meaningful functional outcomes for patients and clients, a therapist must understand the relationship between physical function and disability and appreciate how the application of the process of disablement to patient/client management facilitates the provision of effective and efficient healthcare services. Finally, a therapist as a patient/client educator must know and apply principles of motor learning to the process of exercise instruction. Therefore, the purpose of this chapter is to present an overview of the scope of therapeutic exercise interventions used by physical therapists, to discuss models of disablement and patient/client management as they relate to therapeutic exercise, and to explore strategies for exercise instruction.

Therapeutic Exercise: Impact on Physical Function

Of the many procedures used by physical therapists in the continuum of care of patients and clients, therapeutic exercise takes its place as one of the key elements that lie at the center of programs designed to improve or restore an individual's function or prevent dysfunction.[2]

Definition

Therapeutic exercise[2] is the systematic and planned performance of bodily movements, postures, or physical activities intended to provide a patient or client with the means to

- Remediate or prevent impairments
- Improve, restore, or enhance physical function
- Prevent or reduce health-related risk factors
- Optimize overall health status, fitness, or sense of well-being

Therapeutic exercise programs designed by physical therapists are *individualized* to the unique needs of each patient or client. A *patient* is an individual with impairments and functional limitations diagnosed by a physical therapist and is receiving physical therapy care to improve function and prevent disability.[2] A *client* is an individual without diagnosed dysfunction who engages in physical therapy services to promote health and wellness and to prevent dysfunction.[2] Because the focus of this textbook is on management of individuals with physical impairments and functional limitations, the authors have chosen to use the term "patient" rather than "client" or "patient/client" throughout this text. The authors believe that all individuals receiving physical therapy services must be active participants rather than passive recipients in the rehabilitation process to learn how to self-manage their health needs.

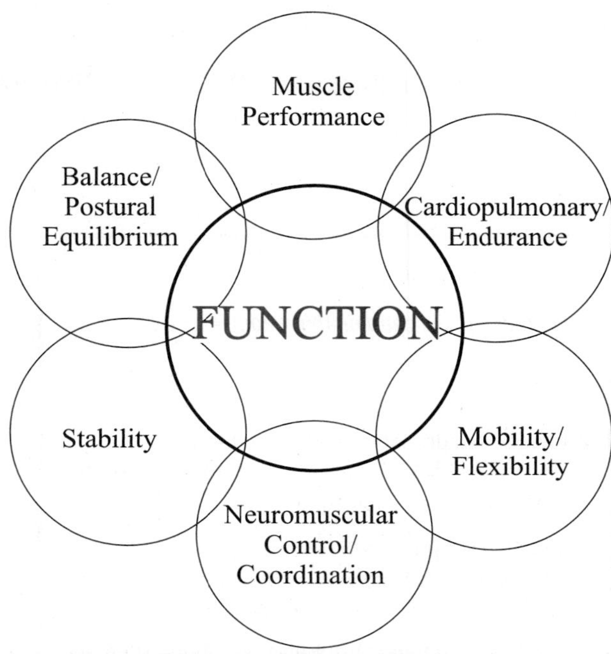

Figure 1–1 Inter-related aspects of physical function.

Aspects of Physical Function: Definition of Key Terms

The ability to function independently at home, in the workplace, within the community, or during leisure and recreational activities is contingent upon physical as well as psychological and social function. The multidimensional aspects of physical function encompass the diverse yet interrelated areas of performance that are depicted in Figure 1–1. These aspects of function are characterized by the following definitions:

Balance. The ability to align body segments against gravity to maintain or move the body (center of mass) within the available base of support without falling; the ability to move the body in equilibrium with gravity via interaction of the sensory and motor systems.[2,45,53,64,88]

Cardiopulmonary fitness. The ability to perform low-intensity, repetitive, total body movements (walking, jogging, cycling, swimming) over an extended period of time;[1,59] a synonymous term is *cardiopulmonary endurance.*

Coordination. The correct timing and sequencing of muscle firing combined with the appropriate intensity of muscular contraction leading to the effective initiation, guiding, and grading of movement. It is the basis of smooth, accurate, and efficient movement and occurs at a conscious or automatic level.[85,86]

Flexibility. Used interchangeably with mobility.

Mobility. The ability of structures or segments of the body to move or be moved in order to allow the occurrence of range of motion (ROM) for functional activities (functional ROM).[2,90] Passive mobility is dependent on soft tissue (contractile and noncontractile) extensibility; in addition, active mobility requires neuromuscular activation.

Muscle performance. The capacity of muscle to produce tension and do physical work. Muscle performance encompasses strength, power, and muscular endurance.[2]

Neuromuscular control. Interaction of the sensory and motor systems that enables synergists, agonists and antagonists, as well as stabilizers and neutralizers to anticipate or respond to proprioceptive and kinesthetic information and, subsequently, to work in correct sequence to create coordinated movement.[51]

Postural control, postural stability, and equilibrium. Used interchangeably with static or dynamic balance.

Stability. The ability of the neuromuscular system through synergistic muscle actions to hold a proximal or distal body segment in a stationary position or to control a stable base during superimposed movement.[90]

The systems of the body that control these aspects of physical function react, adapt, and develop in response to forces and stresses placed upon them.[59] Gravity, for example, is a constant force that affects the musculoskeletal, neuromuscular, and circulatory systems. Additional forces, incurred during routine physical activities, help the body maintain a functional level of strength, cardiopulmonary fitness, and mobility. Imposed forces and stresses that are excessive can cause acute injuries, such as sprains and fractures, or chronic conditions, such as repetitive motion disorders. The absence of typical forces on the body can also cause degeneration, degradation, or deformity. For example, the absence of normal weight bearing associated with prolonged bed rest or immobilization weakens muscle and bone.[10,48,60,77] Prolonged inactivity also leads to decreased efficiency of the circulatory and pulmonary systems.[1] Impairment of any one or more of the body systems and subsequent impairment of any aspect of physical function, separately or jointly, can result in functional limitation and disability. Therapeutic exercise interventions involve the application of carefully graded stresses and forces that are imposed on impaired body systems or individual structures in a controlled, progressive, and appropriately executed manner to reduce physical impairments and improve function.

Types of Therapeutic Exercise Interventions

Therapeutic exercise procedures embody a wide variety of activities, actions, and techniques. The techniques selected for an individualized therapeutic exercise program are based on a therapist's determination of the underlying cause or causes of a patient's functional limitations or disability. The types of therapeutic exercise interventions presented in this textbook are listed in Box 1–1. Additional exercise interventions are used by therapists for patients with neuromuscular or developmental conditions.[2]

Box 1–1 Therapeutic Exercise Interventions

- Aerobic conditioning and reconditioning
- Muscle performance exercises: Strength, power, and endurance training
- Stretching techniques including muscle lengthening procedures and joint mobilization techniques
- Neuromuscular control, inhibition, and facilitation techniques and posture awareness training
- Postural control, body mechanics, and stabilization exercises
- Balance exercises and agility training
- Relaxation exercises
- Breathing exercises and ventilatory muscle training
- Task-specific functional training

Note: Although joint mobilization techniques are often classified as manual therapy procedures and not therapeutic exercise,[2] the authors of this textbook have chosen to include joint mobilization procedures under the broad definition of therapeutic exercise in order to address the full scope of soft tissue stretching techniques.

Process and Models of Disablement

It has been said that the physical therapy profession is defined by a body of knowledge and clinical applications that are directed toward the elimination or resolution of disability.[79] Understanding the disabling consequences of disease, injury, and abnormalities of development and how the risk of potential disability can be reduced, therefore, must be fundamental to the provision of effective care and services geared to the restoration of meaningful function for patients and their families, significant others, and caregivers.

The Disablement Process

Definition

Disablement is a term that refers to the impact(s) and functional consequences of acute or chronic conditions, such as disease, injury, and congenital or developmental abnormalities, on specific body systems that compromise an individual's ability to meet necessary, customary, expected, and desired societal functions and roles.[41,97] Physical therapists most commonly provide care and services to people with *physical* disability. Social, emotional, and cognitive disablement can affect physical function and vice versa and, therefore, should not be disregarded or dismissed.[39,41]

Application in Healthcare

Knowledge of the process of disablement provides a foundation for healthcare professionals to develop an appreciation of the complex relationship between pathology and function. This knowledge, in turn, provides a theoretical framework upon which practice can be organized, thus facilitating effective management and care of patients that is reflected by meaningful functional outcomes.[2,26]

Inherent in the integration and application of knowledge of the disablement process in healthcare delivery is an understanding that the process is *not unidirectional;* that is, it is not necessarily unpreventable or irreversible.[6] Furthermore, it is assumed that in most instances, depending on factors such as the severity and duration of the pathologic condition, a patient's access to quality healthcare as well as the motivation and desires of the patient, the progression of the process can, indeed, be altered and the patient's function improved.[2,6]

An understanding and application of the disablement process shifts the focus of patient management from strict treatment of a disease or injury to treatment of the *impact* that a disease, injury, or disorder has on a patient's *function* as well as the identification of the underlying causes of the patient's dysfunction. This perspective puts the person, not solely the disease or disorder, at the center of efforts to prevent or halt the progression of disablement by use of interventions that improve a patient's functional abilities while simultaneously reducing or eliminating the causes of disability.[25]

Models of Disablement

Several models that depict the process of disablement have been proposed over the past 30 years. The first two models developed were the Nagi model[62,63] and the International Classification of Impairments, Disabilities and Handicaps (ICIDH) model for the World Health Organization.[33] The ICIDH model was recently revised with adjustments made in the descriptions of the classification criteria of the model based on input from healthcare practitioners as they became familiar with the original model.[31] This revised version is now referred to as the ICIDH-2 model.[34] The National Center for Medical Rehabilitation Research (NCMRR) integrated components of the Nagi model with the original ICIDH model to develop their own model.[65] Although each of these models uses slightly different terminology in their classification systems, each reflects a spectrum of disablement. Several sources in the literature have discussed or compared and contrasted the terminology and descriptors used in these and other models.[2,25,33,40,41,62,63,65] Despite the variations in these models, each taxonomy reflects the complex *interrelationships* among the following:

- Acute or chronic pathology
- Impairments
- Functional limitations
- Disabilities, handicaps, or societal limitations

More than a decade ago, physical therapists began to suggest that disablement schema and related terminology provided an appropriate framework on which clinical decision making in practice and research could be based and a mechanism by which terminology for documentation and communication in the clinical and research settings could be standardized.[26,29,40,84] The American Physical Therapy Association (APTA) has subsequently incorporated a disablement model and related terminology into the *Guide to Physical Therapist Practice,*[2] its evolving consensus document designed to reflect "best practice" from the initial examination to the outcomes of intervention. The document also uses the concept of disablement as a framework for organizing and prioritizing clinical decisions made during the continuum of physical therapy care and services. Figure 1–2 depicts a model of the disablement process relevant to the potential impacts of therapeutic exercise interventions on disablement. The impact of risk factors has also been included in this depiction of the process. Incorporating these factors into the model underscores the assumption that disability can be prevented, eliminated, or reduced if the risk of occurrence or severity of pathology, impairment, or functional limitation is reduced. The model also shows that effective interventions, in particular, therapeutic exercise interventions, can have a positive impact on every aspect of the disablement process.

By choosing to use a model of disablement as part of the theoretical framework of practice, physical therapists have a responsibility to provide evidence that there are indeed links among the elements of the disablement process that can be

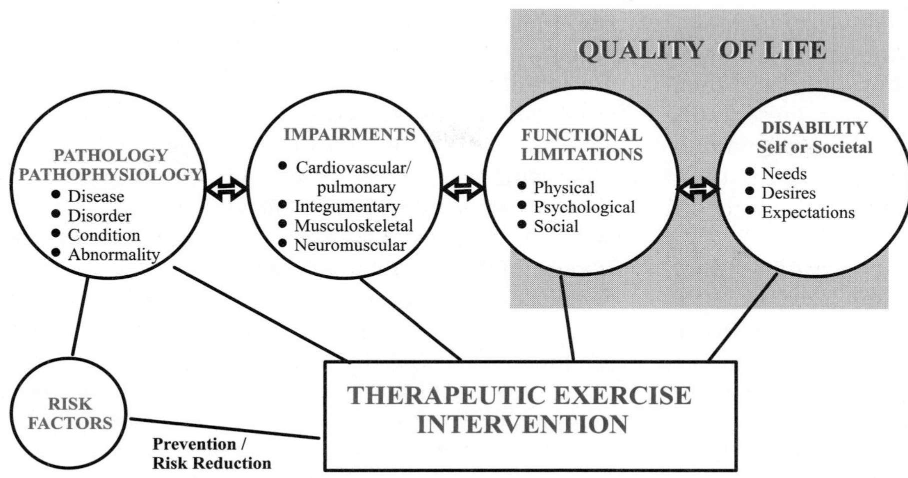

Figure 1–2 Impact of therapeutic exercise on the disablement process.

identified by physical therapy tests and measures. It is also the profession's responsibility to demonstrate that not only can physical impairments be reduced but that functional abilities can be significantly enhanced by physical therapy interventions. This body of evidence has just begun to emerge in the past decade. Examples of some of this evidence are integrated into this chapter and interspersed throughout the textbook.

An overview of the key components of the process of disablement is presented in the following sections of this chapter, with additional discussion of risk factors and their potential impacts on disability. The relationship of the disablement model to patient management and physical therapy interventions, specifically, therapeutic exercise, is also discussed.

Pathology/Pathophysiology

This first major component of the disablement model refers to disruptions of the body's homeostasis as the result of acute or chronic diseases, disorders, or conditions characterized by a set of abnormal findings (clusters of signs and symptoms) that are indicative of alterations or interruptions of structure or function of the body primarily identified at the cellular level.[2,22] Identification and classification of these abnormalities of *anatomic, physiologic,* or *psychological* structure or process generally trigger medical intervention based on a medical diagnosis.

Physical therapists in all areas of practice treat patients with a multitude of pathologies. Knowledge of pathologies (medical diagnoses) is important background information, but it does not tell the therapist how to assess and treat a patient's dysfunction that arises from the pathologic condition. Despite an accurate medical diagnosis and a therapist's thorough knowledge of specific pathologies, the experienced therapist knows full well that two patients with the same medical diagnosis, such as rheumatoid arthritis, and the same extent of joint destruction (confirmed on x-ray) may have very different severities of impairments and functional limitations and, consequently, very different degrees of disablement. This emphasizes the need for physical therapists to always pay close attention to the impact(s) of a particular pathology on function when designing meaningful management strategies to improve functional abilities.

Impairments

Impairments are the *consequences* of pathologic conditions; that is, they are the signs and symptoms that reflect abnormalities at the body system, organ, or tissue level.[2,39]

Types of Impairments

Impairments can be categorized as arising from *anatomic, physiologic,* or *psychological* alterations; losses; or abnormalities of *structure* or *function* of a body system. Physical therapists typically provide care and services to patients with impairments that affect the following systems:

- Musculoskeletal
- Neuromuscular
- Cardiovascular/pulmonary
- Integumentary

Most impairments of these body systems identified and managed by physical therapists primarily are the result of abnormalities of physiologic function or anatomic structure. Some representative examples of physical impairments commonly identified by physical therapists and managed with therapeutic exercise interventions are noted in Box 1–2.

Impairments may arise directly from the pathology **(direct/primary impairments)** or may be the result of a pre-existing impairment(s) **(indirect/secondary impairments).** A patient, for example, who has sustained a minor tear of the rotator cuff (pathology) will exhibit primary impairments, such as pain, limited ROM of the shoulder, and weakness of specific shoulder musculature. The patient may subsequently develop faulty alignment of the shoulder girdle and spine as well as weakness in all shoulder girdle musculature as a result of these primary impairments and altered use of the upper extremity.

Furthermore, when an impairment is the result of multiple underlying causes and arises from a combination of primary or secondary impairments, the term **composite impairment** is sometimes used.[84] For example, a patient who has sustained a severe inversion sprain of the ankle resulting in a tear of the talofibular ligament and whose ankle was immobilized for several weeks is likely to exhibit a balance impairment of the involved lower extremity. This composite impairment could be the result of chronic ligamentous laxity and impaired ankle proprioception from the injury or muscle weakness from immobilization and disuse.

Box 1–2 Common Physical Impairments Managed with Therapeutic Exercise

Musculoskeletal
- Pain
- Muscle weakness/reduced torque production
- Decreased muscular endurance
- Limited range of motion due to:
  - Restriction of the joint capsule
  - Restriction of periarticular connective tissue
  - Decreased muscle length
- Joint hypermobility
- Faulty posture
- Muscle imbalances

Neuromuscular
- Pain
- Impaired balance, postural stability, or control
- Incoordination, faulty timing
- Delayed motor development
- Abnormal tone (hypotonia, hypertonia, dystonia)
- Ineffective/inefficient functional movement strategies

Cardiovascular/Pulmonary
- Decreased aerobic capacity (cardiopulmonary endurance)
- Impaired circulation (lymphatic, venous, arterial)
- Pain with sustained physical activity (intermittent claudication)

Integumentary
- Skin hypomobility (ex. immobile or adherent scarring)

Regardless of the types of impairments exhibited by a patient, a therapist must keep in mind that not all impairments are necessarily linked to functional limitations or disability. An important key to effective management of a patient's problems is to recognize *functionally relevant impairments,* in other words, impairments that directly contribute to functional limitations. Impairments that could contribute to functional limitations and disability in the future or could predispose a patient to secondary pathologies or impairments must also be identified. Equally crucial for the effective management of a patient's dysfunction is the need to analyze and determine, or at least infer and certainly not ignore, the *underlying causes* of the identified physical impairments particularly those related to impaired movement.[83] For example, are biomechanical abnormalities of soft tissues the source of restricted ROM? If so, which soft tissues are restricted and why are they restricted? This information then assists the therapist in the selection of appropriate and effective therapeutic interventions that target the underlying causes of the impairments, the impairments themselves, and the resulting functional limitations.

Although most physical therapy interventions, including therapeutic exercise, are designed to correct or reduce physical impairments, such as decreased ROM or strength, poor balance, or limited cardiopulmonary endurance, the focus of treatment must still be on restoration of function and prevention of dysfunction. Elimination or reduction of functionally relevant impairments is certainly necessary during treatment, but *successful outcomes* of treatment are determined by a reduction or resolution of functional limitations or disabilities and the restoration or improvement of function. A therapist cannot simply assume that intervening at the impairment level (for example, with strengthening or stretching exercises) and subsequently reducing physical impairments (by increasing strength and ROM) necessarily generalizes to remediation of functional limitations and restoration of functional motor abilities for daily living. Mechanisms for integrating correction of physical impairments and restoration of functional abilities through task-specific training are explored in a model of effective patient management later in this chapter.

Functional Limitations

Functional limitations, the third component of the disablement model, occur at the level of the *whole person*. They are the result of impairments and are characterized by the reduced ability of a person to perform actions or activities in an efficient or typically expected manner.[2,62,63,65] As noted in Figure 1–2, functional limitations may be *physical, social, or psychological* in nature. The focus of physical therapy interventions is on the management of limitations of physical functioning while respecting the needs of the whole person and recognizing that social and psychological influences can also limit a person's ability to function. In addition, the focus must be on those functional limitations that are most important to the patient and those that are or could be directly causing disability. When impairments cause functional limitations, a person's *quality of life* may begin to deteriorate (see Fig. 1–2). It should also be noted that a single or even several mild impairments often do not cause loss of function. Evidence suggests that the severity and complexity of impairments must reach a critical level, which is different for each patient, before degradation of function begins to occur.[71,74]

Types of Functional Limitations

Functional limitations in the physical domain deal with the performance of sensorimotor tasks, that is, total body actions that are typically *components or aspects* of activities of everyday life.[2,65] These activities include basic activities of daily living (ADL), such as bathing, dressing, or feeding, and the more complex tasks known as instrumental activities of daily living (IADL), such as occupational tasks, school-related skills, housekeeping, and recreational activities, or community mobility (driving, using public transportation), just to name a few. Box 1–3 lists a number of functional limitations that can arise from physical impairments, involve *whole-body movements,* and are necessary component motions of simple to complex daily living skills. Defining functional limitations in this way underscores the importance of identifying abnormal or absent component motions of motor skills by the process of task analysis during the physical therapy examination and practicing functional motions during treatment.

Note: Not all sources in the literature define functional limitations in this way. For example, some sources[28,29,68] classify all aspects of individual functioning, including basic ADL (personal hygiene and grooming, feeding transfers, and locomotion) as functional limitations.

When a person is unable or has only limited ability to perform any of these whole-body sensorimotor tasks, decreased independence in ADL and IADL may occur, quality of life may become compromised, and hence, disability may ensue. The following is an example of this relationship between functional limitations and potential disability. To perform a basic home maintenance task (IADL), such as painting a room, a person must be able to grasp a brush or roller, climb a ladder, reach overhead, kneel, or stoop down to the floor. If any one of these functional movements is limited, it may not be possible to perform the overall task of painting the room. An essential aspect of a physical therapy examination and evaluation is the analysis of motor tasks to identify the components of tasks that are difficult for a patient to perform. This analysis helps the therapist determine why a patient is unable to perform specific daily living tasks. This information coupled with an identification and measurement of the impairments that are the source of the altered or absent component movement patterns, in turn, is used in treatment planning and selection of interventions to restore function and prevent potential disability.

Box 1–3 Common Functional Limitations Related to Physical Tasks

Limitation of:
- Reaching and grasping
- Lifting and carrying
- Pushing and pulling
- Bending and stooping
- Turning and twisting
- Throwing and catching
- Rolling
- Standing
- Squatting and kneeling
- Standing up and sitting down
- Getting in and out of bed
- Crawling, walking, and running
- Ascending and descending stairs
- Hopping and jumping
- Kicking

Disability

The final category of the disablement continuum is disability. An approach to management that focuses on restoring or improving function may prevent or reduce disability. A disability is the inability to perform or participate in activities or tasks related to one's self, the home, work, recreation, or the community in a manner or to the extent that the individual or the community as a whole (family, friends, co-workers, etc.) perceive as "normal."[2] An individual's roles or functions in life are placed in *the context of the physical environment as well as societal expectations.*[26,41] Social expectations or roles involve interactions with others and participation in activities that are a part of who each of us is. These roles are specific to age, gender, sex, and cultural background. This is a broad definition of disability and encompasses *individual functioning* in the context of the environment that includes basic ADL and more complex daily living skills as well as *societal functioning.* These functions or roles fall into several categories summarized in Box 1–4.

Note: Some sources in the literature[28,29,68] classify only difficulty with societal functioning as a disability.

Understanding the relationships *among* pathology, impairments, functional limitations, and perceived disability is fundamental to the *prevention* or reduction of disability.[6,25,41] Because disability is such a complex process, the extent to which each component of the disablement process affects one's perceived level of disability is not clearly understood. An assumption is made that when impairments and functional limitations are so severe or of such long duration that they cannot be overcome to a degree acceptable to an individual, a family, or society, the perception of "being disabled" then occurs.[2,74] The perception of disability is highly dependent on a person's or society's expectations of how or by whom certain roles or tasks *should* be performed.

Box 1–4 General Categories of Activities Relevant to Disability

- Self-care
- Mobility in the community
- Occupational tasks
- School-related tasks
- Home management (indoor and outdoor)
- Caring for dependents
- Recreational and leisure activities
- Community responsibilities and service

The presence of functional limitations may or may not lead to loss of independence and result in disability. Take for example a relatively inactive person with long-standing osteoarthritis of the knees. The inability to get up from the floor or from a low seat (functional limitation) because of limited flexion of the knees and reduced strength of the quadriceps (impairments) could indeed lead to disability in several areas of everyday function. Disability could be expressed by problems in self-care (inability to get in and out of a tub or stand up from a standard height toilet seat), home management (inability to perform selected housekeeping, gardening, or yard maintenance tasks), or community mobility (inability to get into or out of a car or van independently). The perception of disability can be minimized if the patient's functional ROM and strength can be improved with an exercise program and the increased ROM and strength is incorporated into progressively more challenging functional activities or if the physical environment can be altered sufficiently with the use of adaptive equipment and assistive devices. Adjusting expected roles or tasks within the family may also have a positive impact on the prevention or reduction of disability. Factors within the individual also can have an impact on the prevention, reduction, or progression of disablement. Those factors include level of motivation or willingness to make lifestyle changes and accommodations as well as the ability to understand and cope with an adjusted lifestyle.[97]

This example highlights that inherent in any discussion of disability is the assumption that it can be prevented or remediated.[6] Prevention falls into three categories:[2,60]

- ***Primary prevention.*** Activities such as health promotion designed to prevent disease in an at-risk population
- ***Secondary prevention.*** Early diagnosis and the reduction of the severity or duration of existing disease and sequelae
- ***Tertiary prevention.*** Use of rehabilitation to reduce the degree or limit the progression of existing disability and improve multiple aspects of function in persons with chronic, irreversible disease

Therapeutic exercise, the most frequently implemented physical therapy intervention, has merit at all three levels of prevention. For example, the use of resistance exercises and aerobic conditioning exercises in weight-bearing postures is often advocated for the primary and secondary prevention of age-related osteoporosis,[10,48,60] whereas therapists who work with patients with chronic musculoskeletal or neuromuscular diseases or disorders routinely are involved with tertiary prevention of disability.

Risk Factors

Modifying risk factors is an important tool for reducing or preventing disablement. **Risk factors** related to disablement are influences or characteristics that *predispose* a person to disability. As such, they exist prior to the onset of pathology, impairments, functional limitations, or disability.[6,41,97] Some factors that increase the risk of disability are: biological characteristics, lifestyle behaviors, psychological characteristics, and the impact of the physical and social environments. Some examples of each of these types of risk factors are summarized in Box 1–5.

Some of these risk factors, in particular, lifestyle characteristics and behaviors, and their impact on the potential for disease or injury, have become reasonably well known because of public service announcements and distribution of educational materials in conjunction with health promotion campaigns, such as *Healthy People 2000*, which emphasized primary prevention of specific heart and lung diseases.[72] For instance, information on the adverse influences of health-related risk factors, such as a sedentary lifestyle, obesity, and smoking, has been widely disseminated in this health promotion and disease prevention initiative. Although the benefits of a healthy lifestyle, which includes regular exercise and physical activity, are well founded and widely documented,[1,72] initial outcomes of the *Healthy People 2000* campaign suggest that an increased awareness of risk factors has not necessarily translated into dramatic changes in lifestyle behaviors to actually reduce the risk of disease or injury.[18] This demonstrates that increased knowledge does not necessarily change behaviors.

When active pathology exists, reduction of risk factors by means of *buffers* (interventions aimed at reducing the progression of pathology, impairments, functional limitations, or disability)[41] is appropriate. This focus of intervention is categorized as secondary or tertiary prevention of disability. Initiating a regular exercise program and increasing the level of physical activity on a daily basis or altering the physical environment by removing architectural barriers or by using assistive devices for ADL are all examples of buffers that can reduce the risk of disability.

This summary of the process of disablement has highlighted key elements of this complex process. A basic understanding of this process provides a framework for practice, a foundation for sound clinical decision-making, and sets the stage for delivery of effective, efficient, and meaningful physical therapy care and services for patients.

Box 1–5 Disablement Risk Factors

- **Biological Factors**
  - Age, sex, race
  - Height/weight relationship
  - Congenital abnormalities or disorders, such as skeletal deformities, neuromuscular disorders, or cardiopulmonary diseases or anomalies
  - Family history of disease; genetic predisposition
- **Behavioral/Psychological/Lifestyle Factors**
  - Sedentary lifestyle
  - Use of tobacco, alcohol, and other drugs
  - Poor nutrition
  - Low level of motivation
  - Inadequate coping skills
  - Difficulty dealing with change
  - Negative affect
- **Physical Environment Characteristics**
  - Architectural barriers in the home, community, and workplace
  - Ergonomic characteristics of the home, work, or school environments
- **Socioeconomic Factors**
  - Low economic status
  - Low level of education
  - Inadequate access to healthcare
  - Limited family or social support

Patient Management and Clinical Decision Making: An Interactive Relationship

An understanding of the disablement process as well as knowledge of the process of making informed clinical decisions are necessary foundations of comprehensive management of patients seeking and receiving physical therapy services. Provision for quality patient care involves the ability to make sound clinical judgments, solve problems that are important to a patient, and apply knowledge of the interrelationships among pathology, impairments, functional limitations, and disability throughout each phase of management. The primary purpose of this

Box 1–6 Requirements for Skilled Clinical Decision Making During Patient Management

- Knowledge of pertinent information about the problem(s)
- Prior clinical experience with the same or similar problems
- Ability to recall relevant information
- Cognitive and psychomotor skills to obtain necessary knowledge of an unfamiliar problem
- Ability to integrate new and prior knowledge
- An efficient information-gathering and information-processing style
- Ability to critically organize, categorize, prioritize, and synthesize information
- Ability to recognize clinical patterns
- Ability to form working hypotheses about presenting problems and how they might be solved
- An understanding of the patient's values and goals
- Ability to determine options and make strategic plans
- Use of reflective thinking and self-monitoring strategies to make necessary adjustments

section of the chapter is to describe a model of patient management used in physical therapy practice. Inasmuch as clinical reasoning is imbedded in each phase of patient management, a brief overview of the concepts and processes involved in clinical decision making is presented before exploration of a systematic process of patient management in physical therapy. Relevant examples of the types of clinical decisions that a therapist must make are then highlighted within the context of the patient management model.

Clinical Decision Making

Clinical decision making refers to a dynamic and complex process of reasoning and analytical (critical) thinking that involves making judgments and determinations in the context of patient care.[44] To make effective decisions, a merging of clarification and understanding with critical and creative thinking is necessary.[50] There are a number of requisite attributes that are required for making informed, efficient, and effective clinical decisions.[50,57,87] Those requirements are listed in Box 1–6.

There is a substantial body of knowledge in the literature that describes various models of clinical decision-making in physical therapy.* Several methods of teaching effective clinical decision making have also been proposed.[12,50,87,89] Other articles have focused on comparisons of clinical reasoning of expert versus novice therapists.[16,35,36,43,58,76] In addition, the use of clinical decision making in the diagnostic process has generated substantial interest and has been discussed extensively.† Key points from some of these studies and reports are addressed throughout this section of the chapter.

As healthcare moves in the direction that physical therapists become first contact practitioners and consumers gain access to physical therapy services without physician referral, the need to make sound clinical judgments during the continuum of patient management becomes more and more essential for physical therapy practitioners. Examples of how to incorporate the ongoing process of clinical decision making into each phase of patient management is highlighted in the following discussion of a model for patient management.

A Patient Management Model

The physical therapy profession has developed a comprehensive approach to patient management designed to guide a practitioner through a systematic series of steps and decisions for the purpose of helping a patient achieve the highest level of function possible. This model is illustrated in Figure 1–3.

The process of patient management has five basic components:[2,5]

- A comprehensive *examination*
- *Evaluation* of data collected
- Determination of *a diagnosis* based on impairments, functional limitations, and disability
- Establishment of a *prognosis* and plan of care based on patient-oriented goals
- Implementation of appropriate *interventions*

The patient management process culminates in the attainment of meaningful, functional *outcomes* by the patient, which then must be re-examined and re-evaluated before a patient's discharge. As the model indicates, the *re-examination* and *re-evaluation* process occurs not only at the conclusion of treatment but throughout each phase of patient management. The ability to make timely decisions and appropriate judgments and develop or adjust an ongoing series of working hypotheses makes transition from one phase of management to the next occur in an effective and efficient manner.

Examination

The first component of the patient management model is examination of the patient. Examination is the systematic process by which a therapist obtains

*See references 14, 28, 29, 35, 36, 43, 44, 55, 58, 70, 80, 84, 93.

†See references 5, 12, 13, 24, 26, 40, 55, 78, 83, 93, 96, 102.

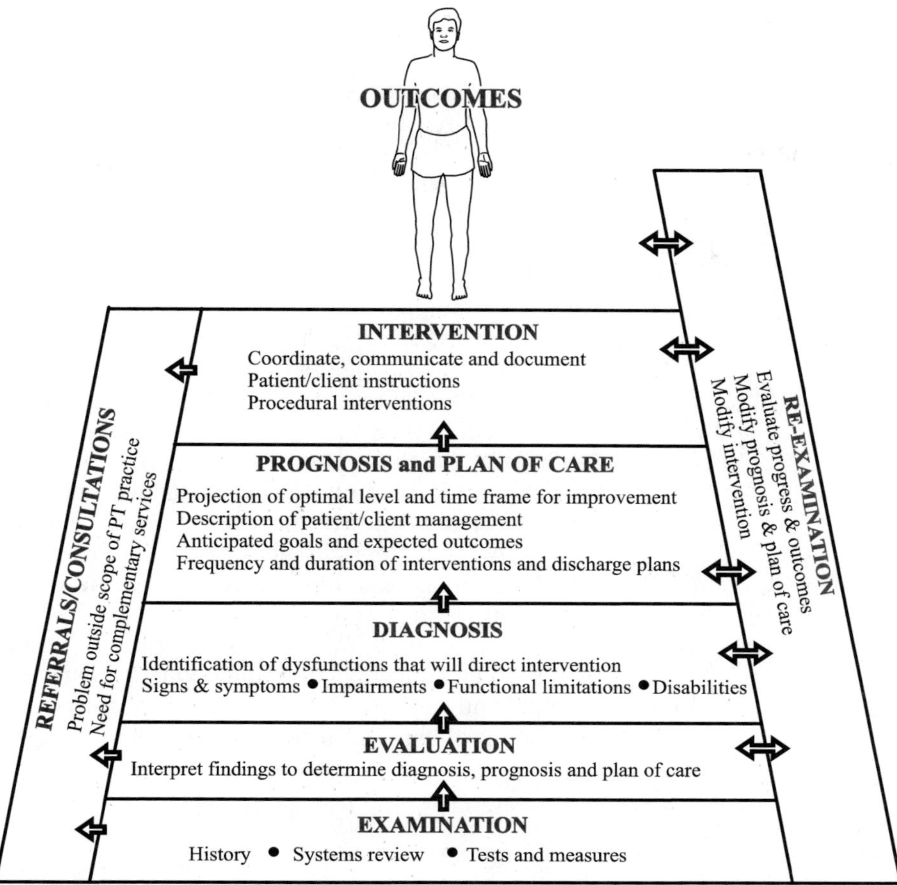

Figure 1–3 A comprehensive outcomes-oriented model of patient management.

information about a patient's problem(s) and reasons for seeking physical therapy services. During this initial data collection, the therapist acquires information from a variety of sources. The examination process involves both comprehensive screening and specific testing. It is the means by which the therapist gathers sufficient information about the patient's problems (pathologic conditions, impairments, functional limitations, and disabilities) to ultimately make a diagnosis and determine whether or not these problems can be appropriately treated by physical therapy interventions. If treatment of the identified problems does not fall within the scope of physical therapy practice, then referral to another healthcare practitioner or resource is warranted. The examination is also the means by which baseline measurements of current impairments, functional limitations, and abilities are established as a reference point from which the results of therapeutic interventions can be measured and documented.

There are three distinct elements within a comprehensive examination.[2] They are:

- The patient's history
- A relevant systems review
- Specific tests and measures

Throughout the examination process, a therapist seeks answers to a number of questions and concurrently makes a series of clinical decisions that shape and guide the examination process. Examples of some questions to be asked and decisions to be made are noted in Box 1–7.

History

The history is the mechanism by which a therapist obtains an *overview* of current and past information (both subjective and objective) about a patient's present condition(s), general health status (health risk factors and coexisting health problems), and why the patient has sought physical therapy services. The types of data that can be generated from

Box 1–7 Key Questions to Consider During the Initial Examination

- What are the most complete and readily available sources for obtaining the patient's history?
- Is there a need to obtain additional information about the patient's presenting pathology or medical diagnosis if one is available?
- Based on initial working hypotheses, which of the patient's signs and symptoms warrant additional testing by physical therapy or by referral to another healthcare practitioner?
- Do the patient's problems seem to fall within or outside the scope of physical therapy practice?
- What types of specific tests and measures should be selected to gather data about the patient's impairments, functional limitations, or disability?
- What are the most important tests to do first? Which could be postponed until a later visit with the patient?

a patient's history are summarized in Box 1–8.[2,5] The therapist determines which aspects of the patient's history are more relevant than others and what data need to be gathered from the history.

Sources of information about the patient's history include:

- Interviews with the patient, family, or other significant individuals involved in patient care
- Review of the medical record
- Reports from the referral source, consultants, or other healthcare team members

The extent of information about the patient's history that is necessary or available may be extensive or very limited and may or may not be readily accessible prior to the first contact with the patient. Compare, for example, the information available to the therapist working in an acute care facility who has ready access to a patient's medical record versus the home health therapist who may have only a patient's medical diagnosis or brief surgical history. Regardless of the extent of written reports or medical/surgical history that is available, reviewing this information prior to the initial contact with the patient helps a therapist prioritize the questions asked and areas explored during the interview with the patient.

The interview is crucial for determining a patient's chief concerns and functional status: past, current, and desired. It also helps a therapist see a patient's problems from the patient's own perspec-

Box 1–8 Information Generated from the Initial History

Demographic Data
- Age, sex, race, ethnicity
- Primary language
- Education

Social History
- Family and caregiver resources
- Cultural background
- Social interactions/support systems

Occupation/Leisure
- Current and previous employment Job/school-related activities
- Recreational, community activities/tasks

Growth and Development
- Developmental history
- Hand and foot dominance

Living Environment
- Current living environment
- Expected destination after discharge
- Community accessibility

General Health Status & Lifestyle Habits and Behaviors: Past/Present (based on self or family report)
- Perception of health/disability
- Lifestyle health risks (smoking, substance abuse,
- Diet, exercise, sleep habits

Medical/Surgical/Psychological History

Medications: Current and Past

Family History
- Health risk factors
- Family illnesses

Cognitive/Social/Emotional Status
- Orientation, memory
- Communication
- Social/emotional interactions

Current Conditions/Chief Complaints/Concerns
- Conditions, reasons PT services sought
- Patient's perceived level of disability
- Patient's needs, goals
- History, onset (date and course), mechanism of injury, pattern and behavior of symptoms
- Family or caregiver needs, goals, perception of patient's problems
- Current or past therapeutic interventions
- Previous outcome of chief complaint(s)

Functional Status and Activity Level
- Current/prior functional status: basic ADL, IADL related to self-care and home
- Current/prior functional status in work, school, community-related IADL

Other Laboratory and Diagnostic Tests

tive, specifically with regard to the perception of functional limitations or disability. A patient will almost always describe a current problem in terms of functional limitations or disabilities, not impairments. For example, a patient might report, "My elbow really hurts when I pick up something heavy", or "I'm really having trouble playing tennis (or bowling or unloading groceries from the car)." Questions that relate to symptoms (in this case, elbow pain) should identify location, intensity, description, and factors that aggravate or alleviate symptoms in a 24-hour period. Depending on a patient's condition and individual situation, the perceptions of family members, significant others, caregivers, or employers are often as important to the overall picture as the patient's own assessment of the current problems.

While taking the history, it is useful to group the interview questions into categories to keep the information organized. Gathering and evaluating data simultaneously makes it easier to recognize and identify *patterns or clusters of signs and symptoms* and even to begin to formulate one or more initial or "working" hypotheses, which later will be supported or rejected. Making these kinds of judgments helps organize and structure the examination.[80] Experienced therapists tend to form working hypotheses quite early in the examination process, even while reviewing a patient's chart before the initial contact with the patient.[35,36,43,58] This enables a therapist to determine and prioritize which definitive tests and measures should be selected for the later portion of the examination.[36]

Systems Review

A brief but relevant screening of the body systems is performed as a part of the examination process after organizing and prioritizing data gathered from the history. The greater the number of health-related risk factors identified during the history, the greater the importance of the review of systems. The systems typically screened by therapists are the cardiovascular and pulmonary, integumentary, musculoskeletal, and neuromuscular systems, but problems in the gastrointestinal and genitourinary systems may also be relevant.[5] This screening process also gives a general overview of a patient's cognition, communication, and social/emotional responses. Only limited information on the anatomic and physiologic status or function of each system is obtained. Table 1–1 identifies each system and gives examples of customary screening procedures used by physical therapists.

Note: Some of this information, such as the patient's psychosocial status, may have been gathered previously while reviewing and taking the patient's history and need not be addressed again.

The purpose of screening each system is to identify any abnormalities or deficits that require further or more specific testing by a therapist or another healthcare practitioner.[2,5] Findings from the systems review coupled with information about a patient's chief complaints secured from the patient's history enable a therapist to begin to make decisions about the possible causes of a patient's impairments and

Table 1–1 Areas of Screening for the Systems Review

System	Screening
Cardiovascular/pulmonary	Heart rate, respiratory rate, and blood pressure; pain or heaviness in the chest or pulsating pain; lightheadedness; peripheral edema
Integumentary	Skin temperature, color, texture, integrity, scars, lumps, growths
Musculoskeletal	Height, weight, symmetry, gross ROM, and strength
Neuromuscular	General aspects of motor control (balance, locomotion, coordination); sensation, changes in hearing or vision; severe headaches
Gastrointestinal/genitourinary	Heartburn, diarrhea, vomiting, severe abdominal pain, problems with swallowing, problems with bladder function, unusual menstrual cycles, pregnancy
Cognitive and social/emotional	Communication abilities (expressive and receptive), cognition, affect, level of arousal, orientation, ability to follow directions or learn, behavioral/emotional stressors and responses
General/miscellaneous	Persistent fatigue, malaise, unexplained weight gain or loss, fever, chills, sweats

functional limitations and to distinguish between problems that can and cannot be managed effectively by physical therapy interventions. If a therapist determines that a patient's problems lie outside the scope of physical therapy practice, no additional testing is warranted and referral to another health-care practitioner is appropriate.[2,5,24]

Specific Tests and Measures

Once it is decided that a patient's problems are most likely amenable to physical therapy intervention, the next decision a therapist must make in the examination process is to decide which aspects of physical function require further investigation through the use of specific tests and measures.

Specific (definitive) tests and measures used by physical therapists provide in-depth information about impairments, functional limitations, and disabilities. The specificity of these tests enables a therapist to support or refute the working hypotheses formulated while taking the patient's history and performing the systems review. The data generated from these definitive tests are the means by which the therapist determines the possible *underlying causes* of a patient's impairments and functional limitations. These tests also give the therapist a clearer picture of a patient's current condition(s) and may reveal information about the patient not previously identified during the history and systems review. If treatment is initiated, the results of these specific tests and measures establish *objective baselines* from which changes in a patient's physical status as the result of interventions then are measured.

Given the array of specific tests available to a therapist for a comprehensive physical therapy examination, the guidelines summarized in Box 1–9 should be considered when determining which examination procedures need to be selected and administered.

There are more than 20 general categories of specific tests and measures commonly performed by physical therapists.[2,92] Tests are selected and administered to target specific impairments of body systems. Typically, testing involves multiple body systems to identify the scope of a patient's impairments. When examining a patient, with chronic knee pain, for example, in addition to performing a thorough musculoskeletal examination, it would also be appropriate to administer tests that identify the impact of the patient's knee pain on the neuromuscular system (by assessing balance and proprioception) and the cardiopulmonary system (by assessing aerobic capacity). Because many of the pathologic conditions discussed in this textbook involve the musculoskeletal system, some examples of specific tests and measures that identify *musculoskeletal impairments* are noted here. They include but are not limited to:

- Assessment of pain
- Goniometry
- Joint mobility, stability, and integrity tests (including ligamentous testing)
- Tests of muscle performance (manual muscle testing, dynamometry)
- Posture analysis
- Gait analysis
- Assessment of assistive, adaptive, or orthotic devices

Note: An outline of a comprehensive and systematic musculoskeletal examination organized to yield data for identification of impairments and functional limitations is described in Appendix A of this textbook.

An in-depth examination of impairments provides valuable information about the extent and nature of the impairments and is the foundation of the diagnosis(es) made by a physical therapist. A thorough examination of impairments also helps a therapist select the most appropriate types of exercise and other forms of intervention for the treatment plan.

Box 1–9 Guidelines for Selection of Specific Tests and Measures

- Select tests and measures that are valid and reliable.
- Administer tests that target multiple levels of disablement: impairments, functional limitations, and the patient's perceived level of disability.
- Prioritize tests and measures selected to gather in-depth information about key problems identified during the history and systems review.
- Decide whether to administer generic tests or tests that are specific to a particular region of the body.
- Choose tests that provide data that are specific enough to support or reject working hypotheses formulated during the history and systems review and to determine a diagnosis, prognosis, and plan of care when the data are evaluated.
- Select tests and measures that help determine the types of interventions that most likely will be appropriate and effective.
- To complete the examination in a timely manner, avoid collecting more information than is necessary to make informed decisions during the evaluation and treatment planning phases of management.

Although specific testing of impairments is crucial, these tests do not tell the therapist how the impairments are affecting the patient's functional capabilities. Therefore, every examination should also include use of instruments that specifically measure *functional limitations and disability.* These tools, often referred to as *functional outcome measures,* are designed to reflect the impact of a patient's pathologic condition and resulting impairments on functional abilities and health-related quality of life. These instruments typically supply baseline measurements of subjective information against which changes in a patient's function or a patient's perceived level of disability are documented over the course of treatment. The tests may be generic, covering a wide range of functional abilities, or specific to a particular body region, such as the upper or lower extremities or spine. Generic instruments can be used to assess the global function of patients with a wide array of pathologies and impairments but yield less site-specific data than regional tests of functional abilities or limitations.[75]

The format of functional testing procedures and instruments varies. Some tests gather information by *self-report* (by the patient or family member);[46] others require *observation and rating of the patient's performance* by a therapist as various functional tasks are carried out. Some instruments measure a patient's ease or difficulty of performing specific physical tasks. Other instruments incorporate temporal (time-based) or spatial (distance-based) criteria, such as measurement of walking speed or distance, in the format. Test scores can also be based on the level of assistance (with assistive devices or by another person) needed to complete a variety of functional tasks.

Indices of disability measure a patient's perception of his or her degree of disability. These self-report instruments usually focus on ADL, such as the ability or inability to care for one's own needs (physical, social, or emotional) or the level of participation in the community that is currently possible, desired, expected, or required. Information gathered with these tools may indicate that the patient requires consultation and possible intervention by other healthcare professionals to deal with some of the social or psychological aspects of disability.

Note: It is well beyond the scope or purpose of this text to identify and describe the many instruments that measure physical function or disability. The reader is referred to several resources in the literature that provide this information.[4,7,23,54,91]

Evaluation

Evaluation is a process that is characterized by the *interpretation of collected data.* The process involves analysis and synthesis of information to form opinions by means of a series of sound clinical decisions.[2] Although evaluation is depicted as a distinct entity or phase of the patient management model (see Fig. 1–3), some degree of evaluation goes on at every phase of patient management, from examination through outcomes. Interpretation of relevant data, one of the more challenging aspects of patient management, is fundamental to the determination of a diagnosis of dysfunction and prognosis of functional outcomes. By pulling together and sorting out subjective and objective data from the examination, a therapist should be able to determine the following:

- A patient's general health status and its impact on current and potential function
- The chronicity and severity of the current condition(s)
- The extent of impairments of body systems and impact on functional abilities
- A patient's current, overall level of physical function (limitations *and* abilities) compared with the functional abilities needed, expected, or desired by the patient
- The impact of physical dysfunction on social/emotional function
- The impact of the physical environment on a patient's function
- A patient's social support systems and their impact on current and potential function

The determinations made during the evaluation process may also suggest that additional testing by the therapist or another practitioner is necessary before the therapist can determine a patient's diagnosis and prognosis. For example, a patient whose chief complaints are related to episodic shoulder pain but who also indicated during the history that bouts of depression sometimes make it difficult to work or socialize should be referred for a psychological consultation and possible treatment.[5] Results of the psychological evaluation could be quite relevant to the success of physical therapy intervention.

Addressing the questions posed in Box 1–10 during the evaluation of data enables a therapist to make pertinent clinical decisions that lead to the

Box 1–10 Key Questions to Consider During the Evaluation and Diagnostic Processes

- What is the extent, degree, or severity of impairments, functional limitations, or disability?
- What is the stability or progression of dysfunction?
- Is the current condition(s) acute or chronic?
- What actions/events change (relieve or worsen) the patient's signs and symptoms?
- How do pre-existing conditions (co-morbidities) affect the current condition?
- How does the information from the patient's medical/surgical history and tests and measures done by other healthcare practitioners relate to the findings of the physical therapy examination?
- Have identifiable clusters of findings, i.e., patterns, emerged relevant to the patient's dysfunction?
- Is there an understandable relationship between the patient's extent of impairments and the degree of functional limitation or disability?
- What are the causal factors that seem to be contributing to the patient's impairments, functional limitations, or disability?

determination of a diagnosis and prognosis and the selection of potential intervention strategies for the plan of care.

During the evaluation it is particularly useful to ascertain if and to what extent relationships exist among measurements of impairments, functional limitations, and the patient's level of disability. These relationships often are not straightforward. In a recent study of patients with cervical spine disorders,[32] investigators reported a strong correlation between measurements of impairments (pain, ROM, and cervical muscle strength) and functional limitations (functional axial rotation and lifting capacity) but a relatively weak correlation between measurements of functional limitations and the patient's perceived level of disability as determined by 3 self-report measures. In another study[94] that compared shoulder ROM with the ability of patients to perform basic self-care activities, a strong correlation was noted between the degree of difficulty of performing these tasks and the extent of limitation of shoulder motion. Although the results of these studies to some extent are related to the choice of measurement tools, these findings highlight the complexity of disablement and suggest that identification of the strength or weakness of the links among the levels of disablement may help a therapist more accurately predict a patient's prognosis and the likelihood of functional improvement as the result of treatment. Evaluating these relationships and answering the other questions noted in Box 1-10 lays the foundation for ascertaining a diagnosis and prognosis and developing an effective plan of care.

Diagnosis

The term diagnosis can be used in two ways; it refers to either a *process* or a *category* (label) within a classification system.[26] Both usages of the word are relevant to physical therapy practice. Diagnosis is an essential element of patient management because diagnosis directs physical therapy prognosis (including the plan of care) and interventions.[2,83]

Diagnostic Process

The diagnostic process is a complex *sequence* of actions and decisions that begins with: (1) the collection of data (examination); (2) the analysis and interpretation of all relevant data collected, leading to the generation of working hypotheses (evaluation); and (3) organization of data, recognition of clustering of data (a pattern of findings), formation of a diagnostic hypothesis, and subsequent classification of data into categories (diagnosis).[2,14,78,83]

This process is necessary to develop a prognosis (including a plan of care) and is a prerequisite for treatment.[13,40,78,83] Through the diagnostic process, a *physical therapist classifies dysfunction* (most often, movement dysfunction), whereas a physician identifies disease[40,78] For the physical therapist, the diagnostic process is a mechanism by which discrepancies and consistencies between a patient's desired level of function and the patient's capacity to achieve that level of function are identified.[2]

Diagnostic Category

A diagnostic classification system, recently developed by physical therapists, is useful in delineating the knowledge base and scope of practice of physical therapy.[2,13,26,40,78,83] The use of a common diagnostic classification scheme also fosters clarity of communication in practice and clinical research.[40,83]

A diagnostic category is a grouping that identifies and describes patterns or clusters of physical findings (signs and symptoms of impairment, functional limitation and disability). A diagnostic category also describes the impact of a condition on function at the system level (musculoskeletal, neuromuscular, cardiovascular/pulmonary, or integumentary) and at the level of the whole person.[2] Within each body system are a number of broad-based diagnostic categories *defined by the primary impairments* exhibited by a patient. Box 1–11 lists the diagnostic categories developed by consensus by physical therapists for the musculoskeletal system.[2]

Most of the conditions discussed in this textbook can be classified in at least one of these categories. These diagnoses and complete descriptions of all diagnostic categories for each system can be found in the *Guide to Physical Therapist Practice.*[2]

Preferred practice patterns, which are identified by the diagnostic categories, represent consensus-based opinions that outline broad patient management guidelines and strategies for each diagnostic category.[2,11,27] These patterns are *not* designed to indicate a specific pathway of care, such as an exercise protocol for a specific postoperative condition, but rather a description of all components of patient management from examination through discharge for which physical therapists are responsible. In other words, the preferred practice patterns describe what it is that physical therapists do. For a detailed description of each preferred practice pattern for the musculoskeletal neuromuscular, cardiovascular/pulmonary, and integumentary systems, refer to *The Guide to Physical Therapist Practice.*[2]

Prognosis and Plan of Care

After the initial examination has been completed, data have been evaluated and an impairment-based diagnosis has been established, a prognosis (see Fig. 1–3), including a plan of care, must be determined before initiating any interventions. A prognosis is a prediction of the patient's optimal level of function expected as the result of a course of treatment and the anticipated length of time needed to reach specified functional outcomes.[2] Some factors that influence a patient's prognosis and functional outcomes are noted in Box 1–12.

Determining an accurate prognosis is, indeed, challenging even for experienced therapists. The more complex a patient's problems, the more difficult it is to project the patient's optimal level of function, particularly at the onset of treatment. For example, if an otherwise healthy and fit 70-year-old patient, who was just discharged from the hospital after a total knee replacement, is referred for home-based physical therapy services, it is relatively easy to predict the timeframe that will be needed to prepare the patient to return to independence in the home and community. In contrast, it may only be possible to predict incremental levels of functional improvement at various stages of rehabilitation for a patient who has sustained multiple fractures and soft tissue injuries as the result of an automobile accident. In these two examples of establishing prognoses for patients with musculoskeletal conditions, as with most other patient problems, the accuracy of the prognosis is, in part, affected by the therapist's clinical decision-making ability based on:[57]

- Familiarity with the patient's condition including pathology and surgical interventions
- A thorough knowledge of the process and timeframes of tissue healing
- Experience managing patients with similar pathologies, impairments, and functional limitations
- Knowledge of the efficacy of tests and measures and physical therapy interventions

Box 1–11 Diagnostic Classifications for the Musculoskeletal System

- Primary prevention/risk reduction for skeletal demineralization
- Impaired posture
- Impaired muscle performance
- Impaired joint mobility, motor function, muscle performance, and range of motion associated with connective tissue dysfunction
- Impaired joint mobility, motor function, muscle performance, and range of motion associated with localized inflammation
- Impaired joint mobility, motor function, muscle performance, range of motion, and reflex integrity associated with spinal disorders
- Impaired joint mobility, muscle performance, and range of motion associated with fracture
- Impaired joint mobility, motor function, muscle performance, and range of motion associated with joint arthroplasty
- Impaired joint mobility, motor function, muscle performance, and range of motion associated with bony or soft tissue surgery
- Impaired motor function, muscle performance, range of motion, gait, locomotion, and balance associated with amputation

Box 1–12 Factors that Influence a Patient's Prognosis/Expected Outcomes

- Complexity, severity, acuity, or chronicity and expected course of the patient's condition(s) (pathology), impairments, and functional limitations
- Patient's general health status and presence of comorbidities and risk factors
- Patient's and/or family's goals
- Patient's motivation and adherence and responses to previous interventions
- Safety issues and concerns
- Extent of support (physical, emotional, and social)

The **plan of care** is an integral component of the prognosis. It delineates the following:[2]

- Anticipated goals
- Expected functional outcomes that are meaningful, utilitarian, sustainable, and measurable
- The extent of improvement predicted and the length of time necessary to reach that level
- Specific interventions
- Proposed frequency and duration of interventions
- Specific discharge plans

Developing a plan of care involves *collaboration* and *negotiation* between the patient (and, when appropriate, the family) and the therapist.[38] The *anticipated goals* and *expected outcomes* documented in the plan of care must be patient-centered. That is, the goals and outcomes must be meaningful to the patient. These goals and outcomes must also be measurable and linked to each other. Goals are directed at the reduction or elimination of the physical signs and symptoms of pathology and impairments that seem to be limiting the patient's functional abilities.[2] Outcomes are associated with the amelioration of functional limitations and disability to the greatest extent possible, coupled with the achievement of the optimal level possible of general health and patient satisfaction.[2]

Establishing meaningful, functionally relevant goals and outcomes requires engaging the patient and/or family in the decision-making process from a therapist's first contact with a patient. Patients come to physical therapy not to get stronger or more flexible, but rather to be able to perform physical activities with ease and comfort that they enjoy doing or must do in their lives. Knowing what a patient wants to be able to accomplish as the result of treatment helps a therapist determine and prioritize intervention strategies that will target the patient's functional limitations and functionally related impairments. This, in turn, increases the likelihood of successful outcomes from treatment.[69,73] Several resources in the literature identify ways to develop goals and outcomes that are functionally relevant and meaningful to the patient.[3,68,69,73] Some key questions that a therapist often asks a patient or the patient's extended support system early in the examination while taking the history but that are also critical for establishing anticipated goals and expected outcomes in the plan of care are listed in Box 1–13.

An integral aspect of effective goal and outcome setting is explaining to a patient how the pathology and identified impairments are associated with the patient's functional limitations and why specific interventions will be used. Discussing an expected timeframe for achieving the negotiated goals and outcomes puts the treatment plan and the patient's perception of progress in a realistic context. This type of information helps a patient and family members set goals that are not just meaningful, but also realistic and attainable. Setting up *short-term and long-term goals,* particularly for patients with severe or complex problems, is also a way to help a patient recognize incremental improvements and progress during treatment.

The plan of care also indicates the optimal level of improvement that will be reflected by the functional outcomes as well as how those outcomes will be measured. An outline of the specific interventions, their frequency and duration of use, and how the interventions are directly related to the attainment of the stated goals and outcomes must also appear in the plan. Finally, the plan of care concludes with the criteria for discharge. These criteria are addressed following a discussion of elements of intervention in the patient management process.

Box 1–13 Key Questions to Establish Patient-Centered Goals and Outcomes in the Plan of Care

- What activities are most important to you at home, school, work, or during your leisure time?
- What activities do you need help with that you would like to be able to do independently?
- Of the activities you are finding difficult to do or cannot do at all at this time, which ones would you like to be able to do better or do again?
- Of the problems you are having, which ones do you want to try to eliminate or minimize first?
- In what areas do you think you have the biggest problems during the activities you would like to do on your own?
- What are your goals for coming to physical therapy? What would you like to be able to accomplish through therapy?
- What would make you feel that you were making progress in achieving your goals?
- How soon do you want to reach your goals?

Note: Periodic re-examination of a patient and re-evaluation of a patient's response to treatment may necessitate modification of the initial prognosis and plan of care.

Intervention

Intervention refers to any *purposeful interaction* a therapist has that directly relates to a patient's care[2] (see Fig. 1–3). There are three broad areas of intervention that occur during the course of patient management:[2]

- Coordination, communication, and documentation
- Procedural interventions
- Patient-related instruction

Each of these areas is an essential aspect of the intervention phase of patient management. Absence of just one of these elements can adversely affect outcomes. For example, inclusion of the most appropriate exercises (procedural intervention) in a treatment program will not lead to successful outcomes if the therapist has not communicated with the necessary parties for an approval or extension of physical therapy services (communication) or if the patient has not learned how to perform the exercises in the program correctly (patient-related instruction). A brief discussion of the three major components of intervention is presented in this section with additional information on exercise instruction, an aspect of patient-related instruction that is most relevant to the focus of this textbook.

Coordination, Communication, and Documentation

The physical therapist is the coordinator of physical therapy care and services and must continually communicate verbally and through written documentation with all individuals involved in the care of a patient. This aspect of intervention encompasses many different patient-related administrative tasks and supportive processes, such as writing reports (evaluations, plans of care, discharge summaries), designing home exercise programs, keeping records, contacting community-based resources, and participating in team conferences.

Note: Even during the intervention phase of patient management, a therapist might decide that referral to another practitioner during the course of physical therapy intervention is appropriate and complementary to the physical therapy interventions. This requires coordination and communication with other healthcare practitioners. For example, a therapist might refer a patient, who is generally deconditioned from a sedentary lifestyle and who is also obese, to a nutritionist for dietary counseling to complement the physical therapy program designed to improve the patient's aerobic capacity (cardiorespiratory endurance) and general level of fitness.

Procedural Interventions

This aspect of intervention pertains to the use of specific procedures used in treatment, such as therapeutic exercise, functional training, or adjunctive modalities (physical agents and electrotherapy). Procedural interventions are identified in the plan of care. Most procedural interventions used by physical therapists, including types of therapeutic exercise, are designed to reduce or correct impairments. If these interventions are to be considered effective, they must also result in a reduction or elimination of functional limitations and, whenever possible, should reduce the risk of future dysfunction.

Although the intended outcome of therapeutic exercise programs has always been to enhance a patient's functional capabilities or prevent loss of function, until the past decade the focus of exercise programs was on the resolution of impairments with success measured primarily by the reduction of the identified impairments or improvements in various aspects of physical performance, such as strength, mobility, or balance. It was assumed that if impairments were resolved, improvements in functional abilities would subsequently follow. Physical therapists now recognize that this assumption should not be made. To reduce functional limitations and improve a patient's health-related quality of life, not only should therapeutic exercise interventions be implemented that correct functionally relevant impairments but, whenever possible, exercises should be performed using movement patterns that closely match a patient's intended functional activities. This point is exemplified in a study of the effects of a resistance exercise program on the stair-climbing abilities of ambulatory older women.[9] Rather than having the subjects perform open-chain, resisted hip, and knee extension exercises, they trained by ascending and descending stairs while wearing a weighted backpack. This activity not only improved muscle performance (strength and endurance), it directly enhanced the subjects' efficiency in stair-climbing.

Another way to effectively use therapeutic exercise interventions to improve functional abilities is to integrate safe but progressively more challenging functional activities that utilize incremental improvements in strength, endurance, and mobility into a patient's daily routine as early as possible in the treatment program. With this functionally oriented approach to exercise, the activities in the treatment program are specific to and directly support the expected functional outcomes. Selection and use of exercise procedures that target more than one goal or outcome is also an appropriate and efficient way to maximize improvements in a patient's function in the shortest time possible.

Effective use of any procedural intervention must include determining the appropriate *frequency* and *duration* of each intervention and periodic re-examination of a patient's responses to the interventions. While implementing therapeutic exercise interventions, a patient's response to exercise is continually monitored to decide when and to what extent to progress the difficulty of the exercise program or when to discontinue specific exercises. Each of the chapters of this textbook provides detailed information on factors that influence selection, application, and progression of therapeutic exercise interventions.

Patient-Related Instruction

There is no question that physical therapists perceive themselves as patient educators, facilitators of change, and motivators.[8,20,38,52,66] Patient education spans all three domains of learning: the cognitive, affective, and psychomotor domains. Education ideally begins during a patient's initial contact with a therapist. Patient-related instruction, the third aspect of intervention during the patient management process, is the means by which a therapist helps a patient *learn* how to get better[8] by becoming an active participant in the rehabilitation process. Patient-related instruction may first focus on providing a patient with background information, such as the interrelationships among the primary condition (pathology) and the resulting impairments and functional limitations or explaining the purpose of specific interventions in the plan of care. Instruction may also center on specific aspects of the treatment program, such as teaching a patient, family member, or caregiver a series of exercises to be carried out in a home program, reviewing health and wellness materials, or clarifying directions for safe use of equipment that is to be used at home. Therapist-directed instruction has benefits for patients. For instance, it has been shown that patients who were taught exercises by a therapist performed their exercises more accurately in a home program than patients whose sole source of information about their exercises was from reading a brochure.[19]

To be an effective patient educator a therapist must possess an understanding of the process of learning, which most often is directed toward learning or adapting motor skills. As a patient educator a therapist must also be able to recognize a patient's learning style, implement effective teaching strategies, and motivate a patient to *want* to learn new skills, adhere to an exercise program, or change health-related behaviors. Because this textbook deals with therapeutic exercise, strategies for effective *exercise instruction,* based on concepts of motor learning and methods of promoting a patient's adherence to an exercise program, are discussed in the final section of this chapter.

A therapist's skillful and creative use of all three components of intervention, coupled with vigilant re-examination and re-evaluation of the interventions selected, paves the way for successful outcomes and a patient's discharge from physical therapy services.

Outcomes

Simply stated, outcomes are results. Collection and analysis of outcome data related to healthcare services is a necessity, not an option.[30] Measurement of outcomes is a means by which quality, efficacy, and cost-effectiveness of services can be assessed. Outcomes are monitored *throughout* an episode of physical therapy care, that is, intermittently during treatment and at the conclusion of treatment.[69] Evaluation of information generated from periodic re-examination and re-evaluation of a patient's response to treatment enables a therapist to ascertain if the anticipated goals and expected outcomes in the plan of care are being met and if the interventions that have been implemented are producing the intended results. It may well be that the goals and outcomes must be adjusted based on the extent of change or lack of change in a patient's function as determined by the measurement of interim outcomes. This information also helps the therapist decide if, when, and to what extent to modify the goals, outcomes, and interventions in the patient's plan of care.

There are several broad areas of outcomes commonly assessed by physical therapists during the continuum of patient care. They are

- The level of a patient's physical function, including impairments, functional limitations, and perceived disability
- The extent of prevention or reduced risk of occurrence or recurrence of future dysfunction related to pathology, impairments, functional limitations, or disability
- The patient's general health status or level of wellness and fitness
- The degree of patient satisfaction

Functional Outcomes

The key to justification of physical therapy services in today's cost-conscious healthcare system is the identification and documentation of successful functional outcomes that can be attributed to interventions.[2,4,7,91] Functional outcomes must be *meaningful, practical, and sustainable.*[91] Outcomes that have an impact on a patient's ability to function at work, in the home, or in the community in ways that have been identified as important by the patient, family, significant others, caregivers, or employers are considered *meaningful.* If the formulation of anticipated goals and expected outcome has been a collaborative effort between patient and therapist, the outcomes will be meaningful to the patient. The *practical* aspect of functional outcomes implies that improvements in function have been achieved in an efficient and cost-effective manner. Improvements in function that are maintained over time after discharge from treatment (to the extent possible given the nature of the pathology) are considered *sustainable.*

Measuring the Impact of Physical Therapy Interventions

The expected outcomes identified in a physical therapy plan of care must be *measurable.* More specifically, changes in a patient's status over time must be *quantifiable.* As noted in the previous discussion of the examination component of the patient management model, many of the specific tests and measures used by physical therapists have traditionally measured impairments (i.e., ROM, muscle performance, joint mobility, or balance). Reduction of impairments may reflect the impact of interventions on the pathological condition but may or may not translate into improvements in health-related quality of life (safety, functional limitations, and disability). Hence, there is the need not only for measurement of impairments but also functional limitations and the level of perceived disability to accurately assess outcomes in physical function and the effectiveness of interventions, such as therapeutic exercise. Some recent studies that have investigated the benefits of exercise programs for individuals with impaired functional abilities[42,47,82] reflect the trend in research for the inclusion of the assessment of changes in a patient's health-related quality of life as the result of intervention.

Assessment of outcomes related to the reduction of risks of future injury or further impairment, prevention of further functional limitations or disability, adherence to a home program, or the use of knowledge that promotes optimal health and fitness may also determine the effectiveness of the services provided. Physical therapists are finding that it is important to collect follow-up data that demonstrate a reduced need for future physical therapy services as the result of interventions directed toward prevention and health promotion activities to substantiate that the use of physical therapy services for prevention is cost-effective.

Another area of outcome assessment that has become increasingly important in physical therapy practice is that of *patient satisfaction.* An assessment of patient satisfaction during or at the conclusion of treatment is one method to measure quality of care. Instruments, such as the Physical Therapy Outpatient Satisfaction Survey (PTOPS),[81] measure a patient's perception of many areas of care including access, the therapist's skills (interpersonal and clinical) and administrative issues, such as scheduling and continuity of care. Patient satisfaction surveys also seek to determine the impact of treatment based on the patient's own assessment of his or her status at the conclusion in comparison to the onset of treatment.[81]

Discharge Planning

Planning for discharge begins early in the rehabilitation process. As previously noted, criteria for discharge are identified in a patient's plan of care. Ongoing assessment of outcomes is the mechanism by which a therapist determines when discharge from care is warranted. A patient is discharged from physical therapy services when the anticipated goals and expected outcomes have been attained.[2] The discharge plan often includes some type of home program, appropriate follow-up, possible referral to community resources, or re-initiation of physical therapy services (an additional episode of care) if the patient's needs change over time and if additional services are approved.

Discontinuation of services is differentiated from discharge.[2] *Discontinuation* refers to the ending of services prior to the achievement of anticipated goals and expected outcomes. Several factors may necessitate discontinuation of services, which may include a decision by a patient to stop services, a change in a patient's medical status such that progress is no longer possible, or the need for further services cannot be justified to the payer.

In conclusion, the patient management model discussed in this section establishes a comprehensive and systematic approach to the provision of effective and efficient physical therapy care and services to patients and clients. The model is a mechanism to demonstrate the interrelationships among each of the phases of the continuum of patient care which is set in a conceptual framework of disablement and is aimed at improving a patient's function and health-related quality of life. The management model also places an emphasis on reducing risk factors for disease, injury, or disability and promoting health and wellness in patients and clients seeking and receiving physical therapy services.

Strategies for Effective Exercise Instruction

As discussed in the previous section of this chapter, patient-related instruction is an essential element of the intervention phase of patient management. As a patient educator, a therapist spends a substantial amount of time teaching patients or their families how to perform exercises correctly and safely. Effective strategies to help patients learn an exercise program under therapist supervision and then carry it out on an independent basis over a necessary period of time contribute to successful outcomes for the patient. Box 1–14 summarizes some practical suggestions for effective exercise instruction.

Box 1–14 Practical Suggestions for Effective Exercise Instruction

- Select a nondistracting environment for exercise instruction.
- Demonstrate proper performance of an exercise (safe vs. unsafe movements; correct vs. incorrect movements). Then have the patient model your movements.
- If appropriate or feasible, initially guide the patient through the desired movement.
- Use clear and concise verbal and written directions.
- Complement written instructions for a home exercise program with illustrations (sketches) of the exercise.
- Have the patient demonstrate an exercise to you as you supervise and provide feedback.
- Provide specific, action-related feedback rather than general, nondescriptive feedback. For example, explain *why* the exercise was performed correctly or incorrectly.
- Teach an entire exercise program in small increments to allow time for a patient to practice and learn components of the program over several visits.

Preparation for Exercise Instruction

When preparing to teach a patient a series of exercises, a therapist should have a plan that will facilitate learning prior to and during exercise interventions. A positive relationship between therapist and patient is a fundamental aspect for creating a motivating environment that fosters learning. A collaborative relationship should be established when the goals for the plan of care are negotiated. This, of course, occurs before exercise instruction begins. Effective exercise instruction is also based on knowing a patient's learning style; that is, if he or she prefers to learn by watching, reading about, or doing an activity. This may not be known early in treatment, so several methods of instruction may be necessary.

Identifying a patient's attitude toward exercise helps a therapist determine how receptive a patient is likely to be about learning and adhering to an exercise program. Does the patient believe exercise will lessen symptoms or improve function? Is the patient concerned that exercising will be uncomfortable? Is the patient accustomed to engaging in regular exercise? Answers to these questions help a therapist formulate a strategy for enhancing a patient's motivation to exercise. One method to promote motivation is to design the exercise program so that the least complicated or stressful exercises are taught first, thus ensuring early success. Always ending an exercise session with a successful effort also helps maintain a patient's level of motivation. Additional suggestions to enhance motivation and promote adherence to an exercise program are discussed in this section after a review of concepts of motor learning.

Concepts of Motor Learning: A Foundation of Exercise Instruction

Integration of motor learning principles into exercise instruction optimizes learning an exercise or functional task. An exercise is simply a motor task (a psychomotor skill) that a therapist teaches and a patient is expected to learn.

Motor learning is a complex set of internal processes that involves the *relatively permanent* acquisition and retention of a skilled movement or task through practice.[85,98] It is thought that motor learning probably modifies the way that sensory information within the central nervous system is organized and processed and affects how motor actions are produced. Motor learning is not directly observable; therefore, it must be measured by observation and analysis of motor performance.

Types of Motor Tasks

There are three basic types of motor tasks: discrete, serial, and continuous.[85] A *discrete task* involves a movement with a recognizable beginning and end. Grasping an object, doing a push-up or locking a wheelchair are examples of discrete motor tasks. Almost all exercises, such as lifting and lowering a weight or performing a self-stretching maneuver, can be categorized as discrete motor tasks. A *serial task* is composed of a series of discrete movements that are combined together in a particular sequence. For example, in order to eat with a fork, a person must be able to grasp the fork, hold it in the correct position, scoop up the food, and lift the fork to the mouth. Many functional tasks in the work setting, for instance, are serial tasks with simple as well as complex components. Some serial tasks require specific timing between each segment of the task or momentum during the task. Wheelchair transfers are serial tasks. A patient must learn how to position the chair, lock the chair, possibly remove an armrest, scoot forward in the chair, and then transfer from the chair to another surface. Some transfers require momentum whereas others do not. A *continuous task* involves repetitive, uninterrupted movements that have no distinct beginning and ending. Examples include walking, ascending and descending stairs, and cycling. Being able to recognize the type of skilled movements that a patient must learn helps a therapist decide which instructional strategies will be most beneficial for acquiring specific functional skills.

Consider what must be learned in the following motor tasks of an exercise program. To self-stretch the hamstrings, a patient must learn how to position and align his or her body and how much stretch force to apply to perform the stretching maneuver correctly. As flexibility improves, the patient must then learn how to safely control active movements in the newly gained portion of the range during functional activities. This requires muscles to contract with correct intensity at an unaccustomed length. In another scenario, to prevent recurrence of a shoulder impingement syndrome or back pain, a patient may need to learn through posture training how to maintain correct alignment of the trunk during a variety of reaching or lifting tasks that place slightly different demands on the patient. In both of these situations motor learning must occur for the exercise program and functional training to be effective. By viewing exercise interventions from this perspective, it becomes apparent why application of strategies to promote motor learning are an integral component of an effective exercise program.

Stages of Motor Learning

There are three stages of motor learning: the cognitive, associative, and autonomous stages.[17] The characteristics of the learner are different at each stage of learning and, consequently, affect the type of instructional strategies selected by a therapist.

Cognitive Stage

When learning a motor skill, a patient first must figure out *what* to do, that is, the patient must learn the goal or purpose and the requirements of the exercise or functional task. Then the patient must learn *how* to do the motor task safely and correctly. At this stage, the patient needs to think about each component or sequence of the exercise.[15,21,67,85] The patient often focuses on how his or her body is aligned and how far and with what intensity to move. In other words, the patient tries to get the "feel" of the exercise. Since all of the patient's attention is often directed to the correct performance of the motor task, distractions in the environment, such as a busy, noisy exercise room, may initially interfere with learning. During this stage of learning errors in performance are common, but with practice, the patient gradually learns to differentiate correct from incorrect performance, initially with frequent feedback from a therapist and eventually by monitoring his or her own performance (self-evaluation).

Associative Stage

The patient makes infrequent errors and concentrates on fine-tuning the motor task during the associative stage of learning. Learning centers on producing the most consistent and efficient movements. The timing of the movements and the distances moved also may be refined. The patient explores slight variations and modifications of movement strategies while doing the task under different environmental conditions. The patient also uses problem solving to correct errors when they do occur. At this stage the patient requires infrequent feedback from the therapist and instead begins to anticipate necessary adjustments and make corrections even before errors occur.

Autonomous Stage

Movements are automatic in this final stage of learning. The patient does not have to pay attention to the movements in the task, thus making it possible to do other tasks simultaneously. The patient also easily adapts to variations in task demands and environmental conditions. Very little, if any, instruction goes on in this phase of learning unless the patient encounters a recurrence of symptoms or other problems. In fact, most patients are discharged before reaching this stage of learning.

Variables that Influence Motor Learning During Exercise Instruction

Motor learning is influenced by many variables, some of which can be manipulated by a therapist during exercise instruction to facilitate learning. Some of these variables include *pre-practice considerations, practice, and feedback.* An understanding of these variables and their impacts on motor learning is necessary to develop strategies for successful exercise instruction and functional training. A brief overview of these key variables that influence the acquisition and retention of skilled movements during each stage of motor learning is presented in this section. Because concepts and principles of motor learning encompass an extensive body of knowledge, the reader is referred to several in-depth resources for additional information.[21,67,85]

Pre-Practice Considerations

A number of variables can influence motor learning in an exercise session even before practice begins. A patient's *understanding* of the purpose of an exercise or task as well as interest in the task affect skill acquisition and retention. The more meaningful a task is to a patient, the more likely that learning will occur. *Attention* to the task at hand also affects learning. The ability to focus on the skill to be learned without distracting influences in the environment promotes learning. Instructions that are given to a patient prior to practice about where his or her attention should be directed during practice may also affect learning. There is evidence in studies of nonimpaired individuals that learning is enhanced if a person attends to the outcomes of performing a task rather than to the details of the task itself.[61,101] This finding is addressed in more detail in a later discussion of feedback and motor learning. *Demonstration* of a task prior to commencing practice also enhances learning. It is often helpful for a patient to observe another person, usually the therapist or possibly another patient, perform the exercise or functional task correctly and then model those actions. *Pre-practice verbal instructions* that describe the task may also facilitate skill acquisition but should be succinct. Extensive information about the task requirements early in the learning process may actually confuse a patient rather than enhance the learning process.

Practice

Motor learning occurs as the direct result of repeatedly performing a movement or series of movements within a task.[49,85] It is probably the single most important variable in learning a motor skill. The *amount, type,* and *variability* of practice directly affects the extent of skill acquisition and retention.[67,85] In general, the more a patient practices a motor task, the more readily it is learned. In today's healthcare environment most of a patient's time spent performing exercises or practicing functional tasks occurs independent of therapist supervision as the patient carries out an exercise program at home or participates in group exercise sessions. Therefore, a therapist must be certain that new motor skills initially are practiced under therapist supervision and learned in an efficient manner. A therapist often sets the practice conditions for a home program prior to a patient's discharge by making suggestions about how to progress the newly acquired skills (exercises or functional tasks) in the later stages of learning to make them more difficult but still safe.

The type of practice strategy selected also has a significant impact on how readily a motor task is learned.[49,67,85,98] Several types of practice are described in Box 1–15.

The type of skill to be learned (discrete, serial, or continuous) and the patient's stage of motor learning determine which practice strategies are more appropriate than others. *Part practice,* for example, has been shown to be most effective in the early stage of learning for acquisition of complex serial skills that have simple and difficult components. Usually it is only necessary to practice the difficult dimensions of the task before practicing the task as a whole. Part practice is less effective than *whole practice* for acquiring continuous skills, such as walking and climbing stairs, or serial tasks in which momentum or timing of the components is the central focus of the learning process. Whole practice is obviously used for acquisition of discrete tasks, such as an ex-

Box 1–15 Types of Practice for Motor Learning

Part Versus Whole Practice

- *Part practice.* A task is broken down into separate dimensions; individual and usually the more difficult components of the task are practiced; after mastery of the individual segments, they are combined in sequence so that the whole task can be practiced
- *Whole practice.* The entire task is performed from beginning to end and is not practiced in separate segments

Blocked, Random, and Random-Blocked Practice

- *Blocked practice.* The same task or series of exercises or tasks is performed repeatedly under the same conditions and in a predictable order; for example, the patient may consistently practice walking in the same environment, standing up from the same height chair, or lifting the same size weight or container; therefore, the task does not change from one repetition to the next
- *Random practice.* Slight variations of the same task are carried out in an unpredictable order; for example, a patient could practice standing up from chairs of different heights or styles in a random order; therefore the task changes with each repetition
- *Random-blocked practice.* Variations of the same task are performed in random order, but each variation of the task is performed more than once; for example, the patient rises from a particular height or style chair, and then repeats the same task a second time before moving on to a different height or style chair

Physical Versus Mental Practice

- *Physical practice.* The movements of an exercise or functional task are actually performed
- *Mental practice.* A cognitive rehearsal of how a motor task is to be performed occurs prior to actually doing the task; the terms *visualization* and *imagery* are used synonymously with mental practice

ercise that involves repetitions of a single movement pattern.

During the initial phase of rehabilitation practice is usually directed toward learning just a few exercises or tasks. In the cognitive stage of learning a new task, *blocked practice* is the appropriate choice because it rapidly improves performance of skilled movements. A transition to *random* or *random-blocked practice* should be made as soon as possible to introduce *variability* into the learning process. Although blocked practice initially improves performance at a faster rate than random practice, random practice leads to better skill retention and generalizability of skills than blocked practice.[67,85] It is thought that varying tasks just slightly, as is done in random practice, requires more cognitive processing and problem solving than blocked practice and, subsequently, culminates in greater retention. Random-blocked practice results in faster skill acquisition than random practice and better retention than blocked practice. Because random-blocked practice enables a patient to perform a task at least twice before changing to another variation of the task, this form of practice gives a patient the opportunity to identify and then immediately correct errors in a movement sequence before proceeding to the next task.

Although physical practice of motor skills by overtly performing the task is considerably superior to mental practice alone for learning motor tasks, mental practice, when used in conjunction with physical practice, has been shown to enhance motor skill acquisition at a faster rate than use of only physical practice.[56,67,85] It is thought that mental rehearsal of a motor task reinforces the cognitive component of motor learning, that is, learning what to do when performing a task.

Feedback

Second only to practice, feedback is considered to be the next most important variable that influences learning.[67] Feedback is sensory information that is received by the learner during or after performance of a movement or task.[67,85,99,100] There are two broad categories of feedback: *intrinsic* (internal) and *augmented* (external). Feedback is also classified by how and when it is given. Box 1–16 describes the different categories of feedback.

Both intrinsic and augmented forms of feedback are useful tools for facilitating motor learning. To use feedback effectively during exercise instruction and functional training, a therapist must decide the *type* of feedback to provide or bring to a patient's attention as well as the most appropriate *amount* and *timing* of feedback during the practice sessions in each stage of motor learning. A therapist should also encourage a patient to provide input on the amount, type, and timing of feedback particularly once the patient has achieved a beginning level of skill acquisition. This participation promotes a sense of self-control in the patient and is thought to have a positive impact on learning.[61]

The types of feedback selected during instruction are often dependent on the status of the patient's sensory system identified during the examination. If, for example, the proprioceptive system is impaired, a therapist may decide to initially use visual feedback so that the patient receives accurate information when a task or exercise is new. Later, the use of proprioceptive feedback may be emphasized to challenge the impaired sensory system. The type of

Box 1–16 Types of Feedback Associated with Motor Learning

Intrinsic Feedback

- A sensory cue or set of cues that are inherent in the execution of a motor task
- Arises directly from performance of the task
- May immediately follow completion of a task or may occur even before a task has been completed
- Most often involves proprioceptive, kinesthetic, tactile, visual, or auditory cues

Augmented Feedback

- Sensory cues from an external source that are supplemental to intrinsic feedback; they are not inherent in the execution of the task
- May arise from a mechanical source or from another person

Concurrent Versus Terminal Feedback

- *Concurrent.* Occurs during the performance of a task
- *Terminal.* Occurs after completion of a task

Immediate, Delayed, and Summary Feedback

- *Immediate.* Occurs or is given directly after a task is completed
- *Delayed.* An interval of time elapses before information is given, which allows time for the learner to reflect on how well or poorly a task was done
- *Summary.* Information is given about the average performance of several repetitions of a movement or task

Knowledge of Performance (KP) Versus Knowledge of Results (KR)

- *KP.* Immediate, post-task, augmented feedback (usually verbal) about the *nature* or *quality* of the performance of a motor task
- *KR.* Immediate, post-task, augmented feedback about the *outcome* of a motor task

feedback chosen is also dependent on the stage of motor learning regardless of whether the sensory systems are impaired or intact. A patient may be instructed to respond to either internal feedback or to external feedback when first learning a task. If the patient is instructed to focus on internal feedback, attention is directed to the movements themselves, such as how the movements are to be performed or sequenced or how the movements feel. If the patient is told to focus on external feedback, attention is directed toward the outcomes of movements.[61] Although research, primarily with non-impaired subjects, has shown that directing a person's attention to the effects of movements rather than to the details of the movements themselves enhances learning,[101] in the clinical setting, traditionally therapists have had patients use an internal focus to first learn the movements inherent in an exercise or motor task, such as the sequence of movements required to weight shift from side to side to maintain standing balance. Therapists are now becoming more familiar with principles of motor learning and recognize the benefits of having a patient perform weight-shifting activities by reaching for objects placed in various positions around the patient, thus focusing on the outcome of the movement. The patient then learns to judge the effectiveness of his or her movements based on feedback received from external cues. Using feedback in this manner is more likely to facilitate motor learning.[61,101]

Therapists have many forms of augmented feedback from which to select for use during exercise instruction and functional training.[100] Some forms of augmented feedback enhance skill acquisition (performance) but are less effective for achieving retention. For example, when nonimpaired subjects practiced a partial weight-bearing activity, those who received concurrent visual feedback (by looking at a scale) achieved the skill more quickly than the subjects who received either immediate or summary *postresponse* feedback (KR). However, subjects who received concurrent feedback performed least well on a retention test 2 days after practice ended than the subjects in the two other groups who received postresponse feedback.[99] Manual guidance, another form of augmented concurrent feedback used extensively in the clinical setting, also may do little to enhance skill acquisition or retention of a motor skill. In fact, as with other forms of augmented concurrent feedback, manual guidance is thought to be detrimental to learning (skill retention) because it fosters dependency on feedback to do the task correctly.[67,85]

The greatest amount or frequency of feedback is necessary in the cognitive stage of learning when a patient is first learning how to perform an exercise or a functional task. Extended use of any form of augmented feedback can create dependency on the feedback and has been shown to be a deterrent to self-detection and correction of errors.[85] Use of *summary feedback,* particularly in the associative stage of learning, is an effective strategy to reduce the total amount of feedback given in a practice session. As augmented feedback is reduced, a patient must explore slight modifications of a movement strategy and analyze the results. This promotes problem solving, self-monitoring, and self-correction, which enable a patient to perform tasks independently and safely.

The timing of feedback also affects learning and should be adjusted during the learning process. Initially, immediate feedback may be necessary for patient safety, but immediate feedback does little to promote self-detection of errors and problem solving to prevent or correct errors. Use of *delayed feedback* after each repetition of a task or exercise or use of summary feedback gives the patient time for problem solving during practice. This process promotes retention and generalizability of the learned skills. In the study previously noted in which subjects practiced a partial weight-bearing task, summary feedback was found to enhance retention to a greater extent than immediate, postresponse feedback.[99]

Box 1–17 summarizes the information discussed in this section with regard to qualities of the learner and effective strategies for exercise instruction and functional training founded on the principles and stages of motor learning.

Adherence

Effective exercise instruction must include considerations for fostering *adherence* to a functionally oriented exercise program. This is particularly challenging when an exercise program must be carried out for an extended period of time. Positive outcomes from treatment are contingent not so much on designing the optimal exercise program for a patient but rather designing a program that a patient or family will actually follow.[36,37,95]

Box 1–17 Qualities of the Learner and Instructional Strategies for the Three Stages of Motor Learning

Cognitive Stage

Qualities of the Learner

Must attend only to the task at hand; must think about each step or component; easily distractible; starts to get a "feel" for the exercise; makes errors and alters performance, particularly when given augmented feedback; begins to differentiate correct vs. incorrect and safe vs. unsafe performance.

Instructional Strategies

- Identify the purpose of the exercise or functional task.
- Demonstrate the movements (modeling).
- Initially, guide or assist the patient through the movements. Reduce this form of feedback as soon as a patient can safely control movements.
- Point out the distance and speed of the movement (how far or fast to move).
- Break complex movements into parts when appropriate.
- Practice only a few motor tasks. Keep repetitions low and alternate tasks to ensure safety and avoid fatigue.
- Provide frequent and explicit positive feedback.
- Use a variety of forms of feedback (verbal, tactile, visual).
- Introduce the concept of self-evaluation and self-correction of movements.
- Allow trial and error to occur within safe limits.

Associative Stage

Qualities of the Learner

Performs tasks more consistently with fewer errors; executes movements in a well-organized manner; refines the movements in the exercise or functional task; detects and self-corrects movement errors when they occur; is less dependent on visual feedback or verbal feedback from the therapist; uses prospective cues and anticipates errors before they occur

Instructional Strategies

- Emphasize practice of a greater number and variety of movements or tasks.
- Increase the complexity of the exercise or task.
- Emphasize problem solving.
- Avoid manual guidance.
- Vary the sequence of exercise or tasks practiced.
- Allow the patient to practice independently, emphasizing problem solving.
- Introduce simulation of functional tasks into the practice session.
- Decrease the total amount of feedback but increase specificity; allow the learner to perform a full set of exercises or several repetitions of a functional task before providing feedback (summary feedback).
- Delay feedback to give the learner an opportunity to detect errors and self-correct them.
- Increase the level of distraction in the exercise environment.

Autonomous Stage

Qualities of the Learner

Performs the task consistently and automatically and while doing other tasks; applies the learned movement strategies to increasingly more difficult or new environmental situations; if appropriate, performs the task more quickly or for an extended period of time at a lower energy cost

Instructional Strategies

- Set up a series of progressively more difficult activities the learner can do independently such as increasing the speed, distance, and complexity of the exercises or task.
- Suggest ways the learner can vary the original exercise or task and use the task in more challenging situations encountered in everyday activities.
- If the patient is still in therapy ,which at most is usually for just a recheck, use little to no feedback unless a potentially unsafe situation arises.

*Adapted from Dennis, JK and McKeough, DM: Mobility. In May, BJ (ed): Home Health and Rehabilitation—Concepts of Care, ed 2. FA Davis, Philadelphia, 1999, pp 121–123 with permission.

Note: Although the terms *adherence* and *compliance* are often used interchangeably by clinicians and in the literature, the term *adherence* has been selected for this discussion because it has a stronger connotation of active involvement of the patient, whereas *compliance* tends to have a more passive connotation.

Many factors influence adherence to an exercise program.[37,38,61,66,95] Some of these factors include:

- Characteristics of the patient: memory, willingness and receptivity to change, fatigue, stress, understanding of the situation, self-perception of the degree of control of the exercise program, cultural background and beliefs about exercise, the value the patient places on the exercise program, and the patient's access to resources
- Factors related to the disease, disorder, injury, or condition: acuity, chronicity, or stability of the pathology; impact of comorbidities
- Treatment-related variables: continuity of care, complexity, and necessary duration of the exercise program, adequacy of instruction and feedback from the therapist, and whether or not the patient has had input into the treatment plan

Box 1–18 Ways to Foster Adherence to an Exercise Program

- Explore and try to appreciate the patient's beliefs about exercising or the value the patient places on exercising as a means to "get better."
- Help the patient identify personal benefits derived from adhering to the exercise program.
- Explain the rationale and importance of each exercise and functional activity.
- Identify how specific exercises are designed to meet specific patient-centered goals or functional outcomes.
- Allow and encourage the patient to have input into the nature and scope of the exercise program, the selection and scheduling of practice and feedback, and decisions of when and to what extent exercises are progressed to enhance a patient's sense of self-control.
- Keep the exercise program as brief as possible.
- Identify practical and functionally oriented ways to do selected exercises during everyday tasks.
- Have the patient keep an exercise log.
- If possible, schedule follow-up visit(s) to review or modify exercises.
- Point out specific exercise-related progress.
- Identify barriers to adherence (not enough time in the day to do the exercises; discomfort during the exercises; lack of necessary equipment); then suggest solutions or modify the exercise program.

Therapists should expect that most patients will not dutifully adhere to any treatment program, particularly if regular exercise has not been a part of the patient's life prior to the occurrence of disease or injury. The most the therapist can hope to do is implement strategies that foster adherence. Some suggestions from a number of resources in the literature[37,38,61,66,95] are noted in Box 1–18.

Independent Learning Activities

CRITICAL THINKING AND DISCUSSION

1. Critically analyze your own, an acquaintance's, or a family member's exercise history. Then identify how a regular regimen of exercise could improve your quality of life or theirs.
2. Research four different pathological conditions, diseases, injuries, or disorders that result in primary impairments of the (1) musculoskeletal, (2) neuromuscular, (3) cardiovascular/pulmonary, and (4) integumentary systems. Identify characteristic impairments (signs and symptoms) associated with each pathology and hypothesize what functional limitations and disabilities are most likely to develop.
3. Why is it essential for a physical therapist to understand and be able to articulate (verbally or in written form) the interrelationships among pathology, impairments, functional limitations, and disability?
4. Last month you sprained your ankle (inversion sprain). You had to use crutches for several days, but since then you've been walking independently. Pain and swelling still return after vigorous activity, and your ankle feels unstable on uneven terrain. Using the disablement model as your frame of reference, identify specific functional limitations that would most likely develop in your life as the result of your history and current problems.
5. Using your current knowledge of examination procedures, develop a list of specific tests and measures you would most likely choose to use when examining a patient whose primary impairments affect the (1) musculoskeletal, (2) neuromuscular, (3) cardiovascular and/or pulmonary and (4) integumentary systems.
6. You have been asked to make recommendations for the adoption of one or more new measure-

ment instruments to be used at your facility for data collection and analysis of functional outcomes. Review the literature on musculoskeletal assessment and identify and summarize key features of five instruments that measure functional limitations associated with musculoskeletal impairments of the extremities, neck, or trunk. In addition, identify and summarize key features of five measurement instruments that assess a patient's perceived level of disability.

7. Three different individuals just recently sustained a similar fracture of the hip. All underwent an open reduction with internal fixation. The patients are: an otherwise healthy 19-year-old college student who was in an automobile accident and wants to return to campus after discharge from the hospital; a 60-year-old person with a somewhat sedentary lifestyle who plans to return home after postoperative rehabilitation and wishes to return to work in an office as soon as possible; and an 80-year-old individual with severe age-related osteoporosis who has been residing in an assisted living facility for the past year. What issues must be considered when identifying anticipated goals and expected outcomes and determining appropriate interventions in the plans of care for these patients? In what ways would goals and expected outcomes differ for these patients?

8. Identify the key components of the patient management model described in this chapter and discuss how each of those components relates to the potential use of therapeutic exercise interventions.

REFERENCES

1. American College of Sports Medicine: ACSM's Guidelines for Exercise Testing and Prescription, ed. 6. Lippincott Williams & Wilkins, Philadelphia, 2000.
2. American Physical Therapy Association: Guide to Physical Therapist Practice, ed 2. Phys Ther 81:9–744, 2001.
3. Baker, SM, et al: Patient participation in physical therapy goal setting. Phys Ther 81: 1118, 2001.
4. Basmajian, J (ed): Physical Rehabilitation Outcome Measures. Canadian Physiotherapy Association in cooperation with Health and Welfare Canada and Canada Communications Group, Toronto, 1994.
5. Boissonnault, W: Differential diagnosis: taking a step back before stepping forward. PT Magazine of Physical Therapy 8:46, 2000.
6. Brandt, EN Jr., and Pope, AM (eds): Enabling America: Assesing the Role of Rehabilitation Science and Engineering. Institute of Medicine, National Academy Press, Washington, DC, 1997, p 62.
7. Charness, AL: Outcomes measurement: intervention versus outcomes. In Cirullo, JA (ed): Orthop Phys Ther Clin North Am 3:147, 1994.
8. Chase, L, et al: Perceptions of physical therapists toward patient education. In Shepard, KF and Jensen, GM (eds): Handbook of Teaching for Physical Therapists. Butterworth Heinemann, Boston, 1997, p 225.
9. Cress, ME, et al: Functional training: muscle structure, function and performance in older women. J Orthop Sports Phys Ther 24:4, 1996.
10. Croakin, E: Osteopenia: implications for physical therapists managing patients of all ages. PT Magazine of Physical Therapy 9:80, 2001.
11. Dalton, D: The Guide to Physical Therapist Practice: Incorporating preferred practice patterns into orthopedic practice. Orthop Phys Ther Prac 11:15, 1999.
12. Davis, CM: Model for teaching physical therapy diagnosis at the post-entry level. J Phys Ther Educ 9:54, 1995.
13. Dekker, J, et al: Diagnosis and treatment in physical therapy. An investigation of their relationship. Phys Ther 73:568, 1993.
14. DeLitto, A, and Snyder-Mackler, L: The diagnostic process: examples in orthopedic physical therapy. Phys Ther 75:203, 1995.
15. Dennis, JK, and McKeough, DM: Mobility. In May BJ (ed): Home Health and Rehabilitation: Concepts of Care, ed 2. FA Davis, Philadelphia, 1999, p 109.
16. Embrey, DG, et al: Clinical decision making by experienced and inexperienced pediatric physical therapists for children with diplegic cerebral palsy. Phys Ther 76:20, 1996.
17. Fitts, PM, and Posner, MI: Human Performance. Brooks/Cole, Belmont, CA, 1967.
18. Francis, KT: Status of the year 2000 health goals for physical activity and fitness. Phys Ther 79:405, 1999.
19. Friedrich, M, Cernak, T, and Maderbacher, P: The effect of brochure use versus therapist teaching on patients' performing therapeutic exercise and on changes in impairment status. Phys Ther 76:1082, 1996.
20. Gahimer, JE, and Domboldt, E: Amount of patient education in physical therapy practice and perceived effects. Phys Ther 76:1089, 1996.
21. Gentile, AM: Skill acquisition: Action, movement, and neuromotor processes. In Carr, J, et al: Movement Science: Foundations for Physical Therapy in Rehabilitation. Aspen Publishers, Rockville, MD, 1987, p 93.
22. Giallonardo, L: The Guide to Physical Therapist Practice: An overview for the orthopedic physical therapist. Orthopedic Physical Therapy Practice 10:10, 1998.
23. Goldstein, TS: Functional Rehabilitation in Orthopaedics. Aspen Publishers, Gaithersburg, MD, 1995.

24. Goodman, CC, and Snyder, TEK: Differential Diagnosis in Physical Therapy, ed 3. WB Saunders, Philadelphia, 2000.
25. Guccione, A: Arthritis and the process of disablement. Phys Ther 74:408, 1994.
26. Guccione, A: Physical therapy diagnosis and the relationship between impairment and function. Phys Ther 71:449, 1991.
27. Hack, LM: History, purpose and structure of part two: Preferred practice patterns. PT Magazine of Physical Therapy 6:72, 1998.
28. Harris, BA, and Dyrek, DA: A model of orthopedic dysfunction for clinical decision making in physical therapy practice. Phys Ther 69:548, 1989.
29. Harris, BA: Building documentation using a clinical decision making model. In Stewart, DL and Abeln, SH: Documenting Functional Outcomes in Physical Therapy. Mosby-Year Book, St Louis, 1993, p 81.
30. Hart, DL, Geril, AC, and Pfohl, RL: Outcomes process in daily practice. PT Magazine of Physical Therapy 5: 68, 1997.
31. Heerkens, YF, et al: Impairments and disabilities—the difference: Proposal for the adjustment of the International Classification of Impairments, Disabilities and Handicaps. Phys Ther 74:430, 1994.
32. Herman, KM, and Reese, CS: Relationship among selected measures of impairment, functional limitation and disability in patients with cervical spine disorders. Phys Ther 81:903, 2001.
33. ICIDH: International Classification of Impairments, Disabilities and Handicaps: A Manual of Classification Relating to Consequences of Disease. World Health Organization, Geneva, 1980.
34. ICIDH-2: International Classification of Functioning, Disability and Health. World Health Organization, Geneva, 2000.
35. Jensen, GM, Shepard, KF, and Hack, LM: The novice versus the experienced clinician: insights into the work of the physical therapist. Phys Ther 70:314, 1990.
36. Jensen, GM, Shepard, KF, Gwyer, J, and Hack, LM: Attribute dimensions that distinguish master and novice physical therapy clinicians in orthopedic settings. Phys Ther 72:711, 1992.
37. Jensen, GM, and Lorish, C: Promoting patient cooperation with exercise programs: linking research, theory and practice. Arthritis Care and Research 7:181, 1994.
38. Jensen, GM, Lorish C, and Shepard, KF: Understanding patient receptivity to change: Teaching for treatment adherence. In Shepard, KF, and Jensen, GM: Handbook of Teaching for Physical Therapists. Butterworth-Heinemann, Boston, 1997, p 241.
39. Jetle, AM, Branch, LG, and Berlin, J: Musculoskeletal impairment and physical disablement among the aged. J Gerontol 45:M203, 1990.
40. Jette, AM: Diagnosis and classification by physical therapists: A special communication. Phys Ther 69:967, 1989.
41. Jette, AM: Physical disablement concepts for physical therapy research and practice. Phys Ther 74:380, 1994.
42. Jette, AM, et al: Exercise—It's never too late: the Strong for Life Program. Am J Public Health 89:66, 1999.
43. Jones, MA: Clinical reasoning in manual therapy. Phys Ther 72:875, 1992.
44. Jones, M, Jensen, G, and Rothstein, J: Clinical reasoning in physiotherapy. In Higgs, J, and Jones, M (eds): Clinical Reasoning in the Health Professions. Butterworth—Heinemann, Oxford, 1995, p 72.
45. Kauffman, TL, Nashner, LM, and Allison, LK: Balance is a critical parameter in orthopedic rehabilitation. Orthopedic Physical Therapy Clinics North America 6:43, 1997.
46. Kelo, MJ: Use of self-report disability measures in daily practice. Orthopedic Physical Therapy Practice 11:22, 1999.
47. Krebs, DE, Jetle, AM, and Assmann, SF: Moderate exercise improves gait stability in disabled elders. Arch Phys Med Rehabil 79:1489, 1998.
48. Lane, JN, Riley, EH, and Wirgnowicz, PZ: Osteoporosis: diagnosis and treatment J Bone Joint Surg 78A:618, 1996.
49. Lee, T, and Swanson, L: What is repeated in a repetition: Effects of practice conditions on motor skill acquisition. Phys Ther 71:150, 1991.
50. Leighton, RD, and Sheldon, MR: Model for teaching clinical decision making in a physical therapy professional curriculum. J Phys Ther Educ 11:23, Fall 1997.
51. Lephart, S, Swanik, CB, and Fu, F: Reestablishing neuromuscular control. In Prentice, WE (ed): Rehabilitation Techniques in Sports Medicine, ed 3. WCB/McGraw-Hill, Boston, 1999, p 88.
52. Lorish, C, and Gale, JR: Facilitating behavior change: strategies for education and practice. J Phys Ther Educ 13:31, 1999.
53. Lusardi, MM: Mobility and balance in later life. Orthopedic Physical Therapy Clinics of North America 6:305, 1997.
54. Magee, DJ: Orthopedic Physical Assessment. WB Saunders, Philadelphia, 1997.
55. Magistro, CM: Clinical decision making in physical therapy: A practitioner's perspective. Phys Ther 69:525, 1989.
56. Maring, J: Effects of mental practice on rate of skill acquisition. Phys Ther 70:165, 1990.
57. May, BJ, and Dennis, JK: Clinical decision making. In May, BJ (ed): Home Health and Rehabilitation—Concepts of Care, ed 2. FA Davis, Philadelphia, 1999, p 21.
58. May, BJ, and Dennis, JK: Expert decision making in physical therapy. A survey of practitioners. Phys Ther 71:190, 1991.
59. McArdle, WD, Katch, FI, and Katch, VL: Essentials of Exercise Physiology, ed 2. Lippincott Williams & Wilkins, Philadelphia, 2000.
60. McCloy, CM: Prevention and health promotion strategies in osteoporosis management. Orthopedic Physical Therapy Clinics of North America 7:235, 1998.
61. McNevin, NH, Wulf, G, and Carlson, C: Effects of attentional focus, self-control and dyad training on motor learning: implications for physical rehabilitation. Phys Ther 80:373, 2000.
62. Nagi, SZ: Disability and Rehabilitation. The Ohio State University Press, Columbus, 1969.
63. Nagi, SZ: Disability concepts revisited: implications for prevention. In Pope, AM, and Tarlov, AR (eds): Disability in America. National Academy Press Washington, DC, 1991.
64. Nashner, L: Sensory, neuromuscular and biomechanical contributions to human balance. In Duncan, P (ed): Balance. American Physical Therapy Association, Alexandria, VA, 1990, p 5.
65. National Advisory Board on Medical Rehabilitation Research, Draft V: Report and Plan for Medical Rehabilitation Research. National Institutes of Health, Bethesda, MD, 1992.

66. Nemshick, MT: Designing educational interventions for patients and families. In Shepard, KF, and Jensen, GM (eds): Handbook of Teaching for Physical Therapists. Butterworth-Heinemann, Boston, 1997, p 303.
67. Nicholson, DE: Teaching psychomotor skills. In Shepard, KF, and Jensen, GM (eds): Handbook of Teaching for Physical Therapists. Butterworth-Heinemann, Boston, 1997, p.271.
68. O'Sullivan, SB: Clinical decision making: Planning effective treatments. In O'Sullivan, SB and Schmitz, TJ: Physical Rehabilitation: Assessment and Treatment, ed 4. FA Davis, Philadelphia, 2001, p1.
69. Ozer, MN, Payton, OD, and Nelson, CE: Treatment Planning for Rehabilitation: A Patient-Centered Approach. McGraw-Hill, New York, 2000.
70. Payton, O: Clinical reasoning process in physical therapy. Phys Ther 65:924, 1985.
71. Posner, JD, et al: Physical determinants in independence in mature women. Arch Phys Med and Rehabil 76:373, 1995.
72. Public Health Service: Healthy People 2000: National Health Promotion and Disease Prevention Objectives. U.S. Department of Heath and Human Services, Washington, DC, 1991, DHHS Publication No. (PHS) 91-50212.
73. Randall, KE, and McEwen, IR: Writing patient-centered functional goals. Phys Ther 80:1197, 2000.
74. Rantanen, T, et al: Disability, physical activity and muscle strength in older women: The Women's Health and Aging Study. Arch Phys Med Rehabil 80:130, 1999.
75. Riddle, DL, and Stratford, PW: Use of generic vs region-specific functional status measures on patients with cervical spine disorders. Phys Ther 78:951, 1998.
76. Rivett, DA, and Higgs, J: Hypothesis generation in the clinical reasoning behavior of manual therapists. J Phys Ther Educ 11:40, 1997.
77. Rose, SJ, and Rothstein, JM: Muscle mutability, part 1: general concepts and adaptations to altered patterns of use. Phys Ther 62:1773, 1982.
78. Rose, SJ: Physical therapy diagnosis: Role and function. Phys Ther 69:535, 1989.
79. Rothstein, JM: Disability and our identity. (Editorial) Phys Ther 74:374, 1994.
80. Rothstein, JM, and Echternach, JL: Hypothesis-oriented algorithm for clinicians: a method for evaluation and treatment planning. Phys Ther 66:1388, 1986.
81. Roush, SE, and Sonstroen, RJ: Development of the Physical Therapy Outpatient Satisfaction Survey (PTOPS). Phys Ther 79:159, 1999.
82. Ruhland, JL, and Shields, RK: The effects of a home exercise program on impairment and health-related quality of life in persons with chronic peripheral neuropathies. Phys Ther 77:1026, 1997.
83. Sahrmann, SA: Diagnosis by physical therapists: A prerequisite for treatment. Phys Ther 68:1703, 1988.
84. Schenkman, M, and Butler, R: A model for multisystem evaluation, interpretation and treatment of individuals with neurologic dysfunction. Phys Ther 69:538, 1989.
85. Schmidt, RA, and Lee, TD: Motor Control and Learning: A Behavioral Emphasis, ed 3. Human Kinetics Pub, Champaign, IL, 1999.
86. Schmitz, TJ: Coordination assessment. In O'Sullivan, SB and Schmitz, TJ: Physical Rehabilitation: Assessment and Treatment, ed 4. FA Davis, Philadelphia, 2001, p 157.
87. Seymour, CJ, and Dybel, GJ: Developing skillful clinical decision making: Evaluation of two classroom teaching strategies. J Phys Ther Educ 10:77, 1996.
88. Shumway-Cook, A, et al: The effect of multidimensional exercises on balance, mobility and fall risk in community-dwelling older adults. Phys Ther 77:46, 1997.
89. Stith, JS, Sahrmann, SA, et al: Curriculum to prepare diagnosticians in physical therapy. J Phys Ther Educ 9: 46, 1995.
90. Sullivan, PE, and Markos, PD: Clinical Decision Making in Therapeutic Exercise. Appleton and Lange, Norwalk, CT, 1995.
91. Swanson, G: Functional outcome report: The next generation in physical therapy reporting. In Stewart, DL, and Abeln, SH: Documenting Functional Outcomes in Physical Therapy. Mosby-Year Book, St Louis, 1993, p 101.
92. Task Force for Standards of Measurement in Physical Therapy: Standards for tests and measurements in physical therapy practice. Phys Ther 71:589, 1991.
93. Tichenor, CJ, Davidson, J, and Jensen, GM: Cases as shared inquiry: Model of clinical reasoning. J Phys Ther Educ 9:57, 1995.
94. Triffett, MA: The relationship between motion of the shoulder and the stated ability to perform activities of daily living. J Bone Joint Surg 80A:41, 1998.
95. Turk, D: Correlates of exercise compliance in physical therapy (commentary). Phys Ther 73:783, 1993.
96. Umphried, D: Physical therapy differential diagnosis in the clinical setting. J Phys Ther Educ 9:39, 1995.
97. Verbrugge, L, and Jetle, A: The disablement process. Soc Sci Med 38:1, 1994.
98. Winstein, C, and Sullivan, K: Some distinctions on the motor learning/motor control distinction. Neurology Report 21:42, 1997.
99. Winstein, C, et al: Learning a partial-weight-bearing skill effectiveness of two forms of feedback. Phys Ther 76:985, 1996.
100. Winstein, C: Knowledge of results and motor learning: Implications for physical therapy. Phys Ther 71:140, 1991.
101. Wulf, G, Hob, M, and Prinz, W: Instructions for motor learning: differential effects of internal vs. external focus of attention. Journal of Motor Behavior 30:169, 1998.
102. Zinny, NJ: Physical therapy management from physical therapy diagnosis: Necessary but insufficient. J Phys Ther Educ 9:36, 1995.

Chapter 2

Range of Motion

OBJECTIVES

After studying this chapter, the reader will be able to:

1 Describe ROM and what affects it.

2 Differentiate among types of ROM exercises, their limitations and benefits, and their indications and contraindications.

3 Discriminate between the indications and goals for passive and active ROM activities.

4 Describe procedures for applying ROM techniques.

5 Apply techniques for joint and muscle ROM using anatomic planes of motion.

6 Apply techniques of ROM using self-assistance and mechanical assistance including wand, finger ladder, pulley, and powder (skate) board.

7 Describe the benefits and procedures for use of continuous passive motion (CPM) equipment.

Range of motion (ROM) is a basic technique used for examination of movement and for initiating movement into a program of therapeutic intervention. Movement that is necessary to accomplish functional activities can be viewed, in its simplest form, as muscles or external forces moving bones in various patterns or ranges of motions. When a person moves, the intricate control of the muscle activity that causes or controls the motion comes from the central nervous system. Bones move with respect to each other at the connecting joints. The structure of the joints, as well as the integrity and flexibility of the soft tissues that pass over the joints, affects the amount of motion that can occur between any two bones. The full motion possible is called the range of motion (ROM). When moving a segment through its ROM, all structures in the region are affected: muscles, joint surfaces, capsules, ligaments, fasciae, vessels, and nerves. ROM activities are most easily described in terms of joint range and muscle range. To describe joint range, terms such as flexion, extension, abduction, adduction, and rotation are used. Ranges of available joint motion are usually measured with a goniometer and recorded in degrees.[15] Muscle range is related to the functional excursion of muscles.

Functional excursion is the distance that a muscle is capable of shortening after it has been elongated to its maximum.[25] In some cases the functional excursion, or range of a muscle, is directly influenced by the joint it crosses. For example, the range for the brachialis muscle is limited by the range available at the elbow joint. This is true of one-joint muscles (muscles with their proximal and distal attachments on the bones on either side of one joint). For two-joint or multijoint muscles (those muscles that cross over two or more joints), their range goes beyond the limits of any one joint they cross. An example of a two-joint muscle functioning at the elbow is the biceps brachii muscle. If it contracts and moves the elbow into flexion and the forearm into supination while simultaneously moving the shoulder into flexion, it will shorten to a point known as *active insufficiency,* where it can shorten no more. This is one end of its range. The muscle is lengthened full range by extending the elbow, pronating the forearm, and simultaneously extending the shoulder. When fully elongated it is in a position known as *passive insufficiency.* Two-joint or multijoint muscles normally function in the midportion of their functional excursion, where ideal length-tension relationships exist.[25]

To maintain normal ROM, the segments must be moved through their available ranges periodically, whether it be the available joint range or muscle range. It is recognized that many factors can lead to decreased ROM, such as systemic, joint, neurologic, or muscular diseases; surgical or traumatic insults; or simply inactivity or immobilization for any reason. Therapeutically, ROM activities are administered to maintain joint and soft tissue mobility in order to minimize loss of tissue flexibility and contracture formation.[5] Extensive research by Salter has provided evidence of the benefits of movement on the healing of tissues in various pathological conditions both in the laboratory and in clinical settings.[19–24]

The principles of ROM that are described in this chapter do not encompass stretching to increase range. Principles and techniques of stretching and joint mobilization are described in Chapters 5 and 6.

Types of Range of Motion (ROM) Exercises

- ***Passive ROM (PROM).*** PROM movement is within the unrestricted ROM for a segment that is produced entirely by an *external force;* there is little to or no voluntary muscle contraction. The external force may be from gravity, a machine, another individual, or another part of the individual's own body.[7] PROM and passive stretching are not synonymous; see Chapter 5 for definitions and descriptions of passive stretching.
- ***Active ROM (AROM).*** AROM is movement within the unrestricted ROM for a segment that is produced by an active contraction of the *muscles* crossing that joint.
- ***Active-Assistive ROM (A-AROM).*** A-AROM is a type of AROM in which assistance is provided by an outside force, either manually or mechanically, because the prime mover muscles need assistance to complete the motion.

Indications and Goals for Range of Motion

Passive Range of Motion

Indications for PROM

- In the region where there is acute, inflamed tissue, passive motion is beneficial; active motion would be detrimental to the healing process. Inflammation after injury or surgery usually lasts 2 to 6 days.
- When a patient is not able to or not supposed to actively move a segment or segments of the body as when comatose, paralyzed, or on complete bed rest, movement is provided by an external source.

Goals for PROM

The primary goal for PROM is to decrease the complications that would occur with immobilization such as cartilage degeneration, adhesion and contracture formation, and sluggish circulation.[7,19,24] Specifically, the goals are to:

- Maintain joint and connective tissue mobility
- Minimize the effects of the formation of **contractures**
- Maintain mechanical elasticity of muscle
- Assist circulation and vascular dynamics
- Enhance synovial movement for cartilage nutrition and diffusion of materials in the joint
- Decrease or inhibit pain
- Assist with the healing process after injury or surgery
- Help maintain the patient's awareness of movement

Other Uses for PROM

- When a therapist is examining inert structures, PROM is used to determine limitations of motion, to determine joint stability, and to determine muscle and other soft tissue elasticity.
- When a therapist is teaching an active exercise program, PROM is used to demonstrate the desired motion.
- When a therapist is preparing a patient for stretching, PROM is often used preceding the passive stretching techniques. Techniques to increase the ROM when motion is restricted are described in Chapters 5 and 6.

Active and Active-Assistive ROM

Indications for AROM

- Whenever a patient is able to actively contract the muscles and move a segment either with or without assistance, AROM is used.
- When a patient has weak musculature and is unable to move a joint through the desired range (usually against gravity), A-AROM is used to provide enough assistance to the muscles in a carefully controlled manner so that the muscle can function at its maximum level and progressively be strengthened. Once the patient gains control of the full ROM, he or she may then be progressed to manual or mechanical resistance exercises if more strength is necessary to return to functional activities (see Chapter 3).
- AROM can be used for aerobic conditioning programs (see Chapter 4).
- When a segment of the body is immobilized for a period of time, AROM is used on the regions

above and below the immobilized segment to maintain the areas in as normal a condition as possible and to prepare for new activities, such as walking with crutches.

Goals for AROM

If there is no inflammation or contraindication to active motion, the same goals of PROM can be met with AROM. In addition, there are physiological benefits that result from an active muscle contraction and motor learning from voluntary muscle control. Specific goals include:

- Maintain physiologic elasticity and contractility of the participating muscles.
- Provide sensory feedback from the contracting muscles.
- Provide a stimulus for bone and joint tissue integrity.
- Increase circulation and prevent thrombus formation.
- Develop coordination and motor skills for functional activities.

Box 2–1 Summary of Precautions and Contraindications to Range of Motion Exercises

ROM should not be done when motion is disruptive to the healing process.

- Carefully controlled motion within the limits of pain-free motion during early phases of healing have been shown to benefit healing and early recovery.
- Signs of too much or the wrong motion include increased pain and inflammation.

ROM should not be done when patient response or the condition is life-threatening.

- PROM may be carefully initiated to major joints and AROM to ankles and feet to minimize venous stasis and thrombus formation.
- After myocardial infarction, coronary artery bypass surgery, or percutaneous transluminal coronary angioplasty, AROM of upper extremities and limited walking are usually tolerated under careful monitoring of symptoms.

Note: ROM is not synonymous with stretching. For precautions and contraindications to passive and active stretching techniques, see Chapters 5 and 6.

Limitations of Range of Motion Exercises

Limitations of Passive Motion

True passive, relaxed ROM may be difficult to obtain when muscle is innervated and the patient is conscious.

Passive motion *will not:*

- Prevent muscle atrophy
- Increase strength or endurance
- Assist circulation to the extent that active, voluntary muscle contraction does

Limitations of Active ROM

For strong muscles, *it will not* maintain or increase strength (see Chapter 3). *It will not* develop skill or coordination except in the movement patterns used.

Precautions and Contraindications to Range of Motion

Although both PROM and AROM are contraindicated under any circumstance when motion to a part is disruptive to the healing process (Box 2–1), complete immobility leads to adhesion and contracture formation, sluggish circulation, and prolonged recovery time. In light of research by Salter[21] and others,[13] early, continuous PROM within a pain-free range has been shown to be beneficial to the healing and early recovery of many soft tissue and joint lesions (this is discussed later in this chapter). Historically, ROM has been contraindicated immediately after acute tears, fractures, and surgery, but because the benefits of controlled motion have demonstrated decreased pain and an increased rate of recovery, early controlled motion is used as long as the patient's tolerance is monitored. It is imperative that the therapist recognizes the value as well as potential abuse of motion and stay within the range, speed, and tolerance of the patient during the acute recovery stage.[7] Additional trauma to the part is contraindicated. Signs of too much or the wrong motion include increased pain and increased inflammation (greater swelling, heat, and redness). (See Chapter 8 for principles of when to use various types of passive and active motion therapeutically.)

Usually, AROM of the upper extremities and limited walking near the bed are tolerated as early exercises after myocardial infarction, coronary artery bypass surgery, or percutaneous transluminal coronary angioplasty.[6,9] Careful monitoring of symptoms, perceived exertion, and blood pressure is necessary. If patient response or the condition is life-threatening, PROM may be carefully initiated to the major joints along with some AROM to the ankles and feet to avoid venous stasis and thrombus formation. Individualized activities are initiated and progress gradually as the patient tolerates (Box 2–1).[6,9]

▶ Principles and Procedures for Applying Range of Motion Techniques

Examination, Evaluation, and Treatment Planning

1. Examine and evaluate the patient's impairments and level of function, determine any precautions and prognosis, and plan the intervention.
2. Determine the ability of the patient to participate in the ROM activity and whether or not PROM, A-AROM, or AROM will meet the immediate goals.
3. Determine the amount of motion that can be safely applied for the condition of the tissues and health of the individual.
4. Decide what patterns will best meet the goals. ROM techniques may be performed in the
   - Anatomic planes of motion: frontal, sagittal, transverse
   - Muscle range of elongation: antagonistic to the line of pull of the muscle
   - Combined patterns: diagonal motions or movements that incorporate several planes of motion
   - Functional patterns: motions used in activities of daily living (ADL)
5. Monitor the patient's general condition and responses during and after the examination and intervention; note any change in vital signs, any change in the warmth and color of the segment, and any change in the ROM, pain, or quality of movement.
6. Document and communicate findings and intervention.
7. Re-evaluate and modify the intervention as necessary.

Prepare the Patient

1. Communicate with the patient. Describe the plan and method of intervention to meet the goals.
2. Free the region from restrictive clothing, linen, splints, and dressings. Drape the patient as necessary.
3. Position the patient in a comfortable position. With proper body alignment and stabilization, and that will allow you to move the segment through the available ROM.
4. Position yourself so that proper body mechanics can be used.

Application of Techniques

1. To control movement, grasp the extremity around the joints. If the joints are painful, modify the grip, still providing support necessary for control.
2. Support areas of poor structural integrity such as a hypermobile joint, recent fracture site, or paralyzed limb segment.
3. Move the segment through its complete pain-free range to point of tissue resistance. Do not force beyond the available range. If you force motion, it becomes a stretching technique.
4. Perform the motions smoothly and rhythmically, 5 to 10 repetitions. The number of repetitions depends on the objectives of the program and the patient's condition and response to the treatment.

To Apply PROM

1. The force for movement is external, being provided by a therapist or mechanical device. When appropriate, a patient may provide the force and be taught to move the part with a normal extremity.
2. No active resistance or assistance is given by the patient's muscles crossing the joint. If so, it becomes an active exercise.
3. The motion is carried out within the free ROM, that is, the range that is available without forced motion or pain.

To Apply AROM

1. Demonstrate to the patient the motion desired using PROM, then ask the patient to perform the motion. Have your hands in position to assist or guide the patient if needed.
2. Assistance is given only as needed for smooth motion. When there is weakness, assistance may

be required only at the beginning or end of the ROM, or when the effect of gravity has the greatest moment arm (torque).

3. The motion is performed within the available ROM.

Techniques for Joint and Muscle Range of Motion

The descriptions of positions and ROM in this section may be used for PROM as well as A-AROM and AROM. When making the transition from PROM to AROM, gravity will have a significant impact especially in individuals with weak musculature. When the segment moves up against gravity, it may be necessary to provide assistance to the patient whereas moving parallel to the ground (gravity eliminated or gravity neutral), the part may only need to be supported while the muscles take the part through the range. When the part moves downward, with gravity causing the motion, muscles antagonist to the motion will become active and may need assistance in controlling the descent of the part. The therapist must be aware of these effects and modify the patient position if needed to meet desired goals for A-AROM and AROM. Principles and techniques for progression to manual and mechanical resistance ROM for developing strength are described in Chapter 3.

The following descriptions are, for the most part, with the patient in the supine position. Alternate positions for many motions are possible and, for some motions, are necessary. For efficiency, perform all motions possible in one position, then change the patient's position and perform all appropriate motions in that position, progressing the treatment with minimal turning of the patient. Individual body types or environmental limitations might necessitate variations of the suggested hand placements. Use of good body mechanics by the therapist while applying proper stabilization and motion to the patient to accomplish the goals and avoid injury to weakened structures is the primary consideration.

Note: The term *upper or top hand* means the hand of the therapist that is toward the patient's head; *bottom or lower hand* refers to the hand toward the patient's foot. Antagonistic ROMs are grouped together for ease of application.

Upper Extremity

Shoulder: Flexion and Extension (Fig. 2–1*A* and *B*)

Hand Placement and Procedure

- Grasp the patient's arm under the elbow with your lower hand.
- With the top hand, cross over and grasp the wrist and palm of the patient's hand.
- Lift the arm through the available range and return.

Note: For normal motion, the scapula should be free to rotate upward as the shoulder flexes. If motion of only the glenohumeral joint is desired, the scapula is stabilized as described in the chapter on stretching (Chapter 5).

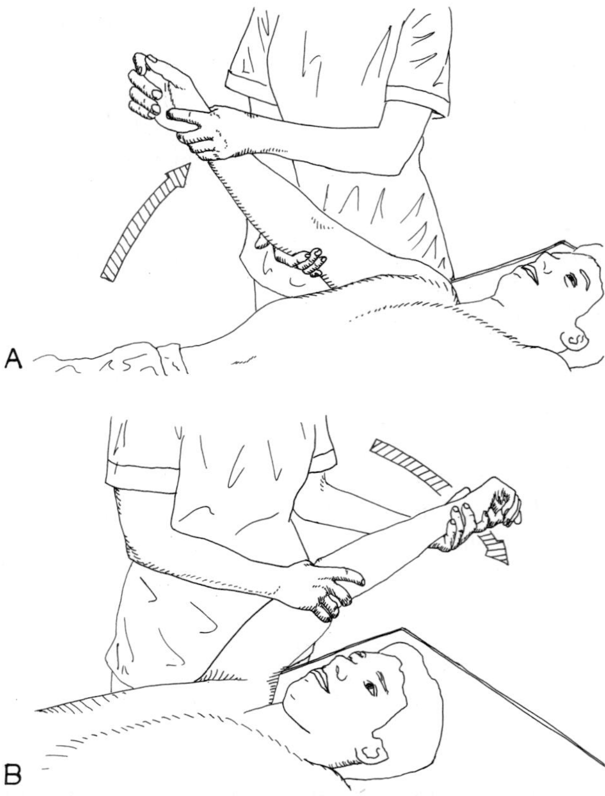

Figure 2–1 Hand placement and positions for (*A*) initiating and (*B*) completing shoulder flexion.

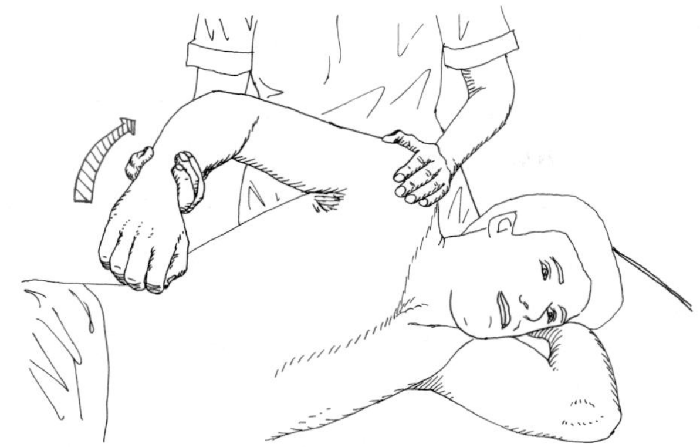

Figure 2–2 Hyperextension of the shoulder with the patient side-lying.

Shoulder: Extension (Hyperextension) (Fig. 2–2)

Alternate Positions

Extension past zero is possible if the patient's shoulder is at the edge of the bed when supine or if the patient is positioned side-lying, prone, or sitting.

Shoulder: Abduction and Adduction (Fig. 2–3)

Hand Placement and Procedure

Use the same hand placement as with flexion, but move the arm out to the side. The elbow may be flexed.

Note: To reach full range of abduction, there must be external rotation of the humerus and upward rotation of the scapula.

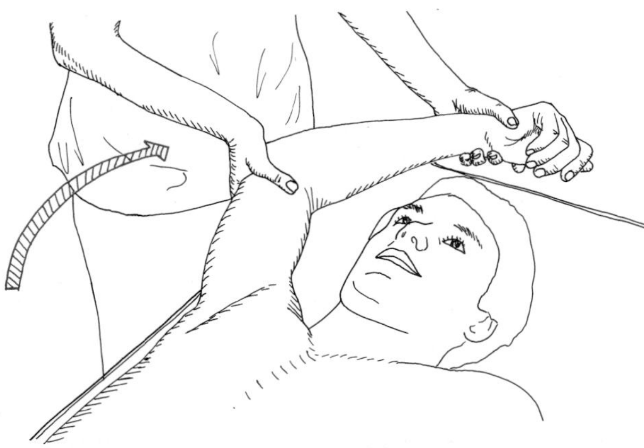

Figure 2–3 Abduction of the shoulder with the elbow flexed.

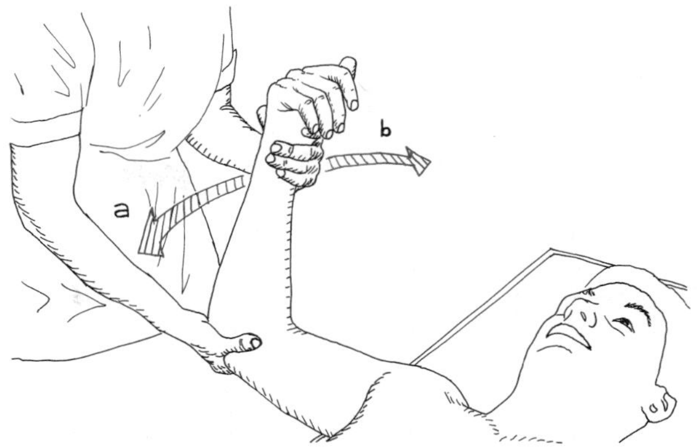

Figure 2–4 Position for initiating (*a*) internal and (*b*) external rotation of the shoulder.

Shoulder: Internal (Medial) and External (Lateral) Rotation (Fig. 2–4)

Initial Position of the Arm

If possible, the arm is abducted to 90 degrees, the elbow is flexed to 90 degrees, and the forearm is held in neutral position. Rotation may also be performed with the patient's arm at the side of thorax, but full internal rotation will not be possible.

Hand Placement and Procedure

- Grasp the hand and the wrist with your index finger between the patient's thumb and index finger.
- Place your thumb and the rest of your fingers on either side of the patient's wrist, thus stabilizing the wrist.
- With the other hand, stabilize the elbow.
- Rotate the humerus by moving the forearm like a spoke on a wheel.

Shoulder: Horizontal Abduction (Extension) and Adduction (Flexion) (Fig. 2–5 *A* and *B*)

Position of the Arm

To reach full horizontal abduction, the shoulder must be at the edge of the table. Begin with the arm either flexed or abducted 90 degrees.

Hand Placement and Procedure

Hand placement is the same as with flexion, but turn your body and face the patient's head as you move the patient's arm out to the side and then across the body.

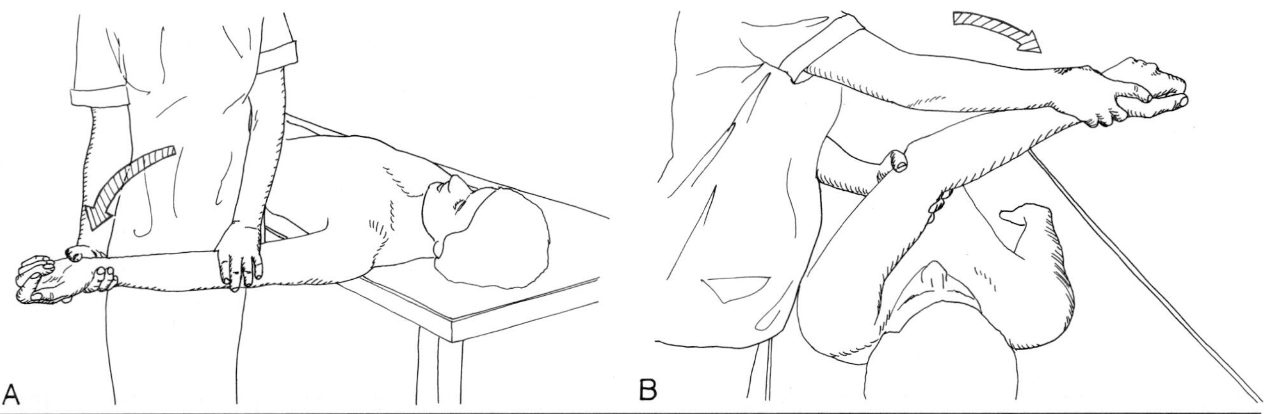

Figure 2–5 Horizontal (*A*) abduction and (*B*) adduction of the shoulder.

Scapula: Elevation/Depression, Protraction/Retraction, and Upward/Downward Rotation (Fig. 2–6)

Alternate Positions

The patient should be prone, with his or her arm at the side, or side-lying, with the patient facing the therapist and the patient's arm draped over the therapist's bottom arm.

Hand Placement and Procedure

- Cup the top hand over the acromion process, and place the other hand around the inferior angle of the scapula.
- For elevation, depression, protraction, and retraction, the clavicle also moves as the scapular motions are directed at the acromion process.
- For rotation, direct the scapular motions at the inferior angle of the scapula while simultaneously pushing the acromion in the opposite direction to create a force couple turning effect.

Elbow: Flexion and Extension (Fig. 2–7)

Hand Placement and Procedure

Hand placement is the same as with shoulder flexion except the motion occurs at the elbow as it is flexed and extended.

Note: Control forearm supination and pronation with your fingers around the distal forearm. Perform elbow flexion and extension with the forearm pronated as well as supinated. The scapula should not tip forward when the elbow extends; this disguises the true range.

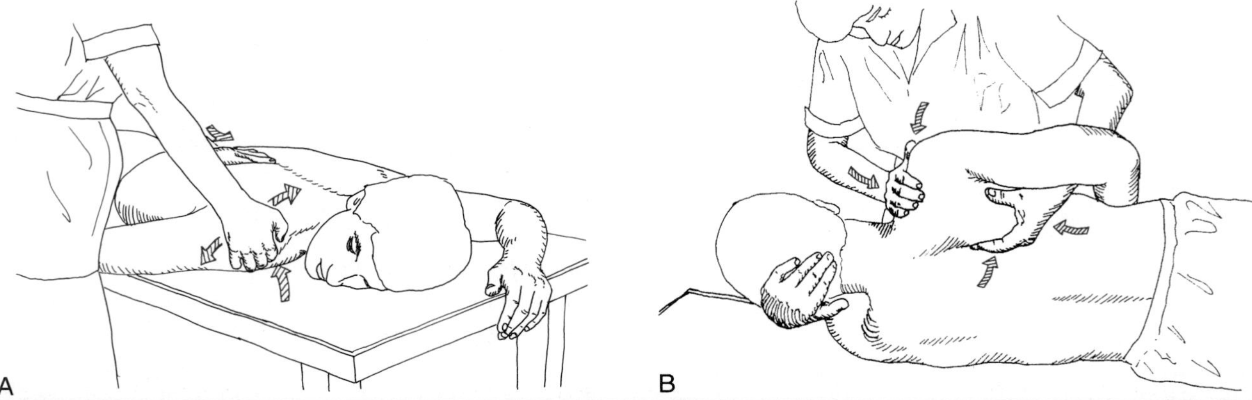

Figure 2–6 Scapular motions with the patient (*A*) prone, and with the patient (*B*) side-lying.

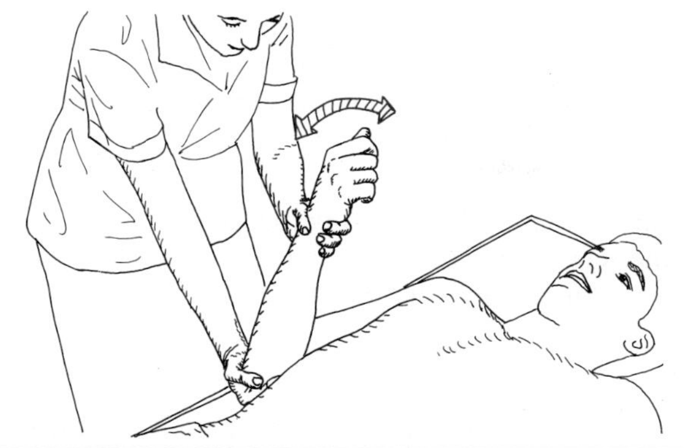

Figure 2–7 Elbow motions with the forearm supinated.

Elongation of Two-Joint Biceps Brachii Muscle (Fig. 2–8)

Position of Patient

The patient should be placed supine, with the shoulder at the edge of the treatment table so that the shoulder can be extended past the neutral position, prone lying, sitting or standing.

Hand Placement and Procedure

- First pronate the patient's forearm by grasping around the wrist, and extend the elbow by supporting under the elbow.
- Then extend (hyperextended) the shoulder to the point of tissue resistance in the anterior arm region. At this point, full available lengthening of the two-joint muscle is reached.

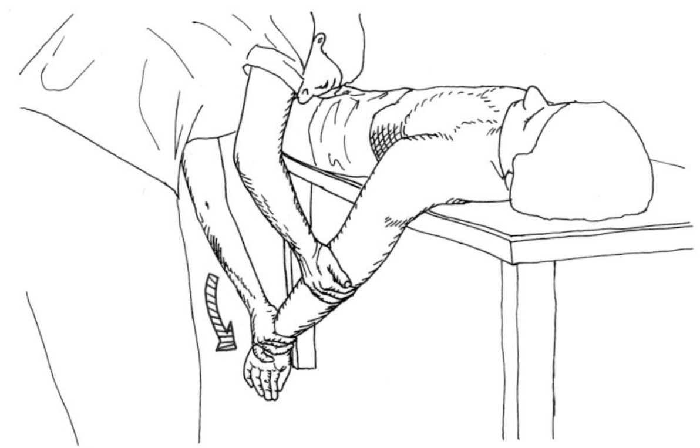

Figure 2–8 End ROM for the biceps brachii muscle.

Elongation of Two-Joint Long Head of the Triceps Brachii Muscle (Fig. 2–9)

Alternate Positions

When near-normal range of this muscle is available, the patient must be sitting or standing to reach the full ROM. With marked limitation in muscle range, ROM can be performed in the supine position.

Hand Placement and Procedure

- First, fully flex the patient's elbow with one hand on the distal forearm.
- Then flex the shoulder by lifting up on the humerus with the other hand under the elbow.
- Full available range is reached when discomfort is experienced in the posterior arm region.

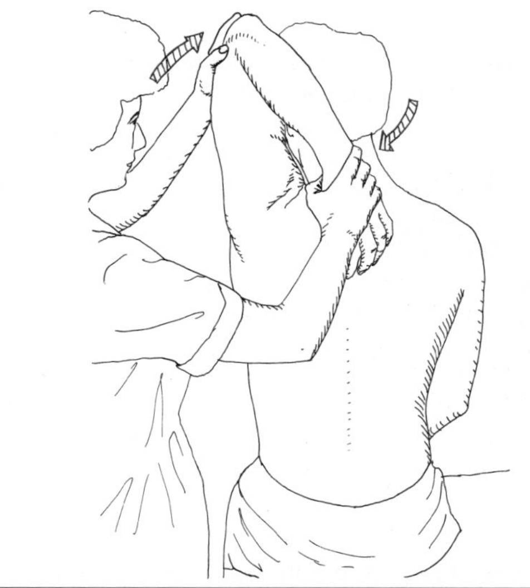

Figure 2–9 End ROM for the long head of the triceps brachii muscle.

Forearm: Pronation and Supination (Fig. 2–10)

Hand Placement and Procedure

- Grasp the patient's wrist, supporting the hand with the index finger and placing the thumb and the rest of the fingers on either side of the distal forearm.
- Stabilize the elbow with the other hand.
- The motion is a rolling of the radius around the ulna at the distal radius.

Alternate Hand Placement

Sandwich the patient's distal forearm between the palms of both hands.

Note: Pronation and supination should be performed with the elbow both flexed and extended.

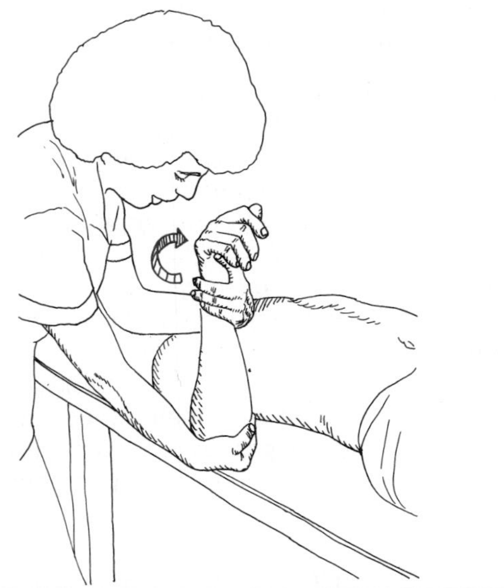

Figure 2–10 Pronation of the forearm.

Precaution: Do not stress the wrist by twisting the hand; control the pronation and supination motion by moving the radius around the ulna.

Wrist: Flexion (Palmar Flexion) and Extension (Dorsiflexion), Radial (Abduction) and Ulnar (Adduction) Deviation (Fig. 2–11)

Hand Placement and Procedure

For all wrist motions, grasp the patient's hand just distal to the joint with one hand, and stabilize the forearm with your other hand.

Note: The range of the extrinsic muscles to the fingers will affect the range at the wrist if tension is placed on them. To get full range of the wrist joint, allow the fingers to move freely as you move the wrist.

Hand: Cupping and Flattening the Arch of the Hand at the Carpometacarpal and Intermetacarpal Joints (Fig. 2–12)

Hand Placement and Procedure

- Face the patient's hand; place the fingers of both your hands in the palms of the patient's hand and your thenar eminences on the posterior aspect.
- Roll the metacarpals palmarward to increase the arch, and dorsalward to flatten it.

Alternate Hand Placement

One hand is placed on the posterior aspect of the patient's hand with the fingers and thumb cupping around the metacarpals.

Note: Extension and abduction of the thumb at the carpometacarpal joint are important in maintaining the web space for functional movement of the hand. Isolated flexion-extension and abduction-adduction ROM of this joint should be performed by moving the first metacarpal while stabilizing the trapezium.

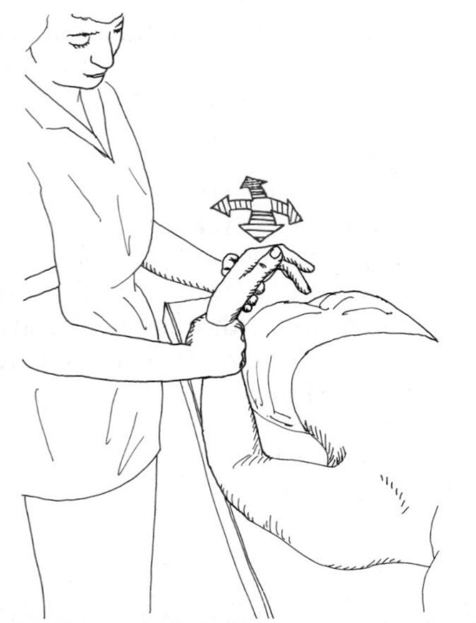

Figure 2–11 ROM at the wrist.

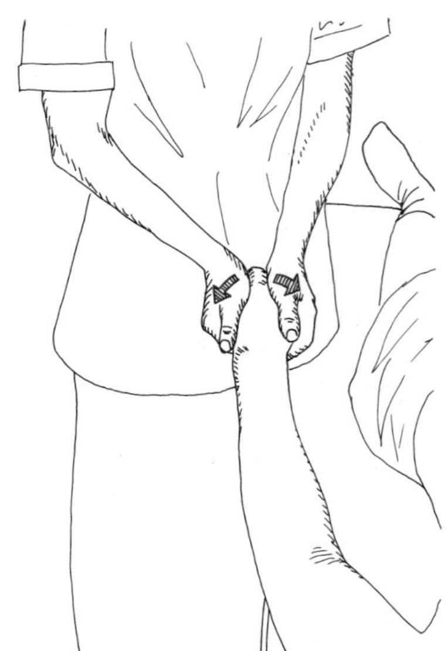

Figure 2–12 ROM to the arch of the hand.

Joints of the Thumb and Fingers: Flexion and Extension and Abduction and Adduction (Metacarpophalangeal Joints and Interphalangeal Joints of the Digits) (Fig. 2–13*A* and *B*)

Hand Placement and Procedure

- Depending on the position of the patient, stabilize the forearm and hand on the bed or table or against your body.
- Move each joint of the patient's hand individually by stabilizing the proximal bone with the index finger and thumb of one hand and moving the distal bone with the index finger and thumb of the other hand.

Alternate Procedure

Several joints can be moved simultaneously if proper stabilization is provided. Example: To move all the metacarpophalangeal joints of digits 2 through 5, stabilize the metacarpals with one hand and move all the proximal phalanges with the other hand.

Note: To accomplish full joint ROM, do not place tension on the extrinsic muscles going to the fingers. Tension on the muscles can be relieved by altering the wrist position as the fingers are moved.

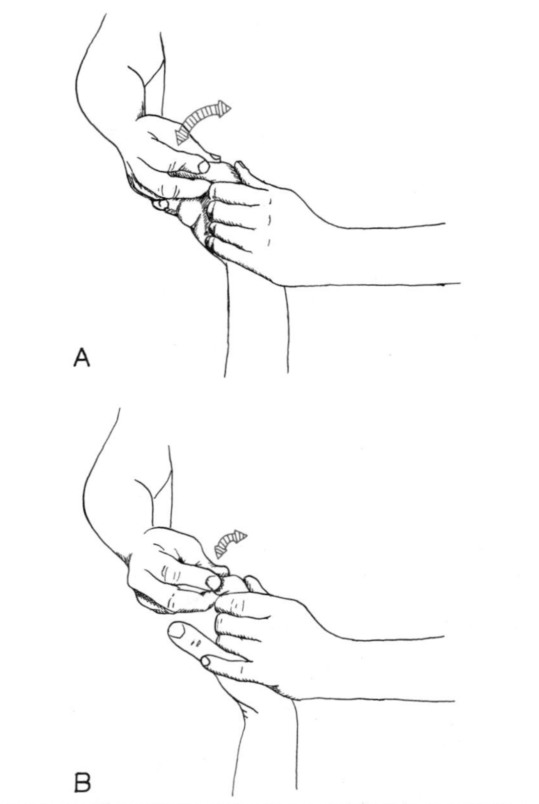

Figure 2–13 ROM to the (*A*) metacarpophalangeal joint of the thumb and (*B*) interphalangeal joint of a finger.

Elongation of Extrinsic Muscles of the Wrist and Hand

General Technique

Elongate the muscles over one joint at a time, stabilize that joint, then elongate the muscle over the next joint until the multijoint muscles are at maximum length. To minimize compression of the small joints of the fingers, begin the motion with the distal-most joint.

Flexor Digitorum Profundus and Superficialis Muscles (Fig. 2–14*A*)

Hand Placement and Procedure

- First extend the distal interphalangeal joints, stabilize them in extension, then extend the proximal interphalangeal joints.
- Hold both these joints in extension, then extend the metacarpophalangeal joints.
- Stabilize all the finger joints and begin to extend the wrist. When the patient feels discomfort in the forearm, the muscles are fully elongated.

Extensor Digitorum Muscles (Fig. 2–14*B*)

Hand Placement and Procedure

- First flex the patient's distal interphalangeal joints and stabilize them in flexion, then flex the proximal interphalangeal joints.
- Hold all these joints in flexion, then flex the metacarpophalangeal joints.
- While stabilizing all these joints in the flexed position, begin to flex the wrist until the patient feels discomfort on the dorsum of the hand.

Lower Extremity

Combined Hip and Knee: Flexion and Extension (Fig. 2–15*A* and *B*)

Hand Placement and Procedure

- Support and lift the patient's leg with the palm and fingers of the top hand under the patient's knee and the lower hand under the heel.
- As the knee flexes full range, swing the fingers to the side of the thigh.

Note: To reach full range of hip flexion, the knee must also be flexed to release tension on the hamstring muscle group. To reach full range of knee flexion, the hip must be flexed to release tension on the rectus femoris muscle.

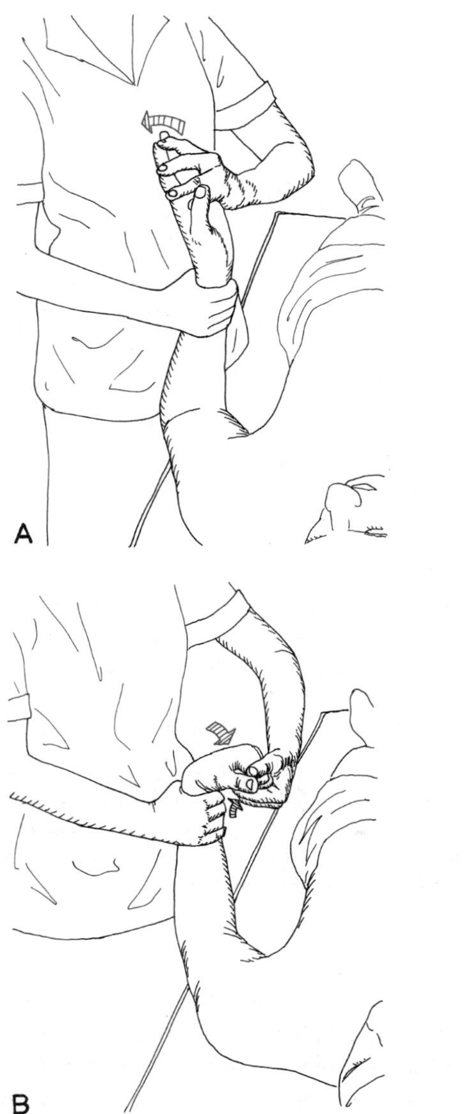

Figure 2–14 End of range for the (*A*) extrinsic finger flexors and (*B*) extensors.

Hip: Extension (Hyperextension) (Fig. 2–16)

Alternate Positions

Prone or side-lying must be used if the patient has near-normal or normal motion.

Hand Placement and Procedure

- If the patient is prone, lift the thigh with the bottom hand under the patient's knee; stabilize the pelvis with the top hand or arm.

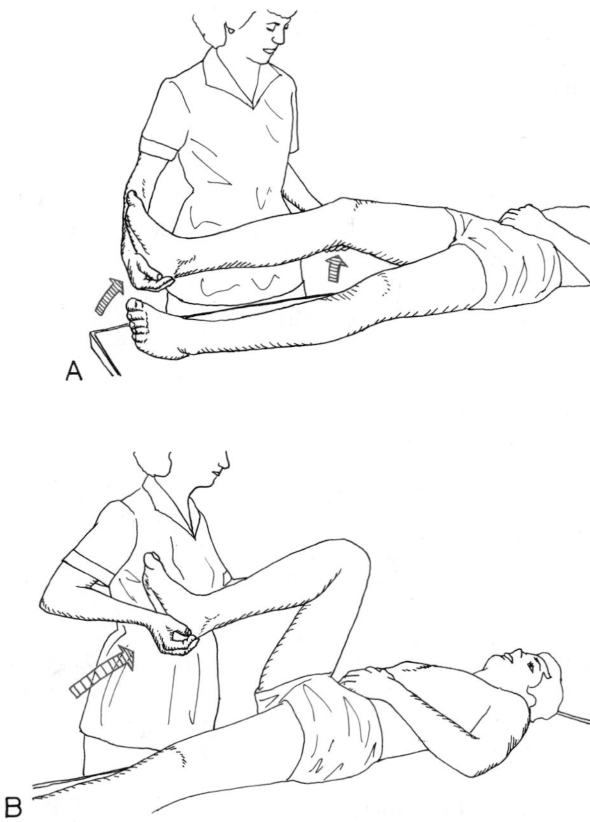

Figure 2–15 (*A*) Initiating and (*B*) completing combined hip and knee flexion.

- If the patient is side-lying, bring the bottom hand under the thigh and place the hand on the anterior surface; stabilize the pelvis with the top hand. For full range of hip extension do not flex the knee full range or the two-joint rectus femoris will restrict the range.

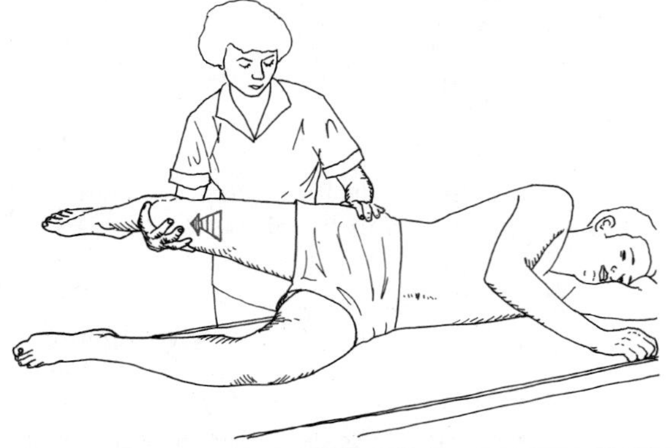

Figure 2–16 Hand placements to complete full range of hip extension with the patient side-lying.

Elongation of the Two-Joint Hamstring Muscle Group (Fig 2–17)

Hand Placement and Procedure

- Place the lower hand under the patient's heel and the upper hand across the anterior aspect of the patient's knee.
- Keep the knee in extension as the hip is flexed.
- If the knee requires support, cradle the patient's leg in your lower arm with your elbow flexed under the calf and your hand across the anterior aspect of the patient's knee. The other hand provides support or stabilization where needed.

Variation

If the hamstrings are so tight as to limit the knee from going into extension, the available range of the muscle is reached simply by extending the knee as far as the muscle allows and not moving the hip.

Elongation of the Two-Joint Rectus Femoris Muscle

Alternate Hand Positions

Supine, with knee flexed over the edge of the treatment table or prone.

Hand Placement and Procedure

- When supine, stabilize the lumbar spine by flexing the hip and knee of the opposite lower extremity and placing the foot on the treatment table (hook lying).
- When prone, stabilize the pelvis with the top hand (see Fig. 5–25).

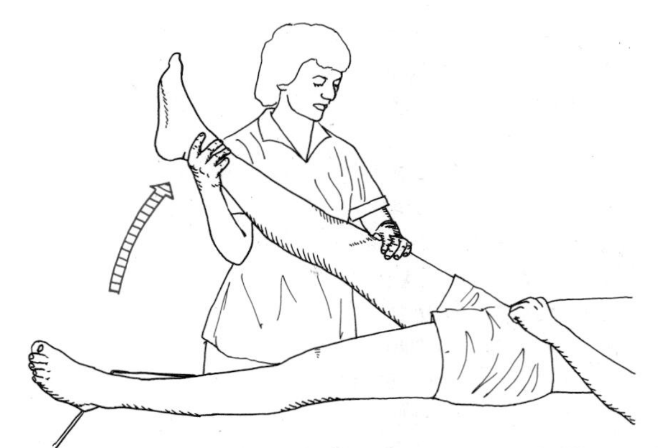

Figure 2–17 ROM to the hamstring muscle group.

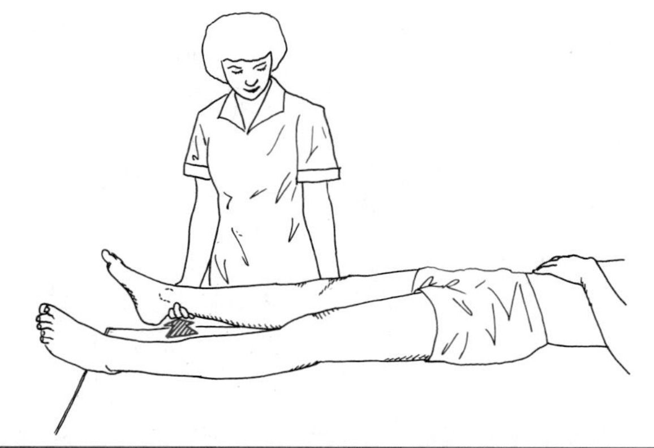

Figure 2–18 Abduction of the hip, maintaining the hip in extension and neutral to rotation.

- Flex the patient's knee until tissue resistance is felt in the anterior thigh, which means the full available range is reached.

Hip: Abduction and Adduction (Fig. 2–18)

Hand Placement and Procedure

- Support the patient's leg with the upper hand under the knee and the lower hand under the ankle.
- For full range of adduction, the opposite leg needs to be in a partially abducted position.
- Keep the patient's hip and knee in extension and neutral to rotation as abduction and adduction are performed.

Hip: Internal (Medial) and External (Lateral) Rotation

Hand Placement and Procedure with the Hip and Knee Extended

- Grasp just proximal to the patient's knee with the top hand and just proximal to the ankle with the bottom hand.
- Roll the thigh inward and outward.

Hand Placement and Procedure with the Hip and Knee Flexed (Fig. 2–19)

- Flex the patient's hip and knee to 90 degrees; support the knee with the top hand.
- Cradle the thigh with the bottom arm, and also support the proximal calf with the bottom hand.
- Rotate the femur by moving the leg like a pendulum.

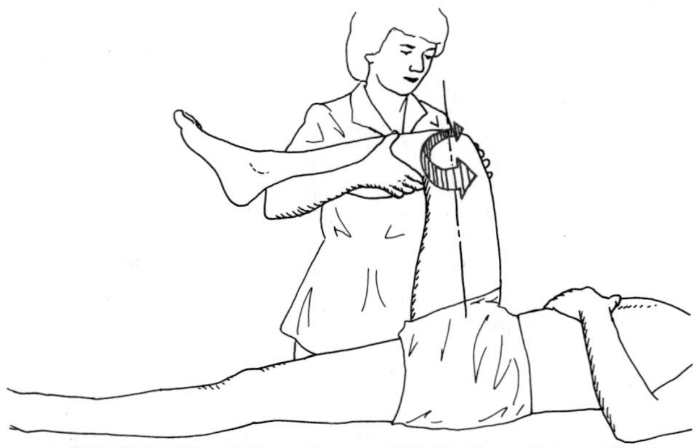

Figure 2–19 Rotation of the hip with the hip positioned in 90 degrees of flexion.

- This hand placement provides some support to the knee but still should be used with caution if there is knee instability.

Ankle: Dorsiflexion (Fig. 2–20)

Hand Placement and Procedure

- Stabilize around the malleoli with the top hand.
- Cup the patient's heel with the bottom hand and place the forearm along the bottom of the foot.
- Pull the calcaneus distalward with the thumb and fingers while pushing upward with the forearm.

Note: If the knee is flexed, full range of the ankle joint can be obtained. If the knee is extended, the lengthened range of the two-joint gastrocnemius muscle can be obtained, but the gastrocnemius will limit full range of dorsiflexion. Apply dorsiflexion in both positions of the knee to provide range to both the joint and the muscle.

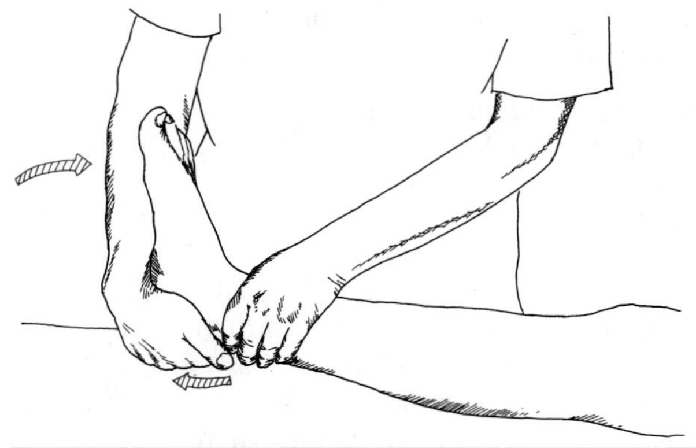

Figure 2–20 Dorsiflexion of the ankle.

Ankle: Plantarflexion

Hand Placement and Procedure

- Support the heel with the bottom hand.
- Place the top hand on the dorsum of the foot and push it into plantarflexion.

Note: In bed-bound patients the ankle tends to assume a plantarflexed position from the weight of the blankets and pull of gravity, so this motion may not need to be performed.

Subtalar (Lower Ankle) Joint: Inversion and Eversion (Fig. 2–21*A* and *B*)

Hand Placement and Procedure

- Using the bottom hand, place the thumb medial and the fingers lateral to the joint on either side of the heel.
- Turn the heel inward and outward.

Note: Supination of the foot may be combined with inversion, and pronation may be combined with eversion.

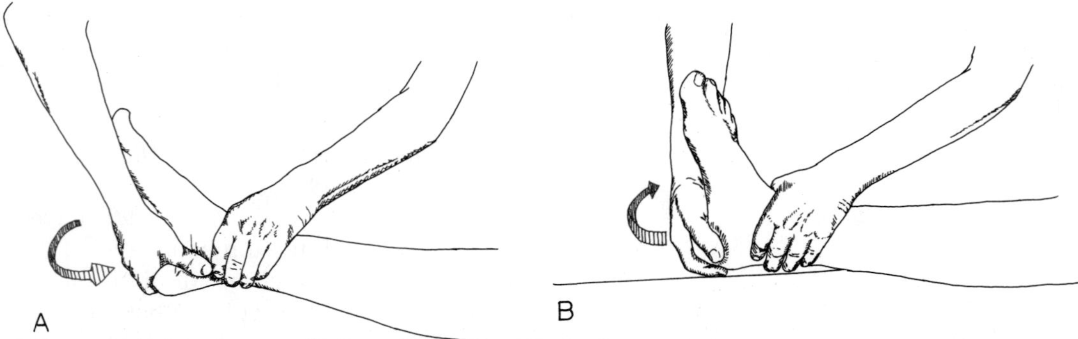

Figure 2–21 End position for (*A*) inversion and (*B*) eversion of the subtalar joint.

Transverse Tarsal Joint: Supination and Pronation (Fig. 2–22)

Hand Placement and Procedure

- Stabilize the patient's talus and calcaneus with the top hand.
- With the bottom hand, grasp around the navicular and cuboid.
- Gently raise and lower the arch.

Joints of the Toes: Flexion and Extension and Abduction and Adduction (Metatarsophalangeal and Interphalangeal Joints) (Fig. 2–23)

Hand Placement and Procedure

- With one hand, stabilize the bone proximal to the joint that is to be moved and move the distal bone with the other hand.
- The technique is the same as with ROM of the fingers.

Alternate Procedure

Several joints of the toes can be moved simultaneously if care is taken not to stress any structure.

Cervical Spine

Position of Therapist and Hand Placement

Standing at the end of the treatment table, securely grasp the patient's head by placing both hands under the occipital region (Fig. 2–24).

Flexion (Forward Bending)

Procedure

- Lift the head as though it were nodding (chin towards larynx) to flex the head on the neck.
- Once full nodding is complete, continue to flex the cervical spine and lift the head toward the sternum.

Extension (Backward Bending or Hyperextension)

Procedure

Tip the head backward.

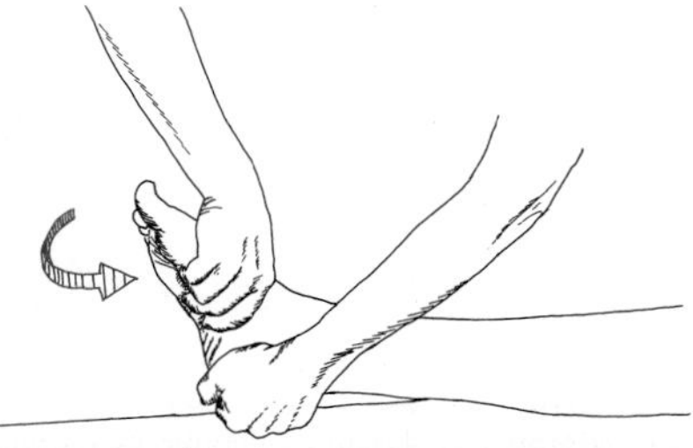

Figure 2–22 End position for supination of the transverse tarsal joint.

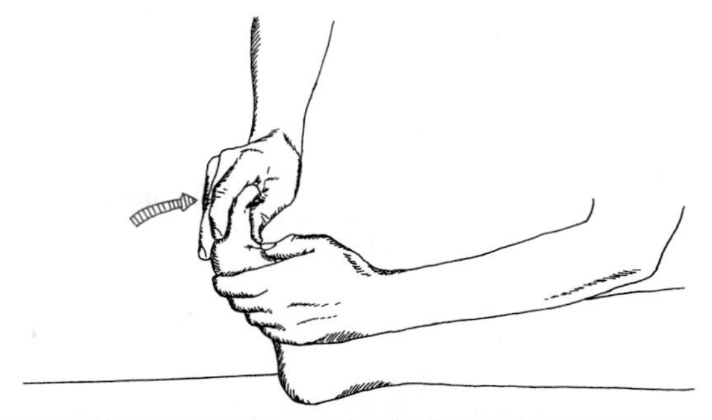

Figure 2–23 Extension of the metatarsophalangeal joint of the large toe.

Note: If the patient is supine, the head must clear the end of the table. The patient may also be prone or sitting.

Lateral Flexion (Side Bending)

Procedure

Maintain the cervical spine neutral to flexion and extension as you direct it into side bending and approximate the ear toward the shoulder.

Rotation (Fig. 2–25)

Motion

Rotate the head from side to side.

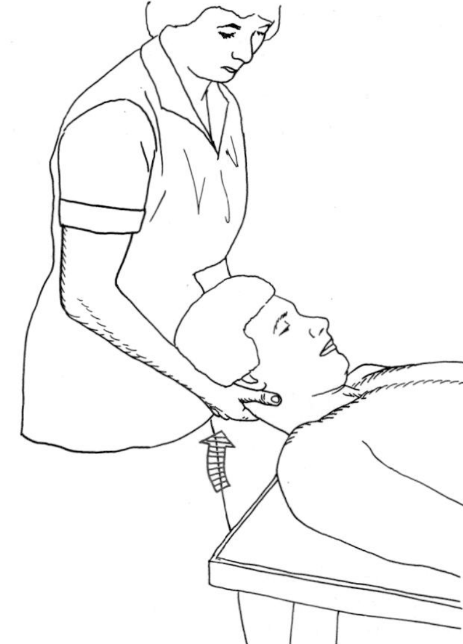

Figure 2–24 Hand placement for cervical motions, illustrating flexion.

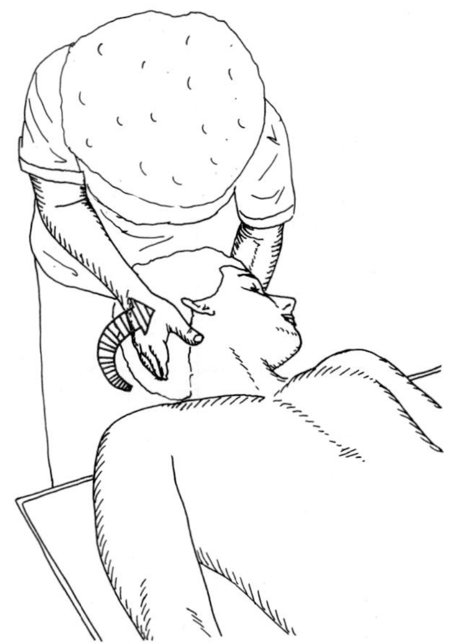

Figure 2–25 Hand placement and end-range for cervical rotation to the left.

Lumbar Spine

Flexion (Fig. 2–26)

Hand Placement and Procedure

- Bring both of the patient's knees to the chest by lifting under the knees (hip and knee flexion).
- Flexion of the spine occurs as the hips are flexed full range and the pelvis starts to rotate posteriorly.
- Greater range of flexion can be obtained by lifting under the patient's sacrum with the lower hand.

Extension

Position of Patient
Prone.

Hand Placement and Procedure
With hands under the thighs, lift the thighs upward until the pelvis rotates anteriorly and the lumbar spine extends.

Rotation (Fig. 2–27)

Position of Patient
Hook-lying.

Hand Placement and Procedure

- Push both of the patient's knees laterally in one direction until the pelvis on the opposite side comes up off the treatment table.
- Stabilize the patient's thorax with the top hand.
- Repeat in the opposite direction.

Combined Patterns of Motion

Effective and efficient ROM can be administered by combining several joint motions that transect several planes resulting in oblique or diagonal patterns. For example, wrist flexion may be combined with ulnar deviation, or shoulder flexion may be combined with abduction and lateral rotation so that movement follows functional patterns. Proprioceptive neuromuscular facilitation (PNF) patterns of move-

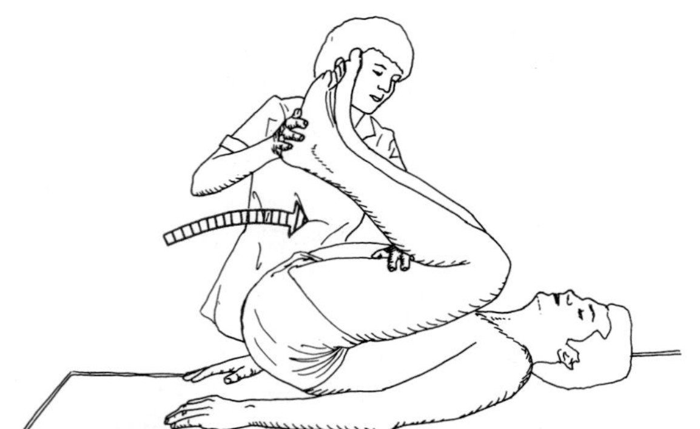

Figure 2–26 Lumbar flexion is achieved by bringing the patient's hips into flexion until the pelvis rotates posteriorly.

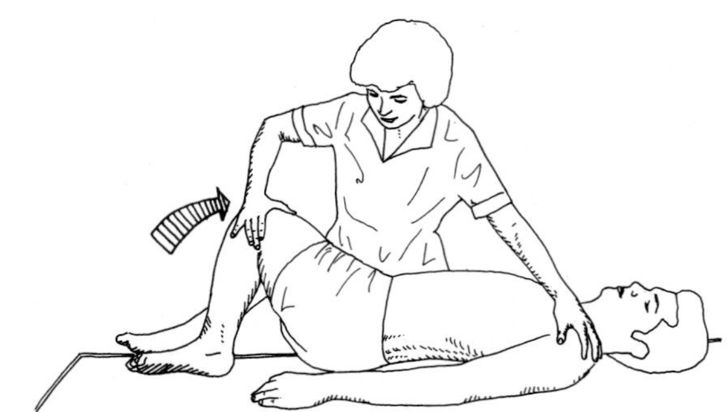

Figure 2–27 Rotation of the lumbar spine results when the thorax is stabilized and the pelvis lifts off the table as far as allowed.

ment follow specific guidelines and may be effectively used for PROM, A-AROM or AROM techniques (see Chapter 3 for descriptions of these patterns).

▶ Self-Assisted ROM (S-AROM)

Patient involvement in self-care should begin as soon as the individual is able to understand and learn what to do. Even with weakness or paralysis, the patient can learn how to move the involved part and be instructed in the importance of movement within safe parameters. After surgery or traumatic injury, S-AROM is used to protect the healing tissues when a more intensive muscle contraction is contraindicated. A variety of devices as well as use of a normal extremity may be used to meet the goals of PROM or A-AROM. Incorporation of S-AROM then becomes a part of the home exercise program (Box 2–2).

Self-Assistance

With cases of unilateral weakness of paralysis, or during early stages of recovery after trauma or surgery, the patient can be taught to use the normal extremity to move the involved extremity through ranges of motion. These exercises may be done supine, sitting, or standing. The effects of gravity will change with patient positioning, so that when lifting the part against gravity, gravity will provide a resistive force against the prime motion and therefore the prime mover will require assistance. When the extremity moves downward, gravity will cause the motion and the antagonists will need assistance to eccentrically control the motion.

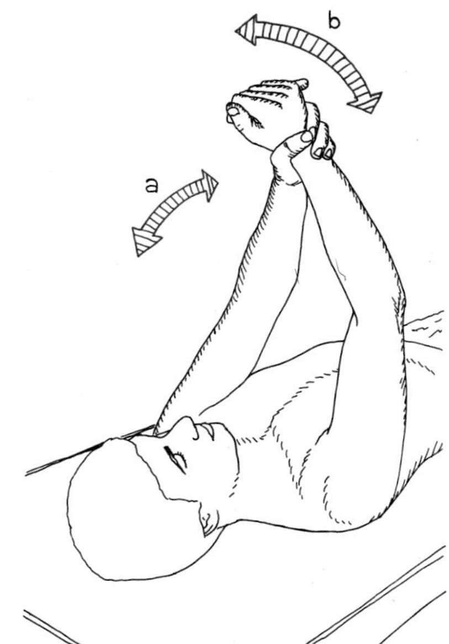

Figure 2–28 Patient giving self-assisted ROM to (*A*) shoulder flexion and extension or (*B*) horizontal abduction and adduction.

Box 2–2 Self-Assisted Range of Motion Techniques

Forms of Self-Assisted ROM
- Manual
- Equipment
  - Wand or T-bar
  - Finger ladder, wall climbing, ball rolling
  - Pulleys
  - Skate board/powder board
  - Reciprocal exercise devices

Guidelines for Teaching Self-Assisted ROM
- Educate the patient on the value of the motion.
- Teach the patient correct body alignment and stabilization.
- Observe patient performance and correct any substitute or unsafe motions.
- If equipment is used, be sure all hazards are eliminated for application to be safe.
- Provide drawings and clear guidelines for number of repetitions and frequency.

Review the exercises at a follow-up session. Modify or progress the exercise program based on the patient response and treatment plan for meeting the outcome goals.

Arm and Forearm

Instruct the patient to reach across the body with the normal extremity and grasp the involved extremity around the wrist, supporting the wrist and hand.

- ***Shoulder flexion and extension.*** The patient lifts the involved extremity over the head and returns it to the side (Fig. 2–28*A*).
- ***Shoulder horizontal abduction and adduction.*** Beginning with the arm abducted 90 degrees, the patient pulls the extremity across the chest and returns it out to the side (Fig. 2–28*B*).

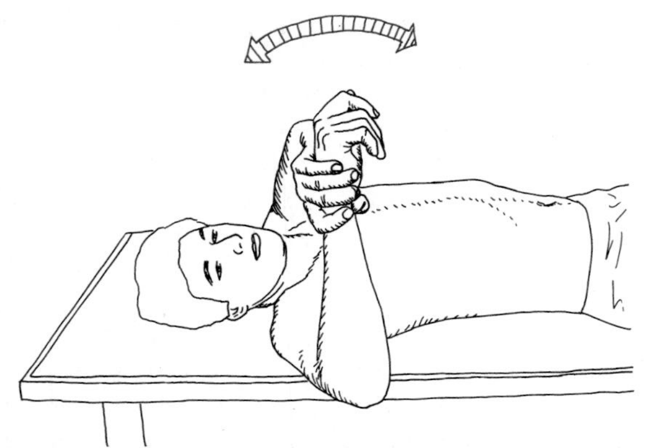

Figure 2–29 Arm position of patient for giving self-assisted ROM to internal and external rotation of shoulder.

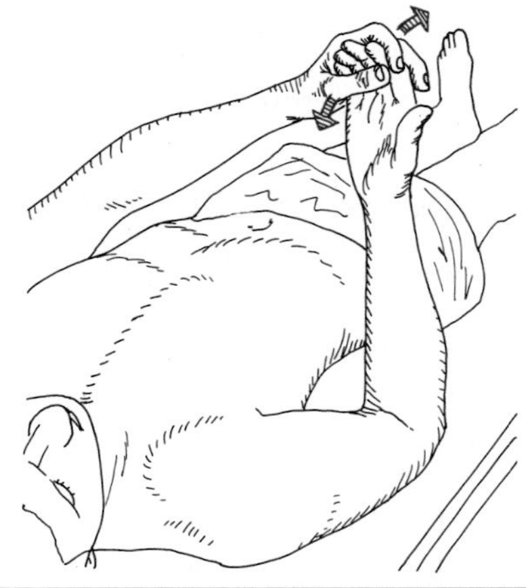

Figure 2–31 Patient applying self-assisted finger flexion and extension.

- ***Shoulder rotation.*** Beginning with the arm at the patient's side, in slight abduction or abducted 90 degrees and elbow flexed 90 degrees, the patient rotates the forearm (Fig. 2–29).
- ***Elbow flexion and extension.*** The patient bends the elbow until the hand is near the shoulder and then moves the hand down toward the side of the leg.
- ***Pronation and supination of the forearm.*** Beginning with the forearm resting across the body, the patient rotates the radius around the ulna; emphasize to the patient not to twist the hand at the wrist joint.

Wrist and Hand

The patient's normal thumb is moved to the involved hand with the normal fingers along the dorsum of the hand.

- ***Wrist flexion and extension and radial and ulnar deviation.*** The patient moves the wrist in all directions, applying no pressure against the fingers (Fig. 2–30).
- ***Finger flexion and extension.*** The patient uses the normal thumb to extend the involved fingers and cups the normal fingers over the dorsum of the involved fingers to flex them (Fig. 2–31).
- ***Thumb flexion with opposition and extension with reposition.*** The patient cups the normal fingers around the radial border of the thenar eminence of the involved thumb and places the normal thumb along the palmar surface of the involved thumb to extend it (Fig. 2–32). To flex and oppose the thumb, the patient cups the normal hand around the dorsal surface of the in-

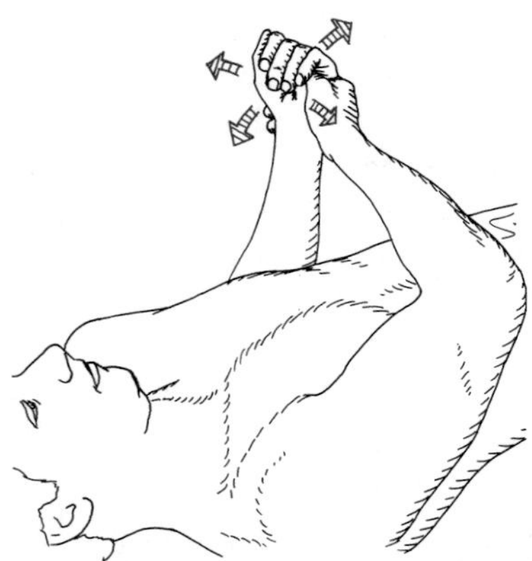

Figure 2–30 Patient applying self-assisted wrist motions.

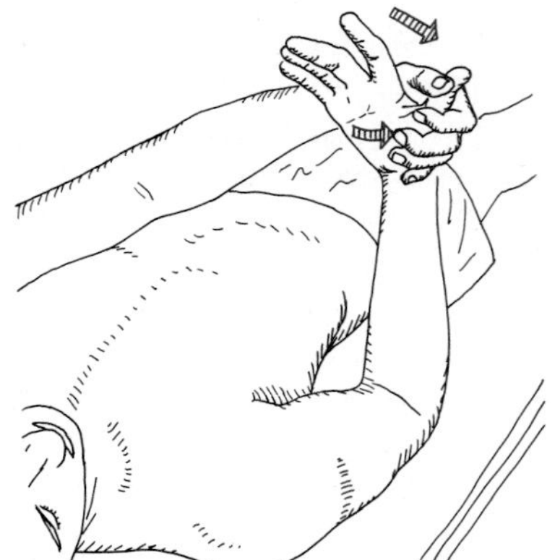

Figure 2–32 Patient applying self-assisted thumb extension.

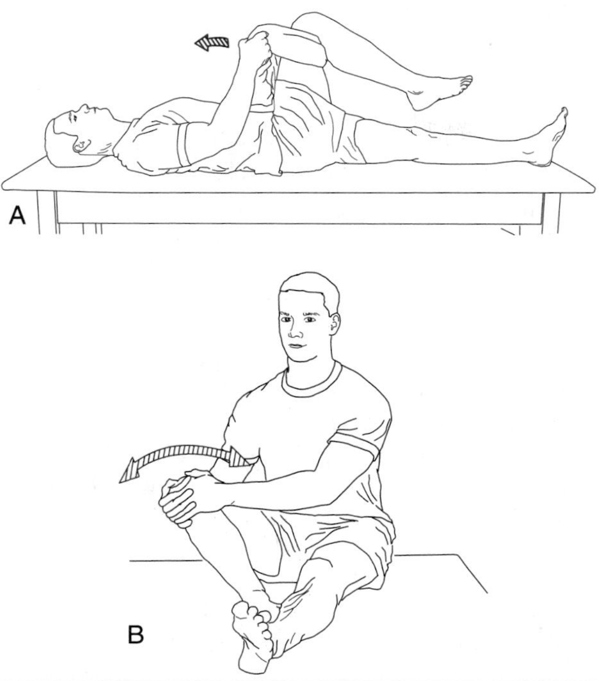

Figure 2–33 Self-assisted ROM of the hip: (*A*) flexion, (*B*) abduction and external rotation.

volved hand and pushes the first metacarpal toward the little finger.

Hip and Knee (Fig. 2–33)

- ***Hip and knee flexion.*** With the patient supine, instruct the patient to initiate the motion by lifting up the involved knee with a strap or belt under the involved knee. He or she can then grasp the knee with one or both hands to bring the knee up toward the chest to complete the range (Fig. 2–32*A*). With the patient sitting, he or she may lift the thigh with the hands and flex the knee to the end of its available range.
- ***Hip abduction and adduction.*** It is difficult for the weak patient to assist the lower extremities into abduction and adduction when supine due to the weight of the leg and friction of the bed surface. It is necessary, though for the individual to move a weak lower extremity from side to side for bed mobility. To practice this functional activity as an exercise, instruct the patient to slide the normal foot from the knee down to the ankle and then move the involved extremity from side to side. S-AROM can be performed sitting by using the hands to assist moving the thigh outward and inward.
- ***Combined hip abduction with external rotation.*** The patient is sitting on the floor or on a bed with the back supported and the involved hip and knee flexed and foot resting on the surface. The knee is moved outward (toward the table/bed) and back inward, with assistance from the upper extremity (Fig. 2–33*B*).

Ankle and Toes

The patient sits with the involved extremity crossed over the normal one so that the distal leg rests on the normal knee. With the normal hand, the involved ankle can be moved into dorsiflexion and plantarflexion, inversion and eversion, and toe flexion and extension (Fig. 2–34).

Wand (T-bar) Exercises

When a patient has voluntary muscle control in an involved upper extremity but needs guidance or motivation to complete the ranges of motion in the shoulder or elbow, a wand (dowel rod, cane, wooden stick, T-bar, or similar object) can be used to provide assistance.

Patient Position

The choice of position is based on the patient's level of function. Most of the techniques can be performed supine if maximum protection is needed. Sitting or standing requires greater control. Choice of position is also guided by the effects of gravity on the weak muscles.

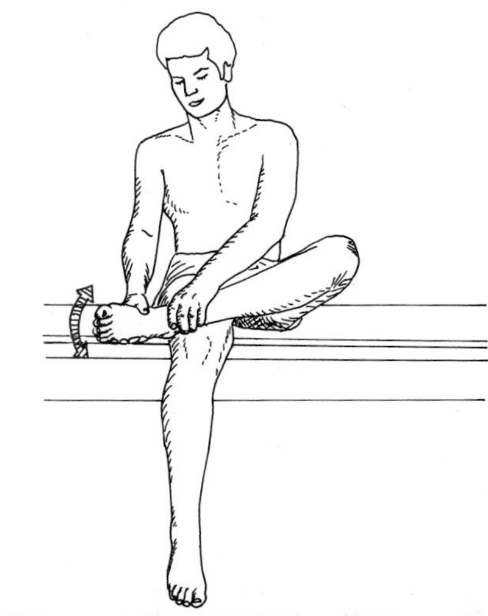

Figure 2–34 Position of patient and hand placement for self-assisted ankle motions.

Procedure

Initially, guide the patient through the proper motion for each activity to ensure that he or she does not use substitute motions. The patient grasps the wand with both hands; the normal extremity guides and controls the motions.

- ***Shoulder flexion and return (Fig. 2–35).*** The wand is grasped with the hands a shoulder-width apart. The wand is lifted forward and upward through the available range, with the elbows kept in extension if possible. Scapulohumeral motion should be smooth; do not allow scapular elevation or trunk movement.
- ***Shoulder horizontal abduction and adduction.*** The wand is lifted to 90 degrees flexion (same as in Fig. 2–35). Keeping the elbows in extension, the patient pushes and pulls the wand back and forth across the chest through the available range. Do not allow trunk rotation.
- ***Shoulder internal and external rotation (Fig. 2–36).*** The patient's arms are at the sides and the elbows are flexed 90 degrees. Rotation of the arms is accomplished by moving the wand from side to side across the trunk while maintaining the elbows at the side. The rotation should occur in the humerus; do not allow elbow flexion and extension. To prevent substitute motions in the humerus as well as provide a slight distraction force to the glenohumeral joint, a small towel roll may be placed in the axilla with instruction to the patient to "keep the roll in place."

Alternate Position

The patient's shoulders are abducted 90 degrees and the elbows flexed 90 degrees. For external rotation, the wand is moved toward the patient's head; for internal rotation, the wand is moved toward the waistline.

- ***Elbow flexion and extension.*** The patient's forearms may be pronated or supinated; the hands grasp the wand, a shoulder-width apart. Instruct the patient to flex and extend the elbows.
- ***Shoulder hyperextension.*** The patient may be standing or prone. He or she places the wand behind the buttocks, grasps the wand with hands, a shoulder-width apart, and then lifts the wand backward away from the trunk. The patient should avoid trunk motion.
- ***Variations and combinations of movements.*** For example, the patient begins with the wand behind

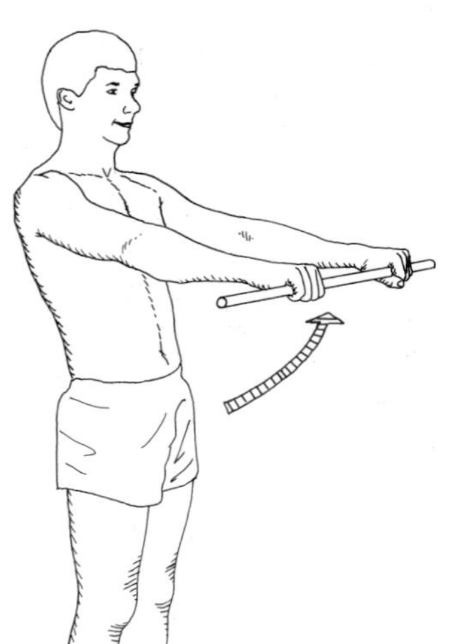

Figure 2–35 Patient using a wand for self-assisted shoulder flexion. This exercise may be done supine to change the effects of gravity and provide support for the trunk.

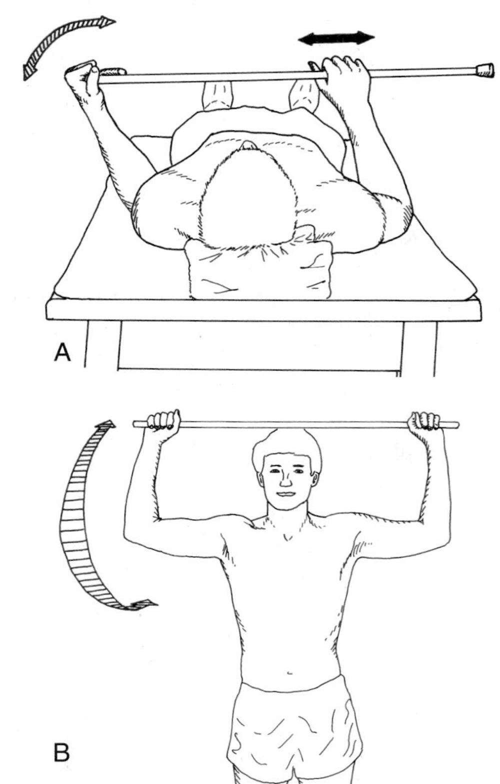

Figure 2–36 Self-assisted shoulder rotation (*A*) with the shoulder at the side, and (*B*) with the shoulder abducted to 90°.

the buttocks and then moves the wand up the back to achieve scapular winging, shoulder internal rotation, and elbow flexion.

Finger Ladder/Wall Climbing

The finger ladder (or wall climbing) is a device that can provide the patient with objective reinforcement and, therefore, motivation for performing shoulder ROM. Wall markings may also be used to provide visual feedback for height reached with "wall climbing."

Precaution: The patient must be taught the proper motions and not allowed to substitute with trunk side bending, toe raising, or shoulder shrugging.

- ***Shoulder flexion.*** The patient stands, facing the finger ladder or wall an arm's length away, and places the index or middle finger on a step of the ladder. The arm is moved into flexion by climbing with the fingers. The patient steps closer to the ladder as the arm is elevated.
- ***Shoulder abduction (Fig. 2–37).*** The patient stands sideways, with the affected shoulder toward the ladder an arm's length away. The patient needs to externally rotate the shoulder while abducting the arm in ranges greater than 90 degrees.

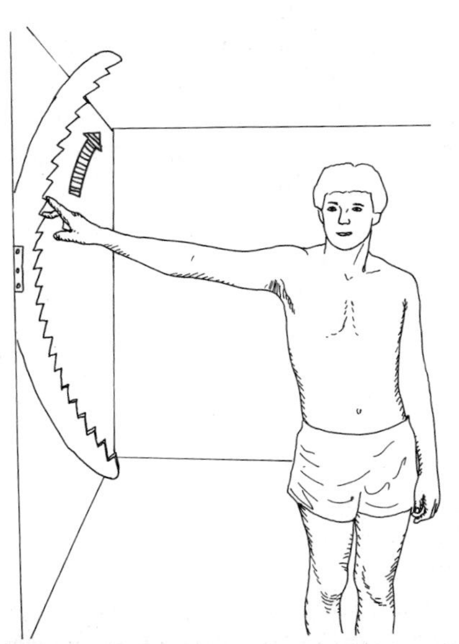

Figure 2–37 Shoulder abduction using a finger ladder.

Overhead Pulleys

If properly taught, pulley systems can be effectively used to assist an involved extremity in performing ROM. The pulley has been demonstrated to utilize significantly more muscle activity than therapist-assisted ROM and continuous passive motion machines (described later in the chapter) so this form of assistance should only be used when muscle activity is desired.[4]

For home use, a single pulley may be attached to a strap that is held in place by closing the strap in a door. A pulley may also be attached to an overhead bar or affixed to the ceiling. The patient should be set up so that the pulley is directly over the joint that is moving or so that the line of pull is effectively moving the extremity and not just compressing the joint surfaces together. The patient may be sitting, standing, or supine.

Shoulder Flexion (Fig. 2–38*A*), Abduction (Fig. 2–38*B*), and Scaption

Instruct the patient to hold one handle in each hand and, with the normal hand, pull the rope and lift the involved extremity either forward (flexion), out to the side (abduction), or in the plane of the scapula (scaption is 30 degrees forward of the frontal plane). The patient should not shrug the shoulder (scapular

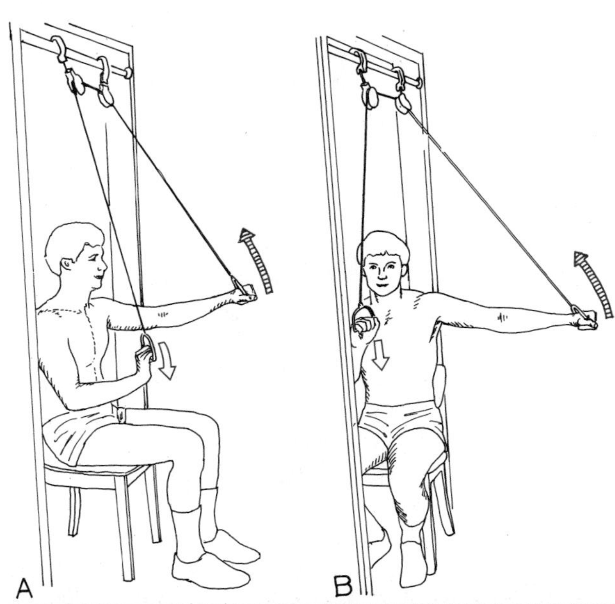

Figure 2–38 (*A*) Shoulder flexion and (*B*) abduction using overhead pulleys to assist the motion.

elevation) or lean the trunk. Guide and instruct the patient so there is smooth motion.

Precaution: Assistive pulley activities for the shoulder are easily misused by the patient, resulting in compression of the humerus against the acromion process. Continual compression will lead to pain and decreased function. Proper patient selection and appropriate instruction can avoid this problem. If a patient cannot learn to use the pulley with proper shoulder mechanics, these exercises should not be performed. With increased pain or decreased mobility, discontinue this activity (see Chapter 9).

Shoulder Internal and External Rotation (Fig. 2–39)

Position the patient with the shoulder abducted 90 degrees and the elbow flexed 90 degrees. Have the arm supported on the back of a chair if the patient is sitting or on the treatment table if the patient is supine. The patient then lifts the forearm with the pulley, causing rotation in the arm.

Elbow Flexion

With the arm stabilized along the side of the trunk, the patient lifts the forearm and bends the elbow.

Skate Board/Powder Board

Use of a friction-free surface may encourage movement without the resistance of gravity or friction. If available, a skate with rollers may be used. Other methods include using powder on the surface or placing a towel under the extremity so that it can slide along the smooth surface of the board. Any motion can be done, but most common are abduction/adduction of the hip while supine, and horizontal abduction/adduction of the shoulder while sitting.

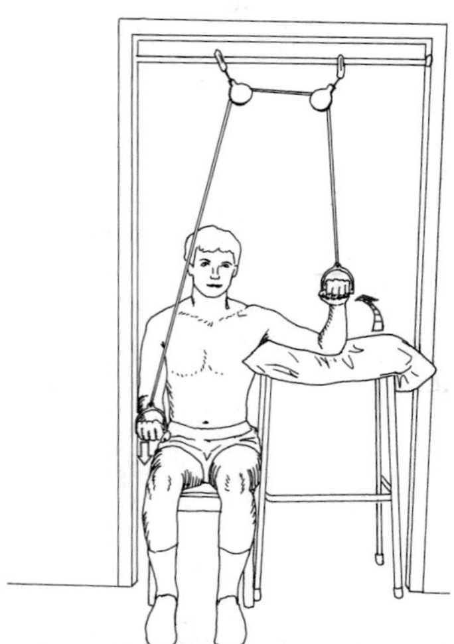

Figure 2–39 Position for shoulder rotation using overhead pulleys to assist the motion.

Reciprocal Exercise Unit

Several devices such as a bicycle, upper body, or lower body ergometer, or reciprocal exercise unit can be set up to provide some flexion and extension to an involved extremity by using the strength of a normal extremity. Moveable devices are available that can be attached to a patient's bed, wheelchair, or standard chair. The circumference of motion as well as excursion of the extremities can be adjusted. A reciprocal exercise unit has additional exercise benefits in that it can be used for reciprocal patterning, endurance training, and strengthening by changing the parameters of the exercise and monitoring the heart rate and fatigue (see Chapter 3 for principles of resistance exercise and Chapter 6 for principles of aerobic exercise).

▶ Continuous Passive Motion

Continuous passive motion (CPM) refers to passive motion that is performed by a mechanical device that moves a joint slowly and continuously through a controlled range of motion. The mechanical devices that exist for nearly every joint in the body (Fig. 2–40) were developed as a result of the research by Robert Salter, who demonstrated that continual passive motion has beneficial healing effects on diseased or injured joint structures and soft tissues in animal and clinical studies.[19–24] Since the development of CPM, many studies have been done to determine the parameters of application, but because the devices are used for many conditions, and studies have used various protocols with varying research designs, no definitive delineation has been established.[3,12,16]

Recent studies have compared short- and long-term outcomes of CPM use after various types of surgeries using different parameters as well as compared CPM with other methods of early movement and positioning.[1,4,10,11,16–18,27,29] Some studies have shown no significant difference between patients receiving CPM and those receiving PROM or other forms of early motion.[10,11,18,28] Many studies support

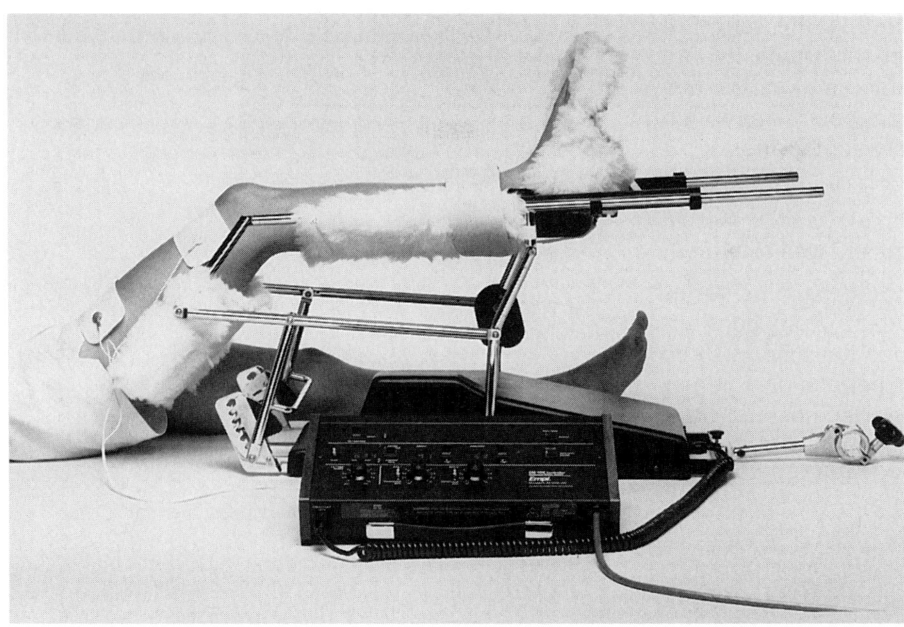

Figure 2–40 CM-100 Continuous Motion Device. (Courtesy of Empi Inc., St. Paul, MN.)

the short-term benefits of CPM use after surgery in that patients gain ROM more quickly and, therefore, may experience earlier discharge from the hospital when CPM is used compared with other forms of intervention, but long-term functional gains are reported to be no different from those patients who received other forms of early motion.[3,27,29] Some studies have identified detrimental effects such as need for greater analgesic intervention and increased postoperative blood drainage when using CPM[17,28] in contrast to claims that CPM decreases postoperative pain and postoperative complications.[20–24,26] Cost-effectiveness of the CPM equipment, patient compliance, utilization and supervision of equipment by trained personnel, length of hospital stay, speed of recovery, and determination of appropriate patient populations all become issues to consider when making the choice whether or not to utilize CPM devices.[11,14]

Benefits of CPM

CPM has been reported to be effective in lessening the negative effects of joint immobilization in conditions such as arthritis, contractures, and intra-articular fractures; and in improving the recovery rate and ROM after a variety of surgical procedures.[12,16,19–24,26] Basic research and clinical studies reported by Salter have demonstrated the effectiveness of CPM in:

- Preventing development of adhesions and contractures and thus joint stiffness
- Providing a stimulating effect on the healing of tendons and ligaments
- Enhancing healing of incisions over the moving joint
- Increasing synovial fluid lubrication of the joint, and thus increasing the rate of intra-articular cartilage healing and regeneration
- Preventing the degradating effects of immobilization
- Providing a quicker return of ROM
- Decreasing postoperative pain

General Guidelines

General guidelines are as follows.[2,3,8,12,13,19,24]

1. The device may be applied to the involved extremity immediately after surgery while the patient is still under anesthesia or as soon as possible if bulky dressings prevent early motion.
2. The arc of motion for the joint is determined. Often a low arc of 20 to 30 degrees is used initially and progressed 10 to 15 degrees per day as tolerated. The portion of the range used initially is based on range available and patient tolerance.

One study looked at accelerating the range of knee flexion post total knee arthroplasty and found greater range was attained and earlier discharge for that group of patients,[29] although there was no difference between groups at 4 weeks.

3. The rate of motion is determined; usually 1 cycle per 45 seconds or per 2 minutes is well tolerated.
4. The amount of time on the CPM machine varies for different protocols; anywhere from continuous for 24 hours to continuous for 1 hour, three times a day.[8,13,24] The longer periods of time per day reportedly result in a shorter hospital stay, fewer postoperative complications, and greater range of motion at discharge,[8] although no significant difference was found in a study comparing 5 hours per day with 20 hours per day of CPM.[2] A recent study compared short duration (3–5 hours/day) with long duration (10–12 hours/day) CPM application and found that patient compliance and the most gained range occurred with a CPM duration between 4 to 8 hours.[3]
5. Physical therapy treatments are usually initiated during periods when the patient is not on CPM, including active-assistive and muscle setting exercises. It is important that patients learn to use and develop motor control of the ROM as motion improves.
6. Duration minimum for CPM is usually less than 1 week or when a satisfactory range of motion is reached. Because CPM devices are portable, home use is possible in cases where the therapist or physician deems additional time would be beneficial. In these cases, the patient, a family member, or caregiver is instructed in proper application.
7. CPM machines are designed to be adjustable, easily controlled, versatile, and portable. Some are battery operated (with rechargeable batteries) to allow the individual to wear the device for up to 8 hours while functioning with daily activities.

▶ Range of Motion Through Functional Patterns

To accomplish motion through functional patterns, first determine what pattern of movement is desired, then move the extremity through that pattern using manual assistance, mechanical assistance if it is appropriate, or self-assistance from the patient. Functional patterning can be beneficial in initiating the teaching of activities of daily living (ADL), and instrumental activities of daily living (IADL) as well as in instructing patients with visual impairments in functional activities. Utilizing functional patterns helps the patient recognize the purpose and value of ROM exercises as well as develop motor patterns that can be used in daily activities as strength and endurance improves. Box 2–3 identifies some examples and the basic motions that are utilized. When the patient no longer requires assistance to perform the pattern safely and correctly, the activity is incorporated into his or her daily activities so that motor learning is reinforced and the motion becomes functional.

Box 2–3 Functional Range of Motion Activities

Early ROM training for functional upper extremity and neck patterns may include activities such as

- Grasping an eating utensil; utilizing finger extension and flexion
- Eating (hand to mouth); utilizing elbow flexion and forearm supination and some shoulder flexion, abduction, and lateral rotation
- Reaching to various shelf heights; utilizing shoulder flexion and elbow extension
- Brushing or combing back of hair; utilizing shoulder abduction and lateral rotation, elbow flexion, and cervical rotation
- Holding a phone to the ear; shoulder lateral rotation, forearm supination, and cervical side bend
- Donning or doffing a shirt or jacket; utilizing shoulder extension, lateral rotation, elbow flexion and extension
- Reaching out a car window to an ATM machine; utilizing shoulder abduction, lateral rotation, elbow extension, and some lateral bending of the trunk

Early ROM training for functional lower extremity and trunk patterns may include activities such as

- Going from supine to sitting at the side of a bed; utilizing hip abduction and adduction followed by hip and knee flexion
- Standing up/sitting down and walking; utilizing hip and knee flexion and extension, ankle dorsi and plantar flexion and some hip rotation
- Putting on socks and shoes; utilizing hip external rotation and abduction, knee flexion and ankle dorsi and plantar flexion, and trunk flexion

Independent Learning Activities

CRITICAL THINKING AND DISCUSSION

1. Analyze a variety of functional activities such as grooming, dressing, and bathing, and determine the functional ranges that are needed to perform each task.

2. Look at the effects of gravity or other forces on the range of motion for each activity in #1. If you had a patient who was unable to do the activity because of inability to control the range needed, determine how you would establish an exercise program to begin preparing the individual to develop the desired function.

LABORATORY PRACTICE

1. Perform PROM of the upper and lower extremities with your partner placed in the following positions: prone, side-lying, sitting.

a. What are the advantages and disadvantages of each of the positions for some of the ranges, such as shoulder and hip extension, knee flexion with the hip extended, rotation of the hip?

b. Progress the PROM to A-AROM and AROM and determine the effects of gravity and the effort required in these positions compared with the supine position.

2. Compare the ranges of motion of the hip, knee, and ankle when each of the two joint muscles is elongated over their respective joints versus when each of the muscles is on a slack.

REFERENCES

1. Alfredson, H, and Lorentzon, R: Superior results with continuous passive motion compared to active motion after periosteal transplantation. A retrospective study of human patella cartilage defect treatment. Knee Surg Sports Traumatol Arthrosc 7 (4):232, 1999.
2. Basso, DM, and Knapp, L: Comparison of two continuous passive motion protocols for patients with total knee implants. Phys Ther 67:360, 1987.
3. Chiarello, CM, Gunersen, L, and O'Halloran, T: The effect of continuous passive motion duration and increment on range of motion in total knee arthroplasty patients. J Orthop Sports Phys Ther 25 (2):119, 1997
4. Dockery, ML, Wright, TW, and LaStayo, P: Electromyography of the shoulder: an analysis of passive modes of exercise. Orthopedics 11:1181, 1998.
5. Donatelli, R, and Owens-Burckhart, H: Effects of immobilization on the extensibility of periarticular connective tissue. J Orthop Sports Phys Ther 3:67, 1981.
6. Fletcher, GF, et al: Exercise Standards: A Statement for Health Professionals. American Heart Association, Dallas, 1991.
7. Frank, C, et al: Physiology and therapeutic value of passive joint motion. Clin Orthop 185:113, 1984.
8. Gose, J: Continuous passive motion in the postoperative treatment of patients with total knee replacement. Phys Ther 67:39, 1987.
9. Guidelines for Exercise Testing and Prescription, ed 4. American College of Sports Medicine, Lea & Febiger, Philadelphia, 1991.
10. Kumar, PJ, McPherson, EJ, et al: Rehabilitation after total knee arthroplasty: a comparison of 2 rehabilitation techniques. Clin Orthop 331:93, 1996.
11. LaStayo, PC, Wright T, et al: Continuous passive motion after repair of the rotator cuff. A prospective outcome study. J Bone Joint Surg Am 80(7):1002, 1998.
12. LaStayo, PC: Continuous passive motion for the upper extremity. In Hunter, JM, MacKin, EJ and Callahan AD (eds). Rehabilitation of the Hand: Surgery and Therapy, ed 4. Mosby, St Louis, 1995.
13. McCarthy, MR, et al: The clinical use of continuous passive motion in physical therapy. J Ortho Sports Phys Ther 15:132, 1992.
14. Nadler, SF, Malanga, GA, and Jimmerman, JR: Continuous passive motion in the rehabilitation setting. A retrospective study. Am J Phys Med Rehabil 72(3):162, 1993.
15. Norkin, CC, and White, DJ: Measurement of Joint Motion: A Guide to Goniometry, ed 2. FA Davis, Philadelphia, 1995.
16. O'Driscoll, SW, and Giori, NJ: Continuous passive motion (CPM) theory and principles of clinical application. J Rehabil Res Dev 37(2):179, 2000.
17. Pope, RO, Corcoran, S, et al: Continuous passive motion after primary total knee arthroplasty. Does it offer any benefits? J Bone Joint Surg Br 79(6):914, 1997.
18. Rosen, MA, Jackson, DW, and Atwell, EA: The efficacy of continuous passive motion in the rehabilitation of anterior crucuate ligament reconstructions. Am J Sports Med 20(2):122, 1992.
19. Salter, RB: History of rest and motion and the scientific basis for early continuous passive motion. Hand Clin 12(1):1, 1996.
20. Salter, RB, Simmens, DF, and Malcolm, BW: The biological effects of continuous passive motion on the healing of full thickness defects in articular cartilage. J Bone Joint Surg Am 62:1232, 1980.
21. Salter, RB: The prevention of arthritis through the preservation of cartilage. Journal of the Canadian Association of Radiology 31:5, 1981.
22. Salter, RB, Bell, RS, and Keely, FW: The protective effect of continuous passive motion on living cartilage in acute septic arthritis. Clin Orthop 159:223, 1981.
23. Salter, RB: Textbook of Disorders and Injuries of the Musculoskeletal System, ed 3. Williams & Wilkins, Baltimore, 1999.
24. Salter, RB, et al: Clinical application of basic research on continuous passive motion for disorders and injuries of synovial joints. J Orthop Res 1:325, 1984.
25. Smith, LK, Weiss, EL and Lehmkuhl, LD: Brunnstrom's Clinical Kinesiology, ed 5. FA Davis, Philadelphia, 1996.
26. Stap, LJ, and Woodfin, PM: Continuous passive motion in the treatment of knee flexion contractures: A case report. Phys Ther 66:1720, 1986.
27. Wasilewski, SA, Woods, LC, et al: Value of continuous passive motion in total knee arthroplasty. Orthopedics 13(3):291, 1990.
28. Witherow, GE, Bollen, SR, and Pinczewski, LA: The use of continuous passive motion after arthroscopically assisted anterior cruciate ligament reconstruction: help or hindrance? Knee Surg Sports Traumatol Arthrosc 1(2):68, 1993.
29. Yashar, AA, Venn Watson, E, et al: Continuous passive motion with accelerated flexion after total knee arthroplasty. Clin Orthop 345:38, 1997.

Chapter 3

Resistance Exercise

OBJECTIVES

After studying this chapter, the reader will be able to:

1. Define and differentiate between the key elements of muscle performance: strength, power, and muscle endurance.
2. Explain the principles and concepts of specificity of exercise, transfer of training overload, and reversibility as they relate to resistance exercise.
3. Identify key factors that influence the tension-producing capacity of normal skeletal muscle.
4. Explain the relationships among muscle fatigue, recovery from exercise, and overtraining.
5. Summarize the age-related changes in muscle structure and function that occur from early childhood to advanced age.
6. Discuss the adaptation of muscle, connective tissue, and bone to resistance exercise.
7. Identify key elements of resistance exercise programs and explain their interrelationship and impact on training-induced changes in muscle performance.
8. Analyze and describe the similarities and differences among isometric, dynamic exercise against constant and variable loads, isokinetic exercise, and open- and closed-chain exercises.
9. Describe common precautions and contraindications for resistance exercise.
10. State the general principles for application and implementation of resistance exercises.
11. Identify commonalities and differences in the guidelines for resistance training for the healthy adult, the child, and the older adult.
12. Explain the principles of and appropriate application of manual resistance exercise for the extremities in anatomic planes of movement.
13. Describe the principles and procedures for the application of proprioceptive neuromuscular facilitation exercises for the extremities.
14. Compare common systems or regimens of mechanical resistance exercise including progressive resistive exercise, circuit weight training, plyometric exercise, and velocity spectrum rehabilitation, and discuss their use in rehabilitation.
15. Compare the use, benefits, and limitations of various types of resistance equipment.

Muscle performance refers to the capacity of a muscle to do work (force × distance).[9] Despite the simplicity of the definition, muscle performance is a complex component of functional movement. It is affected by all of the body systems, more specifically, by factors such as the morphological qualities of muscle, neurological, biochemical, and biomechanical influences as well as metabolic, cardiovascular, respiratory, cognitive, and emotional function. For a person to anticipate, respond to, and control the forces applied to the body and carry out the physical demands of everyday life in a safe and efficient manner, his or her muscles must be able to produce, sustain, and regulate muscle tension to meet these demands.

The key elements of muscle performance are **strength, power,** and **endurance.** If any one or more of these areas of muscle performance is impaired, functional limitations and disability or increased risk of dysfunction may ensue. Many factors such as injury, disease, immobilization, disuse, or inactivity may result in impaired muscle performance, leading to weakness and muscle atrophy.[176,189,211] When deficits in muscle performance place a person at risk for injury or hinder function, the use of resistance exercise is an appropriate therapeutic intervention to improve the integrated use of strength, power, and muscular endurance during functional movements, to reduce the risk of injury or reinjury, and to enhance physical performance.

Resistance exercise is any form of active exercise in which a dynamic or static muscle contraction is resisted by an outside force, applied either manually or mechanically.[95,229] Resistance exercise, also referred to as **resistance training,**[8,30,154] is an essential element of rehabilitation programs for persons with impaired function and an integral component of conditioning programs for those who wish to promote or maintain health and physical well-being, potentially enhance performance of motor skills, and prevent or reduce the risk of injury and disease.[8,97,110]

A comprehensive examination and evaluation of a patient or client is the basis upon which a therapist determines whether or not a program of resistance exercise is warranted and will improve a person's current level of function or prevent potential dysfunction. Many factors influence how appropriate, effective, or safe resistance training is and how the exercises are designed, implemented, and progressed. Factors such as the underlying pathology, the extent and severity of muscle performance impairments, the presence of other deficits, the stage of tissue healing after injury or surgery, as well as a patient's or client's age, overall level of fitness, and the ability to cooperate and learn all must be considered. Once a program of resistance exercise is developed and prescribed to meet specific functional goals and outcomes, direct intervention by a therapist to initially implement the exercise program or to begin to teach and supervise the prescribed exercises for a smooth transition to an independent, home-based program is imperative.

This chapter provides a foundation of information on resistance exercise and summarizes the many determinants of resistance training programs and the principles and guidelines for application of resistance exercise techniques. It also explores the scientific evidence, when available, of the relationship between improvements in muscle performance and enhanced functional abilities. The techniques described and illustrated in this chapter focus on manual resistance exercise for the extremities. Specific techniques for improving muscle performance, primarily using mechanical resistance during exercises performed independently by the patient or client, are described and illustrated in Chapters 9 to 14. The use of resistance exercise for spinal conditions is presented in Chapters 15 and 16.

Muscle Performance and Resistance Exercise—Definitions and Guiding Principles

As noted in the introduction to this chapter, the three elements of muscle performance, that is, strength, power, and endurance, all can be enhanced by some form of resistance exercise. To what extent each of these elements is altered by exercise depends on how the principles of resistance training are applied and how factors such as the intensity, frequency, and duration of exercise are manipulated. Because the physical demands of work, recreation and everyday living usually involve all three aspects of muscle performance, most resistance training programs seek to achieve a balance of strength, power, and muscular endurance to suit an individual's needs and goals. In addition to having a positive impact on muscle performance, resistance training can produce many other benefits. These potential benefits are listed in Box 3–1. After a brief description of the three elements of muscle performance, guiding principles of exercise prescription and training are discussed in this section.

Strength

Muscle strength is a broad term that refers to the ability of contractile tissue to produce tension and a resultant force based on the demands placed upon

Box 3–1 Benefits of Resistance Exercise

- Enhanced muscle performance: restoration, improvement or maintenance of muscle strength, power, and endurance
- Increased strength of connective tissues: tendons, ligaments, intramuscular connective tissue
- Greater bone mineral density or less bone demineralization
- Decreased stress on joints during physical activity
- Reduced risk of soft-tissue injury during physical activity
- Possible improvement in capacity to repair and heal damaged soft tissues due to positive impact on tissue remodeling
- Possible improvement in balance
- Enhanced physical performance during daily living, occupational, and recreational activities
- Positive changes in body composition: ↑ lean muscle mass or ↓ body fat
- Enhanced feeling of physical well-being
- Possible improvement in perception of disability and quality of life

the muscle.[169,176,201,213,219,229] More specifically, muscle strength is the greatest measurable force that can be exerted by a muscle or muscle group to overcome resistance during a *single,* maximum effort.[9,114] *Functional strength* relates to the ability of the neuromuscular system to produce, reduce, or control forces, contemplated or imposed, during functional activities, in a smooth, coordinated manner.[37,199] Insufficient muscular strength can contribute to major functional losses of even the most basic activities of daily living.

The development of muscle strength is an integral component of most rehabilitation or conditioning programs for individuals of all ages and all ability levels.[8,86,204,206] *Strengthening exercise (strength training)* is defined as systematic procedure of a muscle or muscle group lifting, lowering, or controlling heavy loads (resistance) for a relatively low number of repetitions or over a short period of time.[30,95,201] The most common adaptation to heavy resistance exercise is an increase in the maximum force producing capacity of muscle, that is, an increase in muscle strength, primarily as the result of neural adaptations and an increase in muscle fiber size.[30,95,176,188]

Power

Muscle power, another aspect of muscle performance, is related to the strength and speed of movement and is defined as the work (force × distance) produced by a muscle per unit of time (force × distance/time).[9,169,176,184,218] In other words, it is the *rate* of performing work. The rate at which a muscle contracts and produces a resultant force and the relationship of force and velocity are both factors that affect muscle power.[184,258] Because work can be produced over a very brief or extended period of time, power can be expressed by either a single burst of high-intensity activity (such as lifting a heavy piece of luggage onto an overhead rack or performing a high jump) or by repeated bursts of less intense muscle activity (such as climbing a flight of stairs). The terms *anaerobic power* and *aerobic power,* respectively, are sometimes used to differentiate these two aspects of power.[176,218,222]

Many motor skills in our lives are composed of movements that are explosive and involve both strength and speed. Therefore, re-establishing muscle power may be an important priority in a rehabilitation program. Muscle strength is a necessary foundation for developing muscle power. Power can be enhanced by either increasing the work a muscle must perform in a specified period of time or by reducing the amount of time required to produce a given force. The greater the intensity of the exercise and the shorter the time period taken to generate force, the greater the muscle power.[184,218] In power training regimens, such as *plyometric training,* the speed of movement is the variable that is most often manipulated.[19,176,257,259] *Stretch-shortening drills* is a term used synonymously with plyometric training[258,276] (see discussion later in this chapter).

Endurance

Endurance is a broad term that refers to the ability to perform low-intensity, repetitive, or sustained activities over a prolonged period of time. *Cardiorespiratory endurance (total body endurance)* is associated with repetitive, dynamic motor activities such as walking, cycling, swimming, or upper extremity ergometry that involve the use of the large muscles of the body.[8,30] This aspect of endurance is explored in Chapter 4.

Muscle endurance (sometimes referred to as *local endurance*) is the ability of a muscle to contract repeatedly against a load (resistance), generate and sustain tension, and resist fatigue over an extended period of time.[8,9,14,176,213,216] The term *aerobic power* is sometimes used interchangeably with muscle endurance.[218] Maintenance of balance and proper alignment of the body segments require sustained control (endurance) by the postural muscles. In fact, almost all daily living tasks require some degree of muscle and cardiorespiratory endurance.

Although strength and muscle endurance, as elements of muscle performance, are associated, they do not always correlate well with each other. Just because a muscle group is strong, it does not preclude the possibility that muscular endurance is impaired. For example, an individual in the workplace who is strong will have no difficulty lifting a 10-pound object several times, but does the worker have sufficient muscle endurance in the upper extremities and the stabilizing muscles of the trunk and lower extremities to lift 10-pound objects several hundred times in the course of a day's work without excessive fatigue or potential injury?

Endurance exercise (endurance training) is characterized by having a muscle contract and lift or lower a light load for many repetitions or sustain a muscle contraction for an extended period of time.[30,77,94,176,243] The key elements are always low-intensity muscle contractions, high repetitions, and a prolonged time period. Unlike strength training, muscles adapt to endurance training by increases in their oxidative and metabolic capacities, which allow better delivery and use of oxygen. For many patients with impaired muscle performance, endurance training will have a more positive impact on improving function than strength training. In addition, using low levels of resistance in an exercise program minimizes adverse forces on joints, produces less irritation to soft tissues, and is more comfortable for the patient than heavy resistance training.

Overload Principle

Description

A guiding principle of exercise prescription that has been one of the foundations upon which the use of resistance exercise to improve muscle performance has been based is the **overload principle.** Simply stated, if muscle performance is to improve, a load that exceeds the metabolic capacity of the muscle must be applied, that is, the muscle must be challenged to perform at a level greater than that to which it is accustomed.[8,120,176] If the demands remain constant after the muscle has adapted, the level of muscle performance can be maintained, but not increased.

Application of the Overload Principle

This principle focuses on the progressive loading of muscle by manipulating the intensity or volume of exercise. Intensity of resistance exercise refers to how much weight (resistance) is imposed on the muscle, whereas volume encompasses variables such as repetitions, sets, or frequency of exercise, any one or more of which can be gradually adjusted to increase the demands on the muscle.

- In a strength training program, the *amount of resistance* applied to the muscle is incrementally and progressively increased.
- In endurance training, more emphasis is placed on increasing the *time* a muscle contraction is sustained or the *number of repetitions* performed than on increasing resistance.

Precaution: To ensure safety, the extent and progression of overload must always be applied in the context of the underlying pathology, age of the patient, stage of healing of tissues, fatigue, and the overall abilities and goals of the patient. The muscle and related body systems must be given time to *adapt* to the demands of an increased load or repetitions before the load or number of repetitions is again increased.

SAID Principle

Background

The SAID principle (Specific Adaptation to Imposed Demands)[176] suggests that a framework of specificity is a necessary foundation upon which exercise programs should be built. This principle applies to all body systems and is an extension of Wolff's Law (body systems adapt over time to the stresses placed upon them). The SAID principle helps therapists determine the exercise prescription and which parameters of exercise should be selected to create specific training effects and best meet specific functional needs and goals.

Specificity of Training

Specificity of training, also referred to as **specificity of exercise,** is a widely accepted concept that suggests that the adaptive effects of training, such as the improvement of strength, power, and endurance, are highly specific to the training method employed.[30,77,176] Whenever possible, exercises incorporated in a training program should mimic the anticipated function. For example, if the desired functional activity requires greater muscular endurance than strength, then the intensity and duration of exercises should be geared to improve muscular endurance.

Specificity of training should also be considered relative to mode (type) and velocity of exercise[22,76,139,183,187,202] as well as patient or limb position (joint angle)[148,149,265,267] and movement pattern during exercise. For example, if the desired functional outcome is the ability to ascend and descend stairs, then exercise should be performed eccentrically and concentrically in a closed-chain pattern and progressed to the desired speed. Regardless of the simplicity or complexity of the motor task to be learned, task-specific practice must always be emphasized. It has been suggested that the basis of specificity of training is related to morphological and metabolic changes within muscle as well as neural adaptations to the training stimulus associated with motor learning.[198]

Transfer of Training

Contrary to the SAID principle, carryover of training effects from one variation of exercise or task to another has also been reported. This phenomenon is called **transfer of training, overflow,** or **cross-training.** Transfer of training has been reported to occur on a *very limited* basis with respect to velocity of training,[133,183,253] and type or mode of exercise.[76] It has also been suggested that a cross-training effect can occur from an exercised limb to a nonexercised contralateral limb in a resistance training program.[63,265,266]

A program of exercises designed to develop muscle strength has also been shown to at least moderately improve muscular endurance. In contrast, endurance training has little to no cross-training effect on strength.[16,77,95] Strength training at one speed of exercise has been shown to provide some improvement in strength at higher or lower speeds of exercise. In almost all instances the overflow effects are substantially less than the training effects resulting from specificity of training.

Despite the evidence that a small degree of transfer of training does occur in resistance exercise programs, most studies support the importance of designing an exercise program that most closely replicates the desired functional activities. As many variables as possible in the exercise program should match the requirements and demands placed on a patient during specific functional activities.

Reversibility Principle

Adaptive changes in the body's systems, such as increased strength or endurance, in response to a resistance exercise program are transient unless training-induced improvements are regularly used for functional activities or unless an individual participates in a maintenance program of resistance exercises.[8,39,85,176]

Detraining, reflected by a reduction in muscle performance, begins within a week or two after the cessation of resistance exercises and continues until training effects are lost.[8,154] For this reason, it is imperative that gains in strength and endurance are incorporated into daily activities as early as possible in a rehabilitation program. It may also be advisable for patients to participate in a maintenance program of resistance exercises as an integral component of a lifelong fitness program.

► Skeletal Muscle Function and Adaptation to Resistance Exercise

Knowledge of the factors that influence the force-producing capacity of normal muscle during an active contraction is the foundation upon which an understanding of how the neuromuscular system adapts as the result of resistance training. This knowledge, in turn, provides a basis upon which a therapist is able to make sound clinical decisions when designing a resistance exercise program to improve muscle performance in patients with weakness and functional limitations as the result of injury or disease or to enhance physical performance and prevent or reduce the risk of injury in healthy individuals.

Factors that Influence Tension Generation in Normal Skeletal Muscle

Diverse but interrelated factors affect the capacity of *normal* skeletal muscle to generate tension to control the body and perform motor tasks. Determinants and correlates include morphological, biomechanical, neurologic, metabolic, and biochemical factors. All contribute to the *magnitude, duration,* and *speed* of force production as well as how resistant or susceptible a muscle is to fatigue. Properties of muscle itself as well as key neural factors and their impact on tension generation during an active muscle contraction are summarized in Table 3–1.[153,169,176,229,233]

Additional factors such as the energy stores available to muscle, the influence of fatigue and recovery from exercise, and a person's age, gender, and psychological/cognitive status as well as many other factors affect a muscle's ability to develop and sustain tension. A therapist must recognize that these factors will affect a patient's performance during exercise and the potential outcomes of the exercise program.

Energy Stores, Blood Supply

Muscle needs adequate sources of energy (fuel) to contract, generate tension, and resist fatigue. The predominant fiber type found in the muscle and the adequacy of blood supply, which transports oxygen and nutrients to muscle and removes waste products, affect the tension-producing capacity of a muscle and its ability to resist fatigue.[153,176] A review of

Table 3–1 Determinants and Correlates that Affect Tension Generation of Skeletal Muscle

Factor	Influence
Cross-section and size of the muscle (includes muscle fiber number and size)	The larger the muscle diameter, the greater its tension-producing capacity
Fiber arrangement and fiber length (also relates to cross-sectional diameter of the muscle)	Short fibers with pinnate and multipinnate design in high force producing muscles (ex. quadriceps, gastrocnemius, deltoid, biceps brachii) Long parallel design in muscles with high rate of shortening but less force production (ex. sartorius, lumbricals)
Fiber-type distribution of muscle: type I (tonic, slow-twitch) and type IIA & IIB (phasic, fast-twitch)	High percentage of type I fibers: low force production, slow rate of maximum force development, resistant to fatigue High percentage of type IIA and IIB fibers: rapid high force production; rapid fatigue
Length-tension relationship of muscle at time of contraction	Muscle produces greatest tension when it is near or at the physiological resting position at the time of contraction
Recruitment of motor units	The greater the number and synchronization of motor units firing, the greater the force production
Frequency of firing of motor units	The higher the frequency of firing, the greater the tension
Type of muscle contraction	Force output from greatest to least: eccentric, isometric, concentric muscle contraction
Speed of muscle contraction (force-velocity relationship)	Concentric contraction: ↑speed→↓tension. Eccentric contraction: ↑speed→↑tension

the three main energy systems (the ATP-PC system, the anaerobic/glycolytic/lactic acid system, and the aerobic system) is discussed in Chapter 4.

Fatigue

Fatigue is a complex phenomenon that affects muscle performance and must be considered in a resistance training program. Fatigue has a variety of definitions that are based on the type of fatigue being addressed.

Muscle (local) fatigue. Muscle (local) fatigue is the diminished response of muscle to repeated stimulus and is reflected by a progressive decrement in the amplitude of the motor unit potentials.[157] This occurs during exercise when a muscle repeatedly contracts either statically or dynamically, against an imposed load.[176]

This *acute* physiologic response to exercise is *normal* and *reversible*. It is characterized by a gradual decline in the force-producing capacity of the neuromuscular system, that is, a *temporary* state of exhaustion (failure), leading to a decrease in muscle strength.[14,49,57,153]

The diminished response of the muscle is caused by a combination of factors, which include

- Disturbances in the contractile mechanism of the muscle itself because of a decrease in energy stores, insufficient oxygen, and a build-up of lactic acid
- Inhibitory (protective) influences from the central nervous system
- Possibly a decrease in the conduction of impulses at the myoneural junction, particularly in fast-twitch fibers

The fiber-type distribution of a muscle affects how resistant it is to fatigue.[169,176,213] Type II (phasic, fast-twitch) muscle fibers, which generate a great amount of tension in a short period of time, are geared toward anaerobic metabolic activity and tend to fatigue quickly. Type I (tonic, slow-twitch) muscle fibers generate a low level of muscle tension but can sustain the contraction for a long time. These fibers are geared toward aerobic metabolism and are very slow to fatigue.

Because different muscles are composed of varying proportions of tonic and phasic fibers, the function of muscles becomes specialized. For example, a heavy distribution of type I (tonic) fibers is found in postural muscles, which allows these muscles to sustain a low level of tension for extended periods of time to hold the body erect against gravity or stabilize against repetitive loads. On the other end of the fatigue spectrum, muscles with a large distribution of type II (phasic) fibers produce a great burst of tension to enable a person to lift the entire body weight or to lift, lower, push or pull a heavy load but fatigue very quickly.

Clinical signs of muscular fatigue during exercise are summarized in Box 3–2.

When these signs and symptoms develop during resistance exercise, it is time to decrease the load on that muscle or stop the exercise and shift to another muscle group to allow time for the muscle to rest and recover.

Cardiorespiratory (general) fatigue. This is the diminished response of an individual (the entire body) as the result of prolonged physical activity, such as walking; jogging, cycling, or repetitive lifting or digging. It is related to the body's ability to use oxygen efficiently. Cardiorespiratory fatigue associated with endurance training is probably caused by a combination of the following factors.[21,57,106,176]

- A decrease in blood sugar (glucose) levels
- A decrease in glycogen stores in muscle and liver
- A depletion of potassium, especially in the elderly patient

Threshold for fatigue. Threshold for fatigue is that level of exercise that cannot be sustained indefinitely.[21] A patient's threshold for fatigue could be noted as the length of time a contraction is maintained or the number of repetitions of an exercise that initially can be performed. This sets a baseline from which adaptive changes in physical performance can be measured.

Factors that influence fatigue. Factors that influence fatigue are diverse. A patient's health status, diet, or lifestyle (sedentary or active) all influence fatigue. In patients with neuromuscular, cardiorespiratory, oncological, inflammatory, or psychological disorders, the onset of fatigue is often abnormal.[4,49,91] For instance, it may occur abruptly, more rapidly or at predictable intervals. It is advisable for a therapist to become familiar with the patterns of fatigue associated with different diseases and medications. In multiple sclerosis, the patient usually awakens rested and functions well in the early morning. By mid-afternoon, however, the patient reaches a peak of fatigue and becomes notably weak. Then by early evening, fatigue diminishes and strength again returns. Patients with cardiac, peripheral vascular, and pulmonary diseases, as well as patients with cancer undergoing chemotherapy or radiation therapy, all have deficits that compromise the oxygen transport system. Therefore, these patients fatigue more rapidly and require a longer period of time for recovery from exercise.[4,91] Environmental factors, such as outside or room temperature, air quality, and altitude, also influence how quickly the onset of fatigue occurs and how much time is required for recovery from exercise.[14,155,176]

Box 3–2 Signs and Symptoms of Muscle Fatigue

- An uncomfortable sensation within the muscle, even pain and cramping
- Tremulousness in the contracting muscle
- Active movements jerky, not smooth
- Inability to complete the movement pattern through the full range of available motion during dynamic exercise against the same level of resistance
- Use of substitute motions, that is, incorrect movement patterns, to complete the movement pattern
- Inability to continue low-intensity physical activity
- Decline in peak torque during isokinetic testing

Recovery from Exercise

Adequate time for recovery from fatiguing exercise must be built into every resistance training program. This applies to both intrasession and intersession recovery. After vigorous exercise, the body must be given time to restore itself to a state that existed prior to the exhaustive exercise. Recovery from acute exercise, where the force-producing capacity of muscle returns to 90 to 95% of the pre-exercise capacity, usually takes 3 to 4 minutes, with the greatest proportion of recovery occurring in the first minute.[44,57,176,225]

Changes that occur in muscle during recovery are:

- Energy stores are replenished.
- Lactic acid is removed from skeletal muscle and blood within approximately 1 hour after exercise.
- Oxygen stores are replenished in muscles.
- Glycogen is replaced over several days.

It has been shown that if light exercise is performed during the recovery period *(active recovery)*, recovery from exercise will occur more rapidly than with total rest *(passive recovery)*.[26,44,57,105,225] Faster recovery with light exercise is probably the result of neural as well as circulatory influences.[44,57,225]

Precautions: Only if a patient is allowed adequate time to recover from fatigue after each exercise session will long-term muscle performance (strength, power, or endurance) improve.[26,105] If a sufficient rest interval is not an integral component of a resistance exercise program, patient's performance will plateau or deteriorate. Evidence of overtraining or overwork weakness may become apparent (see additional discussion later in this chapter). It has also been shown that fatigued muscles are more susceptible to acute strains.[174]

Age

Muscle performance changes throughout the lifespan. Whether the goal of a resistance training program is to remediate impairments and functional limitations or enhance fitness and performance of physical activities, an understanding of "typical" changes in muscle performance and response to exercise during each phase of life from early childhood through the advanced years of life is necessary to prescribe effective and safe resistance exercises for individuals of all ages. Key aspects of how muscle performance changes throughout life are discussed in this section and summarized in Box 3–3.

Early Childhood and Preadolescence

In absolute terms, muscle performance (specifically strength), which in part is related to the development of muscle mass, increases *linearly* with chronological age in both boys and girls from birth, through early and middle childhood to puberty.[175,244,272] Muscle endurance also increases linearly during the childhood years.[272] Muscle fiber number is essentially determined prior to or shortly after birth,[222] although there is speculation that fiber number may continue to increase into early childhood.[272] The rate of fiber growth (increase in cross-sectional area) is relatively consistent from birth to puberty. Change in fiber type distribution is relatively complete by the age of 1, shifting from a predominance of type II fibers to a more balanced distribution of type I and type II fibers.[272]

Box 3–3 Summary of Age-Related Changes in Muscle and Muscle Performance

Infancy, Early Childhood, and Preadolescence

- At birth, muscle accounts for about 25% of body weight.
- Total number of muscle fibers is established prior to or early in infancy.
- Postnatal changes in distribution of type I and type II fibers within muscle are relatively complete by end of first year of life.
- Muscle fiber size and muscle mass increase linearly from infancy to puberty.
- Muscle strength and muscle endurance increase linearly with chronological age in boys and girls throughout childhood until puberty.
- Muscle mass (absolute and relative) and muscle strength is just slightly greater (approximately 10%) in boys than girls from early childhood to puberty.
- Training-induced strength gains occur equally in both sexes during childhood without evidence of hypertrophy until puberty.

Puberty

- Rapid acceleration in muscle fiber size and muscle mass, especially in boys. During puberty, muscle mass increases more than 30% per year.
- Rapid increase in muscle strength in both sexes.
- Marked difference in strength levels develops in boys and girls.
- In boys, muscle mass and body height and weight peak before muscle strength; in girls, strength peaks before body weight.
- Relative strength gains as the result of resistance training are comparable between the sexes, with significantly greater muscle hypertrophy in boys.

Young and Middle Adulthood

- Muscle mass peaks in women between 16 and 20 years of age; muscle mass in men peaks between 18 and 25 years of age.
- Muscle mass constitutes approximately 40% of total body weight in early adulthood, with men having slightly more muscle mass than women.
- Strength continues to develop into the second decade, especially in men.
- Muscle strength and endurance reach a peak in the second decade, earlier for women than men.
- By sometime in the third decade, strength declines between 8 and 10% per decade through the fifth or sixth decade.
- Strength and muscle endurance deteriorate less rapidly in physically active versus sedentary adults.
- Improvements in strength and endurance are possible with only a modest increase in physical activity.

Late Adulthood

- Rate of decline of muscle strength accelerates to 2 to 4% per year beginning in the sixth to seventh decade.
- Muscle mass, fiber size and fiber number, and number of alpha motoneurons all decrease.
- Loss of flexibility reduces the force-producing capacity of muscle.
- Decrease in the speed of muscle contractions.
- Minimal decline in performance of functional skills in the sixth decade; significant deterioration by the eighth decade.
- Significant improvement in muscle strength is possible in late adulthood with a resistance training program.
- Impact of resistance training on the level of performance of functional motor skills is not clear.

Throughout childhood, boys have slightly greater absolute and relative muscle mass (kg of muscle per kg of body weight) than girls.[25,175] Boys are approximately 10% stronger than girls from early childhood to puberty.[176] This difference may be associated with differences in relative muscle mass, although social expectations especially by mid-childhood also may contribute to the observed difference in muscle strength.

There is no question that an appropriately designed resistance exercise program can improve muscle strength in children above and beyond gains attributable to typical growth and development. A recent review of the literature[86] cites many studies that support this statement. The American Academy of Pediatrics[6] and the American College of Sports Medicine[8] support youth participation in resistance training programs, if they are designed appropriately and carefully supervised. With this in mind, two important questions need to be addressed: (1) At what point in childhood is a resistance training program appropriate? and (2) What constitutes a safe training program?

During the toddler, preschool, and even during the early school years, initially play and then organized but age-appropriate physical activities are effective methods to promote fitness and improve muscle performance, not structured resistance training programs. In the past decade it has become popular for preadolescent boys and girls to participate in resistance training programs to reduce the risk of injury and enhance athletic performance. In addition, prepubescent children often sustain injuries during everyday activities and, therefore, may become candidates for rehabilitation that may include resistance exercises. In this age group many studies have shown that improvements in strength and muscular endurance occur on a relative basis that are similar to training-induced gains in young adults.[25,87,138] It should be noted that, although only a few studies have looked at the effects of detraining in children, as with adults when training ceases, strength levels gradually return to a pretraining level.[85] This suggests that some maintenance level of training could be useful in children as with adults.[86]

Although there is only limited evidence to suggest that a structured resistance training program for children, in addition to a general sports conditioning program, reduces injuries or enhances sports performance, other health-related benefits have been noted including increased cardiorespiratory fitness, decreased blood lipids levels, and improved psychological well-being.[25,85,138] These findings suggest that participation in a resistance training program during the childhood years may, indeed, be of value if the program is performed at an appropriate level and is closely supervised.

Puberty

At puberty, as hormonal levels change, there is a rapid acceleration in the development of muscle strength, especially in boys. During this phase of development, typical strength levels become markedly different in boys and girls, which, in part, are caused by hormonal differences between the sexes. Longitudinal studies[31,175] of adolescent boys indicate that strength increases about 30% per year between ages 10 and 16 with muscle mass peaking before muscle strength. In adolescent girls, peak strength develops before peak weight.[89] Overall, during the adolescent years, muscle mass increases more than 5 times in boys and approximately 3.5 times in girls.[31,175] Although most longitudinal studies of growth stop at age 18, strength continues to develop, particularly in males, well into the second and even into the third decade of life.[272]

As with prepubescent children, resistance training during puberty also results in significant strength gains. During puberty these gains average 30 to 40% above that which is expected as the result of normal growth and maturation.[86] Similar benefits of strength training have been noted during puberty as those noted in prepubescent children.[85,87]

Young and Middle Adulthood

Although data on typical strength and endurance levels during the second through the fifth decades of life are more often from studies of men than women, a few generalizations can be made that appear to apply to both sexes.[171] Strength reaches a maximal level earlier in women than men, with women reaching a peak in the second decade and most men by age 30. Strength then declines approximately 1% per year[272] or 8% per decade.[101] This decline in strength appears to occur later or at a slower rate in active adults versus those who are sedentary.[103,272] The potential for improving muscle performance with a resistance training program or by adding even moderately demanding activities several times a week is high during this phase of life.

Late Adulthood

The rate of decline in the torque-generating capacity of muscle in most cases accelerates to approximately

2 to 4% per year in men and women in their 60s, 70s, and beyond.[11,103,171] However, the rate of decline may be significantly less (only .3% decrease per year) in elderly men and women who maintain a high level of physical activity.[111] These disparate findings and others suggest that loss of muscle strength during the advanced years may be due, in part, to progressively greater inactivity and disuse.[33] Loss of muscle strength during late adulthood, particularly in the 80s and beyond, is associated with a gradual increase in functional limitations as well as an increase in the frequency of falling.[33]

The decline in muscle strength and endurance in the elderly is associated with many factors in addition to progressive disuse and inactivity. It is difficult to determine if these factors are causes or effects of age-related deterioration in strength. Neuromuscular factors include a decrease in muscle mass, decrease in the number of type I and type II fibers, decrease in the cross-sectional size of muscle, particularly of type II fibers, change in the length-tension relationship of muscle associated with loss of flexibility, and a decrease in the number of alpha motoneurons in the spinal cord, as well as axonal deterioration in the peripheral nerves.[11,33,101,131] The decline in the number of motor units appears to begin after age 60.[131] All of these changes have an impact on strength and physical performance.

In addition to decreases in muscle strength, declines in speed of muscle contraction, muscle endurance, and the ability to recover from muscular fatigue also occur with advanced age.[131] The time needed to produce the same absolute and relative levels of torque output and the time necessary to achieve relaxation after a voluntary contraction are both lengthened in the elderly compared to younger adults.[101] Consequently, as velocity of movement declines, so does the ability to generate muscle power during activities that require quick responses, such as rising from a low chair or adjusting balance to prevent a fall. Information on changes in muscle endurance with aging is limited. There is some evidence to suggest that the ability to sustain low-intensity muscular effort also declines with age, in part because of reduced blood supply and capillary density in muscle, decreased mitochondrial density, changes in enzymatic activity level, and decreased glucose transport.[101] As a result, muscle fatigue may tend to occur more readily in the elderly. In the healthy and active (community-dwelling) elderly population, the decline in muscle endurance appears to be minimal well into the 70s.[131]

A review of the literature indicates that when healthy or frail elderly individuals participate in a resistance training program of appropriate duration and intensity, muscle strength and endurance increase.* Only some of the studies on strength or endurance training have also measured pre- and post-training levels of functional abilities, such as balance, stair climbing, walking speed, and chair rise. The effect of strength and endurance training on functional abilities is promising but still in question with most investigations demonstrating a positive impact[3,34,40,90,194,204,248] and a few showing no significant improvement in function.[33] This disparity of outcomes among investigations underscores the point that resistance training has a direct impact on muscle performance but only an indirect impact on functional performance, a more complex variable. Studies of elderly individuals have also shown that if resistance training is discontinued, detraining gradually occurs and, subsequently, strength and functional capabilities deteriorate close to pre-training levels.[39,164] Overall, the evidence indicates that the decline in muscle strength and functional abilities that occurs in late adulthood is at least partially reversible with a resistance training program, but if these training-induced improvements are to be maintained, some degree of resistance training must continue.

Psychological Factors

An array of psychological factors can positively or negatively influence muscle performance and how easily, vigorously, or cautiously a person moves. Just as injury and disease adversely affect muscle performance, so can one's mental status. For example, a fear of pain, injury or reinjury, depression related to physical illness, or impaired attention or memory as the result of age, head injury, or the side-effects of medication all can adversely affect the ability to develop or sustain sufficient muscle tension for execution or acquisition of functional motor tasks. In contrast, psychological factors can also positively influence physical performance. Principles and methods to maximize motor performance and learning as functions of effective patient education were discussed in Chapter 1. These principles and methods should be applied in a resistance training program to

*See references 33, 34, 40, 112, 164, 186, 193, 227, 248.

develop a requisite level of muscle strength, power, and endurance for functional activities.

The following interrelated psychological factors as well as other aspects of motor learning may influence muscle performance and the effectiveness of a resistance training program.

Attention

A patient must be able to focus on a given task (exercise) to learn how to perform it correctly. Attention involves the ability to process relevant data while screening out irrelevant information from the environment and to respond to internal cues from the body. Both are necessary when first learning an exercise and later when carrying out an exercise program independently. Attention to form and technique during a resistance exercise is necessary for patient safety and optimal long-term training effects.

Motivation

If a resistance exercise program is to be effective, a patient must be willing to put forth and maintain sufficient effort and adhere to an exercise program over time to improve muscle performance for functional activities. Use of activities that are meaningful and are perceived as having potential usefulness or periodically modifying an exercise routine help maintain a patient's interest in resistance training. Charting or graphing a patient's improvement also helps sustain motivation. Incorporating gains in muscle performance into functional activities as early as possible in a resistance exercise program puts improvements in strength to practical use, thereby making those improvements meaningful.

Feedback

The importance of feedback for learning an exercise or a motor skill was discussed in Chapter 1. In addition, feedback can have a positive impact on a patient's motivation and subsequent adherence to an exercise program. For example, some computerized equipment, such as isokinetic dynamometers, provide visual or auditory signals that let the patient know if each muscle contraction during a particular exercise is within a zone that will cause a training-effect. Documenting improvements over time, such as the amount of weight used during various exercises or changes in walking distance or speed, also provides positive feedback to sustain a patient's motivation in a resistance exercise program.

Physiologic Adaptations Associated with Resistance Exercise

The use of resistance exercise in rehabilitation and conditioning programs has a substantial impact on all systems of the body. Resistance training is equally important for patients with deficits in motor performance or for individuals who wish to improve or maintain their level of fitness, enhance performance, or reduce the risk of injury. When body systems are exposed to a greater than usual but appropriate level of resistance in an exercise program, they initially react with a number of *acute* physiologic responses[153] and then later adapt. That is, body systems accommodate over time to the newly imposed physical demands.[8,159,176] Training-induced adaptations to resistance exercise, known as *chronic* physiologic responses, that affect muscle performance are summarized in Table 3–2 and discussed in this section.[8,30,159] Key differences in adaptations from strength training versus endurance training are noted.

Adaptations to overload create changes in muscle performance and, in part, determine the effectiveness of a resistance training program. The time course for these adaptations to occur varies from one individual to another and is dependent on a person's health status and previous level of participation in a resistance exercise program.

Neural Adaptations

It is well accepted that in a resistance training program the initial, rapid gain in the tension-generating capacity of skeletal muscle is largely attributed to neural responses, not adaptive changes in muscle itself.[188,214,215] This is reflected by an increase in EMG activity during the first 4 to 8 weeks of training with little to no evidence of muscle fiber hypertrophy. It is also possible that increased neural activity is the source of additional gains in strength late in a resistance training program even after muscle hypertrophy has reached a plateau.[176]

Neural adaptations are attributed to motor learning and improved coordination[154,155,159,176] and include *increased recruitment* in the number of motor units firing as well as an *increased rate and synchronization* of firing.[154,176,214] It is speculated that these changes are caused by a decrease in the inhibitory function of the CNS, decreased sensitivity of the Golgi tendon organ (GTO) or changes at the myoneural junction of the motor unit.[159,176,214]

Table 3–2 Physiologic Adaptations to Resistance Exercise

Variable	Strength Training Adaptations	Endurance Training Adaptations
Skeletal muscle structure	Hypertrophy of muscle fibers; greater in type II fibers Hyperplasia (possibly) of muscle fibers Fiber type composition: remodeling of type IIB to type IIA; No change in type I to type II distribution (i.e., no conversion) Capillary bed density: ↓ or no change Mitochondrial density and volume: ↓	Hypertrophy: minimal or no change Capillary bed density: ↑ Mitochondrial density and volume: ↑
Neural system	Motor unit recruitment: ↑ # motor units firing Rate of firing: ↑ (↓ twitch contraction time) Synchronization of firing: ↑	
Metabolic system	ATP and CP storage: ↑ Myoglobin storage: ↑ Stored triglycerides: not known	ATP and CP storage: ↑ Myoglobin storage: ↑ Stored triglycerides: ↑
Enzymes	Creatine phosphokinase: ↑ Myokinase: ↑	Similar ↑ Similar ↑
Body composition	Lean body (fat-free) mass: ↑ % body fat: ↓	Lean body (fat-free) mass: no change % body fat: ↓
Connective tissue	Tensile strength of tendons, ligaments, and connective tissue in muscle: ↑ Bone: ↑ bone mineral density; no change or possible ↑ in bone mass	Tensile strength of tendons, ligaments, and connective tissue in muscle: ↑ Bone: ↑ mineralization with weight-bearing activities

Skeletal Muscle Adaptations

Hypertrophy

As noted previously, the tension-producing capacity of muscle is directly related to the physiological cross-sectional area of the individual muscle fibers. **Hypertrophy** is an increase in the size of an individual muscle fiber caused by an increase in myofibrillar volume. After an extended period of moderate- to high-intensity resistance training, usually by 4 to 8 weeks,[1,159,176,269] but possibly as early as 2 to 3 weeks with very high-intensity resistance training,[237] hypertrophy becomes an increasingly important adaptation that accounts for strength gains in muscle.

Although the mechanism of hypertrophy is complex and the stimulus for growth is not clearly understood, hypertrophy of skeletal muscle appears to be the result of an increase in protein (actin and myosin) synthesis and a decrease in protein degradation. Hypertrophy is also associated with biochemical changes that stimulate uptake of amino acids.[154,176]

The greatest increases in protein synthesis and, therefore, hypertrophy are associated with high-volume, moderate-resistance exercise performed eccentrically.[154] In addition, it is the type IIB muscle fibers that appear to increase in size most readily with resistance training.[159,176]

Hyperplasia

Although the topic has been debated for many years and evidence of the phenomenon is sparse, there is some thought that a portion of the increase in muscle size that occurs with heavy resistance training is caused by **hyperplasia**, an increase in the *number* of muscle fibers. It has been suggested that this increase in fiber number, observed in laboratory animals, is the result of longitudinal splitting of fibers.[12,108,109,130,181] It has been postulated that fiber splitting occurs when individual muscle fibers increase in size to a point where they are inefficient, then subsequently split to form two distinct fibers.[108]

Critics of the concept of hyperplasia suggest that evidence of fiber splitting may actually be caused by inappropriate tissue preparation in the laboratory.[107] The general opinion in the literature is that hyperplasia either does not occur or, if it does occur to a slight degree, its impact is insignificant.[30,177] In a recent review article it was the author's opinion that if hyperplasia is a valid finding, it probably accounts for a very small proportion (less than 5%) of the increase in muscle size that occurs with resistance training.[155]

Muscle Fiber Type Adaptation

As previously mentioned, type II (phasic) muscle fibers preferentially hypertrophy with heavy resistance training. In addition, a substantial degree of plasticity exists in muscle fibers. Transformation of type IIB to type IIA is common in the early weeks of resistance training, making the type II fibers more fatigue resistant.[156,176,237] But it is doubtful, despite a few reported occurrences of fiber type conversion in laboratory animals,[196,283] that conversion from one muscle fiber type to another (type II to I or I to II) occurs under training conditions in rehabilitation or fitness programs.[156,176]

Vascular and Metabolic Adaptations

Adaptations of the cardiovascular and respiratory systems as the result of low-intensity, high-volume resistance training are discussed in Chapter 4. Opposite to what occurs with endurance training, when muscles hypertrophy with high-intensity, low-volume training, capillary bed density actually decreases because of an increase in the number of myofilaments per fiber.[159] Athletes who participate in heavy resistance training actually have fewer capillaries per muscle fiber than endurance athletes and even untrained individuals.[143,251] Other changes associated with metabolism, such as a decrease in mitochondrial density, also occur with high-intensity resistance training.[154,159] This is associated with a reduced oxidative capacity of muscle.

Adaptations of Connective Tissues

Although evidence is limited it appears that the tensile strength of tendons and ligaments as well as bone increases with resistance training designed to improve the strength or power of muscles.[41,241,242,284]

Tendons, Ligaments, and Connective Tissue in Muscle

Strength improvement in tendons probably occurs at the musculotendinous junction whereas increased ligament strength may occur at the ligament-bone interface. It is believed that tendon and ligament tensile strength increases to support the adaptive strength and size changes in muscle. The connective tissue within muscle (around muscle fibers) also thickens, giving more support to the enlarged fibers.[176] Noncontractile soft tissue strength may develop more rapidly with eccentric resistance training than with other types of resistance exercises.[241,242] Consequently, strong ligaments and tendons may be less prone to injury.

Bone

Numerous sources indicate there is a high correlation between muscle strength and level of physical activity across the life span with bone mineral density.[220,223] Consequently, physical activities and exercises, particularly those performed in weight-bearing positions, are typically recommended to minimize or to prevent age-related bone loss.[203] They are also commonly prescribed to reduce the risk of fractures or improve bone density when osteopenia or osteoporosis is already present.[104,220]

Although the evidence from prospective studies is limited and mixed, resistance exercises, performed with adequate intensity and with site-specific loading through weight bearing of the bony area to be tested, has been shown to increase or maintain bone mineral density.[162,180,190] In contrast, a number of studies in young healthy women[210] and post-menopausal women[207,226] have reported there was no significant increase in bone mineral density with resistance training, but the resistance exercises in these studies were not combined with site-specific weight bearing. In addition, the intensity of the weight training programs may not have been intense enough to have an impact on bone density.[162,220] The time course of the exercise program also may not have been long enough. It has been suggested that it may take as long as 9 months to a year of exercise for detectable and significant increases in bone mass to occur.[223] In the spine, although studies to date have not shown that resistance training prevents spinal fractures, there is some evidence to suggest that strength of the back extensors closely correlates with bone mineral density of the spine.[226] Research continues to determine the most effective forms of exercise to enhance bone density and prevent age-related bone loss and fractures.

▶ Determinants of Resistance Exercise

Many elements (variables) determine whether or not a resistance exercise program is appropriate, effective, and safe. This holds true when resistance training is a part of a rehabilitative program for individuals with known or potential impairments in muscle performance or when it is incorporated into a general conditioning program to improve the level of fitness of healthy individuals.

Each of the inter-related elements discussed in this section must be addressed in order to improve one or more aspects of muscle performance and achieve the desired functional outcomes. Appropriate *alignment* and *stabilization* are always basic elements of any exercise designed to improve muscle performance. A suitable *dosage* of exercise must also be determined. In resistance training, dosage includes *intensity, volume, frequency,* and *duration* of exercise and *rest interval.* Each are mechanisms by which the muscle can be progressively overloaded to improve muscle performance. The *speed* of exercise and the *mode* of exercise must also be considered. These elements are summarized in Box 3–4.

Consistent with the SAID principle, these elements of resistance exercise must be specific to the patient's desired functional goals. Other factors such as the underlying cause or causes of the deficits in muscle performance, the extent of impairment, as well as the patient's age, medical history, mental status, and social situation also affect the design and implementation of a resistance exercise program.

Alignment and Stabilization

Just as correct alignment and effective stabilization are basic elements of manual muscle testing and dynamometry, they are also crucial in resistance exercise. To effectively strengthen a specific muscle or muscle group and avoid substitute motions, appropriate positioning of the body and alignment of a limb or body segment are requisite. **Substitute motions** are compensatory movement patterns caused by muscle action of a stronger adjacent agonist or of a muscle group that normally serves as a stabilizer (fixator).[146] If principles of alignment and stabilization used in manual muscle testing[127,146] are applied during resistance exercise, substitute motions can usually be avoided.

Box 3–4 Elements of a Resistance Exercise Program

- *Alignment* of segments of the body during exercise
- *Stabilization* of proximal or distal joints to prevent substitution
- *Intensity:* the exercise load (level of resistance)
- *Volume:* number of repetitions and sets; number of exercises per session
- *Frequency:* the number of exercise sessions per day or per week
- *Rest interval:* time allotted for recuperation between sets and sessions of exercise
- *Duration:* total time frame of a resistance training program
- *Mode* of exercise: type of muscle contraction, position of the patient, application of resistance, arc of movement, or the primary energy system utilized
- *Speed* of exercise
- *Periodization:* variation of intensity and volume during specific periods of resistance training
- *Integration of function:* use of resistance exercises that replicate functional demands

Alignment

Proper alignment is determined by the direction of muscle fibers and the line of pull of the muscle to be strengthened. The patient or a body segment must be positioned so that the direction of movement of a limb or segment of the body replicates the action of the muscle or muscle groups to be strengthened. For example, to strengthen the gluteus medius, the hip must remain slightly extended, not flexed, and the pelvis must be rotated slightly forward as the patient abducts the lower extremity against the applied resistance. If the hip is flexed as the leg abducts, the adjacent tensor fasciae latae becomes the prime mover and is strengthened.

The alignment or position of the patient or the limb with respect to gravity may also be important during some forms of resistance exercises, particularly if body weight or free weights (dumbbells, barbells, or cuff weights) are the source of resistance. The patient or limb should be positioned so that the muscle being strengthened acts against the resistance of gravity and the weight. This, of course, is contingent upon the comfort and mobility of the patient.

Staying with the example of strengthening the gluteus medius, if a cuff weight is placed around the lower leg, the patient must assume the side-lying position so that abduction occurs through the full ROM against gravity and the additional resistance of the cuff weight. If the patient rolls toward the supine position, the resistance force is applied primarily to the hip flexors, not the abductors.

Stabilization

Stabilization refers to holding down a body segment or holding the body steady.[146] To maintain appropriate alignment, ensure correct muscle action and movement pattern, and avoid unwanted substitute motions during resistance exercise, effective stabilization is imperative. Exercising on a *stable surface,* such as a firm treatment table, helps hold the body steady. *Body weight* may also provide a source of stability during exercise, particularly in the horizontal position. It is most common to stabilize the proximal attachment of the muscle being strengthened, but sometimes the distal attachment is stabilized as the muscle contracts. Stabilization can be achieved either externally or internally.

External stabilization can be applied manually by a therapist or sometimes by the patient, with equipment, such as belts and straps, or by a firm support surface, such as the back of a chair or the surface of the treatment table.

Internal stabilization is achieved by an isometric contraction of an adjacent muscle group that does not enter into the movement pattern but holds the body segment of the proximal attachment of the muscle being strengthened firmly in place. For example, when performing a bilateral straight leg raise, the abdominals contract to stabilize the pelvis and lumbar spine as the hip flexors raise the legs. This form of stabilization is effective only if the fixating muscle group is strong enough or not fatigued.

Intensity

The **intensity** of exercise in a resistance training program is the amount of resistance (weight) imposed on the contracting muscle during each repetition of an exercise. The amount of resistance is also referred to as the **exercise load** (training load), that is, the extent to which the muscle is loaded, or how much weight is lifted, lowered, or held.

Remember, consistent with the overload principle, to improve muscle performance the muscle must be loaded to an extent greater than loads usually incurred. One way to progressively overload a muscle is to gradually increase the amount of resistance used in the exercise program.[14,95,155] The intensity of exercise and the degree to which the muscle is overloaded is also dependent on the volume, frequency and order of exercise, or the length of rest intervals.

Submaximal Versus Maximal Exercise Loads

Many factors, including the goals and expected functional outcomes of the exercise program, the cause of deficits in muscle performance, the extent of impairment, the stage of healing of injured tissues, the patient's age, general health and fitness level, as well as other factors determine whether the exercise will be carried out against submaximal or maximal muscle loading. In general, the level of resistance is lower in rehabilitative programs for persons with impairments versus conditioning programs for healthy individuals.

Submaximal loading (exercise at moderate to low intensities) is indicated:

- At the beginning of an exercise program to evaluate the patient's response to resistance exercise
- In the early stages of soft tissue healing when injured tissues must be protected
- After periods of immobilization when the articular cartilage is not able to withstand large compressive forces or when bone demineralization may have occurred, increasing the risk of pathologic fracture
- For most children or older adults
- When the goal of exercise is to improve muscle endurance
- To warm up and cool down prior to and after a session of exercise; or
- During slow-velocity isokinetic training to minimize compressive forces on joints

Near maximal or maximal loading (high-intensity exercise) is indicated:

- When the goal of exercise is to increase muscle strength and power and possibly increase muscle size
- For otherwise healthy adults in the *last phase* of a *rehabilitation* program after a musculoskeletal injury in preparation for returning to high-demand occupational or recreational activities
- In a conditioning program for individuals with no known pathology
- For individuals training for competitive weight lifting or body building

Precaution: The intensity of exercise should never be so great as to cause pain. As the intensity of exercise increases and a patient exerts a maximum or near-maximum effort, cardiovascular risks will substantially increase. A patient needs to be continually reminded to incorporate rhythmic breathing into each repetition of an exercise to minimize these risks.

Initial Level of Resistance (Load) and Documentation of Training Effects

It is always challenging to estimate how much resistance to apply manually or how much weight a patient should use during resistance exercises to improve muscle strength particularly at the beginning of a strengthening program. With manual resistance exercise the decision is entirely subjective, based on the therapist's judgment during exercise. In an exercise program using mechanical resistance the determination can be made quantitatively.

Repetition Maximum

One method of documenting the effectiveness of a resistance exercise program and calculating an appropriate exercise load is to determine a repetition maximum. This method was developed decades ago by DeLorme[59,60,61] who was investigating the use of heavy resistance in weight-training programs with healthy subjects. **A repetition maximum (RM)** is the greatest amount of weight (load) a muscle can move through the available ROM a specific number of times. A repetition maximum can be used in a number of ways. DeLorme reported determination of a 1 RM (the greatest amount of weight a subject could lift through the full ROM just one time) as a useful baseline measurement of a subject's maximum effort.[60,206] This measurement of strength is consistent with the definition of muscular strength discussed at the beginning of this chapter.[9] From the 1 RM measurement a beginning load for exercise can then be calculated. DeLorme, for example, used a 10 RM (the amount of weight that could be lifted and lowered just 10 times) as the training load in his studies.[60,61]

The use of a 1 RM to measure the dynamic strength of a muscle group or groups and to determine a baseline against which training-induced improvements in muscle strength can be documented is common and has been shown to be a safe and reliable measurement tool with healthy young adults and athletes.[95,155,176,261] Conversely, its use, which requires one maximum effort, is not appropriate for some patient populations. It certainly is not safe for patients, for example, with joint impairments, patients who are recovering from or who are at risk for soft tissue injury, or patients with known or who are at risk for osteoporosis or cardiovascular pathology. However, the 1 RM should not be categorically eliminated as a viable method of determining a baseline measurement of strength in all populations other than young athletes. In a number of studies that investigated the efficacy of resistance training as a component of a conditioning program in the elderly population, the 1 RM was, indeed, found to be safe and reliable.[186,193,248,256]

In addition to questions of safety, critics suggest that determination of a 1 RM for a particular muscle group involves a lot of trial and error and, therefore, may not be accurate if the patient fatigues before the 1 RM is identified. In addition, some patients may not understand or may be apprehensive about exerting one maximum effort. In the clinical setting a safe and more efficient approach to using a repetition maximum as a baseline measurement of strength or determining a training load is for a therapist to select a specific amount of resistance for the patient to lift, say for the knee flexors, and document how many repetitions the patient can complete before fatiguing. That measurement can then be used in two ways: the higher RM value can be used as the baseline or a 1 RM can be calculated from a conversion table. If the patient was able to lift the selected weight 10 times, then the baseline measurement for future comparisons is a 10 RM. If the therapist prefers to use a 1 RM as the baseline measurement, the number of repetitions and weight can be cross-referenced in a published conversion table to determine a calculated 1 RM. According to one such conversion table, a 10 RM is approximately 75% of a 1 RM.[16] Using this conversion method, if the patient lifted 40 pounds 10 times (the 10 RM), the calculated 1 RM would be 55 pounds.

Note: Validity and reliability of this conversion table was not specified.

Given these options, a therapist has several different practical and safe ways to use a repetition maximum (RM) as baseline and outcome measurement of strength and as a guideline (reference point) for selecting an initial training load in a strengthening program.

The Strength-Training Zone

After an RM is ascertained, the exercise load (amount of resistance) to be used at the initiation of resistance training is calculated as a *percentage* of the RM. This percentage can range from as low as 30 to 40% or as high as 90 to 100% to achieve training-induced adaptations. For healthy but untrained adults, the strength training zone usually falls between 70 to 80% of the RM.[176] The lower percentages of this range are safer at the beginning of a strength-training program. Low exercise loads are also recommended for children and the elderly.[8,286] For patients with significant deficits in muscle strength or to train for muscular endurance, using a lower load, possibly at the 30 to 50% level, is safe yet challenging.

Additional Methods of Determining Baseline Strength and a Beginning Exercise Load

Alternative to the use of a repetition maximum have also been suggested. They include:

- Cable tensiometry.[176]
- Isokinetic or handheld dynamometry.[50]
- Percentage of body weight;[206,216,217] the percentages are meant as guidelines and are based on 10 repetitions of each exercise at the beginning of the exercise program; percentages vary for different muscle groups.[216,217]
- Examples are:
  - Universal bench press: 30% body weight
  - Universal leg extension: 20% body weight
  - Universal leg curl: 10 to 15% body weight
  - Universal leg press: 50% body weight

Volume

In resistance training the **volume** of exercise is the summation of the total number of repetitions and sets of a particular exercise during a single exercise session.[155,157] The same combination of repetitions and sets does not and probably should not have to be used for all muscle groups.

There is an inverse relationship between the volume and intensity of resistance exercise. The higher the intensity (load), the lower the volume must be, and the converse is true. Therefore, the exercise load directly dictates how many repetitions and sets are possible. The volume of exercise is also influenced by the frequency of exercise sessions, the type of muscle contraction, the order of exercise, and rest intervals.

Repetitions and Sets

The number of *repetitions* in a dynamic exercise program refers to the number of times a specific movement is repeated. More specifically, it is the number of muscle contractions performed to move the limb through a series of continuous and complete excursions against a specific exercise load.

If the RM designation is used, the number of repetitions at a specific exercise load is reflected in the designation. For example, 10 repetitions at a particular exercise load is a 10 RM. If a 1 RM has been established as a baseline level of strength, the percentage of the 1 RM used as the exercise load determines the number of repetitions that a patient will be able to perform. The "average" untrained adult, when exercising with a load that is equivalent to 75% of the 1 RM, will be able to complete approximately 10 repetitions before needing to rest.[16,176] At 60% intensity about 15 repetitions are possible and at 90% intensity only 4 to 5 repetitions are usually possible.

For practical reasons, after a beginning exercise load is selected, the target number of repetitions performed for each exercise before a brief rest is often within a range rather than an exact number of repetitions. For example, a patient might be able to complete between 8 and 10 repetitions against a specified load before resting. This is sometimes referred to as a *RM zone;*[176] it gives the patient a goal, but builds in some flexibility.

The number of repetitions selected depends on whether the patient's status and goal of the exercise is to improve muscle strength or endurance. No optimal number for strength training or endurance training has been identified. Training effects (greater strength) have been reported with the use of a 2 to 3 RM to 15 RM.[16,157,176]

Sets are a predetermined number of repetitions grouped together; sets are also known as *bouts.* After each set of a specified number of repetitions there is a brief interval of rest. For example, in a single exercise session to strengthen a particular muscle group, a patient might be directed to lift a particular load 8 to 10 times, rest, and then lift the load 8 to 10 more times. That would be two sets of an 8 to 10 RM

As with repetitions, there is no optimal number of sets per exercise session. As few as one set and as many as six sets have yielded positive training effects. Single-set exercises at low intensities are most common in the very early phases of a resistance exercise program or in a maintenance program. Multiple-set exercises are used to progress the program and have been shown to be superior to single-set regimens in advanced training.[157]

Training to Improve Strength or Endurance: Impact of Exercise Load and Repetitions

Overall, since many variations of intensity and volume cause positive training-induced adaptations in muscle performance, there is a substantial amount of latitude for selecting an exercise load/repetition and set scheme for each exercise. The question is, is the goal to improve strength, muscular endurance, or both?

To Improve Muscle Strength

In DeLorme's early studies[59,60,61] three sets of a 10 RM performed for 10 repetitions over the training period led to gains in strength. Since these reports, gains in strength have been shown to occur using as little as a 1 RM to as much as a 15 RM. Current recommendations are to use an exercise load that cause fatigue after 6 to 12 repetitions for two to three sets (6–12 RM).[95,206,243] When fatigue no longer occurs after the target number of repetitions has been completed, the level of resistance is increased to once again overload the muscle.

To Improve Muscle Endurance

Training to improve local endurance involves performing many repetitions of an exercise against a submaximal load.[30,243] For example, as many as three to five sets of 40 to 50 or more repetitions against a light grade of elastic resistance might be used.

Endurance training can also be accomplished by maintaining a muscle contraction for incrementally longer periods of time. Endurance training, because it is performed against very low levels of resistance, can and should be initiated very early in a rehabilitation program without risk of injury to healing tissues. Remember, when injured muscles are immobilized, type I (slow twitch) fibers atrophy at a faster rate than type II (fast twitch) fibers.[211] This underscores the necessity for early initiation of endurance training. When increasing the number of repetitions or sets becomes inefficient, the load can be increased slightly.

Frequency

Frequency in a resistance exercise program refers to the number of exercise sessions per day or per week.[206,217] As with other aspects of dosage, frequency is dependent on other determinants, such as intensity and volume as well as the patient's goals, general health status, previous participation in a resistance exercise program, and response to training. The greater the intensity and volume of exercise, the more time needed between exercise sessions to recover from the temporarily fatiguing effects of exercise. A common cause of a decline in performance from overtraining (see discussion later in this chapter) is excessive frequency, inadequate rest, and progressive fatigue. Some forms of exercise should be performed less frequently than others because they require greater recovery time. For example, high-intensity eccentric exercise is associated with greater microtrauma to soft tissues and a higher incidence of delayed-onset muscle soreness than other modes of exercise.[13,100,192]

Although an optimal frequency per week has not been determined, a few generalizations can be made. Initially in an exercise program as long as the *volume and intensity are low,* short sessions of exercises sometimes can be performed on a daily basis several times per day. This frequency is often indicated for early postsurgical patients when the extent of exercise may be limited to low-intensity isometric exercises to prevent or minimize atrophy. As the intensity and volume of exercise increases, every other day or up to five exercise sessions per week is common.[8,154,268] Frequency is again reduced for a maintenance program, usually to two times per week. With prepubescent children and the very elderly, frequency is usually limited to two to three sessions per week.[8,286] Highly trained athletes involved in body building, power lifting, and weight lifting who know their own response to exercise often train at a high intensity and volume up to 6 days per week.[157]

Duration

Exercise **duration** is the total number of weeks or months during which a resistance exercise program is carried out. Depending on the cause of an impairment in muscle performance, some patients may require only a month or two of training to return to the desired level of function or activity. Other patients may need to continue the exercise program for a lifetime to maintain optimal function.

As noted earlier in this chapter, strength gains, observed early in a resistance training program (after 2 to 3 weeks) are the result of neural adaptations. For significant changes to occur in muscle, such as hypertrophy or increased vascularization, at least 6 to 12 weeks of resistance training is required.[1,8,176]

Rest Interval (Recovery Period)

Purpose of Rest Intervals

Rest is a critical element of a resistance training program and is necessary to allow time for the body to recuperate from the acute effects of exercise, associated with muscle fatigue or to offset adverse responses, such as exercise-induced, delayed-onset muscle soreness. Only with an appropriate balance of progressive loading and adequate rest intervals will muscle performance improve.

Integration of Rest into Exercise

Although not consistently addressed in the literature or by clinicians, a very brief rest occurs when a muscle relaxes between each repetition of reciprocal muscle contractions, which helps maintain blood supply to contracting muscles and wards off muscular spasm and fatigue.

Rest intervals for each exercising muscle group are dependent on the intensity and volume of exercise. For example, between sets of moderate intensity and volume exercise (at an 8- to 12-RM level), a 30- to 60-second rest period is common.[57] While the muscle group that was just exercised is resting, resistance exercises can be performed by another muscle group in the same extremity or the same muscle group in the opposite extremity. With higher intensity, near-maximal loading (at a 3- to 5-RM level), a longer rest period before performing another set of the same exercise is necessary. Patients with pathological conditions that make them more susceptible to fatigue, as well as children and the elderly, should rest from 1 to 2 minutes between sets by performing an unresisted exercise such as low-intensity cycling; or performing the same exercise with the opposite extremity. Remember, active recovery is more efficient than passive recovery for neutralizing the effects of muscle fatigue.[57]

Rest between exercise sessions must also be considered. When strength training is initiated at moderate intensities usually in the intermediate phase of a rehabilitation program after soft tissue injury, a 48-hour rest interval between resistance exercise sessions allows the patient adequate time for recovery.

Decreasing the rest period between bouts of exercise during the same exercise session or "taking off" less time between exercise sessions are both possible strategies to increase the dosage of the resistance training program. This application of the overload principle is sometimes used by healthy individuals who have been participating in a high-intensity conditioning program for some period of time. However, even the elite athlete must be cautious that decreasing rest intervals does not lead to progressive fatigue, overtraining, staleness, and a deterioration in performance.[154,160] This approach is not recommended for children or older adults or for patients with strength and endurance deficits caused by or associated with acute or chronic disease. Even for an otherwise healthy, young adult recovering from a musculoskeletal injury, shortening the rest interval, while increasing the intensity or volume of exercise, does not give healing tissues adequate time to recuperate and can lead to chronic inflammation (see Chapter 8).

Mode

The **mode** of exercise in a resistance exercise program refers to the form or type of exercise or the manner in which the exercise is carried out. Mode of exercise also encompasses the form of resistance, that is, how the exercise load is applied. For example, a patient may perform an exercise dynamically or statically or in a weight-bearing or nonweight-bearing position. The resistance could be applied manually or mechanically.

As with other determinants of resistance training, the modes of exercise selected are based upon a multitude of factors already highlighted throughout this section.

A brief overview of the various modes of exercise is presented in this section. An in-depth explanation and analysis of each of these types of exercise can be found in the next section of this chapter and in Chapter 4.

Forms of Resistance

- *Manual* resistance and *mechanical* resistance are the two broad methods by which resistance can be applied.
- A *constant* or *variable* load can also be imposed by use of mechanical resistance, for example free weights or weight machines.
- *Accommodating* resistance[128] can be implemented by use of an isokinetic dynamometer that controls the velocity of active movement during exercise.
- *Body weight* or partial body weight is always a source of resistance if the exercise occurs in an antigravity position; as defined in Chapter 2, exercise against gravity with no additional source of external resistance is considered active, not active-resistive, exercise.

Type of Muscle Contraction

Figure 3–1 schematically depicts the types of muscle contractions that may be performed in a resistance

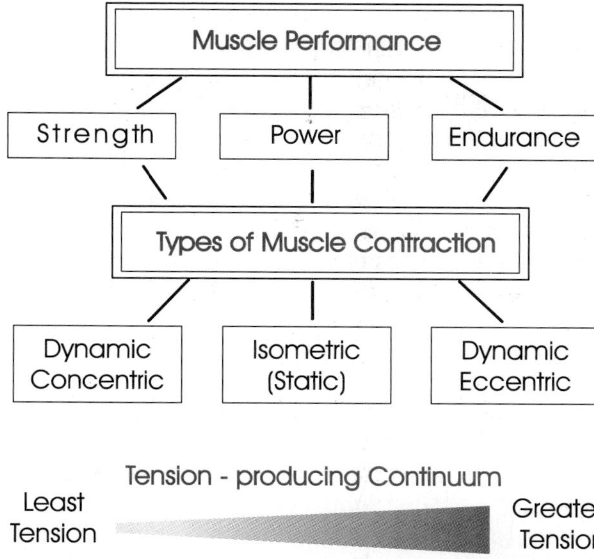

Figure 3–1 Types of muscle contractions: their relationships to muscle performance and their tension-generating capacities.

training program and their relationships to each other and to muscle performance.[169,229]

- Use of *isometric* (static) or *dynamic* muscle contractions are the two basic options for mode exercise.
- Dynamic resistance exercises can be performed using *concentric* (shortening), *eccentric* (lengthening) contractions, or both.
- When the speed of limb movement is held consistent by a rate-controlling device, the term *isokinetic* contraction is sometimes used.[229] An alternative perspective is that this is simply a dynamic (shortening or lengthening) contraction that occurs under controlled conditions.[169]

Position During Exercise: Weight-Bearing or Nonweight-Bearing

The patient's body position or the position of a limb in nonweight-bearing or weight-bearing positions also alters the mode of resistance exercise. When a nonweight-bearing position is assumed and the distal segment (foot or hand) moves freely during exercise, the term *open-chain* exercise is often used.[169,229] When a weight-bearing position is assumed and the body moves over a fixed distal segment, the term *closed-chain* exercise is commonly used.[169,229]

Energy Systems

Modes of exercise can also be classified by the energy systems used during the exercise. *Anaerobic* exercise involves high-intensity (near-maximal) exercise carried out for a very few number of repetitions because of rapid muscular fatigue. Strengthening exercises fall into this category. *Aerobic* exercise is associated with low-intensity, repetitive exercise of large muscle groups, performed over an extended period of time. This mode of exercise primarily increases muscular and cardiorespiratory endurance (refer to Chapter 4 for in-depth explanation).

Range of Movement: Short-Arc or Full-Arc Exercise

Resistance through the full, available range of movement *(full-arc exercise)* is necessary to develop strength through the ROM. Sometimes resistance exercises are executed through only a portion of the available range. This is known as *short-arc exercise.* This form of exercise is used to avoid a painful arc of motion or a portion of the range where the joint is unstable or to protect healing tissues after injury or surgery.

Mode of Exercise and Application to Function

Mode-specific training is essential if a resistance training program is to have a positive effect on function. When tissue healing allows, the type of muscle contractions performed or the position in which an exercise is performed must mimic the desired functional activity.[187]

Speed of Exercise

The speed at which a muscle contracts significantly affects the tension that the muscle produces and subsequently affects muscular strength and power.[169,176,197,229] The speed of exercise is frequently manipulated in a resistance training program to prepare the patient for a variety of functional activities that are performed across a range of slow to fast speeds.

Force-Velocity Relationship

The velocity at which an exercise is performed significantly affects the tension generated by the muscle. The force-velocity relationship is different during concentric and eccentric muscle contractions (Fig. 3–2).

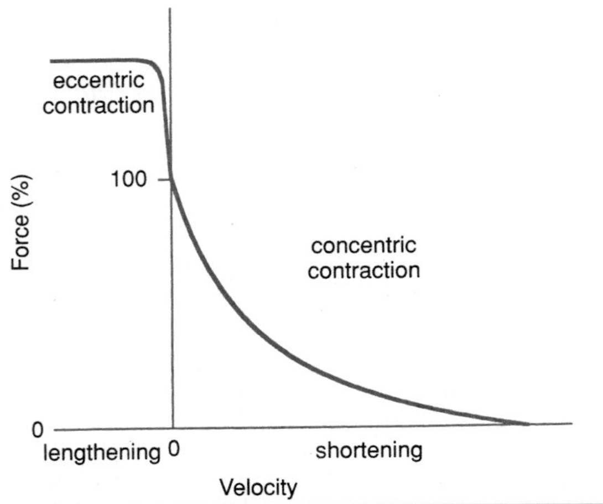

Figure 3–2 Force-velocity curve for concentric and eccentric exercise. (From Levangie, PK, and Norkin, CC: Joint Structure and Function—A Comprehensive Analysis, ed. 3. FA Davis, Philadelphia, 2001, p 97, with permission.)

Concentric Muscle Contraction

As the velocity of muscle *shortening* increases, the force that the muscle can generate *decreases.* Electromyogram (EMG) activity and torque decrease as a muscle shortens at faster contractile velocities, because the muscle may not have sufficient time to develop peak tension.[45,169,229,277]

Eccentric Muscle Contraction

Although findings are less consistent for eccentric than concentric muscle activity, during an eccentric contraction as the velocity of active muscle *lengthening* increases, initially force production in the muscle also *increases* but then *quickly levels off.*[32,58,169,229] The initial increase in force production may be a protective response of the muscle when it is first overloaded. It is thought that this may be important for shock absorption or rapid deceleration of a limb during quick changes of direction.[74,229] The rise in tension may also be caused by a stretch of the noncontractile tissue within muscle.[58] Other research indicates that eccentric force production is essentially unaffected by velocity and remains constant at slow and fast velocities.[45,113]

Application to Resistance Training

A range of slow to fast exercise velocities has a place in an exercise program. Resistance training with free weights is only safe and effective at slow to medium speeds of limb movement so that the patient can maintain control of the moving weight. Because many functional activities involve reasonably fast velocities of limb movement, training at only slow velocities is inadequate. The development of the isokinetic dynamometer in the late 1960s[128,182] gave clinicians a tool to implement resistance training at fast as well as slow velocities. In recent years, some variable resistance exercise units (pneumatic and hydraulic) as well as elastic resistance products also have afforded additional options for safely training at fast velocities.

Speed-specific training is fundamental to a successful rehabilitation program. Results of numerous studies since the 1970s have shown that training-induced strength gains in a resistance exercise program primarily occur at the training speeds,[22,61,76,139,183] with very limited transfer of training (physiological overflow) to other speeds of movement.[133,253] Accordingly, training speeds for resistance exercises should be geared to match or approach the demands of the desired functional activities.[50,139]

Isokinetic training, using **velocity spectrum rehabilitation** regimens and **plyometric training,** also known as **stretch-shortening drills,** often emphasize high speed training. These approaches to resistance exercise are discussed later in this chapter.

Periodization

Periodization, also known as **periodized training,** is an approach to resistance training that builds *systematic variation* in exercise intensity and volume at regular intervals over a specified period of time.[94,240] This approach to training was developed for highly trained athletes preparing for competitive weightlifting or power-lifting events.[240] The concept was designed to prevent overtraining and psychologic staleness prior to competition and maximize performance during competition.

The training calendar is broken down into cycles or phases that sometimes extend over an entire year. The idea is to prepare for a "peak" performance at the time of competition. Different types of exercises at varying intensities, volume, frequency, and rest intervals are done over a specific time period. Table 3–3 summarizes the characteristics of each cycle.

Although periodized training is commonly implemented prior to a competitive event, evidence to support the efficacy of periodization is very limited.[94,157,176] Its use has not been applied or investigated with patients in the clinical setting.

Table 3–3 Characteristics of Periodized Training

Period of Training	Intensity of Exercise	Volume and Frequency of Exercise
Preparation	Lower loads	High number of reps and sets More exercises per session More frequent exercise sessions per day and per week
Competition	Higher loads (peaking just prior to competition)	Decreased reps and sets Fewer exercises per session Less frequent exercise sessions per day and per week
Recuperation	Gradual decrease in exercise loads	Additional decrease in reps, sets, number of exercises and frequency

Integration of Function into a Resistance Exercise Program

A Balance of Stability and Active Mobility

Control of the body during functional movement and the ability to perform functional tasks require a balance of active movement superimposed over a stable background of neuromuscular control. Sufficient performance of agonist and antagonist muscles about a joint contributes to the dynamic stability of individual joints. For example, a person must be able to hold the trunk erect and stabilize the spine while lifting a heavy object. Stability is also necessary to control quick changes of direction during functional movements. Hence, a resistance exercise program must address static as well as dynamic strength of the trunk and extremities.

A Balance of Strength, Power, and Endurance

Functional tasks related to daily living, occupational, or recreational activities require various combinations of muscle strength, power, and endurance. Various motor tasks require slow and controlled movements, rapid movements, repeated movements, or long-term positioning. Analysis of the tasks a patient would like to be able to do provides the framework for a task-specific resistance exercise program.

Progression of Movement Patterns During Resistance Exercise

There is a place in a resistance exercise program for strengthening isolated muscle groups as well as strengthening muscles in combined patterns. Applying resistance during exercise in anatomic planes, diagonal patterns and combined, task-oriented movement patterns all should be integral components of a carefully progressed resistance exercise program. Use of simulated functional movements under controlled, supervised conditions is a means to return a patient safely to independent functional activities. Pushing, pulling, lifting, and holding activities, for example, can first be done against a low level of resistance for a limited number of repetitions. Over time, a patient can gradually return to use of the same movements during functional activities in an unsupervised work or home setting. The key to successful self-management is to teach a patient how to judge the speed, level, and duration of tension generation in muscle as well as appropriate timing that is necessary to safely perform a motor task.

▶ Types of Resistance Exercise

The types of exercise selected for a resistance training program are contingent upon many factors including the cause and extent of primary and secondary impairments, particularly deficits in muscle performance, the stage of tissue healing, the condition of joints and their tolerance to compression and movement, the general abilities (physical and cognitive) of the patient, the availability of equipment and, of course, the patient's goals and the intended functional outcomes of the program. The therapist has an array of forms of exercises from which to choose to design a resistance exercise program to meet the individual needs of each patient. There is no one best form or type of resistance training. Prior to selecting specific types of resistance exercises for a patient's rehabilitation program, the therapist may want to consider the questions listed in Box 3–5.

Application of the SAID principle and the concept of specificity of training are two of the foundations upon which these decisions are made. In addition to

Box 3–5 Considerations for Selection of Modes of Resistance Exercise

- Based on the results of your examination and evaluation, what is the type and extent of the deficits in muscle performance?
- Based on the underlying pathology causing the deficits in muscle performance, would one form of resistance training be more appropriate or effective than another?
- What are the goals and anticipated functional outcomes of the resistance training program? Which types of resistance exercise are more compatible with those goals?
- Are there any limitations on how the patient is permitted or able to be positioned during exercise?
  - Is weight bearing contraindicated, restricted, or fully permissible?
  - Is there hypomobility of affected or adjacent joints (due to pain or contracture) that could affect how the patient is positioned during resistance exercise?
  - Is there a portion of the ROM in which the patient cannot safely or comfortably perform resistance exercises due to hypermobility?
  - Are there cardiorespiratory impairments that could affect positioning during exercise?
- Will the patient be expected to perform the exercises independently using mechanical resistance or would manual resistance applied by the therapist be more appropriate at this point in the rehabilitation program?
- What types of equipment will be available or needed for exercises?

selecting the most appropriate types of exercise, the therapist must also make decisions about the intensity, volume, order, frequency, rest interval, and other factors discussed in the previous section to effectively progress selected resistance exercises. Table 3–4 summarizes general guidelines for progression of exercise.

Variations of exercise presented in this section are: static (isometric) and dynamic, concentric and eccentric, isokinetic, and open- and closed-chain exercise as well as manual and mechanical and constant and variable resistance exercises. The benefits, limitations, and applications of each of these forms of resistance exercise are analyzed and discussed. When available, supporting evidence from the scientific literature is also summarized. Specific regimens or systems of resistance training such as progressive resistive exercise (PRE), circuit weight training, velocity spectrum rehabilitation, and plyometric training are addressed later in this chapter.

Manual and Mechanical Resistance Exercise

From a very broad perspective a load can be applied to a contracting muscle in two ways: manually or mechanically. The benefits and limitations of these two forms of resistance training are summarized in Boxes 3–9 and 3–11 later in this chapter.

Manual Resistance Exercise

Manual resistance exercise is a type of active exercise in which resistance is provided by a therapist or other health professional, or a patient can be taught how to apply self-resistance to selected muscle groups. Although the amount of resistance cannot be measured quantitatively, this technique is useful in the early stages of an exercise program when the muscle to be strengthened is weak and can overcome only minimal to moderate resistance. It is also useful when the range of joint movements needs to be carefully controlled. The amount of resistance given is limited only by the strength of the therapist. Techniques for application of manual resistance exercises in anatomic planes and diagonal patterns are presented in later sections of this chapter.

Mechanical Resistance Exercise

Mechanical resistance exercise is a form of active exercise in which resistance is applied through the use of equipment or mechanical apparatus. The amount of resistance can be measured quantitatively and progressed over time. It is often used in specific resistance exercise regimens. It is also useful when amounts of resistance greater than the therapist can apply manually are necessary. Systems and regimens of resistance training that use mechanical resistance and advantages and disadvantages of different types of mechanical resistance equipment are addressed later in this chapter.

Isometric Exercise (Static Exercise)

Isometric exercise is a static form of exercise in which a muscle contracts and produces force without an appreciable change in the length of the muscle and without visible joint motion.[129,169,229,233] Although there is no mechanical work done (force × distance), a measurable amount of tension and force output are produced by the muscle.[169,229] Sources of resistance for isometric exercise include holding against a force applied manually, holding a weight in a particular position, maintaining a position against the resistance of body weight, or pushing or pulling an immovable object.

In the 1950s and 1960s, isometric resistance training became popular as an alternative to dynamic re-

Table 3–4 Progression of a Resistance Training Program: Factors for Consideration

Factors	Progression
Intensity (exercise load)	Submaximal → maximal (or near-maximal) intensity Low load → high load
Body position (nonweight- or weight-bearing)	Variable: depending on pathology and impairments, weight-bearing restrictions (pain, swelling, instability) and goals of the rehabilitation program
Repetitions and sets	Low volume → high volume
Frequency	Variable: depends on intensity and volume of exercise
Type of muscle contraction	Static → dynamic Concentric and eccentric: variable progression
Range of motion	Short arc → full arc Stable portion of range → unstable portion of range
Plane of movement	Uniplanar → multiplanar
Speed of movement	Slow → fast velocities
Neuromuscular control	Proximal → distal control
Functional movement patterns	Simple → complex Single joint → multijoint Proximal control → distal control

sistance exercise and initially was considered a more effective and efficient method of muscle strengthening.[122,170] In the early research it was reported that isometric strength gains of 5% per week occurred when healthy subjects performed a single, near-maximal isometric contraction everyday over a 6-week period of time.[122] Although replications of this study refuted some of the original findings, particularly the very rapid rate of strength gain, additional studies in the 1960s showed that *repetitive* isometric contractions (a set of 20 per day) held for 6 seconds each against near-maximal resistance consistently improved isometric strength.[170] A cross-exercise effect (a limited increase in strength of the contralateral, unexercised muscle group), as the result of transfer of training, has also been observed with maximum isometric training.[63] Each of these early investigations documented that isometric training was a viable means of improving muscle strength.

Rationale for Use of Isometric Exercise

The need for static strength and endurance is apparent in almost all aspects of control of the body during functional activities. Functional control involves the ability to hold a position against either a high level of resistance for a short period of time or a low-intensity load over a prolonged period of time. Of these two aspects of muscle performance, it has been suggested that muscular endurance plays a more important role than muscle strength in maintaining sufficient postural stability and in preventing injury during daily living tasks.[179] For example, the postural muscles of the trunk and lower extremities must contract isometrically to hold the body erect against gravity and provide a background of stability for balance and functional movements in an upright position.[198,247] Dynamic stability of joints is achieved by activating and maintaining a low level of co-contraction, that is, the isometric contraction of antagonist muscles that surround joints. The importance of isometric strength and endurance, for example, in the elbow, wrist and finger musculature is apparent when a person holds and carries a heavy object for an extended period of time. With these examples in mind, there can be no doubt that isometric exercises are an important part of a rehabilitation program designed to improve functional abilities. The rationale and indications for isometric exercise in rehabilitation are summarized in Box 3–6.

Types of Isometric Exercise

Several forms of isometric exercise with varying degrees of resistance and intensity of muscle contractions are used during successive phases of rehabilitation to serve different purposes. All but one type (muscle setting) incorporate some form of

Box 3–6 Isometric Exercise: Rationale and Indications

- To prevent or minimize muscle atrophy when joint movement is not possible due to external immobilization (casts, splints, skeletal traction)
- To activate muscles (facilitate muscle firing) to begin to re-establish neuromuscular control but protect healing tissues when joint movement is not advisable after soft tissue injury or surgery
- To develop postural or joint stability
- To improve muscle strength when use of dynamic resistance exercise could compromise joint integrity or cause joint pain
- To develop static muscle strength at particular points in the ROM consistent with specific task-related needs

significant resistance and, therefore, are used to improve static strength or sustained muscular control (endurance). Since no appreciable resistance is applied, muscle setting technically is not a form of resistance exercise but is included in this discussion to show the variations of isometric exercise that can be used for multifaceted purposes in a rehabilitation program.

Muscle-setting exercises are low-intensity isometric exercises performed against little to no resistance. They are used to promote muscle relaxation and circulation and to decrease muscle pain and spasm after injury to soft tissues during the *acute* stage of healing. Muscle setting also maintains mobility between muscle fibers as they heal. Two common examples of muscle setting are to the quadriceps and gluteal muscles. Because muscle setting is not performed against any appreciable resistance, it will not improve muscle strength except in very weak muscles, but setting exercises can retard muscle atrophy in the very early stages of rehabilitation of a muscle or joint when immobilization is necessary to protect healing structures.

Stabilization exercises are used to develop a submaximal but sustained level of co-contraction[79] to reduce instability and enhance joint or postural stability by means of midrange isometric contractions against resistance in antigravity positions and in weight-bearing postures if weight bearing is permissible. Body weight or manual resistance often are the sources of resistance. Variations of stabilization exercises include **rhythmic stabilization** and **alternating isometrics,** two techniques associated with proprioceptive neuromuscular facilitation (PNF)[247,260] described later in this chapter, and **dynamic stabilization** exercises[37] described in Chapter 16.

Multiple-angle isometrics is a system of isometric exercise where resistance is applied, manually or mechanically, at multiple joint positions within the available ROM.[50] This approach is used when the goal of exercise is to improve strength throughout the ROM when joint motion is permissible but dynamic resistance exercise is painful or inadvisable.

Special Considerations for Isometric Training

Effective use of isometric exercise in a resistance training program is contingent upon the following considerations.

Intensity of Muscle Contraction

The amount of tension that can be generated during an isometric muscle contraction, in part, depends upon joint position and as such the length of the muscle at the time of contraction.[129,267] It is sufficient to use an exercise load (resistance) of 60 to 80% of a muscle's force-developing capacity to gain strength.[149,267] Therefore, the amount of resistance against which the muscle is able to hold varies and needs to be adjusted at different points in the range. Resistance must be progressively increased to continue to overload the muscle as it becomes stronger.

Duration of Muscle Activation

To achieve adaptive changes in static muscle performance, an isometric contraction should be held for 6 to 10 seconds. This allows time for peak tension to develop and for metabolic changes to occur in the muscle.[50,179] A 10-second contraction allows a 2-second rise time, a 6-second hold time, and a 2-second fall time.

Repetitive Contractions

Use of repetitive contractions, held for 6 to 10 seconds each, decreases muscle cramping and increases the effectiveness of the isometric regimen.[50,170,176]

Joint Angle and Mode Specificity

Gains in muscle strength only occur at or closely adjacent to the training angle.[148,149,267] Physiologic overflow is minimal, occurring no more than 10 degrees in either direction in the ROM from the training angle.[149] Therefore, resistance at four to six points in the range of motion is usually recommended. Isometric resistance training is also mode-specific. It increases static strength but has little to no impact on dynamic strength (concentric or eccentric).[159]

Limitations of Isometrics

Strength improvements occur only at or closely adjacent to the training angle, with little to no carryover to dynamic exercise. Resisted isometric exercise is not as effective for developing muscle endurance as resisted dynamic exercise.

Precautions: To avoid potential injury to the contracting muscle, apply and release the resistance gradually. This helps to grade the muscle tension and ensures that the muscle contraction is pain-free. It also minimizes the risk of uncontrolled joint movement.

Individuals have a tendency to hold their breath during isometric exercise, particularly when performed against substantial resistance. This is likely to cause a pressor response as the result of the Valsalva maneuver, causing a rapid increase in blood pressure.[88] Rhythmic breathing, emphasizing exhalation during the contraction, should always be performed during isometric exercise to minimize this response. High-intensity isometric exercises may be contraindicated for patients with a history of cardiac or vascular disorders.

Dynamic Exercise: Concentric and Eccentric

A dynamic muscle contraction causes joint movement and excursion of a body segment as the muscle contracts and shortens (concentric contraction) or lengthens under tension (eccentric contraction).

Note: Although the term *isotonic* (meaning equal tension) has been used for many years to describe a dynamic muscle contraction against resistance that causes joint movement, application of this terminology is incorrect. In fact, when a body segment moves through a range of motion, the tension that the muscle is capable of generating varies through the range as the muscle shortens or lengthens due to the changing length-tension relationship of the muscle and the changing torque of the load; thus, force-output does not remain constant.[169,229] Therefore, "isotonic" is not used in this textbook to describe dynamic resistance exercise.

Concentric muscle contractions accelerate body segments, whereas eccentric contractions decelerate body segments, such as during sudden changes of direction or momentum. Eccentric contractions act as a source of shock absorption during high-impact activities.[58,233] A combination of concentric and eccentric muscle action is evident in countless tasks of daily life, such as ascending and descending stairs, rising from a chair and sitting back down, or picking up or setting down an object. Consequently, concentric and eccentric exercises are fundamental components of a resistance training program designed to increase muscle strength, power, or endurance for necessary functional abilities.

Concentric exercise in resistance training refers to a form of dynamic muscle loading where tension in a muscle develops, physical shortening of the muscle occurs and an external force (resistance) is overcome as in lifting a weight. Conversely, **eccentric exercise** involves dynamic loading of a muscle beyond its force-producing capacity causing physical lengthening of the muscle as it attempts to control the load. Eccentric exercise is a form of negative work,[58] as in lowering a weight (Fig. 3–3).

During concentric and eccentric exercise resistance can be applied in several ways: (1) constant resistance, such as body weight, a free weight, or a simple weight-pulley system; (2) a weight machine that provides variable resistance; or (3) an isokinetic device that controls the velocity of limb movement.

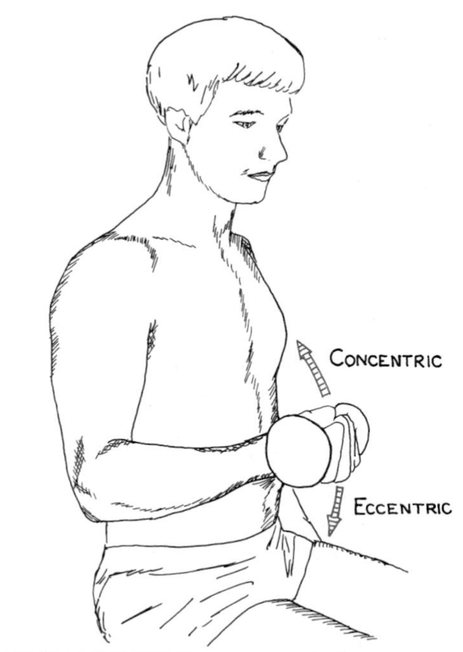

Figure 3–3 Concentric and eccentric strengthening of the elbow flexors occurs as the patient lifts and lowers the weight.

The qualities and use of each of these forms of mechanical resistance during dynamic exercise follows a comparison of concentric and eccentric exercise.

Characteristics of Concentric and Eccentric Contractions During Exercise

A maximum concentric contraction produces less force than a maximum eccentric contraction under the same conditions (see Fig. 3–1). In other words, greater loads can be lowered than lifted. This difference in the magnitude of loads that can be controlled by concentric and eccentric muscle contractions may be associated with the contributions of the contractile *and* noncontractile components of muscle. When a load is lowered, the forces exerted by the load are controlled, not only by the active, contractile components of muscle, but also by the noncontractile components of the muscle. When a weight is lifted, only the contractile components of the muscle lift the load.[58]

With a concentric contraction, greater numbers of motor units must be recruited to control the same load as compared to an eccentric contraction, suggesting that concentric exercise has less mechanical efficiency than eccentric exercise.[58,74,76] Consequently, it requires more effort by a patient to control the same load during concentric exercise as opposed to eccentric exercise. As a result, maximum resistance during the concentric phase of an exercise will not provide a maximum load during the eccentric phase. Although not practical, for maximum resistance during the eccentric phase, an additional load must be applied. In addition, concentric muscle contractions consume more oxygen and require greater use of energy stores than eccentric muscle contractions against the same loads.[36,58,74]

The velocity at which concentric or eccentric exercises are performed directly affects the force-generating capacity of the neuromuscular unit.[45,74,197] At slow velocities with a maximum load an eccentric contraction generates greater tension than a concentric contraction. At slow speeds, therefore, a greater load (weight) can be lowered (with control) than lifted. As the velocity of exercise increases, concentric contraction tension rapidly and consistently decreases whereas eccentric contraction forces increase slightly but then rapidly reach a plateau under maximum load conditions (see Fig. 3–2).

A common error made by some weight-lifters during high-intensity resistance training is to assume that if a weight is lifted quickly (concentric contraction) and lowered slowly (eccentric contraction), the slow eccentric contraction will generate greater tension. In fact, if the load is constant, less tension is generated during the eccentric phase. The only way that greater tension can be developed is to increase the applied load during the eccentric phase of each exercise cycle. This usually requires assistance from an exercise partner to help lift the load during each concentric contraction. This is a very intense form of exercise and should only be used by healthy individuals training for high-demand sports or weight-lifting competition. This technique is not appropriate for individuals recovering from musculoskeletal injuries.

Repeated and rapidly progressed eccentric muscle contractions against heavy resistance are associated with a significantly higher incidence and severity of delayed-onset muscle soreness (DOMS) than resisted concentric exercise. Why DOMS occurs more readily with eccentric exercise is speculative, possibly the result of greater damage to muscle and connective tissue when heavy loads are controlled and lowered.[58,84,176] It should be noted that there is some evidence to suggest that if the intensity and volume of concentric and eccentric exercise are equal, there is no significant difference in the degree of DOMS after exercise.[92]

Rationale for Use of Concentric and Eccentric Exercise

Most resistance training programs involve a combination of eccentric and concentric exercises at various speeds and with the patient or body segment in a variety of positions. Both concentric and eccentric exercises have distinct value. Their use depends on the strength capacity of muscles and the functional needs of the patient. Opinions and results of studies vary on whether or not the effects of training with concentric and eccentric contractions in the exercised muscle group are mode-specific. Although there is substantial evidence to support specificity of training,[10,22,96,187,255] there is also some evidence to suggest that training in one mode leads to strength gains, although less significant, in the other mode.[81,221] Because transfer of training is quite limited, selection of exercises that simulate the functional movements needed by a patient is a prudent choice. In addition, because many functional activities require both concentric and eccentric strength, power, or muscle endurance, incorporating concentric and eccentric training in the rehabilitation progression is advisable.

Concentric[265] and eccentric[266] training has been shown to cause a *cross-training effect,* that is, a slight increase in strength in the same muscle group of the opposite, unexercised extremity. This effect, sometimes referred to as **cross-exercise,** also occurs with high-intensity exercise that involves a combination of concentric and eccentric contractions (lifting and lowering a weight). This effect in the unexercised muscle group may be caused by repeated contractions of the unexercised extremity in an attempt to stabilize the body during high-effort exercise. Although cross-training is an interesting phenomenon, there is no evidence to suggest that a cross-training effect has a positive impact on a patient's functional capabilities.

Given that eccentric exercise requires recruitment of fewer motor units to control a load than concentric exercise, when a muscle is very weak (less than a Fair [3/5] muscle grade), active eccentric muscle contractions against no external resistance (other than gravity) may be easier for a patient to perform than concentric contractions in the early phase of a rehabilitation program. In other words, it may be easier to control lowering a limb against gravity than lifting the limb. This would technically be considered a form of active ROM, not active-resistive ROM, but still bears mention in this discussion.

Eccentric training is also thought to be an essential component of an exercise program for prevention of injury or reinjury during activities that involve high-intensity deceleration and quick changes of direction.[236] As previously mentioned, eccentric contractions act as muscular shock absorbers.[74] In the last stage of rehabilitation, the progressive use of eccentric exercise is indicated at high speeds against large amounts of resistance. Because the greatest amount of muscle tension can be generated with an eccentric contraction, the greatest loads can be controlled and absorbed during eccentric exercise. As a patient begins to return to functional activities, high-speed eccentric exercise against resistance in the form of eccentric isokinetic training and plyometric training (stretch-shortening drills) prepares a patient for high-intensity sports or work-related activities that require eccentric muscle control for deceleration or quick changes of direction during movement.

Although greater loads can be used with eccentric exercise than concentric exercise, the relative adaptive gains in eccentric and concentric strength appear to be similar at the conclusion of an concentric or eccentric resistance training program.[58,76,100] The higher incidence of DOMS with high-intensity eccentric exercise may influence the outcome of these two modes of training.

Because eccentric exercise consumes less oxygen and energy stores than concentric exercise against similar loads, the use of eccentric activities such as downhill running may improve muscular endurance more efficiently than similar concentric activities because muscle fatigue occurs less quickly with eccentric exercise.[58,176]

Precautions: During eccentric exercise there is greater stress on the cardiovascular system (i.e., increased heart rate and arterial blood pressure) than with concentric exercise,[58] possibly because greater loads can be used during eccentric training. This underscores the need for rhythmic breathing during high-intensity exercise.

Because there is a higher incidence of exercise-induced, delayed-onset muscle soreness (DOMS) with high-intensity, rapidly progressed eccentric more so than concentric exercise,[8,13,98,100,192] it is advisable to progress the intensity of eccentric exercise slowly and decrease the frequency of exercise sessions per week to allow additional time for soft tissue recovery.

Dynamic Exercise: Constant Versus Variable Resistance

Dynamic Constant External Resistance (DCER) Exercise

This is a form of resistance training where a limb moves through a ROM against a *constant external load,* provided by free weights, such as a handheld or cuff weight, torque arm units (Fig. 3–4), weight machines, or pulley systems.[176] This terminology (DCER exercise) is used in lieu of the term "isotonic exercise" because, although the imposed load (weight) does not change, the torque imposed by the weight and the tension generated by the muscle do change throughout the range of movement.[169,229] If the load is less than the torque generated by the muscle, the muscle contracts concentrically and accelerates the load; if the load exceeds the muscle's torque production, the muscle contracts eccentrically to decelerate the load.

DCER exercise has an inherent limitation. When lifting or lowering a constant load, the contracting muscle is only challenged maximally at one point in

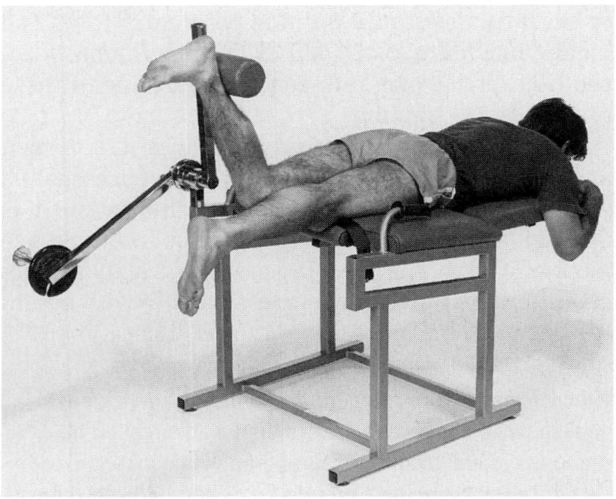

Figure 3–4 N-K Exercise Unit with torque arm and interchangeable weights provides constant external resistance. (Courtesy of N-K Products Company, Inc., Soquel, CA)

the ROM where the maximum torque of the resistance matches the maximum torque output of the muscle. The therapist must be aware of the changing torque of the exercise and the changing length-tension relationship of the muscle and modify body position and resistance to match where in the range the maximum load needs to be applied. Despite this limitation constant external resistance has been and continues to be an effective form of muscle loading for training-induced improvements in muscle performance and a mainstay of resistance exercise programs.

Variable Resistance Exercise

This form of dynamic exercise addresses the primary limitation of dynamic exercise against a constant external load. Specially designed resistance equipment imposes varying levels of resistance to the contracting muscles to load the muscle more effectively at multiple points in the ROM. The resistance is altered throughout the range by means of a weight-cable system that moves over an irregularly shaped cam, a lever arm system, or hydraulic or pneumatic mechanisms.[165,230] Dynamic exercise with elastic resistance products (bands and tubing) can also be classified as variable resistance exercise because of the inherent properties of the material and its response to stretch.[135,142,224]

Dynamic exercise performed against manual resistance also varies the load applied to the contracting muscle through the ROM. When manual resistance is selected, the therapist adjusts the resistance based on the patient's response so that the muscle is loaded maximally at all portions of the range.

Special Considerations for DCER and Variable Resistance Training

During either of these forms of resistance training, the velocity and excursion of limb movement is controlled exclusively by the patient (with the exception of manual resistance exercise and performing exercises on units that have range-limiting devices). Exercises must also be performed at a relatively *slow velocity* to avoid momentum and uncontrolled movements that could jeopardize the safety of the patient.

Note: Hydraulic and pneumatic variable resistance equipment and elastic resistance products do allow safe, high-velocity resistance training. Since most daily living and occupational activities occur at moderate to fast velocities, the training-induced improvements in strength and muscular endurance that occur only at slow velocities may not prepare the patient for activities that require rapid bursts of strength or quick changes of direction. The most common system of resistance training used with DCER and variable resistance exercises is *progressive resistance exercise* (PRE). A later section of this chapter, which covers systems of training using mechanical resistance, addresses PRE.

Isokinetic Exercise

Isokinetic exercise is a form of dynamic exercise in which the velocity of muscle shortening or lengthening and the angular limb velocity is predetermined and held constant by a rate-limiting device (an isokinetic dynamometer).[50,79,128,182] The term *isokinetic* refers to movement that occurs at an equal (constant) speed. Unlike other forms of dynamic resistance exercise, specifically DCER exercise or variable resistance exercise with weight machines, where a specific weight (amount of resistance) is selected and superimposed on the contracting muscle, in isokinetic resistance training the *speed* of limb movement, not the load, is manipulated. The force encountered by the muscle depends on the extent of force applied to the equipment.[128,169] When isokinetic dynamometers were first developed in the 1960s, the units were passive (the unit only provided resistance if the patient moved the arm of the dynamometer), and only concentric, reciprocal exercise was possible. Contemporary isokinetic dynamometers are now active, computerized units that allow concentric and eccentric testing and training as well as other modes of exercise including multiple-angle isometric training and passive ROM (see Fig. 3–49).

Isokinetic exercise is also called **accommodating resistance exercise.**[128] Theoretically, if an individual is putting forth a maximum effort during each repetition of exercise, the contracting muscle produces variable but *maximum* force output, consistent with the muscle's variable tension-generating capabilities at all portions of the range of movement, not at only one small portion of the range as occurs with DCER training. This is why early advocates of isokinetic training[128,182] held the opinion, although not well supported by evidence, that isokinetic training strengthened muscles more efficiently than training against constant loads or even variable resistance machines. Today, isokinetic training is simply regarded as one of many effective forms of resistance training that can be integrated into the later stages rehabilitation to improve muscle performance.[5,50,52,79]

Characteristics of Isokinetic Training

Constant Velocity

Fundamental to the concept of isokinetic exercise is that the velocity of muscle shortening or lengthening is preset and controlled by the unit and remains constant through the ROM.

Range of Training Velocities

Isokinetic training affords a wide range of exercise velocities in rehabilitation from very slow speeds to fast speeds. Current dynamometers manipulate the speed of limb movement from 0 degrees/sec up to 500 degrees/sec. As noted in Table 3–5, these training velocities are classified as slow, medium, and fast with the fastest velocities similar to or approaching the speeds of limb movements inherent in many functional motor skills such as walking or lifting.[5,280] For example, the average angular velocity of the lower extremity during walking has been calculated at 230 to 240 degrees/sec.[5,50,280]

Fiber Type Recruitment

It is speculated that training at slow to fast velocities recruits both type I and type II fibers depending on the effort exerted during the exercise.[5,79,176]

Table 3–5 Classification of Velocity of Training in Concentric Isokinetic Exercises*

Classification	Angular Velocity
Isometric	0 degrees/sec
Slow	30–60 degrees/sec
Medium	60–180 degrees/sec
Fast	180–360 degrees/sec and above**

*Training velocities tend to be substantially slower for eccentric training, ranging from 30–120 degrees/sec with most eccentric training usually initiated between 60 and 120 degrees/sec.[5,114]

**Although isokinetic equipment offers speed settings up to 500 degrees/sec, training at velocities above 300–360 degrees/sec are not frequently used because the patient must accelerate the limb to the predetermined setting before "catching" the machine, that is, before meeting resistance from the unit.

Specificity of Isokinetic Training

Isokinetic training for the most part is *speed-specific,*[22,50,114,139] with only limited evidence of significant overflows from one training speed to another.[133,253] Evidence of mode-specificity (concentric vs. eccentric) with isokinetic exercise is less clear.*

Compressive Forces on Joints

At faster angular velocities during concentric exercise as force output decreases, the compressive forces across the moving joint are less than with slow-velocity training.[5,50,79]

Accommodation to Muscle Fatigue

Since the resistance encountered is directly proportional to the force applied to the resistance arm of the isokinetic unit, as the contracting muscle fatigues, the patient will still be able to perform additional repetitions even though the force output of the muscle temporarily diminishes.

Accommodation for a Painful Arc

During isokinetic exercise, if a patient experiences transient pain at some portion of the arc of motion, this form of training accommodates for the painful arc. The patient simply pushes less vigorously against the resistance arm to move through that portion of the range without pain. If a patient needs to stop a resisted motion because of a sudden onset of pain, the resistance is eliminated as soon as the patient stops pushing against the torque arm of the dynamometer.

Muscle Coactivation

There is some evidence that brief coactivation of the agonist and its antagonist occurs when training

*See references 10, 50, 79, 113, 114, 187, 221.

reciprocally at high speeds of limb movement.[17,73] It has been reported that during fast-velocity, concentric training of the knee extensors, the knee flexors eccentrically contract and develop tension near the end of the range of knee extension to begin to decelerate the limb before contact is made with the ROM stop.[115] It is speculated that this coactivation could contribute to dynamic stability of the exercised joint. With the recent development of an isokinetic dynamometer specifically designed for closed-chain lower extremity testing and training, isokinetic training can now be performed in gradations of weight bearing to enhance coactivation of lower extremity musculature.[54]

Special Considerations for Isokinetic Training

Selection of Training Velocities

Isokinetic training enables a patient to train safely and effectively to improve muscle performance at slow, medium, and fast velocities and, therefore, provides a mechanism for a patient to prepare for the demands of functional activities that occur at a range of velocities of limb movement. Because isokinetic exercise tends to be speed-specific, **velocity spectrum rehabilitation** is advocated.[50,79] This approach to isokinetic training is discussed later in this chapter. Generally, medium to fast velocities (60 or 90–360 degrees/sec) are selected. In addition, selection of training speeds should be as specific as possible to the demands of the anticipated functional tasks. Selection of training speeds may also be based on evidence of strength deficits at specific speeds which have been identified by isokinetic testing. As noted in Table 3–5, the range of training speeds advocated for concentric exercise is substantially greater than for eccentric training.[79,114]

Initiation of Isokinetic Training

Isokinetic training is begun in the later stages of rehabilitation when active motion through the full (or partial) ROM is pain free.

Progression

- Submaximal isokinetic exercise is implemented before isokinetic exercise with maximal effort to keep resistance low initially.
- Short-arc movements are used before full-arc motions when necessary to avoid movement in an unstable or painful portion of the range. This can be accomplished by a mechanical range-limiting device or with a computerized dynamometer.
- Slow to medium training velocities (60–180 degrees/sec) are incorporated into the exercise program before progressing to faster velocities.
- A patient should be able to perform maximal concentric motions at various speeds before introducing eccentric isokinetics for several reasons[5,50,79,114] The concentric mode of training on an isokinetic unit is easier to learn and is fully under the control of the patient. During eccentric isokinetic exercise the velocity of movement of the resistance arm is robotically controlled by the dynamometer, not the patient.

Selecting the Appropriate Set-Up

The set-ups recommended in the product manuals often must be altered to ensure that the exercise occurs in a position that is safe for a particular joint. For example, even though a manufacturer may describe a 90/90 degree position of the shoulder and elbow for strengthening the shoulder rotators, exercising with the arm at the side may be a safer, more comfortable position (Fig. 3–5).

Reciprocal Versus Isolated Muscle Training

Use of reciprocal training of agonist and antagonist muscles is possible on an isokinetic dynamometer emphasizing quick reversals of motion. For example, the training parameter can be set so that the patient performs a concentric contraction of the quadriceps followed by a concentric contraction of the hamstrings. An alternative approach is to target the same muscle in a concentric, followed by an eccentric mode, thus strengthening only one muscle group at a time as occurs during many functional activities.[279] Both of these approaches have merit.

Limitations of Isokinetic Training

From a pragmatic perspective one limitation of isokinetic exercise is that a patient can only incorporate this form of exercise into a rehabilitation program by going to a facility where the equipment is available. In addition, a patient must be given assistance to set up the equipment and often requires supervision during exercise. All of these considerations contribute to high costs for a long-term rehabilitation program.

Although isokinetic training affords a spectrum of velocities for training, the speed of limb movement during many functional and sports-related activities far exceeds the maximum speed settings available on isokinetic equipment. Despite this limitation, the

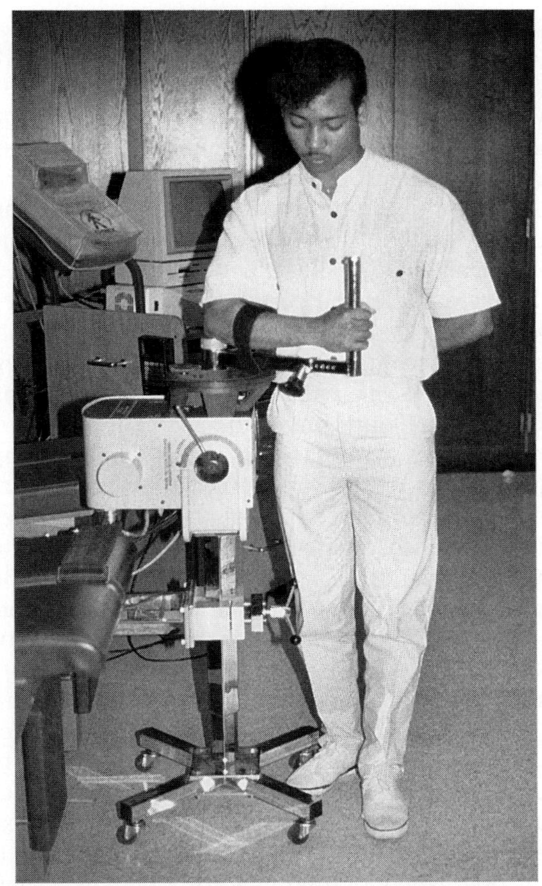

Figure 3–5 Set-up for isokinetic strengthening of the internal and external rotators of the shoulder with the arm at the side to protect a potentially unstable glenohumeral joint.

use of concentric and eccentric isokinetic training has been associated with increases in functional performance, such as throwing and tennis serve velocities.[81,185]

Several factors inherent in the design of most types of isokinetic equipment may limit the extent to which isokinetic exercises carry over to improvements in functional performance. Isokinetic exercise usually isolates a single muscle or opposite muscle groups, involves movement of a single joint, is uniplanar and occurs in an open-chain. Although isolation of a single muscle can be beneficial in remediating strength deficits in specific muscle groups, most functional activities require contractions of multiple muscle groups and movement of multiple joints in several planes of motion, some in weight-bearing positions. In addition, limb movement during most functional tasks occurs at multiple velocities, depending on the conditions of the task, not at a constant velocity. Some of these limitations can be addressed by adapting the set-up of the equipment to allow multiaxis movements in diagonal planes. As noted earlier, the recent introduction of closed-chain features opens up additional options for isokinetic training.

Open-Chain and Closed-Chain Exercise

In the clinical setting and in the rehabilitation literature, human motions or exercises are often described or classified as occurring in "open or closed *kinetic* chains" and "open or closed *kinematic* chains." When the concepts of *kinetic* chains and *kinematic* chains were introduced in the human biomechanics and kinesiology literature by Steindler[238] and Brunnstrom,[29] respectively, these terms were used to describe how forces occur during human motion and how segments (structures) of the body are linked together, not to categorize resistance exercises.

In his analysis of human motion, Steindler[238] proposed that motion in an open kinetic chain applies to completely unrestricted movement in space of a peripheral segment of the body, as in waving the hand or swinging the leg. In contrast, he suggested that in closed kinetic chain movements the peripheral segment meets with considerable external resistance. He stated that if the terminal segment remains fixed, the encountered resistance moves the proximal segments over the stationary distal segments. Brunnstrom[29] concurred but used the term "closed kinematic chain." Both noted that the action of a muscle changes when the distal segment is free to move versus when it is fixed in place. For example, the tibialis posterior functions in an open-chain to invert and plantarflex the foot and ankle. In the stance phase of gait, when the foot is planted on the ground in a closed-chain, the tibialis posterior contracts to decelerate pronation of the subtalar joint during loading and to supinate the foot as well as to externally rotate the lower leg during mid- and terminal stance. Both authors also pointed out that in a closed-chain, motion in one joint is accompanied by motions of adjacent joints that occur in reasonably predictable patterns. Examples of open- and closed-chain classifications of motion are evident in the lower extremities when walking, climbing stairs, or getting into or out of a car.

Unlike Brunnstrom, Steindler[238] also included another condition under the classification of closed kinetic chain motions that is often overlooked in the current literature. He pointed out that if the external resistance is overcome in the closed kinetic chain, it results in movement of the peripheral segment. The examples Steindler cited were lifting a load and pushing a cart. It is the interpretation and application of this condition of his definition of closed kinetic chain motions that is the source of considerable inconsistency and ambiguity in today's literature on resistance training. For example, a bench press exercise, a seated or reclining leg press exercise, or cycling, all of which are similar to pushing a cart away from the body, are often classified as closed kinetic chain exercises or activities.[23,53] In contrast, lifting a handheld weight or pushing against the force arm of an isokinetic dynamometer are consistently cited as examples of open kinetic chain exercises.* In all instances, the distal segment is moving and meeting with considerable external resistance but only the former examples not the latter usually are classified as closed kinetic chain exercises. In the literature even the stated parameters of closed-chain exercises are inconsistent. Must the distal segment be absolutely fixed to be classified as a closed kinetic chain motion? If the peripheral component remains in contact with but slides across the support surface as it meets resistance, does this motion qualify as a closed kinetic chain motion? Herein lies one of several problems when clinicians try to sort out the often vague or confusing descriptions of open- and closed-chain exercises in the literature.[23,67,68,116,232,273]

Another source of inconsistency is whether or not weight bearing is an inherent component of closed kinetic chain motions. Steindler[238] does not specify that weight-bearing must occur for a motion to be categorized as closed kinetic chain, but many of his examples of closed-chain movements particularly in the lower extremity involve weight bearing. In the current literature, descriptions of a closed kinetic chain often do[55,93] but sometimes do not[119,232] include weight bearing as a necessary element of closed-chain exercises. One author suggests that all weight-bearing exercises involve some elements of closed-chain motions, but not all closed-chain exercises are performed in weight-bearing positions.[232]

Several authors and clinicians have offered additional or alternative categories for classification of resistance activities to eliminate the ambiguity. One suggestion is to add a category dubbed *partial kinetic chain*[273,275] to describe exercises in which the distal segment (hand or foot) meets resistance but is not absolutely stationary, such as using a stepping machine or slide board. The term closed kinetic chain is then reserved for instances when the terminal segment does not move. To date, this additional term has not been widely used in the literature or in the clinical setting.

To avoid use of the concepts of closed kinetic or kinematic chains, other classification systems have been proposed and described. One system categorizes exercises as either *joint isolation exercises* (movement of only one joint segment) or *kinetic chain exercises* (simultaneous movement of multiple segments that are linked together).[147,200] Boundaries of movement of the peripheral segment (movable or stationary) or loading conditions are not parameters of these classifications. Other systems of classification of motions or exercises that have been proposed are based on boundaries of motion *and* external loads.[68,168] Despite evidence that EMG activity is similar in exercises with a comparable level of loading, regardless of whether or not the boundary (distal segment) is fixed or movable,[23,68] combined boundary/loading systems also have not been widely accepted as yet to classify or describe exercises. Instead most authors continue to use the terms open and closed kinetic (or kinematic) chains to describe exercises.†

Therefore, despite the many inconsistencies and shortcomings of the kinetic or kinematic chain terminology, and recognizing that many exercises and functional activities involve a combination of open- and closed-chain motions and cannot be classified as exclusively one type of motion or the other, the authors of this textbook have chosen to continue to describe resistance exercises as occurring in either an open- or a closed-chain or both. Following operational definitions and descriptions of commonly accepted characteristics of open- and closed-chain exercises, the rationale and methods of application of these categories of exercise are discussed. Whenever possible, presumed benefits and limitations or comparisons of both forms of exercise are analyzed in light of existing scientific evidence. It should also be noted that most reports and investigations comparing or analyzing closed- or open-chain exercises to date have focused on the knee, in particular, the ACL

*See references 53, 55, 93, 119, 137, 209, 239, 273.

†See references 24, 50, 71, 80, 93, 116, 119, 137, 140, 178, 209, 239, 245, 250, 254, 274.

or patellofemoral joint. Far fewer articles have addressed the application or reported the impact of open- vs. closed-chain exercises on the upper extremities.

Selection and use of specific open- or closed-chain exercises mentioned in this chapter or the regional chapters of this textbook depends entirely on the status and functional goals of an individual patient. Since functional activities involve many combinations and considerable variations of open- and closed-chain motions, inclusion and integration of task-specific open-chain as well as closed-chain exercises into a rehabilitation or conditioning program is both appropriate and prudent.

Characteristics of Open- and Closed-Chain Exercises

For the purpose of clarity of discussion of the exercise interventions described in this textbook, the following definitions and characteristics of open- and closed-chain exercises in a resistance training program are delineated. Although the characteristics of open- and closed-chain exercises included under each classification vary from source to source, there is agreement that isometric, concentric, and eccentric muscle contractions may be employed during open- and closed-chain exercises. The parameters of the definitions set forth in this section reflect the most common usage in the current literature. Common characteristics of open- and closed-chain exercises are compared in Table 3–6.

Open-Chain Exercises

Open-chain exercises involve motions in which the distal segment (hand or foot) is free to move in space, without necessarily causing simultaneous motions at adjacent joints.[53,80,93,147] Limb movement only occurs *distal* to the moving joint. Muscle activation occurs in the muscles that cross the moving joint. For example, during knee flexion in an open-chain (Fig. 3–6), the action of the hamstrings is independent of recruitment of either hip or ankle musculature. Open-chain exercises also are typically performed in nonweight-bearing positions.[55,93,282] In addition, during resistance training, the exercise load (resistance) is applied to the moving distal segment.

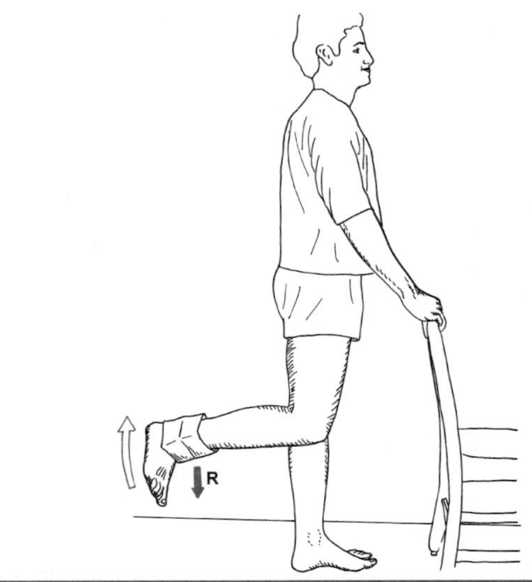

Figure 3–6 Open-chain resisted knee flexion.

Table 3–6 Characteristics of Open- and Closed-Chain Exercises

Open-Chain Exercises	Closed-Chain Exercises
Distal segment moves in space	Distal segment remains stationary (fixed in place)
Independent joint movement; no predictable joint motion in adjacent joints	Interdependent joint movements; relatively predictable movement patterns in adjacent joints
Movement of body segments only distal to the moving joint	Movement of body segments may occur distal and/or proximal to the moving point
Muscle activation occurs predominantly in the prime mover and is isolated to muscles of the moving joint	Muscle activation occurs in multiple muscle groups, both distal and proximal to the moving joint
Typically performed in nonweight-bearing positions	Typically performed in weight-bearing positions
Resistance is applied to the moving distal segment	Resistance is applied simultaneously to multiple moving segments
Use to external rotary loading	Use of axial loading
External stabilization (manually or with equipment) usually required	Internal stabilization by means of muscle action, joint compression, and congruency and postural control

Closed-Chain Exercises

Closed-chain exercises involve motions in which the body moves on a distal segment that is fixed or stabilized on a support surface.[55,80,93,119,137,147,232,273] Movement at one joint causes simultaneous motions at distal as well as proximal joints in a relatively predictable manner. For example when a patient is performing a bilateral short-arc squatting motion (Fig. 3–7) and then returning to an erect position, as the knees flex and extend, the hips and ankles move in a predictable pattern along with the knees.

Closed-chain exercises are primarily performed in weight-bearing positions.[56,93,119,282] Examples in the upper extremities include balance activities in quadruped, sitting press-ups, or prone push-ups; examples in the lower extremities are lunges, squats, step-up or step-down exercises, or heel rises.

Note: In this textbook as in some other publications[80,119,245] inclusive in the scope of closed-chain exercises are *weight-bearing activities* where the distal segment *moves but remains in contact with the support surface,* as when using a slide board or a stepping machine. In the upper extremities a few nonweight-bearing activities qualify as closed-chain exercises, such as pull-ups on a trapeze in bed or chin-ups at an overhead bar.

Rationale for Open- and Closed-Chain Exercises

The rationale for selecting open- vs. closed-chain exercises for the rehabilitation of extremity dysfunction is based on the goals of the rehabilitation program and the potential benefits and limitations inherent in either form of exercise. There is no evidence to support the global assumption that closed-chain exercises are "more functional" than open-chain exercises. In contrast, there is substantial evidence that both open- and closed-chain exercises are effective for reducing deficits in muscle performance in the upper and lower extremities. Of the extensive number of studies summarized in a recent review very few are randomized, controlled studies that associate improvements in muscle strength, power, or endurance as the result of open- or closed-chain training with a reduction of functional limitations or an improvement in physical performance.[51]

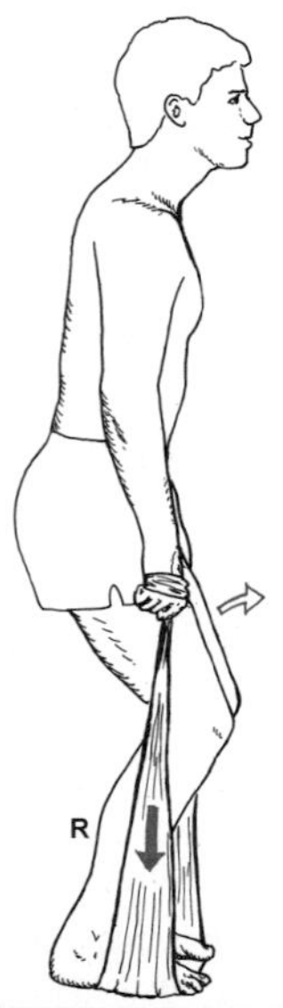

Figure 3–7 Bilateral closed-chain resisted hip and knee extension.

Some of the reported benefits or limitations of either open- or closed-chain exercises are supported by scientific evidence, whereas others are often founded on opinion or anecdotal reports. That which is viewed as a benefit from one perspective in some instances is perceived as a limitation from another perspective. Research that has compared benefits or limitations of specific exercises is described in the regional chapters of this textbook.

Isolation of Muscle Groups

Open-chain testing and training identifies strength deficits and improves muscle performance of individual muscles or muscle groups more effectively than closed-chain exercises. The possible occurrence of substitute motions that compensate for and mask strength deficits of individual muscles is greater with closed-chain exercise than open-chain exercise. In a study of the effectiveness of a closed-chain-only resistance training program after ACL reconstruction, residual muscle weakness of the quadriceps femoris was identified.[231] The investigators suggested that this residual strength deficit, which altered gait, might have been avoided with the inclusion of open-chain quadriceps training in the postoperative rehabilitation program.

Control of Movements

During open-chain resisted exercises a greater level of control is possible with a *single* moving joint than with multiple moving joints as occurs during closed-chain training. In open-chain exercises stabilization is usually applied externally by a therapist's manual contacts or with belts or straps. In contrast, during closed-chain exercises the patient most often uses muscular stabilization to control joints or structures proximal and distal to the targeted joint. Greater levels of control afforded by open-chain training are often advantageous in the early phases of rehabilitation.

Joint Approximation

Almost all muscle contractions have a compressive component, which approximates the joint surfaces and provides stability to the joint whether in open- or closed-chain situations.[169,229] Joint approximation also occurs during weight bearing and is associated with lower levels of shear forces. This has been demonstrated in the knee (decreased anterior or posterior tibiofemoral translation)[281,282] and possibly the glenohumeral joint.[263] The joint approximation that occurs with the axial loading during weight bearing is thought to cause an increase in joint congruency which, in turn, contributes to stability.[53,80,247,260]

Coactivation and Dynamic Stabilization

Although not to the degree that occurs with closed-chain exercises, coactivation (co-contraction) of agonist and antagonist muscle groups may occur with some open-chain exercises. For example, rhythmic stabilization against manual resistance, use of a Bodyblade® (see Fig. 3–48), high-velocity isokinetic training, and stretch-shortening drills (plyometric training), all of which can be performed in an open-chain, are thought to stimulate coactivation of muscle groups. To date, there is only limited evidence to support this purported benefit of open-chain exercise. As already noted, during high-velocity, concentric training as the agonist contracts to accelerate the limb, the antagonist contracts to decelerate the limb at the end of the ROM, thus causing a brief window of co-contraction that can contribute to end-range dynamic stability of the moving joint.[17,73,115] Coactivation of agonist and antagonist muscle groups is not evident at slow-velocity (60 degrees/sec) open-chain training.[161] Some types of open-chain training may have an adverse effect on unstable, injured, or recently repaired joints as demonstrated in the ACL-deficient knee.[82,140,274,281]

Since most closed-chain exercises are performed in weight-bearing positions, it has been assumed and commonly reported that closed-chain exercises stimulate joint and muscle mechanoreceptors, facilitate coactivation of agonists and antagonists (co-contraction) and subsequently promote dynamic stability.[246,247,260] During a standing squat, for example, the quadriceps and hamstrings are thought to contract concurrently to control the knee and hip respectively. In studies of lower extremity closed-chain exercises and activity of knee musculature, this assumption has been supported,[28,42,235,274] and refuted.[82]

In the upper extremity, closed-chain exercises in weight-bearing positions are thought to cause coactivation of the scapular and glenohumeral stabilizers and, therefore, to improve dynamic stability of the shoulder complex.[80,273] To date, evidence of co-contraction of muscles of the shoulder girdle during weight-bearing exercises, such as a prone push-up or a press-up in a chair, is just beginning to emerge,[163] making it difficult for clinicians to make evidence-based decisions at this time.

Proprioception, Kinesthesia, Neuromuscular Control, and Balance

Conscious awareness of joint position or movement is one of the foundations of motor learning during the early phase of training for neuromuscular control of functional movements. After soft tissue or joint injury, proprioception and kinesthesia are disrupted and alter neuromuscular control. Re-establishing the effective and efficient use of sensory information to initiate and control movement is a high priority in rehabilitation. Studies have shown that proprioception and kinesthesia do improve after rehabilitation.[18,165]

It is thought that closed-chain training provides greater proprioceptive and kinesthetic feedback than open-chain training. Theoretically, because multiple muscle groups that cross multiple joints are activated during closed-chain exercise, to control motion more sensory receptors in more muscles and intra-articular and extra-articular structures are activated than during open-chain exercises. The weight-bearing element (axial loading) of closed-chain exercises, which causes joint approximation, is believed to stimulate mechanoreceptors in muscles and in and around joints to enhance sensory input for the control of movement.*

Despite the assumption that joint position or movement sense is enhanced to a greater extent under closed-chain than open-chain conditions, evidence is mixed. The results of one study[166] indicated

*See references 119, 165, 166, 167, 168, 209, 232, 274.

that in patients with unstable shoulders kinesthesia improved to a greater extent with a program of closed-chain and open-chain exercises as compared with only open-chain exercises. In contrast, in a recent comparison of the ability to detect knee position during closed-chain vs. open-chain conditions, no significant difference was reported.[250]

Finally, closed-chain positioning is the obvious choice to improve balance and postural control in the upright position. Balance training is an essential element of the comprehensive rehabilitation of patients after musculoskeletal injuries or surgery, particularly in the lower extremities to restore functional abilities and prevent reinjury.[144,261] The parameters for the progression of closed-chain exercises (see Table 3–7) are the same as those used for balance training to challenge the body's balance mechanisms.

Carry-Over to Function

Functional activities in the upper extremity predominantly involve movement of the distal segment (the hand) in space, but closed-chain demands also occur in the upper extremity such as scooting across a bed or car seat, pushing oneself up from a chair, or pushing a cart or stroller. Similarly, many lower extremity functional tasks are composed of a combination of open-chain and closed-chain movement patterns, such as walking and climbing stairs, and getting into a car.

Consistent with the principle of task-specific training, exercises should be incorporated into a rehabilitation program that simulates the desired functions and prepares the patient for the functional tasks.[53] For example, squatting exercises in standing have been shown to enhance performance of a jumping task more effectively than open-chain iso-

Table 3–7 Parameters and Progression of Closed-Chain Exercises

Parameters	Progression
% Body weight	Partial → full weight-bearing (LE: Aquatic exercise, parallel bars, overhead harnessing; UE: wall push-up → modified prone push-up → prone push-up) Full weight-bearing + additional weight (Weighted vest or belt, handheld or cuff weights, elastic resistance)
Base of support	Wide → narrow Bilateral → unilateral Fixed on support surface → sliding on support surface
Support surface	Stable → unstable/moving (LE: Floor → rocker board, wobble board, sideboard, treadmill) (UE: Floor, table or wall → rocker or side board, ball) Right → soft (Floor, table → carpet, foam) Height: ground level → increasing height (Low step → high step)
Balance	With external support → no external support Eyes open → eyes closed
Exclusion of limb movement	Small → large ranges Short-arc → full-arc (if appropriate)
Plane or direction of movement	Uniplanar → multiplanar Anterior → posterior → diagonal (Forward walking → retrowalking; forward step-up → backward step-up) Sagittal → frontal or transverse (forward-backward sliding → side to side sliding; forward or backward step-up → lateral step-up)
Speed of movement or directional changes	Slow → fast

kinetic knee extension exercises.[15] Similar studies that demonstrate an association between closed-chain training and improved performance of upper extremity functional tasks to date have not been published.[80]

Implementation and Progression of Open- and Closed-Chain Exercises

Note: Principles and general guidelines for the implementation and progression of open-chain and closed-chain exercises are similar in a resistance training program with respect to variables such as intensity, volume, frequency, and rest intervals. These variables were discussed earlier in this chapter.

Introduction of Open-Chain Training

Because open-chain training typically is performed in nonweight-bearing postures, open-chain exercises may be the only option when weight bearing is either contraindicated or must be severely restricted or when unloading in a closed-chain position is not possible. soft tissue pain and swelling or restricted motion of any segment of the chain may also necessitate the use of open-chain exercises at adjacent joints. After a fracture of the tibia, for example, the lower extremity is commonly immobilized in a long leg cast, and weight bearing is restricted for at least a few weeks. During this period, hip strengthening exercises in an open-chain can still be initiated and gradually progressed until partial weight bearing and closed-chain activities are permissible.

Any activity that involves open-chain motions can easily be replicated with open-chain exercises, first by developing isolated control and strength of the weak musculature, then combining motions to simulate functional patterns.

Special Consideration for Use of Closed-Chain Exercises—Weight-Bearing Restrictions/Unloading

If weight bearing must be restricted, a safe alternative to open-chain exercises may be to perform closed-chain exercises while partial weight bearing. This is simple to achieve in the upper extremity, but in the lower extremity, because the patient is in an upright position during closed-chain exercises, axial loading in one or both lower extremities must be reduced. Use of aquatic exercises or decreasing the percentage of body weight borne on the involved lower extremity in parallel bars are both feasible strategies even though each has its own limitations. It is difficult to control the extent of weight bearing when performing closed-chain exercises in parallel bars. In addition, lower limb movements while weight bearing in the parallel bars or in water tend to be slower than what typically occurs during functional tasks. An alternative is the use of a harnessing system to unload the lower extremities.[145] This system enables a patient to perform a variety of closed-chain exercises and to begin ambulation on a treadmill at functional speeds early in rehabilitation.

Note: Relevant features of closed-chain exercises and guidelines for progression are listed in Table 3–7. The examples of parameters and suggestions for progressions are not all-inclusive and are certainly very flexible. The selection and progression of activities should always be based on the discretion of the therapist and the patient's functional needs and response to intervention.

Resistance Exercise: Principles, Precautions, and Contraindications

General Principles of Resistance Training

As with all forms of therapeutic exercise a comprehensive examination and evaluation is the foundation of an individualized resistance training program. The principles presented in this section apply to the use of both manual and mechanical resistance exercises for persons of all ages, but they are not "set in stone." There are many instances when these principles may or should be modified based on the judgment of the therapist. Additional guidelines specific to the application of manual resistance exercise, proprioceptive neuromuscular facilitation, and mechanical resistance exercise are addressed in later sections of this chapter.

Examination and Evaluation

1. Prior to initiating any exercise intervention, perform a comprehensive examination of the patient, including a thorough history, a systems review, and selected tests and measurements.
   - Determine qualitative and quantitative baselines of strength, muscular endurance, ROM, and overall level of functional performance against which progress can be measured.
   - Implement testing procedures, such as manual muscle testing, determination of a repetition

maximum, dynamometry, goniometry, quantitative functional performance tests, and assessment of the patient's perceived level of disability.

2. Evaluate the findings to determine if the use of resistance exercises is appropriate or inappropriate. Some questions that may need to be answered are noted in Box 3–7. Be sure to identify the goals the patient is seeking to achieve and the expected functional outcomes of the exercise program.
3. Based on the interpretation of the findings, determine if a program of resistance exercises is a suitable intervention at this time to meet the goals of rehabilitation and achieve, at least in part, the desired functional outcomes.
4. Establish how resistance training should be integrated into the plan of care with other therapeutic interventions, such as stretching, joint mobilization techniques, balance training, and cardiorespiratory fitness exercises.
5. Re-evaluate periodically to document progress and determine if and how the dosage of exercises (intensity, volume, frequency, rest) and the types of resistance training should be adjusted to continue to challenge the patient.

Box 3–7 Is Resistance Training Appropriate? Questions to Consider

- Were deficits in muscle performance identified? If so, do these deficits appear to be contributing to limitations of functional abilities that you have observed or the patient or family has reported?
- Could identified deficits cause future impairment of function?
- What is the irritability and current stage of healing of involved tissues?
- Is there evidence of tissue swelling?
- Is there pain? (At rest or with movement? At what portion of the ROM? In what tissues?)
- Are there other deficits, such as impaired mobility, balance, sensation, coordination, or cognition, that are adversely affecting much performance?
- What are the patient's goals or desired functional outcomes? Are they realistic in light of the findings of the examination?
- Given the patient's current status, are resistance exercises indicated? Contraindicated?
- Can the identified deficits in muscle performance be eliminated or minimized with resistance exercises?
- If a decision is made to prescribe resistance exercises in the treatment plan, what types of resistance exercises are expected to be most effective?
- Should one area of muscle performance be emphasized over another?
- Will the patient require supervision or assistance over the course of the exercise program or can the program be carried out independently?
- What is the expected frequency and duration of the resistance training program? Will a maintenance program be necessary?
- Are there any precautions specific to the patient's physical status, general health, or age that may warrant special consideration?

Preparation for Resistance Exercises

1. Select and prescribe the forms of exercise and resistance that are appropriate and expected to be effective.
2. Decide whether to implement manual or mechanical resistance exercises or both. Determine what equipment is needed and available.
3. Review the anticipated goals and expected functional outcomes.
4. Explain the exercise plan and procedures. Be sure that the patient and/or family understands and gives consent.
5. Have the patient wear nonrestrictive clothing and supportive shoes appropriate for exercise. If the patient is wearing a hospital gown, use a sheet to drape for modesty.
6. If possible, select a firm but comfortable support surface for exercise.
7. *Warm up* prior to initiation of resistance exercises with light, repetitive, dynamic, site-specific movements. For example prior to lower extremity resistance exercise, have the patient walk on a treadmill, if possible, for 5 to 10 minutes followed by flexibility exercises for the trunk and lower extremities.
8. Demonstrate each exercise and the desired movement pattern.

Application of Resistance Exercises

Note: These general guidelines apply to the use of *dynamic* exercises against manual *or* mechanical resistance. In addition to these guidelines, refer to special considerations and guidelines unique to the application of manual and mechanical resistance exercises in sections of this chapter that follow.

Placement of Resistance

1. Resistance is typically applied to the distal end of the segment in which the muscle to be strength-

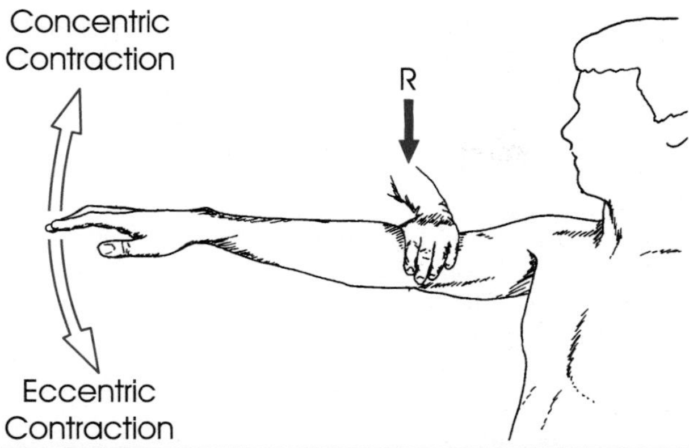

Figure 3–8 Resistance (R) is applied to the distal end of the segment being strengthened. Resistance is applied in the *opposite direction* as limb movement to resist an eccentric muscle contraction.

ened attaches. Distal placement of resistance generates the greatest amount of external torque with the least amount of manual or mechanical resistance (load). For example, to strengthen the anterior deltoid, resistance is applied to the distal humerus as the patient flexes the shoulder (Fig. 3–8).

2. Resistance may be applied across an intermediate joint if that joint is stable and pain free and if there is adequate muscle strength supporting the joint. For example, to strengthen the anterior deltoid using mechanical resistance, a handheld weight is a common source of resistance.
3. Revise the placement of resistance if pressure from the load is uncomfortable.

Direction of Resistance

During *concentric* exercise resistance is applied in the direction *directly opposite* to the desired motion. During *eccentric* exercise resistance is applied in the *same* direction as the desired motion (see Fig. 3–8).

Stabilization

Stabilization is necessary to avoid unwanted, substitute motions.

1. In open-chain resisted exercises external stabilization of a segment is usually applied at the proximal attachment of the muscle to be strengthened. In the case of the biceps brachii muscle, for example, stabilization should occur at the anterior shoulder as elbow flexion is resisted (Fig. 3–9). Equipment such as belts or straps are effective sources of stabilization.

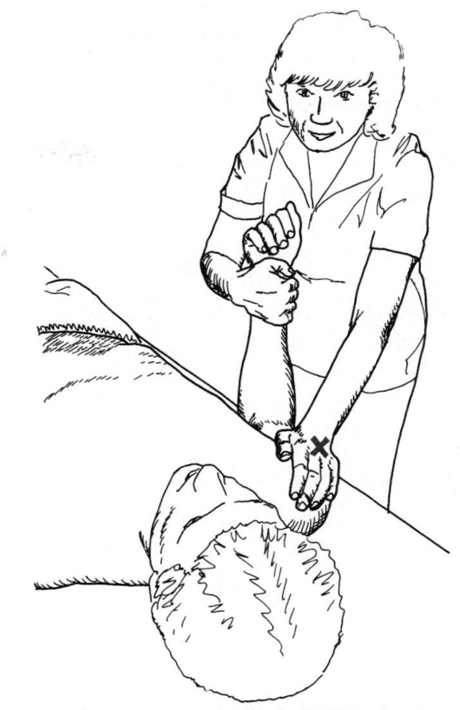

Figure 3–9 Stabilization is applied at the proximal attachment of the muscle being strengthened. In this illustration, the proximal humerus and scapula are stabilized as elbow flexion is resisted.

2. During closed-chain, multijoint resisted exercises, the patient must use muscle control (internal stabilization) to hold nonmoving segments in alignment.

Intensity of Exercise/Amount of Resistance

Note: The intensity of the exercise (submaximal to near-maximal) must be consistent with the intended goals of resistance training, the type of muscle contraction as well as other aspects of dosage.

1. Initially, have the patient practice the movement pattern against a minimal load to learn the correct pattern and the exercise technique.
2. Have the patient exert a forceful but controlled and pain-free effort. The level of resistance

should be such that movements are smooth and nonballistic or tremulous.

3. Adjust the alignment, stabilization, or the amount of resistance if the patient is unable to complete the available ROM, muscular tremor develops, or substitute motions occur.

Volume/Number of Repetitions and Sets; Rest Intervals

1. In general, for most adults, use 8 to 12 repetitions of a specific motion against a moderate exercise load. This volume induces typical acute and chronic responses: muscular fatigue and adaptive gains in muscular strength, respectively.
2. Decrease the amount of resistance if the patient cannot complete 8 to 12 repetitions.
3. After a brief rest, perform additional repetitions, a second set of 8 to 12 repetitions, if possible.
4. For progressive overloading, initially increase the number of repetitions or sets; at a later point in the exercise program, gradually increase the resistance.

Verbal or Written Instructions

When teaching an exercise using mechanical resistance or when applying manual resistance, use simple instructions that are easily understood. Do not use medical terminology or jargon. For example, tell the patient to "Bend and straighten your elbow" rather than "Flex and extend your elbow." Be sure that descriptions of resistance exercises to be performed in a home program are written and clearly illustrated.

Monitoring the Patient

Assess the patient's responses before, during, and after exercise. It may be advisable to monitor the patient's vital signs. Adhere to relevant precautions in the discussion of precautions that follows.

Cool Down

Cool down after a series of resistance exercises with rhythmic, unresisted movements, such as arm swinging, walking, or cycling. Gentle stretching is also appropriate after resistance exercises.

Precautions During Resistance Training

Regardless of the goals of a resistance exercise program and the types of exercises prescribed and implemented, the exercises should not only be effective, but *safe.* The therapist's interpretation of the findings of the examination determine the exercise prescription. Regardless of the types of resistance exercise selected, following a number of general precautions maximizes patient safety. General precautions for resistance training are summarized in Box 3–8.

Several of these precautions are discussed in detail in this section. Special considerations and precautions for children and older adults who participate in weight-training programs are addressed later in this chapter.

Valsalva Maneuver

The **Valsalva maneuver (phenomenon),** which is an expiratory effort against a closed glottis, must be avoided during resistance exercise. When a person is exerting a strenuous and prolonged effort, the phenomenon occurs. The Valsalva maneuver is characterized by the following sequence. A deep inspiration is followed by closure of the glottis and contraction of the abdominal muscles. This increases intra-abdominal and intrathoracic pressures which, in turn, forces blood from the heart, causing

Box 3–8 General Precautions During Resistance Training

- Keep the ambient temperature of the exercise setting comfortable for vigorous exercise. Select clothing for exercise that facilitates heat dissipation and does not impede sweat evaporation.
- Caution the patient that pain should *not* occur *during* exercise.
- Do not initiate resistance training at a maximal level of resistance, particularly with eccentric exercise to minimize delayed-onset muscle soreness (DOMS). Use light to moderate exercise during the recovery period.
- Avoid use of heavy resistance during exercise for children, older adults, and in patients with osteoporosis.
- Do not apply resistance across an unstable joint or distal to a fracture site that is not completely healed.
- Have the patient avoid breath-holding during resisted exercises to prevent the Valsalva maneuver; emphasize exhalation during exertion.
- Avoid uncontrolled, ballistic movements as they compromise safety and effectiveness.
- Prevent incorrect or substitute motions by adequate stabilization and an appropriate level of resistance.
- Avoid exercises that place excessive, unintended secondary stresses on the back.
- Be aware of medications a patient is using that can alter acute and chronic responses to exercise.
- Avoid cumulative fatigue from excessive frequency of exercise and the effects of overtraining or overwork by incorporating adequate rest intervals between exercise sessions to allow adequate time for recovery after exercise.
- Discontinue exercises if the patient experiences pain, dizziness, or unusual or precipitous shortness of breath.

an abrupt, but temporary increase in arterial blood pressure.

During exercise the Valsalva phenomenon occurs most often with *high-effort* isometric[88] and dynamic[172] muscle contractions. It has been shown that the rise in blood pressure induced by an isometric muscle contraction is proportional to the percentage of maximum voluntary force that is exerted.[172] During isokinetic (concentric) testing, if a patient exerts maximum effort at increasing velocities, the rise in blood pressure appears to be the same at all velocities of movement despite the fact that the force output of the muscle decreases.[72] Although occurrence of the Valsalva phenomenon is more often thought to be associated with isometric[88,141] and eccentric[58] resistance exercise, a recent study[172] indicates that the rise in blood pressure appears to be based more on extent of effort not strictly on the mode of muscle contraction.

High-Risk Patients

The risk of complications from the rapid rise in blood pressure is particularly high in patients with a history of coronary artery disease, myocardial infarction, cerebrovascular disorders, or hypertension. Also at risk are patients who have had neurosurgery or eye surgery or who have intervertebral disk pathology. High-risk patients must be monitored closely.

Note: Although resistance training is often recommended for individuals with a history of or high risk for cardiovascular disorders,[7,8] it is important to distinguish those individuals for whom resistance training is and is not safe and appropriate. Guidelines are available to assist with this screening process.[7,8]

Prevention During Exercise

- Caution the patient about breath-holding.
- Ask the patient to breathe rhythmically, count, or talk during exercise.
- Have the patient exhale with each resisted effort.
- Be certain that high-risk patients avoid high-intensity resistance exercises.

Substitute Motions

If too much resistance is applied to a contracting muscle during exercise, substitute motions can occur. When muscles are weak because of fatigue, paralysis, or pain, a patient will attempt to carry out the desired movements that the weak muscles normally perform by any means possible. For example, if the deltoid or supraspinatus muscles are weak or abduction of the arm is painful, a patient will elevate the scapula (shrug the shoulder) and laterally flex the trunk to the opposite side to elevate the arm. It may appear that the patient is abducting the arm, but in fact he or she is not. To avoid substitute motions during exercise, an appropriate amount of resistance must be applied, and correct stabilization must be used with manual contacts, with equipment, or by means of muscular stabilization.

Overtraining and Overwork

Exercise programs in which heavy resistance is applied or exhaustive training is performed repeatedly must be progressed cautiously to avoid a problem known as overtraining or overwork. These terms reflect deterioration in muscle performance and physical capabilities (either temporary or permanent) that can occur in either healthy individuals or in patients with certain neuromuscular disorders. In most instances, the uncomfortable sensation associated with acute muscle fatigue induces individuals to cease exercising. This is not necessarily the case in highly motivated athletes who are said to be *overreaching* in their training program or in patients who may not adequately sense fatigue because of a neuromuscular disorder.

Overtraining is the term more commonly used to describe a decline in physical performance in healthy individuals participating in a high-intensity, high-volume strength and endurance training program.[14,102,160] The terms *chronic fatigue, staleness,* and *burnout* are also used to describe this phenomenon. When overtraining occurs, the individual progressively fatigues more quickly and requires more time to recover from strenuous exercise, because of physiologic and psychologic factors.

Overtraining is brought on by inadequate rest intervals between exercise sessions, too rapid progression of exercises, and inadequate diet and fluid intake. Fortunately, in healthy individuals, overtraining is a preventable and reversible phenomenon that can be resolved by tapering the training program for a period of time by periodically decreasing the volume and frequency of exercise (periodization).[102,157,160]

Overwork, sometimes called **overwork weakness,** refers to progressive deterioration of strength in muscles already weakened by non-progressive neuromuscular disease.[199] It was first observed in patients recovering from polio who were actively involved in rehabilitation.[20] In many instances the decrement in strength that was noted was permanent or very prolonged. More recently, overwork weakness has been reported in patients with other nonprogressive neuromuscular diseases, such as Guillain-Barré syndrome.[121] Postpolio syndrome is also thought to be related to long-term overuse of weak muscles.[91]

This phenomenon has been produced in laboratory animals,[121] which provides some insight to its cause. When strenuous exercise was initiated soon after a peripheral nerve lesion, the return of functional motor strength was retarded. It was suggested that this could be caused by excessive protein breakdown in the denervated muscle.

Prevention is the key to dealing with overwork weakness. Resistance exercise programs for patients with impaired neuromuscular function or who have some systemic, metabolic, or inflammatory diseases, which increase susceptibility to muscle fatigue, must be progressed slowly and cautiously. These patients should not exercise to exhaustion and should be given longer and more frequent rest intervals during and in between exercise sessions.[4,49] For example, a patient might rest 2 days between exercise sessions rather than just 1 day. Patients who are at risk for overwork weakness must be monitored very closely to evaluate ongoing responses to exercise and to determine if adjustments need to be made in the intensity or volume of the exercise program.

Exercise-Induced Muscle Soreness

Acute Muscle Soreness

Acute muscle soreness often develops during or directly after strenuous exercise performed to the point of muscle exhaustion.[38,84] This response occurs as a muscle becomes fatigued during acute exercise because of lack of adequate blood flow and oxygen (ischemia) and a temporary buildup of metabolites, such as lactic acid and potassium, in the exercised muscle.[38,153,176] The sensation is characterized as a burning or aching sensation within the muscle. It is thought that the noxious metabolic waste products may stimulate free nerve endings and cause pain. The muscle pain experienced during intense exercise is transient and subsides quickly after exercise when adequate blood flow and oxygen are restored to the muscle. An appropriate cool-down period of low-intensity exercise (active recovery) can facilitate this process.[44]

Delayed-Onset Muscle Soreness (DOMS)

After vigorous and unaccustomed resistance training or any form of muscular overexertion, delayed-onset muscle soreness, which is noticeable in the muscle belly or at the myotendinous junction,[66,96,134] begins to develop approximately 12 to 24 hours after the completion of exercise. As was already pointed out in the discussion of concentric and eccentric exercise, high-intensity eccentric exercise activities consistently cause the most severe DOMS symptoms.[13,58,74,92,96,195] Box 3–9 lists the signs and symptoms over the time-course of DOMS.*

Gradually, the DOMS sensation intensifies and usually peaks 24 to 48 hours after exercise. Although the time course varies, the signs and symptoms, which can last up to 10 to 14 days, gradually dissipate.[74,96,176]

Etiology of DOMS. Despite years of research dating back to the early 1900s,[132] the underlying cause of DOMS is still unclear. Several theories have been proposed and some have subsequently been refuted. Early investigators proposed the *metabolic waste accumulation theory,* which suggested that both acute and delayed-onset muscle soreness was caused by a buildup of lactic acid in muscle after exercise. Although this is a source of muscle pain with acute exercise, this theory has been disproved as a cause of DOMS.[262] Multiple studies have shown that it requires only about 1 hour of recovery after exercise to exhaustion to remove almost all lactic acid from skeletal muscle and blood.[96]

The *muscle spasm theory* also was proposed as the cause of DOMS, suggesting that a feedback cycle

Box 3–9 Delayed-onset Muscle Soreness: Clinical Signs and Symptoms

- Muscle soreness and aching beginning 12 to 48 hours after exercise and peaking at 48 to 72 hours
- Tenderness with palpation throughout the involved muscle belly or at the myotendinous junction
- Muscle soreness increases with passive stretching or an active contraction of the involved muscle
- Local edema and warmth
- Muscle stiffness reflected by spontaneous muscle shortening[66] before the onset of pain
- Decreased ROM during time-course of muscle soreness
- Decreased muscle strength prior to onset of muscle soreness that persists for up to 1 to 2 weeks after soreness has remitted[38,117,229]

*See references 13, 38, 66, 79, 96, 117, 134, 229.

of pain caused by ischemia and a buildup of metabolic waste products during exercise led to muscle spasm.[65] This, in turn, it was hypothesized, caused the DOMS sensation and an ongoing reflex pain-spasm cycle that lasted for several days after exercise. The muscle spasm theory has not been supported in subsequent research that showed no increase in EMG activity and, therefore, no evidence of spasm in muscles with delayed soreness.[2]

Although studies on the specific etiology of DOMS continue, current research seems to suggest that DOMS is linked to some form of contraction-induced microtrauma to muscle fibers and/or connective tissues that results in degeneration of these tissues. The damage, which is evident for several days after exercise, is accompanied by inflammation and edema.[2,84,98,100]

The temporary loss of strength and the perception of muscle soreness associated with DOMS appear to occur independently and follow different time courses. Strength deficits develop prior to the onset of soreness and persist after soreness has remitted.[62,192] Thus, force production deficits appear to be the result of muscle damage, specifically myofibrillar damage at the Z bands,[191] which directly affects the structural integrity of the contractile units of muscle, not neuromuscular inhibition as the result of pain.[191,192]

Prevention and treatment of DOMS. Prevention and treatment of DOMS at the initiation of an exercise program after a short or long period of inactivity has been either ineffective or at best only marginally successful. It is a commonly held opinion in clinical and fitness settings that the initial onset of DOMS may be prevented or at least limited by progressing the intensity and volume of exercise *gradually,*[8,74] by performing low-intensity warm-up and cool-down activities,[8,64,74,176,228] or by gently stretching the exercised muscles before and after strenuous exercise.[64,228] Although these techniques are regularly advocated and employed, little to no evidence in the literature supports their efficacy in the prevention of DOMS.

There is some evidence to suggest that the use of repetitive concentric exercise prior to DOMS-inducing eccentric exercise does not prevent but reduces the severity of muscle soreness and other markers of muscle damage.[194] Vitamin C and E supplements taken every day for approximately 1 week prior to the initiation of vigorous eccentric exercise has also been shown to minimize postexercise muscle damage and significantly decrease the severity of DOMS.[176] Paradoxically, the best prevention of DOMS is a regular routine exercise after an initial episode of DOMS has developed and remitted.[38,159,228]

Effective treatment of DOMS once it has occurred is continually being sought because, to date, the efficacy of DOMS treatment has been mixed. Evidence shows that continuation of a training program that has induced DOMS does not worsen the muscle damage or slow the recovery process.[195] Light, high-speed (isokinetic), concentric exercise has been reported to reduce muscle soreness and hasten the remediation of strength deficits associated with DOMS,[117] but other reports suggest no significant improvement in strength or relief of muscle soreness with light exercise.[70,264]

The value of therapeutic modalities and massage techniques is also questionable. Electrical stimulation to reduce soreness has been reported to be effective[62] and ineffective.[264] Although cryotherapy (cold water immersion) after vigorous eccentric exercise reduces signs of muscle damage (creatine kinase activity), it has been reported to have no effect on the perpetuation of muscle tenderness or strength deficit.[83] There is also no significant evidence that postexercise massage, despite its widespread use in sports settings, reduces the signs and symptoms of DOMS.[252,264] In a recent prospective study[158] of DOMS that was induced by maximal eccentric exercise, the use of a compression sleeve over the exercised muscle group resulted in no increase in circumferential measurements of the upper arm (which could suggest a prevention of soft tissue swelling), a more rapid reduction in the perception of muscle soreness, and a more rapid amelioration of deficits in peak torque than recovery from DOMS without the use of compression. Finally, topical salicylate creams, which provide an analgesic effect, may also reduce the severity of and hasten the recovery from DOMS-related symptoms.[124] In summary, although some interventions for the treatment of DOMS appear to have potential, definitive treatment has yet to be determined.

Pathologic Fracture

When a patient with osteoporosis participates in a resistance exercise program, the risk of pathologic fracture must be considered. *Osteoporosis* is a systemic skeletal disease characterized by a reduction of mineralized bone mass that is associated with an imbalance between bone resorption and bone formation leading to fragility of bones. In addition to the loss of bone mass, there is also a narrowing of the bone shaft and widening of the medullary canal.[27,78,162,223] A differentiation is made between *osteoporosis* (−2.5 or more standard deviations in bone mineral density [BMD] below the young adult mean) and *osteopenia* (−1.0 to −2.5 standard deviations below the mean).[46]

The changes in bone associated with osteoporosis make the bone less able to withstand physical stresses and highly susceptible to pathologic fracture (fragility fracture). A **pathologic fracture** is a fracture of bone already weakened by disease that occurs as the result of very minor stresses to the skeletal system.[27,78,104,173,190] Pathologic fractures most commonly occur in the vertebrae, hips, wrists, and ribs.[78,162] Therefore, to design and implement a safe exercise program a therapist needs to know if a patient has a history of osteoporosis and subsequently an increased risk of pathologic fracture. If there is no known history of osteoporosis, the therapist must be able to recognize those factors that place a patient at risk for osteoporosis.[27,46,47,78,104,162,173] Special precautions to prevent pathologic fracture can then be taken during resistance exercises.

Risk Factors for Type I (Primary) Osteoporosis

- ***Normal aging.*** Affects men and women
- ***Hormonal imbalance or deficiency.*** Postmenopausal decrease in estrogen secretion
- ***Hereditary factors.*** Family history; racial and ethnic background (example: higher incidence in white women)
- ***Idiopathic factors.*** Usually associated with prepubertal onset

Risk Factors for Type II (Secondary) Osteoporosis

- ***Prolonged immobilization.*** Postfracture; soft tissue or joint pain; swelling or joint effusion
- ***Prolonged disuse and inability to bear weight.*** Sedentary lifestyle, paralysis associated with neuromuscular disorders; inflammatory diseases
- ***Long-term use of medications.*** Systemic corticosteroids for patients with inflammatory diseases or post-transplant patients; immunosuppressants for patients with cancer or inflammatory diseases; anticoagulants; anticonvulsants and others

Malignancy and radiation therapy. Both the pathology and the treatment weaken bone.

Prevention of Pathologic Fracture

As noted earlier in this chapter, evidence of the positive osteogenic effects of resistance exercise is promising but not yet clear. Despite this, resistance exercises have become an essential element of rehabilitation and conditioning programs for patients with known or who are at risk for osteoporosis.[46,203,220,223] Therefore, patients who are also at risk for pathologic fracture often engage in resistance training.[190]

A successful resistance exercise program for these patients imposes enough load (greater than what regularly occurs with ADL) to achieve the goals of the exercise program (which might include increasing bone density) but not too heavy a load that could cause a pathologic fracture. To prevent or reduce the risk of pathologic fracture the following precautions are suggested:[46,104,190,203,220,223]

- Avoid high-intensity (high-load), high-volume weight training. Depending on the severity of osteoporosis, begin weight training at low intensities and perform only one set of several exercises. Keep intensity low for 6 to 8 weeks.
- Progress intensity and volume very gradually: eventually up to three to four sets of each exercise at moderate levels of intensity, if appropriate.
- Avoid high-impact activities such as jumping or hopping. Perform most strengthening exercises in weight-bearing postures that involve low impact to no impact, such as lunges or step-ups/step-downs against additional resistance (handheld weights, weighted vest, or elastic resistance).
- Avoid high-velocity movements of the spine or extremities.
- Avoid trunk flexion with rotation and end-range resisted flexion of the spine that could place excessive loading on the anterior portion of vertebrae, which could result in anterior compression fracture, wedging of the vertebral body, and loss of height.
- Avoid lower extremity weight-bearing activities that involve torsional movements of the hips, particularly if there is evidence of osteoporosis of the proximal femur.
- To avoid loss of balance or falling during lower extremity closed-chain exercises, have the patient hold onto a stable surface such as a countertop for balance. If the patient is at high risk for falling

or has a history of falls, perform exercises in a chair to provide weight bearing through the spine.

- In group exercise classes keep participant-instructor ratios low; for patients with high risk for falling or a history of previous fracture, consider direct supervision on a 1 to 1 basis from another trained person.

Contraindications to Resistance Training

There are only a few instances when resistance exercises are contraindicated. Resistance training is most often contraindicated during periods of acute inflammation and with some acute diseases and disorders.[30] By carefully selecting the appropriate mode of exercise (state vs. dynamic; weight-bearing vs. nonweight-bearing) and keeping the intensity of the exercise at a very low to moderate level, adverse effects from resistance training can be avoided.

Pain

If a patient experiences severe joint or muscle pain during active-free (unresisted) movements, dynamic resistance exercises should not be initiated. During testing, if a patient experiences acute muscle pain during a resisted isometric contraction, resistance exercises (static or dynamic) should not be initiated. If a patient experiences pain that cannot be eliminated by redoing the resistance, the exercise should be stopped.

Inflammation

Dynamic and static resistance training is absolutely contraindicated in the presence of inflammatory neuromuscular disease. For example, in patients with acute anterior horn cell disease (Guillain-Barré) or inflammatory muscle disease (polymyositis, dermatomyositis) resistance exercises may actually cause irreversible deterioration of strength as the result of damage to muscle. *Dynamic* resistance exercises are contraindicated in the presence of acute inflammation of a joint. The use of resisted dynamic exercise will irritate the joint and cause more inflammation. Gentle setting (static) exercises against negligible resistance is appropriate.

Severe Cardiopulmonary Disease

Severe cardiac or respiratory diseases or disorders associated with acute symptoms contraindicate resistance training. For example, patients with severe coronary artery disease, carditis, or cardiac myopathy should not participate in vigorous physical activities, including a resistance training program.[7,8] Resistance training should be postponed for up to 12 weeks postmyocardial infarction or coronary artery bypass graft surgery or until the patient has clearance from a physician.[30]

▶ Manual Resistance Exercise

Definition and Use in Rehabilitation

Manual resistance exercise is a form of active resistive exercise in which the resistance force is applied by the therapist to either a dynamic or a static muscular contraction.

- When joint motion is permissible, resistance is usually applied throughout the available ROM as the muscle contracts and shortens or lengthens under tension.
- Exercise is carried out in the anatomic planes of motion, in diagonal patterns associated with proprioceptive neuromuscular facilitation (PNF) techniques,[260] or in combined patterns of movement that simulate functional activities.
- A specific muscle may also be strengthened by resisting the action of that muscle, as described in manual muscle-testing procedures.[15,57]
- In rehabilitation programs manual resistance exercise is part of the continuum of active exercises available to the therapist for the improvement or restoration of muscular strength and endurance. There are many advantages to the use of manual resistance exercises, but there are also disadvantages and limitations to this form of resistance exercises. These issues are summarized in Box 3–10.

Guidelines and Special Considerations for Manual Resistance Exercise

The general principles for the application of resistance exercises discussed in the preceding section of this chapter apply to manual resistance exercise. In addition, there are some special guidelines that are unique to manual resistance exercises that also should be followed when using this form of resistance exercise. These guidelines apply to manual resistance applied in anatomic planes of motion discussed in this section and to manual resistance used in association with PNF, discussed in the following section of this chapter.

Box 3–10 Manual Resistance Exercise: Advantages and Disadvantages

Advantages

- Most effective in early stages of rehabilitation when muscles are weak (4/5 or less).
- Effective form of exercise for transition from assisted to mechanically resisted movements.
- More finely graded resistance than mechanical resistance.
- Resistance is adjusted throughout the ROM as the therapist responds to the patient's efforts or a painful arc.
- Muscle works maximally at all portions of the ROM.
- The range of joint movement can be carefully controlled by the therapist to protect healing tissues or to prevent movement into an unstable portion of the range.
- Useful for dynamic or static strengthening.
- Direct manual stabilization prevents substitute motions.
- Can be performed in a variety of patient positions.
- Placement of resistance easily adjusted.
- Gives the therapist an opportunity for direct interaction with the patient to continually monitor the patient's performance.

Disadvantages

- Exercise load (amount of resistance) is subjective; it cannot be measured or quantitatively documented.
- Amount of resistance limited to the strength of the therapist; therefore, resistance imposed is not adequate to strengthen already strong muscle groups.
- Little value for strong muscle groups.
- Speed of movement is slow to moderate, which may not carry over to most functional activities.
- Cannot be performed independently by the patient to strengthen most muscle groups.
- Not useful in home program unless caregiver assistance is available.
- Labor- and time-intensive for the therapist.
- Impractical for improving muscular endurance; too time-consuming.

Body Mechanics of the Therapist

1. Select a treatment table on which to position the patient that is a suitable height or adjust the height of the patient's bed, if possible, to enhance use of proper body mechanics.
2. Assume a position close to the patient to avoid stresses on your low back and maximize control of the patient's upper or lower extremity.
3. Use a wide base of support to maintain a stable posture while manually applying resistance; shift your weight to move as the patient moves his or her limb.

Application of Manual Resistance and Stabilization

1. Review the principles and guidelines for placement and direction of resistance and stabilization depicted in Figures 3–8 and 3–9. Stabilize the proximal attachment of the contracting muscle with one hand when necessary while applying resistance distally to the moving segment. Use appropriate hand placements (manual contacts) to provide tactile and proprioceptive cues to help the patient better understand in which direction to move.[247]
2. Grade and vary the amount of resistance to equal the abilities of the muscle through all portions of the available ROM.

Note: It requires well-developed skills on the part of the therapist to provide enough resistance to challenge but not overpower the patient's efforts, especially when the patient has significant weakness.

3. Gradually apply and release the resistance so that movements are smooth, not unexpected or uncontrolled.
4. Hold the extremity close to your body so that some of the force applied is from the weight of your body not just the strength of your upper extremities. This allows you to apply a greater amount of resistance, particularly as the patient's strength increases.
5. When applying manual resistance to alternating isometric contractions of agonist and antagonist muscles to develop joint stability, maintain manual contacts at all times as the isometric contractions are repeated. As a transition is made from one muscle contraction to another, no distinct relaxation phase or joint movements should occur between the opposing contractions.

Verbal Commands

1. Coordinate the *timing* of the verbal commands with the application of resistance to maintain control when the patient initiates a movement.
2. Use simple direct verbal commands.
3. Use different verbal commands to facilitate isometric, concentric, or eccentric contractions.
4. To resist an *isometric* contraction, tell the patient to "Hold" or "Don't let me move you" or "Match my resistance."
5. To resist a *concentric* contraction, tell the patient to "Push" or "Pull."
6. To resist an *eccentric* contraction, tell the patient to "Slowly let go as I push or pull you."

Number of Repetitions and Sets; Rest Intervals

- As with all forms of resistance exercise, the number of repetitions is dependent upon the response of the patient.
- In manual resistance exercise the volume of exercise is also contingent upon strength and endurance of the therapist.
- Build in adequate rest intervals for the patient *and* the therapist; after 8 to 12 repetitions both the patient and the therapist will begin to experience some degree of fatigue.

Techniques of Manual Resistance Exercise for the Extremities: General Background

The manual resistance exercise techniques described in this section are for the upper and lower extremities, performed concentrically in the anatomic planes of motion. The direction of limb movement, of course, would be the opposite if manual resistance were applied to an eccentric contraction (see Fig. 3–8). The exercises described are performed in nonweight-bearing positions and involve open-chain movements to isolate individual muscles or muscle groups.

Consistent with Chapter 2, most of the exercises described and illustrated in this section are performed with the patient in a *supine position*. Variations in the therapist's position and hand placements may be necessary, depending on the size and strength of the therapist and patient. Alternate positions are described when appropriate or necessary. Ultimately a therapist must be versatile and able to apply manual resistance with the patient in all positions, to meet the needs of many patients with significant differences in abilities, limitations, and pathologies.

Note: In all illustrations the direction in which resistance (R) is applied is indicated with a solid arrow.

Opposite motions, such as flexion/extension and abduction/adduction, are often alternately resisted in an exercise program in which strength and balanced neuromuscular control in both an agonist and an antagonist is desired. Resistance to reciprocal movement patterns also enhances a patient's ability to reverse the direction of movement smoothly and quickly, a neuromuscular skill that is necessary in many functional activities. Reversal of direction requires muscular control of both prime movers and stabilizers and combines concentric and eccentric contractions to decrease momentum and make a controlled transition from one direction to the opposite direction of movement.

The use of manual resistance in diagonal patterns of motion associated with PNF are described and illustrated in the next section of this chapter. Additional exercises to increase strength, endurance, and neuromuscular control in the extremities can be found in Chapters 9 through 14. In these chapters many examples and illustrations of resisted eccentric exercises, closed-chain exercises, and exercises in functional movement patterns are included. Resistance exercises for the cervical, thoracic, and lumbar spine are described and illustrated in Chapters 15 and 16.

The Upper Extremity

Flexion of the Shoulder

Hand Placement and Procedure

- Apply resistance to the anterior aspect of the distal arm or to the distal portion of the forearm if the elbow is stable and pain free (Fig. 3–10).
- Stabilization of the scapula and trunk is provided by the treatment table.

Extension of the Shoulder

Hand Placement and Procedure

- Apply resistance to the posterior aspect of the distal arm or the distal portion of the forearm.
- Stabilization of the scapula is provided by the table.

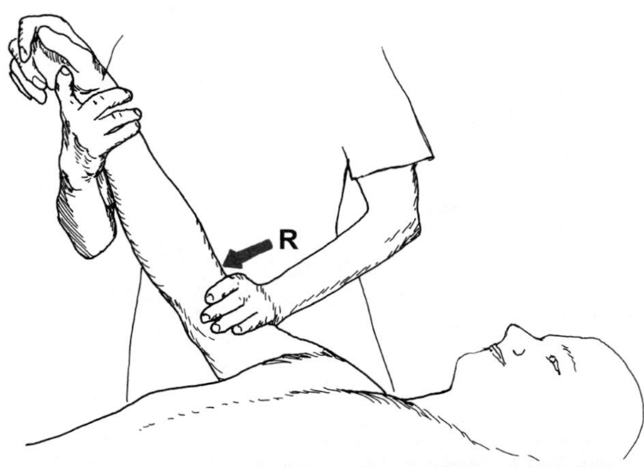

Figure 3–10 Resisted shoulder flexion.

Hyperextension of the Shoulder

The patient may be in the supine position, close to the edge of the table, side-lying, or prone so that hyperextension can occur.

Hand Placement and Procedure

- Apply resistance in the same manner as with extension of the shoulder.
- Stabilize the anterior aspect of the shoulder if the patient is supine.
- If the patient is side-lying, adequate stabilization must be given to the trunk and scapula. This can usually be done if the therapist places the patient close to the edge of the table and stabilizes the patient with the lower trunk.
- If the patient is lying prone, manually stabilize the scapula.

Abduction and Adduction of the Shoulder

Hand Placement and Procedure

- Apply resistance to the distal portion of the arm with the patient's elbow flexed to 90 degrees. To resist abduction (Fig. 3–11), give resistance to the lateral aspect of the arm. To resist adduction, give resistance to the medial aspect of the arm.
- Stabilization (although not pictured in Fig. 3–11) is applied to the superior aspect of the shoulder, if necessary, to prevent the patient from *initiating* abduction by shrugging the shoulder (elevation of the scapula).

Precaution: Allow the GH joint to externally rotate when resisting abduction above 90 degrees to prevent impingement.

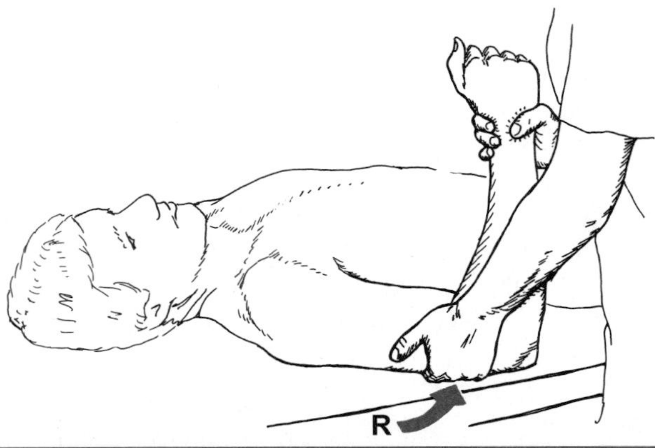

Figure 3–11 Resisted shoulder abduction.

Elevation of the Arm in the Plane of the Scapula ("Scaption")

Hand Placement and Procedure

- Same as previously described for shoulder flexion.
- Apply resistance as the patient elevates the arm in the plane of the scapula (30–40 degrees anterior to the frontal plane of the body).[48,69,169]

Although "scaption" is not a motion of the shoulder that occurs in one of the anatomic planes of the body, resistance in the scapular plane is thought to have its merits. Although evidence is inconclusive[48,271] as to whether or not the torque-producing capabilities of the key muscle groups of the glenohumeral joint are greater when the arm elevates in the plane of the scapula versus the frontal or sagittal planes, the glenohumeral joint has been shown to be more stable, and there is less risk of impingement of soft tissues when strength training is performed in the scapular plane.[69] (See additional discussion in Chapter 9.)

Internal and External Rotation of the Shoulder

Hand Placement and Procedure

- Flex the elbow to 90 degrees and position the shoulder in the plane of the scapula.
- Apply resistance to the distal portion of the forearm during internal rotation and external rotation (Fig. 3–12*A*).
- Stabilize at the level of the clavicle during internal rotation; the back and scapula are stabilized by the table during external rotation.

Alternate Procedure

Alternate alignment of the humerus (Fig. 3–12*B*). If mobility and stability of the glenohumeral joint permit, the shoulder can be positioned in 90 degrees of abduction during resisted rotation.

Horizontal Abduction and Adduction of the Shoulder

Hand Placement and Procedure

- Flex the shoulder and elbow to 90 degrees and place the shoulder in neutral rotation.
- Apply resistance to the distal portion of the arm just above the elbow during horizontal adduction and abduction.
- Stabilize the anterior aspect of the shoulder during horizontal adduction. The table stabilizes the scapula and trunk during horizontal abduction.
- To resist horizontal abduction from 0 to 45 de-

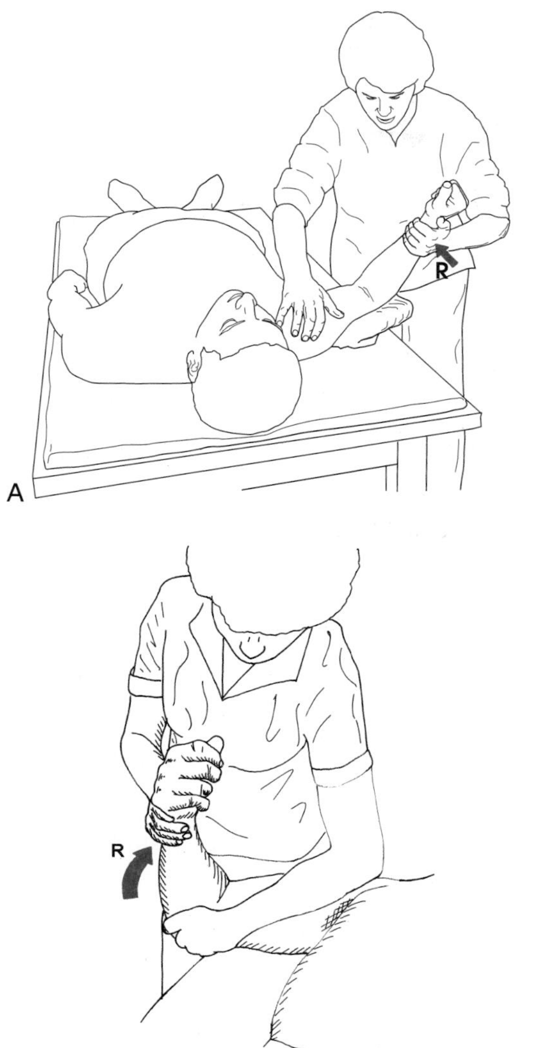

Figure 3–12 *(A)* Initially place the humerus in the plane of the scapula (POS) when resisting internal and external rotation of the shoulder; resisted shoulder external rotation in the POS. *(B)* Resisted shoulder internal rotation with the shoulder in 90 degrees of abduction.

grees, the patient must be close to the edge of the table while supine or be placed side-lying or prone.

Elevation and Depression of the Scapula

Hand Placement and Procedure

- Have the patient assume a supine, side-lying, or sitting position.
- Apply resistance along the superior aspect of the shoulder girdle just above the clavicle during scapular elevation (Fig. 3–13).

Alternate Procedures: Scapular Depression

To resist unilateral scapular depression in supine have the patient attempt to reach down toward the feet and push the hand into the therapist's hand. When the patient has adequate strength, the exercise can be done in a closed-chain by having the patient sit on the edge of a low table and lift the body weight with both hands.

Protraction and Retraction of the Scapula

Hand Placement and Procedure

- Apply resistance to the anterior portion of the shoulder at the head of the humerus to resist protraction and to the posterior aspect of the shoulder to resist retraction.
- Resistance may also be applied directly to the scapula if the patient sits or lies on the side, facing the therapist.
- Stabilize the trunk to prevent trunk rotation.

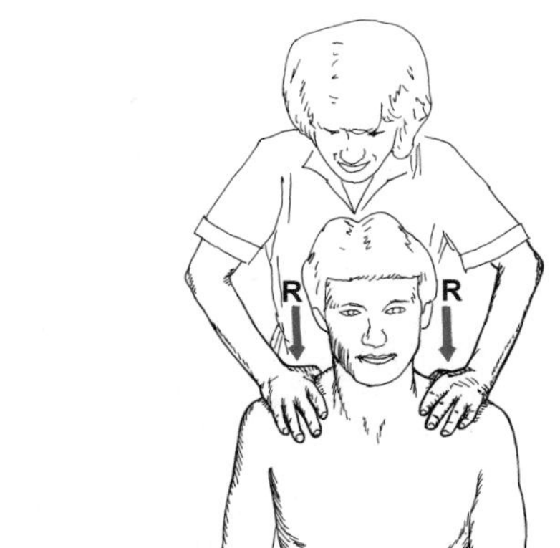

Figure 3–13 Elevation of the shoulders (scapulae), resisted bilaterally.

Flexion and Extension of the Elbow

Hand Placement and Procedure

- To strengthen the elbow flexors, apply resistance to the anterior aspect of the distal forearm (Fig. 3–14).
- The forearm may be positioned in supination, pronation, and neutral to resist individual flexor muscles of the elbow.
- To strengthen the elbow extensors, place the patient prone (Fig. 3–15) or supine and apply resistance to the distal aspect of the forearm.
- Stabilize the upper portion of the humerus during both motions.

Pronation and Supination of the Forearm

Hand Placement and Procedure

- Apply resistance to the radius of the distal forearm with the patient's elbow flexed to 90 degrees (Fig. 3–16) to prevent rotation of the humerus.
- Do not apply resistance to the hand to avoid twisting forces at the wrist.

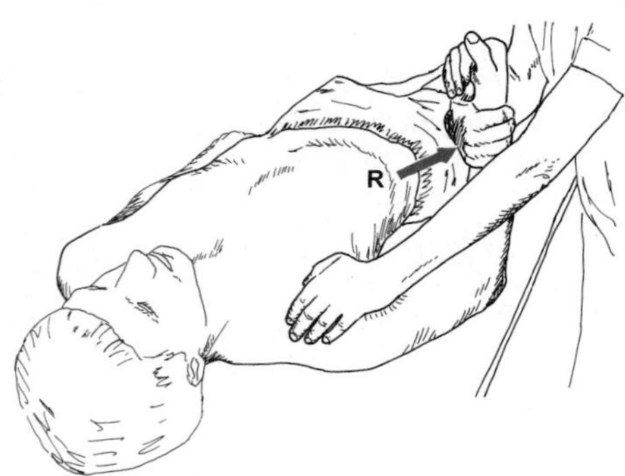

Figure 3–14 Resisted elbow flexion with proximal stabilization.

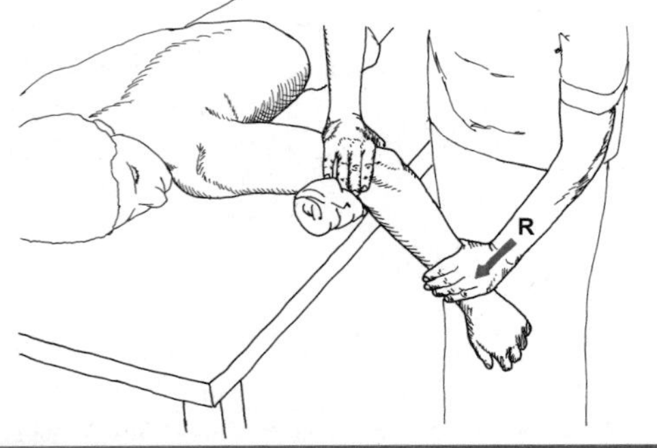

Figure 3–15 Resisted elbow extension.

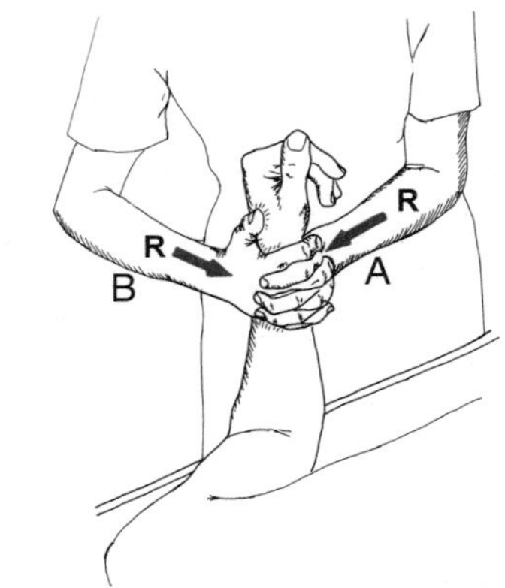

Figure 3–16 *(A)* Resisted pronation. *(B)* Resisted supination of the forearm.

Flexion and Extension of the Wrist

Hand Placement and Procedure

- Apply resistance to the volar and dorsal aspects of the hand at the level of the metacarpals to resist flexion and extension, respectively (Fig. 3–17).
- Stabilize the volar or dorsal aspect of the distal forearm.

Radial and Ulnar Deviation of the Wrist

Hand Placement and Procedure

- Apply resistance to second and fifth metacarpals alternately to resist radial and ulnar deviation.
- Stabilize the distal forearm.

Motions of the Fingers and Thumb

Hand Placement and Procedure

- Apply resistance just distal to the joint that is moving. Resistance is applied to one joint motion at a time (Figs. 3–18 and 3–19).
- Stabilize the joints proximal and distal to the moving joint.

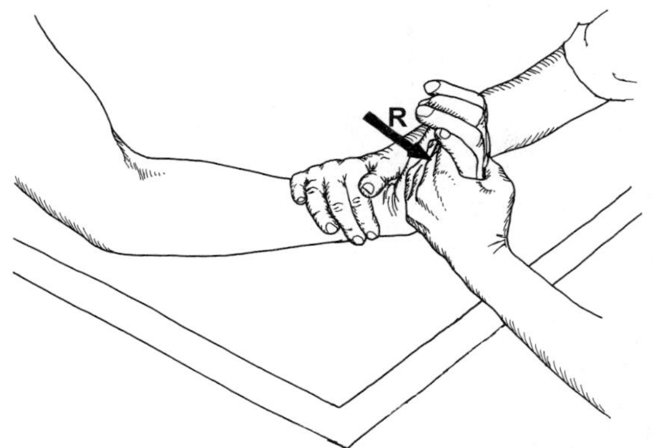

Figure 3–17 Resisted wrist flexion and stabilization of the forearm.

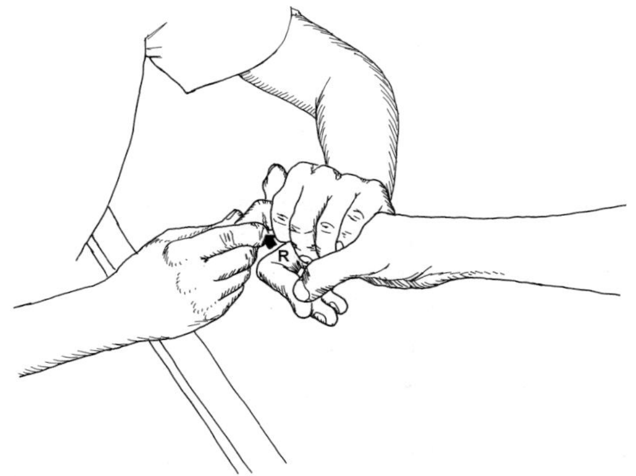

Figure 3–18 Resisted flexion of the proximal interphalangeal (PIP) joint of the index finger with stabilization of the MCP and DIP joints.

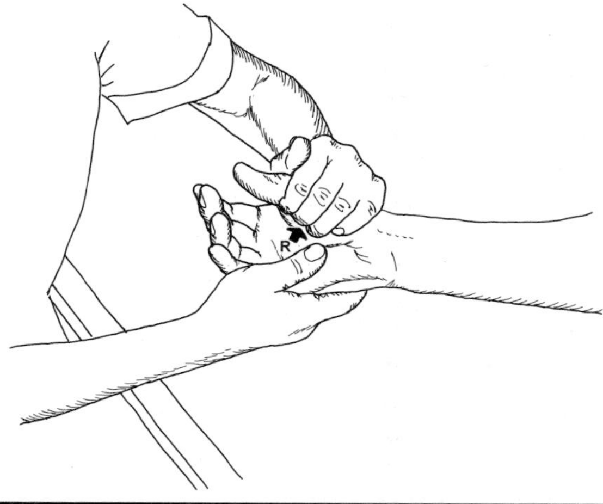

Figure 3–19 Resisted opposition of the thumb.

The Lower Extremity

Flexion of the Hip with Knee Flexion

Hand Placement and Procedure

- Apply resistance to the anterior portion of the distal thigh (Fig. 3–20). Simultaneous resistance to knee flexion may be applied at the distal and posterior aspect of the lower leg, just above the ankle.
- Stabilization of the pelvis and lumbar spine is provided by adequate strength of the abdominal muscles.

Precaution: If, when the opposite hip is extended, the pelvis rotates anteriorly and lordosis in the lumbar spine increases during resisted hip flexion, have the patient flex the opposite hip and knee and plant the foot on the table to stabilize the pelvis and protect the low back region.

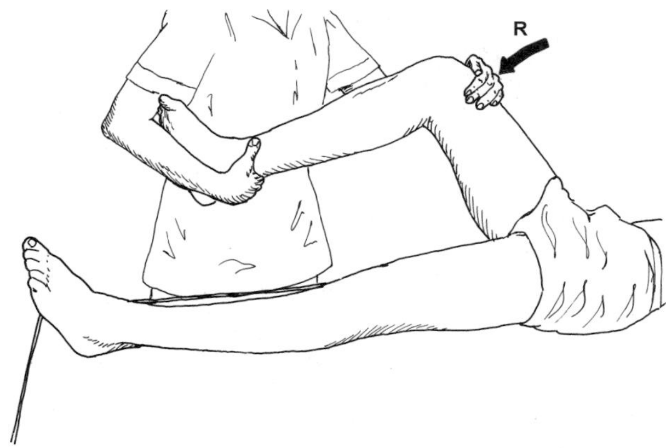

Figure 3–20 Resisted flexion of the hip with the knee flexed.

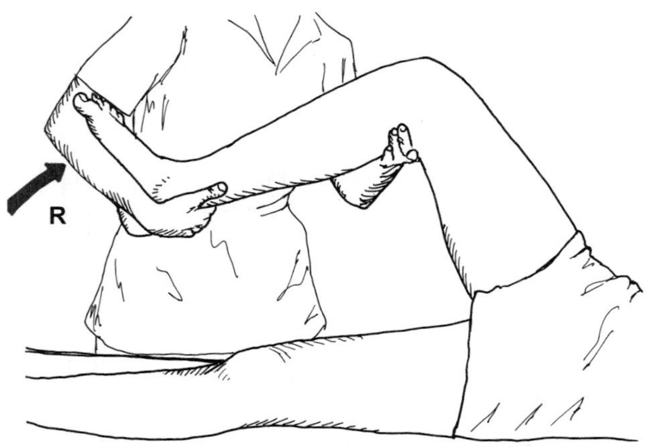

Figure 3–21 Resisted hip and knee extension with hand placement at the popliteal space to prevent hyperextension of the knee.

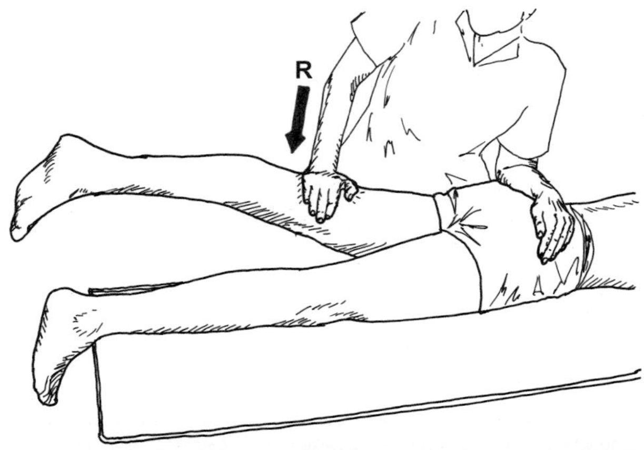

Figure 3–22 Resisted hyperextension of the hip with stabilization of the pelvis.

Extension of the Hip

Hand Placement and Procedure

- Apply resistance to the posterior aspect of the distal thigh with one hand and to the inferior and distal aspect of the heel with the other hand (Fig. 3–21).
- Stabilization of the pelvis and lumbar spine is provided by the table.

Hyperextension of the Hip

Patient position: Prone.

Hand Placement and Procedure

- Apply resistance to the posterior aspect of the distal thigh (Fig. 3–22).
- Stabilize the posterior aspect of the pelvis to avoid motion of the lumbar spine.

Abduction and Adduction of the Hip

Hand Placement and Procedure

- Apply resistance to the lateral and the medial aspects of the distal thigh to resist abduction (Fig. 3–23) and adduction, respectively, or to the lateral and medial aspects of the distal leg just above the malleoli if the knee is stable and pain-free.
- Stabilization is applied:
  - To the pelvis to avoid hip-hiking from substitute action of the quadratus lumborum
  - To keep the thigh in neutral position to prevent external rotation of the femur and subsequent substitution by the iliopsoas

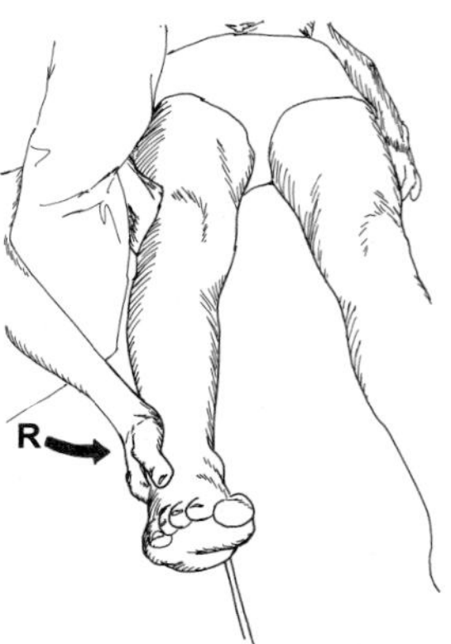

Figure 3–23 Resisted hip abduction.

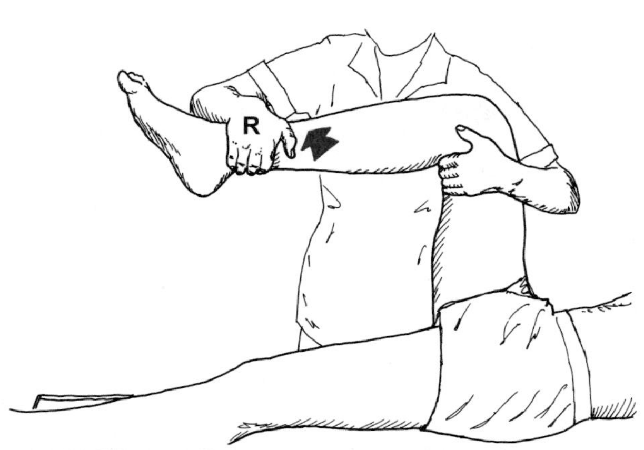

Figure 3–24 Resisted external rotation of the hip with the patient supine.

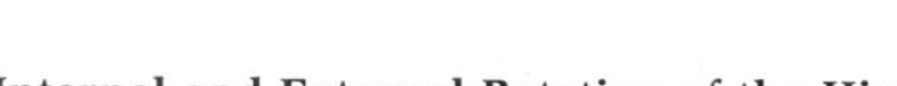

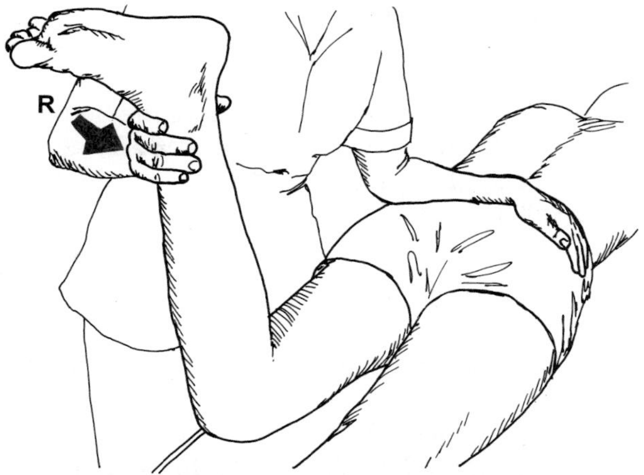

Figure 3–25 Resisted internal rotation of the hip with the patient prone.

Internal and External Rotation of the Hip

Patient position: Supine with the hip and knee extended.

Hand Placement and Procedure

- Apply resistance to the lateral aspect of the distal thigh to resist external rotation and to the medial aspect of the thigh to resist internal rotation.
- Stabilize the pelvis.

Patient position: Supine with the hip and knee flexed (Fig. 3–24).

Hand Placement and Procedure

- Apply resistance to the medial aspect of the lower leg just above the malleolus during external rotation and to the lateral aspect of the lower leg during internal rotation.
- Stabilize the anterior aspect of the pelvis as the thigh is supported to keep the hip in 90 degrees flexion.

Patient position: Prone, with the hip extended and the knee flexed (Fig. 3–25).

Hand Placement and Procedure

- Apply resistance to the medial and lateral aspects of the lower leg.
- Stabilize the pelvis by applying pressure across the buttocks.

Flexion of the Knee

Resistance to knee flexion may be combined with resistance to hip flexion as described earlier with the patient supine.

Patient position: Prone with the hip extended (Fig. 3–26).

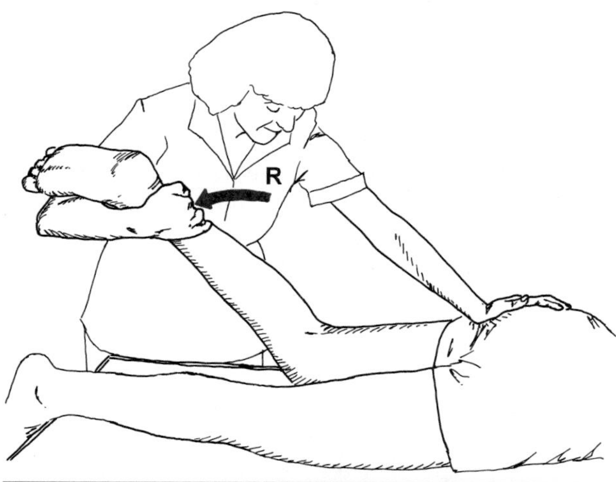

Figure 3–26 Resisted knee flexion with stabilization of the hip.

Hand Placement and Procedure

- Apply resistance to the posterior aspect of the lower leg just above the heel.
- Stabilize the posterior pelvis across the buttocks.

The patient may also be sitting at the edge of a table with the hips and knees flexed and the trunk supported and stabilized.

Extension of the Knee

Patient Position

- If the patient is lying supine on a table, the hip must be abducted and the knee flexed so the lower leg is over the side of the table. This position should not be used if the rectus femoris or iliopsoas is tight, because it will cause an anterior tilt of the pelvis and place stress on the low back.
- If the patient is prone, place a rolled towel under the anterior aspect of the distal thigh; this will allow the patella to glide normally during knee extension.

Hand Placement and Procedure

- Apply resistance to the anterior aspect of the lower leg.
- Stabilize the femur and pelvis.

The sitting position is often used for vigorous strengthening of the knee extensors. If this position is used, trunk and back stabilization is necessary for optimum performance.

Dorsiflexion and Plantarflexion of the Ankle

Hand Placement and Procedure

- Apply resistance to the dorsum of the foot just above the toes to resist dorsiflexion (Fig. 3–27*A*) and to the plantar surface of the foot at the metatarsals to resist plantarflexion (Fig. 3–27*B*).
- Stabilize the lower leg.

Inversion and Eversion of the Ankle

Hand Placement and Procedure

- Apply resistance to the medial aspect of the first metatarsal to resist inversion and to the lateral aspect of the fifth metatarsal to resist eversion.
- Stabilize the lower leg.

Flexion and Extension of the Toes

Hand Placement and Procedure

- Apply resistance to the plantar and dorsal surfaces of the toes as the patient flexes and extends the toes.
- Stabilize the joints above and below the joint that is moving.

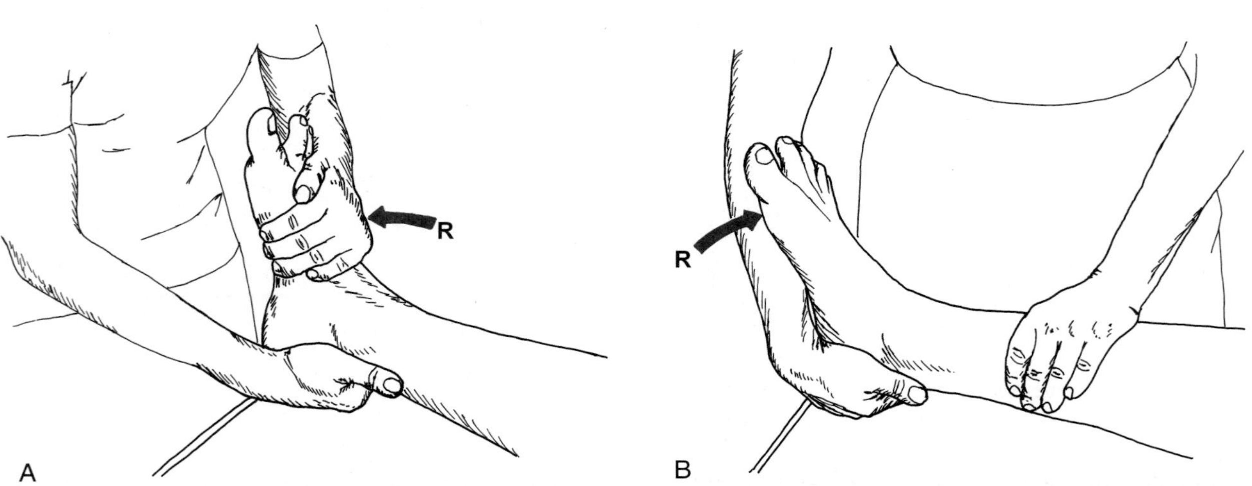

Figure 3–27 *(A)* Resisted dorsiflexion. *(B)* Resisted plantarflexion of the ankle.

Proprioceptive Neuromuscular Facilitation: Principles and Techniques

Proprioceptive neuromuscular facilitation (PNF) is an approach to therapeutic exercise that combines functionally based diagonal patterns of movement with techniques of neuromuscular facilitation to evoke motor responses and improve neuromuscular control and function. This widely used approach to exercise was developed in the 1940s and 1950s by the pioneering work of Kabat, Knott, and Voss.[152,260] Their work integrated the analysis of movement during functional activities with then-current theories of motor development, control, and learning and principles of neurophysiology as the foundations of their approach to exercise and rehabilitation. Long associated with neurorehabilitation, PNF techniques also have widespread application for rehabilitation of patients with musculoskeletal conditions that result in altered neuromuscular control of the extremities, neck, and trunk.[14,205,247]

PNF techniques can be used to develop muscular strength and endurance; facilitate stability, mobility, neuromuscular control, and coordinated movements; and lay a foundation for the restoration of function. PNF techniques are useful throughout the continuum of rehabilitation from the early phase of tissue healing when isometric techniques are appropriate to the final phase of rehabilitation when high-speed, diagonal movements can be performed against maximum resistance. Hallmarks of this approach to therapeutic exercise are the use of diagonal patterns and the application of sensory cues, specifically proprioceptive, cutaneous, visual, and auditory stimuli, to elicit or augment motor responses. Imbedded in this philosophy and approach to exercise is that the strong muscle groups of a diagonal pattern facilitate the responsiveness of the weaker muscle groups. The focus of discussion of PNF in this chapter deals with the use of PNF patterns and techniques as an important form of resistance exercise for the development of strength, muscular endurance, and dynamic stability. Although PNF patterns for the extremities can be performed unilaterally or bilaterally and in a variety of open- and closed-chain positions, only unilateral patterns with the patient in a supine position are described and illustrated. In Chapter 5 of this text, the use of PNF techniques, specifically contract-relax or hold-relax techniques or other variations, to increase flexibility are described. As noted in Chapter 2, PNF patterns can also be used for passive and active ROM. Additional application of PNF techniques for the extremities and trunk, some using resistance equipment, are described in the regional chapters later in this text.

The Diagonal Patterns

The patterns of movement associated with PNF are composed of *multijoint, multiplanar, diagonal,* and *rotational* movements of the extremities, trunk, and neck. Multiple muscle groups contract simultaneously. There are two pairs of diagonal patterns for the upper and lower extremities: Diagonal 1(D_1) and Diagonal 2(D_2). Each of these patterns can be performed in either flexion or extension. Hence, the terminology used is D_1Flexion or Extension and D_2Flexion or Extension of the upper or lower extremities. The patterns are identified by the motions occurring at proximal pivot points, either the shoulder or the hip joints. In other words, a pattern is named by *the position of the shoulder or hip when the diagonal pattern has been **completed.*** Flexion or extension of the shoulder or hip is coupled with abduction or adduction as well as external or internal rotation. Motions of body segments distal to the shoulder or hip also occur simultaneously during each diagonal pattern. Table 3–8 summarizes the component motions of each of the diagonal patterns. As mentioned, the diagonal patterns can be carried out unilaterally or bilaterally. Bilateral patterns can be done *symmetrically* (e.g., D_1Flexion of both extremities); *asymmetrically* (D_1Flexion of one extremity coupled with D_2Flexion of the other extremity); or *reciprocally* (D_1Flexion of one extremity and D_1 Extension of the opposite extremity). In addition, there are patterns specifically for the scapula or pelvis and techniques that integrate diagonal movements into functional activities such as rolling, crawling, and walking. There are several in-depth resources that describe and illustrate the many variations and applications of PNF techniques.[247,260]

Basic Procedures and Principles Used with PNF Patterns

A number of basic procedures that involve the application of multiple types of sensory cues are superimposed on the diagonal patterns to elicit the

Table 3–8 Component Motions of PNF Patterns: Upper and Lower Extremities

Joints or Segments	Diagonal 1: Flexion (D_1 Flx)	Diagonal 1: Extension (D_1 Ext)	Diagonal 2: Flexion (D_2 Flx)	Diagonal 2: Extension (D_2 Ext)
	UPPER EXTREMITY COMPONENT MOTIONS			
Shoulder	*Flexion-Adduction External Rotation*	*Extension-Abduction Internal Rotation*	*Flexion-Abduction External Rotation*	*Extension-Adduction Internal Rotation*
Scapula	Elevation, abduction, upward rotation	Depression, adduction, downward rotation	Elevation, abduction, upward rotation	Depression, adduction downward rotation
Elbow	Flexion or extension	Flexion or extension	Flexion or extension	Flexion or extension
Forearm	Supination	Pronation	Supination	Pronation
Wrist	Flexion, radial deviation	Extension, ulnar deviation	Extension, radial deviation	Flexion, ulnar deviation
Fingers and Thumb	Flexion, adduction	Extension, abduction	Extension, abduction	Flexion, adduction
	LOWER EXTREMITY COMPONENT MOTIONS			
Hip	*Flexion-Adduction External Rotation*	*Extension-Abduction Internal Rotation*	*Flexion-Abduction Internal Rotation*	*Extension-Adduction External Rotation*
Knee	Flexion or extension	Flexion or extension	Flexion or extension	Flexion or extension
Ankle	Dorsiflexion, inversion	Plantarflexion, eversion	Dorsiflexion, eversion	Plantarflexion, inversion
Toes	Extension	Flexion	Extension	Flexion

best possible neuromuscular responses. Although the diagonal patterns can be used with various forms of mechanical resistance, such as free weights, simple weight-pulley systems, elastic resistance, or even an isokinetic unit, the interaction between the patient and therapist, a prominent feature of PNF, particularly in the early phases of re-establishing neuromuscular control, provides the greatest amount and variety of sensory input.

Manual Contacts

This refers to how and where the therapist's hands are placed on the patient. Whenever possible, manual contacts are placed over the agonist muscle groups or their tendinous insertions. These contacts allow the therapist to apply resistance to the appropriate muscle groups and cue the patient as to the desired direction of movement. For example, if wrist and finger extension is to be facilitated, then manual contact is on the dorsal surface of the hand and wrist. In the extremity patterns one manual contact is placed distally (where movement begins). The other manual contact can be placed more proximally, for example, at the shoulder or scapula. Placement of manual contacts is adjusted based on the patient's response and level of control.

Maximal Resistance

The amount of resistance applied during dynamic concentric muscle contractions is the greatest amount possible that still allows the patient to move smoothly and without pain through the available range. Resistance should be adjusted throughout the pattern to accommodate to strong and weak portions of the pattern. Maximal resistance is the means by which *irradiation (overflow)* from strong to weak muscle groups occurs.

Position and Movement of the Therapist

The therapist remains positioned and aligned along the diagonal planes of movement with shoulders and trunk facing in the direction of the moving limb. Use of effective body mechanics is essential. Resistance should be applied through body weight, not only through the upper extremities. The therapist must use a wide base of support, move with the patient and pivot over the base of support to allow rotation to occur in the diagonal pattern.

Stretch

The *stretch stimulus* is the placing of body segments in positions that lengthen the muscles that are to contract during the diagonal movement pattern. For example, prior to initiating D_1Flexion of the lower extremity, the lower limb is placed in D_1Extension.

Rotation is of utmost consideration because it is the rotational component that elongates the muscle fibers and spindles of the agonist muscles of a given pattern and increases the excitability and responsiveness of those muscles. The stretch stimulus is sometimes described as "winding up the part" or "taking up the slack."

The *stretch reflex* is facilitated by a rapid stretch (overpressure) just past the point of tension to an already elongated agonist muscle. The stretch reflex is usually directed to a distal muscle group to elicit a phasic muscle contraction to initiate a given diagonal movement pattern. The quick stretch is followed by sustained resistance to the agonist muscles to keep the contracting muscles under tension. For example, to initiate D_1Flexion of the upper extremity, a quick stretch is applied to the already elongated wrist and finger flexors followed by application of resistance. A quick stretch can also be applied to any agonist muscle group at any point in the execution of a diagonal pattern to further stimulate an agonist muscle contraction or direct a patient's attention to a weak component of a pattern. (See additional discussion of the use of repeated contractions in the next section which describes special PNF techniques.)

Precaution: Use of a stretch reflex, even prior to resisted isometric muscle contractions, is not advisable in the early stages of soft tissue healing after injury or surgery. It is also inappropriate with acute or active arthritic conditions.

Normal Timing

A *sequence* of distal to proximal, coordinated muscle contractions occurs during the diagonal movement patterns. The distal component motions of the pattern should be completed halfway through the pattern. Correct sequencing of movements promotes neuromuscular control and coordinated movement.

Traction

Traction is the slight separation of joint surfaces and appears to inhibit pain and facilitate movement during execution of the movement patterns. Traction is most often applied during flexion (antigravity) patterns.

Approximation

The gentle compression of joint surfaces, by means of manual compression or weight-bearing, stimulates co-contraction of agonists and antagonists to enhance dynamic stability and postural control via joint and muscle mechanoreceptors.

Verbal Commands

Auditory cues are given to enhance motor output. The tone and volume of the verbal commands are varied to help maintain the patient's attention. A sharp verbal command is given simultaneously with the application of the stretch reflex to synchronize the phasic, reflexive motor response with a sustained volitional effort by the patient. Verbal cues then direct the patient throughout the movement patterns. As the patient learns the sequence of movements, verbal cues can be more succinct.

Visual Cues

The patient is asked to follow the movement of a limb to further enhance control of movement throughout the ROM.

Upper Extremity Patterns

Note: All descriptions for hand placements are for the patient's (R) upper extremity. During each pattern tell the patient to watch the moving hand. Be sure that rotation shifts *gradually* from internal to external rotation (or vice versa) throughout the range. By midrange, the arm should be in neutral rotation. Manual contacts (hand placements) may be altered from the suggested placements as long as contact remains on the appropriate surfaces. Resist all patterns through the full, available ROM.

D_1Flexion

Starting Position (Fig. 3–28A)
Position the upper extremity in shoulder extension, abduction, and internal rotation; elbow extension; forearm pronation and wrist and finger extension with the hand about 8 to 12 inches from the hip.

Hand Placement
Place the index and middle fingers of your (R) hand in the palm of the patient's hand and your (L) hand on the volar surface of the distal forearm or at the cubital fossa of the elbow.

Verbal Commands
As you apply a quick stretch to the wrist and finger flexors, tell the patient "Squeeze my fingers, turn your palm up; pull your arm up and across your face," as you resist the pattern.

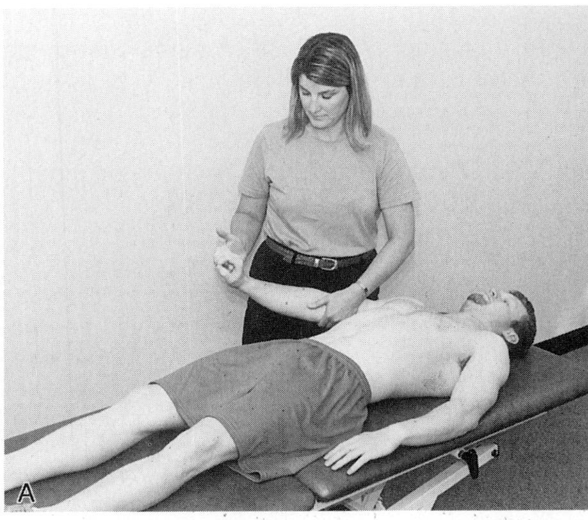

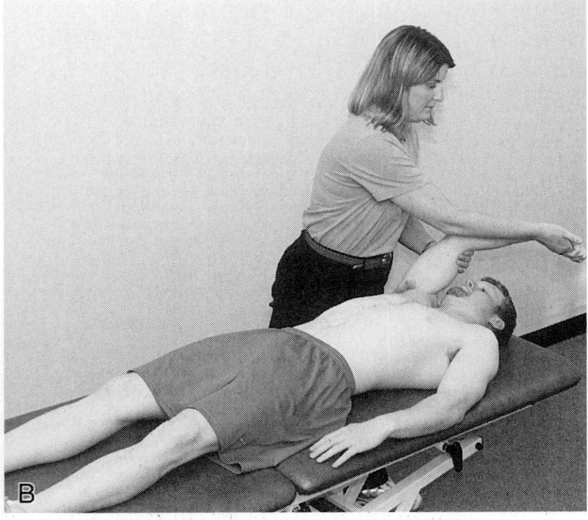

Figure 3–28 *(A)* Starting position and *(B)* ending position for D_1 Flexion of the upper extremity.

Ending Position (Fig. 3–28B)
Complete the pattern with the arm across the face in shoulder flexion, adduction, external rotation; partial elbow flexion; forearm supination and wrist and finger flexion.

D_1Extension

Starting Position (Fig. 3–29A)
Begin as described for completion of D_1Flexion.

Hand Placements
Grasp the dorsal surface of the patient's hand and fingers with your (R) hand using a *lumbrical grip.* Place your (L) hand on the extensor surface of the arm just proximal to the elbow.

Verbal Commands
As you apply a quick stretch to the wrist and finger extensors, tell the patient, "Open your hand" (or "Wrist and fingers up"); "Push your arm down and out."

Ending Position (Fig. 3–29B)
Finish the pattern in shoulder extension, abduction, internal rotation; elbow extension; forearm pronation and wrist and finger extension.

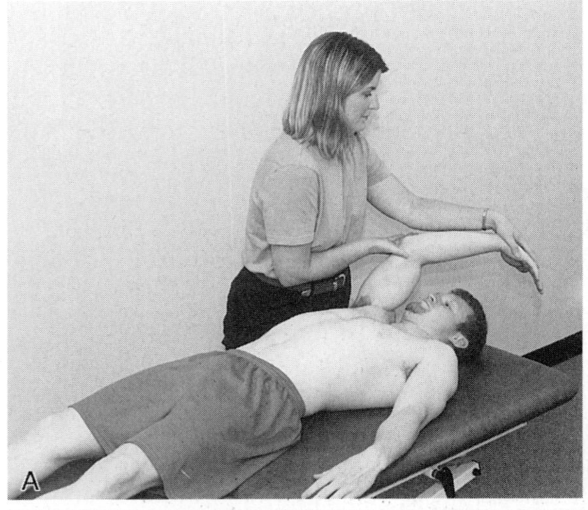

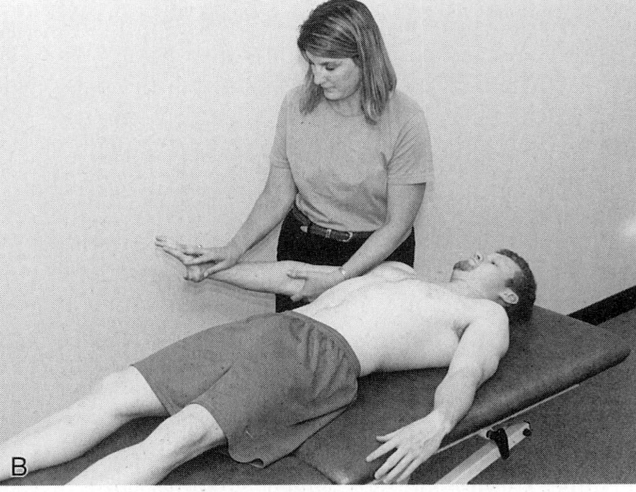

Figure 3–29 *(A)* Starting position and *(B)* ending position for D_1 Extension of the upper extremity.

D_2Flexion

Starting Position (Fig. 3–30A)
Position the upper extremity in shoulder extension, adduction and internal rotation; elbow extension; forearm pronation and wrist and finger flexion. The forearm should lie across the umbilicus.

Hand Placement
Grasp the dorsum of the patient's hand with your (L) hand using a lumbrical grip. Grasp the dorsal surface of the patient's forearm close to the elbow with your (R) hand.

Verbal Commands
As you apply a quick stretch to the wrist and finger extensors, tell the patient, "Open your hand and turn it to your face"; "Lift your arm up and out"; "Point your thumb out."

Ending Position (Fig. 3–30B)
Finish the pattern in shoulder flexion, abduction, and external rotation; elbow extension; forearm supination and wrist and finger extension. The arm should be 8 to 10 inches from the ear; the thumb should be pointing to the floor.

D_2Extension

Starting Position (Fig. 3–31A)
Begin as described for completion of D_2Flexion.

Hand Placement
Place the index and middle fingers of your (R) hand in the palm of the patient's hand and your (L) hand on the volar surface of the forearm or distal humerus.

Verbal Commands
As you apply a quick stretch to the wrist and finger flexors, tell the patient, "Squeeze my fingers, and pull down and across your chest."

Ending Position (Fig. 3–31B)
Complete the pattern in shoulder extension, adduction, and internal rotation; elbow extension; forearm pronation and wrist and finger flexion. The forearm should cross the umbilicus.

Lower Extremity Patterns

Note: Follow the same guidelines with regard to rotation and resistance as previously described for the upper extremity. All descriptions of hand placements are for the patient's (R) lower extremity.

D_1Flexion

Starting Position (Fig. 3–32A)
Position the lower extremity in hip extension abduction and internal rotation; knee extension; plantar flexion and eversion of the ankle; and toe flexion.

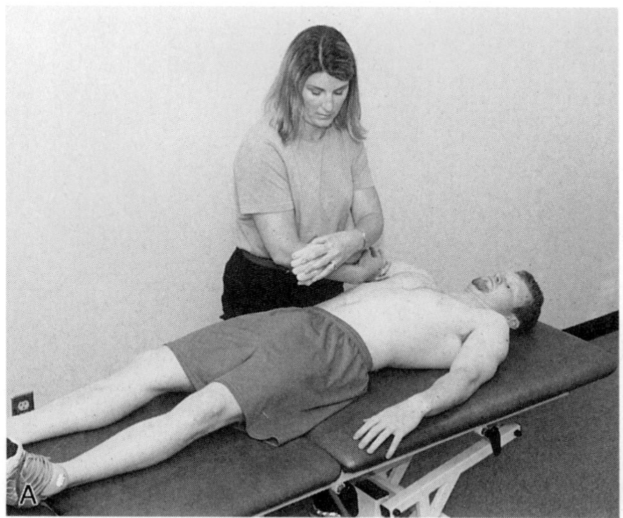

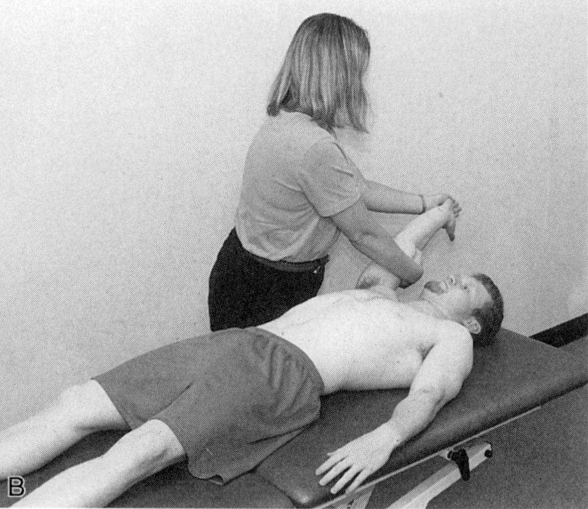

Figure 3–30 *(A)* Starting position and *(B)* ending position for D_2 Flexion of the upper extremity.

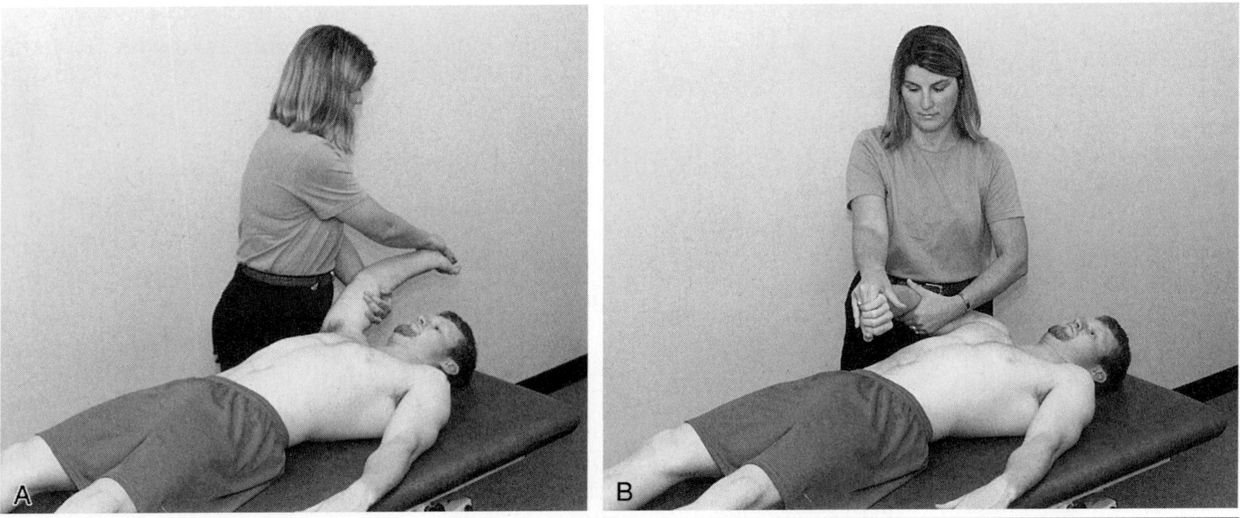

Figure 3–31 *(A)* Starting position and *(B)* ending position for D_2 Extension of the upper extremity.

Note: This pattern may also be initiated with the knee flexed and the lower leg over the edge of the table.

Hand Placement

Place your (R) hand on the dorsal and medial surface of the foot and toes and your (L) hand on the anteromedial aspect of the thigh just proximal to the knee.

Verbal Commands

As you apply a quick stretch to the ankle dorsiflexors and invertors and toe extensors, tell the patient, "Foot and toes up and in; bend your knee; pull your leg over and across."

Ending Position (Fig. 3–32B)

Complete the pattern in hip flexion, adduction, and external rotation; knee flexion (or extension); ankle dorsiflexion and inversion; toe extension. The hip should be adducted across the midline, creating lower trunk rotation to the patient's (L) side.

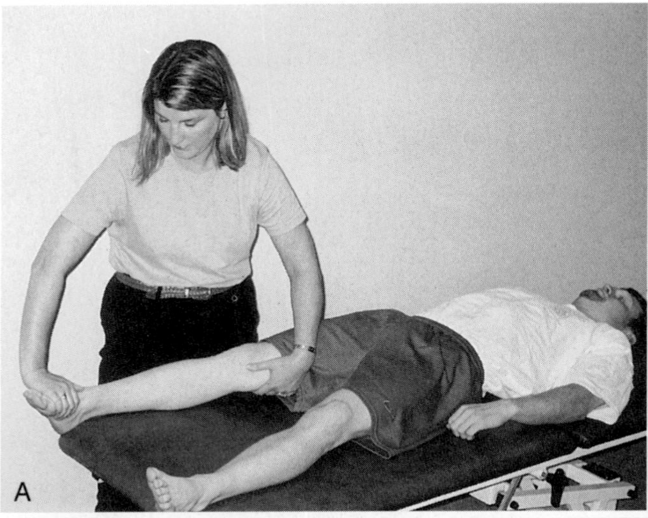

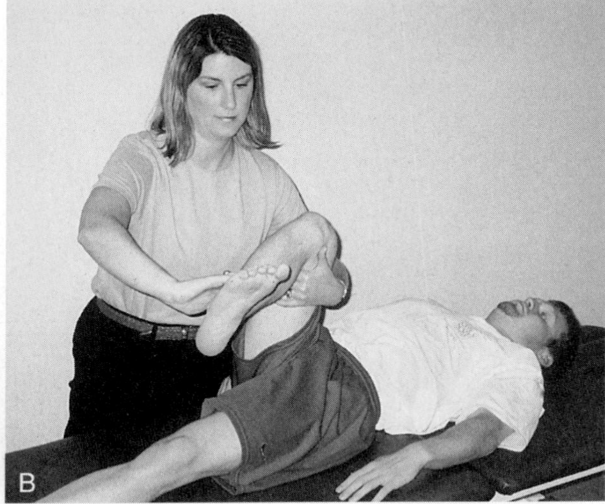

Figure 3–32 *(A)* Starting position and *(B)* ending position for D_1 Flexion of the lower extremity.

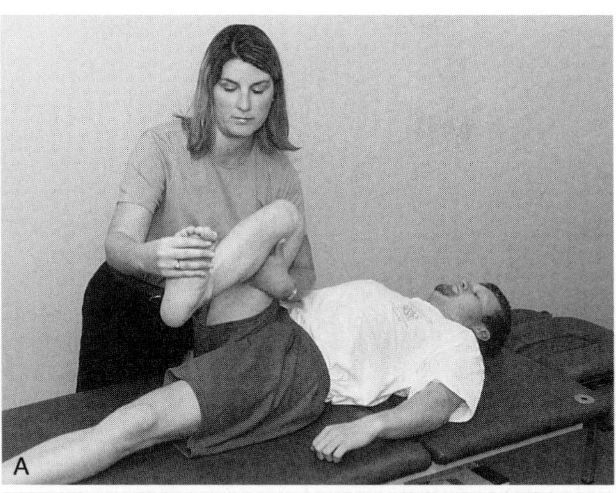

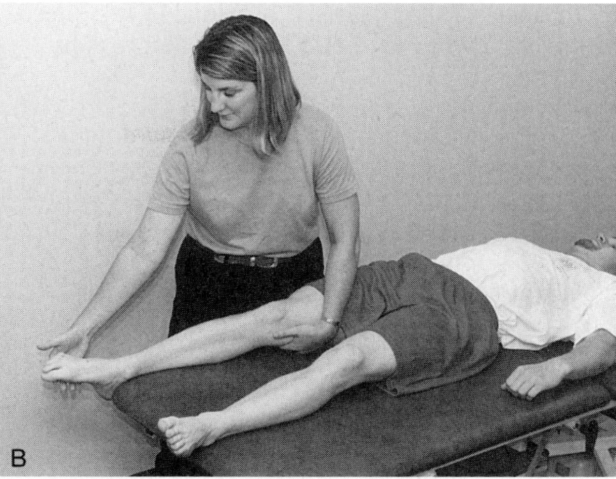

Figure 3–33 *(A)* Starting position and *(B)* ending position for D_1 Extension of the lower extremity.

D_1Extension

Starting Position (Fig. 3–33A)
Begin as described for completion of D_1Flexion.

Hand Placement
Place your (R) hand on the plantar and lateral surface of the foot at the base of the toes. Place your (L) hand (palm up) at the posterior aspect of the knee at the popliteal fossa.

Verbal Commands
As you apply a quick stretch to the plantarflexors of the ankle and toes, tell the patient, "Curl (point) your toes; push down and out."

Ending Position (Fig. 3–33B)
Finish the pattern in hip extension, abduction, and internal rotation; knee extension or flexion; ankle plantarflexion and eversion and toe flexion.

D_2Flexion

Starting Position (Fig. 3–34A)
Place the lower extremity in hip extension, adduction, and external rotation; knee extension; ankle plantarflexion and inversion; and toe flexion.

Hand Placement
Place your (R) hand along the dorsal and lateral surfaces of the foot and your (L) hand on the antero-

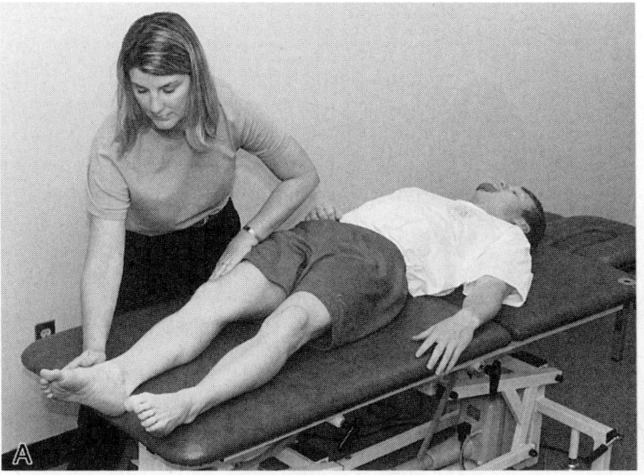

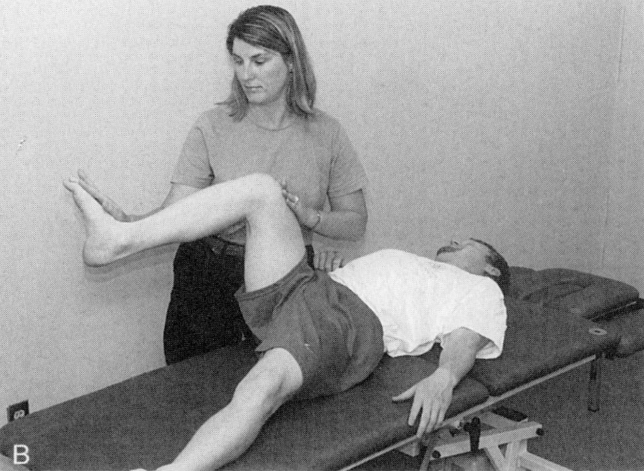

Figure 3–34 *(A)* Starting position and *(B)* ending position for D_2 Flexion of the lower extremity.

lateral aspect of the thigh just proximal to the knee. The fingers of your (L) hand should point distally.

Verbal Commands
As you apply a quick stretch to the ankle dorsiflexors and evertors and toe extensors, tell the patient, "Foot and toes up and out; lift your leg up and out."

Ending Position (Fig. 3–34B)
Complete the pattern in hip flexion, abduction, and internal rotation; knee flexion (or extension); ankle dorsiflexion and eversion and toe extension.

D_2Extension

Starting Position (Fig. 3–35A)
Begin as described for the completion of D_2Flexion.

Hand Placement
Place your (R) hand on the plantar and medial surface of the foot at the base of the toes and your (L) hand at the posteromedial aspect of the thigh, just proximal to the knee.

Verbal Commands
As you apply a quick stretch to the plantarflexors and invertors of the ankle and toe flexors, tell the patient, "Curl (point) your toes down and in; push your leg down and in."

Ending Position (Fig. 3–35B)
Complete the pattern in hip extension, adduction, and external rotation; knee extension; ankle plantarflexion and inversion and toe flexion.

Specific Techniques Associated with PNF

There are a number of specific techniques that may be used during the execution of a PNF pattern to further stimulate weak muscles and enhance movement or stability. These techniques are implemented selectively by the therapist to evoke the best possible response from the patient and focus on specific treatment goals.

Rhythmic Initiation

This technique is used to promote the ability to initiate a movement pattern. After the patient voluntarily relaxes, the therapist moves the patient's limb *passively* through the *available range* of the desired movement pattern several times so that the patient becomes familiar with the sequence of movements within the pattern. It also helps the patient understand the *rate* at which movement is to occur. Practicing assisted or active movements (without resistance) also helps the patient learn a movement pattern.

Repeated Contractions

Repeated, dynamic contractions, initiated with repeated quick stretches followed by resistance are applied at any point in the ROM to strengthen a weak agonist component of a diagonal pattern.

Reversal of Antagonists

Many functional activities involve quick reversals of the direction of movement. This is evident in diverse

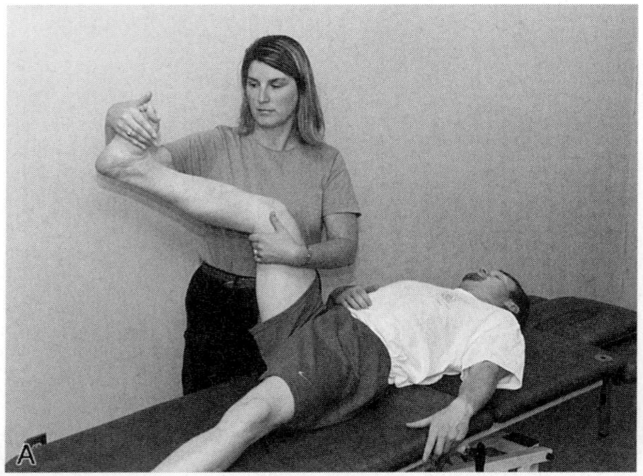

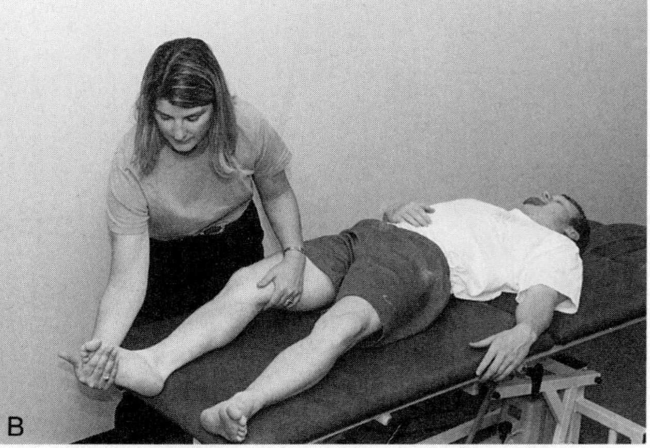

Figure 3–35 *(A)* Starting position and *(B)* ending position for D_2 Extension of the lower extremity.

activities such as sawing or chopping wood, dancing, playing tennis, or grasping and releasing objects. The reversal of antagonists technique involves stimulation of a weak agonist pattern by first resisting static or dynamic contractions of the antagonist pattern. The reversals of a movement pattern are instituted *just before* the previous pattern has been fully completed. The reversal of antagonists technique is based on Sherrington's law of *successive induction*.[247,260] There are two categories of reversal techniques available to strengthen weak muscle groups.

Slow reversal. Slow reversal involves a dynamic concentric contraction of a stronger agonist pattern immediately followed by a dynamic concentric contraction of the weaker antagonist pattern. There is no voluntary relaxation between patterns. This promotes rapid, reciprocal action of agonists and antagonists.

Slow reversal hold. Slow reversal hold adds an *isometric* contraction at the end of the range of a pattern to enhance end-range holding of a weakened muscle. With no period of relaxation, the direction of movement is then rapidly reversed by means of a *dynamic* contraction of the agonist muscle groups quickly followed by an isometric contraction of those same muscles. This is one of several techniques used to enhance dynamic stability, particularly in proximal muscle groups.

Alternating Isometrics

Another technique to improve isometric strength and stability of the postural muscles of the trunk or proximal stabilizing muscles of the shoulder girdle and hip is alternating isometrics. Manual resistance is applied in a single plane on one side of a body segment and then on the other. The patient is instructed to "Hold" his or her position as resistance is alternated from one direction to the opposite direction. No joint movement should occur. This procedure isometrically strengthens agonists and antagonists. This technique can be applied to one extremity, both extremities simultaneously, or to the trunk. Alternating isometrics can be applied with the extremities in open- or closed-chain positions.

For example, if a patient assumes a side-lying position, manual contacts are alternately placed on the anterior aspect of the trunk and then on the posterior aspect of the trunk. The patient is told to maintain (hold) the side-lying position as the therapist first attempts to push the trunk posteriorly and then anteriorly (Fig. 3–36*A*). Manual contacts are maintained on the patient as the therapist's hands are moved alternately from the anterior to posterior surfaces. Resistance is gradually applied and released. The same can be done unilaterally or bilaterally in the extremities (Fig. 3–36*B*).

Rhythmic Stabilization

This technique is used as a progression of alternating isometrics and is designed to promote stability

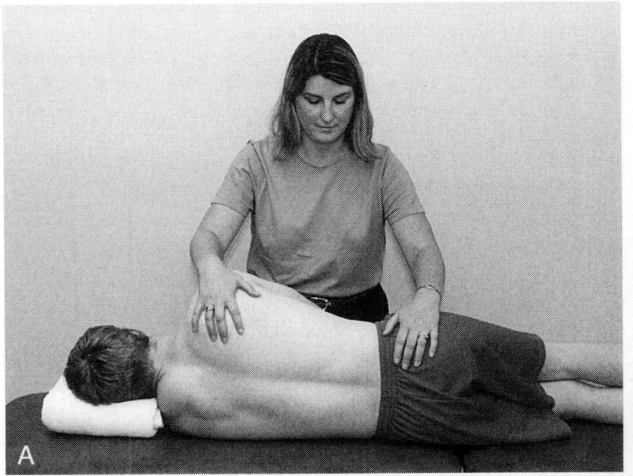

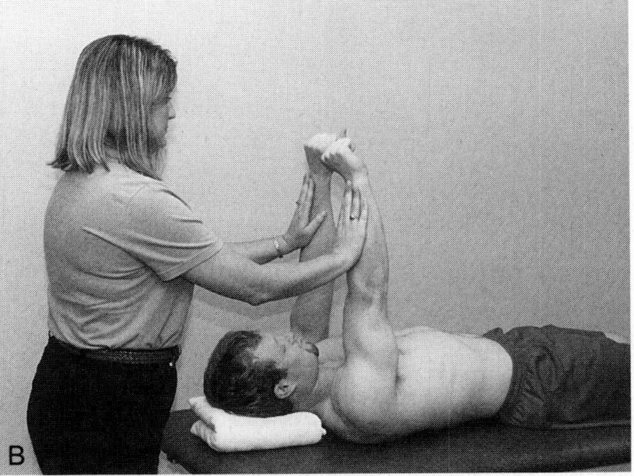

Figure 3–36 *(A)* Use of alternating isometrics to improve static strength of the proximal musculature by alternately placing both hands and applying resistance on the anterior aspect of the body and then on the posterior aspect of the body. *(B)* Use of alternating isometrics in the upper extremities.

through co-contraction of the proximal stabilizing musculature of the trunk as well as shoulder and pelvic girdle regions of the body. Rhythmic stabilization is typically performed in weight-bearing positions to incorporate joint approximation into the procedure, hence further facilitating co-contraction. The therapist applies multidirectional, rather than unidirectional, resistance by placing manual contacts on opposite sides of the body and applying resistance *simultaneously* in opposite directions as the patient holds the selected position. Multiple muscle groups around joints must contract, most importantly the rotators, to hold the position.

For example, in the selected position, the patient is told to hold that position as one hand pushes against the posterior aspect of the body and the other hand simultaneously pushes against the anterior aspect of the body (Fig. 3–37). Manual contacts are then shifted to the opposite surfaces and isometric holding against resistance is repeated. There is no voluntary relaxation between contractions.

Use of these special techniques, as well as others associated with PNF gives the therapist a significant variety of manual resistance exercise techniques to promote dynamic stability and controlled mobility as the foundation of and in preparation for learning task-specific skilled movements.

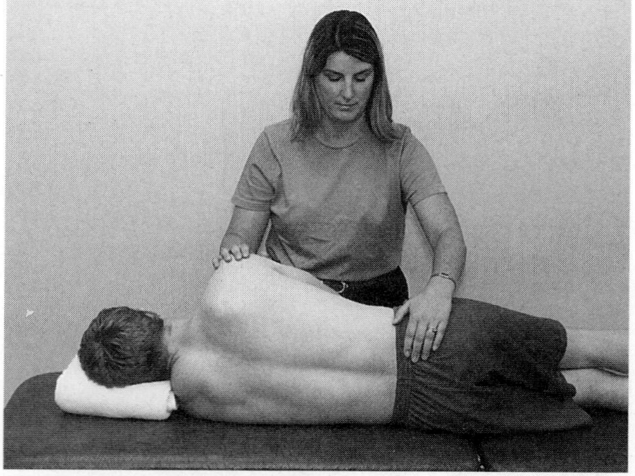

Figure 3–37 Use of rhythmic stabilization to improve stability of the trunk by simultaneously applying resistance in opposite directions to the anterior and posterior surfaces of the trunk emphasizing isometric contractions of the trunk rotators.

▶ Mechanical Resistance Exercise

Definition and Use

Mechanical resistance exercise is any form of exercise in which resistance (the exercise load) is applied by the use of some type of equipment. Terms synonymous with mechanical resistance exercise are *weight training*[8,16,110,217,286] and *load-resisting exercise.*[60,61] The many advantages as well as limitations of mechanical resistance exercises are listed in Box 3–11.

Box 3–11 Mechanical Resistance Exercise: Advantages and Disadvantages

Advantages

- Establishes a quantitative baseline measurement of muscle performance against which improvement can be judged.
- Most appropriate during intermediate and advanced phases of rehabilitation when muscle strength is 4/5 or greater or when the strength of the patient exceeds the therapist's strength.
- Heavy exercise loads, far beyond that which can be applied manually by a therapist, can be used to induce a training effect for already strong muscle groups.
- Increases in level of resistance can be incrementally and quantitatively documented.
- Quantitative improvement is an effective source of motivation for the patient.
- Useful for improving dynamic or static muscular strength.
- Adds variety to a resistance training program.
- Practical for improving muscular endurance.
- Some equipment provides variable resistance through the ROM.
- High-velocity resistance training is possible and safe with some forms of mechanical resistance (hydraulic and pneumatic variable resistance machines, isokinetic units, elastic resistance). Potentially better carry over to functional activities than relatively slow-velocity manual resistance exercises.
- Appropriate for independent exercise in a home program after careful patient education and a period of supervision.

Disadvantages

- Not appropriate when muscles are very weak or soft tissues are in the very early stages of healing with the exception of some equipment that provides assistance, support, or control against gravity.
- Equipment that provides constant external resistance maximally loads the muscle at only one point in the ROM.
- No accommodation for painful arc (except with hydraulic, pneumatic, or isokinetic equipment).
- Expense for purchase and maintenance of equipment.
- With free weights and weight machines gradation in resistance dependent on the manufacturer's increments of resistance.

Use in Rehabilitation

Mechanical resistance exercise is commonly implemented in rehabilitation to eliminate or minimize impairments in muscular strength, power, and endurance caused by an array of pathologic conditions and to restore or improve functional abilities. Guidelines for integration of mechanical resistance exercises into an individualized rehabilitation program for patients with specific conditions are detailed in Chapters 9 through 16.

Use in Conditioning Programs

There is a growing awareness through health promotion and disease prevention campaigns[208] that training with weights or other forms of mechanical resistance is an important component of comprehensive conditioning programs to improve or maintain physical fitness and health throughout most of the lifespan. As with rehabilitation, resistance training complements aerobic conditioning and flexibility exercises in conditioning programs. Guidelines for a balanced weight-training program for the healthy, but untrained adult (<50–60 years of age) recommended by the American College of Sports Medicine[8] and other authors[16,30,176] are summarized in Box 3–12. Many of these guidelines have already been discussed earlier in this chapter. They are highlighted here as a basis for comparison to guidelines for weight training for children and older adults.

Box 3–12 Summary of Guidelines for Resistance Training for Use in Conditioning Programs for Healthy Aduls (<50–60 years old)[8,16,30,176]

- Prior to resistance training, perform warm-up activities followed by flexibility exercises.
- Perform dynamic exercises that target the major muscle groups of the body (approximately 8–10 different muscle groups of the upper and lower extremities and trunk) for total body muscular fitness.
- Balance flexion-dominant (pulling) exercises with extension-dominant (pushing) exercises.
- Move through the full, available, and pain-free ROM.
- Include both concentric (lifting) and eccentric (lowering) muscle actions.
- Use *moderate*-intensity exercises: *at least* 8 to 12 repetitions per set.
- Perform a minimum of one set of each exercise for 8 to 12 repetitions per set.
- Use slow to moderate speeds of movement.
- Use rhythmic, controlled, nonballistic movements.
- Exercises should not interfere with normal breathing.
- Include rest intervals of 30 to 60 seconds between sets.
- Frequency: two to three times per week.
- Increase intensity gradually (increments of approximately 5%) to progress the program as strength and muscular endurance improve.
- Whenever possible, train with a partner for feedback and assistance.
- Cool down after completion of exercises.
- After a layoff of more than 1 to 2 weeks, reduce the resistance and volume when reinitiating weight training.

Special Considerations for Children and Older Adults

As noted previously, children and older adults often wish to incorporate resistance training in a conditioning program to improve physical fitness or in many cases for children to enhance performance in sports. Resistance training can be safe and effective if guidelines are modified to meet the unique needs of both of these groups.

Children and Weight Training

Until the past decade, health professionals have been reluctant to support preadolescent youth participation in resistance training as a part of fitness programs because of concerns about possible adverse stress and injury to the immature musculoskeletal system, in particular, growth-plate injuries. In addition, a common assumption was that the benefits of a weight-training program were questionable for growing children.[25,85,86,87]

There is now a growing body of evidence that demonstrates that children do achieve health-related benefits from weight training and can safely engage in closely supervised weight-training programs.[249] Training-induced strength gains in prepubescent children have been documented,[86,99,278] but sports-related injury prevention still remains of questionable benefit.[86,278] As with adults, the information on the impact of strength training on functional motor skills is limited. Research has also shown that although some acute and chronic responses of children to exercise are similar to those of adults, other responses are quite different. For example, children dissipate heat less easily and fatigue more quickly than adults.[278,286] Those differences in response to resistance exercise must be addressed when designing and implementing strength training programs for children. Accordingly, the American Academy of Pediatrics[6] and the American College of Sports Medicine[8] and many health professionals now support youth involvement in resistance training, but only if a number of special guidelines and precautions are consistently followed.[8,25,86,286] Although the risk of injury from resistance training is quite low,[30,87] exercise-induced soft tissue or growth-plate injuries have been noted if guidelines and precautions are not followed.[75] Special guidelines are summarized in Box 3–13.[8,30,86,99,249,286] Consistent with adult guidelines, a balanced program of dynamic exercise for major muscle groups includes warm-up and cool-down periods.

Older Adults and Weight Training

It is well known that muscle performance diminishes with age,[11,43,101,270] and deficits in muscle strength, power, and endurance are associated with a higher incidence of functional limitations.[30] The extent to which decreasing muscle strength is caused by the normal aging process versus a sedentary lifestyle or an increasing incidence of age-related diseases, such as osteoarthritis, is not clear.

A major goal of resistance training in older adults is to maintain or improve their levels of functional independence.[8,30,43,190] As with young and middle-age adults, older adults (>age 60–65) benefit from regular exercise that includes aerobic activity, flexibility exercises, and resistance training. Even in previously sedentary older adults, a program of weight training has resulted in training-induced gains in muscle strength.* and improvements in a number of parameters of physical function, such as balance, speed of walking, and the ability to rise from a chair.[34,90,190,204] It has also been suggested that strength training in the elderly population may minimize the incidence of falls.[30]

Box 3–13 Resistance Training for Children: Special Guidelines and Considerations

- No formal resistance training for children less than 6 to 7 years of age.
- At age 6 to 7 introduce the concept of an exercise session initially using exercises without weights, then with light (only 1 or 2 lb) weights.
- Maintain *close* and *continuous supervision* by trained personnel or a parent who has received instruction.
- Focus on proper form, exercise technique, and safety (alignment, stabilization, controlled motion).
- Keep the level of resistance low throughout childhood to avoid potential injury to a child's growing skeletal system and as well as joints and supportive soft tissues.
- Emphasize a variety of low-intensity, short-duration, play-oriented exercises to prevent boredom, overheating, and muscle fatigue.
- Select low exercise loads that allow a *minimum* of 8 to 12[30] or 12 to 15[86] repetitions. Emphasize multijoint, combined movements.
- Perform only one to two sets of each exercise; rest at least 1 to 2 minutes between sets of exercises.
- Initially progress resistance training by increasing repetitions, not resistance, or by increasing the total number of exercises. Later, increase weight by no more than 5% at a time.[30,86]
- Limit frequency to two sessions per week.
- Use properly fitting equipment that is designed or can be adapted for a child's size. Many weight machines cannot be adequately adjusted to fit a child's stature.

Note: The positive impact of resistance training on bone mineral density and slowing bone loss in older adults and exercise precautions for persons with or who are at risk for osteoporosis have already been discussed in previous sections of this chapter.

Although many of the guidelines for weight training that apply to young and middle-aged adults (see Box 3–12) also apply to older adults, in general, resistance training for older adults should be more closely supervised and less rigorous than for younger populations of adults for many reasons. For example, impaired balance, age-related postural changes and vision may compromise safety. Also, because of age-related changes in connective tissue, there is a higher incidence of DOMS and greater muscle fiber damage in older vs. young adults after heavy-resistance, high-volume strength training.[212] Guidelines for safe but effective resistance training for older adults are listed in Box 3–14.[8,30,43,270] As with young adult guidelines and exercise guidelines for youth, proper warm-up and cool-down periods, a balanced program of dynamic exercises, controlled movements, and proper form and technique are equally important for older adults.

Specific Exercise Regimens

Investigators have developed and studied many systems of resistance training all of which are based on the overload principle and use some form of mechanical resistance to load the muscle. The ultimate rationale for the development of each different system of training seems to be to design the most effective and efficient method to improve muscular performance and functional abilities. The most commonly used regimens of resistance training in rehabilitation and conditioning programs and those that are discussed in this section are **progressive resis-**

*See references 40, 43, 90, 112, 164, 186, 193, 212, 227, 248, 256.

Box 3–14 Resistance Training for Older Adults (>60–65 Years): Special Guidelines and Considerations

- Secure approval to initiate exercise from the participant's physician.
- Institute close supervision in the early phases of training to ensure safety.
- Monitor vital signs, particularly when the program is progressed.
- Begin with low-resistance, low-repetition exercises, especially for eccentric exercises to minimize loads on joints and to allow time for connective tissue as well as muscle to adapt.
- Keep resistance low (at a level that permits 10–12 repetitions) for 6 to 8 weeks. Progress the program during this time by increasing repetitions. Later, increase resistance by small increments.
- Throughout the program avoid high-resistance exercises to avoid excessive stresses on joints.
- Perform resistance training two to three times weekly, allowing a 48-hour rest interval between sessions.
- Modify exercises for age-related postural changes, such as excessive kyphosis, that can alter the biomechanics of an exercise.
- Avoid flexion-dominant resistance training that could emphasize postural changes.
- When possible, use weight machines that allow the participant to perform exercises in a seated position to avoid loss of balance.
- Reduce the intensity and volume of weight training by 50% after a 1- to 2-week layoff.

tive exercise (PRE), circuit weight training, plyometric training, and isokinetic regimens. Dynamic exercises rather than isometric exercises are emphasized in each of these systems. **Multiple-angle isometrics,** which is considered by some to be a system of resistance training using static exercise,[50,56] can be easily implemented using manual resistance but is cumbersome and rather impractical with most forms of mechanical resistance. This application of resistance training was already described in the discussion of isometric exercise in an earlier section of this chapter and will not be readdressed in this section.

Progressive Resistive Exercise (PRE)

PRE is a system of dynamic resistance training in which a constant external load is applied to the contracting muscle by some mechanical means (usually a free weight or weight machine) and incrementally progressed. The **repetition maximum** is used as the basis for determining and progressing the resistance.

The concept of PRE was introduced by DeLorme,[59,60,61] who originally used the term *heavy resistance training,*[59] to describe a new system of strength training. DeLorme proposed and studied the use of three sets of a 10 RM with *progressive loading* during each set. Other investigators[285] developed a regimen, the Oxford technique, with *regressive loading* in each set (Table 3–9).

Table 3–9 Comparison of Two PRE Regimens

DeLorme Regimen	Oxford Regimen
Determination of a 10RM	Determination of a 10 RM
10 reps @ 50% of the 10 RM	10 reps @ 100% of the 10 RM
10 reps @ 75% of the 10 RM	10 reps @ 75% of the 10 RM
10 reps @ 100% of the 10 RM	10 reps @ 50% of the 10 RM

The DeLorme technique builds a warm-up period into the protocol, whereas the Oxford technique diminishes the resistance as the muscle fatigues. Both regimens incorporate a rest interval between sets; both gradually increase the resistance over time; and both have been shown to result in training-induced strength gains over time.

Since these early investigations, numerous variations of PRE protocols have been proposed and studied to determine an optimal intensity of resistance training, an optimal number of repetitions and sets, an optimal frequency, and an optimal progression of loading. In reality an ideal combination of these variables does not exist. Extensive research has shown that many combinations of exercise load, repetitions and sets, frequency, and rest intervals significantly improve strength.[14,16,95,155] In general, training-induced strength gains occur with two to three sets of 6 to 12 repetitions of a 6 to 12 RM.[8,14,16,30,95,110,155] This gives a therapist wide latitude when designing an effective weight-training program.

Knowing when and by how much to increase the resistance in a PRE program to progressively overload the muscle is often imprecise and arbitrary. A common guideline is to increase the weight by 5 to 10% when all prescribed repetitions and sets can be completed easily without significant fatigue.[14,30,206] The Daily Adjustable Progressive Resistive Exercise (DAPRE) technique[150,151] is more systematic and takes into account the different rates at which individuals progress in a rehabilitation or conditioning programs. The system is based on a 6 RM *working weight* (Table 3–10). The *adjusted working weight,* which is based on the maximum number of repetitions possible using the working weight in set three of the regimen, determines the working weight for the next exercise session (Table 3–11). It should be

Table 3–10 DAPRE Technique

Sets	Repetitions	Amount of Resistance
1	10	50% 6 RM*
2	6	75% 6 RM
3	maximum possible	100% 6 RM
4	maximum possible	100% *adjusted working weight***

*6 RM = working weight
**See Table 3–11 for calculation of the *adjusted working weight.*

Table 3–11 Calculation of the Adjusted Working Weight for the DAPRE Regimen

Adjustment of Working Weight		
Repetitions in Set 3	Set 4	Next exercise session 3
0-2	↓ 5-10 lb	↓ 5-10 lb
3-4	↓ 0-5 lb	Same weight
5-6	Keep same weight	↑ 5-10 lb
7-10	↑ 5-10 lb	↑ 5-15 lb
11 or more	↑ 10-15 lb	↑ 10-20 lb

pointed out that the recommended increases or decrease in the adjusted working weight are based on progressive loading of the quadriceps.

Circuit Weight Training

Another system of training that employs mechanical resistance exercise is **circuit weight training.**[110,155,176,216] A pre-established sequence (circuit) of continuous exercises are performed in succession at individual exercise stations that target a variety of major muscle groups (usually 8–12) as an aspect of total body conditioning. Each resistance exercise is performed at an exercise station for a specified number of repetitions and sets; for example, two to three sets of 8 to 12 repetitions of 100% 10 RM or 10 to 20 repetitions of 40 to 50% 1 RM,[176] with a minimum amount of rest (15–30 seconds) between sets and stations. The program is progressed by increasing the number of sets or repetitions, the resistance, the number of exercise stations, and the number of circuit revolutions.

Exercise order is an important consideration in setting up a weight training circuit.[16,153] Exercises with free weights or weight machines should alternate among upper extremity, lower extremity, and trunk musculature. This enables one part of the body to recover from exercise while exercising another area, and therefore minimizes muscle fatigue. Larger muscle groups should be exercised before smaller muscle groups. Multijoint exercises that recruit multiple muscle groups should be performed before exercises that recruit an isolated muscle group to minimize the risk of injury from fatigue.

A circuit might include the following sequence of exercises:

1. bench press
2. leg press or squats
3. sit-ups
4. upright rowing
5. hamstring curls
6. trunk extension
7. shoulder press
8. heel raises
9. push-ups
10. leg lifts or lowering

When the use of successive exercise stations is approached more broadly to encompass flexibility exercises and aerobic activities, such as calisthenics as well as weight training, the term *circuit training* is used.[14,206]

Plyometric Training—Stretch-Shortening Drills

High-intensity, high-velocity exercises emphasize the development of muscular power and coordination. Quick bursts of force in functional movement patterns are often necessary if a patient is to return to high-demand occupational, recreational, or sports-related activities. Plyometric training can also be considered as a mechanism to prepare some carefully selected patients for everyday activities that require rapid starting and stopping movements.

Definition and Characteristics

Plyometric training,[176,257] often called plyometrics,[35,259] or **stretch-shortening drills,**[276] employs high velocity eccentric to concentric muscle loading, reflexive reactions, and functional movement patterns. More specifically, these exercises utilize the series-elastic and stretch reflex properties of the neuromuscular unit. It is thought that the stretch-shortening cycle stimulates the proprioceptors of muscles, tendons, ligaments, and joints, increases the excitability of the neuromuscular receptors, and improves the reactivity of the neuromuscular system. The term *reactive neuromuscular training* has also been used to describe this approach to exercise. Plyometric training is defined as a system of high-velocity resistance training characterized by a rapid eccentric contraction during which the muscle elongates, followed immediately by a rapid reversal of movement with a resisted shortening contraction of the same muscle.[258,259,276] The rapid eccentric loading phase is the stretch cycle and the concentric phase is the shortening cycle. The period of time between the stretch and shortening cycles is known as the *amortization phase*. It is important that the amortization phase is kept very brief by a rapid reversal of movements to capitalize on the increased tension in the muscle.

Body weight or an external form of loading, such as elastic bands or tubing or a weighted ball, are possible sources of resistance. An example of a stretch-shortening drill against the resistance of body weight is represented in the following activity: A patient jumps off a low platform to the floor, controlling impact with a loaded, lengthening contraction of the hip and knee extensors and plantarflexors—the stretch phase—and then without delay jumps back on the platform using a concentric contraction of the same muscle group—the shortening phase. Examples of plyometric training for the upper and lower extremities are noted in Box 3–15.

Neurologic and Biomechanical Influences

It is thought that the loaded, eccentric contraction (stretch cycle) prepares the contractile elements of the muscle for a concentric contraction (shortening cycle) by stimulation and activation of the monosynaptic stretch reflex.[35,74,257] Muscle spindles, the receptors that lie in parallel with muscle fibers, sense the length of a muscle and the velocity of stretch of a muscle and transmit this information to the CNS via afferent pathways. Impulses are then sent back to the muscle from the CNS, which facilitates a reflexive shortening contraction of the stretched muscle (the shortening cycle).[169,176,229] Theoretically, the more rapid the eccentric muscle contraction (the stretch), the more likely the stretch reflex is activated. It is also speculated that because of the elastic, spring-like properties of the noncontractile series-elastic components of muscle, elastic energy may be created by the loaded lengthening of the muscle, temporarily stored and then retrieved and used to augment the concentric (shortening) contraction.[35,176,257]

It has been suggested that the ability to use this stored elastic energy and neural facilitation is contingent upon the velocity and magnitude of the stretch and the transition time between the stretch and shortening phases (the amortization phase).[35] During the amortization phase the muscle must reverse its action, switching from deceleration to acceleration of the load. A decrease in the amortization phase theoretically increases the force output during the shortening phase.[35,257,259]

To date, evidence to support the claims of effectiveness of plyometric training is very limited with most resources citing opinion and anecdotal evidence. There is some evidence that indicates that plyometric training is associated with an increase in a muscle's ability to resist stretch, which may enhance the muscle's dynamic restraint capabilities.[19] As yet there is only emerging evidence to suggest that use of plyometric training in a rehabilitation program is associated with a decrease in the incidence of lower extremity injury when a patient returns to full activity.[123,236]

Box 3–15 Plyometric Activities for the Upper and Lower Extremities

Upper Extremities

- Catching and throwing a weighted ball with a partner or against a wall: bilaterally, then unilaterally.
- Stretch-shortening drills with elastic tubing using anatomic and diagonal motions.
- Dribbling a ball on the floor or against a wall.
- Drop push-ups: from boxes to floor and back to boxes.
- Clap push-ups.

Lower Extremities

- Repetitive jumping on the floor: in place; forward/backward; side to side; diagonally to four corners; jump with rotation; zig-zag jumping; later, jump on foam.
- Vertical jumps and reaches.
- Multiple jumps across a floor (bounding).
- Box jumping: initially off and freeze; then off and back on box increasing speed and height.
- Side to side jumps (box to floor to box).
- Jumping over objects on the floor.
- Hopping activities: in place; across a surface; over objects on the floor.
- Depth jumps (advanced): jump from a box, squat to absorb shock, and then jump and reach as high as possible.

Application and Progression of Plyometric Exercises

Plyometric training is appropriate only in the later stages of rehabilitation of active individuals who must achieve a high level of physical performance in specific, high-demand activities. Prior to initiation of plyometric training, the patient should have an adequate base of muscle strength and endurance as well as flexibility of the muscle to be exercised. Criteria to begin plyometric training usually include an 80 to 85% level of strength and 90 to 95% ROM.[35]

The plyometric program should be designed with specific functional activities in mind and include movement patterns in a closed or open-chain that replicate the desired activity. The stretch-shortening activity should be performed as quickly as possible. The rate of stretch of the contracting muscle is more important than the length of the stretch.[257] Emphasis should be placed on decreasing the reversal time from an eccentric to a concentric contraction (decreasing the amortization phase). This trains the muscle to generate tension in the shortest time possible. If a jumping activity is performed, for example, progression of the plyometric activity should center on reducing the time on the ground between the eccentric and concentric contractions.

Understandably, the methods of progression are different when training for increased power versus increased muscular endurance.

- ***Intensity.*** Increase the resistance applied, but not enough to slow down the activity. Examples include: use of a weighted vest, heavier Plyoballs (weighted balls), heavier grade elastic resistance, double-leg to single-leg jumping or hopping, or using higher height platforms. Intensity also involves progressing from simple to complex movements.
- ***Volume and frequency.*** Increase the number of repetitions of an activity *a long as proper form (technique) is maintained,* increase the number of plyometric exercises in a session or increase the number of plyometric sessions in a week. A 48- to 72-hour recovery period is recommended.[35,257]

Precautions: As with other forms of high-intensity resistance training, special precautions must be followed to ensure patient safety. These precautions are listed in Box 3–16.

Box 3–17 summarizes sample activities for upper extremity plyometric training.[35,257,259,276] Programs, of course, must be individually designed and progressed to meet each patient's needs and goals. Note that prior to initiating plyometric activities a series of warm-up exercises must be performed.

Isokinetic Regimens

It is well established that isokinetic training improves muscle performance. Its effectiveness in carryover to functional abilities is less clear. Studies support[81,185] and refute[118,209] that isokinetic training improves function. Ideally, when isokinetic training is implemented in a rehabilitation program, to have the most positive impact on function, it should be performed at velocities that closely match the expected velocities of movement associated with specific functional tasks. Since many ADL occur at a variety of medium to fast speeds, isokinetic training is also typically performed at medium and fast velocities.[5,50,56,79]

Current isokinetic technology makes it reasonably possible to match training speeds to velocities of movement during many lower extremity functions, such as walking.[50,280] In the upper extremity this is far less possible. Some functional movements in the

Box 3–16 Precautions for Plyometric Training

- If high-stress, shock-absorbing activities are not permissible, do not incorporate plyometric training into a patient's rehabilitation program.
- If a decision is made to include plyometric activities in a rehabilitation program for children or elderly patients, select only beginning level stretch-shortening drills against light resistance. Do not include high-impact, heavy-load exercises that could place excessive stress on joints.
- Be sure the patient has adequate flexibility and strength before initiating plyometric exercises.
- Wear shoes that provide support for lower extremity plyometrics.
- *Always* warm-up prior to plyometric training with a series of active, dynamic trunk and extremity exercises.
- During jumping activities, emphasize learning techniques for a safe landing before progressing to rebounding.
- Progress repetitions of an exercise before increasing the level of resistance used or the height or length of jumps.
- Stop an exercise if a patient can no longer perform the plyometric activity with good form and technique because of fatigue.

Box 3–17 Sample Plyometric Sequence for the Upper Extremities

- Warm-up activities
  - Trunk exercises holding lightweight ball: rotation, side-bending, wood-chopping
  - Upper extremity exercises in anatomic and diagonal planes of motion with light-grade elastic tubing
  - Prone push-ups
- Throwing motions with a weighted ball to and from a partner: bilateral chest press; bilateral overhead throw; bilateral side throw
- ER/IR against elastic tubing (90/90 position of shoulder and elbow)
- Diagonal patterns against elastic resistance
- Unilateral throwing motions with weighted ball: baseball throw; side throws
- Additional exercises
  - Trunk exercises holding weighted ball: abdominal curl-ups; back extension; sit-up and bilateral throw; long sitting throws
  - Clap push-ups
  - Prone push-ups from box to floor and back to box

upper extremities occur at exceedingly rapid velocities, for instance, over 1000 degrees per second for overhead throwing, that far exceed the capabilities of isokinetic dynamometers.[79]

It is also widely accepted that isokinetic training is relatively speed specific with only limited transfer of training (physiologic overflow causing improvements in muscle performance at speeds other than the training speed.)[253] Therefore, *speed-specific isokinetic training,* similar to the velocity of a specific functional task, is advocated.[5,50,52,76,79,139,253]

Velocity Spectrum Rehabilitation

To deal with the problem of limited physiological overflow of training effects from one training speed to another, a regimen called **velocity spectrum rehabilitation (VSR)** has been advocated.[50,79,95,239,209] In this approach to training, exercises are performed across a wide range of velocities.[234]

Note: Most guidelines for VSR have been directed to concentric isokinetic training. The principles of velocity spectrum training can also be applied to eccentric isokinetic training, but literature documenting guidelines or effectiveness is still limited.[114]

Selection of training velocities. Typically, medium (60 or 90–180 degrees/sec) and fast (180–360 degrees/sec) angular velocities are selected. Although isokinetic units are designed for testing and training at velocities faster than 360 degrees per second, the fastest velocities usually are not used. This is because the limb must accelerate to the very fast, preset speed before encountering resistance from the torque arm of the dynamometer. Therefore, the contracting muscles are only resisted through a small portion of the ROM.

It has been suggested that the effects of isokinetic training (improvements in muscle strength, power or endurance) carry over only 15 degrees per second from the training velocity.[50,139] Therefore, some VSR protocols use 30 degrees per second increments for medium and fast speed training. Of course, if a patient trains at medium and fast velocities (from 60 or 90–360 degrees/sec) in one exercise session, this strategy necessitates nine different training velocities, giving rise to a very time-consuming exercise session for one agonist/antagonist combination of muscle groups. Other protocols, typically with a minimum of three or more widely spaced training velocities, have also been shown to improve strength.[5,76,234]

Repetitions, sets, and rest. One of the most commonly described VSR protocols involves one or two sets of 8 to 10 or as many as 20 repetitions of concentric contractions of antagonist muscle groups (reciprocal training) at multiple velocities.[5,50,52,79,239] For example, at medium velocities training could occur at 90, 120, 150, and 180 degrees per second. A second series would then be performed at decreasing velocities: 180, 150, 120, and 90 degrees per second. Because many combinations of repetitions, sets, and different training speeds lead to improvement in muscle performance, the clinician has many options when designing a VSR program. A 15- to 20-second rest between sets and a 60-second rest between exercise speeds has also been recommended.[239] VSR training should be performed a maximum of three times per week.[5]

Intensity. Submaximal effort is used for a brief warm-up period on the dynamometer. This is not a replacement for a more general form of upper or lower body warm-up exercises, such as cycling or upper-extremity ergometry. When training to improve endurance, exercises are carried out at a submaximal intensity (effort) but at a maximal intensity to improve dynamic strength.

In the early stages of an isokinetic exercise program, it is useful to begin with *submaximal* isokinetic exercise in a concentric mode at intermediate and slow speeds so the patient gets the "feel" of the isokinetic equipment and still protects the muscle. As the patient progresses, he or she may exert maximum effort at intermediate speeds. Slow-speed training is usually eliminated when the patient begins to exert maximum effort. In the advanced stage of rehabilitation, maximum-effort, fast-velocity training is emphasized, as long as exercises are pain free.[56] Additional aspects to a progression of isokinetic exercises include short-arc to full-arc exercises (if necessary) and concentric to eccentric movements.[56]

Precaution: Maximum-effort, slow-velocity training is rarely indicated because of the excessive shear forces produced across joint surfaces.[50,234]

Eccentric Isokinetic Training: Special Considerations

As isokinetic technology evolved over the past few decades, eccentric isokinetic training became

Box 3–18 Key Differences in Eccentric Versus Concentric Isokinetic Training

Eccentric isokinetic exercise is:

- Introduced only *after maximal* effort concentric isokinetic exercise can be performed without pain
- Implemented only after functional ROM has been restored
- Performed at slower velocities across a narrower velocity spectrum than concentric isokinetic exercise: usually between 60 and 120 degrees per second for the general population and up to 180 degrees per second for athletes
- Carried out at submaximal levels for a longer time frame to avoid extensive torque production and lessen the risk of DOMS
- Most commonly performed in a continuous concentric-eccentric pattern for a muscle group during training

possible,[50,76,81,113,114] but guidelines for eccentric isokinetic training and evidence of their efficacy remains limited. Guidelines for eccentric isokinetic training developed to date are primarily based on clinical opinion or anecdotal evidence. Key differences in eccentric isokinetic guidelines (intensity, repetitions, frequency, rest) as compared with commonly implemented guidelines for concentric isokinetic training are listed in Box 3–18. Several resources describe pathology-specific guidelines for eccentric isokinetic training based on clinical experience.[50,79,113,114]

Precautions: Eccentric isokinetic exercises are only appropriate in the final phase of a rehabilitation program to continue to challenge individual muscle groups when isolated deficits in strength and power persist. Because of the robotic nature of eccentric isokinetic training, medium rather than fast training velocities are considered safer. A sudden, rapid, motor-driven movement of the dynamometer's torque arm against a limb could cause an injury to healing tissue.

Use of Equipment with Resistance Exercise

There seems to be an almost limitless selection of exercise equipment on the market that is designed for resistance training. The equipment ranges from simple to complex, compact to space-consuming, or inexpensive to expensive. An assortment of simple but versatile handheld and cuff weights or elastic resistance products is useful in clinical and home settings, whereas a computerized isokinetic dynamometer may be useful for an in-depth evaluation of muscle performance or advanced-level resistance training. The best sources of information on new products on the market and equipment design and capabilities are from literature distributed by manufacturers, product demonstrations at professional meetings, and studies of these products reported in the research literature.

Although most equipment is *load resisting* (augments the resistance of gravity), a few pieces of equipment are *load assisting* (eliminates or diminishes the resistance of gravity) to improve the strength of weak muscles. Equipment can be used for static or dynamic, concentric or eccentric, and open-chain or closed-chain exercises to improve muscular strength, power or endurance, neuromuscular stability or control, as well as cardiorespiratory fitness.

In the final analysis, the choice of equipment depends primarily on the individual needs, abilities, and goals of the person using the equipment. Other factors that influence the choice of equipment are: the *availability;* the *cost* of purchase or maintenance by a facility or a patient; the *ease of use* (application or set-up) of the equipment; the *versatility* of the equipment; and the *space requirements* of the equipment. Once the appropriate equipment has been selected, its safe and effective use is the highest priority. General principles for use of equipment are listed in Box 3–19.

Free Weights and Simple Weight-Pulley Systems

Types of Free Weights

Free weights are graduated weights that are handheld or applied to the upper and lower extremities or trunk. They include commercially available dumbbells, barbells, cuff weights, weighted vests, and even sandbags. Free weights can also be fashioned for a home exercise program from readily available materials and objects found around the home.

Simple Weight-Pulley Systems

Free-standing or wall-mounted simple weight-pulley systems with weight-plates are commonly used for resisted upper and lower extremity or trunk exercises (Fig. 3–38).

Note: The simple weight-pulley systems described here are those that impose a relatively constant (fixed) load. Variable resistance weight machines, some of which incorporate pulleys into their designs, are discussed later in this section. Permanent or interchangeable weights are available. Per-

Box 3–19 General Principles for the Selection and Use of Equipment

- Base the selection of equipment on a comprehensive examination and evaluation of the patient.
- Determine when in the exercise program the use of equipment should be introduced and when it should be altered or discontinued.
- Determine if the equipment could or should be set up and used independently by a patient.
- Teach appropriate exercise form before adding resistance with the equipment.
- Teach and supervise the application and use of the equipment before allowing a patient to use the equipment independently.
- Adhere to all safety precautions when applying and using the equipment.
  - Be sure all attachments, cuffs, collars, and straps are securely fastened and that the equipment is appropriately adjusted to the individual patient prior to the exercise.
  - Apply padding for comfort, if necessary, especially over bony prominences.
  - Stabilize or support appropriate structures to prevent unwanted movement and to prevent undue stress on body parts.
  - If exercise machines are used independently, be certain that set-up and safety instructions are clearly illustrated and affixed directly to the equipment.
- If compatible with the selected equipment, use range-limiting attachments if ROM must be restricted to protect healing tissues or unstable structures.
- If the patient is using the equipment in a home program, give explicit instructions on how, when and to what extent to change or adapt the equipment to provide a progressive overload.
- When making a transition from use of one type of resistance equipment to another, be certain that the newly selected equipment and method of set-up initially provides a similar level of torque production to the equipment previously employed to avoid insufficient or excessive loads.
- When the exercise has been completed:
  - Disengage the equipment and leave it in proper condition for future use.
  - Never leave broken or potentially hazardous equipment for future use.
- Set up a regular routine of maintenance, replacement or safety checks for all equipment.

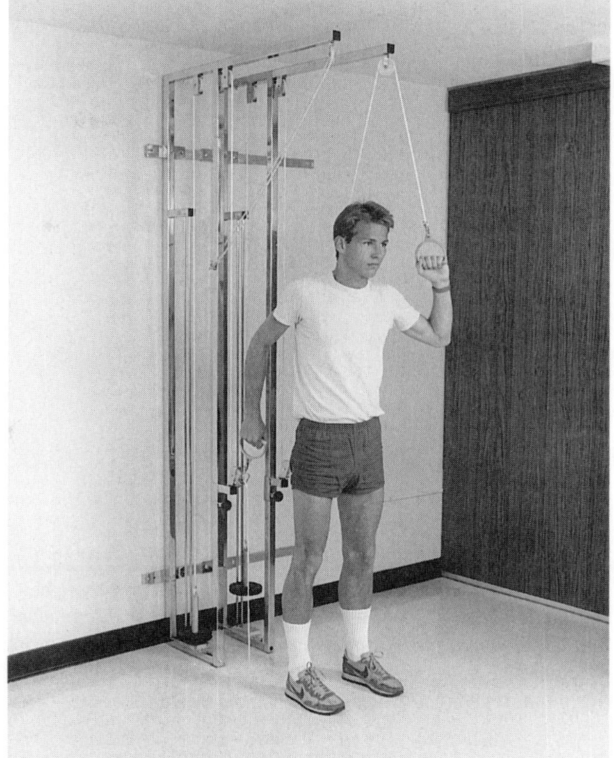

Figure 3–38 The Multi Exercise Pulley Unit can be used to strengthen a variety of muscle groups. (Courtesy of N-K Products Company, Inc., Soquel, CA.)

manent weights are usually stacked with individual weight-plates of 5- to 10-lb increments that can be easily adjusted by changing the placement of a single weight key.

Characteristics of Free Weights and Simple Weight-Pulley Systems

This resistance equipment imposes a fixed (constant) load. The weight selected, therefore, maximally challenges the contacting muscle at only one portion of the ROM when a patient is in a particular position. The weight that is lifted or lowered can be no greater than what the muscle can control at the point in the ROM where the load provides the maximum torque. In addition, there is no accommodation for a painful arc.

When using free weights, it is possible to vary the point in the ROM at which the maximum resistance load is experienced by changing the patient's position with respect to gravity or the direction of the resistance load. For example, shoulder flexion may be resisted with the patient standing or supine and holding a weight in the hand.

- Patient position: Standing (Fig. 3–39)

Maximum resistance is experienced and maximum torque is produced when the shoulder is at 90 degrees of flexion. Zero torque is produced when the shoulder is at 0 degrees of flexion. Torque again decreases as the patient lifts the weight from 90 to 180 degrees of flexion. In addition, when the weight is at the side (in the 0 degree position of the shoulder), it causes a traction force on the humerus, and when

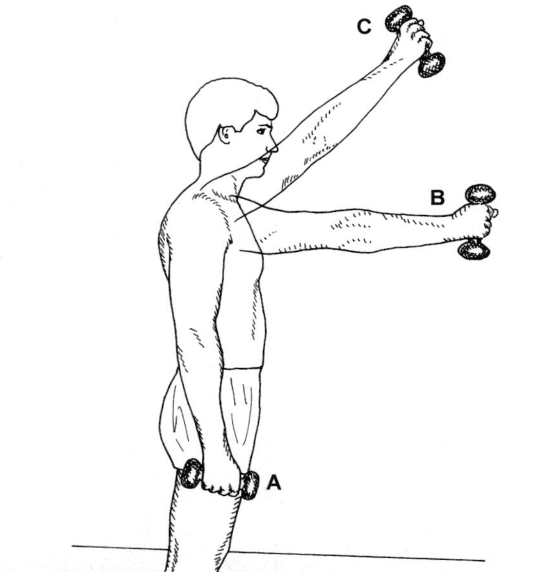

Figure 3–39 When the patient is standing and lifting a weight. *(A)* Zero torque is produced in the shoulder flexors when the shoulder is at 0 degrees flexion. *(B)* Maximum torque is produced when the shoulder is at 90 degrees flexion. *(C)* Torque again decreases as the arm moves from 90–180 degrees of shoulder flexion.

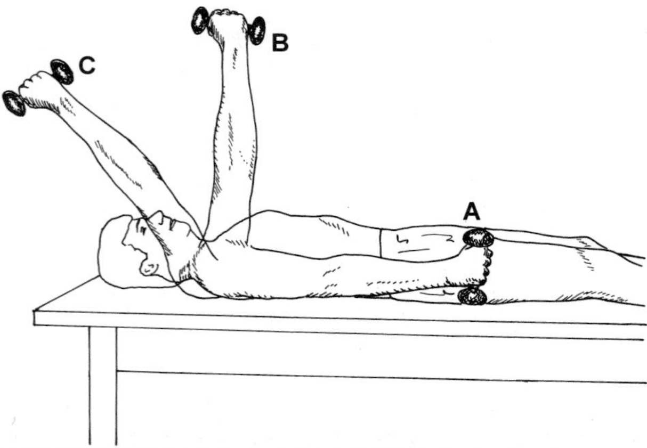

Figure 3–40 When the patient is supine and lifting a weight. *(A)* Maximum torque is produced at 0 degrees of shoulder flexion. *(B)* Zero torque is produced at 90 degrees shoulder flexion. *(C)* The shoulder extensors are active and contract eccentrically against resistance from 90–180 degrees shoulder flexion.

overhead, it causes a compression force through the upper extremity.

- Patient position: Supine (Fig. 3–40)

Maximum resistance is experienced and maximum torque is produced when the shoulder is at 0 degrees of flexion. Zero torque is produced at 90 degrees of shoulder flexion. In this position the entire load creates a compression force. The shoulder flexors are not active between 90 and 180 degrees of shoulder flexion. Instead, the shoulder extensors must contract eccentrically to control the descent of the arm and weight.

The therapist must determine at which portion of the patient's ROM maximum strength is needed and must choose the optimum position in which the exercise should be performed to gain maximum benefit from the exercise.

Simple weight-pulley systems provide maximum resistance when the angle of the pulley is at right angles to the moving bone. As the angle of the pulley becomes more acute, the load creates more compression through the moving bones and joints and less effective resistance.

Unlike many weight machines, neither free weights nor pulleys provide external stabilization to guide the moving segment or restrict ROM. When a patient lifts or lowers a weight to an overhead position as in Figures 3–39 and 3–40, shoulder abductors, adductors, and rotators must synergistically contract to keep the arm aligned in the sagittal plane during shoulder flexion. The necessity for concurrent contraction of adjacent stabilizing muscle groups can be viewed as an advantage or disadvantage. Because muscular stabilization is necessary to control the plane or pattern of movement, the patient will be able to control less resistance with free weights than with weight machine during the same movement pattern.

Advantages and Disadvantages of Free Weights and Simple Weight-Pulley Systems

- Exercises can be set up in many different positions, such as supine, side-lying, or prone in bed or on a cart, sitting in a chair or on a bench, or standing. Many muscle groups can be strengthened by simply repositioning the patient.
- Free weights and simple weight-pulley systems typically are used for dynamic, nonweight-bearing exercises but also can be set up for iso-

metric exercise and for use during weight-bearing activities.

- A variety of movement patterns is possible incorporating single plane or multiplanar motions. An exercise can be highly specific to one muscle or generalized to several muscle groups.
- If a large enough assortment of graduated free weights is available, resistance can be increased by very small increments, as little as 1 lb at a time. The weight plates of pulley systems have larger increments of resistance, usually a minimum of 5 lb per plate.
- Exercises with free weights and weight-pulley systems must be performed slowly to minimize acceleration and momentum and prevent uncontrolled, end-range movements that could compromise patient safety. It is thought that the use of exclusively slow movements during strengthening activities has less carry over to many daily living activities than incorporating slow- and fast-speed exercises into a rehabilitation program.
- Free weights with interchangeable disks, such as a barbell, are versatile and can be used for patients with many different levels of strength, but require patient or personnel time for proper assembly.
- Bilateral lifting exercises with free weights often require the assistance of a spotter to ensure patient safety, thus increasing personnel time.

Variable Resistance Machines

Variable-resistance exercise equipment falls into two broad categories: specially designed weight-cable (weight-pulley) machines or hydraulic or pneumatic units. Both categories of equipment impose a variable load on the contracting muscles consistent with the changing torque-producing capabilities of the muscles throughout the available ROM.

Variable Resistance Weight-Cable Systems

Variable resistance weight-cable machines (Fig. 3–41) use a cam in their design. The cam (an elliptical or kidney-shaped disk) in the weight-cable system is designed to vary the load (torque) applied to the contracting muscle even though the weight selected remains the same. In theory, the cam is configured to replicate the length-tension relationship and resultant torque curve of the contracting muscle with the greatest amount of torque applied in the mid-range. This system varies the external load imposed on the contracting muscle based on the physical dimensions of the "average" individual. How effectively this design provides truly accommodating resistance throughout the full ROM is debatable. With each repetition of an exercise, the same muscle contracts concentrically and eccentrically. As with simple weight-pulley systems and free weights, exercises must be performed at relatively slow velocities, thus compromising carry over to many functional activities.

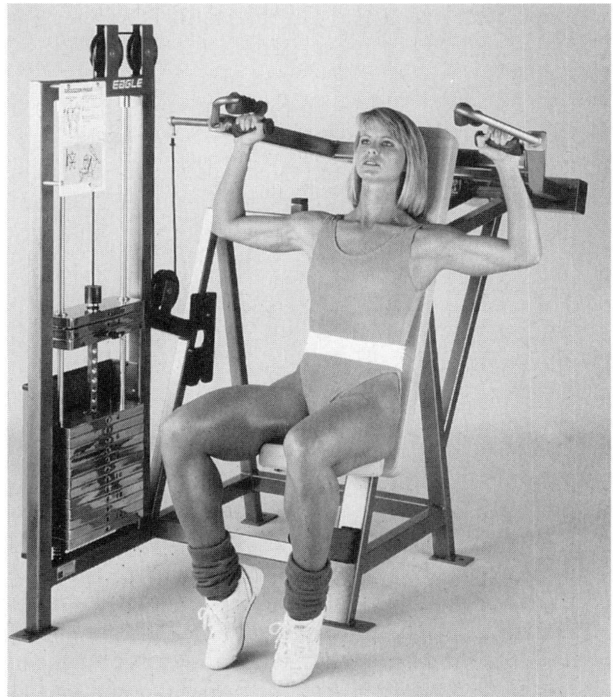

Figure 3–41 The Cybex/Eagle Fitness Systems shoulder press provides variable resistance throughout the range of motion. (Courtesy of Cybex, Division of Lumex, Ronkonkoma, NY.)

Hydraulic and Pneumatic Variable Resistance Exercise Units

Other variable resistance machines employ hydraulic or pressurized pneumatic resistance to vary the resistance throughout the ROM. These units allow concentric reciprocal, muscle work to agonist and antagonist muscle groups. Patients can safely exercise at higher velocities with these units.

Advantages and Disadvantages of Variable Resistance Machines

- The obvious advantage of these machines to constant load equipment is that the effective resistance, at least to some extent, is adjusted to a muscle's tension-generating capabilities throughout the ROM. The contracting muscle is loaded maximally at multiple points in the ROM, rather than just one small portion of the range.

- Most pieces of equipment are designed to isolate and exercise a specific muscle group. For example, resisted squats are performed on one machine and hamstring curls on another. Some units, such as a leg press or shoulder press, strengthen multiple muscle groups simultaneously.
- Most machines only allow single-plane movements although some newer units now offer a dual axis design allowing multiplanar motions that strengthen multiple muscle groups and more closely resemble functional movement patterns.
- The equipment is adjustable to a certain extent to allow individuals of varying heights to perform each exercise in a well-aligned position.
- Each unit provides substantial external stabilization to guide or limit movements. This makes it easier for the patient to learn how to perform the exercise correctly and safely and helps the patient maintain appropriate alignment without assistance or supervision.
- One of the main disadvantages of weight machines is the initial expense and ongoing maintenance costs. Multiple machines, usually 8 to 10 or more, must be purchased to target multiple major muscle groups. Multiple machines also require a large amount of space in a facility.

Elastic Resistance

The use of elastic resistance products for therapeutic exercise has become widespread in rehabilitation and has been shown to be an effective method of improving muscle strength.[135] However, unlike graduated weights, there is only limited quantitative information on the actual or relative resistance supplied by elastic material or the level of muscle activation during use.[125,126,136,142,224] These studies suggest that the effective use of elastic products for resistance training requires not only the application of biomechanical principles but also an understanding of the physical properties of elastic material.

Types of Elastic Resistance

Elastic bands and elastic tubing produced by several manufacturers specifically for use during exercise are available in an assortment of grades or thicknesses that provide multiple levels of resistance. Grades of resistance are denoted by color.

Application of Elastic Resistance

Elastic bands or tubing can be cut in varying lengths depending on the specific exercise to be performed and the height of a patient or the length of the extremities. The length of the elastic material should be sufficient to attach it *securely* at both ends. It should be taut but not stretched at the beginning position of the exercise. This is known as the *resting length* of the material.[135,224] One end is often tied or attached to a fixed object (doorknob, table leg, or D-ring) or secured by having the patient stand on one end of the band or tubing. The other end is grasped or fastened to a nylon loop, which is then placed around a limb segment. The band or tubing can also be held in both hands or looped under both feet for bilateral exercise. Figs. 3–42*A*, *B*, and *C* depict upper or lower extremity or trunk strengthening activities using elastic resistance.

With elastic resistance the muscle will receive the maximum resistive force when the material is on a stretch and angled 90 degrees to the moving bone. The therapist should determine the limb position at which maximum resistance is desired and anchor the elastic material so it is at right angles at that portion of the range. When the material is at an acute angle to the moving bone, there will be less resistance but a greater joint compressive force.

Characteristics of Elastic Resistance and Effect on Exercise

Elastic resistance can be classified as a form of variable resistance because the level of resistance changes as the material is stretched.[135] The amount of tension (force) generated by a piece of elastic band or tubing as it is stretched depends on the *relative change* in the length of the material *(percentage of elongation or deformation)* from start to finish of the exercise. There is a relatively linear relationship between the percentage of deformation and the tensile force of the material.[126,127,135,142,224] The method of calculating the percentage of elongation (deformation) is:[135,224]

Percentage of elongation =

$$\frac{(\text{final length} - \text{resting length})}{\text{resting length}} \times 100$$

Consequently, the same exercise performed with a long and a short piece of elastic will impose differ-

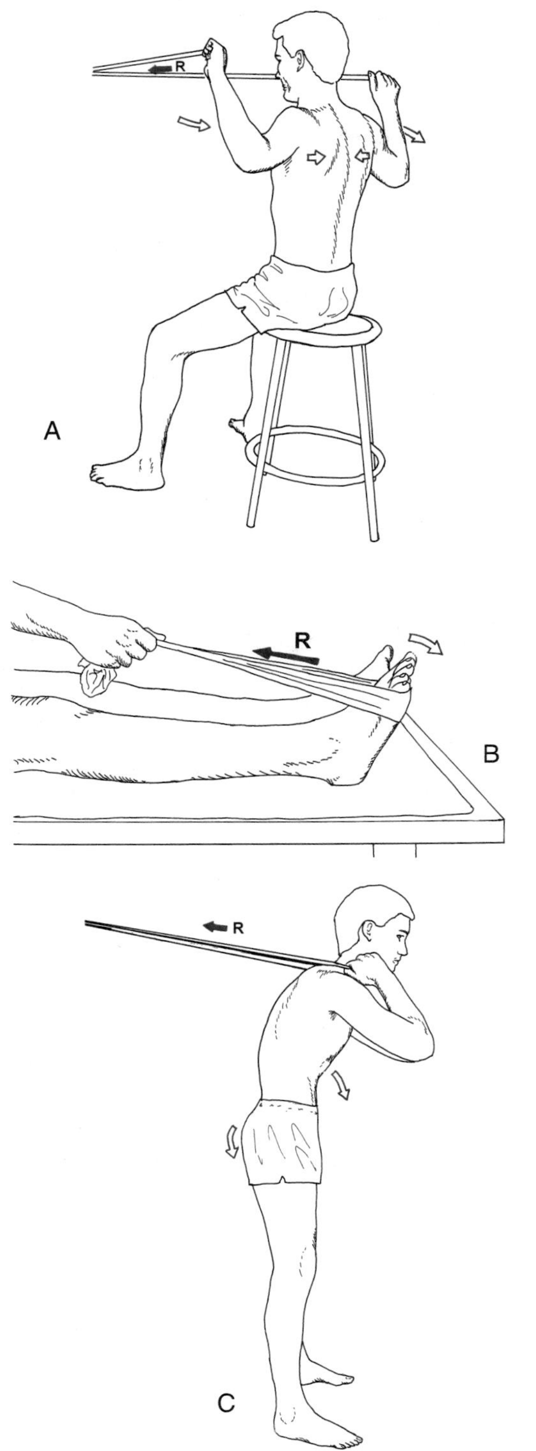

Figure 3–42 Use of elastic resistance to strengthen *(A)* upper or *(B)* lower extremity or *(C)* trunk musculature.

ent amounts of resistance. Therefore, it is important to consistently set up the exercise in the same manner from one exercise session to the next.

Percentage of deformation of the material is not the only factor that determines the amount of torque imposed by the elastic on a contracting muscle. Just because the tension produced by an elastic band or tubing increases as it is stretched does not mean that the torque imposed on the contracting muscle necessarily increases from the beginning to the end of an exercise. Other factors, such as the change in length of the moment arm and the angle of the elastic to the moving limb, affect the torque imparted by the elastic material.[135,136] The thickness (stiffness) of the material also affects the level of resistance. A heavier grade of elastic generates greater tension when stretched and therefore imparts a greater level of resistance.[126,135,224] Tubing tends to be thicker than bands and consequently generates greater tension. Therefore, the two should not be used interchangeably.

Elastic material tends to fatigue over time, which causes the material to lose some of its tension-generating property.[135] The extent of *material fatigue* is dependent on the number of times the elastic band or tubing has been stretched (number of stretch cycles) and the amount of deformation with each stretch.[224] Significant material fatigue of tubing and bands has been reported to occur within 500 stretch cycles with much of the decrease in tensile force occurring within the first 50 cycles. Elastic materials also display a property called *viscoelastic creep*. If a constant load is placed on elastic material, for example, when being stored, in time it will become brittle and eventually rupture.[135]

Advantages and Disadvantages of Exercise with Elastic Resistance

- Elastic resistance products are extremely versatile exercise tools. Exercises can be performed in many different positions because elastic resistance is not significantly gravity dependent;[135,136] rather, resistance is dependent primarily on the percentage of deformation of the material.
- Despite its versatility, remember, the percentage of elongation of the material effects the tension produced. Accordingly, it is essential that the same length of elastic resistance is used each time a particular exercise is performed. Otherwise, the imposed load may be too little or too much from one exercise session to the next even though the same grade (thickness) of elastic is used.

- Elastic bands and tubing are inexpensive, portable and practical for a home-based, independent exercise program.
- It is safe to exercise at moderate to high speeds with elastic resistance because the patient does not have to overcome the inertia of a rapidly moving weight. As such, it is appropriate for plyometric training.
- One of the most significant drawbacks with elastic resistance is the difficulty in quantifying the resistance level, making it difficult to know which grade to initially select and to what extent changing the grade of the band or tubing changes the level of resistance.
- As with free weights there is no source of stabilization or control of extraneous movements when an elastic band or tubing is used for resistance. The patient must use muscular stabilization to ensure that the correct movement pattern occurs.
- Because of the properties of viscoelastic creep and fatigue displayed by elastic material, bands and tubing should be replaced frequently.[135,224]

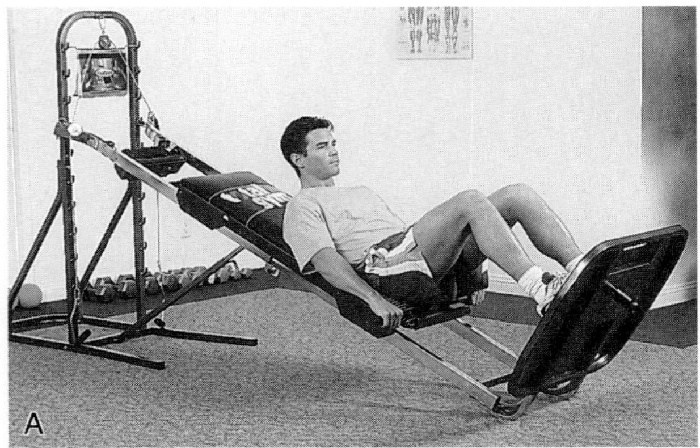

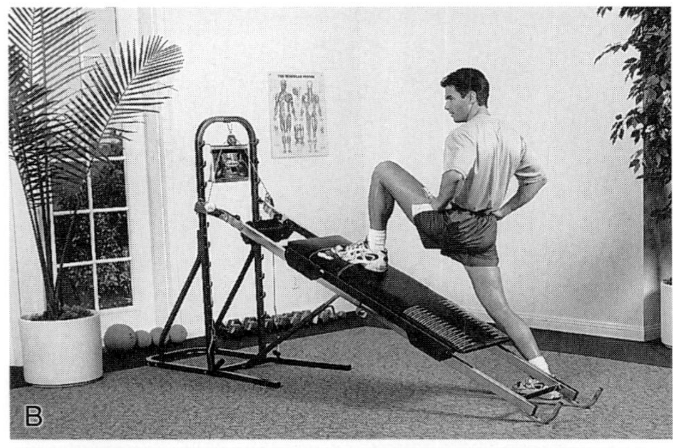

Figure 3–43 Closed-chain training: *(A)* in the semi-reclining position and *(B)* standing position using the Total Gym system. (Courtesy of Total Gym, San Diego, CA.)

Equipment for Closed-Chain Training

As discussed earlier in this chapter, most closed-chain exercises are performed in weight-bearing postures to develop strength, endurance, and stability across multiple joints. Often these exercises are begun using only the resistance of partial or full body weight and then progressed by simply adding resistance with handheld weights, a weighted vest or elastic resistance. The following equipment is designed specifically for closed-chain resistance exercises and has closed-chain features to improve muscle performance across multiple joints.

Multipurpose Exercise Units

With some multipurpose equipment it is possible to perform closed-chain exercises in a variety of positions to strengthen many different muscle groups in the upper or lower extremities and the trunk. The Total Gym® system, for example, uses a glideboard that enables a patient to perform bilateral or unilateral closed-chain strengthening and endurance exercises in positions that range from partially reclining to standing (Fig. 3–43*A* and *B*). The level of resistance on the Total Gym apparatus is adjusted by varying the angle of the glideboard on the incline.

Performance of bilateral and later unilateral squatting exercises in a semi-reclining position allows the patient to begin closed-chain training in a partially unloaded (partial weight-bearing) position early in the rehabilitation program. Later, the patient can progress to forward lunges (where the foot slides forward on the glideboard) while in a standing position.

Note: The Total Gym® system can also be set up for trunk exercises and open-chain exercises for the upper or lower extremities.

Balance Boards

The balance board is used for proprioceptive training in the upper or lower extremities. One example is the BAPS system (Biomechanical Ankle Platform System). The system can be used in the standing position (see Fig. 14–7), the seated position for the ankle, or in the quadriped position for upper extremity activities. Progressively increasing the size of the half spheres under the board or placing weights on the board makes the balance activity more challenging.

Slide Boards

The ProFitter® (Fig. 3–44) consists of a moving platform that slides side to side across an elliptical surface against adjustable resistance. Although it is most often used with the patient standing for lower extremity rehabilitation, it can also provide upper extremity closed-chain resisted movements and trunk stability. Medial-lateral or anterior-posterior movements are possible.

Stepping Machines

The StairMaster® is an example of a stepping machine that allows the patient to perform reciprocal pushing movements against adjustable resistance to make the closed-chain activity more difficult. Stepping machines provide nonimpact, closed-chain strengthening as an alternative to walking or jogging on a treadmill. A patient can also kneel next to the unit to use this equipment for upper extremity closed-chain exercises.

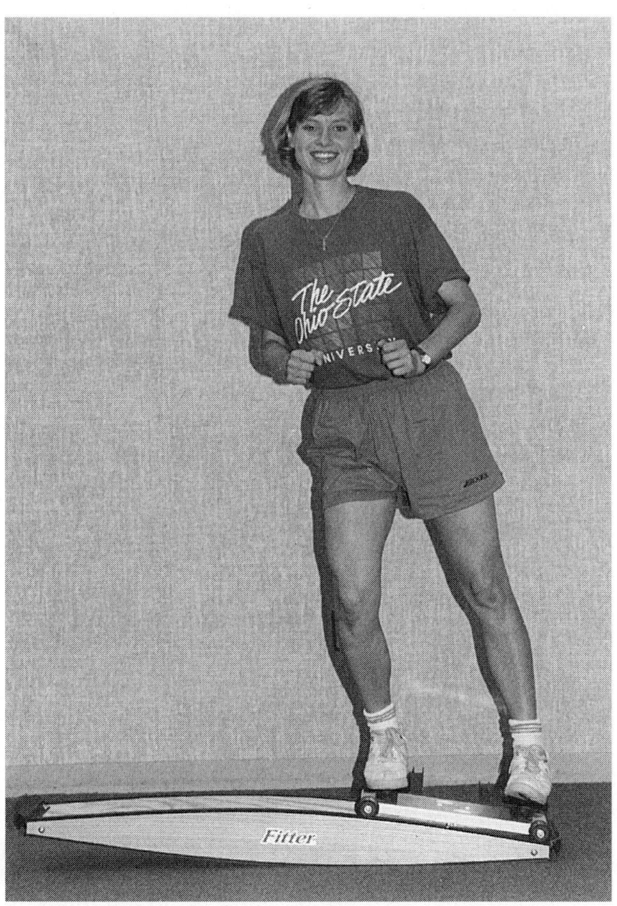

Figure 3–44 The ProFitter provides closed-chain resistance to lower extremity musculature in preparation for functional activities.

Elliptical Trainers and Cross-Country Ski Machines

These units also provide nonimpact, reciprocal resistance to the lower extremities in an upright, weight-bearing position. Variable incline adjustments of these units further supplement resistance options. In addition, both types of equipment also incorporate sources of reciprocal resistance to the upper extremities into their designs.

Mini-Trampolines

These devices enable the patient to begin gentle, bilateral or unilateral bouncing activities on a resilient surface to decrease the impact on joints. The patient can jog, jump, or hop in place.

Reciprocal Exercise Equipment

In addition to the closed-chain, reciprocal exercise devices already described, such as stepping machines and cross-country ski machines, other types of reciprocal exercise devices are appropriate for low-intensity, high-repetition resistance training to increase muscular endurance and reciprocal coordination of the upper or lower extremities and cardiorespiratory fitness. They also are often used for ROM exercises or warm-up or cool-down exercises prior to and after more intense resistance training. Resistance is imparted by an adjustable friction device or hydraulic or pneumatic resistance.

Exercise Cycle

The stationary exercise cycle (upright or recumbent) is used to increase lower extremity strength and endurance (Fig. 3–45). An upright cycle requires greater trunk control and balance than a recumbent cycle. A few exercise cycles provide resistance to both the upper and lower extremities. Resistance can be graded to progressively challenge the patient. Distance, speed, or duration of exercise can also be monitored.

The exercise cycle provides resistance to muscles during repetitive, nonimpact, reciprocal and usually nonweight-bearing movements of the extremities. Passive devices resist only concentric muscle activity as the patient performs either pushing or pulling movements. Motor-driven exercise cycles can be

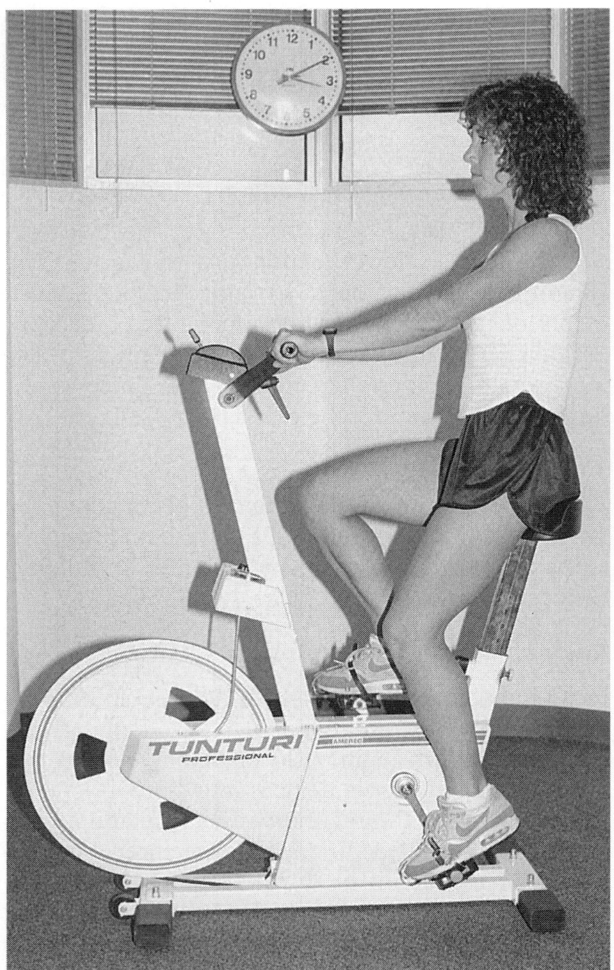

Figure 3–45 Exercise bicycles are used to increase muscular endurance and cardiopulmonary fitness.

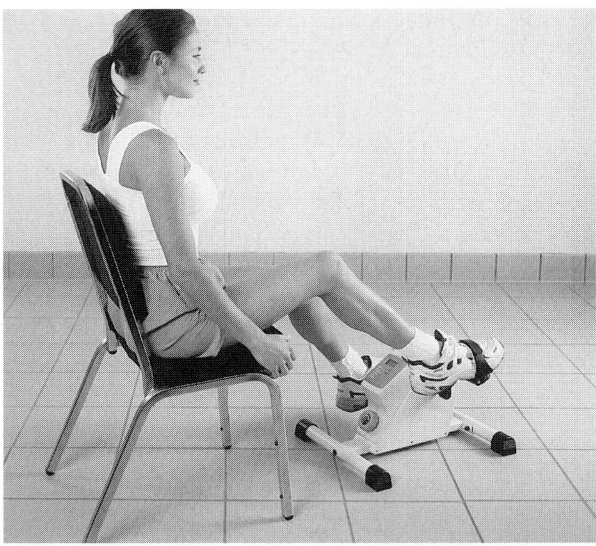

Figure 3–46 Resisted reciprocal exercise using the Chattanooga Exerciser. (Courtesy of Chattanooga Group, Inc., Hixon, TN.)

adjusted to provide eccentric as well as concentric resistance. The placement of the seat can also be adjusted to alter the arc of motion that occurs in the lower extremities.

Portable Resistive Reciprocal Exercise Units

A number of portable resistive exercisers are effective alternatives to an exercise bicycle for repetitive, reciprocal exercise. One such product, the Chattanooga Group Exerciser® (Fig. 3–46), can be used for lower extremity exercise by placing the unit on the floor in front of a chair or wheelchair. This is particularly appropriate for a patient who is unable to get on and off an exercise cycle. In addition, it can be placed on a table for upper extremity exercise. Resistance can be adjusted to meet the abilities of individual patients.

Upper Extremity Ergometer

The Upper Body Exerciser® (UBE) provides accommodating resistance exclusively for the upper extremities (Fig. 3–47). Typically the patient is seated, but the UBE can also be used with the patient in a standing position to lessen the extent of elevation of the arms necessary with each revolution. This is particularly helpful for patients with impingement syndromes of the shoulder.

Equipment for Dynamic Stabilization Training

The Bodyblade® (Fig. 3–48) is a dynamic, reactive form of resistance equipment that uses the principle of inertia as the source of resistance. While the patient drives the Bodyblade, rapidly, alternating contractions of agonist and antagonist muscle groups occur in an attempt to control the instability in three planes of motion dictated by movements of the blade, thus producing dynamic stability. The greater the amplitude or flex of the blade, the greater the resistance. This provides progressive resistance that the patient controls.

Initially, the oscillating blade is maintained in various positions in space, particularly those positions in which dynamic stability is required for func-

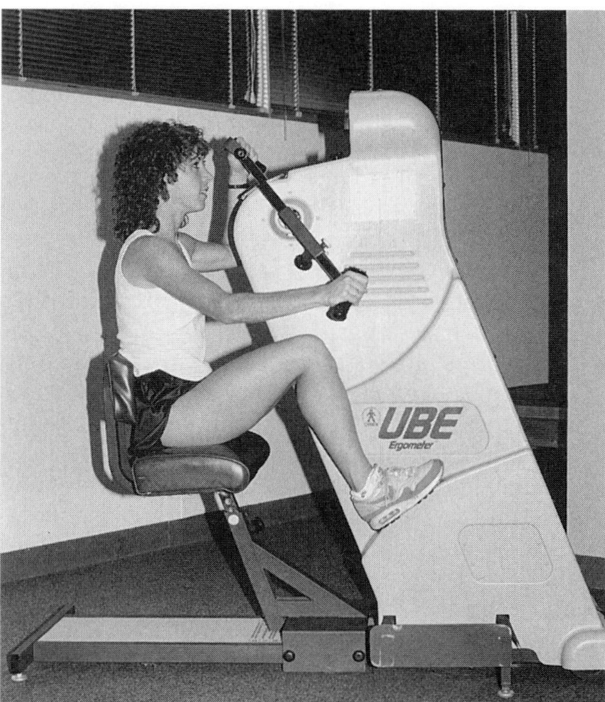

Figure 3–47 The Upper Body Exerciser (UBE) is used for upper extremity strength and endurance training.

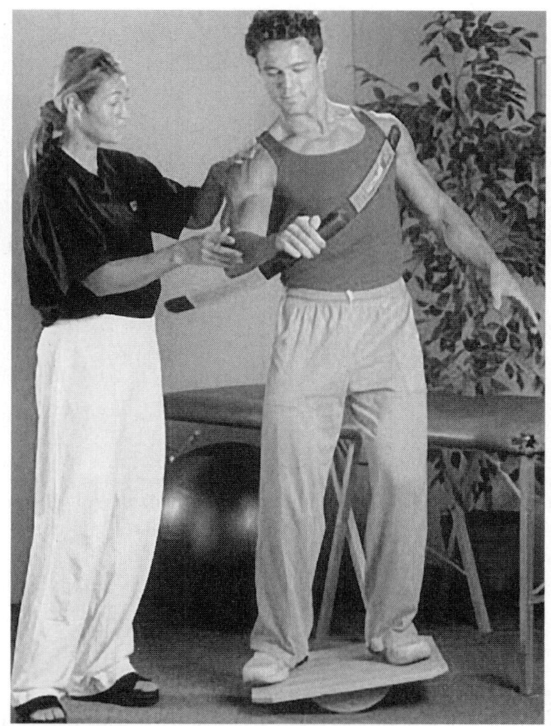

Figure 3–48 Dynamic stabilization exercises of the upper extremity and trunk using the Bodyblade. (Courtesy of Bodyblade/Hymanson, Inc., Los Angeles, CA. 1-800-77BLADE (25233); www.Bodyblade.com.)

tional activities. The patient can progress the difficulty of the stabilization exercises by moving the upper extremity through various planes of motion (from sagittal to frontal and ultimately to transverse) as the blade oscillates. The goal is to develop proximal stability (a stable core) as a foundation of controlled mobility.

Isokinetic Testing and Training Equipment

Several manufacturers produce isokinetic dynamometers (rate-limiting devices that control the velocity of motion) that provide accommodating resistance during dynamic exercise to the extremities or trunk. The equipment supplies resistance proportional to the force generated by the person using the machine. The preset rate (degrees per second) cannot be exceeded no matter how vigorously the person pushes against the force arm. Therefore, the muscle contracts to its maximum capacity at all points in the ROM.

Features of Isokinetic Dynamometers

New product lines of isokinetic equipment and improvements in existing equipment are continually being developed. The Biodex isokinetic dynamometer (Fig. 3–49) is an example of a unit currently on the market. Other product lines include the Cybex 6000 and the Kin-Com units. The specifications of the various manufacturers' dynamometers differ somewhat. Features include: computerized testing capabilities; passive and active modes that permit open-chain, concentric and eccentric testing and training; and velocity settings from 0 degrees per second up to 500 degrees per second for the concentric mode and up to 120 to 250 degrees per second for the eccentric mode. All units can be used for continuous passive motion. Computer programming allows limb movement within a specified range. Single-joint, uniplanar movements are most common, but some multiplanar movement patterns are possible. The Biodex dynamometer has attachments for multijoint exercises. Reciprocal training of agonist and antagonist and concentric/eccentric training of the same muscle group are both possible.

A relatively new product, marketed as the Lido Linea® closed kinetic chain dynamometer, is de-

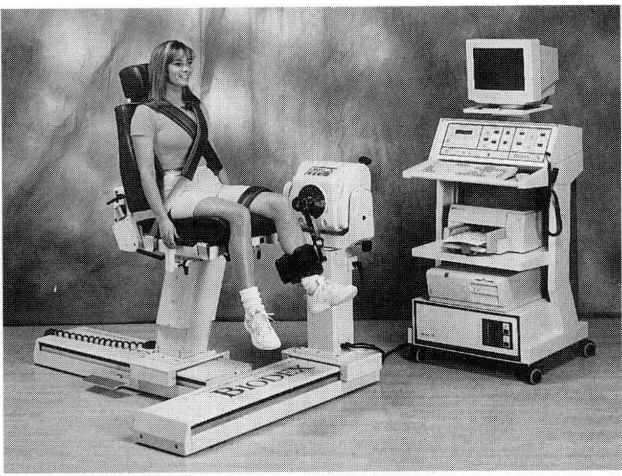

Figure 3–49 The Biodex isokinetic dynamometer is used for testing and training. (Courtesy of Biodex Medical Systems, Inc., Shirley, NY.)

signed exclusively for multijoint testing and training. The movement pattern performed on this apparatus is a seated or supine leg press; the unit can also be placed in a vertical position so that double- or single-leg squats can be performed. It can be used in concentric, eccentric and isometric modes. In an initial study[54] of the seated leg press, test-retest reliability was found to be high.

Advantages and Disadvantages of Isokinetic Equipment

Advantages

- Isokinetic equipment can provide maximum resistance at all points in the range of motion as a muscle contracts.
- Both high- and low-velocity training can be done safely and effectively.
- The equipment accommodates for a painful arc of motion.
- As a patient fatigues, exercise can still continue.
- Isolated strengthening of muscle groups is possible to correct specific strength deficits.
- External stabilization keeps the patient and moving segment well aligned.
- Concentric and eccentric contractions of the same muscle group can be performed repeatedly, or reciprocal exercise of opposite muscle groups can be performed, allowing one muscle group to rest while its antagonist contracts; the latter minimizes muscle ischemia.
- Computer-based visual or auditory cues provide feedback to the patient so that submaximal to maximal work can be carried out more consistently.

Disadvantages

- The equipment is large and expensive.
- Set-up time and assistance from personnel are necessary if a patient is to exercise multiple muscle groups.
- The equipment cannot be incorporated into a home exercise program.
- Most units allow only open-chain (nonweight-bearing) movement patterns, which do not simulate most lower extremity functions and some upper extremity functions.
- Although functional movements typically occur in combined patterns and at many different velocities, most exercises are performed in a single plane and at a constant velocity.
- Although the range of concentric training velocities (up to 500 degrees/sec) is comparable to lower extremity limb speeds during many functional activities, even the upper limits of this range cannot begin to match the very rapid limb speeds that are necessary during some sports-related motions such as throwing. In addition, the eccentric velocities available, at best, only begin to approach medium-range speeds, far slower than the velocity of movement associated with quick changes of direction and deceleration. Both of these limitations in the range of training velocities compromise carry over to functional goals.

Equipment for Isometric Training

To complete the total picture of the importance of equipment for effective resistance training, isometric resistance exercises must also be addressed. One of the advantages of isometric training is that it is possible to perform a variety of exercises *without* equipment. For example, multiple-angle isometrics can be carried out by simply having the patient push against an immovable object, such as a doorframe, a heavy table, a sofa, or a wall. Of course, manual resistance is also an effective means of strengthening muscles isometrically, particularly early in a rehabilitation program.

Many pieces of equipment designed for dynamic exercise can be adapted for isometric exercise. A weight-pulley system that provides resistance greater than the force-generating capacity of a muscle will result in a static muscle contraction Most isokinetic devices can be set up with the speed set at 0 degrees per second at multiple joint angles for isometric resistance at multiple points in the ROM. If elastic resistance or a pulley system is applied to the sound lower extremity, as the patient stands and bears full weight on the involved lower extremity, the muscles of the involved extremity will have to contract isometrically to hold the body in a stable, upright position as the sound extremity moves against the resistance.

Independent Learning Activities

CRITICAL THINKING AND DISCUSSION

1. What physical findings from an examination and evaluation of a patient would lead you to determine that resistance exercises were an appropriate intervention?
2. What are the benefits and limitations of isometric, dynamic (against constant or variable resistance), and isokinetic exercises?
3. What are the key changes that occur in muscle strength and endurance throughout the life span?
4. You have been asked to design a resistance exercise program as part of a total fitness program for a group of 7- to 9-year old soccer players (boys and girls). Indicate the exercises you would include, the equipment you will need, and the guidelines for intensity, volume, frequency, and rest.
5. Analyze five daily living tasks or recreational activities that you currently perform or would like to be able to perform effectively and efficiently. Identify what aspects of muscle performance (strength, power, and endurance) as well as other parameters of function, such as mobility (flexibility), stability, balance, and coordinated movement are involved in each of these tasks.
6. Develop an in-service instructional presentation that deals with the appropriate and effective use of elastic resistance products.
7. You have been asked to help design a circuit weight training sequence at a soon-to-open fitness facility at the outpatient treatment center where you work. Select equipment to meet the needs of beginning and advanced individuals. Establish general guidelines for intensity, repetitions and sets, order of exercise, rest intervals, and frequency.
8. Analyze the plyometric training activities listed in Box 3–15 and determine in which muscle groups training-induced gains in strength and power will occur and what functional tasks could each of the activities enhance.
9. Design a resistance-training program as part of a total fitness program for a group of older adults who participate in activities at a community-based senior citizen center. All participants are ambulatory and range in age from 65 to 85 years. Each has received clearance from his or her physician to participate in the program. What types of resistance equipment and levels of resistance would you recommend? Identify special precautions you would want to take.

LABORATORY PRACTICE

1. Perform manual resistance exercise to all muscle groups of the upper and lower extremities in the following positions: supine, prone, side-lying, and sitting. What are the major limitations to effective, full range strengthening in each of these positions?
2. Apply manual resistance exercises to each of the muscles of the wrist, fingers, and thumb.
3. Practice upper extremity and lower extremity D_1 and D_2 PNF exercises on your lab partner's right *and* left extremities.
4. Determine a 1 RM and 10 RM for the following muscle groups: shoulder flexors, shoulder abductors, shoulder external rotators, elbow flexors and extensors, hip abductors, hip flexors, knee flexors and extensors. Select one upper and one lower extremity muscle group. Determine a 1 RM or 10 RM with free weights in two different positions. Determine where in the ROM maximum resistance is encountered. Then determine a 1 RM or 10 RM with a pulley system. Compare your results.
5. Set up and safely apply exercises with elastic bands or tubing to strengthen the major muscle groups of the upper and lower extremities. Include a dynamic open-chain, a dynamic closed-chain, and an isometric exercise for each muscle group.
6. Demonstrate a series of simulated functional activities that could be used in the final stages of rehabilitation to continue to improve muscle performance as a transition into independent functional activities for a mail carrier, a nurse's aide who works in a skilled nursing facility, a ski instructor, a baseball player, and a daycare worker who cares for a group of active toddlers (each weighing approximately 25 pounds).

REFERENCES

1. Abe, T, DeHoyos, DV, Pollock, ML, and Garzarella, L: Time course for strength and muscle thickness changes following upper and lower body resistance training in men and women. Eur J Appl Physiol 81:174, 2000.
2. Abraham, WM: Factors in delayed muscle soreness. Med Sci Sports Exerc 9:11, 1977.
3. Ades, PA, et al: Weight training improves walking endurance in healthy elderly persons. Am J Internal Med 124:568, 1996.
4. Aitkens, S, et al: Moderate resistance exercise program. Its effects in slowly progressive neuromuscular disease. Arch Phys Med Rehabil 74:711, 1993.
5. Albert, MS, and Wooden, MJ: Isokinetic evaluation and treatment. In Donatelli, RA (ed): Physical Therapy of the Shoulder, ed 3. Churchill Livingstone, New York, 1997, p 401.
6. American Academy of Pediatrics: Strength training, weight and power lifting and body building by children and adolescents. Pediatrics 86:801, 1990.
7. American Association of Cardiovascular and Pulmonary Rehabilitation: Guidelines for cardiac rehabilitation programs, ed 3. Human Kinetics, Champaign, IL, 1999.
8. American College of Sports Medicine: ACSM's Guidelines for Exercise Testing and Prescription, ed 6, Lippincott Williams & Wilkins, Philadelphia, 2000.
9. American Physical Therapy Association: Guide to Physical Therapist Practice, ed 2. Phys Ther 81:9–744, 2001.
10. Amiridis, IG, et al: Concentric and/or eccentric training-induced alterations in shoulder flexor and extensor strength. J Orthop Sports Phys Ther 25:26, 1997.
11. Aniansson, A, et al: Muscle morphology enzymatic activity and muscle strength in elderly men. A follow-up study. Muscle Nerve 9:585, 1986.
12. Antonio, J, and Gonyea, WJ: Skeletal muscle fiber hyperplasia. Med Sci Sports Exerc 25:1333, 1993.
13. Armstrong, RB: Mechanisms of exercise-induced delayed onset muscular soreness: A brief review. Med Sci Sports Exerc 15:529–538, 1984.
14. Arnheim, DD, and Prentice, WE: Principles of Athletic Training, ed 9. McGraw-Hill, Boston, 1997.
15. Augustsson, J, et al: Weight training of the thigh muscles using closed vs. open kinetic chain exercises: A comparison of performance enhancement. J Orthop Sports Phys Ther 27:3, 1998.
16. Baechle, TR, Earle, RW, and Wathen, D: Resistance training. In Baechle, TR and Earle, RW (eds): Essentials of Strength Training and Conditioning, ed 2. Human Kinetics, Champaign, IL, 2000, p 395.
17. Baratta, R, et al: Muscular coactivation. The role of the antagonist musculature in maintaining knee stability. Am J Sports Med 16:113, 1988.
18. Barrett, DS: Proprioception and function after anterior cruciate ligament reconstruction. J Bone Joint Surg 73:83, 1991.
19. Benn, C, et al: The effects of serial stretch loading on stretch work and stretch-shorten cycle performance in the knee musculature. J Orthop Sports Phys Ther 27:412, 1998.
20. Bennett, R, and Knowlton, G: Overwork weakness in partially denervated skeletal muscle. Clin Orthop 12:22, 1958.
21. Bigland-Richie, B, and Woods, J: Changes in muscle contractile properties and neural control during human muscle fatigue. Muscle Nerve 7:691, 1984.
22. Bishop, KN, et al: The effect of eccentric strength training at various speeds on concentric strength of the quadriceps and hamstring muscles. J Orthop Sports Phys Ther 13:226–229, 1991.
23. Blackard, DO, Jensen, RL, and Ebben, WP: Use of EMG analysis in challenging kinetic chain terminology. Med Sci Sports Exerc 31:443, 1999.
24. Blackburn, JR, and Morrissey, MC: The relationship between open and closed kinetic chain strength of the lower limb and jumping performance. J Orthop Sports Phys Ther 27:430, 1998.
25. Blimkie, C: Benefits and risks of resistance training in youth. In Cahill, B, Pearl, A (eds): Intensive Participation in Children's Sports. Human Kinetics, Champaign, IL, 1993, p 133.
26. Bonen, A, and Belcastro, AN: Comparison of self-directed recovery methods on lactic acid removal rates. Med Sci Sports Exerc 8:176, 1976.
27. Bottomley, JM: Age-related bone health and pathophysiology of osteoporosis. Orthop Phys Ther Clin North Am 7:117, 1998.
28. Brask, B, Lueke, R, and Sodeberg, G: Electromyographic analysis of selected muscles during the lateral step-up exercise. Phys Ther 64:324, 1984.
29. Brunnstrom, S: Clinical Kinesiology. FA Davis, Philadelphia, 1962.
30. Bryant, CX, Peterson, JA, and Graves, JE: Muscular strength and endurance. In Roitman, JL (ed): ACSM's Resource Manual for Exercise Testing and Prescription, ed 4. Lippincott Williams & Wilkins, Philadelphia, 2001, p 460.
31. Carron, AV, and Bailey, DA: Strength development in boys from 10–16 years. Monographs of the Society for Research in Child Development, 39:1, 1974.
32. Chandler, JM, and Duncan, PW: Eccentric versus concentric force-velocity relationships of the quadriceps femoris muscle. Phys Ther 68:800, 1988.
33. Chandler, JM: Understanding the relationship between strength and mobility in frail older persons: A review of the literature. Topics in Geriatr Rehabil 11:20, 1996.
34. Chandler, JM, et al: Is lower extremity strength gain associated with improvement in physical performance and disability in frail, community-dwelling elders? Arch Phys Med Rehabil 79:24, 1998.
35. Chu, DA, and Cordier, DJ: Plyometrics in rehabilitation. In Ellenbecker, TS: Knee Ligament Rehabilitation. Churchill-Livingstone, New York, 2000, p 321.
36. Chung, F, Dean, E, and Ross, J: Cardiopulmonary responses of middle-aged men without cardiopulmonary disease to steady-rate positive and negative work performed on a cycle ergometer. Phys Ther 79:476, 1999.
37. Clark, MA, Foster, D, and Reuteman, P: Core (trunk) stabilization and its importance for closed kinetic chain performance. Orthop Phys Ther Clin North Am 9:119, 2000.
38. Clarkson, PM, and Tremblay, I: Exercise induced muscle damage, repair and adaptation in humans. J Appl Physiol 65:1–6, 1988.

39. Connelly, DM, and Vandervoort, AA: Effects of detraining on knee extensor strength and functional mobility in a group of elderly women. J Orthop Sports Phys Ther 26:340, 1997.
40. Connelly, DM, and Vandervoort, AA: Improvement in knee extensor strength of institutionalized elderly women after exercise with ankle weights. Physiother Can 47:15, 1995.
41. Conroy, BP, and Earle, RW: Bone, muscle and connective tissue adaptations to physical activity. In Beachle, TR (ed): Essentials of Strength Training and Conditioning. Human Kinetics, Champaign, IL, 1994, p 51.
42. Cook, TM, et al: EMG comparison of lateral step-up and stepping machine exercise. J Orthop Sports Phys Ther 16:108, 1992.
43. Corbin, DE: Exercise programming for older adults. In Roitman, JL (ed): ACSM's Resource Manual for Guidelines for Exercise Testing and Prescription, ed 4. Lippincott Williams & Wilkins, Philadelphia, 2001, p 529.
44. Corder, KP, et al: Effects of active and passive recovery conditions on blood lactate, rating of perceived exertion, and performance during resistance exercise. J Strength and Conditioning Research 14:151, 2000.
45. Cress, NM, Peters, KS, and Chandler, JM: Eccentric and concentric force-velocity relationships of the quadriceps femoris muscle. J Orthop Sports Phys Ther 16:82–86, 1992.
46. Croarkin, E: Osteopenia: Implications for physical therapists managing patients of all ages. PT Magazine of Physical Therapy 9:80, 2001.
47. Croarkin, E: Osteopenia in the patient with cancer. Phys Ther 79:196, 1999.
48. Cullan, E, and Peat, M: Functional anatomy of the shoulder complex. J Orthop Sports Phys Ther 18:342, 1993.
49. Curtis, C, and Weir, J: Overview of exercise responses in healthy and impaired states. Neurology Report 20:13, 1996.
50. Davies, GJ: A Compendium of Isokinetics in Clinical Usage and Rehabilitation Techniques, ed 4. S & S Publishing, Onalaska, WI, 1992.
51. Davies, GJ: The need for critical thinking in rehabilitation. J Sports Rehabil 4:1, 1995.
52. Davies, GJ, and Ellenbecker, TS: Application of isokinetics in testing and rehabilitation. In Andrews, JR, Harrelson, GL, Wilk, KE (eds): Physical Rehabilitation of the Injured Athlete, ed 2. WB Saunders, Philadelphia, 1998, p 219.
53. Davies, GJ, et al: The scientific and clinical rationale for the integrated approach to open and closed kinetic chain rehabilitation. Orthop Phys Ther Clin North Am 9:247, 2000.
54. Davies, GJ, and Heiderscheit, BC: Reliability of the Lido Linea closed kinetic chain isokinetic dynamometer. J Orthop Sports Phys Ther 25:133, 1997.
55. Davies, GJ, Heiderscheit, BC, and Clark, M: Open and closed kinetic chain rehabilitation. In Ellenbecker, TS: Knee Ligament Rehabilitation. Churchill Livingstone, New York, 2000, p 219.
56. Davies, GJ, and Zillmer, DA: Functional progression of a patient through a rehabilitation program. Orthop Phys Ther Clin North Am 9:103, 2000.
57. Davis, M, and Fitts, R: Mechanisms of muscular fatigue. In Roitman, JL (ed): ACSM's Resource Manual for Guidelines for Exercise Testing and Prescription, ed 4. Lippincott Williams & Wilkins, Philadelphia, 2001, p 184.
58. Dean, E: Physiology and therapeutic implications of negative work: A review. Phys Ther 68:233, 1988.
59. DeLorme, TL: Heavy resistance exercise. Arch Phys Med Rehabil 27:607, 1946.
60. DeLorme, TL, and Watkins, A: Progressive Resistance Exercise. Appleton-Century, New York, 1951.
61. DeLorme, T, and Watkins, A: Technics of progressive resistance exercise. Arch Phys Med Rehabil 29:263, 1948.
62. Denegar, CR, et al: Influence of transcutaneous electrical nerve stimulation on pain, range of motion and serum cortisol concentration in females experiencing delayed onset muscle soreness. J Orthop Sports Phys Ther 11:100–103, 1989.
63. DeVine, K: EMG activity recorded from an unexercised muscle during maximum isometric exercise of contralateral agonists and antagonists. Phys Ther 61:898, 1981.
64. DeVries, HA: Electromyographic observations on the effects static stretching has on muscular distress. Res Quarterly 32:468, 1961.
65. Devries, HA: Quantitative electromyographic investigation of the spasm theory of muscle pain. Am J Phys Med Rehabil 45:119, 1966.
66. Dierking, JK, et al: Validity of diagnostic ultrasound as a measure of delayed onset muscle soreness. J Orthop Sports Phys Ther 30:116, 2000.
67. DiFabio, RP: Editorial: Making jargon from kinetic and kinematic chains. J Orthop Sports Phys Ther 29:142, 1999.
68. Dillman CJ, Murray, TA, and Hintermeister, RA: Biomechanical differences of open and closed-chain exercises with respect to the shoulder. J Sport Rehabil 3:228, 1994.
69. Donatelli, RA: Functional anatomy and mechanics. In Donatelli, RA (ed): Physical Therapy of the Shoulder, ed 3. Churchill Livingstone, Philadelphia, 1997, p 1.
70. Donnelly, AE, Clarkson, PM, and Maughan, RJ: Exercise-induced damage: Effects of light exercise on damaged muscle. Eur J Appl Physiol 64:350, 1992.
71. Doucette, SA, and Child, DD: The effect of open and closed-chain exercise and knee joint position on patellar tracking in lateral patellar compression syndrome. J Orthop Sports Phys Ther 23:104, 1996.
72. Douris, PC: Cardiovascular response to velocity-specific isokinetic exercises. J Orthop Sports Phys Ther 13:28–32, 1991.
73. Draganich, LF, Jaeger, RJ, and Kraji, AR: Coactivation of the hamstrings and quadriceps during extension of the knee. J Bone Joint Surg 71A:1075, 1989.
74. Drury, DG: The role of eccentric exercise in strengthening muscle. Orthop Phys Ther Clin North Am 9:515, 2000.
75. Duarte, JA, et al: Exercise-induced signs of muscle overuse in children. Int. J Sports Med 20:103, 1999.
76. Duncan, PW, et al: Mode and speed specificity of eccentric and concentric exercise training. J Orthop Sports Phys Ther 11:70–75, 1989.
77. Durstine, JL, and Davis, PG: Specificity of exercise training and testing. In Roitman, JL (ed): ACSM's Resource Manual for Guidelines for Exercise Testing and Prescription, ed 4. Lippincott Williams & Wilkins, Philadelphia, 2001, p 484.
78. Edwards, BJ, and Perry, HM: Age-related osteoporosis. Clin Geriatr Med 10:575, 1994.
79. Ellenbecker, TS: Isokinetics in rehabilitation. In Ellenbecker, TS: Knee Ligament Rehabilitation. Churchill Livingstone, New York, 2000, p 277.
80. Ellenbecker, TS, and Cappel, K: Clinical application of closed kinetic chain exercises in the upper extremities. Orthop Phys Ther Clin North Am 9:231, 2000.
81. Ellenbecker, TS, Davies, GJ, and Rowinski, MJ: Concentric

versus eccentric isokinetic strengthening of the rotator cuff. Am J Sports Med 16:64, 1988.
82. Escamilla, RF, et al: Biomechanics of the knee during closed kinetic chain and open kinetic chain exercises. Med Sci Sports Exerc 30:556, 1998.
83. Eston, R, and Peters, D: Effects of cold water immersion symptoms of exercise-induced muscle damage. J Sports Sci 17:231, 1999.
84. Evans, WJ: Exercise-induced skeletal muscle damage. Phys Sportsmed 15:89, 1987.
85. Faigenbaum, A, et al: The effects of strength training and detraining on children. J Strength and Conditioning Research, 10:109, 1996.
86. Faigenbaum, AD, and Bradley, DF: Strength training for the young athlete. Orthop Phys Ther Clin North Am 7:67, 1998.
87. Falk, B, and Tenenbaum, G: The effectiveness of resistance training in children: a meta-analysis. Sports Medicine 22: 176, 1996.
88. Fardy, P: Isometric exercise and the cardiovascular system. Phys Sportsmed 9:43, 1981.
89. Faust, MS: Somatic development of adolescent girls. Soc Res Child Develop 42:1, 1977.
90. Fiatarone, MA, et al: High-intensity strength training in nonagenarians. JAMA 263:3029, 1990.
91. Fillyaw, M, et al: The effects of long-term nonfatiguing resistance exercise in subjects with post-polio syndrome. Orthopedics 14:1252, 1991.
92. Fitzgerald, GK, et al: Exercise induced muscle soreness after concentric and eccentric isokinetic contractions. Phys Ther 7:505–513, 1991.
93. Fitzgerald, GK: Open versus closed kinetic chain exercise: Issues in rehabilitation after anterior cruciate ligament surgery. Phys Ther 77:1747, 1997.
94. Fleck, SJ: Periodized strength training: A critical review. J Strength Condition Res 13:82, 1999.
95. Fleck, SJ, and Kraemer, WJ: Designing Resistance Training Programs, ed 2. Human Kinetics, Champaign, IL, 1997.
96. Francis, KT: Delayed muscle soreness: A review. J Orthop Sports Phys Ther 5:10, 1983.
97. Francis, KT: Status of the year 2000 health goals for physical activity and fitness. Phys Ther 79:405, 1999.
98. Franklin, ME, et al: Effect of isokinetic soreness-inducing exercise on blood levels of creatine protein and creatine kinase. J Orthop Sports Phys Ther 16:208–214, 1992.
99. Freedson, PS, Ward, A, and Rippe, JM: Resistance training for youth. In Grana, WA, et al (eds). Advances in Sports Medicine and Fitness, Vol 3. Year Book Medical Publishers, Chicago, 1990, p 57.
100. Friden, J, Sjostrom, M, and Ekblom, B: Myofibrillar damage following intense eccentric exercise in man. Int J Sports Med 4:170, 1983.
101. Frontera, WR, and Larsson, L: Skeletal muscle function in older people. In Kauffman, TL (ed): Geriatric Rehabilitation Manual. Churchill Livingstone, New York, 1999, p 8.
102. Fry, AC: The role of training intensity in resistance exercise, overtraining and overreaching. In Kreider R, Fry, A, and O'Toole M (eds): Overtraining in Sport. Human Kinetics, Champaign, IL, 1998, p 107.
103. Gajdosik, RL, Vander Linden, DW, and Williams, AK: Concentric isokinetic torque characteristics of the calf muscles of active women aged 20 to 84 years. J Orthop Sports Phys Ther 29:181, 1999.
104. Gilligan, C, Checovich, MN, and Smith, EL: Osteoporosis. In Skinner, JS (ed): Testing and Exercise Prescription in Special Cases, ed 2. Lea & Febiger, Philadelphia, 1993, p 127.
105. Gisolti, C, Robinson, S, and Turrell, ES: Effects of aerobic work performed during recovery from exhausting work. J Appl Physiol 21:1767, 1966.
106. Gollnick, P, et al: Glycogen depletion patterns in human skeletal muscle fibers during prolonged work. J Appl Physiol 34:615, 1973.
107. Gollnick, PD, et al: Muscular enlargement and number of fibers in skeletal muscle of rats. J Appl Physiol 50:936, 1981.
108. Gonyea, WJ: Role of exercise in inducing increases in skeletal muscle fibre number. J Appl Physiol 48:424, 1980.
109. Gonyea, WJ, Ericson, GC, and Bonde-Petersen, F: Skeletal muscle fiber splitting induced by weightlifting in cats. Acta Physiol Scand 99:105, 1977.
110. Graves, JE, Pollock, ML, and Bryant, CX: Assessment of muscular strength and endurance. In: Roitman, JL (ed): ACSM's Resource Manual for Guidelines for Exercise Testing and Prescription, ed 4. Lippincott Williams & Wilkins, Philadelphia, 2001, p 376.
111. Greig, CA, Botella, J, and Young, A: The quadriceps strength of healthy elderly people remeasured after 8 years. Muscle and Nerve 16:6, 1993.
112. Grimby, G, et al: Training can improve muscle strength and endurance in 78–84 year old men. J Appl Physiol 73:2517, 1992.
113. Hageman, PA, Gillaspie, and Hall, LD: Effects of speed and limb dominance on eccentric and concentric isokinetic testing of the knee. J Orthop Sports Phys Ther 10:59, 1988.
114. Hageman, PA, and Sorensen, TA: Eccentric isokinetics. In Albert, M: Eccentric Muscle Training in Sports and Orthopedics, ed 2. Churchill Livingstone, New York, 1995, p 115.
115. Hagood, S, et al: The effect of joint velocity on the contribution of the antagonist musculature to knee stiffness and laxity. Am J Sports Med 18:182, 1990.
116. Harbst, KB, and Wilder, PA: Neurophysiologic, motor control and motor learning basis of closed kinetic chain exercises. Orthop Phys Ther Clin North Am 9:137, 2000.
117. Hasson, S, et al: Therapeutic effect of high speed voluntary muscle contractions on muscle soreness and muscle performance. J Orthop Sports Phys Ther 10:499, 1989.
118. Heiderscheit, BC, McLean, KP, and Davies, GJ: The effects of isokinetic vs. plyometric training on the shoulder internal rotators. J Orthop Sports Phys Ther 23:125, 1996.
119. Heiderscheit, BC, and Rucinski, TJ: Biomechanical and physiologic basis of closed kinetic chain exercises in the upper extremities. Orthop Phys Ther Clin North Am 9:209, 2000.
120. Hellebrandt, FA, and Houtz, SJ: Mechanisms of muscle training in man: Experimental demonstration of the overload principle. Phys Ther Rev 36:371, 1956.
121. Herbison, GJ, Jaweed, MM, Ditunno, JF, et al: Effect of overwork during reinnervation of rat muscle. Exp Neurol 41:1, 1973.
122. Hettinger, T, and Muller, EA: Muskelliestung and Muskeltraining. Arbeitsphysiol 15:111, 1953.
123. Hewett, TE: The effect neuromuscular training on the incidence of knee injury in female athletes. A prospective study. Am J Sports Med 27:699, 1999.
124. Hill, DW, and Richardson, JD: Effectiveness of 10% tro-

lamine salicylate cream on muscular soreness induced by a reproducible program of weight training. J Orthop Sports Phys Ther 11:19–23, 1989.
125. Hintermeister, RA, et al: Electromyographic activity and applied load during shoulder rehabilitation exercises using elastic resistance. Am J Sports Med 26:210, 1998.
126. Hintermeister, RA, et al: Quantification of elastic resistance knee rehabilitation exercises. J Orthop Sports Phys Ther 28:40, 1998.
127. Hislop, HJ, and Montgomery, J: Daniels and Worthingham's Muscle Testing: Techniques of Manual Examination, ed 6. WB Saunders, Philadelphia, 1995.
128. Hislop, HJ, and Perrine, J: The isokinetic concept of exercise. Phys Ther 41:114, 1967.
129. Hislop, HJ: Quantitative changes in human muscular strength during isometric exercise. Phys Ther 43:21, 1963.
130. Ho, K, et al: Muscle fiber splitting with weight lifting exercise. Med Sci Sports Exerc 9:65, 1977.
131. Hopp, JF: Effects of age and resistance training on skeletal muscle: A review. Phys Ther 73:361, 1993.
132. Hought, T: Ergographic studies in muscular soreness. Am J Physiol 7:76, 1902.
133. Housh, D, and Housh T: The effects of unilateral velocity-specific concentric strength training. J Orthop Sports Phys Ther 17:252–256, 1993.
134. Howell, JN, Chleboun, G, and Conaster, R: Muscle stiffness, strength loss, swelling and soreness following exercise-induced injury in humans. J Physiol 464:183, 1993.
135. Hughes, C, and Maurice, D: Elastic exercise training. Orthop Phys Ther Clin North Am 9:581, 2000.
136. Hughes, CJ, et al: Resistance properties of Thera-Band® tubing during shoulder abduction exercise. J Orthop Sports Phys Ther 29:413, 1999.
137. Irrgang, JJ, Safran, MR, and Fu, FH: The knee ligaments and meniscus injuries. In Zachazewski, JE, Magee, DJ and Quillen, WS (eds): Athletic Injuries and Rehabilitation. WB Saunders, Philadelphia, 1996, p 623.
138. Issacs, L, Pohlman, R, and Craig, B: Effects of resistance training on strength development in prepubescent females. Med Sci Sports Exerc 265:210, 1994.
139. Jenkins, WL, Thackaberry, M, and Killan, C: Speed-specific isokinetic training. J Orthop Sports Phys Ther 6:181, 1984.
140. Jenkins, WL, et al: A measurement of anterior tibial displacement in the closed and open kinetic chain. J Orthop Sports Phys Ther 25:49, 1997.
141. Jones, H: The Valsalva procedure: Its clinical importance to the physical therapist. Phys Ther 45:570, 1965.
142. Jones, KW, et al: Predicting forces applied by Thera-Band® tubing during resistive exercises [abstr]. J Orthop Sports Phys Ther 27:65, 1998.
143. Kadi, F, et al: Cellular adaptation of the trapezius muscle in strength-trained athletes. Histochem Cell Biol 111:189, 1999.
144. Kauffman, TL, Nashner, LM, and Allison, LK: Balance is a critical parameter in orthopedic rehabilitation. Orthop Phys Ther Clin North Am 6:43, 1997.
145. Kelsey, DD, and Tyson, E: A new method of training for the lower extremity using unloading. J Orthop Sports Phys Ther 19:218–223, 1994.
146. Kendall, FP, McCreary, EK, and Provance, PG: Muscles: Testing and Function with Posture and Pain, ed 4. Lippincott Williams & Wilkins, Philadelphia, 1993.
147. Kernozck, TW, McLean, KP, and McLean, DP: Biomechanical and physiologic factors of kinetic chain exercise in the lower extremity. Orthop Phys Ther Clin North Am 9:151, 2000.
148. Kitai, TA, and Sale, DG: Specificity of joint angle in isometric training. Eur J Appl Physiol 58:741, 1989.
149. Knapik, JJ, Mawadsley, RH, and Ramos, MU: Angular specificity and test mode specificity of isometric and isokinetic strength training. J Orthop Sports Phys Ther 5:58, 1983.
150. Knight, KL: Knee rehabilitation by the daily adjustable progressive resistive exercise technique. Am J Sports Med 7:336, 1979.
151. Knight, KL: Quadriceps strengthening with DAPRE technique: Case studies with neurological implications. Med Sci Sports Exerc 17:636, 1985.
152. Knott, M, and Voss, DE: Proprioceptive Neuromuscular Facilitation, Patterns and Techniques, ed 2. Harper and Row, Philadelphia, 1968.
153. Kraemer, WJ, and Bush, JA: Factors affecting the acute neuromuscular responses to resistance exercise. In Rotman, JL (ed): ACSM's Resource Manual for Guidelines for Exercise Testing and Prescription, ed 4. Lippincott Williams & Wilkins, Philadelphia, 2001, p 167.
154. Kraemer, WJ, and Ratamess, NA: Physiology of resistance training: current issues. Orthop Phys Ther Clin North Am 9:467, 2000.
155. Kraemer, WJ, Duncan, ND, and Volek, JS: Resistance training and elite athletes: adaptations and program considerations. J Orthop Sports Phys Ther 28:110, 1998.
156. Kraemer, WJ, et al: Compatibility of high intensity strength and endurance training on hormonal and skeletal muscle adaptations. J Appl Physiol 78:976, 1995.
157. Kraemer, WJ, et al: Influence of resistance training volume and periodization on physiological and performance adaptations in collegiate women tennis players. Am J Sports Med 28:626, 2000.
158. Kraemer, W, et al: Influence of compression therapy on symptoms following soft tissue injury from maximal eccentric exercise. J Orthop Sports Phys Ther 31:282, 2001.
159. Kraemer, WJ, Volek, JS, and Fleck, SJ: Chronic musculoskeletal adaptations to resistance training. In Roitman, JL (ed): ACSM's Resource Manual for Guidelines for Exercise Testing and Prescription, ed 4. Lippincott Williams & Wilkins, Philadelphia, 2001, p 176.
160. Kuipers, H: Training and overtraining: An introduction. Med Sci Sports Exerc 30:1137, 1998.
161. Kvist, J, et al: Anterior tibial translation during different isokinetic quadriceps torque in anterior cruciate ligament deficient and nonimpaired individuals. J Orthop Sports Phys Ther 31:4, 2001.
162. Lane, JN, Riley, EH, and Wirganowicz, PZ: Osteoporosis: diagnosis and treatment. J Bone Joint Surg 78A:618, 1996.
163. Lear, LJ, and Gross, MT: An electromyographical analysis of the scapular stabilizing synergists during a push-up progression. J Orthop Sports Phys Ther 28:146, 1998.
164. Lemmer, JT, et al: Age and gender responses to strength training and detraining. Med Sci Sports Exerc 32:1505, 2000.
165. Lephart, SM, et al: Proprioception following ACL reconstruction. J Sports Rehabil 1:188, 1992.
166. Lephart, SM, et al: The effects of neuromuscular control exercises on functional stability in the unstable shoulder. J Athletic Training 33S:15, 1998.

167. Lephart SM, et al: The role of proprioception in rehabilitation of athletic injuries. Am J Sports Med 25:130, 1997.
168. Lephart, SM, and Henry, TJ: The physiological basis for open and closed kinetic chain rehabilitation for the upper extremity. J Sport Rehabil 5:71, 1996.
169. Levangie, PK, and Norkin, CC: Joint Structure and Function: A Comprehensive Analysis, ed 3. FA Davis, Philadelphia, 2001.
170. Liberson, WT: Brief isometric exercise. In Basmajian, JV (ed): Therapeutic Exercise, ed 3. Williams & Wilkins, Baltimore, 1978.
171. Lindle, RS, et al: Age and gender comparisons of muscle strength of 654 women and men aged 20–93 yr. J Appl Physiol 83:1581, 1997.
172. MacDougal, J, et al: Arterial pressure responses to heavy resistance exercise. J Appl Physiol 70:2498, 1991.
173. MacKinnon, J: Osteoporosis: A review. Phys Ther 68:1533–1540, 1988.
174. Mair, SD, et al: The role of fatigue in susceptibility to acute muscle strain injury. Am J Sports Med 24:137, 1996.
175. Malina, R, and Bouchard, C: Growth, maturation and physical activity. Human Kinetics, Champaign, IL, 1991.
176. McArdle, WD, Katch, FI, and Katch, VL: Essentials of Exercise Physiology, ed 2. Lippincott Williams & Wilkins, Philadelphia, 2000.
177. McDougall, DJ: Hypertrophy or hyperplasia. In Komi, PV (ed): Strength and Power in Sport. Blackwell Scientific Publications, Oxford, 1992, p 230.
178. McGee, C: Standard rehabilitation vs. standard plus closed kinetic chain rehabilitation for patients with shoulder pathologies: A rehabilitation outcomes study [abstr]. Phys Ther 79:S 65, 1999.
179. McGill, SM, and Cholewicki, J: Biomechanical basis of stability. An explanation to enhance clinical utility. J Orthop Sports Phys Ther 31:96–99, 2001.
180. Menkes, A, et al: Strength training increases regional bone mineral density and bone remodeling in middle-aged and older men. J Appl Physiol 74:2478, 1993.
181. Mikesky, AE, et al: Changes in muscle fiber size and composition in response to heavy resistance exercise. Med Sci Sports Exerc 23:1042, 1991.
182. Moffroid, M, et al: A study of isokinetic exercise. Phys Ther 49:735, 1969.
183. Moffroid, M, and Whipple, R: Specificity of the speed of exercise. Phys Ther 50:1693, 1970.
184. Moffroid, MT, and Kusick, ET: The power struggle: Definition and evaluation of power of muscular performance. Phys Ther 55:1098, 1975.
185. Mont, MA, et al: Isokinetic concentric versus eccentric training of shoulder rotators with functional evaluation of performance enhancement in elite tennis players. Am J Sports Med 22:513, 1994.
186. Morganti, CM, et al: Strength improvements with 1 yr of progressive resistance training in older women. Med Sci Sport Exerc 27:906, 1995.
187. Morrissey, MC, Harman, EA, and Johnson, MJ: Resistance training modes: Specificity and effectiveness. Med Sci Sport Exerc 27:648, 1995.
188. Mortain, T, and Devries, HA: Neural factors vs. hypertrophy in the time course of muscle strength gain. Am J Phys Med Rehabil 58:115, 1979.
189. Muller, EA: Influence of training and inactivity on muscle strength. Arch Phys Med Rehabil 51:449, 1970.
190. Nelson, ME, et al: Effects of high-intensity strength training on multiple risk factors for osteoporotic fractures. JAMA 272:1909, 1994.
191. Newman, D: The consequences of eccentric contractions and their relationship to delayed onset muscle pain. Eur J Appl Physiol 57:353–359, 1988.
192. Newman, D, Jones, D, and Clarkson, P: Repeated high force eccentric exercise effects on muscle pain and damage. J Appl Physiol 63:1381–1386, 1987.
193. Nichols, JF, et al: Efficacy of heavy-resistance training for active women over sixty: muscular strength, body composition and program adherence. J Am Geriatr Soc 41:205, 1993.
194. Nosaka, K, and Clarkson, PM: Influence of previous concentric exercise on eccentric exercise-induced damage. J Sports Sci 15:477, 1997.
195. Nosaka, K, and Clarkson, PM: Muscle damage following repeated bouts of high force eccentric exercise. Med Sci Sports Exerc 27:1263, 1995.
196. Oakley, CR, and Gollnick, PD: Conversion of rat muscle fiber type: A time course study. Histochemistry 83:555, 1985.
197. Osternig, LR, et al: Influence of torque and limb speed on power production in isokinetic exercise. Am J Phys Med Rehabil 62:163–171, 1983.
198. O'Sullivan, SB: Strategies to improve motor control and motor learning. In O'Sullivan, SB, and Schmitz, TJ: Physical Rehabilitation: Assessment and Treatment. FA Davis, Philadelphia, 2001, p 363.
199. O'Sullivan, SB: Assessment of motor function. In O'Sullivan, SB and Schmitz, TJ: Physical Rehabilitation: Assessment and Treatment, ed 4. FA Davis, Philadelphia, 2001, p177.
200. Palmitier, RA, et al: Kinetic chain exercise in knee rehabilitation. Sports Med 11:402, 1991.
201. Pardy W: Strength training. In Basmajian, JV, and Nyberg, R (eds): Rational Manual Therapies. Williams & Wilkins, Baltimore, 1993.
202. Petersen, SR, et al: The effects of concentric resistance training and eccentric peak torque and muscle cross-sectional area. J Orthop Sports Phys Ther 13:132–137, 1991.
203. Pomerantz, EM: Osteoporosis and the female patient. Orthop Phys Ther Clin North Am 3:71, 1996.
204. Porter, MM, and Vandervoort, AA: High-intensity strength training for the older adult—A review. Topics Geriatric Rehabil 10:61, 1995.
205. Prentice, WE: Proprioceptive neuromuscular facilitation techniques in rehabilitation. In Prentice, WE: Rehabilitation Techniques in Sports Medicine, ed 3. WCB McGraw-Hill, Boston, 1999, p 198.
206. Prentice, WE: Restoring muscular strength, endurance, and power. In Prentice, WE: Rehabilitation Techniques in Sports Medicine, ed 3, WCB/McGraw-Hill, Boston, 1999, p 73.
207. Pruitt, LA, et al: Weight-training effects on bone mineral density in early postmenopausal women. J Bone Mineral Res 7:179, 1992.
208. Public Health Service: Healthy People 2000: National Health Promotion and Disease Prevention Objectives. US Department of Health and Human Services, Washington, DC, 1991, DHHS Publication No: (PHS) 91-50212.
209. Rivera, JE: Open versus closed kinetic rehabilitation of the

lower extremity: a functional and biomechanical analysis. J Sports Rehabil 3:154, 1994.
210. Rockwell, JC, et al: Weight training decreases vertebral bone density in premenopausal women: A prospective study. J Clin Endocrinol Metab 71:988, 1990.
211. Rose, SJ, and Rothstein, JM: Muscle mutability. Part 1. General concepts and adaptations to altered patterns of use. Phys Ther 62:1773–1787, 1982.
212. Roth, SM, et al: High-volume, heavy-resistance strength training and muscle damage in young and older women. J Appl Physiol 88:1112, 2000.
213. Rothstein, JM: Muscle biology: Clinical considerations. Phys Ther 62:1823, 1982.
214. Sale, D: Neural adaptation to strength training. In Komi, PV: Strength and Power in Sport. Blackwell Scientific Publications, Boston, 1992, p 249.
215. Sale, DG: Neural adaptation to resistance training. Med Sci Sports Exerc 20:S135, 1988.
216. Sanders, B: Exercise and rehabilitation concepts. In Malone, TR, McPoil, T and Nitz, AJ (eds): Orthopedic and Sports Physical Therapy, ed 3. Mosby, St. Louis, 1997, p 211.
217. Sanders, MT: Weight training and conditioning. In Sanders, B (ed): Sports Physical Therapy. Appleton & Lange, Norwalk, CT, 1990.
218. Sapega, AA, and Drillings, G: The definition and assessment of muscular power. J Orthop Sports Phys Ther 5:7, 1983.
219. Sapega, AA, and Kelley, MJ: Strength testing about the shoulder. J Shoulder Elbow Surg 3:327, 1994.
220. Schueman, SE: The physical therapist's role in the management of osteoporosis. Orthop Phys Ther Clin North Am 7:199, 1998.
221. Seger, J, Arvidsson, B, and Thortensson, A: Specific effects of eccentric and concentric training on muscle strength and morphology. Eur J Appl Physiol 79:49, 1998.
222. Servedio, FJ: Normal growth and development: Physiologic factors associated with exercise and training in children. Orthop Phys Ther Clin North Am 6:417, 1997.
223. Shaw, JM, Witzke, KA, and Winters, KM: Exercise for skeletal health and osteoporosis prevention. In Rotman, JL (ed): ACSM's Resource Manual for Guidelines for Exercise Testing and Prescription, ed 4. Lippincott Williams & Wilkins, Philadelphia, 2001, p 299.
224. Simoneua, GG, et al: Biomechanics of elastic resistance in therapeutic exercise programs. J Orthop Sports Phys Ther 31:16, 2001.
225. Sinacore, DR, Bander, BL, and Delitto, A: Recovery from a 1-minute bout of fatiguing exercise: Characteristics, reliability and responsiveness. Phys Ther 74:234–241, 1994.
226. Sinaki, M, et al: Can strong back extensors prevent vertebral fractures in women with osteoporosis? Mayo Clin Proced 71:951, 1996.
227. Skelton, DA, et al: Effects of resistance training on strength, power and selected functional abilities of women aged 75 and older. J Am Geriatric Soc 43:1081, 1995.
228. Smith, CA: The warm up procedure: To stretch or not to stretch. A brief review. J Orthop Sports Phys Ther 19:12, 1994.
229. Smith, LK, Weiss, EL, and Lehmkuhl, LD: Brunnstrom's Clinical Kinesiology, ed 5. FA Davis, Philadelphia, 1996.
230. Smith, MJ, and Melton, P: Isokinetic vs. isotonic variable-resistance training. Am J Sports Med 9:275, 1981.
231. Snyder-Mackler, L, et al: Strength of the quadriceps femoris muscle and functional recovery after reconstruction of the anterior cruciate ligament. J Bone Joint Surg 77A:1166, 1995.
232. Snyder-Mackler, L: Scientific rationale and physiological basis for the use of closed kinetic chain exercise in the lower extremity. J Sport Rehabil 5:2, 1996.
233. Soderberg, GL: Skeletal muscle function. In Currier, DP and Nelson, RM (eds): Dynamics of Human Biologic Tissues. FA Davis, Philadelphia, 1992, p 74.
234. Soderberg, GJ, and Blaschak, MJ: Shoulder internal and external rotation peak torque through a velocity spectrum in differing positions. J Orthop Sports Phys Ther 8:518, 1987.
235. Solomonow, M, et al: The synergistic action of the anterior cruciate ligament and thigh muscles in maintaining joint stability. Am J Sports Med 15:207, 1987.
236. Stanton, P, and Purdam, C: Hamstring injuries in sprinting. The role of eccentric exercise. J Orthop Sports Phys Ther 10:343, 1989.
237. Staron, RS, et al: Skeletal muscle adaptations during the early phase of heavy-resistance training in men and women. J Appl Physiol 76:1247, 1994.
238. Steindler, A: Kinesiology of the Human Body under Normal and Pathological Conditions. Charles C Thomas, Springfield, IL, 1955.
239. Stiene, HA, et al: A comparison of closed kinetic chain and isokinetic joint isolation exercise in patients with patellofemoral dysfunction. J Orthop Sports Phys Ther 24:136, 1996.
240. Stone, M, et al: A hypothetical model for strength training. J Sports Med Phys Fitness 21:342, 1981.
241. Stone, MH: Connective tissue and bone responses to strength training. In Komi, PV (ed): Strength and Power in Sport. Blackwell Scientific Publishing, Boston, 1992, p 279.
242. Stone, MH: Implications for connective tissue and bone alterations resulting from resistance exercise training. Med Sci Sports Exerc 20:5162, 1988.
243. Stone, WJ, and Coulter, SP: Strength/endurance effects from three resistance training protocols with women. J Strength Conditioning Res 8:231, 1994.
244. Stout, JL: Physical fitness during childhood and adolescence. In Campbell, SK, Vander Linden, DW and Palisano, RJ (eds): Physical Therapy for Children, ed 2. WB Saunders, Philadelphia, 2000, p 141.
245. Straker, JS, and Stuhr, PJ: Clinical application of closed kinetic chain exercises in the lower extremity. Orthop Phys Ther Clin North Am 9:185, 2000.
246. Sulivan, PE, Markos, PD, and Minor, MAD: An Integrated Approach to Therapeutic Exercise, Reston, Reston, VA, 1982.
247. Sullivan, PE, and Markos, PD: Clinical Decision Making in Therapeutic Exercise. Appleton and Lange, Norwalk, CT, 1995.
248. Taaffe, DR, et al: Once-weekly resistance exercise improves muscle strength and neuromuscular performance in older adults. J Am Geriatr Soc 47:1208, 1999.
249. Tanner, SM: Weighing the risks: Strength training for children and adolescents. Phys Sports Med 21:105, 1993.
250. Taylor, RA, et al: Knee position error detection in closed and open kinetic chain tasks during concurrent cognitive distraction. J Orthop Sports Phys Ther 28:81, 1998.
251. Tesch, PA, Thurstensson, A, and Kaiser, P: Muscle capillary

supply and fiber type characteristics in weight and power lifters. J Appl Physiol 56:35, 1984.

252. Tiidus, PM: Manual massage and recovery of muscle function following exercise: A literature review. J Orthop Sports Phys Ther 25:107, 1997.
253. Timm, KE: Investigation of the physiological overflow effect from speed-specific isokinetic activity. J Orthop Sports Phys Ther 9:106, 1987.
254. Tippett, SR: Closed-chain exercise. Orthop Phys Ther Clin North Am 1:253–267, 1992.
255. Tomberlin, JP, et al: Comparative study of isokinetic eccentric and concentric quadriceps training. J Orthop Sports Phys Ther 14:31–36, 1991.
256. Tracy, BL, et al: Muscle quality. II. Effects of strength training in 65- to 75-year old men and women. J Appl Physiol 86:195, 1999.
257. Voight, M, and Tippett, S: Plyometric exercise in rehabilitation. In Prentice, WE: Rehabilitation Techniques in Sports Medicine, ed 3. WCB/McGraw-Hill, Boston, 1999, p 157.
258. Voight, ML: Stretch strengthening: An introduction to plyometrics. Orthop Phys Ther Clin North Am 1:243–252, 1992.
259. Voight, ML, and Draovitch, P: Plyometrics. In Albert, M (ed): Eccentric Muscle Training in Sports and Orthopedics, ed 2. Churchill Livingstone, New York, 1995, p149.
260. Voss, DE, Ionta, MK, and Myers, BJ: Proprioceptive Neuromuscular Facilitation, ed 3. Harper & Row, New York, 1985.
261. Wallace, B: Balance training. In Bandy, WD and Sanders B: Therapeutic Exercise: Techniques for Intervention. Lippincott Williams & Wilkins, Baltimore, 2001, p 239.
262. Waltrous, B, Armstrong, R, and Schwane, J: The role of lactic acid in delayed onset muscular soreness. Med Sci Sports Exerc 1:380, 1981.
263. Warner, JJP, et al: Effect of joint compression on the inferior stability of the glenohumeral joint. J Shoulder Elbow Surg 8:31, 1999.
264. Weber, MD, Servedio, F, and Woodall, WR: The effect of three modalities on delayed onset muscle soreness. J Orthop Sports Phys Ther 20:236–242, 1994.
265. Weir, JP, et al: The effect of unilateral concentric weight training and detraining on joint angle specificity, cross-training and the bilateral deficit. J Orthop Sports Phys Ther 25:264, 199.
266. Weir, JP, et al: The effect of unilateral eccentric weight training and detraining on joint angle specificity, cross-training and the bilateral deficit. J Orthop Sports Phys Ther 22:207, 1995.
267. Weir, JP, Housh, TJ, and Wagner, LI: Electromyographic evaluation of joint angle specificity and cross-training following isometric training. J Appl Physiol 77:197, 1994.
268. Weiss, LW, Clark, FC, and Howard, DG: Effects of heavy-resistance triceps surae muscle training on strength and muscularity of men and women. Phys Ther 68:208, 1988.
269. Weiss, LW, Coney, HD, and Clark, FC: Gross measures of exercise-induced muscular hypertrophy. J Orthop Sports Phys Ther 30:141, 2000.
270. Wescott, WL: Strength Training Past 50. Human Kinetics, Champaign, IL, 1998.
271. Whitcomb, LJ, Kelley, MJ, and Leiper, CI: A comparison of torque production during dynamic strength testing shoulder abduction in the coronal plane and the plane of the scapula. J Orthop Sports Phys Ther 21:227, 1995.
272. Wilder, PA: Muscle development and function. In Cech, D and Martin, S: Functional Movement Development Across the Life Span. WB Saunders, Philadelphia, 1995, p 137.
273. Wilk, K, Arrigo, C, and Andrews, J: Closed and open kinetic chain exercise for the upper extremity. J Sports Rehabil 5:88, 1995.
274. Wilk, KE, et al: A comparison of tibiofemoral joint forces and electromyography during open and closed kinetic chain exercises. Am J Sports Med 24:518, 1996.
275. Wilk, KE, et al: Open and closed kinetic chain exercise for the lower extremity: theory and clinical application. Athletic Training Sports and Health Perspectives 1:336, 1995.
276. Wilk, KE, et al: Stretch-shortening drills for the upper extremities: Theory and clinical application. J Orthop Sports Phys Ther 17:225–239, 1993.
277. Wilke, DV: The relationship between force and velocity in human muscle. J Physiol 110:249, 1950.
278. Woodall, WR, and Weber, MD: Exercise response and thermoregulation. Orthop Phys Ther Clin North Am 7:1, 1998.
279. Wu, Y, et al: Relationship between isokinetic concentric and eccentric contraction modes in the knee flexor and extensor muscle groups. J Orthop Sports Phys Ther 26:143, 1997.
280. Wyatt, MP, and Edwards, AM: Comparison of quadriceps and hamstrings torque values during isokinetic exercise. J Orthop Sports Phys Ther 3:348, 1981.
281. Yack, HJ, Colins, CE, and Whieldon, T: Comparison of closed and open kinetic chain exercise in the anterior cruciate ligament deficient knee. Am J Sports Med 21:49, 1993.
282. Yack, HJ, Riley, LM, and Whieldon, T: Anterior tibial translation during progressive loading the ACL-deficient knee during weight-bearing and nonweight-bearing isometric exercise. J Orthop Sports Phys Ther 20:247, 1994.
283. Yarasheski, KE, Lemon, PW, and Gilloteaux, J: Effect of heavy resistance exercise training on muscle fiber composition in young rats. J Appl Physiol 69:434, 1990.
284. Zernicke, RF, and Loitz, BJ: Exercise-related adaptations in connective tissue. In Komi, PV (ed): Strength and Power in Sport. Blackwell Scientific Publishing, Boston, 1992, p 77.
285. Zinowieff, AN: Heavy resistance exercise: The Oxford technique. Br J Phys Med 14:129, 1951.
286. Zwiren, LD, and Manos, LM: Exercise testing and prescription considerations throughout childhood. In Roitman, JL (ed): ACSM's Resource Manual for Guidelines for Exercise Testing and Prescription, ed 4. Lippincott Williams & Wilkins, Philadelphia, 2001, p 520.

Chapter 4

Principles of Aerobic Exercise

Terri M. Glenn, PhD, PT · Janet A. Mulcare, PhD, FASCM

OBJECTIVES

After studying this chapter, the reader will be able to:

1 Define fitness, endurance, conditioning, adaptation, cardiac output, $\dot{V}O_{2\,max}$, $a - \bar{v}O_2$ difference, training stimulus threshold, metabolic equivalent (MET), telemetry, and efficiency.

2 Describe the determination of fitness and/or endurance levels in humans.

3 Discuss the factors influencing the transport of oxygen.

4 Identify the changes that occur with deconditioning and the implications of these changes.

5 Compare the characteristics of the three energy systems.

6 Describe the determination of energy expenditure.

7 Differentiate high-level and low-level activity in terms of energy cost.

8 Differentiate between stress testing and fitness testing.

9 Identify the end points used to determine if $\dot{V}O_{2\,max}$ is achieved.

10 List the signs and symptoms that determine cessation of the stress test or the exercise session.

11 Identify the appropriate guidelines for determining the intensity, duration, and frequency of an exercise program.

12 Calculate the maximum heart rate for an individual of a certain age and determine the safest way to calculate the target heart rate for individuals of differing physical capacities, using the maximum heart rate or the heart rate reserve.

13 Discuss the overload principle in endurance training or conditioning.

14 Differentiate between high-level and low-level exercise programs (characteristics, activities, and energy expenditure).

15 Identify some special considerations that should be taken into account when setting up an exercise program.

16 List the cardiovascular and biochemical changes that occur with endurance training and the mechanisms for their occurrence.

17 Compare cardiovascular and respiratory parameters and $\dot{V}O_{2\,max}$ in the child, young adult, and aged.

There are numerous sources from which to obtain information on training for endurance in athletes and healthy young people and for individuals with coronary heart disease. But information or emphasis on endurance training and the improvement of fitness in the individual who has other types of chronic disease or disability is only beginning to emerge. The American College of Sports Medicine recently published basic guidelines for several of the more common chronic conditions and is currently in the process of revising that information based upon more recent research.[2] This chapter uses information from well-known sources to demonstrate that the physical therapist can use aerobic-type activity when working with either healthy individuals or patients with a variety of conditions. In addition, some fundamental information about cardiovascular and respiratory parameters in children and the elderly, as well as the young or middle-aged adult, is presented so the physical therapist can be prepared to treat individuals of all ages.

▶ Key Terms

Fitness

Fitness is a general term used to describe the ability to perform physical work. Performing physical work requires cardiorespiratory functioning, muscular strength and endurance, and musculoskeletal flexibility (Box 4–1). Optimum body composition is also included when describing fitness.

To become physically fit, individuals must participate regularly in some form of physical activity that uses large muscle groups and challenges the cardiorespiratory system. Individuals of all ages can improve their general fitness status by participating in activities that include walking, biking, running, swimming, stairclimbing, cross-country skiing, and/or training with weights.

Fitness levels can be described on a continuum from poor to superior based on energy expenditure during a bout of physical work.[7,8,9] These ratings are often based on the direct or indirect measurement of the body's maximal oxygen consumption ($\dot{V}O_{2\ max}$).

- Oxygen consumption is influenced by age, gender, heredity, inactivity, and disease.
- Several methods are available to estimate maximal oxygen consumption from submaximal effort and are summarized in Table 4–1.

Box 4–1 Fitness Goals for the Nation[10]

Did You Know?

The U.S. Dept. of Health and Human Services has identified health promotion and disease prevention objectives for Americans for the 20th century in the publication Healthy People 2000[10] *and are forthcoming with new recommendations as we enter the 21st century. The following objectives address both cardiorespiratory and musculoskeletal fitness:*

- Increase to at least 20% the proportion of people aged 18 and older and to at least 75% the proportion of children and adolescents aged 6 through 17 who engage in vigorous physical activity that promotes the development and maintenance of cardiorespiratory fitness 3 or more days per week for 20 or more minutes per occasion.
- Increase to at least 40% the proportion of people aged 6 and older who regularly perform physical activities that enhance and maintain muscular strength, muscular endurance and flexibility. These same recommendations apply to persons with chronic disability.

Maximum Oxygen Consumption

Maximum oxygen consumption ($\dot{V}O_{2\ max}$) is a measure of the body's capacity to use oxygen.[2,7,8,9] It is usually measured when performing an exercise bout that uses many large muscle groups such as swimming, walking, and running. It is the maximum amount of oxygen consumed per minute when the individual has reached maximal effort. It is usually expressed relative to body weight, as milliliters of oxygen per kilogram of body weight per minute (mL/kg per minute). It is dependent on the transport of oxygen, the oxygen-binding capacity of the blood, cardiac function, oxygen extraction capabilities, and muscular oxidative potential. The $\dot{V}O_2$ can be defined mathematically using the Fick equation (Box 4–2).

At rest, the average person has a cardiac output of 5 liters. (Stroke volume is approximately 70 mL and resting heart rate is approximately 72 beats per minute). Even though circulating arterial blood carries approximately 1000 mL of oxygen, the average resting level of oxygen extraction (i.e., $\dot{V}O_2$) is 250 mL.

Endurance

Endurance (a measure of fitness) is the ability to work for prolonged periods of time and the ability to resist fatigue.[7,8,9] It includes muscular endurance and cardiovascular endurance. Muscular endurance refers to the ability of an isolated muscle group to perform repeated contractions over a period of time, whereas cardiovascular endurance refers to the ability to perform large muscle dynamic exercise, such as walking, swimming, and/or biking for long periods of time.

Aerobic Exercise Training (Conditioning)

Aerobic exercise training or conditioning is an augmentation of the energy utilization of the muscle by means of an exercise program.[7,8,9] The improvement of the muscle's ability to use energy is a direct result of increased levels of oxidative enzymes in the muscles, as well as increased mitochondrial density and size, and an increased muscle fiber capillary supply.

- Training is dependent on exercise of sufficient intensity, duration, and frequency.
- Training produces a cardiovascular and/or muscular adaptation and is reflected in an individual's endurance.

Table 4–1 Summary of Methods to Estimate Maximal Oxygen Consumption from Submaximal Exercise

Method	Patient Population Application	Advantages	Disadvantages
Cycle ergometer tests	Cerebral vascular accident, multiple sclerosis, peripheral vascular disease, obesity, any patient with balance problems	• Eliminates need for balance • Documentable workloads for use with the prediction equations • Nonweight-bearing • Easy, safe, and quick to administer	• Requires ergometer with a calibrated braking mechanism
3-minute step test	General nonlower extremity orthopedic patient; nonobese	• Can be administered to many subjects simultaneously	• Assumes patient locates and counts HR accurately
Distance runs	Active individuals	• Whole body effort • Easy to perform	• Need large measured area • Not feasible with a group
Walking tests	Older, healthy individuals and ambulatory persons with chronic conditions	• Whole body effort • Easy to perform	• Need large measured area • Not feasible with a group

- Training for a particular sport or event is dependent on the *specificity principle;*[7,8,9] that is, the individual improves in the exercise task used for training and may not improve in other tasks. For example, swimming may enhance one's performance in swimming events but may not improve one's performance in treadmill running.

Adaptation

The cardiovascular system and the muscles used will *adapt* to the training stimulus over time.[7,8,9] Significant changes can be measured in as little as 10 to 12 weeks.

Adaptation results in increased efficiency of the cardiovascular system and the active muscles. Adaptation represents a variety of neurologic, physical, and biochemical changes within the cardiovascular and muscular systems. Performance improves in that, the same amount of work can be performed after training, at a lower physiological cost.

Adaptation is dependent on the ability of the organism to change and the training stimulus threshold (the stimulus that elicits a training response).

Box 4–2 Fick Equation

$\dot{V}O_2$ = cardiac output × arteriovenous O_2 difference
= Q × $a - \bar{v}O_2$
Cardiac output (Q) = heart rate (HR) × stroke volume (SV)
Arteriovenous O_2 difference ($a - \bar{v}O_2$)
= arterial oxygen − venous oxygen

- The person with a low level of fitness will have more potential to improve than the one who has a high level of fitness.
- Training stimulus thresholds are variable. The higher the initial level of fitness, the greater the intensity of exercise needed to elicit a significant change.

Myocardial Oxygen Consumption

Myocardial oxygen consumption ($m\dot{V}O_2$) is a measure of the oxygen consumed by the myocardial muscle.[2,3,7,8,9]

- The need or demand for oxygen is determined by heart rate (HR), systemic blood pressure, myocardial contractility, and afterload. Afterload is determined by the left ventricular wall tension and central aortic pressure. It is the ventricular force required to open the aortic valve at the beginning of systole. Left ventricular wall tension is primarily determined by ventricular size and wall thickness.
- The ability to supply the myocardium with oxygen is dependent on the arterial oxygen content (blood substrate), hemoglobin oxygen dissociation, and coronary blood flow, which is determined by aortic diastolic pressure, duration of diastole, coronary artery resistance, and collateral circulation.
- In a healthy individual, a balance between myocardial oxygen supply and demand is maintained during maximal exercise. When the

Box 4–3 Clinical Relevance—Exertional Angina

A person who has coronary occlusion may not present with any type of chest pain (angina) until they need to exert themselves. This is because, when the body works harder, HR increases, diastolic filling time decreases, and increased coronary blood flow is sacrificed by the reduced time for filling the coronary arteries. Without an adequate blood supply, the underlying cardiac tissue no longer receives the oxygen needed for metabolic activity, resulting in anginal pain.

demand for oxygen is greater than the supply, myocardial ischemia results.

- Since the myocardial muscle extracts 70 to 75% of the oxygen from the blood during rest, its main source of supply during exercise is through an increase in coronary blood flow.
- Clinical relevance is described in Box 4–3.

Deconditioning

Deconditioning occurs with prolonged bed rest, and its effects are frequently seen in the patient who has had an extended, acute illness or long-term chronic condition. Decreases in maximal oxygen consumption, cardiac output (stroke volume), and muscular strength occur very rapidly. These effects are also seen, although possibly to a lesser degree, in the individual who has spent a period of time on bed rest without any accompanying disease process and in the individual who is sedentary because of lifestyle and increasing age (Box 4–4).

Energy Systems, Energy Expenditure, and Efficiency

Energy Systems

Energy systems are metabolic systems involving a series of biochemical reactions resulting in the formation of adenosine triphosphate (ATP), carbon dioxide, and water.[7–9] The cell uses the energy produced from the conversion of ATP to adenosine diphosphate (ADP) and phosphate (P) to perform metabolic activities. Muscle cells use this energy for actin-myosin cross-bridge formation when contracting. There are three major energy systems. The intensity and duration of activity determine when and to what extent each metabolic system contributes.

1. ***The phosphagen or ATP-PC system.*** The ATP-PC system (adenosine triphosphate-phosphocreatine) has the following characteristics:
   - Phosphocreatine and ATP are stored in the muscle cell.
   - Phosphocreatine is the chemical fuel source.
   - No oxygen is required.
   - When muscle is rested, the supply of ATP-PC is replenished.
   - The maximum capacity of the system is small (0.7 mol ATP).
   - The maximum power of the system is great (3.7 mol ATP/min).
   - The system provides energy for short, quick bursts of activity.
   - It is the major source of energy during the first 30 seconds of intense exercise.
2. ***The anaerobic glycolytic system.*** The anaerobic glycolytic system has the following characteristics:
   - Glycogen (glucose) is the fuel source (glycolysis).
   - No oxygen is required (anaerobic).
   - ATP is resynthesized in the muscle cell.
   - Lactic acid is produced (by-product of anaerobic glycolysis).
   - The maximum capacity of the system is intermediate (1.2 mol ATP).
   - The maximum power of the system is intermediate (1.6 mol ATP/min).
   - The systems provide energy for activity of moderate intensity and short duration.
   - It is the major source of energy from the 30th to 90th second of exercise.
3. ***The aerobic system.*** The aerobic system has the following characteristics:
   - Glycogen, fats, and proteins are fuel sources and are utilized relative to their availability and the intensity of the exercise.
   - Oxygen is required (aerobic).
   - ATP is resynthesized in the mitochondria of the muscle cell. The ability to metabolize oxygen and

Box 4–4 Deconditioning Effects Associated with Bed Rest[3]

↓ *muscle mass*
↓ *strength*
↓ *cardiovascular function*
↓ *total blood volume*
↓ *plasma volume*
↓ *heart volume*
↓ *orthostatic tolerance*
↓ *exercise tolerance*
↓ *bone mineral density*

other substrates is related to the number and concentration of the mitochondria and cells.

- The maximum capacity of the system is great (90.0 mol ATP).
- The maximum power of the system is small (1.0 mol ATP/min).
- The system predominates over the other energy systems after the second minute of exercise.

4. ***Recruitment of motor units.*** Recruitment of motor units is dependent on rate of work. Fibers are recruited selectively during exercise.[7,8,9]

- Slow-twitch fibers (type I) are characterized by a slow contractile response, are rich in myoglobin and mitochondria, have a high oxidative capacity and a low anaerobic capacity, and are recruited for activities demanding endurance. These fibers are supplied by small neurons with a low threshold of activation and are used preferentially in low-intensity exercise.
- Fast-twitch fibers (type IIB) are characterized by a fast contractile response, have a low myoglobin content and few mitochondria, have a high glycolytic capacity, and are recruited for activities requiring power.
- Fast-twitch fibers (type IIA) have characteristics of both type I and type IIB fibers and are recruited for both anaerobic and aerobic activities.

Functional Implications

- Bursts of intense activity (seconds) develop muscle strength and stronger tendons and ligaments. ATP is supplied by the phosphagen system.
- Intense activity (1 to 2 minutes) repeated after 4 minutes of rest or mild exercise enhances anaerobic power. ATP is supplied by the phosphagen and anaerobic glycolytic system.
- Activity with large muscles, which is less than maximal intensity for 3 to 5 minutes repeated after rest or mild exercise of similar duration, may develop aerobic power and endurance capabilities. ATP is supplied by the phosphagen, anaerobic glycolytic, and aerobic systems.
- Activity that is of submaximal intensity lasting 20 to 30 minutes or more taxes a high percentage of the aerobic system and develops endurance.

Energy Expenditure

Energy is expended by individuals engaging in physical activity and is often expressed in kilocalories. Activities can be categorized as light, moderate or heavy by determining the energy cost. The energy cost of any activity is affected by mechanical efficiency and body mass. Factors that affect both walking and running are terrain, stride length, and air resistance.[7,8,9]

Energy expenditure can be determined easily by open-circuit spirometry or cardiac telemetry. *Open-circuit portable spirometry* requires that the individual breathe into and out of a mouthpiece with a one-way valve.[2,3]

- The expired air passes directly through a gas analyzer that measures volume and analyzes the oxygen and carbon dioxide composition of the expired sample. This occurs automatically on a breath-by-breath basis.
- The energy expenditure is computed from the amount of oxygen consumed.

Telemetry, or physiological radio transmission, allows the individual to move freely. The heart rate of the individual is transmitted to a graphic printout system, producing an electrocardiographic strip.

- Heart rate is linearly related to the work performed.
- Heart rate is therefore linearly related to the amount of oxygen consumed per minute.

Energy expended is computed from the amount of oxygen consumed. Units used to quantify energy expenditure are kilocalories and METs (Box 4–5).

A *kilocalorie* is a measure expressing the energy value of food. It is the amount of heat necessary to raise 1 kilogram (kg) of water 1°C. A kilocalorie (kcal) can be expressed in oxygen equivalents. Five kilocalories equal approximately one liter of oxygen consumed (5 kcal = 1 liter O_2).

A *MET* is defined as the oxygen consumed (milliliters) per kilogram of body weight per minute (mL/kg). It is equal to approximately 3.5 mL/kg per minute.[2]

Activities are classified as light, moderate or heavy according to energy expended or oxygen consumed while accomplishing them.[7,8,9]

Box 4–5 Daily Energy Expenditure

The average individual engaged in normal daily tasks expends 1800 to 3000 kcal per day. Athletes engaged in intense training can use more than 10,000 kcal per day.

Data from Wilmore, JH, and Costill, DL: Physiology of Sport and Exercise. Human Kinetics, Champaign, IL, 1994.

- Light work for the average male (65 kg) requires 2.0 to 4.9 kcal/min, or 6.1 to 15.2 mL O_2/kg per minute, or 1.6 to 3.9 METs. Strolling 1.6 km/h, or 1.0 mph, is considered light work.
- Heavy work for the average male (65 kg) requires 7.5 to 9.9 kcal/min, or 23.0 to 30.6 mL O_2/kg per minute, or 6.0 to 7.9 METs. Jogging 8.0 km/h, or 5.0 mph, is considered heavy work.
- Jogging 8.0 km/h, or 5.0 mph, requires 25 to 28 mL O_2/kg per minute and is considered heavy work. The energy expended is equivalent to 8 to 10 kcal/min, or 7 to 8 METs.

The energy expenditure necessary for most industrial jobs requires more than three times the energy expenditure at rest.

Energy expenditure of certain physical activities can vary, depending on factors such as skill, pace, and fitness level (Box 4–5).

Efficiency

Efficiency is usually expressed as a percentage[7,8,9] (Box 4–6).

Work output equals force times distance ($W = F \times D$). It can be expressed in power units or work per unit of time ($P = w/t$).

- On a treadmill, work equals the weight of the subject times the vertical distance the subject is raised walking up the incline of the treadmill.
- On a bicycle ergometer, work equals the distance (which is the circumference of the flywheel times the number of revolutions) times the bicycle resistance.

Work input equals energy expenditure and is expressed as the net oxygen consumption per unit of time. With aerobic exercise, the resting volume of oxygen used per unit of time ($\dot{V}O_2$ value) is subtracted from the oxygen consumed during 1 minute of the steady-state period.

- Steady state is reached within 3 to 4 minutes after exercise has started if the load or resistance is kept constant.
- In the steady-state period, $\dot{V}O_2$ remains at a constant (steady) value.

Total net oxygen cost is multiplied by the total time in minutes that the exercise is performed.

Box 4–6 Efficiency Expressed as a Percentage

$$\text{Percent efficiency} = \frac{\text{useful work output}}{\text{energy expended or work input}} \times 100$$

The higher the net oxygen cost, the lower the efficiency in performing the activity.

Efficiency of large muscle activities is usually 20 to 25%.

▶ Physiologic Response to Aerobic Exercise

The rapid increase in energy requirements during exercise requires equally rapid circulatory adjustments to meet the increased need for oxygen and nutrients to remove the end products of metabolism such as carbon dioxide and lactic acid and to dissipate excess heat. The shift in body metabolism occurs through a coordinated activity of all the systems of the body; neuromuscular, respiratory, cardiovascular, metabolic, and hormonal (Box 4–7). Oxygen transport and its utilization by the mitochondria of the contracting muscle are dependent on adequate blood flow in conjunction with cellular respiration.[7,8,9]

Cardiovascular Response to Exercise

The Exercise Pressor Response

Stimulation of small myelinated and unmyelinated fibers in skeletal muscle involves a sympathetic nervous system (SNS) response. The central pathways are not known.[2,3,7,8,9]

- The SNS response includes a generalized peripheral vasoconstriction in nonexercising muscles and increased myocardial contractility, an increased heart rate, and an increase in systolic blood pressure. This results in a marked increase and redistribution of the cardiac output.
- The degree of the response equals the muscle mass involved and the intensity of the exercise.

Cardiac Effects

- Frequency of sinoatrial node depolarization increases and heart rate increases. There is a de-

Box 4–7 Factors Affecting the Response to Acute Exercise

Ambient temperature, humidity, and altitude can affect the physiologic responses to acute exercise. Diurnal fluctuations as well as changes associated with a female's menstrual cycle can affect these responses as well. Therefore, researchers control these factors as much as possible when evaluating the response to exercise.

crease in vagal stimuli as well as an increase in SNS stimulation.
- There is an increase in the force development of the cardiac myofibers. A direct inotropic response of the SNS increases myocardial contractility.

Peripheral Effects

- Generalized vasoconstriction occurs that allows blood to be shunted from the nonworking muscles, kidneys, liver, spleen, and splanchnic area to the working muscles.
- A locally mediated reduction in resistance in the working muscle arterial vascular bed, independent of the autonomic nervous system, is produced by metabolites such as Mg^{2+}, Ca^{2+}, ADP, and Pco_2.
- The veins of the working as well as the nonworking muscles remain constricted.
- A *net* reduction in total peripheral resistance results.

The cardiac output increases because of the:
- Increase in myocardial contractility, with a resultant ↑ in stroke volume
- Increase in heart rate
- Increase in the blood flow through the working muscle
- Increase in the constriction of the capacitance vessels on the venous side of the circulation in both the working and nonworking muscles, raising the peripheral venous pressure
- Net reduction in the total peripheral resistance

The increase in the systolic blood pressure is the result of the augmented cardiac output.

Respiratory Response to Exercise

Respiratory changes occur rapidly, even before the initiation of exercise.[7,8,9] Gas exchange (O_2, CO_2) increases across the alveolar-capillary membrane by the first or second breath. Increased muscle metabolism during exercise results in more O_2 extracted from arterial blood resulting in an increase in venous Pco_2 and H^+, an increase in body temperature, increased epinephrine, and an increased stimulation of receptors of the joints and muscles. Any of these factors alone or in combination may stimulate the respiratory system. Baroreceptor reflexes, protective reflexes, pain, emotion, and voluntary control of respiration may also contribute to the increase in respiration.

Minute ventilation increases as respiratory frequency and tidal volume increase.

Alveolar ventilation, occurring with the diffusion of gases across the capillary-alveolar membrane, increases 10-fold to 20-fold in heavy exercise to supply the additional oxygen needed and excrete the excess carbon dioxide produced.

Responses Providing Additional Oxygen to Muscle

The increased blood flow to the working muscle previously discussed provides additional oxygen. There is also extraction of more oxygen from each liter of blood. There are several changes that allow for this.
- A decrease of the local tissue Po_2 occurs because of the use of more oxygen by the working muscle. As the partial pressure of oxygen decreases, the unloading of oxygen from hemoglobin is facilitated.
- The production of more carbon dioxide causes the tissue to become acidotic (the hydrogen ion concentration increases) and the temperature of the tissue to increase. Both situations increase the amount of oxygen released from hemoglobin at any given partial pressure.
- The increase of red blood cell 2,3-diphosphoglycerate (DPG) produced by glycolysis during exercise also contributes to the enhanced release of oxygen.

Factors determining how much of the oxygen is consumed are:
- Vascularity of the muscles.
- Fiber distribution.
- Number of mitochondria.
- Oxidative mitochondrial enzymes present in the fibers. The oxidative capacity of the muscle is reflected in the $a - \bar{v}O_2$ difference, which is the difference between the oxygen content of arterial and venous blood.

▶ Testing as a Basis for Exercise Programs

Testing for physical fitness of healthy individuals should be distinct from graded exercise testing of convalescing patients, individuals with symptoms of coronary heart disease, or individuals who are age 35 years or older but asymptomatic.[1,2] Regardless of the type of testing, the level of performance is based on the submaximal or maximal oxygen uptake ($\dot{V}O_{2\ max}$) or the symptom-limited oxygen uptake. The capacity of the individual to transport and utilize oxygen is reflected in the oxygen uptake. Readers are referred to publications by the American College of Sports Medicine[1,2] for additional information.

Fitness Testing of Healthy Subjects

Field tests for the determination of cardiovascular fitness include time to run 1.5 miles or distance run in 12 minutes. These correlate well with $\dot{V}O_{2\ max}$, but their use is limited to young persons or middle-aged individuals who have been carefully screened and have been jogging or running for some time.[2,3]

Multistage testing can provide a direct measurement of $\dot{V}O_{2\ max}$ by analyzing samples of expired air.[1,2] Testing is usually completed in four to six treadmill stages, which progressively increase in speed and or grade. Each stage is 3 to 6 minutes long. Electrocardiographic (ECG) monitoring is performed during the testing. Maximum oxygen uptake can be determined when the oxygen utilization plateaus despite an increase in workload.

Stress Testing for Convalescing Individuals and Individuals at Risk

Individuals undergoing stress testing should have a physical examination, be monitored by the ECG, and be closely observed at rest, during exercise, and during recovery (Fig. 4–1).

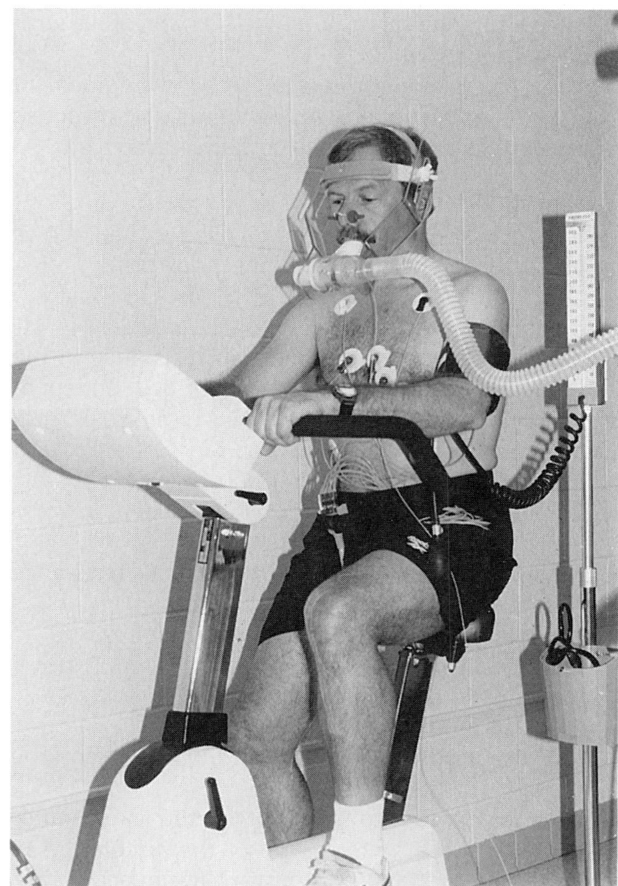

Figure 4–1 Placement of electrodes for the 12-lead exercise electrocardiogram used to determine heart rate and rhythm during the stress test.

1. The *principles of stress testing* include:[2,3]

- Changing the workload by increasing the speed and/or grade of the treadmill or the resistance on the bicycle ergometer.
- An initial workload that is low in terms of the individual's anticipated aerobic threshold.
- Maintenance of each workload for 1 minute or longer.
- Termination of the test at the onset of symptoms or a definable abnormality of the ECG.
- When available, measurement of the individual's maximal oxygen consumption.

2. In addition to serving as a basis for determining exercise levels or the exercise prescription, the stress test:

- Helps establish a diagnosis of overt or latent heart disease.
- Evaluates cardiovascular functional capacity as a means of clearing individuals for strenuous work or exercise programs.
- Determines the physical work capacity in kilogram-meters per minute (kg-m/min) or the functional capacity in METs.
- Evaluates responses to exercise training and/or preventive programs.
- Assists in the selection and evaluation of appropriate modes of treatment for heart disease.
- Increases individual motivation for entering and adhering to exercise programs.
- Is used clinically to evaluate patients with chest sensations or a history of chest pain to establish the probability that such patients have coronary disease. It can also evaluate the functional capacity of patients with chronic disease.

3. All individuals who are taking a stress test should:

- Have had a physical examination.
- Be monitored by the ECG and closely observed at rest, during exercise, and during recovery.
- Sign a consent form.

Box 4–8 Precautions for Stress Testing and Exercise Program

Monitor the pulse to assess abnormal increases in heart rate.

Blood pressure increases with exercise approximately 7 to 10 millimeters (mm) of mercury (Hg) per MET of physical activity.

- Systolic pressure should not exceed 220 to 240 mm Hg.
- Diastolic pressure should not exceed 120 mm Hg.

Rate and depth of respiration increase with exercise.

- Respiration should not be labored.
- The individual should have no perception of shortness of breath.

The increase in blood flow while exercising, which regulates core temperature and meets the demands of the working muscles, results in changes in the skin of the cheeks, nose, and earlobes. They become pink, moist, and warm to the touch.

Precautions: Precautions to be taken are are summarized in Box 4–8. They are applicable for both stress testing and the exercise program.[2,3]

4. End points requiring termination of the test period are[2]:

- Progressive angina.
- A significant drop in systolic pressure in response to an increasing workload.
- Lightheadedness, confusion, pallor, cyanosis, nausea, or peripheral circulatory insufficiency.
- Abnormal ECG responses including ST segment depression greater than 4 mm.
- Excessive rise in blood pressure.
- Subject wishes to stop.

Multistage Testing

Each of the four to six stages is approximately 1 to 6 minutes. Differences in protocols involve the number of stages, magnitude of exercise (intensity), equipment used (bicycle, treadmill), duration of stages, end points, position of body, muscle groups exercised, and types of effort (Box 4–9).[2,3]

Protocols have been developed for multistage testing. The most popular treadmill protocol is the Bruce protocol. Treadmill speed and grade are changed every 3 minutes. Speed increases from 1.7 mph up to 5.0 mph, while the initial grade of 10% increases up to 18% during the five stages.

Box 4–9 Case Example of an Exercise Stress Test

Mr. Smith is a 55-year-old sedentary male with a history of chest pain with exertion. He has undergone a stress test to assist in evaluating his angina. He is not taking any medications at the present time. He has been a smoker for 20 years.

- Resting electrocardiogram (ECG): normal
- Resting heart rate: 75 beats/min
- Age-predicted maximal heart rate: 165 beats/min
- Resting blood pressure: 128/86
- Resting respiration rate: 20 breaths/min
- Treadmill: Bruce protocol

Stage	Heart Rate	Blood Pressure	Comments
1	80		
	84		
	85	138/88	No complaints
2	88		
	90		
	92	142/90	No complaints
3	98		
	100		
	102	156/91	Complaining of leg fatigue
4	114		
	116		
	122	161/90	Complaining of minimal chest pain
5	133		
	135		
	137	174/89	Complaining of severe chest pain; test terminated

Conclusion

The stress test was terminated because of complaints of severe chest pain accompanied by a drop in the ST segment of the ECG to 4 mm. The symptom-limited maximum heart rate was determined to be 137 beats/min. Maximal oxygen consumption was determined to be 32 mL/kg/min.

▶ Determinants of an Exercise Program

Just as testing for fitness should be distinct from stress testing for patients or individuals at high risk, training programs for healthy individuals are distinct from the exercise prescription for individuals with cardiopulmonary disease.

Effective endurance training for any population must produce a conditioning or cardiovascular response. Elicitation of the cardiovascular response is dependent on three critical elements of exercise: *intensity, duration,* and *frequency.*[2,3,7,8,9]

Intensity

Determination of the appropriate intensity of exercise to use is based on the overload principle and the specificity principle.[2,3,7,8,9]

- The *overload principle:* Overload is a stress on an organism that is greater than the one regularly encountered during everyday life. To improve cardiovascular and muscular endurance, an overload must be applied to these systems. The exercise load (overload) must be above the training stimulus threshold (that stimulus that elicits a training or conditioning response) for adaptation to occur.

- Once adaptation to a given load has taken place, for the individual to achieve further improvement, the training intensity (exercise load) must be increased.
- Training stimulus thresholds are variable, depending on the individual's level of health, level of activity, age, and gender.
- The higher the initial level of fitness, the greater the intensity of exercise needed to elicit a change.
- A conditioning response occurs generally at 60 to 90% maximum heart rate (50–85% $\dot{V}O_{2\ max}$) depending on the individual and the initial level of fitness.
  - Seventy percent maximum heart rate is a minimal level stimulus for eliciting a conditioning response in healthy young individuals.
  - Sedentary or "deconditioned" individuals will respond to a low exercise intensity, 40 to 50% of $\dot{V}O_{2\ max}$.
  - The exercise does not have to be exhaustive to achieve a training response.
  - Determining **maximum heart rate** and **exercise heart rate** for training programs provides the basis for the initial intensity of the exercise (Box 4–10).
  - When the individual is young and healthy, the *maximum heart rate* can be determined directly from a maximum performance multistage test, extrapolated from a heart rate achieved on a predetermined submaximal test, or less accurately calculated as 220 minus age.
  - The *exercise heart rate* is determined in one of two ways: (1) as a percentage of the maximum heart rate (the percentage used is dependent on the level of fitness of the individual); and (2) using the heart rate reserve (Karvonen's formula). Karvonen's formula is based on the heart rate reserve (HRR), which is the difference between the resting heart rate (HR_{rest}) and the maximal heart rate (HR_{max}). The exercise heart rate is determined as a percentage (usually 60 to 70%) of the heart rate reserve plus the resting heart rate (see Box 4–10).
  - When using Karvonen's formula, the exercise heart rate is higher than when using maximum heart rate alone.
- Maximum heart rate and exercise heart rate used for the exercise prescription for individuals at risk for coronary artery disease, individuals with coronary artery disease or other chronic disease, and individuals who are elderly are ideally determined from performance on the stress test. Maximum heart rate cannot be determined in the same manner as with the young and healthy.
  - Assuming that an individual has an average maximum heart rate, using the formula 220 minus age will produce substantial errors in prescribing exercise intensity for these individuals.
  - Maximum heart rate, which may be symptom-limited, is considered maximum. At no time should the exercise heart rate exceed the symptom-limited heart rate achieved on the exercise test.
  - Individuals with cardiopulmonary disease may start exercise programs, depending on their diagnosis, as low as 40 to 60% of their maximal heart rate.
- Exercising at a high intensity for a shorter period of time appears to elicit a greater improvement in $\dot{V}O_{2\ max}$ than exercising at a moderate intensity for a longer period of time. However, as exercise approaches the maximum limit, there is an increase in the relative risk of cardiovascular complications and the risk of musculoskeletal injury.
- The higher the intensity and the longer the exercise intervals, the faster the training effect.
- Maximum oxygen consumption ($\dot{V}O_{2\ max}$) is the best measure of exercise intensity. Aerobic capacity and heart rate are linearly related and, therefore, maximum heart rate is a function of intensity.

Box 4–10 Methods to Determine Maximum Heart Rate and Exercise Heart Rate

Determine Maximum Heart Rate (HR)
- From multistage test (for young and healthy)
- HR achieved in predetermined submaximal test
- 220 minus age (less accurate)

Determine Exercise Heart Rate
- Percentage of maximum heart rate (dependent on level of fitness)
- Karvonen's formula (heart rate reserve)

Exercise heart rate $= HR_{rest} + 60\text{–}70\% (HR_{max} - HR_{rest})$

- The *specificity principle* as related to the specificity of training refers to adaptations in metabolic and physiologic systems depending on the demand imposed. There is no overlap when training for strength–power activities and training for endurance activities. Workload and work-rest periods are selected so that training results in:
  - Muscle strength without a significant increase in total oxygen consumption.
  - Aerobic or endurance training without training the anaerobic systems.
  - Anaerobic training without training the aerobic systems.
  - Even when evaluating aerobic or endurance activities, there appears to be little overlap. When training for swimming events, the individual may not demonstrate an improvement in $\dot{V}O_{2\ max}$ when running.

Duration

- The optimal duration of exercise for cardiovascular conditioning is dependent on the total work performed, exercise intensity and frequency, and fitness level.
- Generally speaking, the greater the intensity of the exercise, the shorter the duration needed for adaptation. And the lower the intensity of exercise, the longer the duration needed.
- A 20- to 30-minute session is generally optimal at 60 to 70% maximum heart rate. When the intensity is below the heart rate threshold, a 45-minute continuous exercise period may provide the appropriate overload. With high-intensity exercise, 10- to 15-minute exercise periods are adequate; three 5-minute daily periods may be effective in some deconditioned patients.
- Exercise of longer than 45 minutes duration increases the risk of musculoskeletal complications.

Frequency

- Like duration, there is no clear-cut information provided on the most effective frequency of exercise for adaptation to occur. Frequency may be a less important factor in exercise training than is intensity or duration.
- Frequency varies, dependent on the health and age of the individual. Optimal frequency of training is generally three to four times a week. If training is at a low intensity, greater frequency may be beneficial. A frequency of two times a week does not generally evoke cardiovascular changes, although older individuals and convalescing patients may benefit from a program of that frequency.
- As frequency increases beyond the optimal range, the risk of musculoskeletal complications increases.
- For individuals who are in good general health, exercising 30 to 45 minutes at least three times a week (2000 kcal/week) appears to protect against coronary heart disease.

Mode

- Many types of activities provide the stimulus for improving cardiorespiratory fitness. The important factor is that exercise involve large muscle groups that are activated in a rhythmic, aerobic nature. However, the magnitude of the changes may be determined by the mode used.
- For specific aerobic activities such as cycling and running, the overload must use the muscles required by the activity as well as stress the cardiorespiratory system (specificity principle). If endurance of the upper extremities is needed to perform activities on the job, then the upper extremity muscles must be targeted in the exercise program. The muscles trained develop a greater oxidative capacity with an increase in blood flow to the area. The increase in blood flow is due to increased microcirculation and more effective distribution of the cardiac output.
- Training benefits are optimized when programs are planned to meet the individual needs and capacities of the participants. The skill of the individual, variations among individuals in competitiveness and aggressiveness, and variation in environmental conditions all must be considered.

The Reversibility Principle

The beneficial effects of exercise training are transient and reversible.

- Detraining occurs rapidly when a person stops exercising. After only 2 weeks of detraining, significant reductions in work capacity can be measured, and improvements can be lost within several months. In addition, a similar phenomenon occurs with individuals who are confined to bed with illness or disability: the individual becomes severely deconditioned, with loss of the ability to carry out normal daily activities as a result of inactivity.

- The frequency or duration of physical activity required to maintain a certain level of aerobic fitness is less than that required to improve it.

The Exercise Program

A carefully planned exercise program can result in higher levels of fitness for the healthy individual, slow the decrease in functional capacity of the elderly, and recondition those who have been ill or have chronic disease. There are three components of the exercise program: (1) a warm-up period, (2) the aerobic exercise period, and (3) a cool-down period.

The Warm-Up Period

Physiologically, a time lag exists between the onset of activity and the bodily adjustments needed to meet the physical requirements of the body.

The purpose of the warm-up period is to enhance the numerous adjustments that must take place before physical activity. During this period there is:

- An increase in muscle temperature. The higher temperature increases the efficiency of muscular contraction by reducing muscle viscosity and increasing the rate of nerve conduction.
- An increased need for oxygen to meet the energy demands for the muscle. Extraction from hemoglobin is greater at higher muscle temperatures, facilitating the oxidative processes at work.
- Dilatation of the previously constricted capillaries with increases in the circulation, augmenting oxygen delivery to the active muscles and minimizing the oxygen deficit and the formation of lactic acid.
- Adaptation in sensitivity of the neural respiratory center to various exercise stimulants.
- An increase in venous return. This occurs as blood flow is shifted centrally from the periphery.

The warm-up also prevents or decreases:

- The susceptibility of the musculoskeletal system to injury by increasing flexibility.
- The occurrence of ischemic ECG changes and arrhythmias.

The warm-up should be gradual and sufficient to increase muscle and core temperature without causing fatigue or reducing energy stores. Characteristics of the period include:

- A 10-minute period of total body movement exercises such as calisthenics, static stretching, and walking slowly.
- The attainment of a heart rate within 20 beats per minute of the target heart rate.

The Aerobic Exercise Period

The aerobic exercise period is the conditioning part of the exercise program. Attention to the determinants of intensity, frequency, duration, and mode of the program, as previously discussed, will have an impact on the effectiveness of the program. The main consideration when choosing a specific method of training is that the *intensity* be great enough to stimulate an increase in stroke volume and cardiac output and to enhance local circulation and aerobic metabolism within the appropriate muscle groups. The exercise period must be within the person's tolerance, above the threshold level for adaptation to occur, and below the level of exercise that evokes clinical symptoms.

In aerobic exercise, submaximal, rhythmic, repetitive, dynamic exercise of large muscle groups is emphasized.

There are four methods of training that will challenge the aerobic system: continuous, interval (work relief), circuit, and circuit interval.

Continuous Training

- A submaximal energy requirement, sustained throughout the training period, is imposed.
- Once the steady state is achieved, the muscle obtains energy by means of aerobic metabolism. Stress is placed primarily on the slow-twitch fibers.
- The activity can be prolonged for 20 to 60 minutes without exhausting the oxygen transport system.
- Work rate is increased progressively as training improvements are achieved. Overload can be accomplished by increasing the exercise duration.
- In the healthy individual, continuous training is the most effective way to improve endurance.

Interval Training

In this type of training, the work or exercise is followed by a properly prescribed relief or rest interval. Interval training is perceived to be less demanding than continuous training. In the healthy individual, interval training tends to improve strength and power more than endurance.

- The relief interval is either a rest relief (passive recovery) or a work relief (active recovery), and its duration ranges from a few seconds to several minutes. Work recovery involves continuing the exercise but at a reduced level from the work period. During the relief period, a portion of the muscular stores of ATP and the oxygen associated with myoglobin that were depleted during the work period are replenished by the aerobic system; an increase in $\dot{V}O_{2\ max}$ occurs.

- The longer the work interval, the more the aerobic system is stressed. With a short work interval, the duration of the rest interval is critical if the aerobic system is to be stressed (a work–recovery ratio of 1:1 to 1:5 is appropriate). A rest interval equal to one and a half times the work interval allows the succeeding exercise interval to begin before recovery is complete and stresses the aerobic system. With a longer work interval, the duration of the rest is not as important.
- A significant amount of high-intensity work can be achieved with interval or intermittent work if there is appropriate spacing of the work–relief intervals. The total amount of work that can be completed with intermittent work is greater than the amount of work that can be completed with continuous training.

Circuit Training

Circuit training employs a series of exercise activities. At the end of the last activity, the individual starts from the beginning and again moves through the series. The series of activities is repeated several times.

- Several exercise modes can be used involving large and small muscle groups and a mix of static or dynamic effort.
- Use of circuit training can improve strength and endurance by stressing both the aerobic and anaerobic systems.

Circuit-Interval Training

- Combining circuit and interval training is effective because of the interaction of aerobic and anaerobic production of ATP.
- In addition to the aerobic and anaerobic systems being stressed by the various activities, with the relief interval there is a delay in the need for glycolysis and the production of lactic acid prior to the availability of oxygen supplying the ATP.

The Cool-Down Period

A cool-down period is necessary following the exercise period.

The purpose of the cool-down period is:

- To prevent pooling of the blood in the extremities by continuing to use the muscles to maintain venous return.
- To prevent fainting by increasing the return of blood to the heart and brain as cardiac output and venous return decreases.
- To enhance the recovery period with the oxidation of metabolic waste and replacement of the energy stores.
- To prevent myocardial ischemia, arrhythmias, or other cardiovascular complications.

Characteristics of the cool-down period are similar to those of the warm-up period.

- Total-body exercises such as calisthenics are appropriate.
- The period should last 5 to 10 minutes.

Application

Application of aerobic training is summarized in Box 4–11.

Box 4–11 General Guidelines for an Aerobic Training Program

- Establish the target heart rate and maximum heart rate.
- Warm up gradually for 5 to 10 minutes. Include stretching and repetitive motions at slow speeds, gradually increasing the effort.
- Increase the pace of the activity so that the target heart rate can be maintained for 20 to 30 minutes. Examples include fast walking, running, bicycling, swimming, cross-country skiing, and aerobic dancing.
- Cool down for 5 to 10 minutes with slow, total body repetitive motions and stretching activities.
- The aerobic activity should be three to five times per week.
- To avoid injuries from stress, use appropriate equipment, such as correct footwear, for proper biomechanical support. Avoid running, jogging, or aerobic dancing on hard surfaces such as asphalt and concrete.
- To avoid overuse syndromes to structures of the musculoskeletal system, proper warm-up and stretching of muscles to be used should be performed. Progression of activities should be within the tolerance of the individual. Overuse commonly occurs when there is an increase in time or effort without adequate rest (recovery) time between sessions. Increase repetitions or time by no more than 10% per week. If pain begins while exercising, or lasts longer than 4 hours after exercising, heed the warning and reduce the stress.
- Individualize the program of exercise. All people are not at the same fitness level and therefore cannot perform the same exercises. Any one exercise has the potential to be detrimental if attempted by someone not able to execute it properly. During recovery following an injury or surgery choose an exercise that will not stress the vulnerable tissue. Begin at a safe level for the individual and progress as the individual meets the desired goals.

Physiologic Changes that Occur with Training

Changes in the cardiovascular and respiratory systems as well as changes in muscle metabolism occur following endurance training. These changes are reflected both at rest and with exercise. It is important to note that all of the following training effects cannot result from one training program.

Cardiovascular Changes

Changes at Rest

A reduction in the resting pulse rate in some individuals will occur because of:

- A decrease in sympathetic drive, with decreasing levels of norepinephrine and epinephrine
- A decrease in atrial rate secondary to biochemical changes in the muscles and levels of acetylcholine, norepinephrine, and epinephrine in the atria
- An apparent increase in parasympathetic (vagal) tone secondary to decreased sympathetic tone

A decrease in blood pressure will occur in some individuals.

- This occurs with a decrease in peripheral vascular resistance.
- The largest decrease is in systolic blood pressure.
- This is most apparent in hypertensive individuals.

An increase in blood volume and hemoglobin may occur, which facilitates the oxygen delivery capacity of the system.

Changes During Exercise

A reduction in the pulse rate because of the mechanisms listed earlier in this section may occur in some individuals. An increased stroke volume may occur because of:

- An increase in myocardial contractility
- An increase in ventricular volume

An increased cardiac output may occur.

- The increased cardiac output is a result of the increased stroke volume.
- The increased cardiac output occurs with maximal exercise but not with submaximal exercise.
- The magnitude of the change is directly related to the increase in stroke volume and the magnitude of the reduced heart rate.

An increased extraction of oxygen by the working muscle because of enzymatic and biochemical changes in the muscle may occur in some individuals, as well as an increased maximum oxygen uptake ($\dot{V}O_{2\,max}$).

- Greater $\dot{V}O_{2\,max}$ results in a greater work capacity.
- The increased cardiac output increases the delivery of oxygen to the working muscles.
- The increased ability of the muscle to extract oxygen from the blood increases the utilization of the available oxygen.

A decreased blood flow per kilogram of the working muscle may occur.

- This occurs even though increasing amounts of blood are shunted to the exercising muscle.
- The increase in extraction of oxygen from the blood compensates for this change.

There may be a decreased myocardial oxygen consumption (pulse rate times systolic blood pressure) for any given intensity of exercise.

- This results from a decreased pulse rate, with or without a modest decrease in blood pressure.
- The product can be decreased significantly in the healthy subject without any loss of efficiency at a specific workload.

Respiratory Changes

These changes are observed at rest and with exercise after endurance training.

Changes at Rest

- Larger lung volumes because of improved pulmonary function, with no change in tidal volume
- Larger diffusion capacities because of:
  - Larger lung volumes
  - Greater alveolar-capillary surface area

Changes During Exercise

- Larger diffusion capacities for the same reasons as those listed previously; maximal capacity of ventilation is unchanged.
- A lower amount of air ventilated at the same oxygen consumption; maximum diffusion capacity is unchanged.
- An increased maximal minute ventilation.
- An increased ventilatory efficiency.

Metabolic Changes

These changes are observed at rest and with exercise following endurance training.

Changes at Rest

- Muscle hypertrophy and increased capillary density
- An increased number and size of mitochondria increasing the capacity to generate ATP aerobically
- Increases in muscle myoglobin concentration
  - Myoglobin increases the rate of oxygen transport.
  - Myoglobin possibly increases the rate of oxygen diffusion to the mitochondria.

Changes During Exercise

A decreased rate of depletion of muscle glycogen at submaximal work levels may occur. Another term for this phenomenon is *glycogen sparing*. This is due to:

- An increased capacity to mobilize and oxidize fat
- Increased fat mobilizing and metabolizing enzymes

Lower blood lactate levels at submaximal work may occur.

- The mechanism for this is unclear.
- It does not appear to be related to a decrease in hypoxia of the muscles.

There may be less reliance on phosphocreatine (PC) and ATP in skeletal muscle and an increased capability to oxidize carbohydrate because of:

- An increased oxidative potential of the mitochondria
- An increased glycogen storage in the muscle

Note: Ill health may influence metabolic adaptations to exercise.

Other System Changes

Changes in other systems that occur with training include:

- A decrease in body fat
- A decrease in blood cholesterol and triglyceride levels
- An increase in heat acclimatization
- An increase in the breaking strength of bones and ligaments and the tensile strength of tendons

▶ Application of Principles of an Aerobic Conditioning Program for the Patient with Coronary Disease

The use of the principles of aerobic conditioning in physical therapy has been most dominant in program planning for the individual following a myocardial infarction (MI) or following coronary artery bypass surgery.[4,5,6]

In the past 15 to 20 years, there have been major changes in the medical management of these patients. These changes have included shortened hospital stays, a more aggressive progression of activity for the patient following MI or cardiac surgery, and earlier initiation of an exercise program based on a low-level stress test prior to discharge from the hospital. An aerobic conditioning program, in addition to risk factor modification, is a dominant part of cardiac rehabilitation.

In-Patient Phase (Phase I)

This phase of the program occurs in the hospital following stabilization of the patient's cardiovascular status after MI or coronary bypass surgery. Because the length of hospital care has decreased over the past few years, this time may be limited to 3 to 5 days. When hospital stays were longer, this phase often lasted 7 to 14 days and was referred to as phase 1 of the cardiac rehabilitation program.

The purpose of the early portion of cardiac rehabilitation is to:

- Initiate risk factor education and address future modification of certain behaviors, such as eating habits and smoking.
- Initiate self-care activities and progress from sitting to standing to minimize deconditioning (1 to 3 days postevent).
- Provide an orthostatic challenge to the cardiovascular system (3 to 5 days postevent). This is usually accomplished by supervised ambulation. Ambulation is usually monitored electrocardiographically, as well as manually monitoring the heart rate, ventilation rate, and blood pressure.
- Prepare patients and family for continued rehabilitation and for life at home after a cardiac event.

Out-Patient Phase (Phase II)

This program is initiated either upon discharge from the hospital or, depending on the severity of the diagnosis, 6 to 8 weeks later. This delay will allow time for the myocardium to heal as well as time to monitor the patient's response to a new medical regimen. Participants are monitored via telemetry to determine heart rate and rhythm responses, blood pressure is recorded at rest and during exercise, and ventilation responses are noted. These programs usually last 8 to 12 weeks (Box 4–12).

The purpose of the program is to:

- Increase the person's exercise capacity in a safe and progressive manner so that adaptive cardiovascular and muscular changes occur. The early part of the program is referred to by some as "low-level" exercise training.
- Enhance cardiac functions and reduce the cardiac cost of work. This may help eliminate or delay symptoms such as angina and ST-segment changes in the patient with coronary heart disease.
- Produce favorable metabolic changes.
- Determine the effect of medications on increasing levels of activity.
- Relieve anxiety and depression.
- Progress the patient to an independent exercise program.

A symptom-limited test is performed 6 to 12 weeks after hospital discharge or as early as 2 to 4 weeks following discharge.

The exercise program is predominantly aerobic. Generally, for patients with functional capacities greater than 5 METs, the exercise prescription is based on the results of the symptom-limited exercise stress test.

- The initial level of activity or training intensity may be as low as 40 to 60% of the maximal heart rate or 40 to 70% of the functional capacity defined in METs. The starting intensity is dictated by the severity of the diagnosis in concert with the individual's age and prior fitness level. The intensity is progressed as the individual responds to the training program.
- The duration of the exercise session may be limited to 10 to 15 minutes to start, progressing to 30 to 60 minutes as the patient's status improves. Each session usually includes 8- to 10-minute warm-up and cool-down periods.
- Participants often attend sessions offered three times per week.
- The mode of exercise is usually continuous, using large muscle groups, such as stationary biking or walking. These activities allow for electrocardiographic monitoring via telemetry.
- Circuit-interval exercise is a common method used with the patient in phase II. The patient can exercise on each modality at a defined workload, compared with exercising continuously on a bicycle or treadmill. As a result, the patient can:
  - Perform more physical work.
  - Exercise at a higher intensity. Fitness may improve in a shorter period of time.
  - Maintain lactic acid and the oxygen deficit at minimum levels.
  - Exercise at a lower rate of perceived exertion.
- Low-level weight training may be initiated during the outpatient program, provided the individual has undergone a symptom-limited stress test. Resistive exercises should not produce ischemic symptoms associated with an increase in heart rate and systolic blood pressure. Therefore, heart rate and blood pressure should be monitored periodically throughout the exercise session. Starting weight may be calculated using 40% of a 1-RM effort.
- Progression of the workload occurs when there have been three consecutive sessions (every-other-day sessions) during which the peak heart rate is below the target heart rate.

Box 4–12 Case Example of a Cardiac Rehabilitation Referral

Mr. Smith is referred and undergoes further evaluation to determine the cause of his chest pain. He is diagnosed with single vessel coronary artery disease. He is referred to cardiac rehabilitation.

- ***Medications.*** Nitroglycerin as needed to relieve angina.
  Mr. Smith will attend cardiac rehabilitation three times per week for 8 to 12 weeks to improve his fitness level and attend smoking cessation classes. He will meet with a medical dietitian to discuss meal planning to lower his intake of fat and cholesterol.
- ***Exercise prescription***. Mr. Smith will exercise at an intensity lower than his anginal threshold. This intensity will be initially established at 60 to 65% of his maximal heart rate or 50% of his $\dot{V}O_{2\,max}$. He will exercise three times per week for 20 to 40 minutes, depending on his tolerance.

Out-Patient Program (Phase III)

This phase of cardiac rehabilitation includes a supervised exercise conditioning program, which is often continued in a hospital or community setting. Heart rate and rhythm are no longer monitored via telemetry. Participants are reminded to monitor their own pulse rate, and a supervisory person is available to monitor blood pressure.

The purpose of the program is to continue to improve or maintain fitness levels achieved during the phase II program.

Recreational activities to maintain levels gained in phase II can include:

- Swimming, which incorporates both arms and legs. However, there is a decreased awareness of ischemic symptoms while swimming, especially when skill level is poor.
- Outdoor hiking, which is excellent if on level terrain.

Activities at 8 METs include:

- Jogging approximately 5 miles per hour
- Cycling approximately 12 miles per hour
- Vigorous down-hill skiing

Special Considerations

There are special considerations related to types of exercise and patient needs that must be recognized when developing conditioning programs for patients with coronary disease. Arm exercises elicit different responses than leg exercises.

- Mechanical efficiency based on the ratio between output of external work and caloric expenditure is lower than with leg exercises.
- Oxygen uptake at a given external workload is significantly higher for arm exercises than for leg exercises.
- Myocardial efficiency is lower with leg exercises than with arm exercises.
- Myocardial oxygen consumption (heart rate times systolic blood pressure) is higher with arm exercises than with leg exercises.

Coronary patients complete 35% less work with arm exercises than with leg exercises before symptoms occur.

Adaptive Changes

Adaptive changes following training of individuals with cardiac disease include:

- An increased myocardial aerobic work capacity.
- An increased maximum aerobic or functional capacity by predominantly widening the arteriovenous oxygen ($a - \bar{v}O_2$) difference.
- An increased stroke volume following high-intensity training 6 to 12 months into the training program.
- A decreased myocardial demand for oxygen.
- An increased myocardial supply by the decreased heart rate and prolongation of diastole.
- An increased tolerance to a given physical workload before angina occurs.
- A heart rate significantly lower at each submaximal workload and therefore a greater heart rate reserve. When muscles are used that are not directly involved in the activity, the reduction in heart rate will not be as great.
- An improved psychological orientation and, over time, an impact on depression scores, scores for hysteria, hypochondriasis, and psychoasthenia on the Minnesota Multiphasic Personality Inventory.

Note: Cardiovascular complications will be prevented and/or reduced if the program includes appropriate selection of patients, continuous evaluation of each patient, medical supervision of the exercise throughout the training period, regular communication with the physician, specific instructions to patients about adverse symptoms, class size limitations to 30 patients or fewer, and the maintenance of accurate records related to compliance to the program.

Applications of Aerobic Training for the Deconditioned Individual and the Patient with Chronic Illness

Deconditioned individuals, including those with chronic illness and the elderly, may have major limitations in pulmonary and cardiovascular reserve that severely curtail their daily activities. Implications of the changes due to deconditioning brought on by inactivity, resulting from any illness or chronic disease, are important to remember.

- There is a decreased work capacity, which is a result of a decreased maximum oxygen uptake and decreased ability to use oxygen and perform work. There is also a decreased cardiac output, which is the major limiting factor.
- There is a decreased circulating blood volume that can be as much as 700 to 800 mL. For some individuals, this results in tachycardia along with orthostatic hypotension, dizziness, and episodes of syncope when initially attempting to stand.
- There is a decrease in plasma and red blood cells, which increases the likelihood of life-threatening embothrombolic episodes and the prolongation of the convalescent period.
- There is a decrease in lean body mass, which results in decreased muscle size and decreased muscle strength and ability to perform activities requiring large muscle groups. For example, the individual may have difficulty walking with crutches or climbing stairs.

- There is an increased excretion of urinary calcium, which results from a decrease in the weight-bearing stimulus critical in maintaining bone integrity, in bone loss or osteoporosis, and in an increased likelihood of fractures upon falling due to the osteoporosis.

Through an exercise program, the negative cardiovascular, neuromuscular, and metabolic functions can be reversed. This results in:

- A decrease in resting heart rate, heart rate with any given exercise load, and urinary excretion of calcium
- An increase in stroke volume at rest, stroke volume with exercise, cardiac output with exercise, total heart volume, lung volume (ventilatory volume), vital capacity, maximal oxygen uptake, circulating blood volume, plasma volume and red blood cells, and lean body mass
- A reversal of the negative nitrogen and protein balance
- An increase in levels of mitochondrial enzymes and energy stores
- Less use of the anaerobic systems during activity

Adaptations for Disabilities, Functional Limitations, and Deconditioning

Individuals who have a physical disability or functional limitation should not be excluded from a conditioning program that will increase their fitness level. This includes individuals in wheelchairs or persons who have problems ambulating, such as those with paraplegia, hemiplegia, or amputation, and those with an orthopedic problem, such as arthrodesis.

- Adaptations must be made in testing the physically disabled using a wheelchair treadmill or more frequently using the upper extremity ergometer.
- Exercise protocols may emphasize upper extremities and manipulation of the wheelchair.
- It is important to remember that energy expenditure is increased when the gait is altered, and wheelchair use is less efficient than walking without impairment.

Impairments, Goals, and Plan of Care

The goals of an aerobic exercise program are dependent on the initial level of fitness of the individual and on his or her specific clinical needs. The general goals are to decrease the deconditioning effects of disease and chronic illness and to improve the individual's cardiovascular and muscular fitness.

Common Impairments

- Increased susceptibility to thromboembolic episodes, pneumonia, atelectasis, and the likelihood of fractures
- Tachycardia, dizziness, and orthostatic hypotension when moving from sitting to standing
- A decrease in general muscle strength, with difficulty and shortness of breath in climbing stairs
- A decrease in work capacity that limits distances walked and activities tolerated
- Increased heart rate and blood pressure responses (rate-pressure product) to various activities
- A decrease in the maximum rate-pressure product tolerated with angina or other ischemic symptoms appearing at low levels of exercise

Goals

- Prevention of thromboembolic episodes, pneumonia, atelectasis, and fractures
- Decrease in the magnitude of the orthostatic hypotensive response
- Ability to climb stairs safely and without shortness of breath
- Tolerance for walking longer measured distances and completing activities without fatigue or symptoms
- Decrease in the heart rate and blood pressure (rate-pressure product) at a given level of activity
- An increase in the maximum rate-pressure product tolerated without ischemic symptoms

Box 4–13 Guidelines for Initiating an Aerobic Exercise Program for the Deconditioned Individual and Patient with Chronic Illness

- Determine the exercise heart rate response that can be safely reached using the Karvonen formula as a guide, accounting for medical conditions, medications and the individuals perceived exertion.
- Initiate a program of activities for the patient that will not elicit a cardiovascular response over the exercise heart rate (e.g., walking, repetitive activities, easy calisthenics).
- Provide the patient with clearly written instructions about any activity they perform on their own.
- Initiate an educational program that provides the patient with information about effort symptoms and exercise precautions, monitoring of heart rate, and modification when indicated.

Box 4–14 Guidelines for Progression of an Aerobic Training Program

- Determine the maximum heart rate or symptom-limited heart rate by multistage testing with ECG monitoring.
- Decide on the threshold stimulus (percentage of maximum or symptom-limited heart rate) that will elicit a conditioning response for the individual tested and that will be used as the exercise heart rate.
- Determine the intensity, duration, and frequency of exercise that will result in attainment of the exercise heart rate and a conditioning response.
- Determine the mode of exercise to be used based on the individual's physical capabilities and interest.
- Initiate an exercise program with the patient and provide clearly written instructions regarding the details of the program.
- Educate the patient about:
  - Effort symptoms and the need to cease or modify exercise when these symptoms appear and to communicate with the physical therapist and/or physician about these problems.
  - Monitoring heart rate at rest as well as during and following exercise.
  - The importance of exercising within the guidelines provided by the physical therapist.
  - The importance of consistent long-term follow-up about the exercise program so that it can be progressed within safe limits.
  - The importance of modifying risk factors related to cardiac problems.

Outcomes

- An improved pulmonary, cardiovascular, and metabolic response to various levels of exercise
- An improved ability to complete selected activities with appropriate heart rate and blood responses to exercise

Guidelines

Guidelines for establishing a safe program of intervention for the deconditioned individual and the convalescent patient with chronic illness are summarized in Boxes 4–13 and 4–14.

Age Differences

Differences in endurance and physical work capacity among children, young adults, and middle-aged or elderly individuals are evident. Some comparisons are made between maximal oxygen uptake and the factors influencing it and among blood pressure, respiratory rate, vital capacity, and maximum voluntary ventilation in the different age categories. It is important when developing aerobic conditioning programs that these age-related differences are taken into consideration.

Children

Between the ages of 5 and 15 there is a threefold increase in body weight, lung volume, heart volume, and maximum oxygen uptake.

Heart Rate

- Resting heart rate is on the average above 125 (126 in girls, 135 in boys) at infancy.
- Resting heart rate drops to adult levels at puberty.
- Maximum heart rate is age related (220 minus age).

Stroke Volume

- Stroke volume is closely related to size.
- Children 5 to 16 years of age have a stroke volume of 30 to 40 mL.

Cardiac Output

- Cardiac output is related to size.
- Cardiac output increases with increasing stroke volume.
- The increase in cardiac output for a given increase in oxygen consumption is a constant throughout life: it is the same in the child as in the adult.

Arteriovenous Oxygen Difference

- Children tolerate a larger $a - \bar{v}O_2$ difference than adults.
- The larger $a - \bar{v}O_2$ difference makes up for the smaller stroke volume.

Maximal Oxygen Uptake ($\dot{V}O_{2\,max}$)

- The $\dot{V}O_{2\,max}$ increases with age up to 20 years (expressed as liters per minute).
- Before puberty, girls and boys show no significant difference in maximal aerobic capacity.
- Cardiac output in children is the same as in the adult for any given oxygen consumption.
- Endurance times increase with age until 17 to 18 years.

Blood Pressure

- Systolic blood pressure increases from 40 mm Hg at birth to 80 mm Hg at age 1 month to 100 mm Hg several years before puberty. Adult levels are observed at puberty.
- Diastolic pressure increases from 55 to 70 mm Hg from 4 to 14 years of age, with little change during adolescence.

Respiration

- Respiratory rate decreases from 30 breaths per minute at infancy to 16 breaths per minute at 17 to 18 years of age.
- Vital capacity and maximum voluntary ventilation correlate with height, although the greater increase in boys than girls at puberty may be due to an increase in lung tissue.

Muscle Mass and Strength

- Muscle mass increases through adolescence, primarily from muscle fiber hypertrophy and the development of sarcomeres. Sarcomeres are added at the musculotendinous junction to compensate for the required increase in length.
- Girls develop peak muscle mass between 16 and 20 years, whereas boys develop peak muscle mass between 18 and 25 years.
- Strength gains are associated with increased muscle mass in conjunction with neural maturation.

Anaerobic Ability

- Children generally demonstrate a limited anaerobic capacity. This may be due to a limited amount of phosphofructokinase, a controlling enzyme in the glycolytic pathway.
- Children produce less lactic acid when performing anaerobically. This may be due to a limited glycolytic capacity.

Young Adult

There are more data on the physiologic parameters of fitness for the young and the middle-aged adult than for the child or the elderly.

Heart Rate

- Resting heart rate reaches 60 to 65 beats per minute at 17 to 18 years of age (75 beats per minute in a sitting, sedentary young man).
- Maximum heart rate is age related (190 beats per minute in the same sedentary young man).

Stroke Volume

- The adult values for stroke volume are 60 to 80 mL (75 mL in a sitting, sedentary young man).
- With maximal exercise, stroke volume is 100 mL in that same sedentary young man.

Cardiac Output for the Sedentary Young Man at Rest

- Cardiac output at rest is 75 beats per minute times 75 mL, or 5.6 liters per minute.
- With maximal exercise, cardiac output is 190 beats per minute times 100 mL, or 19 liters per minute.

Arteriovenous Oxygen Difference ($a - \bar{v}O_2$ Difference)

- 25 to 30% of the oxygen is extracted from blood as it runs through the muscles or other tissues at rest.
- In a normal, sedentary young man, it increases threefold (5.2 to 15.8 mL/100 mL blood) with exercise.

Maximum Oxygen Uptake

- The difference in $\dot{V}O_{2\,max}$ between male and female is greatest in the adult.
- Differences in $\dot{V}O_{2\,max}$ between the sexes is minimal when $\dot{V}O_{2\,max}$ is expressed relative to lean body weight.
- In the sedentary young man, maximum oxygen uptake equals 3000 mL/min (oxygen uptake at rest equals 300 mL/min).

Blood Pressure

- Systolic blood pressure is 120 mm Hg (average). At peak effort of exercise, values may range from as low as 190 mm Hg to as high as 240 mm Hg.
- Diastolic blood pressure is 80 mm Hg (average). Diastolic pressure does not change markedly with exercise.

Respiration

- Respiratory rate is 12 to 15 breaths per minute.
- Vital capacity is 4800 mL in a man 20 to 30 years of age.
- Maximum voluntary ventilation varies considerably from laboratory to laboratory and is dependent on age and surface area of the body.

Muscle Mass and Strength

- Muscle mass increases with training as a result of hypertrophy. This hypertrophy can be the result of an increased number of myofibrils, increased actin and myosin, sarcoplasm, and/or connective tissue.
- There is limited evidence that suggests that the number of muscle fibers may increase, referred to as hyperplasia.
- As the nervous system matures, increased recruitment of motor units or decreased autogenic inhibition by Golgi tendon organs appears to also dictate strength gains.

Anaerobic Ability

- Anaerobic training increases the activity of several controlling enzymes in the glycolytic pathway and enhances stored quantities of ATP and phosphocreatine.
- Anaerobic training increases the muscle's ability to buffer the hydrogen ions released when lactic acid is produced. Increased buffering allows the muscle to work anaerobically for longer periods of time.

Older Adult

With increasing interest in the aged, data are appearing in the literature about this age group and their response to exercise.

Heart Rate

- Resting heart rate is not influenced by age.
- Maximum heart rate is age related and decreases with age (in very general terms, 220 minus age). The average maximum heart rate for men 20 to 29 years of age is 190 beats per minute. For men 60 to 69 years of age, it is 164 beats per minute.
- The amount that the heart rate increases in response to static and maximum dynamic exercise (hand grip) decreases in the elderly.

Stroke Volume

Stroke volume decreases in the aged and results in decreased cardiac output.

Cardiac Output

Cardiac output decreases on an average of 7 to 3.4 liters per minute from age 19 to 86 years.

$a - \bar{v}O_2$ Difference

Arteriovenous oxygen difference decreases as a result of decreased lean body mass and low oxygen-carrying capacity.

Maximum Oxygen Uptake

- According to cardiorespiratory fitness classification, if men 60 to 69 years of age of average fitness level are compared with men 20 to 29 years of age of the same fitness level, the maximal oxygen uptake for the older man is lower:
  20 to 29 years 31 to 37 mL/kg per minute
  60 to 69 years 18 to 23 mL/kg per minute
- Aerobic capacity decreases about 10% per decade when evaluating sedentary men. Maximum oxygen consumption decreases on an average from 47.7 mL/kg per minute at age 25 years to 25.5 mL/kg per minute at age 75 years. This decrease is not directly the result of age; athletes who continue exercising have a significantly lesser decrease in $\dot{V}O_{2\ max}$ when evaluated over a 10-year period.

Blood Pressure

Blood pressure increases because of increased peripheral vascular resistance.

- Systolic blood pressure of the aged is 150 mm Hg (average).
- Diastolic blood pressure is 90 mm Hg (average).
- If the definition of high blood pressure is 160/95, then 22% of men and 34% of women 65 to 74 years of age are hypertensive.
- Using 150/95 mm Hg as a cutoff, 25% of individuals are hypertensive at age 50 years and 70% between the ages of 85 and 95 years.

Respiration

- Respiratory rate increases with age.
- Vital capacity decreases with age. There is a 25% decrease in the vital capacity of the 50- to 60-year-old male compared with the 20- to 30-year-old male with the same surface area.
- Maximum voluntary ventilation decreases with age.

Muscle Mass and Strength

- Generally, strength decline with age is associated with a decrease in muscle mass and physical activity.
- The decrease in muscle mass is primarily due to a decrease in protein synthesis, in concert with a decline in the number of fast-twitch muscle fibers.
- Aging may also affect strength by slowing the nervous system's response time. This may alter the ability to effectively recruit motor units.
- Continued training as one ages appears to reduce the effects of aging on the muscular system.

Independent Learning Activities

CRITICAL THINKING AND DISCUSSION

1. A 16-year-old cross-country runner is referred to the clinic where you are employed with a diagnosis of a right ankle sprain. You examine and

evaluate him and develop a treatment plan for the ankle. You must also address his desire to return to competition when able.

- Discuss the energy systems utilized with distance running.
- Discuss the notion of sport specificity.
- What aerobic exercises could the patient do to maintain his aerobic condition while his ankle heals but not stress the ankle?

2. You are an invited speaker at a senior citizen center for a lunch time discussion of lifetime fitness and establishing an appropriate exercise program for individuals within this age category.

- Discuss the definition of fitness.
- Discuss the concept of the exercise prescription.
- Describe the necessary precautions when dealing with the older population (both the older athlete and the untrained individual).

3. Explain the concepts of energy expenditure, oxygen consumption, and efficiency with regard to ambulating with an assistive device with each of these diagnoses: rheumatoid arthritis, post-tibial fracture, and post-total-hip replacement.

4. Design an exercise program for the local fire fighters. Utilize the concepts of the aerobic energy systems, anaerobic energy system, and strength training.

5. You have been invited to speak to a group of elementary and preschool teachers about the importance of aerobic exercise for children. Explain the basic physiological differences between children and adults at rest with regard to heart rate, respiratory rate and metabolism, and their response to exercise.

REFERENCES

1. American College of Sports Medicine: Exercise Management for Persons with Chronic Diseases and Disabilities, ed 2. Lea & Febiger, Philadelphia, 1997.
2. American College of Sports Medicine: ASCM's Guidelines for Exercise Testing and Prescription, ed 6. Lea & Febiger, Philadelphia, 2000.
3. American College of Sports Medicine: Resource Manual for Guidelines for Exercise Testing and Prescription, ed 4. Lea & Febiger, Philadelphia, 2001.
4. Brannon, FJ, Foley, MW, Starr, JA and Black, MG: Cardiopulmonary Rehabilitation: Basic Theory and Application, ed 2. FA Davis Co, Philadelphia, 1993.
5. Hillegass, S and Sadowsky, H: Essentials of Cardiopulmonary Physical Therapy. WB Saunders Co, 1994.
6. Irwin, S and Teckline, JS: Cardiopulmonary Physical Therapy, ed 3. CV Mosby, St. Louis, 1995.
7. McArdle, WD, Katch, FI and Katch VL: Essentials of Exercise Physiology, ed 2. Lippincott Williams & Wilkins, Philadelphia, 1996.
8. McArdle, WD, Katch, FI and Katch, VL: Exercise Physiology: Energy, Nutrition, and Human Performance, ed 4. Lippincott Williams & Wilkins, 1996.
9. Powers, SK and Howley, ET: Exercise Physiology: Theory and Application. McGraw-Hill Co., Boston, 2001.
10. US Department of Health and Human Services, Public Health Service: Healthy People 2000. National Health Promotion and Disease Prevention Objectives. US Government Printing Office, Washington, 1990.

Chapter 5

Stretching

OBJECTIVES

After studying this chapter, the reader will be able to:

1 Discuss the relationship of impaired mobility to functional limitations and disability.

2 Define key terms associated with functional and impaired mobility and therapeutic procedures used to improve mobility.

3 Differentiate between types of soft tissue contractures.

4 Identify pathologic processes and factors that contribute to restrictions in soft tissue mobility and limited ROM.

5 Explain how contractile and noncontractile tissues respond to immobilization and remobilization.

6 Analyze the interrelated determinants of stretching procedures and how they affect the application and outcomes of stretching.

7 Describe the various types of stretching procedures—specifically manual, mechanical, and self-stretching—as well as passive, assisted, and active stretching.

8 Explain the principles upon which stretching and neuromuscular inhibition techniques are based and how they are integrated into a program of exercises to improve functional mobility.

9 Describe the use of adjunctive agents or procedures in a stretching program.

10 Summarize the guidelines and precautions for the application and implementation of stretching exercises as well as the contraindications for stretching.

11 Describe proper positioning, hand placement and stabilization used when applying manual stretching techniques to the upper and lower extremities.

The term **mobility** can be described based on two different but interrelated parameters. It is often defined as the ability of structures or segments of the body to move or be moved to allow the presence of range of motion for functional activities *(functional ROM)*.[1,114] It can also be defined as the ability of an individual to initiate, control, or sustain active movements of the body to perform simple to complex motor skills *(functional mobility)*.[30,100,114] Mobility, as it relates to functional ROM, is associated with joint integrity as well as the *flexibility* or *extensibility* of soft tissues that cross or surround joints, such as muscles, tendons, fascia, joint capsules, and skin, which are necessary for unrestricted, pain-free movements of the body during functional tasks of daily living. The ROM needed for the performance of functional activities does not necessarily mean full or "normal" ROM.

Sufficient mobility of soft tissues and ROM of joints must be supported by a requisite level of neuromuscular control to allow the body to accommodate to imposed stresses placed upon it during functional movement and thus to enable an individual to be functionally mobile. In addition, soft tissue mobility and neuromuscular control consistent with demand are thought to be an important factor in the prevention of injury or reinjury of the musculoskeletal system.[4,56,62,67,71,124]

Hypomobility (restricted motion) caused by adaptive shortening of soft tissues can occur as the result of many disorders or situations.[93] Factors include: (1) prolonged immobilization of a body segment, (2) sedentary lifestyle, (3) postural malalignment and muscle imbalances, (4) impaired muscle performance (weakness) associated with an array of musculoskeletal or neuromuscular disorders, (5) tissue trauma resulting in inflammation and pain, and (6) congenital or acquired deformities. Any factor that impairs mobility, that is, causes restrictions of soft tissues, can also impair muscular performance. These impairments, in turn, can lead to functional limitations and disabilities in a person's life.

Just as strength and endurance exercises are

essential interventions to improve impaired muscle performance or prevent injury, when restricted mobility adversely affects function and increases the risk of injury, stretching exercises become an integral component of individualized intervention or fitness programs.[56] **Stretching** is a general term used to describe any therapeutic maneuver designed to *increase* mobility of soft tissues and subsequently improve ROM by elongating (lengthening) structures that have adaptively shortened and have become hypomobile over time.[8,58,124,133,138]

Only through a systematic examination and evaluation of a patient can a therapist determine what structures are restricting motion and if, when, and what types of stretching procedures are indicated. Early in the rehabilitation process manual stretching and joint mobilization, which involve direct, "hands-on" intervention by a practitioner, may be the most appropriate techniques. Later, self-stretching exercises, performed independently by a patient, after careful instruction and close supervision, may be a more suitable intervention. Sometimes the use of mechanical stretching devices are indicated, particularly when manual therapies have been ineffective. Regardless of the types of stretching procedures selected for an exercise program, if the gain in mobility is to become permanent, it must be complemented by an appropriate level of strength and endurance and used on a regular basis in functional activities.

The stretching procedures described in this chapter are techniques designed to elongate the contractile or noncontractile components of muscle-tendon units and periarticular structures. In addition, neuromuscular inhibition procedures used to relax tight muscles are also described. Techniques focus on manual or mechanical stretching procedures for the extremities. Foundational concepts upon which self-stretching procedures for the extremities are based are also discussed, but specific self-stretching exercises are described or illustrated in Chapters 9 through 14. Joint mobilization and manipulation procedures of extremity joints are described and illustrated in Chapter 6. Procedures to increase mobility of the spine are covered in Chapters 15 and 16.

▶ Definition of Terms Related to Mobility and Stretching

Flexibility

Flexibility is the ability to move a single joint or series of joints smoothly and easily through an unrestricted, pain-free ROM.[4,89,103,126,138] Muscle length in conjunction with joint integrity and the extensibility of periarticular soft tissues determine flexibility.[1] The *extensibility* of musculotendinous units that cross a joint is based on their ability to relax and yield to a stretch force. The arthrokinematics of the moving joint (the ability of the joint surfaces to roll and slide) as well as the ability of periarticular connective tissues to deform also affect joint ROM and an individual's overall flexibility.

Dynamic flexibility (active mobility) refers to the active ROM of a joint. This aspect of flexibility is dependent upon the degree to which a joint can be moved by a muscle contraction and the amount of tissue resistance met during the active movement. *Passive flexibility* (passive mobility) is the degree to which a joint can be passively moved through the available ROM and is dependent upon the extensibility of muscles and connective tissues that cross and surround a joint. Passive flexibility is a prerequisite for but does not ensure dynamic flexibility.

Hypomobility

Hypomobility refers to decreased mobility or restricted motion. A wide range of pathological processes restrict movement and impair mobility. There are many factors that can contribute to hypomobility and stiffness of soft tissues, the potential loss of range of motion and the development of contractures. These factors are summarized in Table 5–1. Restricted motion can range from mild muscle shortening to irreversible contractures.

Contracture

Contracture is defined as the adaptive shortening of the muscle-tendon unit and other soft tissues that cross or surround a joint, which results in significant resistance to passive or active stretch and limitation of ROM.[26,37,71,124]

There is no clear delineation of how much restriction of motion from loss of soft tissue extensibility must exist to designate the limitation of motion as a contracture.[4,26,37,124] In one reference,[71] contracture is defined as an almost complete loss of motion, whereas the term *shortness* is used to denote a partial loss of motion. In the clinical and fitness settings the term *tightness,* albeit a very nonspecific term, is frequently used to describe a mild restriction of motion. However, this term has not been clearly defined in the literature and, therefore, should not be used interchangeably with contracture.

Table 5–1 Factors that Contribute to Restricted Motion

Contributing Factors	Examples
Prolonged immobilization	
Extrinsic:	Fractures, osteotomy, soft tissue trauma or repair
Casts and splints	
Skeletal traction	
Intrinsic:	
Pain	Micro- or macrotrauma; degenerative diseases
Joint inflammation and effusion	Joint diseases or trauma
Muscle, tendon, or fascial disorders	Myositis, tendonitis, fasciitis
Skin disorders	Burns, skin grafts, scleroderma
Bony block	Osteophytes, ankylosis, surgical fusion
Vascular disorders	Peripheral lymphedema
Sedentary lifestyle and habitual faulty or asymmetric postures	Confinement to bed or a wheelchair; prolonged positioning associated with occupation or work environment
Paralysis, tonal abnormalities, and muscle imbalances	Neuromuscular disorders and diseases: CNS or PNS dysfunction (spasticity, rigidity, flaccidity, weakness, muscle guarding, spasm)
Postural malalignment: Congenital or acquired	Scoliosis, kyphosis

Designation of Contractures by Location

Contractures are described by identifying the action of the shortened muscle. If a patient has shortened elbow flexors and cannot fully extend the elbow, he or she is said to have an elbow flexion contracture. When a patient cannot fully abduct the leg because of shortened adductors of the hip, he or she is said to have an adduction contracture of the hip.

Contracture Versus Contraction

The terms *contracture* and *contraction* (the process of tension developing in a muscle during shortening or lengthening) are *not* synonymous and should not be used interchangeably.

Types of Contractures

One way to clarify what is meant by the term *contracture* is to describe contractures by the pathological changes in the different types of soft tissues involved.[25]

Myostatic Contracture

In a myostatic (myogenic) contracture, although the musculotendinous unit has adaptively shortened and there is a significant loss of ROM, there is no specific muscle pathology present.[25] From a morphologic perspective, although there may be a reduction in the number of sarcomere units in series, there is no decrease in individual sarcomere length. Myostatic contractures can be resolved in a relatively short time with stretching exercises.[25,37]

Pseudomyostatic Contracture

Impaired mobility and limited ROM may also be the result of hypertonicity, that is, spasticity or rigidity, associated with a central nervous system lesions such as a cerebral vascular accident, a spinal cord injury, or a traumatic brain injury.[25,37] Muscle spasm or guarding and pain may also cause a pseudomyostatic contracture. In both situations the involved muscles appear to be in a constant state of contraction, giving rise to excessive resistance to passive stretch. Hence, the term pseudomyostatic contracture or *apparent* contracture is used. If inhibition procedures to temporarily relax the hypertonicity or muscle spasm are applied, full, passive elongation of the apparently shortened muscle is then possible.[19]

Arthrogenic and Periarticular Contractures

An arthrogenic contracture is the result of intra-articular pathology. These changes may include adhesions, synovial proliferation, joint effusion, irregularities in articular cartilage, or osteophyte formation.[37] A periarticular contracture develops when connective tissues that cross or attach to a joint or the joint capsule become stiff, thus restricting normal arthrokinematic motion.

Fibrotic Contracture and Irreversible Contracture

Fibrous changes in the connective tissue of muscle and periarticular structures can cause adherence of these tissues and subsequent development of a fibrotic contracture. Although it is possible to stretch a fibrotic contracture and eventually increase ROM, it is often very difficult to re-establish optimal tissue length.[26]

A permanent loss of mobility of soft tissues that cannot be reversed by nonsurgical interventions may occur when normal muscle tissue and organized connective tissue are replaced with a large amount of relatively nonextensible, fibrotic adhesions and scar tissue[26] or even heterotopic bone. These changes can occur after long periods of immobilization of tissues in a shortened position or after tissue trauma and subsequent inflammatory response. The longer a fibrotic contracture exists or the greater the replacement of normal muscle and connective tissue with nonextensible adhesions and scar tissue or bone, the more difficult it becomes to regain optimal mobility of soft tissues and the more likely the contracture will become irreversible.[26,53,123]

Interventions to Increase Mobility of Soft Tissues

There are many types of therapeutic interventions that are designed to improve the mobility of soft tissues and consequently increase ROM. Stretching and mobilization are general terms that describe any therapeutic maneuver that increases the extensibility of restricted soft tissues. Boxes 5-1 and 5-2 list indications and contraindications for the use of stretching procedures.

The following are terms that describe these procedures, only some of which will be covered in depth in this chapter.

Box 5-1 Indications for Use of Stretching

- When ROM is limited because soft tissues have lost their extensibility as the result of adhesions, contractures, and scar tissue formation, causing functional limitations or disabilities
- When restricted motion may lead to structural deformities otherwise preventable
- When there is muscle weakness and shortening of opposing tissue
- As part of a total fitness program designed to prevent musculoskeletal injuries
- Prior to and after vigorous exercise to potentially minimize postexercise muscle soreness

Box 5-2 Contraindications to Stretching

- When a bony block limits joint motion
- After a recent fracture before bony union is complete
- Whenever there is evidence of an acute inflammatory or infectious process (heat and swelling) or when soft tissue healing could be disrupted in the tight tissues and surrounding region
- Whenever there is sharp, acute pain with joint movement or muscle elongation
- When a hematoma or other indication of tissue trauma is observed
- When hypermobility already exists
- When contractures or shortened soft tissues are providing increased joint stability in lieu of normal structural stability or neuromuscular control
- When contractures or shortened soft tissues are the basis for increased functional abilities, particularly in patients with paralysis or severe muscle weakness

Manual or Mechanical/Passive or Assisted Stretching

A sustained or intermittent external, end-range stretch force, applied with overpressure and by manual contact or by a mechanical device, elongates a shortened muscle-tendon unit and periarticular connective tissues by moving a restricted joint just past the available ROM. If the patient is as relaxed as possible, it is called **passive stretching.** If the patient assists in moving the joint through a greater range, it is called **assisted stretching.**

Self-Stretching

Any stretching exercise that is carried out independently by a patient after instruction and supervision by a therapist is referred to as self-stretching. The terms **self-stretching, active stretching,** and **flexibility exercises** are often used interchangeably. Some practitioners prefer to limit the definition of flexibility exercises to ROM exercises that are part of a general conditioning program.

Neuromuscular Inhibition Techniques

These procedures reflexively relax tension in shortened muscles prior to or during stretching. Because the use of inhibition techniques to assist with muscle elongation was originally developed as a component of proprioceptive neuromuscular facilitation (PNF),[127] many clinicians and some authors refer to these combined inhibition/stretching procedures as *PNF stretching*[4,15,93,99] or *facilitated stretching.*[101] (This is an interesting paradox in use of the terms since the techniques inhibit rather than facilitate muscle tension in tight muscles.) *Muscle energy techniques* are manipulative procedures that have evolved out of osteopathic medicine and employ inhibition procedures to stretch muscles and fascia and mobilize joints.[17,50,58,92]

Joint Mobilization/Manipulation

These are stretching techniques specifically applied to joint structures and are used to stretch capsular restrictions or reposition a subluxed or dislocated joint. Techniques are described and illustrated in detail in Chapter 6.

Soft Tissue Mobilization and Manipulation

Various techniques, including *friction massage,*[72,117] *myofascial release,*[16,50,52,83,117] *acupressure,*[58,117,125] and *trigger point therapy,*[83,117,125] are designed to improve tissue mobility by mobilizing and manipulating connective tissue that binds down soft tissues. Although they are useful adjuncts to manual stretching procedures, specific techniques are not described in this textbook.

Neural Tissue Mobilization (Neuromeningeal Mobilization)

After trauma or surgical procedures, adhesions or scar tissue may form around the meninges and nerve roots or at the site of injury at the plexus or peripheral nerves. Tension placed on the adhesions or scar tissue leads to pain or neurologic symptoms. After tests to determine neural tissue mobility are conducted, the neural pathway is mobilized, through selective procedures.[35,58,88] These maneuvers are described in Chapter 9 for the brachial plexus, in Chapter 11 for the median nerve, and in Chapter 15 for nerve roots.

Selective Stretching

Selective stretching is a process whereby the overall function of a patient may be improved by applying stretching techniques selectively to some muscles and joints but allowing limitation of motion to develop in other muscles or joints. When determining which muscles to stretch and which to allow to become slightly tight, the therapist must always keep in mind the functional needs of the patient and the importance of maintaining a balance between mobility and stability for maximum functional performance.

- For example, in the patient with spinal cord injury, stability of the trunk is necessary for independence in sitting. With thoracic and cervical lesions, the patient will not have active control of the back extensors. If the hamstrings are routinely stretched to improve or maintain their extensibility and moderate hypomobility is allowed to develop in the extensors of the low back, the patient will be able to lean into the slightly shortened structures and will have some trunk stability in long-sitting. The patient must still have enough flexibility for independence in dressing and transfers. Too much limitation of motion in the low back can decrease function.
- Allowing slight hypomobility to develop in the long flexors of the fingers while maintaining flexibility of the wrist will enable the patient with spinal cord injury who lacks innervation of the intrinsic finger muscles to develop grasp through a tenodesis action.

Overstretching and Hypermobility

Overstretching is a stretch well beyond the normal ROM of a joint and the surrounding soft tissues, resulting in **hypermobility** (excessive mobility).

- Creating selective hypermobility by overstretching may be necessary for certain healthy individuals with normal strength and stability participating in sports that require extensive flexibility.[103]
- Overstretching becomes detrimental and creates joint *instability* when the supporting structures of a joint and the strength of the muscles around a joint are insufficient and cannot hold a joint in a stable, functional position during activities. Instability of a joint often causes pain and may predispose a person to musculoskeletal injury.

▶ Properties of Soft Tissue that Affect Response to Immobilization and Elongation

The ability of the body to move freely, that is, without restrictions and with control during functional activities, is dependent upon the passive mobility of soft tissues as well as active neuromuscular control. Motion is necessary for the health of tissues in the body. As mentioned previously, the soft tissues that can become restricted and impair mobility are muscles with their contractile and noncontractile elements and various types of connective tissue (tendons, ligaments, articular cartilage, fascia, and skin). Each type of tissue has unique qualities that affect its response to immobilization and its extensibility, that is, its ability to elongate. When stretching procedures are applied to these soft tissues, the velocity, intensity, frequency, and duration of the stretch force as well as temperature of the soft tissues all affect the responses of the different types of soft tissues. Mechanical characteristics of contractile and noncontractile tissue and the neurophysiologic properties of contractile tissue all affect soft tissue lengthening. Most of the information on the biomechanical and biochemical responses of soft tissues is derived from animal studies, but the exact physiologic mechanism by which stretching exercises produce an increase in the extensibility of human tissues is still unclear. Despite this, an understanding of the properties of these tissues and their responses to immobilization and stretch is the basis for selecting the safest and most effective stretching procedures in a therapeutic exercise program for patients with impaired mobility.

When soft tissue is stretched, either elastic or plastic changes occur. **Elasticity** is the ability of soft tissue to return to its resting length after passive stretch.[78] **Plasticity** is the tendency of soft tissue to assume a new and greater length after the stretch force has been removed.[42,107,123] Both contractile and noncontractile tissues have elastic and plastic qualities.

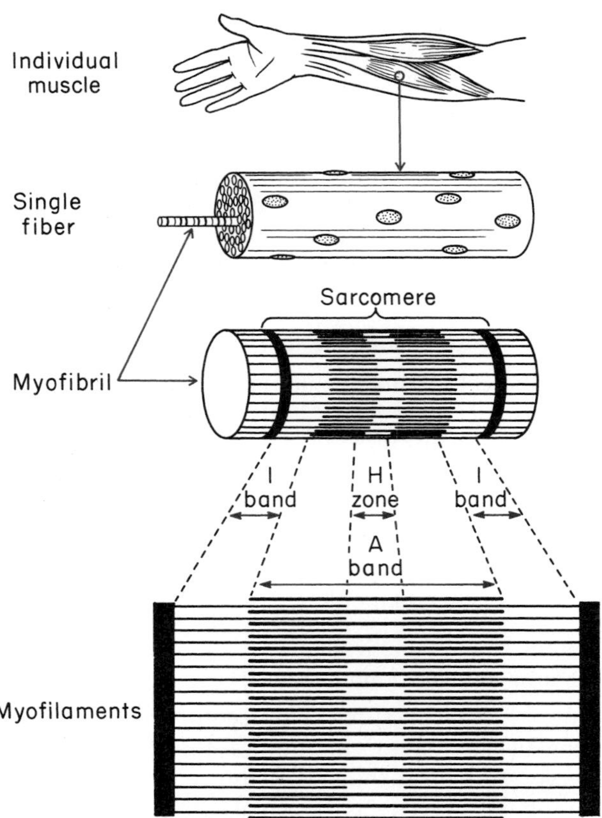

Figure 5–1 Structure of skeletal muscle.

Mechanical Properties of Contractile Tissue

Muscle is composed of both contractile tissue and noncontractile connective tissues. The contractile elements of muscle (Fig. 5–1) give it the characteristics of contractility and irritability. The noncontractile connective tissue within and around muscle (Fig. 5–2) has the same properties as all connective tissue, including the ability to resist deforming forces as well as viscoelasticity.[78,120] The connective tissue structures of the muscle-tendon unit are the *endomysium,* which is the innermost layer that separates individual muscle fibers and myofibrils; the *perimysium,* which encases fiber burrelles; and the *epimysium,* which is the enveloping fascial sheath around the entire muscle. It is the connective tissue framework of muscle that is the primary source of a muscle's resistance to passive elongation.[64,78] When contractures develop, adhesions within and between collagen fibers restrict movement.[26]

Contractile Elements of Muscle

Individual muscles are composed of many *muscle fibers* that lie in parallel with one another. A single muscle fiber is made up of many *myofibrils.* Each myofibril is composed of even smaller structures called *sarcomeres,* which lie in series within a myofibril. The sarcomere is the contractile unit of the myofibril and is composed of overlapping *myofila-*

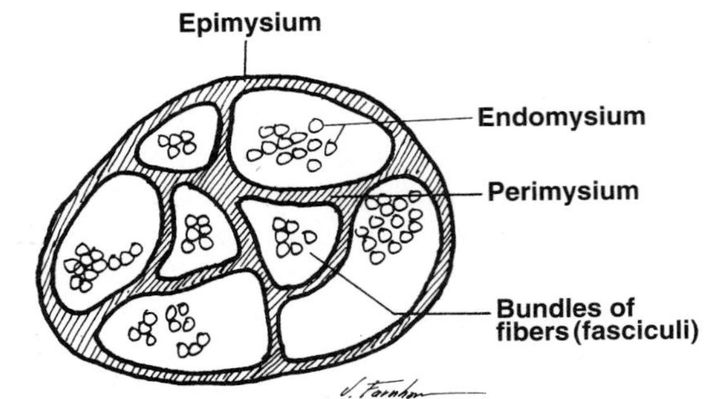

Figure 5–2 Muscular connective tissue. A schematic cross-sectional view of the connective tissue in a muscle shows how the perimysium is continuous with the outer layer of epimysium. (From Levangie and Norkin, p. 93 (78) with permission.)

ments of actin and myosin that form cross-bridges. The sarcomere gives a muscle its ability to contract and relax. When a motor unit stimulates a muscle to contract, the actin-myosin filaments slide together and the muscle actively shortens. When a muscle relaxes, the cross-bridges slide apart slightly, and the muscle returns to its resting length (Fig. 5–3).

Mechanical Response of the Contractile Unit to Stretch and Immobilization

There are a number of changes that occur over time in the anatomic structure and physiologic function of the contractile units (sarcomeres) within muscle if a muscle is stretched during an exercise or if it is immobilized in either a lengthened or shortened position for an extended time period and then remobilized. Of course, the noncontractile structures within and around muscle also affect a muscle's response to stretch and immobilization.[24,120] Those responses and adaptations are discussed later in this chapter.

Response to Stretch

When a muscle is stretched and elongates, the stretch force is transmitted to the muscle fibers via the connective tissue (endomysium and perimysium) in and around the fibers. It is hypothesized that molecular interactions link these noncontractile elements to the contractile unit of muscle, the sarcomere.[28]

During passive stretch both longitudinal and lateral force transduction occurs.[28] When initial lengthening occurs in the series elastic (connective tissue) component, tension rises sharply. After a point there is a mechanical disruption (influenced by neural and biochemical changes) of the cross-bridges as the filaments slide apart, leading to an abrupt lengthening of the sarcomeres,[28,64,80] known as *sarcomere give.*[40] When the stretch force is released, the individual sarcomeres return to their resting length[28,80] (Fig. 5–3). The tendency of muscle to return to its resting length after short-term stretch is called elasticity.[110] If more permanent (plastic) length increases are to occur, the stretch force must be maintained over an extended period of time.[28]

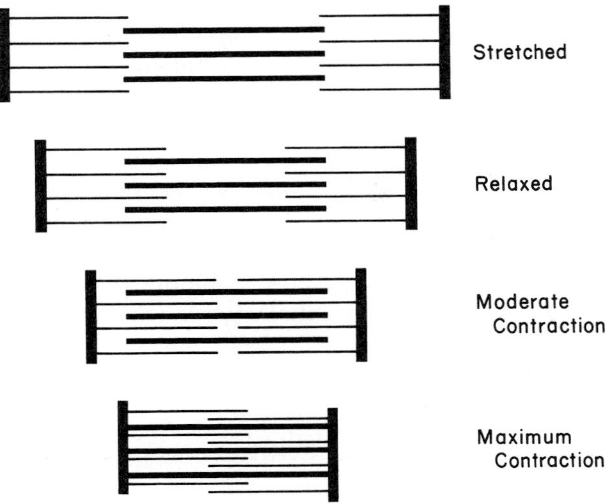

Figure 5–3 A model of myofilament sliding. Elongation and shortening of the sarcomere, the contractile unit of muscle.

Response to Immobilization

If a muscle is immobilized for a prolonged period of time, a decay in contractile protein and a decrease in the number of myofibrils occur, resulting in *atrophy* and *weakness.*[14,25,48,51,69,70,80,111] The duration of time and the position in which a muscle is immobilized affect the extent of atrophy and loss of strength. The composition of muscle also affects its response to immobilization. Atrophy occurs more quickly and more extensively in tonic (slow-twitch) postural muscle fibers than in phasic (fast-twitch) fibers.[80]

The longer the duration of immobilization, the greater the atrophy of muscle and loss of functional strength. Atrophy can begin in as little as a few days to a week.[69,70] Not only is there a decrease in the cross-sectional size of muscle fibers over time, an even more significant deterioration in motor unit recruitment occurs as reflected by EMG activity.[80] Both compromise the force-producing capabilities of the muscle. It has also been suggested that a muscle immobilized in a shortened position atrophies and weakens at a faster rate than if it is held in a lengthened position over time.[14]

If a muscle is immobilized in a *shortened* position for several weeks, which is often necessary after a fracture, muscle tear or tendon rupture, there is a reduction in the length of the muscle and its fibers and in the number of sarcomeres in series within myofibrils as the result of *sarcomere absorption.*[44,68,115,118,134] This absorption occurs at a faster rate than the muscle's ability to regenerate sarcomeres in an attempt to restore itself. The decrease in the overall length of the muscle fibers and their in-series sarcomeres contributes to muscle atrophy and weakness associated with immobilization. A shift to the left in the length-tension curve of the muscle decreases the muscle's capacity to produce maximum tension at its normal resting length as it contracts. A muscle that has been immobilized in a shortened position also produces an increased amount of connective tissue that serves to protect the weakened muscle when it stretches.[26,48] This contributes to its decreased mobility.

Sometimes a muscle is immobilized in a position of maximum available length for a prolonged period of time. This occurs with the application of a series of positional casts (serial casts)[63] or the use of a dynamic splint to stretch a contracture and increase ROM.[55,90] There is some research to suggest[115,118,134] that if a muscle is held in a lengthened position for an extended time period, it will adapt by increasing the number of sarcomeres in series (*myofibrillogenesis*[28]) to maintain the greatest functional overlap of actin and myosin filaments. This may lead to a more permanent (plastic) form of muscle lengthening if the newly gained length is used on a regular basis in functional activities.

The minimum time frame necessary for a stretched muscle (fiber) to become a longer muscle (fiber) by adding sarcomeres in series is not known. In animal studies that have reported increased muscle length as the result of myofibrillogenesis, the stretched muscle was continuously immobilized for several weeks.[115,118,134] There is speculation that this same process not only occurs and contributes to long-term gains in ROM associated with use of serial casts[63] and dynamic splints,[55,90] but also as the result of stretching exercises.[28]

The adaptation of the contractile units of muscle (an increase or decrease in the number of sarcomeres) to prolonged positioning in either lengthened or shortened positions is transient, lasting for only 3 to 5 weeks if the muscle resumes its preimmobilization use and degree of lengthening for functional activities.[70,115] In clinical situations this underscores the need for patients to use full-range motions during a variety of functional activities after removal of immobilization.

Neurophysiologic Properties of Contractile Tissue

The Muscle Spindle (Fig. 5–4)

The muscle spindle is the major sensory organ (stretch receptor) of muscle and is composed of microscopic *intrafusal muscle fibers* that are bundled together and lie parallel to an extrafusal muscle fiber.[48,64,78,84,110] The sensory receptors of the spindle

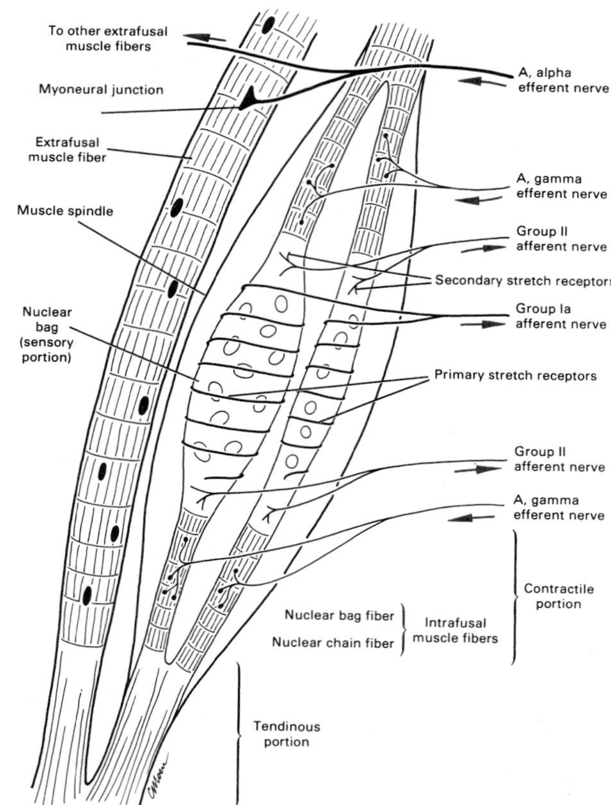

Figure 5–4 Muscle spindle. Diagram shows intrafusal and extrafusal muscle fibers. The muscle spindle acts as a stretch receptor. (From Lemkuhl, LD, and Smith, LK: Brunnstrom's Clinical Kinesiology, ed 4. FA Davis, Philadelphia, 1983, p 97, with permission.)

are located in the central portions called the *nuclear bag* and *nuclear chain.* When stimulated by stretch, information from these receptors about velocity and duration of stretch and length changes in muscle is transmitted via primary (type Ia) and secondary (type II) afferent fibers to the CNS. These fibers also synapse on the alpha or gamma motoneurons and facilitate contraction of their own extrafusal and intrafusal fibers, respectively, and inhibit the muscle's antagonists. There are essentially two ways to stimulate these sensory fibers via stretch; one is by overall lengthening of the muscle, and the other is by stimulating contraction of the intrafusal fibers via the gamma efferent neural pathways.

The Golgi Tendon Organ (GTO)

The GTO is located near the musculotendinous junction, wraps around the ends of the extrafusal fibers of a muscle, and transmits afferent stimuli via II B fibers. It is sensitive to the tension in a muscle caused by either passive stretch or an active muscle contraction. The GTO is a protective mechanism that inhibits tension in the muscle in which it lies. This effect is called *autogenic inhibition*. The GTO has a very low threshold for firing (fires easily) after an active muscle contraction and has a high threshold for firing with passive stretch.[41,64,84]

When excessive tension develops in a muscle the GTO fires, inhibits alpha motoneuron activity, and decreases tension in the muscle. During stretching procedures the tension within the tendon determines if the individual muscle fibers are inhibited and, thus, relaxed and able to be lengthened.

The Neurophysiologic Response of Muscle to Stretch

When a muscle is stretched very quickly, the primary afferent fibers stimulate alpha motoneurons in the spinal cord and facilitate contraction of extrafusal fibers, increasing tension in a muscle. This is called the *monosynaptic stretch reflex*.[78,84,110] Stretching procedures that are performed at too high a velocity may actually increase the tension in a muscle that is to be lengthened.[108,126] If a slow stretch force is applied to muscle, the GTO fires and inhibits the tension in the muscle, allowing the parallel elastic component (the sarcomere) of the muscle to remain relaxed and lengthen.[103,126]

Mechanical Characteristics of Noncontractile Soft Tissue

Noncontractile soft tissue permeates the entire body and is organized into various types of connective tissue to support the structures of the body. Ligaments, tendons, joint capsules, fasciae, noncontractile tissue within muscles (see Fig. 5–2), and skin all have connective tissue characteristics that will lead to the development of adhesions and contractures and thus affect the flexibility of the tissues crossing the joint. When these tissues restrict ROM and require stretching, it is important to understand how they respond to the intensity and duration of stretch forces and to recognize that the only way to increase the extensibility of connective tissue is by remodeling its basic architecture.[26]

Composition of Connective Tissue

Connective tissue is composed of three types of fibers and nonfibrous ground substance.[23,53,123]

- *Collagen fibers* resist tensile deformation and are responsible for the strength and stiffness of tissue. Collagen fibers are composed of tropocollagen crystals, which form the building blocks of collagen microfibrils. Each additional level of composition of the fibers is arranged in an organized relationship and dimension (Fig. 5–5). There are six classes with 19 types[24] of collagen; the fibers of tendons and ligaments mostly contain type I collagen, which is highly resistant to tension.[123] As collagen fibers develop and mature, they bind together, initially with unstable hydrogen bonding, which then converts to stable covalent bonding. The stronger the bonds, the greater the mechanical stability of the tissue.
- *Elastin fibers* provide extensibility. They show a great deal of elongation with small loads and fail abruptly without deformation at higher loads. Tissues with greater amounts of elastin have greater flexibility.
- *Reticulin fibers* provide tissue with bulk.
- *Ground substance* is made up of proteoglycans (PGs) and glycoproteins. The PGs function to

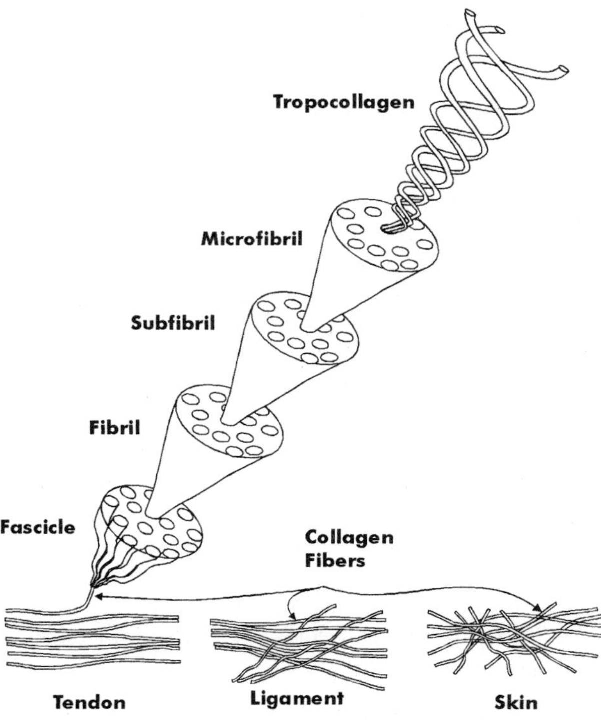

Figure 5–5 Composition of collagen fibers showing the aggregation of tropocollagen crystals as the building blocks of collagen. Organization of the fibers within connective tissue is related to the function of the tissue. Tissues with parallel fiber orientation, such as tendons, are able to withstand greater tensile loads than tissue such as skin where the fiber orientation appears more random.

hydrate the matrix, stabilize the collagen networks, and resist compressive forces (this is most important in cartilage and intervertebral discs). The type and amount of PGs are proportional to the types of compressive and tensile stresses the tissue undergoes.[47] The glycoproteins provide linkage between the matrix components and between the cells and matrix opponents. In essence, the ground substance is mostly an organic gel containing water that reduces friction between fibers, transports nutrients and metabolites, and may help prevent excessive cross-linking between fibers by maintaining space between fibers.[32,123]

Mechanical Behavior of Noncontractile Tissue

The mechanical behavior of the various noncontractile tissues is determined by the proportion of collagen and elastin fibers and by the structural orientation of the fibers. The proportion of proteoglycans (PGs) also influences the mechanical properties of connective tissue. Those high in collagen and low in PGs are designed to resist high tensile loads; those tissues that withstand greater compressive loads have greater concentrations of PGs.[47] Collagen is the structural element that absorbs most of the tensile stress. Collagen fibers elongate quickly under light loads (wavy fibers align and straighten). With increased loads, tension in the fibers increases and fibers stiffen. The fibers strongly resist the deforming force, but with continued loading, the bonds beteen collagen fibers begin to break. When a substantial number of bonds are broken, the fibers fail. Tissue with a greater proportion of collagen provides greater stability. When tensile forces are applied, maximum elongation of collagen is less than 10%, whereas elastin may lengthen 150% and return to its original configuration. Collagen is five times as strong as elastin. The alignment of collagen fibers in various tissues reflects the tensile forces acting on that tissue. (See Fig. 5–5.)

- In tendons, collagen fibers are parallel and can resist the greatest tensile load. They transmit forces to the bone created by the muscle.
- In skin, collagen fibers are random and weakest in resisting tension.
- In ligaments, joint capsules, and fasciae, the collagen fibers vary between the two extremes, and they resist multidirectional forces. Ligaments that resist the major joint stresses have more parallel orientation of collagen fibers and a larger cross-sectional area.[98]

Interpreting Mechanical Behavior of Connective Tissue: The Stress–Strain Curve

The stress–strain curve illustrates the mechanical strength of structures (Fig. 5–6) and is used to interpret what is happening to connective tissue under stress loads.[23,79,121,123,139]

- ***Stress.*** Force per unit area. Mechanical stress is the internal reaction or resistance to an external load. There are three kinds of stress:
  - *Tension:* a force applied perpendicular to the cross-sectional area of the tissue in a direction away from the tissue. A stretching force is a tension stress.
  - *Compression:* a force applied perpendicular to the cross-sectional area of the tissue in a direction toward the tissue. Muscle contraction and loading of a joint during weight bearing cause compression stresses within joints.
  - *Shear:* a force applied parallel to the cross-sectional area of the tissue.
- ***Strain.*** The amount of deformation or lengthening that occurs when a load (stress) or stretch force is applied.
- ***Toe region.*** That area of the stress–strain curve where there is considerable deformation without

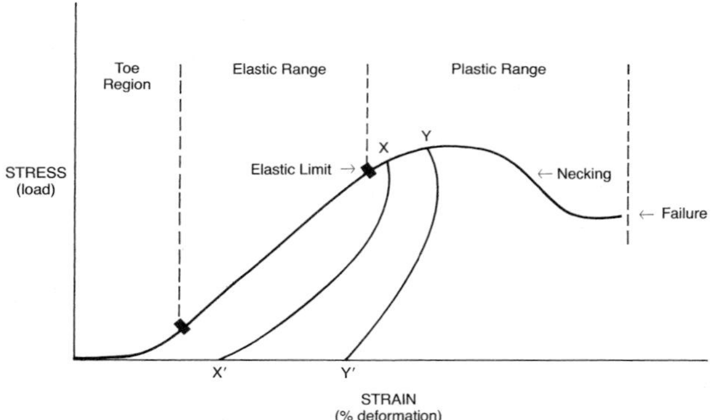

Figure 5–6 Stress–strain curve. When stressed, initially the wavy collagen fibers straighten (toe region). With additional stress, recoverable deformation occurs in the elastic range. Once the elastic limit is reached, sequential failure of the collagen fibers and tissue occurs in the plastic range, resulting in release of heat (hysteresis) and new length when the stress is released. The length from the stress point (X) results in a new length when released (X′); the heat released is represented by the area under the curve between these two points (hysteresis loop). (Y to Y′ represents additional length from additional stress with more heat released.) Necking is the region in which there is considerable weakening of the tissue and less force is needed for deformation. Total failure quickly follows even under smaller loads.

the use of much force. This is the range where most functional activity normally occurs. Collagen fibers at rest are wavy and are situated in a three-dimensional matrix, so some distensibility in the tissue occurs by straightening and aligning the fibers.

- ***Elastic range/the linear phase.*** Strain is directly proportional to the ability of the tissue to resist the force. This occurs when tissue is taken to the end of its ROM and a gentle stretch is applied. With stress in this phase the collagen fibers line up with the applied force, the bonds between fibers and between the surrounding matrix are strained, some microfailure between the collagen bonds begins, and some water may be displaced from the ground substance. There is complete recovery from this deformation, and the tissue returns to its original size and shape when the load is released if the stress is not maintained for any length of time (see the following discussion on creep and stress-relaxation for prolonged stretch).
- ***Elastic limit.*** The point beyond which the tissue will not return to its original shape and size.
- ***Plastic range.*** The range beyond the elastic limit extending to the point of rupture. Tissue strained in this range will have permanent deformation when the stress is released. In this range there is sequential failure of the bonds between collagen fibrils and eventually of collagen fibers. Heat is released and absorbed in the tissue. Because collagen is crystalline, individual fibers do not stretch but instead, they rupture. In the plastic range it is the rupturing of fibers that results in increased length.
- ***Ultimate strength.*** The greatest load the tissue can sustain. Once this load is reached, there is increased strain (deformation) without an increase in stress required. The *region of necking* is reached in which there is considerable weakening of the tissue, and it rapidly fails. The therapist must be cognizant of the tissue feel when stretching, because as the tissue begins necking, if the stress is maintained, there could be complete tearing of the tissue. Experimentally, maximum tensile deformation of isolated collagen fibers prior to failure is 7 to 8%. Whole ligaments may withstand strain of 20 to 40%.[98]
- ***Failure.*** Rupture of the integrity of the tissue.
- ***Structural stiffness.*** Tissues with greater stiffness have a higher slope in the elastic region of the curve, indicating there is less elastic deformation with greater stress. Contractures and scar tissue have greater stiffness, probably because of a greater degree of bonding between collagen fibers and their surrounding matrix.
- ***Creep.*** When a load is applied for an extended period of time, the tissue elongates, resulting in permanent deformation (Fig. 5–7*A*). It is related to the viscosity of the tissue and is, therefore, time-dependent. The amount of deformation depends on the amount of force and the rate at which the force is applied. Low-magnitude loads, usually in the elastic range and applied for long periods, increase the deformation of connective tissue and allow a gradual rearrangement of collagen fiber bonds (remodeling) and redistribution of water to surrounding tissues.[26,112,120,121] Increasing the temperature of the part will increase the creep and, therefore, the distensibility of the tissue.[75,130,132] Complete recovery from creep may occur over time, but not as rapidly as a single strain. Patient reaction dictates the time a specific load is tolerated.
- ***Stress-relaxation.*** When a force (load) is applied to stretch a tissue and the length of the tissue is kept constant, after the initial creep there is a decrease in the force required to maintain that

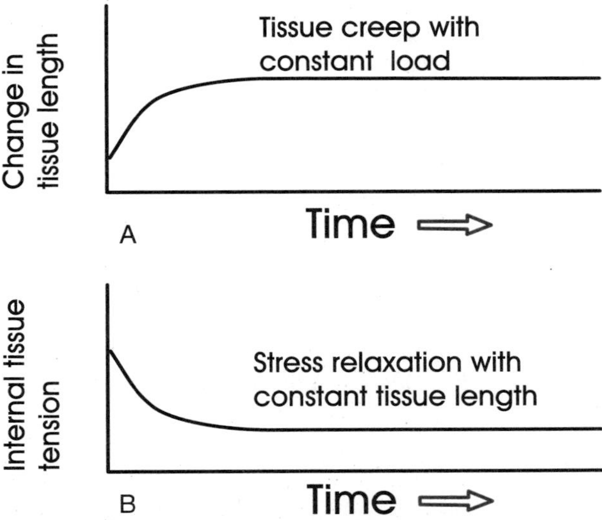

Figure 5-7 Tissue response to prolonged stretch forces as a result of viscoelastic properties. *(A)* Effects of creep. A constant load, applied over time, will result in increased tissue length until equilibrium is reached. *(B)* Effects of stress-relaxation. A load applied with the tissue kept at a constant length will result in decreased internal tension within the tissue until equilibrium is reached.

length, and the tension in the tissue decreases[26] (Fig. 5–7*B*). This, like creep, is related to the viscoelastic qualities of the connective tissue and redistribution of the water content. Stress-relaxation is the underlying principle used in prolonged stretching procedures where the stretch position is maintained for several hours or days. Recovery (i.e., no change) versus permanent changes in length is dependent on the amount of deformation and length of time the deformation is maintained.[26]

- ***Cyclic loading and connective tissue fatigue.*** Repetitive loading of tissue increases heat production and may cause failure below the yield point. The greater the applied load, the fewer number of cycles needed for failure. This principle can be used for stretching by applying repetitive (cyclic) loads at a submaximal level on successive days. The intensity of the load is determined by the patient's tolerance. A minimum load is required for this failure. Below the minimum load an apparent infinite number of cycles will not cause failure. This is the *endurance limit.* Examples of connective tissue fatigue from cyclic loading are stress fractures and overuse syndromes, neither of which is desired as a result of stretching. Therefore, periodically, time is allowed between bouts of cyclic stretching to allow for remodeling and healing in the new range.
- ***Summary of mechanical principles for stretching connective tissue***
  - Connective tissue deformation (stretch) occurs to different degrees at different intensities of force. It requires breaking of collagen bonds and realignment of the fibers for there to be permanent elongation or increased flexibility. Failure of tissue begins as microfailure of fibrils and fibers before complete failure of the tissue occurs. Complete tissue failure can occur as a single maximal event (acute tear from a traumatic injury or manipulation that exceeds the failure point) or from repetitive submaximal stress (fatigue or stress failure from cyclic loading). Microfailure (needed for permanent lengthening) also occurs with creep, stress-relaxation, and controlled cyclic loading.
  - Healing and adaptive remodeling capabilities allow the tissue to respond to repetitive and sustained loads if time is allowed between bouts. This is important for increasing both flexibility and tensile strength of the tissue. If healing and remodeling time is not allowed, a breakdown of tissue (failure) will occur as in overuse syndromes and stress fractures. Intensive stretching is usually not done every day in order to allow time for healing. If the inflammation from the microruptures is excessive, additional scar tissue is laid down, which could become more restrictive.[26]
  - It is imperative that the individual use any newly gained range to allow the remodeling of tissue and to train the muscle to control the new range, or the tissue will eventually return to its shortened length.

Changes in Collagen Affecting Stress–Strain Response

Effects of Immobilization

There is weakening of the tissue because of collagen turnover and weak bonding between the new, nonstressed fibers. There is also adhesion formation because of greater cross-linking between disorganized collagen fibers and because of decreased effectiveness of the ground substance maintaining space and lubrication between the fibers.[32,121] Rate of return to normal tensile strength is slow. For example, after 8 weeks of immobilization the anterior cruciate ligament in monkeys failed at 61% of maximum load; after 5 months of reconditioning, it failed at 79%; after 12 months of reconditioning, it failed at 91%.[96,97] There was also a reduction in energy absorbed and an increase in compliance (decreased stiffness) prior to failure following immobilization. Partial and near-complete recovery followed the same 5-month and 12-month pattern.[97]

Effects of Inactivity (Decrease of Normal Activity)

There is a decrease in size and amount of collagen fibers, resulting in weakening of the tissue. There is a proportional increase in the predominance of elastin fibers, resulting in an increased compliance. Recovery takes about 5 months of regular cyclic loading. Physical activity has a beneficial effect on the strength of connective tissue.

Effects of Age

There is a decrease in the maximum tensile strength and in the elastic modulus, and the rate of adaptation to stress is slower.[98] There is an increased tendency for overuse syndromes, fatigue failures, and tears with stretching.[139]

Effects of Corticosteroids

There is a long-lasting deleterious effect on the mechanical properties of collagen with a decrease in tensile strength.[139] There is fibrocyte death next to the injection site with delay in reappearance up to 15 weeks.[98]

Effects of Injury

Excessive tensile loading can lead to rupture of ligaments and tendons at musculotendinous junctions. Healing follows a predictable pattern (see Chapter 8) with bridging of the rupture site with newly synthesized type III collagen. This is structurally weaker than mature type I collagen. Remodeling progresses and eventually collagen matures to type I. Remodeling usually begins about 3 weeks postinjury and continues for several months to a year, depending on the size of the connective tissue structure and magnitude of the tear.[47]

Determinants of Stretching Exercises

As with other forms of therapeutic exercise, such as strengthening exercises and endurance training, there are a number of essential elements that determine the effectiveness of a stretching program. The elements of stretching, all of which are interrelated, include the *alignment* and *stabilization* of the body during stretching; the *intensity, speed, duration, frequency,* and *mode* of stretch; and the integration of neuromuscular inhibition and functional activities into stretching procedures. The numerous variations and combination of these elements provide the therapist with many options from which to choose when designing stretching exercises that are safe and effective and meet many patients' needs, goals, and capabilities.

Note: Many of the investigations comparing the intensity, duration, frequency, and mode of stretching have been carried out with healthy, young adults as subjects. The findings and recommendations of these studies may be difficult to extrapolate and apply to patients with long-standing contractures or other forms of tissue restriction. Therefore many decisions, particularly those dealing with intensity, duration, and frequency of stretching, must continue to be based on a balance of scientific evidence and sound clinical judgments by the therapist.

Alignment and Stabilization

Just as appropriate alignment and effective stabilization are fundamental components of muscle testing and goniometry as well as ROM and strengthening exercises, they are also essential elements of effective stretching.

Alignment

Proper alignment or positioning of the patient and the specific muscles and joints to be stretched is necessary for patient comfort and stability during stretching. Alignment influences the amount of tension present in soft tissue and consequently affects the range of motion available in joints. Alignment of the muscles and joint to be stretched as well as the alignment of the trunk and adjacent joints must all be considered. For example, to effectively stretch the rectus femoris (a muscle that crosses two joints), as the knee is flexed and the hip extended, the lumbar spine and pelvis should be aligned in a neutral position. The pelvis should not tilt anteriorly nor the low back hyperextend; the hip should not abduct or remain flexed (Fig. 5–8 *A* and *B*). When the patient is self-stretching to increase shoulder flexion, the trunk should be erect, not slumped (Fig. 5–9 *A* and *B*).

Note: Throughout this and later chapters recommendations for appropriate alignment and positioning during stretching procedures are identified. If it is impossible for the patient to be placed in or assume the recommended

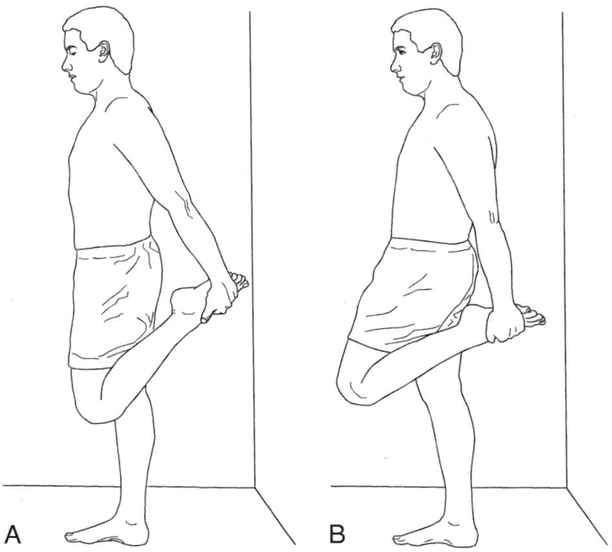

Figure 5-8 *(A)* Correct alignment when stretching the rectus femoris: the lumbar spine, pelvis, and hip are held in a neutral position as the knee is flexed. *(B)* Incorrect position of the hip in flexion. In addition, avoid an anterior pelvic tilt, hyperextension of the lumbar spine, and abduction of the hip.

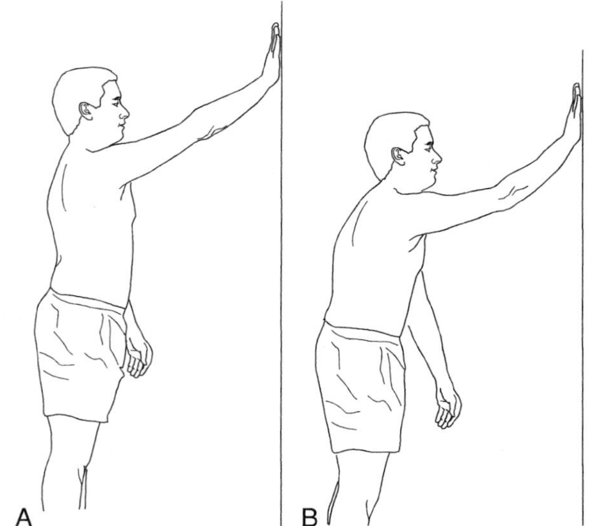

Figure 5-9 *(A)* Correct alignment when stretching to increase shoulder flexion: cervical and thoracic spine is erect. *(B)* Incorrect alignment (forward head and rounded spine).

postures because of discomfort, restrictions of motion of adjacent joints, inadequate neuromuscular control, or cardiorespiratory capacity, the therapist must critically analyze the situation to determine an alternative position.

Stabilization

To achieve an effective stretch of a specific muscle or muscle group and associated periarticular structures, it is imperative to stabilize (fixate) either the proximal or distal attachment site of the muscle-tendon unit being elongated. Either site may be stabilized, but in manual stretching it is more common to stabilize the proximal attachment as the distal segment moves, whereas in some self-stretching procedures, the distal attachment is stabilized as the proximal segment moves. (Compare Figs. 5–25 and 13–7, both of which show a stretch to increase knee flexion.)

Stabilization of multiple segments of a patient's body also helps maintain the proper alignment necessary for an effective stretch. For example, when stretching the iliopsoas the pelvis and lumbar spine must maintain a neutral position as the hip is extended to avoid stress to the low back region. Sources of stabilization include manual contacts, body weight, or firm surfaces such as a table, wall, or floor.

Intensity of Stretch

The intensity of a stretch force is determined by the load placed on soft tissue as it is being elongated. There is general agreement among clinicians and researchers that stretching should be applied gently, that is, at a *low intensity* by means of a *low load.*[10,21,82,102,126,138] Low-intensity stretching in comparison to high-intensity stretching makes the stretching maneuver more comfortable for the patient and minimizes voluntary or involuntary muscle guarding so that the patient can either remain relaxed or assist with the stretching maneuver.

Low-intensity stretching (usually coupled with a long duration of stretch) results in optimal rates of improvement in ROM without exposing tissues, possibly weakened by immobilization, to excessive loads and potential injury. Low-intensity stretching has also been shown to more effectively elongate dense connective tissue, a significant component of chronic contractures, with less soft tissue damage and post-exercise soreness than a high-intensity stretch.[2]

Duration of Stretch

One of the most important decisions a therapist must make when selecting and implementing a stretching intervention (stretching exercises or use of a stretching device) is to determine the duration of stretch that is expected to be safe, effective, and efficient for an individual patient.

The duration of stretch refers to the period of time a stretch force is applied, and shortened tissues are held in a lengthened position. Duration most often refers to how long a *single cycle* of stretch is applied. If more than one repetition of stretch *(stretch cycle)* occurs in a treatment session, the cumulative time of all the stretch cycles is also considered an aspect of duration. The duration of stretch must be put in context with many other factors, including intensity and frequency of stretch. Despite extensive research there continues to be a lack of agreement on how long a single cycle of stretch should be held or how many cycles of stretch should be applied to achieve the most effective, efficient, and sustained stretch-induced gains in ROM. Key findings from the literature are summarized in Box 5–3.

Numerous descriptors are used to differentiate between a long-duration versus a short-duration stretch. Terms such as *static, sustained, maintained,* and *prolonged* are all used to describe a long-duration stretch, whereas terms such as *cyclic, intermittent,* or *ballistic* are used to characterize a short-duration stretch. There is no specific time frame assigned to any of these descriptors, nor is there a time frame that distinguishes a long-duration from a short-duration stretch.

Box 5-3 Intensity, Duration, and Frequency of Stretch: Interrelationships and Impact on Stretching Outcomes

- There is an inverse relationship between intensity and duration as well as intensity and frequency of stretch.
  - The lower the intensity, the longer the time the patient will tolerate stretching and soft tissues can be held in a lengthened position.
  - The higher the intensity, the less frequently the stretching intervention can be applied to allow time for tissue healing.
- A low-load (low-intensity), long-duration stretch is considered the safest form of stretch and yields the most significant, elastic deformation and long-term, plastic changes in soft tissues.[75]
- Manual stretching and self-stretching in hypomobile but healthy subjects[5,6,7,11,38] and prolonged mechanical stretching in patients with chronic contractures[13,63,66,82,91] yield stretch-induced gains in ROM.
- In the well elderly, stretch cycles of 15, 30, and 60 seconds, applied to the hamstrings for four repetitions, have all been shown to produce significant gains in ROM with the greatest and longest-lasting improvements occurring with the use of 60-second stretch cycles.[38]
- In healthy, young adults
  - Stretch durations of 15, 30, 45, or 60 seconds or 2 minutes to lower extremity musculature have produced significant gains in ROM.[5,6,87]
  - Stretch cycles of 30- and 60-second durations of the hamstrings are both more effective than a 15-second stretch cycle but are equally effective when compared to each other.[5] Yet, 15-second and 2-minute static stretches of the hip adductors have produced similar improvements in ROM.[87]
  - There seems to be no additional benefit to holding each stretch cycle beyond 60 seconds.[5,87]
  - Three cycles of 30-second and 1-minute stretches were no more effective than one cycle of each duration of stretch.[6]
- When the total duration of stretch is equal, a cyclic stretch is equally effective and possibly more comfortable than a static stretch.[112]
- In patients with chronic, fibrotic contractures
  - Common durations of manual stretching or self-stretching may not be effective.[82,94]
  - Use of very prolonged static stretch with splints or casts is more effective.[13,66,82,91]
- Frequency of stretching needs to occur a minimum of two times per week[46] with healthy hypomobile individuals, but more frequently for patients with soft tissue pathology to achieve gains in ROM.
- Although stretch-induced gains in ROM often persist for a week after cessation of a stretching intervention, permanent improvement in mobility can be achieved only by use of the newly gained ROM in functional activities and/or with a maintenance stretching program.

Static Stretching

Static stretching* is the most common term used to describe a method by which soft tissues are lengthened just past the point of tissue resistance and then held in the lengthened position for an extended period of time with a sustained stretch force. Other terms used interchangeably are sustained, maintained, or prolonged stretching. The duration of static stretch is either predetermined prior to stretching or is based on the patient's response during the stretching procedure. In the research literature "static stretching" has been linked to durations ranging from as few as 15 seconds to several minutes when a manual stretch or self-stretching procedure is employed.† If a mechanical device provides the static stretch, the time frame can range from almost an hour to several days or weeks[13,55,63,66,82,86,90] (see additional information on mechanical stretching later in this section).

Static stretching has been well accepted as a safer form of stretching than ballistic stretching (described in the next section on speed of stretch) for many years.[31,109] Research has shown that tension created in muscle during static stretching is approximately half that created during ballistic stretching.[128] From a neurophysiologic perspective, during static stretching the GTO, which monitors tension created by stretch of a muscle-tendon unit, may override any facilitative impulses from the primary afferents of the muscle spindle (Ia afferent fibers) and subsequently may inhibit tension in the contractile units of the muscle being stretched. For these reasons clinicians believe that static stretching, if applied at a low intensity, generates less tissue trauma and less postexercise muscle soreness than ballistic stretching.

Static Progressive Stretching

Static progressive stretching is another term that describes how static stretch is applied for maximum effectiveness. The shortened soft tissues are held in a comfortably lengthened position until a degree of relaxation is felt by the patient or therapist. Then the shortened tissues are incrementally lengthened even further and again held in the new end-range position for an additional duration of time.[13,66,94] This approach involves continuous displacement of a limb by varying the stretch force (stretch load). This approach to stretching capitalizes on the stress-relaxation properties of soft tissue[91,93,94,111] (see Fig. 5–7*B*).

Most studies that have explored the merits of static *progressive* stretching have examined the effectiveness of a dynamic orthosis (see Fig. 5–11),

*See references 4, 5, 6, 7, 11, 12, 31, 38, 43, 46, 73, 81, 87, 106, 113, 126, 131, 136, 138.

†See references 5, 6, 7, 11, 12, 38, 82, 106, 131, 136.

which allows the patient to control the degree of displacement of the limb.[13,66] Manual stretching and self-stretching procedures are also routinely applied in this manner.

Cyclic (Intermittent) Stretching

A relatively short-duration stretch force that is repeatedly but gradually applied, released, and then reapplied is described as a cyclic (intermittent)[10,36,112] stretch. Cyclic stretching, by its very nature is applied for multiple repetitions (stretch cycles) in a single treatment session. Each cycle of stretch is held between 5 and 10 seconds,[36,112] but there is no consensus on the optimum number of cycles in a treatment session. This determination is often based on the patient's response to stretching. The end-range stretch force is applied gradually and in a controlled manner and at a relatively low intensity. For these reasons, cyclic stretching is *not* synonymous with ballistic stretching.

Based on clinical experience some therapists hold the opinion that appropriately applied, end-range cyclic stretching is as effective and more comfortable for a patient than a static stretch of comparable intensity. There is some evidence to support this opinion. Although there have been few studies on cyclic or intermittent stretching (aside from those on ballistic stretching), cyclic loading has been shown to cause tissues to yield at slightly lower intensities than static stretch, possibly due to heat production.[112] One such study, comparing cyclic stretching to a single, prolonged static stretch, does support the contention that cyclic stretching is as effective and more comfortable than a prolonged static stretch.[112]

Speed of Stretch

Importance of a Slowly Applied Stretch

To ensure optimal muscle relaxation and prevent injury to restricted tissues, the speed of stretch should be *slow*.[4,31,43,46,84,106,107] The stretch force should be applied and released *gradually*. A slowly applied stretch is less likely to facilitate the stretch reflex and increase tension in the muscle being stretched.[81] Remember, the Ia fibers of the muscle spindle are sensitive to the *velocity* of muscle lengthening. A stretch force applied at a low speed is also easier for the therapist or patient to control and is, therefore, safer than a high-speed stretch. In addition, a low-speed stretch affects the viscoelastic properties of connective tissue, making them more compliant.

Ballistic Stretching

A *rapid, forceful* intermittent stretch, that is, a high-speed *and* high-intensity stretch, is commonly called **ballistic stretching.**[4,6,7,8,106,126,138] It is characterized by the use of vigorous bouncing movements that create momentum to carry the body segment quickly through the ROM to stretch shortened structures. Although ballistic stretching has been shown to increase ROM in young, healthy subjects, who participated in a conditioning program,[54] it is, for the most part, not recommended. It is consistently contraindicated in elderly or sedentary individuals or patients with musculoskeletal pathology or chronic contractures[26] because:

- The high-velocity, high-intensity movements are difficult to control.
- Tissues, weakened by immobilization or disuse, are easily injured.
- Dense connective tissue found in chronic contractures does not yield easily with rapid stretch, rather it becomes more brittle and tears more readily.

High-Velocity Stretching in Advanced Phase Rehabilitation

Although controversial, some practitioners believe there is at least one situation when high-velocity stretching may be appropriate.[4,15] Occasionally in carefully selected individuals—such as a highly trained athlete or a young, active patient in the final phase of rehabilitation, who wishes to return to high-velocity sports—high-speed stretching may be appropriate in a conditioning program or in preparation for plyometric training. If employed, rapid, but *low-load (low-intensity)*, end-range stretches are applied paying close attention to effective stabilization. The stretch force is initiated by having the patient actively contract the muscle group opposite the muscle and connective tissues to be stretched.

Frequency of Stretch

Frequency of stretching refers to the *number of bouts (sessions) per day or per week* a patient carries out a stretching regimen.[6,46] The recommended frequency of stretching is often based on the underlying cause of immobility, the quality and level of healing of tissues, the chronicity and severity of a contracture, as well as the patient's age, use of corticosteroids, and previous response to stretching. Since very few studies have attempted to determine the optimal frequency of stretching within a day or a week,[6,46] it is not possible to draw evidence-based guidelines from the literature. As with decisions on the most appropriate number of repetitions of stretch in an exercise session, most suggestions are based on opinion. Frequency on a weekly basis ranges from two to five sessions, allowing time for rest between sessions for tissue healing and to minimize postexercise soreness. Ultimately the decision is based on the clinical discretion of the therapist and the response and needs of the patient.

The therapist must be aware of any breakdown of tissues with repetitive stretch. A fine balance between collagen tissue breakdown and repair is needed to allow an increase in length. If there is excessive frequency of loading, tissue breakdown will exceed repair and ultimate tissue failure is a possibility. In addition, if there is progressive loss of ROM over time rather than gains in range, continued low-grade inflammation from the stress can cause excessive collagen formation and hypertrophic scarring.

Box 5–4 Considerations for Selection of Methods of Stretching

- Based on the results of your examination, what types of tissues are involved and impairing mobility?
- Is there evidence of pain or inflammation?
- How long has the hypomobility existed?
- What is the stage of healing of restricted tissues?
- What form(s) of stretching have been implemented previously? How did the patient respond?
- Are there any underlying diseases, disorders, or deformities that might affect the choice of stretching procedures?
- Does the patient have the ability to actively participate in, assist with, or independently perform the exercises? Consider the patient's physical capabilities, age, ability to cooperate, or ability to follow and remember instructions.
- Will assistance from a therapist or caregiver be necessary to execute the stretching procedures and appropriate stabilization? If so, what is the size and strength of the therapist or the caregiver who is assisting the patient with a stretching program?

Mode of Stretch

The mode of stretch refers to the form of stretch or the manner in which stretching exercises are carried out. Mode of stretch can be defined by who or what is applying the stretch force or whether or not the patient is actively participating in the stretching maneuver. Categories include but are not limited to **manual, mechanical,** or **self-stretching** as well as **passive, assisted,** or **active stretching.** Regardless of the form of stretching selected and implemented, it is imperative that the shortened muscle remains relaxed and that the restricted connective tissues yield as easily as possible to stretch. To accomplish this, stretching procedures should be preceded by either low-intensity active exercise or therapeutic heat to warm up the tissues that are to be lengthened.

There is no one best form of stretching. What is important is that the therapist and patient have many modes of stretching from which to choose. Box 5–4 lists some questions a therapist will need to answer to determine which forms of stretching are most appropriate and will be most effective for each patient at different stages of a rehabilitation program.

Manual Stretching

A therapist or other trained practitioner or caregiver applies an external force to move the involved body segment *slightly beyond* the point of tissue resistance and available ROM. The therapist manually controls the site of stabilization as well as the direction, speed, intensity, and duration of stretch. Manual stretching usually employs a gentle, controlled, end-range, static, and progressive stretch held for about 30 to 60 seconds and then repeated for several or more cycles.

Manual stretching is indicated in the early stages of a stretching program when a therapist may want to determine how a patient responds to varying intensities or durations of stretch and when optimal stabilization is most critical. Similar to ROM exercises (described in Chapter 2), manual stretching can be performed *passively, with assistance from the patient,* or even *independently by the patient.*

Note: Remember, stretching and ROM exercises are not synonymous terms. Stretching takes soft tissue structures *beyond* their available length to *increase* ROM. ROM exercises stay within the limits of tissue extensibility to *maintain* the available length of tissues.

- Manual stretching performed *passively,* also referred to as **passive stretching,** is the only choice if a patient lacks neuromuscular control of the body segment to be stretched.
- It is often helpful to ask the patient to assist the therapist with the stretching maneuver, particularly if the patient is apprehensive and is having difficulty relaxing. If the patient concentrically contracts the muscle opposite the short muscle and assists with joint movement, the range-limiting muscle will reflexively relax, making

muscle elongation easier. Some clinicians refer to this as a form of neuromuscular inhibition, called *agonist contraction;* this approach to muscle relaxation and elongation will be discussed later in this chapter.

- Using procedures and hand placements similar to those described for self-ROM exercises (Chapter 2), a patient can also independently lengthen range-limiting muscles and periarticular tissues with manual stretching. As such, this form of stretch is usually referred to as **self-stretching** and will be discussed in more detail as the next topic in this section.

Self-Stretching

Self-stretching (also referred to as **flexibility exercises** or **active stretching**) is a type of stretching procedure that a patient can carry out independently after careful instruction and supervised practice. Self-stretching enables a patient to maintain or increase the ROM gained as the result of direct intervention by a therapist. This form of stretching is often an integral component of a home exercise program and is necessary for effective and efficient long-term self-management of many musculoskeletal and neuromuscular disorders. Educating the patient to safely carry out self-stretching procedures is also important for the prevention of reinjury or future dysfunction.

Teaching the patient proper alignment during the stretching maneuver is critical for effective self-stretching. Effective stabilization of either the proximal or distal attachment of a shortened muscle can be difficult to achieve with self-stretching. Every effort should be made to see that shortened structures are stretched specifically and that adjacent structures are not overstretched.

The guidelines for the intensity, speed, duration, and frequency of stretch that apply to manual stretching are also appropriate for self-stretching procedures. Self-stretching exercises can be performed in several ways.

- The patient can passively move a distal segment of a restricted joint with one or both hands.
- Repeated intermittent, end-range active muscle contractions of the muscle opposite the shortened muscle (also referred to as *active stretching, agonist contraction,* or *dynamic ROM*) is considered by some to be another form of self-stretching exercise.[7,95,131]
- If the distal attachment of the shortened muscle is fixed, body weight can be used as the source of the stretch force to passively elongate the shortened muscle-tendon unit.
- Integration of neuromuscular inhibition can also be useful during self-stretching procedures to maintain relaxation in the muscle that is being elongated.

Mechanical Stretching

There are many ways to use equipment to stretch a contracture and increase joint ROM. The equipment can be as simple as a cuff weight or weight-pulley system or as sophisticated as some orthoses or automated stretching machines.*

These mechanical stretching devices either provide a constant load with variable displacement or constant displacement with variable loads. Studies[13,66] about the efficacy of these two categories of mechanical stretching devices base their effectiveness on the soft tissue properties of either creep or stress-relaxation, which occur in a short period of time, as well as plastic deformation, which occurs over a prolonged period of time.

It is often the responsibility of a therapist to recommend the type of stretching device that is most suitable or to teach a patient how to safely use the equipment and to monitor its use in the home setting. A therapist may also be involved in the fabrication of serial casts or splints.

Mechanical stretching devices apply a very low-intensity stretch force (low-load) over a prolonged period of time to create plastic deformation (lengthening) of tissues.

- The stretch load, which can be applied with a cuff weight, is often as low as a few pounds (Fig. 5–10).
- Some devices, such as the Joint Active Systems™ orthosis (Fig. 5–11), allow the patient to control and adjust the load (stretch force) during the stretching session.[13,66] With other devices, such as the Dynasplint™ (Fig. 5–12), the load is preset prior to the application of the splint and the load remains constant while the splint is in place.[55]
- Each of these forms of stretch have been shown to be effective, particularly in reducing long-standing contractures.

The duration of mechanical stretch ranges from 15 to 30 minutes[13,66] or as long as 8 to 10 hours at a time,[55] depending on the type of device employed,

*See references 13, 66, 75, 77, 82, 86, 90, 107, 111, 112, 129, 130.

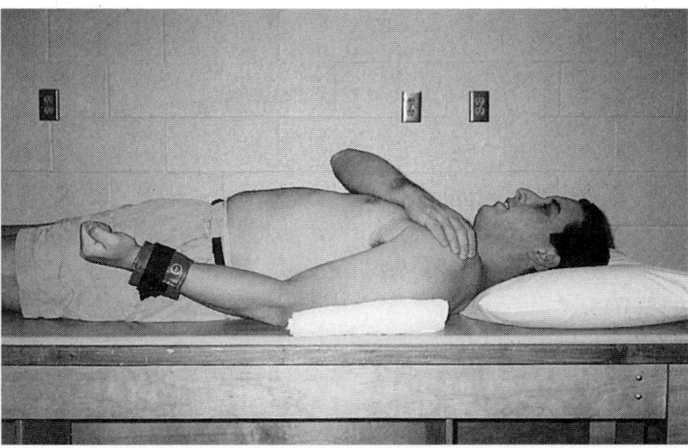

Figure 5-10 Low-load mechanical stretch with a cuff weight and self-stabilization of the proximal humerus to stretch the elbow flexors and increase end-range elbow extension.

the severity of impairment, and patient tolerance. Some devices such as serial casts are worn for days or weeks at a time before being removed and then reapplied.[63] Significantly longer durations of stretch are required for patients with chronic contractures as the result of neurologic or musculoskeletal disorders than healthy subjects with only mild hypomobility as the result of myostatic contractures.[13,63,66,82,86,91,94] In one study low-intensity, prolonged mechanical stretch (5- to 12-lb stretch force applied by hanging a weight from the involved lower extremity 1 hour per day over a 4-week period of time) was shown to be significantly more effective than manual passive stretching over an equal timeframe in patients with long-standing bilateral knee flexion contractures.[82] The duration of stretch

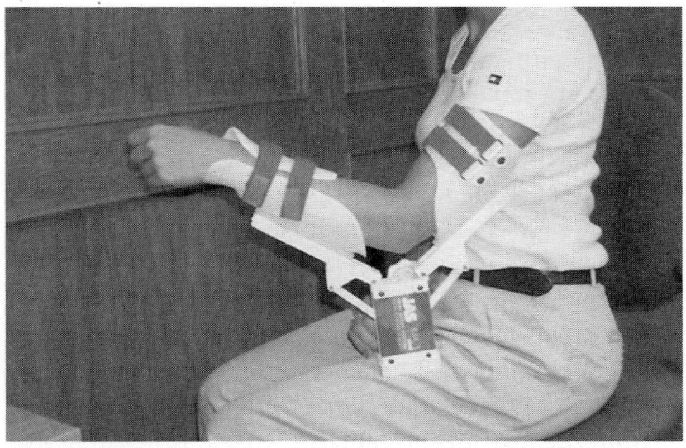

Figure 5-11 JAS orthosis is a patient-directed device that applies a static progressive stretch. (Courtesy of Joint Active Systems, Inc., Effingham, IL)

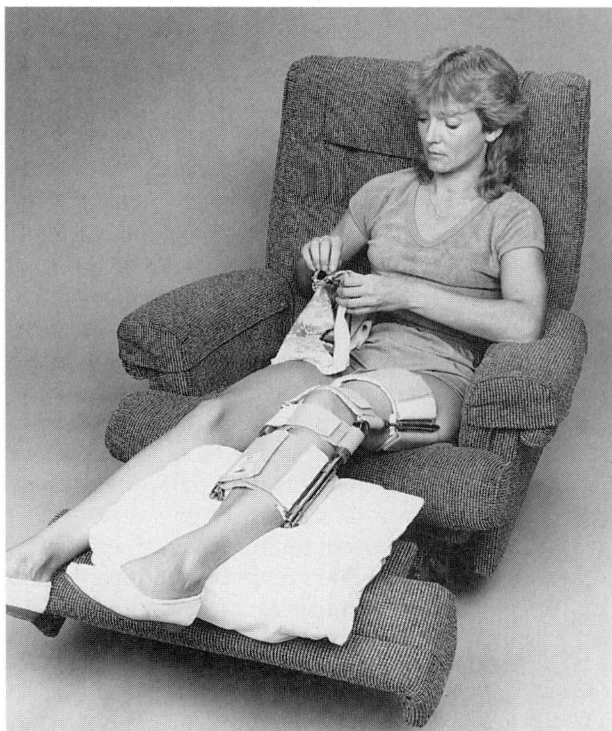

Figure 5–12 The Dynasplint Systems® Unit places a prolonged stretch on soft tissue to reduce a knee flexion contracture. (Reprinted by permission of Dynasplint Systems, Inc., Baltimore, MD.)

for those knees stretched mechanically was much longer than the duration of stretch applied manually. The patients also reported that the prolonged mechanical stretch was more comfortable than the manual stretching procedure, which tended to be applied at a higher intensity.

Note: Be cautious of studies that have reported "permanent lengthening" as the result of the use of some mechanical stretching device that applies a long-term stretch. In some studies permanent lengthening only meant that increased length was maintained for some designated period of time, such as a few days or a week, after the stretch force was removed. Follow-up, after stretching was discontinued, indicated that tissues often returned to their shortened position within a few weeks or even days if the newly gained motion was not used regularly in daily activities.

Neuromuscular Inhibition and Muscle Elongation

With respect to the neuromuscular system, inhibition is a state of decreased neuronal activity and altered synaptic potential, which reflexively diminishes the capacity of a muscle to contract.[61,64,101] The use of neuromuscular inhibition techniques prior to and during stretching increases the likelihood that the muscle will remain relaxed as it is being stretched. When a muscle is reflexively inhibited, there is less resistance to elongation by the contractile units of the muscle. Inhibition techniques relax only the contractile structures within muscle, not the connective tissue within and around shortened muscles. The neuromuscular inhibition techniques described in this section require normal innervation and voluntary control of either the shortened muscle or the muscle on the opposite side of the joint. Consequently, these techniques cannot be used effectively in patients with paralysis or spasticity from neuromuscular diseases or injury.

Therapists have used neuromuscular inhibition techniques, most of which have been adapted from proprioceptive neuromuscular facilitation (PNF) techniques,[114,127] for many years as an adjunct to manual stretching or self-stretching procedures. Inhibition techniques increase muscle length by relaxing and elongating the contractile components of muscle. The assumption is that sarcomere give will occur more easily when the muscle is relaxed, with less active resistance (tension) in the muscle as it is elongated. An advantage to the use of inhibition techniques prior to or during stretching is that muscle elongation is more comfortable for the patient.

Types of Procedures

Several variations of neuromuscular inhibition techniques can be used to relax (inhibit) and elongate shortened muscles if coupled with stretching. They include (1) hold-relax (HR) or contract-relax (CR), (2) agonist contraction (AC), and (3) hold-relax with agonist contraction (HR-AC). In classic PNF, these inhibition techniques are performed using diagonal patterns.[114,127] These techniques have been modified[4,20,52,61,99,103] to stretch isolated muscle groups in patients with musculoskeletal disorders by stretching in anatomic planes or opposite the line of pull of specific muscle groups rather than in combined, diagonal patterns. As mentioned earlier in this chapter, because the use of neuromuscular inhibition for elongating shortened muscles was first discussed by Knott and Voss in their approach to exercise, some therapists refer to the use of inhibition with stretch as *PNF stretching*[4,15,22,99] or *facilitated stretching.*[101]

Hold-Relax (HR) and Contract-Relax (CR)

- In the hold-relax procedure, the range-limiting muscle is first lengthened to the point of limitation or to the extent that is comfortable for the patient. The patient then performs a *prestretch, end-range, isometric contraction* (up to 10 seconds) followed by voluntary relaxation of the tight muscle.[20,35,61,101,114] Then the limb is passively moved into the new range as the range-limiting muscle is elongated. The rationale behind this technique is that after the isometric contraction there is a brief period during which the muscle is reflexively relaxed and, therefore, can be more easily stretched. Because the source of this inhibition may be from the GTO, it is often referred to as *autogenic inhibition.*[101] Postisometric contraction relaxation is also used in *muscle energy techniques* to mobilize joints by overcoming restrictive barriers to specific joint motions.[17,50,56,88,92]

Precaution: Because blood pressure may elevate during the prestretch isometric contraction,[22] it is always advisable to have the patient exhale while performing a *submaximal* isometric contraction.

- Although some investigators and clinicians use the term *contract-relax* (CR) synonymously with hold-relax (HR), the techniques are, in fact, slightly different. In classical PNF, the contract-relax technique is performed in diagonal patterns, and during the prestretch contraction of the restricting muscles, the rotators of the limb contract concentrically while all other muscle groups contract isometrically.[116] In the hold-relax technique, the prestretch contraction is isometric in all muscles of the pattern.
- In the clinical and athletic training settings, practitioners have reported that both techniques (HR and CR) appear to make passive elongation of muscle more comfortable for the patient than do manual passive stretching procedures.[4,61] Practitioners have assumed that the prestretch contraction causes a reflexive relaxation accompanied by a decrease in electromyographic (EMG) activity in the range-limiting muscle. Some investigators[21,34] have refuted this assumption, whereas others have supported it. In one study,[34] a postcontraction sensory discharge (increased EMG activity) was identified in the muscle to be lengthened. This indicated that the muscle to be stretched was not effectively relaxed. In another study, no post-

contraction elevation in EMG activity was found with the use of the contract-relax technique.[21] Obviously clinicians must evaluate the effectiveness of the hold-relax and contract-relax techniques and determine their usefulness with individual patients.

Agonist Contraction (AC)

- Another neuromuscular inhibition technique used to stretch muscles is agonist contraction (AC). This term has been used by several authors but can be misunderstood. The "agonist" refers to the muscle *opposite* the range-limiting muscle. "Antagonist," therefore, refers to the range-limiting muscle.[19] Think of it as the short muscle (the antagonist) preventing the full movement of the prime mover (the agonist).
- During this procedure the patient *concentrically contracts (shortens) the muscle opposite the range-limiting muscle.*[21,38,61] The motion of the limb is completely controlled by the patient. It is deliberate and slow, not ballistic. The shortening contraction either can be performed against a very low level of resistance or actively against no resistance. This causes a *reciprocal inhibition*[101,114,127] of the antagonist, the range-limiting muscle. Consequently, the tight muscle lengthens more easily and ROM increases.
- The terms **dynamic range of motion** (DROM) and **active stretching** are also used to describe the use of an agonist contraction to lengthen a muscle and increase ROM. It has been suggested in the chiropractic literature[95] that DROM is a more effective method to increase ROM than static stretching. Two studies have compared these techniques to stretch the hamstring muscles of healthy subjects who participated in 6-week stretching programs. DROM was found to be as effective as static stretch in one study[131] but far less effective in the other study.[7] In fact, in the latter study it was reported that a 30-second static stretch was almost three times as effective as DROM in increasing hamstring muscle flexibility.[7]
- During use of the AC procedure in clinical situations, therapists have observed that this technique of inhibition is especially effective in increasing ROM if the range-limiting muscle is painful and in the early stages of healing or if significant muscle guarding is restricting muscle lengthening, particularly in the midrange. This technique appears to be less effective if a patient has close to normal flexibility. This may be why in one of the previously discussed studies[7] comparing static stretching and dynamic range of motion, static stretch was far more effective for elongating muscles that exhibited only slight shortening.
- This technique is also useful for initiating neuromuscular control into the new ROM because the patient is actively using the agonist muscle in its newly gained range where it previously could not function because of hypomobility in the antagonist.

Hold-Relax with Agonist Contraction (HR-AC)

- A variation of the hold-relax technique is the use of a prestretch isometric contraction of the range-limiting muscle in a lengthened position, *followed* by a concentric contraction of the muscle *opposite* the range-limiting muscle.[21,38,101,114,127] As the agonist muscle "opposite the tight muscle" contracts, the hypomobile muscle is reciprocally inhibited, making lengthening easier. This technique combines *autogenic inhibition* and *reciprocal inhibition* to lengthen a muscle.
- In one study,[36] the HR-AC technique produced a greater increase in ankle dorsiflexion range than did the HR technique. Both inhibition techniques produced a greater increase in range of ankle dorsiflexion than did manual passive stretching. In another study, there was no significant difference between HR and HR-AC techniques.[61]

Integration of Function into a Stretching Program

Importance of Strength and Muscle Endurance

- As previously discussed, the strength of soft tissues is altered when they become hypomobile.[16,18,47,59] The magnitude of peak tension produced by muscle decreases, and the tensile strength of noncontractile tissues decreases. A muscle group that has been overstretched because its opposing muscle group has been in a shortened state for an extended period of time is also weakened.[71] Therefore, it is critical to begin low-load resistance exercises to improve muscular strength and endurance as early as possible in a mobility program.
- Initially, it is important to place emphasis on developing motor control and strength of the muscle group opposite the muscle that is being stretched. For example, if the elbow flexors are the range-limiting muscle group, emphasize

contraction of the elbow extensors in the gained range. Complement stretching the hamstrings to reduce a knee flexion contracture by using the quadriceps in the new range. Early use of the agonist enables the patient to actively elongate the hypomobile structures and use the recently gained ROM.

- As ROM approaches a "normal" or functional level, the muscles that were shortened and then stretched must also be strengthened to maintain an appropriate balance of strength between agonists and antagonist throughout the ROM.
- Manual and mechanical resistance exercises are certainly effective ways to load and strengthen muscles, but functional weight-bearing activities, such as those mentioned below also strengthen antigravity muscle groups.

Use of Mobility for Functional Activities

- The most effective means of achieving *permanent* increases in ROM is to integrate functional activities into the stretching program to use the gained range. Active movements should be within the pain-free ROM. Functional movements for the upper or lower extremities or spine could involve reaching, grasping, turning, twisting, bending, pushing, pulling, and squatting. As soon as even small increases in tissue extensibility and ROM have been achieved, have the patient use the gained range by performing motions that *simulate* functional activities. Later have the patient use all of the available ROM when actually doing specific functional activities.
- Functional activities that are emphasized should specifically complement the stretching program. For example, if a patient has been performing stretching exercises to increase shoulder mobility, have the patient fully use the available ROM by reaching as far as possible behind the back and overhead when washing or dressing. Have the patient reach for or place objects on a high shelf in the kitchen. Gradually increase the weight of objects placed or removed from the shelf to simultaneously strengthen shoulder musculature.

  If the focus of a stretching program has been to increase knee flexion after removal of a long-leg cast, emphasize flexing both knees as far as possible before standing up from a chair. The motion of rising from the chair will also strengthen the quadriceps that became weak while immobilized in a shortened position.
- Use of functional activities to maintain mobility lends diversity and interest to a stretching program, and it is the most effective way to minimize functional limitations.

▶ Guidelines for Applications of Stretching Procedures

Examination and Evaluation of the Patient Prior to Stretching

1. Carefully review the patient's history and perform a thorough systems review.
2. Select and perform appropriate tests and measurements. Determine the ROM available in involved and adjacent joints, and if either active or passive mobility is impaired.
3. Determine if hypomobility is related to pain, injury, functional limitations, or disabilities.
4. Determine if, and if so, which soft tissues are the source of the impaired mobility. In particular differentiate between joint capsule, periarticular noncontractile tissue, and muscle length restrictions as the cause of limited ROM. Be sure to assess joint play and fascial mobility.
5. Assess the irritability of the involved tissues and determine their stage of healing. When moving the patient's extremities or spine, pay close attention to the patient's reaction to movements. This not only helps identify the stage of healing of involved tissues, it also helps determine the probable dosage (such as intensity and duration) of stretch that stays within the patient's comfort range.
6. Assess the underlying strength of muscles in which there is limitation of motion and realistically consider the value of stretching the range-limiting structures. The individual must have the capability of developing adequate strength to control and safely use the new ROM.
7. Be sure to determine what outcome goals (i.e., functional improvements) the patient is seeking to achieve as the result of the intervention program, and determine if those goals are realistic.
8. Analyze the impact of any factors that could adversely affect the projected outcomes of the stretching program.

Prior to the Initiation of Stretching

1. Review the goals and desired outcomes of the stretching program with the patient. Obtain the patient's consent to initiate treatment.
2. Select the stretching techniques that will be most effective and efficient. Consider manual stretching, self-stretching, or the use of equipment for mechanical stretching.
3. Warm up the soft tissues to be stretched either by the application of local heat or by active, low-intensity exercises. Warming up tight structures increases their extensibility and decreases the possibility of injury.
4. Position the patient in a comfortable and stable position that will allow the best plane of motion in which the stretching procedure can be done. The direction of stretch will be exactly opposite the direction of the joint or muscle restriction.
5. Explain the procedure to the patient, and be certain he or she understands.
6. Free the area to be stretched of any restrictive clothing, bandages, or splints.
7. Explain to the patient that it is important to be as relaxed as possible or assist when requested and that the stretching procedures will be geared to his or her tolerance level.

When Applying Manual Stretching Procedures

1. Move the extremity slowly through the free range to the point of tissue restriction.
2. Then grasp proximally and distally to the joint in which motion is to occur. The grasp should be firm but not uncomfortable to the patient. Use padding, if necessary, in areas with minimal subcutaneous tissue, over a bony surface, or with reduced sensitivity. Use the broad surfaces of the hands to apply all forces.
3. Firmly stabilize the proximal segment (manually or with equipment) and move the distal segment.
   - To stretch a multijoint muscle, stabilize either the proximal or distal segment to which the range-limiting muscle attaches.
   - Stretch the muscle over one joint at a time, then over all joints simultaneously until optimal length of soft tissues is achieved.
   - To minimize compressive forces in small joints, stretch the distal joints first and proceed proximally.
4. Incorporate a prestretch, isometric contraction of the range-limiting muscle to reflexively inhibit the muscle prior to stretching it.
5. To avoid joint compression during the stretching procedure, apply gentle (grade I) traction to the moving joint.
6. Apply the stretch force in a low-intensity, slow, and sustained manner. Remember, the direction of the stretching movement is directly opposite the line of pull of the range-limiting muscle. Ask the patient to assist you with the stretch or apply a passive stretch to lengthen the tissues. Take the hypomobile soft tissues to the point of restriction and then move just beyond. The force must be enough to place tension on the soft tissue structures, but not so great as to cause pain or injure the structures. The patient should experience a pulling sensation within the structures being stretched but not pain. When stretching adhesions of a tendon within its sheath, the patient may experience a "stinging" sensation.
7. Hold the patient in the stretched position for 30 to 60 seconds.
   - During this time, the tension in the tissues should slowly decrease.
   - When tension decreases, move the extremity or joint a little farther to progressively lengthen hypomobile tissues.
8. Gradually release the stretch force.
9. Use several very slow and gentle, intermittent stretches with the muscle in a lengthened position if the patient does not seem to tolerate a sustained stretch.
10. If deemed appropriate, apply selected soft tissue mobilization procedures, such as fascial massage or cross-fiber friction massage, at or near the sites of adhesions during the stretching maneuver.
11. Allow the patient and therapist to rest momentarily while maintaining the range-limiting tissues in a comfortably elongated position, and then repeat the sequence several times.

Note: Do not attempt to gain full range in one or two treatment sessions. Resolving mobility impairments is a slow and gradual process. It may take several weeks of treatment to see significant results.

Special Considerations for Teaching Self-Stretching Exercises

1. Be sure to carefully teach the patient all elements of self-stretching procedures, including appropriate intensity, duration, and frequency of stretching. Since many self-stretching exercises are performed by using a portion of body weight as the stretch force (by moving the body over a fixed distal segment), emphasize the importance of performing a slow and sustained stretch, not a ballistic stretch that creates momentum and may lengthen but can potentially injure hypomobile soft tissues.
2. Make sure that the patient is taught to carry out stretching exercises on a firm and stable but comfortable surface to maintain proper alignment.
3. Supervise the patient and make suggestions or corrections to make sure the patient performs self-stretches using safe biomechanics that protect joints and ligaments especially at the end of the ROM. Pay particular attention to maintaining postural alignment and effective stabilization. For example, if the patient is self-stretching the hamstrings in a long-sitting position or while standing with one leg resting on a table, be sure that the patient knows to keep the thoracolumbar segments of the spine in extension and to bend forward at the hips to prevent a posterior pelvic tilt and an overstretch of the low back.
4. Emphasize the importance of warming up the tissues with gentle rhythmic activities, such as cycling, prior to stretching. Stretching should not be the first activity in an exercise routine because cold tissue is more brittle and more easily torn.
5. If appropriate and possible, teach the patient how to independently incorporate neuromuscular inhibition into specific stretching exercises.
6. Provide written instructions with illustrations that the patient can refer to when performing the self-stretching exercises.
7. Demonstrate how items commonly found around the house, such as a towel, belt, a broomstick, or a homemade weight, can be used to assist with stretching activities.
8. Emphasize the importance of using the gained ROM during appropriately progressed functional activities.

Note: Specific self-stretching exercises are not described or illustrated in this chapter. Illustrations and explanations for many self-stretching exercises can be found in Chapters 9 through 14 for the extremities and Chapters 15 and 16 for the spine.

Special Considerations for Use of Mechanical Stretching Devices

1. Become thoroughly familiar with a manufacturer's product information.
2. Become familiar with stretching protocols recommended by the manufacturer; seek out research studies that provide evidence of the efficacy of the equipment or protocols. Determine if modifications of a suggested protocol are warranted to meet your patient's needs. For example, should the suggested intensity of stretch or recommended wearing time (duration and frequency) be modified?
3. Check the fit of the equipment before sending it home with the patient.
4. Teach the patient how to apply and safely adjust the equipment.
5. Teach the patient how to maintain the equipment in good working order. Be sure that the patient knows whom to contact if equipment appears to be defective.
6. Teach the patient where and how to inspect skin for areas of excessive pressure and potential irritation to skin.
7. If the mechanical stretching device is "homemade," such as a cuff weight, check to see if the equipment is safe and effective.
8. Have the patient keep a daily record of use of the stretching device.
9. Re-examine and re-evaluate the patient and equipment periodically to determine the effectiveness of the mechanical stretching program.
10. Be sure the patient complements the use of mechanical stretching with active exercises.

After Stretching

1. Apply cold to the soft tissues that have been stretched and allow these structures to cool in a

lengthened position. This may minimize post-stretch muscle soreness that can occur as the result of microtrauma during stretching. When soft tissues are cooled in a lengthened position, increases in ROM are more readily maintained.[77,107]

2. Have the patient perform active ROM and strengthening exercises through the gained range immediately after stretching.
3. With your supervision and feedback have the patient use the gained range by performing simulated functional movement patterns that are part of daily living, occupational or recreational tasks.
4. Develop a balance in strength in the antagonistic muscles in the new range so that there is control and stability as flexibility increases.

Application of Inhibition and Relaxation Procedures

Inhibition as well as methods of general and local relaxation can enhance the effectiveness of stretching. The background and rationale for the use of neuromuscular inhibition techniques to reflexively relax the contractile components of shortened muscles have already been discussed in this chapter. The procedures for application of neuromuscular inhibition (active stretching, facilitated stretching) procedures follow.

Relaxation training, using methods of general relaxation (total body relaxation), has been used for many years by a variety of practitioners[39,65,108,135] to help patients learn to relieve or reduce pain, muscle tension, anxiety or stress, and associated physical impairments including tension headaches, high blood pressure, and respiratory distress. Volumes have been written by health professionals from many disciplines on topics such as chronic pain management, progressive relaxation, stress and anxiety management, and imagery. Hertling and Jones[57] provide an extensive listing of references on relaxation training in a recent publication. Therapists managing patients with impairments including chronic pain, muscle guarding or imbalances, and restricted mobility may find it useful to integrate general relaxation procedures into an intervention program to improve mobility. General elements of relaxation training and a sequence of progressive relaxation activities are outlined in this section. Furthermore, the use of other interventions, specifically superficial and deep heat, massage, biofeedback, and joint traction, which promote local muscle relaxation and serve as adjuncts to stretching, are briefly described to highlight their potential use.

Neuromuscular Inhibition Techniques: Procedures for Application

Hold-Relax (HR)

- ***Procedure***

1. Start with the range-limiting muscle in a comfortably lengthened position.
2. Ask the patient to isometrically contract the tight muscle against substantial resistance for up to 10 seconds until the muscle begins to fatigue.
3. Then have the patient voluntarily relax.
4. The therapist then lengthens the muscle by passively moving the extremity through the gained range.
5. Repeat the entire procedure after several seconds of rest. Have the patient rest with the muscle in a comfortably lengthened position.

- ***Precautions***

1. The isometric contraction of the range-limiting muscle should not be painful.
2. It is not necessary for the patient to perform a maximal isometric contraction of the tight muscle prior to stretch. A *submaximal* isometric contraction held for a longer period will adequately inhibit the range-limiting muscle. Postcontraction sensory discharge (lingering tension in muscle after the prestretch contraction) may be a greater problem if a maximum contraction is performed. A submaximal long-duration contraction will also be easier for the therapist to control if the patient is strong.
3. Multiple repetitions of prestretch isometric contractions can lead to an acute increase in arterial blood pressure, most notably after the third repetition.[22] It may be possible to lessen the elevation in blood pressure by using low-intensity isometric contractions and by making sure the patient breathes regularly during this procedure to minimize the effects of the Valsalva maneuver.

- ***Example.*** Shortened ankle plantarflexors

1. Dorsiflex the ankle to a comfortable position to lengthen the range-limiting muscles.
2. Place your hand on the plantar surface of the patient's foot.

3. Have the patient isometrically contract the plantarflexors against your resistance for 5 to 10 seconds.
4. Tell the patient to relax; then passively dorsiflex the patient's ankle to lengthen the plantarflexors.

Hold-Relax with Agonist Contraction (HR-AC)

- ***Procedure***

1. Follow the same procedure as done for hold-relax.
2. After the patient contracts the range-limiting muscle, have the patient perform a concentric contraction of the agonist, the muscle opposite the tight muscle. The patient actively moves the extremity through the increased range.

- ***Precautions.*** Same as for hold-relax.
- ***Example.*** Shortened ankle plantarflexors.

1. Follow the procedures described in hold-relax.
2. After the patient isometrically contracts the plantarflexors, have the patient actively dorsiflex the foot to elongate the plantarflexors.

Agonist Contraction (AC)

- ***Procedure***

1. Passively lengthen the range-limiting muscle to a comfortable position.
2. Have the patient perform a concentric (shortening) contraction of the agonist, the muscle opposite the tight muscle.
3. Apply mild resistance to the contracting muscle, but allow joint movement to occur.
4. The range-limiting muscle will relax and lengthen as the result of reciprocal inhibition as joint movement occurs.

- ***Precautions***

1. Do not apply excessive resistance to the contracting muscle. This may cause irradiation of tension to the hypomobile muscle rather than relaxation and may restrict movement of the joint or cause pain.
2. Remember: This procedure is often used when muscle spasm restricts joint movement. This type of inhibition is very useful if a patient cannot generate a strong, pain-free contraction of the range-limiting muscle, which must be done in the HR procedure. The AC technique is least effective if the patient has already achieved nearly full ROM.

- ***Example.*** Painful and shortened ankle plantarflexors

1. Place the patient's ankle in a comfortable position.
2. Apply low-intensity resistance to the dorsum of the foot as the patient dynamically contracts the dorsiflexors. As joint movement (increased dorsiflexion) occurs, the plantarflexors will relax and elongate.

General Relaxation Training

Common Elements of Relaxation Training

- *Conscious* relaxation of the entire body or the region that is painful or restricted. Tension in muscles can be reduced by conscious effort and thought.
- Deep breathing exercises or visualizing a peaceful scene.
- Quiet environment with low lighting and soothing music or an auditory cue upon which to focus.
- Soft tone of voice by the therapist for instructions.

Examples of Approaches to Relaxation Training

- *Autogenic training* advocated by Schultz[57,108] involves conscious relaxation through autosuggestion and a progression of exercises as well as meditation.
- *Progressive relaxation* developed by Jacobson[57,63] involves a systematic distal to proximal progression of voluntary contraction and relaxation of muscles. This technique is sometimes incorporated into natural childbirth.
- *Awareness through movement,* the Feldenkrais system of therapy,[39] combines sensory awareness, movements of the limbs and trunk, deep breathing, conscious relaxation procedures, and self-massage to alter muscle imbalances and abnormal postural alignment to remediate muscle tension and pain.

Procedure for Progressive Relaxation Training

1. Place the patient in a quiet area and in a comfortable position, and be sure that restrictive clothing is loosened.
2. Have the patient breathe in a deep, relaxed manner.
3. Ask the patient to voluntarily contract the distal musculature in the hands or feet for a few seconds; then have the patient consciously relax those muscles.

4. Suggest that the patient try to feel a sense of heaviness in the hands or feet.
5. Suggest to the patient that he or she feels a sense of warmth in the muscles just relaxed.
6. Progress to a more proximal area of the body and have the patient actively contract and then actively relax the more proximal musculature. Eventually have the patient isometrically contract and then consciously relax the entire extremity.
7. Suggest to the patient that he or she should feel a sense of relaxation and warmth throughout the entire limb and eventually throughout the whole body.

Additional Adjuncts to Stretching Interventions for Local Relaxation

Heat

Warming up soft tissue prior to stretching increases the extensibility of the shortened tissue. Warm muscles relax and lengthen more easily, making stretching more comfortable for the patient. As the temperature of muscle increases, the amount of force required to elongate noncontractile and contractile tissues and the time the stretch force must be applied decrease. As intramuscular temperature increases, connective tissue yields more easily to passive stretch.[33,76,79,105] There is also a decrease in the rate of firing of the type II efferents from the muscle spindles and an increase in the sensitivity of the GTO, which makes it more likely to fire.[41,76,104] Both of these responses inhibit muscle tension.[41,76,104] Heating may also decrease discomfort some patients experience during stretching, which, in turn, decreases muscle guarding and minimizes the chance of microtrauma to soft tissues and, therefore, may decrease postexercise, delayed-onset muscle soreness.[33,76,77,138]

Superficial or deep-heating modalities, such as hot packs, paraffin, or ultrasound, are used primarily to heat small areas such as individual joints or muscle groups. In most situations these modalities are applied prior to stretching but in some instances are applied concurrently with the stretching procedure.[33,105] Low-intensity, active exercise performed prior to stretching also increases circulation and core body temperature,[43,60,103,126] and is an effective way to increase the intramuscular temperature of a large number of muscle groups simultaneously. Some common warm-up exercises are a brief walk, nonfatiguing cycling on a stationary bicycle, or a few minutes of active arm exercises.[45,60,109]

Precaution: Although stretching is often thought of as a warm-up activity and performed prior to vigorous exercise, the clinician and patient must always remember that an appropriate warm-up must also occur in the preparation for stretching. It is debatable whether heating should occur prior to or during the stretching procedure.

The use of heat alone without stretching has been shown to have either little effect or no effect on long-term improvement in muscle flexibility.[54,112] Although a large body of knowledge indicates that a combination of heat and stretching produces greater long-term gains in tissue length than stretching without the application of prestretch heating,[76] the results of a few studies suggest that superficial heat prior to stretch does not have a *significant* impact on the outcomes of stretching programs in healthy individuals.[54,119]

Note: The application of cold prior to stretching (cryostretching) has been advocated to decrease muscle tone and make the muscle less sensitive during stretch in healthy subjects[49] and in patients with spasticity or rigidity secondary to upper motor neuron lesions.[127] The use of cold immediately after soft tissue injury effectively decreases pain and muscle spasm.[74,76,102] Once soft tissue healing and scar formation begin, cold makes healing tissues less extensible and more susceptible to microtrauma during stretching.[26,74,76,79] Cooling soft tissues in a lengthened position after stretching has also been shown to promote more lasting increases in soft tissue length and minimize poststretch muscle soreness.[77,107]

To summarize, it is the authors' recommendation that cold be applied to injured soft tissues in the first 24 to 48 hours after injury to minimize swelling, muscle spasm, and pain. Remember, stretching is contraindicated in the presence of inflammation that occurs during the acute phase of tissue healing (see Chapter 8). When inflammation subsides and when stretching is indicated, soft tissues should be heated prior to or during the stretching maneuver. After stretching, cold should be applied to soft tissues held in a lengthened position to minimize poststretch muscle soreness and to promote longer lasting gains in ROM.

Massage

Local muscle relaxation can be enhanced by massage, particularly with light or deep stroking techniques.[29,117] In some approaches to stress and anxiety or pain management, self-massage, using light stroking techniques (effleurage), is performed during the relaxation process.[39] In sports and conditioning programs[9,117] massage may be implemented for general relaxation purposes or to enhance recovery after strenuous physical activity, although the efficacy of the latter is not well documented.[122] Because massage has been shown to increase circulation to muscles and decrease muscle spasm, it is a useful adjunct to stretching exercises.

Another broad category of massage is soft tissue mobilization. Although soft tissue mobilization and manipulation techniques involve various forms of deep massage, the primary purpose of these massage techniques is not relaxation, but rather to increase mobility of adherent or shortened connective tissues including fascia, tendons, and ligaments.[16] There are many techniques and explanations as to their effects on connective tissues, including the mechanical effects of stress and strain. Stresses are applied long enough for creep and stress-relaxation of tissues to occur. In *myofascial massage*[16,50,83] stretch forces are applied across fascial planes or between muscle and septae. In *friction massage*[27,72,117] deep circular or cross-fiber massage is applied to break up adhesions or minimize rough surfaces between tendons and their synovial sheaths. Friction massage is also used to increase the mobility of scar tissue within muscle as it heals. Theoretically, it applies stresses to scar tissue as it matures to align collagen fibers along the lines of stress for normal mobility. These forms of connective-tissue massage as well as many other approaches and techniques of soft tissue mobilization are useful interventions for patients with restricted mobility.

Biofeedback

A patient, if properly trained, can monitor and reduce the amount of tension in a muscle through biofeedback.[57] Through visual or auditory feedback, a patient can begin to sense or feel what muscle relaxation is. Biofeedback is just one tool that can be useful in helping the patient learn and practice the process of relaxation. By reducing muscle tension, pain can be decreased and flexibility increased.

Joint Traction or Oscillation

Slight manual distraction of joint surfaces prior to or in conjunction with joint mobilization or stretching techniques can be used to inhibit joint pain and spasm of muscles around a joint (see Chapter 6).[38,58] Pendular motions of a joint use the weight of the limb to distract the joint surfaces and simultaneously oscillate and relax the limb. The joint may be further distracted by adding a 1- or 2-lb weight to the extremity, which will cause a stretch force on joint tissues.

▶ Precautions

General Precautions

1. Do not passively force a joint beyond its normal ROM. Remember, normal ROM varies among individuals.
2. Newly united fractures should be protected by stabilization between the fracture site and the joint in which the motion takes place.
3. Use extra caution in patients with known or suspected osteoporosis due to disease, prolonged bed rest, age, and prolonged use of steroids.
4. When treating elderly patients, be aware of age-related changes in flexibility.[2,3]
5. Avoid vigorous stretching of muscles and connective tissues that have been immobilized over a long time. Connective tissues (tendons and ligaments) lose their tensile strength after prolonged immobilization.
   - High-intensity short-duration stretching procedures tend to cause more trauma and resulting weakness of soft tissues than low-intensity long-duration stretch.
   - Strengthening exercises should be concurrently built into a stretching program as ROM increases so that a patient can develop an appropriate balance between flexibility and strength.[18]
6. Progress the dosage (intensity, duration, and frequency) of stretching exercises gradually to minimize soft tissue trauma and postexercise muscle soreness. If a patient experiences joint pain or muscle soreness lasting more than 24 hours after stretching, too much force has been used during stretching and an inflammatory response is occurring that will cause increased scar tissue for-

mation. Patients should experience no more residual discomfort than a transitory feeling of tenderness.

7. Avoid stretching edematous tissue, as it is more susceptible to injury than normal tissue. Continued irritation of edematous tissues usually causes increased pain and edema.
8. Avoid overstretching weak muscles, particularly those that support body structures in relation to gravity.

Special Precautions for Mass-Market Flexibility Programs

In an effort to develop and maintain a desired level of fitness, many people, young and old, participate in physical conditioning programs at home or in the community. Flexibility exercises (self-stretching) are an integral component of these programs. As a result, individuals frequently learn self-stretching procedures in fitness classes or from popular videos or television programs. Although much of the information in these resources is usually safe and accurate, there may be some errors and potential problems that are evident in flexibility programs designed for the mass market.

Common Errors and Potential Problems

- ***Nonselective or poorly balanced stretching activities.*** General flexibility programs may include stretching regions of the body that are already mobile, or even hypermobile, but may neglect regions that are tight from faulty posture or inactivity. For example, in the sedentary population, some degree of hypomobility tends to develop in the hip flexors, trunk flexors, shoulder extensors and internal rotators, and scapular protractors from sitting in a slumped posture. Yet many commercially available flexibility routines overemphasize exercises that stretch posterior muscle groups that already may be overstretched but fail to include exercises to stretch the tight anterior structures. Consequently, faulty postures may worsen rather than improve.
- ***Insufficient warm-up.*** Individuals involved in flexibility programs often fail to warm up prior to stretching.
- ***Ineffective stabilization.*** These programs often lack effective methods of self-stabilization. Therefore, an exercise may fail to stretch the intended tight structures and may transfer the stretch force to structures that are already mobile or even hypermobile.
- ***Use of ballistic stretching.*** Although a less common problem than in the past, some exercise routines still demonstrate some stretches using ballistic maneuvers. Because this form of stretching is not well controlled, it increases the likelihood of postexercise muscle soreness and significant injury to soft tissues.
- ***Excessive intensity.*** The phrase "*No pain, no gain*" is often used inappropriately as the guideline for intensity of stretch. An effective flexibility routine should be progressed gradually and should not cause pain or excessive stress to tissues.
- ***Abnormal biomechanics.*** Some popular stretching exercises do not respect the biomechanics of the region. For example, the "hurdler's" stretch is designed to unilaterally stretch the hamstrings of one lower extremity and the quadriceps of the opposite extremity, but imposes unsafe stresses on the medial capsule and ligaments of the flexed knee.
- ***Insufficient information about age-related differences.*** One flexibility program does not fit all age groups. As a result of the normal aging process, mobility of connective tissues diminishes.[2,3] Consequently, elderly individuals typically exhibit less flexibility than young adults. Even an adolescent after a growth spurt temporarily will exhibit restricted flexibility, particularly in two-joint muscle groups. Flexibility programs marketed to the general public usually are not sensitive to those normal, age-related differences in flexibility and may foster unrealistic expectations.

Strategies for Risk Reduction

- Whenever possible, assess the appropriateness and safety of exercises in a "prepackaged" flexibility program.

1. If a patient you are treating is participating in a community-based fitness class, review the exercises in the program and determine their appropriateness and safety for your patient.
2. Monitor the content and safety and your patient's use of home exercise videotapes.

3. Eliminate or modify those exercises that are inconsistent with the intervention plan you have developed for your patient.

- Teach your patient basic principles of self-stretching and how to apply those principles to select safe and appropriate stretching exercises and to avoid those that perpetuate impairments or have no value.
- Make sure your patient understands the importance of warming up prior to stretching. Give suggestions on how to warm up before stretching.
- Teach your patient how to determine the appropriate intensity of stretch; be sure your patient knows that at most postexercise muscle soreness should be mild and last no more than 24 hours.
- Be sure that the flexibility program maintains a balance of mobility between antagonistic muscle groups.
- See that the program emphasizes stretching those muscle groups that often become tight with age, faulty posture, or sedentary lifestyle.
- Be certain that the patient knows how to provide effective self-stabilization to isolate stretch to specific muscle groups.
- Determine whether or not a class or video is geared for individuals of the same age or with similar pathologic conditions.
- Stay up-to-date on current exercise programs, products, and trends.

▶ Manual Stretching Techniques Using Anatomic Planes of Motion

As with ROM exercises described in Chapter 2, the following techniques are described with the patient in a supine position. Alternate patient positions such as prone or seated are indicated for some motions and are noted when necessary. Manual stretching procedures in an aquatic environment are described in Chapter 7.

Effective manual stretching techniques require adequate stabilization of the patient and sufficient strength and good body mechanics of the therapist. Depending on the size (height and weight) of the therapist and the patient, modifications in the position of the patient and suggested hand placements for stretching or stabilization may have to be made by the therapist.

Each description of a stretching technique is identified by the anatomic plane of motion that is to be increased, followed by a notation of the muscle group being stretched. Although limitations in ROM, as the result of immobilization or injury to soft tissues, usually are caused by restriction of multiple muscle groups and periarticular structures and affect functional movement in combined as well as anatomic planes of motion, stretching multiple muscle groups simultaneously using diagonal patterns (i.e., D_1 and D_2 flexion and extension of the upper or lower extremities as described in Chapter 3) is not recommended, and, therefore, not described in this chapter. The authors believe that combined, diagonal patterns are appropriate for maintaining available ROM with passive and active exercises and increasing strength in multiple muscle groups, but are ineffective for *isolating* a stretch force to specific muscles or muscle groups of the extremities that are restricting functional movements. Special considerations for each region being stretched are also noted in this section.

Prolonged passive stretching techniques using mechanical equipment are applied using the same points of stabilization as manual stretching. The stretch force is applied at a lower intensity and is applied over a much longer period than with manual stretching. The stretch force is provided by weights or splints rather than the strength or endurance of a therapist. The patient is stabilized with belts, straps, or counterweights.

Self-stretching techniques of the extremities and spine, which the patient can do without assistance from the therapist, are not covered in this chapter. These techniques are found for each joint of the extremities in Chapters 9 through 14. Stretching procedures for the musculature of the cervical, thoracic, and lumbar spine are found in Chapter 16.

The Upper Extremity

The Shoulder: Special Considerations

Many muscles involved with shoulder motion attach to the scapula rather than the thorax. Therefore, when most muscles of the shoulder girdle are stretched, it is imperative to stabilize the scapula. Without scapular stabilization the stretch force will be transmitted to those muscles that normally stabilize the scapula during movement of the arm. This subjects these muscles to possible overstretching and disguises the true ROM of the glenohumeral joint.

Remember:

- When the scapula is stabilized and not allowed to abduct or upwardly rotate, only 120 degrees of shoulder flexion and abduction can occur at the glenohumeral joint.

- The humerus must be externally rotated to gain full ROM of abduction.
- Muscles most apt to become shortened are those that *prevent* full shoulder flexion, abduction, and external rotation. It is rare to find restrictions in structures that prevent shoulder adduction and extension to neutral.

Flexion of the Shoulder

To increase flexion of the shoulder (to stretch the shoulder extensors) (Fig. 5–13*A*):

Hand Placement and Procedures

- Grasp the posterior aspect of the distal humerus, just above the elbow.
- Stabilize the axilliary border of the scapula to stretch the teres major, or stabilize the lateral aspect of the thorax and superior aspect of the pelvis to stretch the latissimus dorsi.
- Move the patient's arm into full shoulder flexion to elongate the shoulder extensors.

Hyperextension of the Shoulder

To increase hyperextension of the shoulder (to stretch the shoulder flexors) (Fig. 5–13*B*):

Patient Position

Place the patient in a prone position.

Hand Placement and Procedure

- Support the forearm and grasp the distal humerus.
- Stabilize the posterior aspect of the scapula to prevent substitute movements.
- Move the patient's arm into full hyperextension of the shoulder to elongate the shoulder flexors.

Abduction of the Shoulder

To increase abduction of the shoulder (to stretch the adductors) (Fig. 5–14):

Hand Placement and Procedure

- With the elbow flexed to 90 degrees, grasp the distal humerus.
- Stabilize the axillary border of the scapula.
- Move the patient into full shoulder abduction to lengthen the adductors of the shoulder.

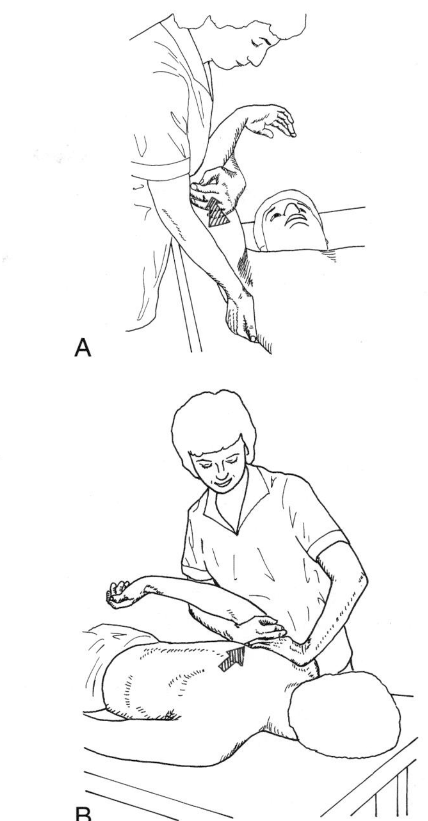

Figure 5–13 *(A)* Hand placement and stabilization of the scapula for stretching procedure to elongate the teres major. *(B)* Hand placement and stabilization of the scapula to increase hyperextension of the shoulder.

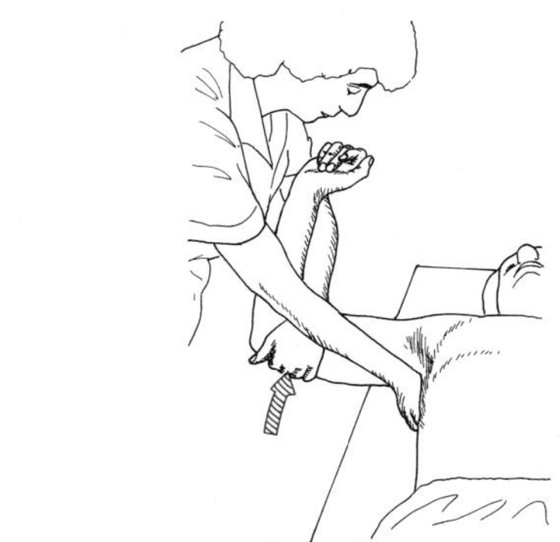

Figure 5–14 Hand placement and stabilization of the scapula for stretching procedure to increase shoulder abduction.

Adduction of the Shoulder

To increase adduction of the shoulder (to stretch the abductors): It is rare that a patient will not be able to fully adduct the shoulder to 0 degrees (so the upper arm is at the patient's side). Even if a patient has worn an abduction splint after a soft tissue or joint injury of the shoulder, when the patient is upright the constant pull of gravity will elongate the shoulder abductors so the patient can adduct to a neutral position.

External Rotation of the Shoulder

To increase external rotation of the shoulder (to stretch the internal rotators) (Fig. 5–15):

Hand Placement and Procedure

- Abduct the shoulder to a comfortable position (initially 30 or 45 degrees, and later to 90 degrees if the GH joint is stable), or place the arm at the patient's side.
- Flex the elbow to 90 degrees so that the forearm can be used as a lever.
- Grasp the volar surface of the mid-forearm with one hand.
- Stabilization of the scapula is provided by the table upon which the patient is lying.
- Externally rotate the patient's shoulder by moving the patient's forearm closer to the table. This will fully lengthen the internal rotators.

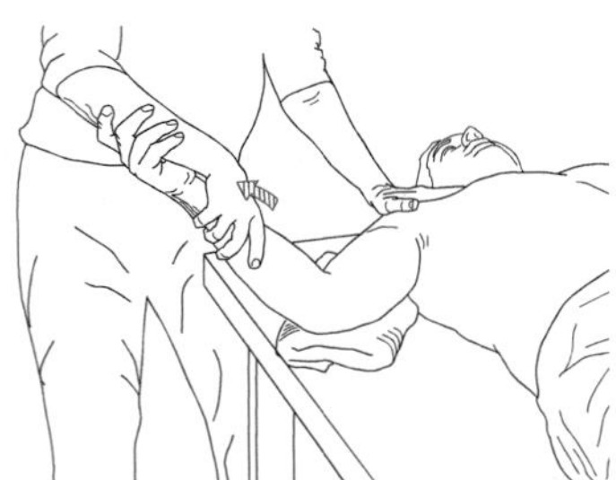

Figure 5-15 Shoulder position (slightly abducted and flexed) and hand placement at the mid to proximal forearm to increase external rotation of the shoulder. A folded towel is place under the distal humerus to maintain the shoulder in slight flexion. The table stabilizes the scapula.

Precaution: Since it is necessary to apply the stretch forces across the intermediate elbow joint when elongating the internal and external rotators of the shoulder, be sure the elbow joint is stable and pain-free. In addition, keep the intensity of the stretch force very low, particularly in patients with osteoporosis.

Internal Rotation of the Shoulder

To increase internal rotation of the shoulder (to stretch the external rotators) (Fig. 5–16):

Hand Placement and Procedure

- Abduct the shoulder to a comfortable position that will allow internal rotation to occur without the thorax blocking the motion (initially to 45 degrees and eventually to 90 degrees).
- Flex the elbow to 90 degrees so that the forearm can be used as a lever.
- Grasp the dorsal surface of the midforearm with one hand, and stabilize the anterior aspect of the shoulder and support the elbow with your other forearm and hand.
- Move the patient's arm into internal rotation to lengthen the external rotators of the shoulder.

Horizontal Abduction of the Shoulder

To increase horizontal abduction of the shoulder (to stretch the pectoralis muscles):

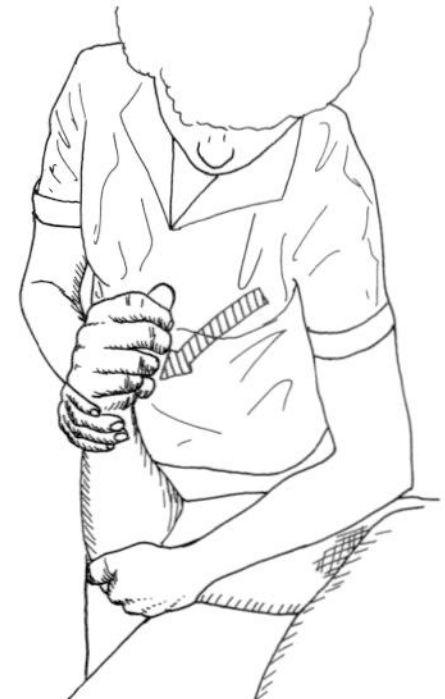

Figure 5–16 Hand placement and stabilization of the shoulder to increase internal rotation of the shoulder.

Patient Position

To reach full horizontal abduction in the supine position, the patient's shoulder must be at the edge of the table. As with passive ROM (see Fig. 2–5*A*), begin with the shoulder in 60 to 90 degrees of abduction. The patient's elbow may also be flexed.

Hand Placement and Procedure

- Grasp the anterior aspect of the distal humerus.
- Stabilize the anterior aspect of the shoulder.
- Move the patient's arm into full horizontal abduction to stretch the horizontal adductors.

Note: The horizontal adductors are usually tight bilaterally. Stretching techniques can be applied bilaterally by the therapist, or a bilateral self-stretch can be done by the patient by using a corner or wand (see Figs. 9–18 through 9–20).

Scapular Mobility

To have full shoulder motion, a patient must have normal scapular mobility. See scapular mobilization techniques in Chapter 6.

The Elbow and Forearm: Special Considerations

Several muscles that cross the elbow, such as the biceps brachii and brachioradialis, also influence supination and pronation of the forearm. Therefore, when stretching the elbow flexors and extensors, the techniques should be performed with the forearm pronated as well as supinated.

Elbow Flexion

To increase elbow flexion (to stretch the elbow extensors):

Hand Placement and Procedure

- Grasp the distal forearm just proximal to the wrist.
- Stabilize the humerus.
- Flex the patient's elbow just past the point of tissue resistance to lengthen the elbow extensors.

Elbow Extension

To increase elbow extension (to stretch the elbow flexors) (Fig. 5–17):

Hand Placement and Procedure

- Grasp the distal forearm.
- Stabilize the scapula and anterior aspect of the proximal humerus.

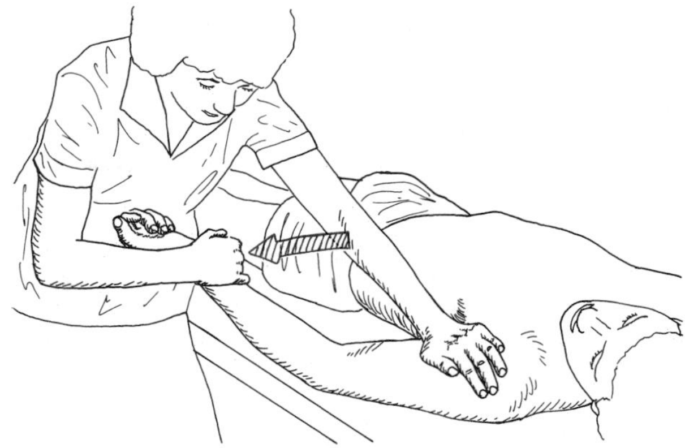

Figure 5–17 Hand placement and stabilization of the scapula and proximal humerus for stretching procedures to increase elbow extension.

- Extend the elbow just past the point of tissue resistance to lengthen the elbow flexors.

Note: Be sure to do this with the forearm in supination, pronation, and a neutral position to stretch each of the elbow flexors.

Precaution: Vigorous stretching of the elbow flexors may cause internal trauma to these muscles. This may precipitate myositis ossificans, especially in children. Passive stretching should be done gently, or the use of neuromuscular inhibition techniques should be considered to minimize tension in these muscles as they are elongated.

Supination or Pronation of the Forearm

To increase supination or pronation of the forearm:

Hand Placement and Procedure

- With the patient's humerus supported on the table and the elbow flexed to 90 degrees, grasp the distal forearm.
- Stabilize the humerus.
- Supinate or pronate the forearm just beyond the point of tissue resistance as indicated.
- Be sure the stretch force is applied to the radius rotating around the ulna. Do not twist the hand to avoid stress to the wrist articulations.
- Repeat the procedure with the elbow extended. Be sure to stabilize the humerus to prevent internal or external rotation of the shoulder.

The Wrist and Hand: Special Considerations

The extrinsic muscles of the fingers cross the wrist joint and, therefore, may influence the ROM of the wrist. Wrist motion may also be influenced by the position of the elbow and forearm because the wrist flexors and extensors attach proximally on the epicondyles of the humerus.

When stretching the musculature of the wrist, the stretch force should be applied proximal to the metacarpophalangeal (MCP) joints, and the fingers should be relaxed.

Patient Position

It may be easier to stabilize and stretch the patient's wrist and hand structures by having the patient sit in a chair adjacent to you with the forearm supported on a table, rather than lying supine.

Wrist Flexion

To increase wrist flexion:

Hand Placement and Procedure

- The forearm may be supinated, in midposition, or pronated.
- Stabilize the forearm against the table and grasp the dorsal aspect of the patient's hand.
- To elongate the wrist extensors, flex the patient's wrist and allow the fingers to extend passively.
- To further elongate the wrist extensors, extend the patient's elbow.

Wrist Extension

To increase wrist extension (Fig. 5–18):

Hand Placement and Procedure

- Pronate the forearm or place it in midposition, and grasp the patient at the palmar aspect of the hand. If there is a severe wrist flexion contracture, it may be necessary to place the patient's hand over the edge of the treatment table.
- Stabilize the forearm against the table.
- To lengthen the wrist flexors, extend the patient's wrist, allowing the fingers to passively flex.

Radial Deviation

To increase radial deviation:

Hand Placement and Procedure

- Grasp the ulnar aspect of the hand along the fifth metacarpal.
- Hold the wrist in midposition.

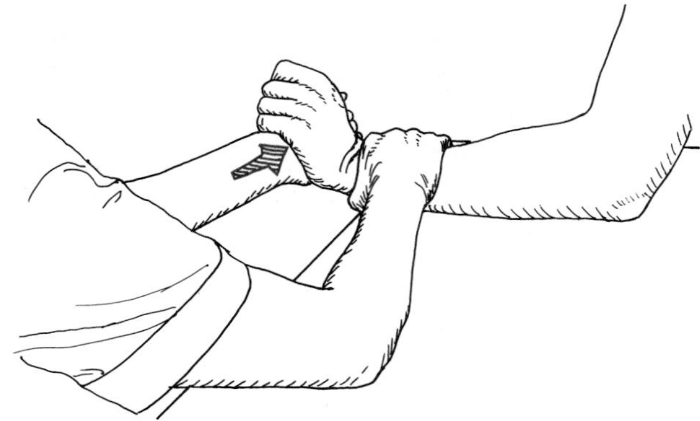

Figure 5–18 Hand placement and stabilization of the forearm for stretching procedure to increase extension of the wrist.

- Stabilize the forearm.
- Radially deviate the wrist to lengthen the ulnar deviators of the wrist.

Ulnar Deviation

To increase ulnar deviation:

Hand Placement and Procedure

- Grasp the radial aspect of the hand along the second metacarpal, not the thumb.
- Stabilize the forearm.
- Ulnarly deviate the wrist to lengthen the radial deviators.

The Digits: Special Considerations

The complexity of the relationships among the joint structures and intrinsic and multijoint extrinsic muscles of the digits requires careful examination and evaluation of the factors that contribute to loss of function in the hand because of limitation of motion. The therapist must determine if a limitation is from restriction of joints, decreased muscle flexibility, or adhesions of tendons or ligaments. Digits should always be stretched individually, not simultaneously. If an extrinsic muscle limits motion, lengthen it over one joint while stabilizing the other joints. Then hold the lengthened position and stretch it over the second joint, and so forth, until normal length is obtained. As noted in Chapter 2, begin the motion with the most distal joint to minimize shearing and compressive stresses to the surfaces of the small joints of the digits. Specific methods of intervention for dealing with adhesions of tendons are described in Chapter 11.

CMC Joint of the Thumb

To increase flexion, extension, abduction or adduction of the CMC joint of the thumb:

Hand Placement and Procedure

- Stabilize the trapezium with your thumb and index finger.
- Grasp the first metacarpal (not the first phalanx) with your other thumb and index finger.
- Move the first metacarpal in the desired direction to increase CMC flexion, extension, abduction and adduction.

MCP Joints of the Digits

To increase flexion, extension, abduction, or adduction of the MCP joints of the digits:

Hand Placement and Procedure

- Stabilize the metacarpal with your thumb and index finger.
- Grasp the proximal phalanx with your other thumb and index finger.
- Keep the wrist in midposition.
- Move the MCP joint in the desired direction for stretch.
- Allow the IP joints to passively flex or extend.

PIP and DIP Joints

To increase flexion or extension of the PIP and DIP joints:

Hand Placement and Procedure

- Grasp the middle or distal phalanx with your thumb and finger.
- Stabilize the proximal or middle phalanx with your other thumb and finger.
- Move the PIP or DIP joint in the desired direction for stretch.

Stretching Specific Extrinsic and Intrinsic Muscles of the Fingers

In Chapter 2 elongation of extrinsic and intrinsic muscles of the hand is described. To stretch these muscles beyond their available range, the same hand placement and stabilization are used as with passive ROM. The only difference in technique is that the therapist moves each segment into the stretch range.

The Lower Extremity

The Hip: Special Considerations

Because muscles of the hip attach to the pelvis or lumbar spine, the pelvis must always be stabilized when lengthening muscles about the hip. If the pelvis is not stabilized, the stretch force will be transferred to the lumbar spine, in which unwanted compensatory motion will occur.

Flexion of the Hip

To increase flexion of the hip with the knee flexed (to stretch the gluteus maximus):

Hand Placement and Procedure

- Flex the hip and knee simultaneously.
- Stabilize the opposite femur in extension to prevent a posterior tilt of the pelvis.
- Move the patient's hip and knee into full flexion to lengthen the one-joint hip extensor.

Flexion of the Hip with Knee Extension

To increase flexion of the hip with the knee extended (to stretch the hamstrings) (Fig. 5–19*A*):

Hand Placement and Procedure

- With the patient's knee fully extended, support the patient's lower leg with your arm or shoulder.
- Stabilize the opposite extremity along the anterior aspect of the thigh with your other hand or a belt or with the assistance of another person.
- With the knee at 0 degrees extension, and the hip in neutral rotation, flex the hip as far as possible.

Note: Externally rotate the hip prior to hip flexion to isolate the stretch force to the medial hamstrings and internally rotate the hip to isolate the stretch force to the lateral hamstrings.

Alternate Therapist Position (Fig. 5–19B)

Kneel on the mat and place the patient's heel or distal tibia against your shoulder. Place both of your hands along the anterior aspect of the distal thigh to keep the knee extended. The opposite extremity is stabilized in extension by a belt or towel and held in place by the therapist's knee.

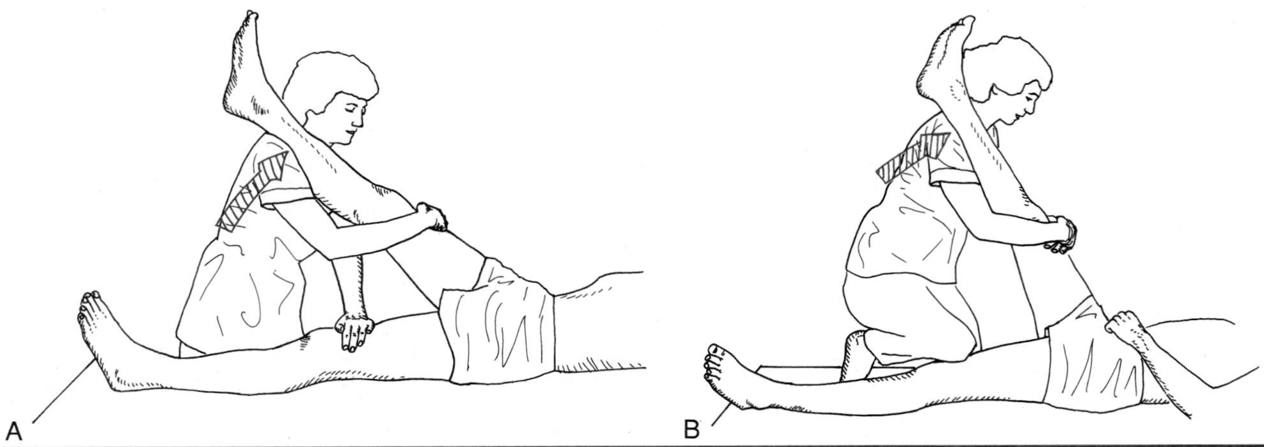

Figure 5–19 (*A* and *B*) Hand placement and stabilization of the pelvis and low back for stretching procedures to increase hip flexion with knee extension (stretch the hamstrings).

Extension of the Hip

To increase hip extension (to stretch the iliopsoas) (Fig. 5–20):

Patient Position

Have the patient close to the edge of the treatment table so that the hip being stretched can be extended beyond neutral. The opposite hip and knee are flexed toward the patient's chest to stabilize the pelvis and spine.

Hand Placement and Procedure

- Stabilize the opposite leg against the patient's chest with one hand, or if possible have the patient assist by grasping around the thigh and holding it to the chest to prevent an anterior tilt of the pelvis during stretching.
- Move the hip to be stretched into extension or hyperextension by placing a downward pressure on the anterior aspect of the distal thigh with your other hand. Allow the knee to extend so that the two-joint rectus femoris does not restrict the range.

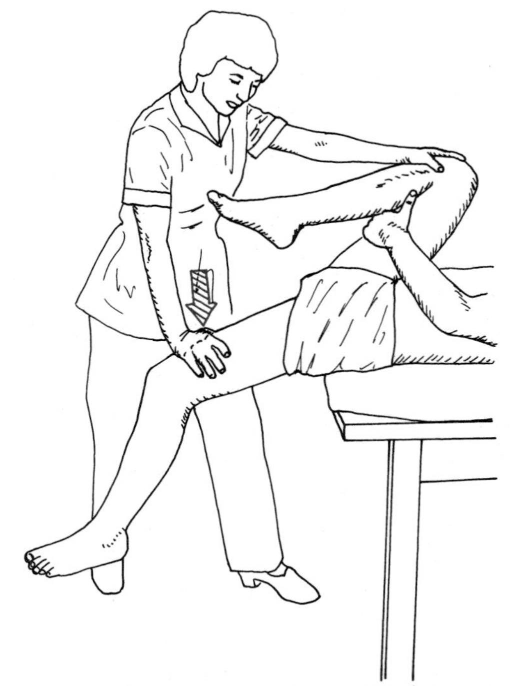

Figure 5–20 Hand placement and stabilization of the pelvis to increase hyperextension of the hip (stretch the iliopsoas) with the patient lying supine. Flexing the knee when in this position also elongates the rectus femoris.

Alternate Position
The patient can lie prone (Fig. 5–21).

Hand Placement and Procedure
- Support and grasp the anterior aspect of the patient's distal femur.
- Stabilize the patient's buttocks to prevent movement of the pelvis.
- Hyperextend the patient's hip by lifting the femur off the table.

Extension of the Hip with Knee Flexion

To increase hip extension and knee flexion simultaneously (to stretch the rectus femoris):

Patient Position
Use either of the positions previously described for increasing hip extension in the supine or prone positions (see Fig. 5–20).

Hand Placement and Procedure
- With the hip held in full extension on the side to be stretched, move your hand to the distal tibia and gently flex the knee of that extremity as far as possible.
- Do not allow the hip to abduct or rotate.

Abduction of the Hip

To increase abduction of the hip (to stretch the adductors) (Fig. 5–22):

Hand Placement and Procedure
- Support the distal thigh with your arm and forearm.
- Stabilize the pelvis by placing pressure on the opposite anterior iliac crest or by maintaining the opposite lower extremity in slight abduction.
- Abduct the hip as far as possible to stretch the adductors.

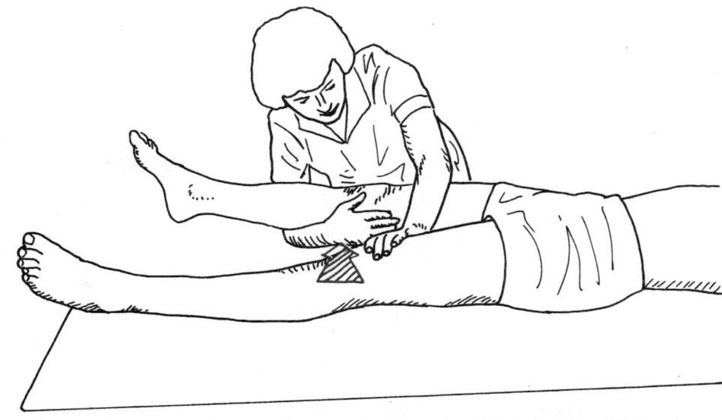

Figure 5–22 Hand placement and stabilization of the opposite extremity and pelvis for stretching procedure to increase abduction of the hip.

Note: You may apply your stretch force cautiously at the medial malleolus only if the knee is stable and pain-free. This creates a great deal of stress to the medial supporting structures of the knee and is generally not recommended by the authors.

Adduction of the Hip

To increase adduction of the hip (to stretch the tensor fasciae latae and IT band) (Fig. 5–23):

Patient Position
Place the patient in a side-lying position with the hip to be stretched uppermost. Flex the bottom hip and knee to stabilize the patient.

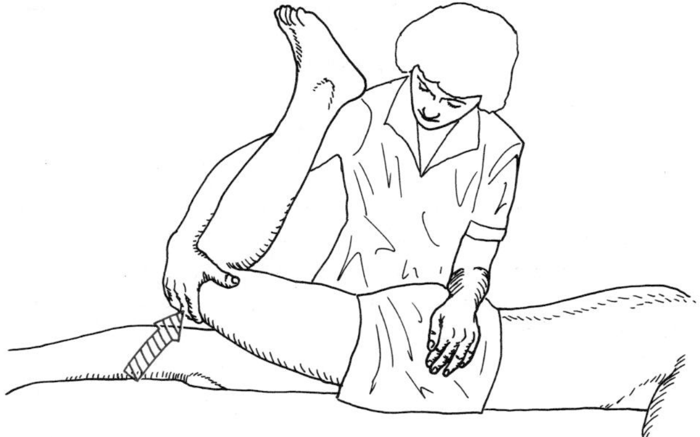

Figure 5–21 Hand placement and stabilization to increase hyperextension of the hip with the patient lying prone.

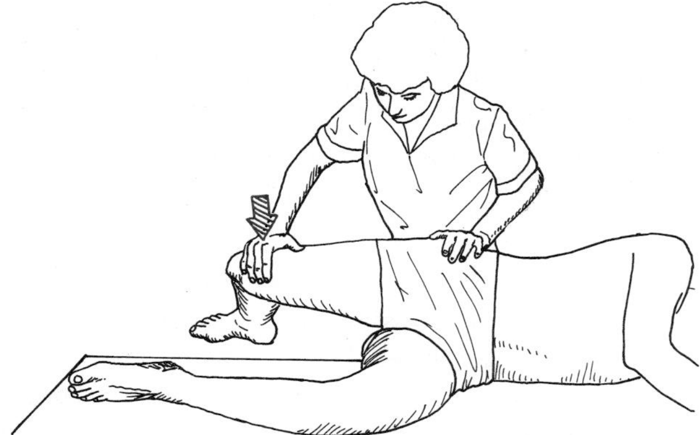

Figure 5–23 Patient positioned side-lying. Hand placement and procedure to stretch the tensor fasciae latae and IT band.

Hand Placement and Procedure

- Stabilize the pelvis at the iliac crest with your proximal hand.
- Flex the knee and extend the patient's hip to neutral or into slight hyperextension, if possible.
- Let the patient's hip adduct with gravity and apply an additional stretch force with your other hand to the lateral aspect of the distal femur to further adduct the hip.

Note: If the patient's hip cannot be extended to neutral, the hip flexors must be stretched before the tensor fasciae latae can be stretched.

External Rotation of the Hip

To increase external rotation of the hip (to stretch the internal rotators) (Fig. 5–24*A*):

Patient Position

Place the patient in a prone position, hips extended and knee flexed to 90 degrees.

Hand Placement and Procedure

- Grasp the distal tibia of the extremity to be stretched.
- Stabilize the pelvis by applying pressure with your other hand across the buttocks.
- Apply pressure to the lateral malleolus or lateral aspect of the tibia, and externally rotate the hip as far as possible.

Alternate Position

Sitting at the edge of a table with hips and knees flexed to 90 degrees

- Stabilize the pelvis by applying pressure to the iliac crest with one hand.
- Apply the stretch force to the lateral malleolus or lateral aspect of the lower leg, and externally rotate the hip.

Note: When you apply the stretch force against the lower leg in this manner, thus crossing the knee joint, the knee must be stable and pain free. If the knee is not stable, it is possible to apply the stretch force by grasping the distal thigh, but the leverage is poor and there is a tendency to twist the skin.

Internal Rotation of the Hip

To increase internal rotation of the hip (to stretch the external rotators) (Fig. 5–24*B*):

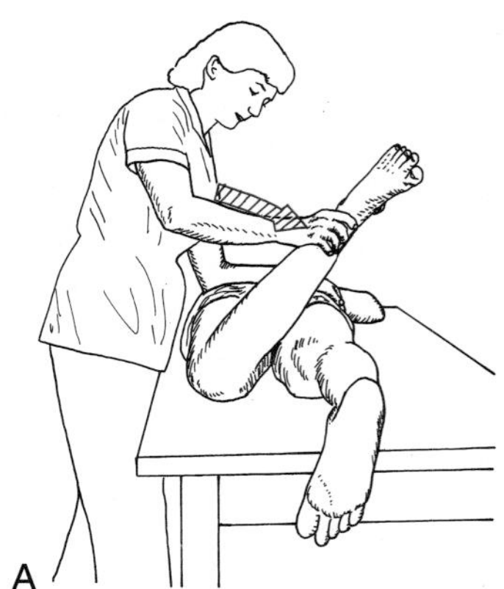

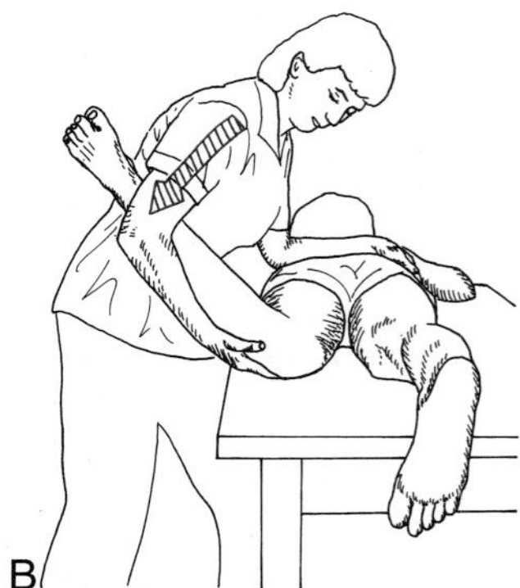

Figure 5–24 (*A* and *B*) Hand placement and stabilization to increase external and internal rotation of the hip with patient prone.

Patient Position and Stabilization
Same as when increasing external rotation, described previously.

Hand Placement and Procedure
Apply pressure to the medial malleolus or medial aspect of the tibia, and internally rotate the hip as far as possible.

The Knee: Special Considerations

The position of the hip during stretching influences the flexibility of the flexors and extensors of the knee. The flexibility of the hamstrings and the rectus femoris must be examined and evaluated separately from the one-joint muscles that affect knee motion.

Knee Flexion

To increase knee flexion (to stretch the knee extensors) (Fig. 5–25):

Patient Position
Have the patient assume a prone position.

Hand Placement and Procedure
- Stabilize the pelvis by applying a downward pressure across the buttocks.
- Grasp the anterior aspect of the distal tibia and flex the patient's knee.

Precaution: Place a rolled towel under the thigh just above the knee to prevent compression of the patella against the table during the stretch. Stretching the knee extensors too vigorously in the prone position can traumatize the knee joint and cause swelling.

Alternate Position and Procedure
- Have the patient sit with the thigh supported on the treatment table and leg flexed over the edge as far as possible.
- Stabilize the anterior aspect of the proximal femur with one hand.
- Apply the stretch force to the anterior aspect of the distal tibia and flex the patient's knee as far as possible.

Note: This position is useful when working in the 0- to 100-degree range of knee flexion. The prone position is best for increasing knee flexion from 90 to 135 degrees.

Knee Extension

To increase knee extension in the midrange (to stretch the knee flexors) (Fig. 5–26):

Patient Position
Place the patient in a prone position and put a small, rolled towel under the patient's distal femur, just above the patella.

Hand Placement and Procedure
- Grasp the distal tibia with one hand and stabilize the buttocks to prevent hip flexion with the other hand.
- Slowly extend the knee to stretch the knee flexors.

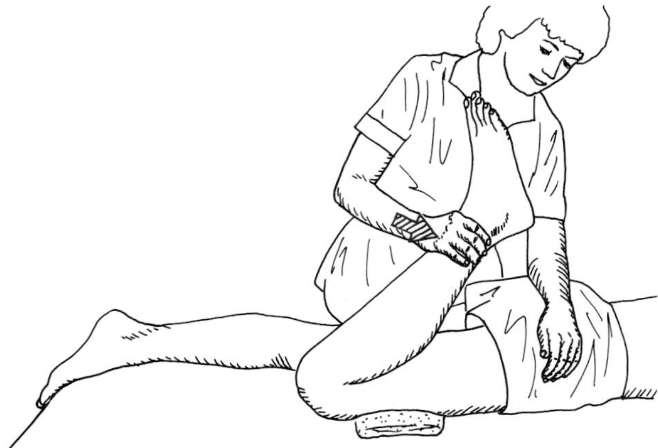

Figure 5–25 Hand placement and stabilization to increase knee flexion (stretch the rectus femoris and quadriceps) with the patient lying prone.

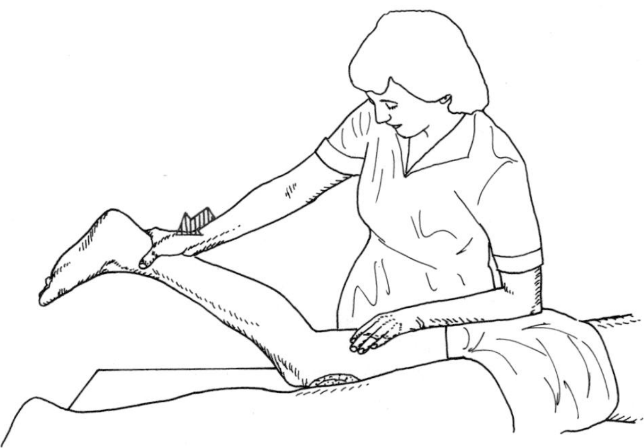

Figure 5–26 Hand placement and stabilization to increase midrange knee extension with the patient lying prone.

End-Range Knee Extension

To increase knee extension at the end of the range (Fig. 5–27):

Patient Position
Have the patient assume a supine position.

Hand Placement and Procedure
- Grasp the distal tibia of the knee to be stretched.
- Stabilize the hip by placing your hand or forearm across the anterior thigh. This will prevent hip flexion during stretching.
- Apply the stretch force to the posterior aspect of the distal tibia, and extend the patient's knee.

The Ankle and Foot: Special Considerations

The ankle and foot are composed of multiple joints. Consider the mobility of these joints (see Chapter 6) as well as the multijoint muscles that cross these joints when increasing ROM of the ankle and foot.

Dorsiflexion of the Ankle

To increase dorsiflexion of the ankle with the knee extended (to stretch the gastrocnemius muscle) (Fig. 5–28):

Hand Placement and Procedure
- Grasp the patient's heel (calcaneus) with one hand, maintain the subtalar joint in a neutral position, and place your forearm along the plantar surface of the foot.
- Stabilize the anterior aspect of the tibia with your other hand.

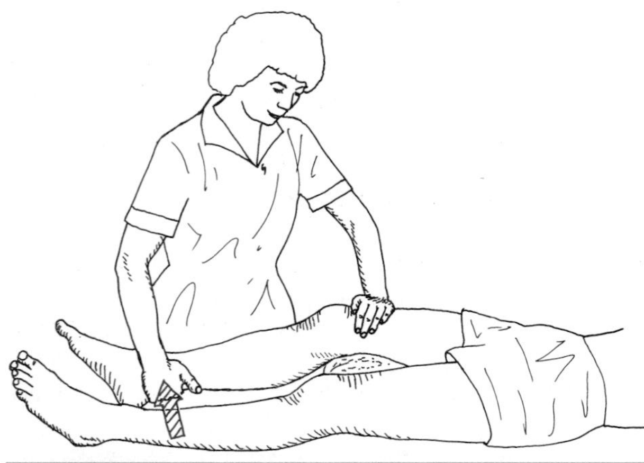

Figure 5–27 Hand placement and stabilization to increase knee extension at the end of the range.

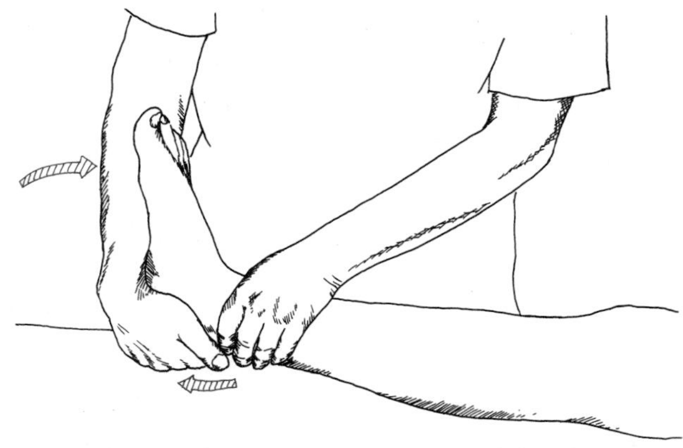

Figure 5–28 Hand placement and procedure to increase dorsiflexion of the ankle with the knee extended (stretch the gastrocnemius).

- Dorsiflex the talocrural joint of the ankle by pulling the calcaneus in an inferior direction with your thumb and fingers while gently applying pressure in a superior direction just proximal to the heads of the metatarsals with your forearm.

Dorsiflexion of the Ankle

To increase dorsiflexion of the ankle with the knee flexed (to stretch the soleus muscle): To eliminate the effect of the two-joint gastrocnemius muscle, the knee must be flexed. Hand placement, stabilization, and stretch force are the same as when stretching the gastrocnemius.

Precaution: When stretching the gastrocnemius or soleus muscles, avoid placing too much pressure against the heads of the metatarsals and stretching the long arch of the foot. Overstretching the long arch of the foot can cause a flat foot or a rocker-bottom foot.

Plantarflexion of the Ankle

To increase plantarflexion of the ankle:

Hand Placement and Procedure
- Support the posterior aspect of the distal tibia with one hand.
- Grasp the foot along the tarsal and metatarsal areas.
- Apply the stretch force to the anterior aspect of the foot, and plantarflex the foot as far as possible.

Inversion and Eversion of the Ankle

To increase inversion and eversion of the ankle: Inversion and eversion of the ankle occur at the subtalar joint as a component of pronation and supination. Mobility of the subtalar joint (with appropriate strength) is particularly important for walking on uneven surfaces.

Hand Placement and Procedure

- Stabilize the talus by grasping just distal to the malleoli with one hand.
- Grasp the calcaneus with your other hand, and move it medially and laterally at the subtalar joint.

Stretching Specific Muscles of the Ankle and Foot

Hand Placement and Procedure

- Stabilize the distal tibia with your proximal hand.
- Grasp around the foot with your other hand and align the motion and force opposite the line of pull of the tendons. Apply the stretch force against the bone to which the muscle attaches distally.
    - To stretch the tibialis anterior (which inverts and dorsiflexes the ankle): Grasp the dorsal aspect of the foot across the tarsals and metatarsals and plantarflex and evert the ankle.
    - To stretch the tibialis posterior (which plantarflexes and inverts the foot): Grasp the plantar surface of the foot around the tarsals and metatarsals and dorsiflex and evert the foot.
    - To stretch the peroneals (which evert the foot): Grasp the lateral aspect of the foot at the tarsals and metatarsals and invert the foot.

Flexion and Extension of the Toes

To increase flexion and extension of the toes: It is best to individually stretch any musculature that limits motion in the toes. With one hand, stabilize the bone proximal to the restricted joint, and with the other hand move the phalanx in the desired direction.

The Neck and Trunk

Stretching techniques to increase motion in the cervical, thoracic, and lumbar spine can be found in Chapter 16.

Self-Stretching Techniques

Examples of self-stretching techniques, performed independently by the patient after appropriate instruction, are found in Chapters 9 through 14 (upper and lower extremities) and Chapter 16 (neck and trunk).

Independent Learning Activities

CRITICAL THINKING AND DISCUSSION

1. What physical findings from an examination of a patient would lead you to decide that stretching exercises were an appropriate intervention?
2. Discuss the advantages and disadvantages of various stretching exercises, specifically manual stretching, self-stretching, and mechanical stretching. Under what circumstances would one form be a more appropriate choice than another?
3. Discuss how the effectiveness of a program of stretching activities is influenced by the responses of contractile and noncontractile soft tissues to stretch. Consider such factors as intensity, speed, duration, and frequency of stretch.
4. Discuss how your approach to and application of stretching would differ when developing stretching exercises for a healthy young adult with limited mobility in the (a) shoulder, (b) knee, or (c) ankle in contrast to an elderly individual with osteoporosis and limited motion in the same regions.
5. Explain the procedures for and rationale behind each of the following types of neuromuscular inhibition: HR, HR-AC, CR, and AC. Under what circumstances would you choose one technique over another?
6. Select a popular exercise videotape. Review and critique the flexibility exercises on the tape. Was there a balance in the flexibility exercises in the program? Were the exercises executed safely and correctly? Were the exercises appropriate for the target population?

LABORATORY PRACTICE

1. Manually stretch as many major muscle groups of the upper and lower extremities as is *safe* and *practical* with the patient in prone-lying, side-lying, or seated positions.
2. While considering individual muscle actions and lines of pull, demonstrate how to specifically and fully elongate the following muscles: pectoralis major, biceps brachii, brachioradialis, and brachialis, triceps, extensor or flexor carpi ulnaris

or radialis, flexor digitorum superficialis or profundus, rectus femoris versus the iliopsoas, gastrocnemius versus soleus, and the tibialis anterior and posterior.

3. Teach your partner how to stretch major muscle groups of the upper and lower extremities using either body weight or a cuff weight as the stretch force. Be sure to include effective stabilization procedures for these stretching techniques whenever possible.
4. Using either the hold-relax or contract-relax and the hold-relax agonist contraction neuromuscular inhibition techniques, elongate at least two major muscle groups at the shoulder, elbow, wrist, hip, knee, and ankle. Be sure to position, align, and stabilize your partner properly.
5. Design an effective and efficient series of self-stretching exercises that a person who works at a desk most of the day should incorporate into a daily home fitness routine. Demonstrate and teach each self-stretching exercise to your laboratory partner.
6. Identify a recreational/sport activity that your partner enjoys (i.e., tennis, golf, cycling, jogging, etc.) and design and demonstrate a program of self-stretching exercises to prepare your partner for the activity and reduce the risk of injury.
7. Design a program of progressive relaxation exercises for total body relaxation. Then implement the relaxation training sequence with your partner.

REFERENCES

1. American Physical Therapy Association: Guide to Physical Therapist Practice, ed 2. Phys Ther 81(1):1–768, 2001.
2. Amundsen, LR: The effect of aging and exercise on joint mobility. Orthop Phys Ther Clin North Am 2:241, 1993.
3. Amundsen, LR: Effects of age on joints and ligaments. In Kauffman, TL (ed): Geriatric Rehabilitation Manual. Churchill Livingstone, New York, 1999, pp. 14–16.
4. Arnheim, DD, and Prentice, WE: Principles of Athletic Training (ed 9), WCB/ McGraw-Hill, Boston, 1997.
5. Bandy, WB, and Irion, JM: The effects of time on static stretch on the flexibility of the hamstring muscles. Phys Ther 74:845–850, 1994.
6. Bandy, W, Irion, J, and Briggler, M: The effect of time and frequency of static stretch on flexibility of the hamstring muscle. Phys Ther 77:1090–1096, 1997.
7. Bandy, W, Irion, J, and Briggler, M: The effect of static stretch and dynamic range of motion training on the flexibility of the hamstring muscles. J Orthop Sports Phys Ther 27(4):295–300, 1998.
8. Beaulieu, JA: Developing a stretching program. The Physician and Sportsmedicine 9:59, 1981.
9. Benjamin, PJ, and Lamp, SP: Understanding Sports Massage. Human Kinetics, Champaign, IL, 1996.
10. Bohannon, RW: Effect of repeated eight minute muscle loading on the angle of straight leg raising. Phys Ther 64:491, 1984.
11. Bohannon, RW, and Larkin, PA: Passive ankle dorsiflexion increases in patients after a regimen of tilt table: Wedge board standing. Phys Ther 65:1676, 1985.
12. Bohannon, R, Tiberio, D, and Zito, M: Effect of 5 minutes of stretch on ankle dorsiflexion range of motion. J Phys Ther Sci 6:2–8, 1994.
13. Bonutti, PM, et al: Static progressive stretch to re-establish elbow range of motion. Clin Orthop Relat Res 303:128, 1994.
14. Booth, FW: Physiologic and biochemical effects of immobilization on muscle. Clin Orthop 219:5, 1987.
15. Brody, LT: Mobility impairment. In Hall, CM and Brody, LT: Therapeutic Exercise–Moving Toward Function. Lippincott Williams & Wilkins, Philadelphia, 1999, pp 87–111.
16. Cantu, RI, and Grodin, AJ: Myofascial Manipulation: Theory and Clinical Application. Aspen Publishers, Gaithersburg, MD, 1992.
17. Chaitow, L, and Liebenson, C: Muscle Energy Techniques; Churchill-Livingstone, New York 1996.
18. Chandler, JM: Understanding the relationship between strength and mobility in frail elder persons: A review of the literature. Topics Geriatr Rehab 11:20, 1996.
19. Cherry, D: Review of physical therapy alternatives for reducing muscle contracture. Phys Ther 60:877, 1980.
20. Clark, S, Christiansen A, Hellman DF, et al: Effects of ipsilateral anterior thigh soft tissue stretching on passive unilateral straight leg raise. J Orthop Sports Phys Ther 29(1):4–9, 1999.
21. Condon, SN, and Hutton, RS: Soleus muscle electromyographic activity and ankle dorsiflexion range of motion during four stretching procedures. Phys Ther 67:24, 1987.
22. Cornelius, WL, Jensen, RL, and Odell, ME: Effects of PNF stretching phases on acute arterial blood pressure. J Appl Physiol 20:222–229, 1995.
23. Cornwall, M: Biomechanics of non-contractile tissue: A review. Phys Ther 64:1869, 1984.
24. Culav, EM, Clark, CH, and Merrilees, MJ: Connective tissue matrix composition and its relevance to physical therapy. J Orthop Sports Phys Ther 79:308–319, 1999.
25. Cummings, GS, Crutchfeld, CA, and Barnes. MR: Soft Tissue Changes in Contractures, Vol 1. Stokesville, Atlanta, 1983.
26. Cummings, GS, and Tillman, LJ: Remodeling of dense connective tissue in normal adult tissues. In Currier, DP, and Nelson, RM (eds): Dynamics of Human Biologic Tissues. FA Davis, Philadelphia, 1992, p 45.
27. Cyriax, J: Textbook of Orthopedic Medicine: Treatment by Manipulation, ed 11. WB Saunders, Philadelphia, 1984.

28. DeDeyne, PG: Application of passive stretch and its implications for muscle fibers. Phys Ther 81(2):819–827, 2001.
29. De Domenico, G, and Wood, EC: Beard's Massage, ed 4: WB Saunders, Philadelphia, 1997.
30. Dennis, JK, and McKeough, DM: Mobility. In May, BJ (ed): Home Health and Rehabilitation: Concepts of Care. FA Davis, Philadelphia, 1999, pp 109–143.
31. de Vries, HA: Evaluation of static stretching procedures for improvement of flexibility. Res Quarterly 33:222–229, 1962.
32. Donatelli, R, and Owens-Burkhart. H: Effects of immobilization on the extensibility of periarticular connective tissue. J Orthop Sports Phys Ther 3:67, 1981.
33. Draper, DO, and Richard, MD: Rate of temperature decay in human muscle following 3MHz ultrasound: the stretching window revealed J Athletic Training 30:304–307, 1996.
34. Eldred, E, Hulton, RS, and Smith, JL: Nature of persisting changes in afferent discharge from muscle following its contraction. Prog Brain Res 44:157, 1976.
35. Elvey, RL: Treatment of arm pain associated with abnormal brachial plexus tension. Austral J Physiother 32:225–230, 1986.
36. Etnyre, BR, and Abraham, LD: Gains in range of ankle dorsiflexion using three popular stretching techniques. Am J Phys Med 65:189, 1986.
37. Euhardy, R: Contracture. In: Kauffman, TL(ed): Geriatric Rehabilitation Manual. Churchill-Livingstone, New York, 1999, pp 77–80.
38. Feland, JB, et al: The effect of duration of stretching of the hamstring muscle group for increasing range of motion in people aged 65 years or older. Phys Ther 81:1110, 2001.
39. Feldenkrais, M: Awareness Through Movement. Harper and Row, New York, 1985.
40. Flitney, FW, and Hirst, DG: Cross bridge detachment and sarcomere "give" during stretch of active frog's muscle. J Physiol 276:449, 1978.
41. Fukami, Y, and Wilkinson, RS: Responses of isolated golgi tendon organs of the cat. J Physiol 265:673–689, 1977.
42. Fung, YC: Biomechanics: Mechanical Properties of Living Tissue, ed 2. Springer-Verlag, New York, 1993.
43. Gajdosik, RL: Effects of static stretching on the maximal length and resistance to passive stretch of short hamstring muscles. J Orthop Sports Phys Ther 14(6):250–255, 1991.
44. Garrett, W, and Tridball, J: Myotendinous junction: structure, function and failure: In Woo, SL-Y, Buchwalter, JA (eds). Injury and Repair of the Musculoskeletal Soft Tissues, American Academy of Orthopedic Surgeons, Park Ridge, IL, 1988.
45. Gillette, TM, et al: Relationship of body core temperature and warm-up to knee range of motion. J Orthop Sports Phys Ther 13(3):126–131, 1991.
46. Godges, JJ, et al: The effects of two stretching procedures on hip range of motion and gait economy. J Orthop Sports Phys Ther 10(9):350–356, 1989.
47. Gossman, M, Sahrmann, S, and Rose, S: Review of length-associated changes in muscle. Phys Ther 62:1799, 1982.
48. Guyton, AC: Human Physiology and Mechanism of Disease (ed 5). WB Saunders, Philadelphia, 1992.
49. Halkovich, LR, et al; Effect of Fluori-Methane® spray on passive hip flexion. Phys Ther 61:185–189, 1981.
50. Hall, RC, and Nitz, AJ: Basic concepts of orthopedic manual therapy. In Malone, TR, McPoil, T, and Nitz, AJ (eds): Orthopedic and Sports Physical Therapy. (ed 3). Mosby-Year Book, Inc., St. Louis, 1997, pp 191–209.
51. Hansen, M: Pathophysiology: Foundations of Disease and Clinical Intervention. WB Saunders, Philadelphia, 1998.
52. Hanten, WP, and Chandler, SD: The effect of myofascial release leg pull and sagittal plane isometric contract-relax technique on passive straight-leg raise angle. J Orthop Sports Phys Ther 20:138–144, 1994.
53. Hardy, MA: The biology of scar formation. Phys Ther 69:1015, 1989.
54. Henricson, AS, et al: The effect of heat and stretching on range of hip motion. J Orthop Sports Phys Ther 6(2): 110–115, 1985.
55. Hepburn, G, and Crivelli, K: Use of elbow Dynasplint for reduction of elbow flexion contracture: A case study. J Orthop Sports Phys Ther 5:269, 1984.
56. Herbert, LA: Preventative stretching exercises for the workplace. Orthop Phys Ther Practice 11:11, 1999.
57. Hertling, D, and Jones, D: Relaxation and related techniques. In Hertling, D, and Kessler, RM: Management of Common Musculoskeletal Disorders, ed 3. Lippincott Raven Publications, Philadelphia, 1996, pp 140–162.
58. Hertling, D, and Kessler, RM: Introduction to manual therapy. In Hertling, D and Kessler, RM: Management of Common Musculoskeletal Disorders, ed 3. Lippincott, Philadelphia, 1996, pp 112–132.
59. Hlasney, J: Effect of flexibility exercises on muscle strength. Phys Ther Forum 7:3, 15, 1988.
60. Hubley, CL, Korzey, JW, and Stansih, WD: The effects of static stretching exercise and stationary cycling on range of motion at the hip joint. J Orthop Sports Phys Ther 6(2):104–109, 1984.
61. Hulton, RS: Nueromuscular basis of stretching exercise. In Komi, PV ed Strength and Power in Sports, Blackwell, Scientific Pub., Boston, 1992, pp 29–38.
62. Isernbagen, SJ: Industrial physical therapy. In Malone, TK, McPoil, T and Nitz, AJ (eds): Orthopedic and Sports Physical Therapy, ed 3. Mosby-Year Book Inc., St. Louis, 1997, pp 597–610.
63. Ito, CS: Conservative management of joint deformities and dynamic posturing. Orthop Phys Ther Clin North Am 2(1): 25–38, 1993.
64. Iyer, MB, Mitz, AR, and Winstein, C: Motor 1: Lower Centers. In Cohen, H: Neuroscience for Rehabilitation. Lippincott Williams & Wilkins, Philadelphia, 1999, pp 209–242.
65. Jacobson, E: Progressive Relaxation. University of Chicago Press, Chicago, 1929.
66. Jansen, CM, et al: Treatment of a knee contracture using a knee orthosis incorporating stress-relaxation techniques. Phys Ther 76(2):182–186, 1996.
67. Johnagen, S, Nemeth, G, and Grikkson, F: Hamstring injuries in sprinters: the role of concentric and eccentric muscle strength and flexibility. An J Sports Med 22:262–266, 1994.
68. Jokl P, and Konstadt, S: The effect of limb immobilization on muscle function and protein composition. Clin Orthop 174:222, 1983.
69. Kannus, P, et al: The effects of training, immobilization and remobilization on musculoskeletal tissue. I. Training and immobilization. Scand J Med Sci Sports 2:100–118, 1992.
70. Kannus, P, et al: The effects of training, immobilization and

remobilization on musculoskeletal tissue. II. Remobilization and prevention of immobilization atrophy. Scand J Med Sci Sports 2:164–176, 1992.

71. Kendall, F, McCreary, EK, and Provance, PG: Muscles, Testing and Function: With Posture and Pain, ed 4. Williams & Wilkins, Baltimore, MD, 1993.
72. Kessler, RM, and Hertling, D: Friction Massage. In Hertling, D, and Kessler, RM: Management of Common Musculoskeletal Disorders ed 3. Lippincott, Philadelphia, 1996, pp 133–140.
73. Kirch, RF, Weiss PL, Dannenbaum, RM, and Kearney, RE: Effect of maintained stretch on the range of motion of the human anklejoint. Clin Biomech 10:166–168, 1995.
74. Knight, KL: Cryotherapy: Theory, Technique and Physiology. Chattanooga Corp. Chattanooga, TN, 1989.
75. Kottke, FJ, Pauley, DL, and Park, KA: The rationale for prolonged stretching for correction of shortening of connective tissue. Arch Phys Med Rehabil 47:345, 1966.
76. Lehmann, JF, and DeLateur, BJ: Therapeutic heat. In Lehmann, JF (ed). Therapeutic Heat and Cold, ed 4, Williams & Wilkins, Baltimore, 1990.
77. Lentell, G, et al: The use of thermal agents to influence the effectiveness of a low-load prolonged stretch. J Orthop Sports Phys Ther 16(5):200–207, 1992.
78. Levangie, PK, and Norkin, CC: Joint Structure and Function: A Comprehensive Analysis, ed 3. FA Davis Philadelphia, 2001.
79. Leveau, B: Basic biomechanics in sports and orthopedic therapy. In Gould, J, and Davies, G (eds): Orthopedic and Sports Physical Therapy. CV Mosby, St Louis, 1985.
80. Lieber, RL, and Boodine-Fowler, SC: Skeletal muscle mechanisms: implications for rehabilitation. Phys Ther 73: 844–856, 1993.
81. Liebesman, JL, and Cafarelli, E: Physiology of range of motion in human joints: A critical review. Crit Rev Phys Rehabil Med 6:131–160, 1994.
82. Light, KE, et al: Low-load prolonged stretch vs. high-load brief stretch in treating knee contractures. Phys Ther 64:330, 1984.
83. Liston, C: Specialized systems of massage. In De Domenico, G and Wood, EC: Beard's Massage, ed 4. WB Saunders, Philadelphia, 1997, pp 163–171.
84. Lundy-Ekman, L: Neuroscience: Fundamentals for Rehabilitation. WB Saunders, Philadelphia, 1998.
85. Macefield, G, Hagbath, KE, Gorman, R, et al: Decline in spindle support to alphamotoneurons during sustained voluntary contractions. J Physiol 440:497–512, 1991.
86. MacKay-Lyons, M: Low-load prolonged stretch in treatment of elbow flexion contractures secondary to head trauma: a case report. Phys Ther 69:292–296, 1989.
87. Madding, SW, et al: Effect of duration of passive stretch on hip abduction range of motion. J Orthop Sports Phys Ther 8:409, 1987.
88. Maitland, GD: Vertebral Manipulation (ed 5). Butterworth, London, 1986.
89. McClure, M: Exercise and training for spinal patients. Part B: Flexibility training. In Basmajian, JV, and Nyberg, R (eds): Rational Manual Therapies. Williams & Wilkins, Baltimore, 1993, p 359.
90. McClure, PW, Blackburn, LG, and Dusold, C: The use of splints in the treatment of stiffness: Biologie ranoncle and an algorithm for making clinical decisions. Phys Ther 74: 1101–1107, 1994.
91. McHugh MP, Magnuson, SP, Gleim, GW, and Nicholas JA: Viscoelastic stress relaxation in human skeletal muscle. Med Sci Sports Exerc 24:1375–1381, 1992.
92. Mitchell, FL: Elements of muscle energy techniques. In Basmagian, JV, and Nyberg, R (eds): Rational Manual Therapies, Williams & Wilkins, Baltimore, 1993.
93. Monroe, LG: Motion restrictions. In Cameron, MH: Physical Agents in Rehabilitation. WB Saunders, Philadelphia, 1999, pp 68–86.
94. Muir, IW, Chesworth, BM, and Vandervoort, AA: Effect of a static calf-stretching exercise on resistive torque during passive ankle dorsiflexion in healthy subjects. J Orthop Sports Phys Ther 29:107–113, 1999.
95. Murphy, DR: Dynamic range of motion training: An alternative to static stretching. Chiroprac Sports Med 8:59–66, 1994.
96. Noyes, FR, et al: Biomechanics of ligament failure. J Bone Joint Surg Am 56:1406, 1974.
97. Noyes, FR: Functional properties of knee ligaments and alterations induced by immobilization. Clin Orthop Rel Res 123:210, 1977.
98. Noyes, FR, Keller, CS, Grood, ES, and Butler, DL: Advances in understanding of knee ligament injury, repair and rehabilitation. Med Sci Sports Exerc 16:427, 1984.
99. Ostering LR, Robertson, R, Troxel, R, and Hansen, R: Differential response to proprioceptive neuromuscular facilitation (PNF) stretch technique. Med Sci Sports Exerc 22:106–111, 1990.
100. O'Sullivan, SB: Assessment of motor function. In O'Sullivan, SB, and Schmitz, TJ (eds): Physical Rehabilitation: Assessment and Treatment, ed 4. FA Davis, Philadelphia, 2001, pp 197–198.
101. O'Sullivan, SB: Strategies to improve motor control and motor learning. In O'Sullivan, SB, and Schmitz, TJ (eds): Physical Rehabilitation: Assessment and Treatment, ed 4. FA Davis, Philadelphia, 2001, pp 363–411.
102. Prentice, WE: A electromyographic analysis of the effectiveness of heat or cold and stretching for inducing relaxation in an injured muscle. J Orthop Sports Phys Ther 3:133–140, 1982.
103. Prentice, WE: Rehabilitation Techniques in Sports Medicine. In Prentice, WE: Restoring range of motion and improving flexibility, ed 3. MCB/McGraw Hill, Boston, 1999, pp 2–72.
104. Rennie, GA, and Michlovitz, SL: Biophysical principles of heating and superficial heating agents. In Michlovitz, SL: Thermal Agents in Rehabilitation. FA Davis, Philadelphia, 1996.
105. Rose, S, Draper, DO, et al: The stretching window, part two: Rate of thermal decay in deep muscle following 1 MHz ultrasound. J Athletic Training 31:139–143, 1996.
106. Sady, SP, Wortman, M, and Blanke, D: Flexibility training: Ballistic, static or proprioceptive neuromuscular facilitation. Arch Phys Med Rehabil 63:261, 1982.
107. Sapega, A, et al: Biophysical factors in range of motion exercises. The Physician and Sportsmedicine 9:57, 1981.
108. Schultz, JH, and Luthe, W: Autogenic Training: A Psychophysiologic Approach in Psychotherapy. Grune & Stratton, New York, 1959.
109. Smith, CA: The warm-up procedure: To stretch or not to

stretch. A brief review. J Orthop Sports Phys Ther 19(1): 12–17, 1994.

110. Smith, LK, Weiss, EL, and Lehmkuhl, LD: Brunnstrom's Clinical Kinesiology, ed 5: FA Davis, Philadelphia, 1995.
111. Sotoberg, GL: Skeletal muscle function. In Currier, DP, and Nelson, RM (eds): Dynamics of Human Biologic Tissues, FA Davis, Philadelphia, 1992, p 74.
112. Starring, DT, et al: Comparison of cyclic and sustained passive stretching using a mechanical device to increase resting length of hamstring muscles. Phys Ther 68:314, 1988.
113. Sullivan, MK, Dejulia, JJ, and Worrell, TW: Effect of pelvic position and stretching method on hamstring muscle flexibility. Med Sci Sports Exerc 24:1383–1389, 1992.
114. Sullivan, PE, and Markos, PD: Clinical Decision Making in Therapeutic Exercise. Appleton and Lange, Norwalk, CT, 1995.
115. Tabary, JC, et al: Physiological and structural changes in the cat soleus muscle due to immobilization at different lengths by plaster casts. J Physiol (Lond) 224:231, 1972.
116. Tannigawa, M: Comparison of the hold-relax procedure and passive mobilization on increasing muscle length. Phys Ther 52:725, 1972.
117. Tappan, FM, and Benjamin, PJ: Tappan's Handbook of Healing Massage Techniques. Appleton and Lange, Stamford CT, 1998.
118. Tardieu, C, et al: Adaptation of connective tissue length to immobilization in the lengthened and shortened position in cat soleus muscle. J Physiol (Paris) 78:214, 1982.
119. Taylor, BF, Waring, CA, and Brashear, TA: The effects of therapeutic heat or cold followed by static stretch on hamstring muscle length. J Orthop Sports Phys Ther 21:283–286, 1995.
120. Taylor, D, Dalton, J, Seaber, A, and Garrett, W: Viscoelastic properties of muscle-tendon units: The biomechanical effects of stretching. Am J Sports Med 18(3):300–309, 1990.
121. Threlkeld, AJ: The effects of manual therapy on connective tissue. Phys Ther 72:893, 1992.
122. Tiidus, PM: Manual massage and recovery of muscle function following exercise: A literature review. J Orthop Sports Phys Ther 25:107–112, 1997.
123. Tillman, LJ, and Cummings, GS: Biologic mechanisms of connective tissue mutability. In Currier, DP, and Nelson, RM (eds): Dynamics of Human Biologic Tissues. FA Davis, Philadelphia, 1992, p 1.
124. Tomberlin, JP, and Saunders, HD: Evaluation, Treatment and Prevention of Musculoskeletal Disorders (ed 2), The Saunders Group, Chaska, MN, 1994.
125. Travell, JG, and Simons, DG: Myofascial Pain and Dysfunction Trigger Point Manuals, Vol. 2. Williams & Wilkins, Baltimore, 1992.
126. Vesco, JJ: Principles of stretching. In Torg, JS, Welsh, RP, and Shephard, RJ (eds): Current Therapy in Sports Medicine, Vol 2. BC Decker, Toronto, 1990.
127. Voss, DE, Ionla, MK, and Myers, BJ: Proprioceptive Neuromuscular Facilitation, ed 3. Harper & Row, Philadelphia, 1985.
128. Walker, SM: Delay of twitch relaxation induced by stress and stress relaxation. J Appl Physiol 16:801, 1961.
129. Warren, CG, Lehmann, JF, and Koblanski, JN: Heat and stretch procedures: An evaluation using rat tail tendon. Arch Phys Med Rehabil 57:122, 1976.
130. Warren, CG, Lehmann, JF, and Koblanski, JN: Elongation of rat tail tendon: Effect of load and temperature. Arch Phys Med Rehabil 51:481, 1970.
131. Webright, WG, Randolph, BJ, and Perin, DH: Comparison of nonballistic active knee extension in neural slump position and static stretch techniques on hamstring flexibility. J Orthop Sports Phys Ther 26:7–13, 1997.
132. Wessling, KC, Derane, DA, and Hylton, CR: Effect of static stretch vs. static stretch and ultrasound combined on triceps surae muscle extensibility in healthy women. Phys Ther 67:674, 1987.
133. Wilkinson, A: Stretching the truth. A review of the literature on muscle stretching. Austral J Physiother 38:283–287, 1992.
134. Wiliams, PR, and Goldspink, G: Changes in sarcomere length and physiological properties in immobilized muscle. J Anat 127:459, 1978.
135. Wolpe, J: Psychotherapy by Reciprocal Inhibition. Stanford University Press, Stanford, 1958.
136. Worrell, T, McCullough, M, and Pfeiffer, A: Effect of foot position on gastrocnemius/soleus stretching in subjects with normal flexibility. J Orthop Sports Phys Ther 19:352–356, 1994.
137. Worrell, TW, Smith, TL, and Winegardner, J: Effect of hamstring stretching on hamstring muscle performance. J Orthop Sports Phys Ther 20:154–159, 1994.
138. Zachazewski, JE: Improving flexibility. In Scully, RM, and Barnes, MR (eds): Physical Therapy. JB Lippincott, Philadelphia, 1989, p 698.
139. Zarins, B: Soft tissue injury and repair: Biomechanical aspects. Int J Sports Med 3:9, 1982.

Chapter 6

Peripheral Joint Mobilization

OBJECTIVES

After studying this chapter, the reader will be able to:

1. Define terminology of joint mobilization.
2. Summarize basic concepts of joint motion.
3. Differentiate between dosages and indications for using various types of joint mobilization procedures on various movement impairments.
4. Discriminate between the usefulness of joint mobilization and other stretching techniques for gaining mobility.
5. Recognize limitations of joint mobilization.
6. Recognize contraindications for joint mobilization.
7. Describe procedures for applying passive joint mobilization and mobilization with movement.
8. Apply basic techniques of joint mobilization to the extremity joints.

Joint mobilization refers to manual therapy techniques that are used to modulate pain and treat joint dysfunctions that limit range of motion (ROM) by specifically addressing the altered mechanics of the joint. The altered joint mechanics may be from pain and muscle guarding, from joint effusion, from contractures or adhesions in the joint capsules or supporting ligaments, or from malalignment or subluxation of the bony surfaces. Joint mobilization stretching techniques differ from other forms of passive or self-stretching (described in Chapter 5) in that they specifically address restricted capsular tissue by replicating normal joint mechanics while minimizing abnormal compressive stresses on the articular cartilage within the joint.[6,17]

To use joint mobilization for treatment effectively, the practitioner must know and be able to examine the anatomy, arthrokinematics, and pathology of the neuromusculoskeletal system and to recognize when the techniques are indicated or when other techniques would be more effective for regaining lost motion. Indiscriminate use of joint mobilization techniques, when not indicated, could lead to potential harm to the patient's joints. We assume that, prior to learning the joint mobilization techniques presented here, the student or therapist will have had (or will be concurrently taking) a course in orthopedic examination and evaluation and, therefore, will be able to choose appropriate, safe techniques for treating the patient's functional limitation. The reader is referred to several resources for additional study of evaluation procedures.[2,6,8,9] When indicated, joint mobilization is a safe and effective means of restoring or maintaining joint play within a joint and can also be used for treating pain.[6,17]

▶ Definitions of Terms

Mobilization/Manipulation

Mobilization and manipulation are two words that have come to have the same meaning[9a] and are, therefore, interchangeable. They are passive, skilled manual therapy techniques applied to joints and related soft tissues at varying speeds and amplitudes using physiologic or accessory motions, for therapeutic purposes. The varying speeds and amplitudes could range from a small-amplitude force applied at a high velocity to a large-amplitude force applied at a slow velocity; that is, there is a continuum of intensities and speeds at which the technique could be applied.

Self-Mobilization (Automobilization)

Self-mobilization refers to self-stretching techniques that specifically use joint traction or glides that direct the stretch force to the joint capsule. Self-mobilization techniques will be described in the chapters on specific regions of the body.

Mobilization with Movement (MWM)

MWM is the concurrent application of a sustained accessory mobilization applied by a therapist and an active physiologic movement to end range applied by the patient. Passive end-of-range overpressure, or stretching, is then able to be delivered without pain as a barrier. The techniques are always applied in a pain-free direction and are described as correcting joint tracking from a positional fault.[11,12] Brian Mulligan of New Zealand originally described these techniques.[12]

Physiologic Movements

Physiologic movements are movements that the patient can do voluntarily; for example, the classic or traditional movements, such as flexion, abduction, and rotation. The term *osteokinematics* is used when these motions of the bones are described.

Accessory Movements

Accessory movements are movements within the joint and surrounding tissues that are necessary for normal ROM but that cannot be actively performed by the patient.[13] Terms that relate to accessory movements are component motions and joint play.

- ***Component motions*** are those motions that accompany active motion but are not under voluntary control. The term is often used synonymously with accessory movement. For example, motions such as upward rotation of the scapula and rotation of the clavicle, which occur with shoulder flexion, and rotation of the fibula, which occurs with ankle motions, are component motions.
- ***Joint play*** describes the motions that occur between the joint surfaces as well as the distensibility or "give" in the joint capsule, which allows the bones to move. The movements are necessary for normal joint functioning through the ROM and can be demonstrated passively, but they cannot be performed actively by the patient.[16] The movements include distraction, sliding, compression, rolling, and spinning of the joint surfaces. The term *arthrokinematics* is used when these motions of the bone surfaces within the joint are described.

Note: Procedures to distract or slide the joint surfaces to decrease pain or restore joint play are the fundamental joint mobilization techniques described in this text.

Thrust

Thrust is a high-velocity, short-amplitude motion such that the patient cannot prevent the motion.[9,16] The motion is performed at the end of the pathologic limit of the joint and is intended to alter positional relationships, to snap adhesions, or to stimulate joint receptors.[16] Pathologic limit means the end of the available ROM when there is restriction. *Thrust techniques are beyond the scope of this text.*

Manipulation Under Anesthesia

This is a medical procedure used to restore full ROM by breaking adhesions around a joint while the patient is anesthetized. The technique may be a rapid thrust or a passive stretch using physiologic or accessory movements.

Muscle Energy

Muscle energy techniques use an active contraction of deep muscles that attached near the joint and whose line of pull can cause the desired accessory motion. The technique requires the therapist to provide stabilization to the segment on which the distal aspect of the muscle attaches. A command for an isometric contraction of the muscle is given, which causes the accessory movement of the joint. These techniques are not described in this text.

▶ Basic Concepts of Joint Motion: Arthrokinematics

Joint Shapes

The type of motion occurring between bony partners within a joint is influenced by the shapes of the joint surfaces. The shapes may be described as *ovoid* or *sellar.*[6,19]

- ***Ovoid.*** One surface is convex, the other is concave (Fig. 6–1*A*).
- ***Sellar (saddle).*** One surface is concave in one direction and convex in the other, with the opposing surface convex and concave, respectively; similar to a horseback rider being in complementary opposition to the shape of a saddle (Fig. 6–1*B*).

Types of Motion

As a bony lever moves about an axis of motion, there is also movement of the bone surface on the opposing bone surface within the joint.

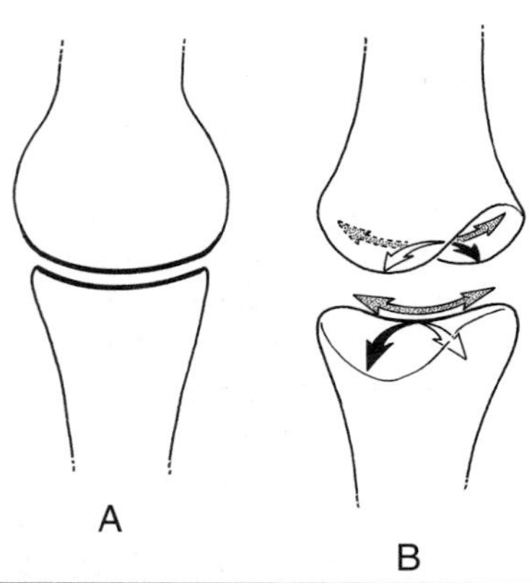

Figure 6–1 *(A)* With ovoid joints, one surface is convex, and the other is concave. *(B)* With sellar joints, one surface is concave in one direction and convex in the other, with the opposing surface convex and concave, respectively.

- The movement of the bony lever is called *swing* and is classically described as flexion, extension, abduction, adduction, and rotation. The amount of movement can be measured in degrees with a goniometer and is called ROM.
- Motion of the bone surfaces within the joint is a variable combination of *rolling, sliding,* or *spinning.*[6,14,19] These accessory motions allow for greater angulation of the bone as it swings. For the rolling, sliding, or spinning to occur, there must be adequate capsule laxity or joint play.

Roll

Characteristics of one bone rolling on another (Fig. 6–2) are as follows:

- The surfaces are incongruent.
- New points on one surface meet new points on the opposing surface.
- Rolling results in angular motion of the bone (swing).
- Rolling is always in the same direction as the swinging bone motion (Figs. 6–3*A* and *B*), whether the surface is convex or concave.
- Rolling, if it occurs alone, causes compression of the surfaces on the side to which the bone is swinging and separation on the other side. Passive stretching using bone angulation alone may cause stressful compressive forces to portions of the joint surface, potentially leading to joint damage.
- In normally functioning joints, pure rolling does not occur alone but in combination with joint sliding and spinning.

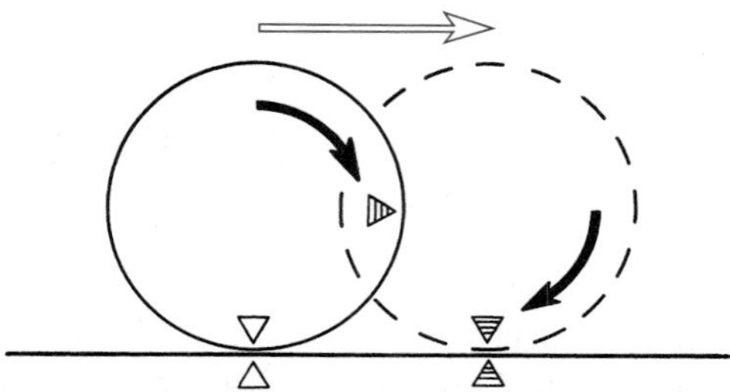

Figure 6–2 Diagrammatic representation of one surface rolling on another. New points on one surface meet new points on the opposing surface.

Slide

Characteristics of one bone sliding across another include the following:

- For a pure slide, the surfaces must be congruent, either flat (Fig. 6–4*A*) or curved (Fig. 6–4*B*).
- The same point on one surface comes into contact with the new points on the opposing surface.
- Pure sliding does not occur in joints, because the surfaces are not completely congruent.

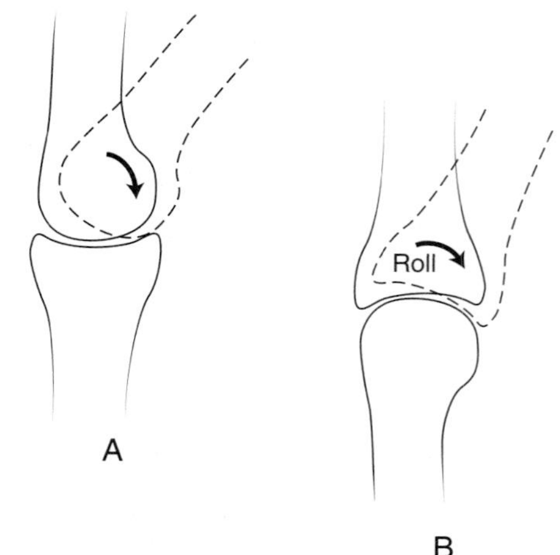

Figure 6–3 Rolling is always in the same direction as bone motion, whether the moving bone is *(A)* convex or *(B)* concave.

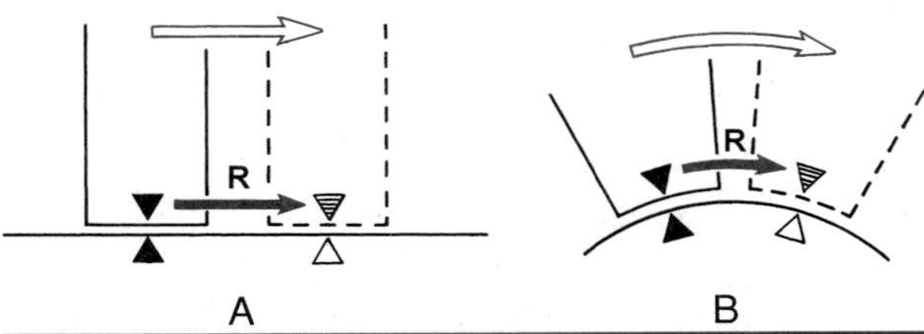

Figure 6–4 Diagrammatic representation of one surface sliding on another, whether *(A)* flat or *(B)* curved. The same point on one surface comes into contact with new points on the opposing surface.

- The direction in which sliding occurs depends on whether the moving surface is concave or convex. Sliding is in the opposite direction of the angular movement of the bone if the moving joint surface is convex (Fig. 6–5*A*). Sliding is in the same direction as the angular movement of the bone if the moving surface is concave (Fig. 6–5*B*).

Note: This mechanical relationship is known as the *convex-concave rule* and is the basis for determining the direction of the mobilizing force when joint mobilization gliding techniques are used.[6]

Combined Roll-Sliding in a Joint

- The more congruent the joint surfaces are, the more sliding there is of one bony partner on the other with movement.

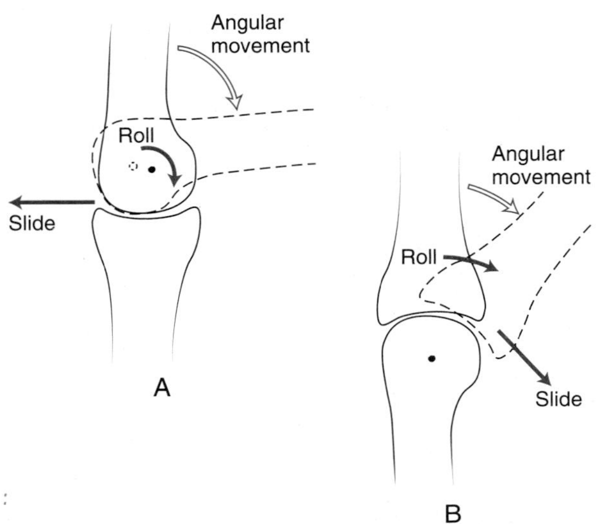

Figure 6–5 Diagrammatic representation of the concave-convex rule. *(A)* If the surface of the moving bone is convex, sliding is in the opposite direction of the angular movement of the bone. *(B)* If the surface of the moving bone is concave, sliding is in the same direction as the angular movement of the bone.

- The more incongruent the joint surfaces are, the more rolling there is of one bony partner on the other with movement.
- When muscles actively contract to move a bone, some of the muscles may cause or control the sliding movement of the joint surfaces. For example, the caudal sliding motion of the humeral head during shoulder abduction is caused by the rotator cuff muscles, and the posterior sliding of the tibia during knee flexion is caused by the hamstring muscles. If this function is lost, the resulting abnormal joint mechanics may cause microtrauma and joint dysfunction.
- The joint mobilization techniques described in this chapter use the sliding component of joint motion to restore joint play and reverse joint hypomobility. Rolling (passive angular stretching) is not used to stretch tight joint capsules because it causes joint compression.

Note: When the therapist passively moves the articulating surface in the direction in which the slide normally occurs, the technique is called translatoric glide or, simply, glide.[6] It is used to control pain when applied gently or to stretch the capsule when applied with a stretch force.

Spin

Characteristics of one bone spinning on another include the following:

- There is rotation of a segment about a stationary mechanical axis (Fig. 6–6).
- The same point on the moving surface creates an arc of a circle as the bone spins.
- Spinning rarely occurs alone in joints but in combination with rolling and sliding.
- Three examples of spin occurring in joints of the body are the shoulder with flexion/extension, the hip with flexion/extension, and the radiohumeral joint with pronation/supination (Fig. 6–7).

Passive-Angular Stretching Versus Joint-Glide Stretching[17]

Passive-angular stretching procedures, as when the bony lever is used to stretch a tight joint capsule, may cause increased pain or joint trauma because:

- The use of a lever significantly magnifies the force at the joint.
- The force causes excessive joint compression in the direction of the rolling bone (see Fig. 6–3).
- The roll without a slide does not replicate normal joint mechanics.

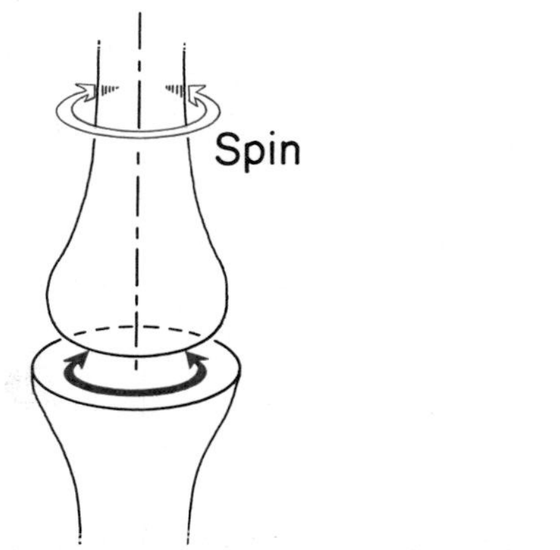

Figure 6–6 Diagrammatic representation of spinning. There is rotation of a segment about a stationary mechanical axis.

Joint glide (mobilization) stretching procedures, as when the translatoric slide component of the bones is used to stretch a tight capsule, are safer and more selective because

- The force is applied close to the joint surface and controlled at an intensity compatible with the pathology.
- The direction of the force replicates the sliding component of the joint mechanics and does not compress the cartilage.
- The amplitude of the motion is small yet specific to the restricted or adhered portion of the capsule or ligaments. Thus, the forces are selectively applied to the desired tissue.

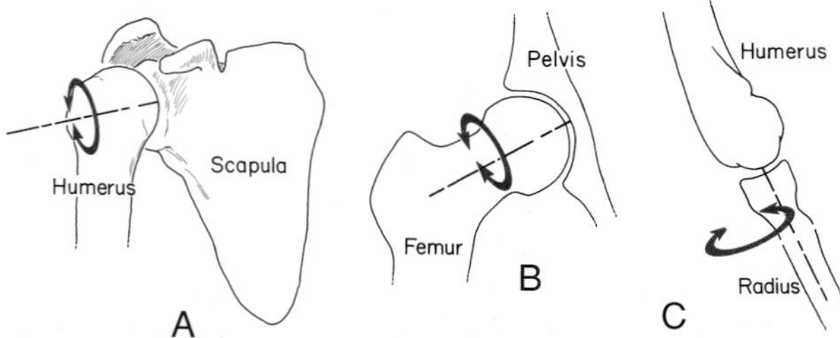

Figure 6–7 Examples of joint spin location in the body. *(A)* Humerus with flexion/extension. *(B)* Femur with flexion/extension. *(C)* Head of the radius with pronation/supination.

Other Accessory Motions that Affect the Joint

Compression

Compression is the decrease in the joint space between bony partners.

- Compression normally occurs in the extremity and spinal joints when weight-bearing.
- Some compression occurs as muscles contract, which provides stability to the joints.
- As one bone rolls on the other (see Fig. 6–3), some compression also occurs on the side to which the bone is angulating.
- Normal intermittent compressive loads help move synovial fluid and thus help maintain cartilage health.
- Abnormally high compression loads may lead to articular cartilage changes and deterioration.[14]

Traction

Traction or distraction is the separation of the joint surfaces.

- For distraction to occur within the joint, the surfaces must be pulled apart. The movement is not always the same as pulling on the long axis of one of the bony partners. For example, if traction is applied to the shaft of the humerus, it will result in a glide of the joint surface (Fig. 6–8*A*). Distraction of the glenohumeral joint requires a pull at right angles to the glenoid fossa (Fig. 6–8*B*).
- For clarity, whenever there is pulling on the long axis of a bone, the term *long-axis traction* will be used. Whenever the surfaces are to be pulled apart at right angles, the terms *distraction, joint traction, or joint separation* will be used.

Note: For joint mobilization techniques, distraction is used to control or relieve pain when applied gently or to stretch the capsule when applied with a stretch force.

Effects of Joint Motion

- Joint motion stimulates biological activity by moving synovial fluid, which brings nutrients to the avascular articular cartilage of the joint surfaces and intra-articular fibrocartilage of the menisci.[14] Atrophy of the articular cartilage begins soon after immobilization is imposed on joints.[1,3,4]
- Joint motion maintains extensibility and tensile strength of the articular and periarticular tissues.

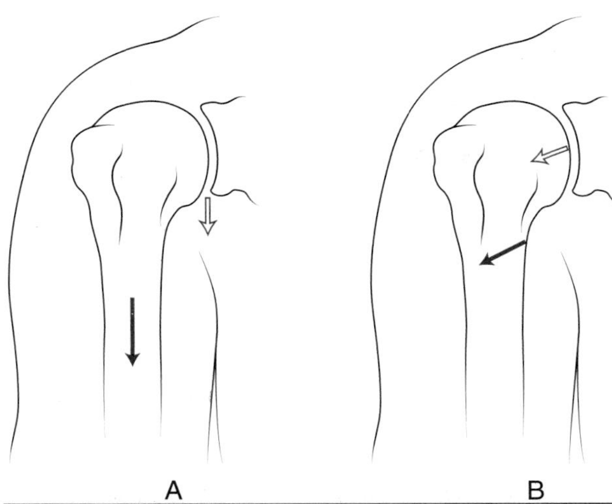

Figure 6–8 *(A)* Traction applied to the shaft of the humerus results in caudal gliding of the joint surface. *(B)* Distraction of the glenohumeral joint requires separation at right angles to the glenoid fossa.

With immobilization there is fibrofatty proliferation, which causes intra-articular adhesions, as well as biochemical changes in tendon, ligament, and joint capsule tissue, which causes joint contractures and ligamentous weakening.[1]

- Afferent nerve impulses from joint receptors transmit information to the central nervous system and, therefore, provide for awareness of position and motion. With injury or joint degeneration, there is a potential decrease in an important source of proprioceptive feedback that may affect an individual's balance response.[20] Joint motion provides sensory input relative to:[22,23]
  - Static position and sense of speed of movement (type I receptors found in the superficial joint capsule)
  - Change of speed of movement (type II receptors found in deep layers of the joint capsule and articular fat pads)
  - Sense of direction of movement (type I and III receptors; type III found in joint ligaments)
  - Regulation of muscle tone (type I, II, and III receptors)
  - Nociceptive stimuli (type IV receptors found in the fibrous capsule, ligaments, articular fat pads, periosteum, and walls of blood vessels)

Indications for Joint Mobilization

Pain, Muscle Guarding, and Spasm

Painful joints, reflex muscle guarding, and muscle spasm can be treated with *gentle joint-play* techniques to stimulate neurophysiologic and mechanical effects.[9]

Neurophysiological Effects

Small-amplitude oscillatory and distraction movements are used to stimulate the mechanoreceptors that may inhibit the transmission of nociceptive stimuli at the spinal cord or brain stem levels.[16,19]

Mechanical Effects

Small-amplitude distraction or gliding movements of the joint are used to cause synovial fluid motion, which is the vehicle for bringing nutrients to the avascular portions of the articular cartilage (and intra-articular fibrocartilage when present). Gentle joint-play techniques help maintain nutrient exchange and thus prevent the painful and degenerating effects of stasis when a joint is swollen or painful and cannot move through a ROM.

Note: The small-amplitude joint techniques used to treat pain, muscle guarding, or muscle spasm should not place a stretch on the reactive tissues (see Contraindications and Precautions).

Reversible Joint Hypomobility

Reversible joint hypomobility can be treated with *progressively vigorous joint-play stretching* techniques to elongate hypomobile capsular and ligamentous connective tissue. Sustained or oscillatory stretch forces are used to mechanically distend the shortened tissue.[6,9]

Positional Faults/Subluxations

A malposition of one bony partner with respect to its opposing surface may result in limited motion or pain. This can occur with a traumatic injury, after periods of immobility, or with muscle imbalances. The malpositioning may be perpetuated with maladapted neuromuscular control across the joint so that whenever attempting active ROM there is faulty tracking of the joint surfaces resulting in pain or limited motion. Mobilization with movement (MWM) techniques attempt to realign the bony partners while the person actively moves the joint through its ROM.[12] Manipulations are used to reposition an obvious subluxation such as a pulled elbow or capitate-lunate subluxation.

Progressive Limitation

Diseases that progressively limit movement can be treated with joint-play techniques to maintain available motion or retard progressive mechanical restrictions. The dosage of distraction or glide is dictated by the patient's response to treatment and the state of the disease.

Functional Immobility

When a patient cannot functionally move a joint for a period of time, the joint can be treated with nonstretch gliding or distraction techniques to maintain available joint play and prevent the degenerating and restricting effects of immobility.

▶ Limitations of Joint Mobilization Techniques

Mobilization techniques cannot change the disease process of disorders such as rheumatoid arthritis or the inflammatory process of injury. In these cases, treatment is directed toward minimizing pain, maintaining available joint play, and reducing the effects of any mechanical limitations (see Chapter 8).

The skill of the therapist will affect the outcome. The techniques described in this text are relatively safe if directions are followed and precautions are heeded, but if these techniques are used indiscriminately on patients not properly evaluated and screened for such maneuvers or if they are applied too vigorously for the condition, joint trauma or hypermobility may result.

▶ Contraindications and Precautions

The only true contraindications to stretching techniques are hypermobility, joint effusion, and inflammation.

Hypermobility

- The joints of patients with potential necrosis of the ligaments or capsule should not be stretched.
- Patients with painful hypermobile joints may benefit from gentle joint-play techniques if kept within the limits of motion; stretching is not done.

Joint Effusion

There may be joint swelling (effusion) from trauma or disease. Rapid swelling of a joint usually indicates bleeding within the joint and may occur with trauma or in diseases such as hemophilia. Medical intervention is required for aspiration of the blood to minimize its necrotizing effect on the articular cartilage. Slow swelling (greater than 4 hours) usually indicates serous effusion (a buildup of excess synovial fluid) or edema within the joint from mild trauma, irritation, or a disease, such as arthritis.

- Never stretch a swollen joint with mobilization or passive stretching techniques. The capsule is already on a stretch by being distended to accommodate the extra fluid. The limited motion is from the extra fluid and muscle response to pain, not from shortened fibers.
- Gentle oscillating motions that do not stress or stretch the capsule may help block the transmission of a pain stimulus so that it is not perceived and may also help improve fluid flow while maintaining available joint play.
- If the patient's response to gentle techniques results in increased pain or joint irritability, the techniques were applied too vigorously or should not be done with the current state of pathology.

Inflammation

Whenever inflammation is present, stretching will increase pain and muscle guarding and will result in greater tissue damage. Gentle oscillating or distraction motions may temporarily inhibit the pain response. See Chapter 8 for an appropriate approach to treatment when inflammation is present.

Conditions Requiring Special Precautions for Stretching

In most cases, joint mobilization techniques are safer than passive angular stretching, in which the bony lever is used to stretch tight tissue and joint compression results. Mobilization may be used with extreme care in the following conditions if signs and the patient's response are favorable:

- Malignancy.
- Bone disease detectable on x-ray.
- Unhealed fracture (depends on the site of the fracture and stabilization provided).
- Excessive pain (determine the cause of pain and modify treatment accordingly).
- Hypermobility in associated joints (associated joints must be properly stabilized so the mobilization force is not transmitted to them).
- Total joint replacements (the mechanism of the replacement is self-limiting, and therefore, the mobilization gliding techniques may be inappropriate).
- Newly formed or weakened connective tissue such as immediately after injury, surgery, or disuse or when the patient is taking certain medications such as corticosteroids (gentle progressive techniques within the tolerance of the tissue help align the developing fibrils, but forceful techniques are destructive).
- Systemic connective tissue diseases such as rheumatoid arthritis, in which the disease weakens the connective tissue (gentle techniques may benefit restricted tissue, but forceful techniques may rupture tissue and result in instabilities).
- Elderly individuals with weakened connective tissue and diminished circulation (gentle techniques within the tolerance of the tissue may be beneficial to increase mobility).

▶ Procedures for Applying Passive Joint Mobilization Techniques

Examination and Evaluation

If the patient has limited or painful motion, examine and decide which tissues are limiting function and the state of pathology. Determine whether treatment will be directed primarily toward relieving pain or stretching a joint or soft tissue limitation.[2,9]

- The quality of pain when testing the ROM helps determine the stage of recovery and the dosage of techniques used for treatment (see Figs. 8–2 and 8–3.)
  - If pain is experienced *before* tissue limitation—such as the pain that occurs with muscle guarding after an acute injury or during the active stage of a disease—gentle pain-inhibiting joint techniques may be used. The same techniques will also help maintain joint play (see next section on Grades or Dosages of Movement). Stretching under these circumstances is contraindicated.
  - If pain is experienced *concurrently* with tissue limitation—such as the pain and limitation that occur when damaged tissue begins to heal—the limitation is treated cautiously. Gentle stretching techniques specific to the tight structure are used to gradually improve movement yet not exacerbate the pain by reinjuring the tissue.
  - If pain is experienced *after* tissue limitation is met because of stretching of tight capsular or periarticular tissue, the stiff joint can be aggressively stretched with joint-play techniques and the periarticular tissue with the stretching techniques described in Chapter 5.
- The joint capsule is limiting motion and should respond to mobilization techniques if the following signs are present:
  - The passive ROM for that joint is limited in a capsular pattern (these patterns are described for each peripheral joint under the respective sections on joint problems in Chapters 9 through 14).
  - There is a firm capsular end-feel when overpressure is applied to the tissues limiting the range.
  - There is decreased joint-play movement when mobility tests (articulations) are performed.
- An adhered or contracted ligament is limiting motion if there is decreased joint play and pain when the fibers of the ligament are stressed; ligaments often respond to joint mobilization techniques if applied specific to their line of stress.
- Subluxation or dislocation of one bony part on another and loose intra-articular structures that block normal motion may respond to thrust techniques. Some of the simpler manipulations are described in appropriate sections in this text. Others require more advanced training and are beyond the scope of this book.

Grades or Dosages of Movement

Two systems of grading dosages for mobilization are used.[9]

Graded Oscillation Techniques (Fig. 6–9)

Dosages

- ***Grade I.*** Small-amplitude rhythmic oscillations are performed at the beginning of the range.

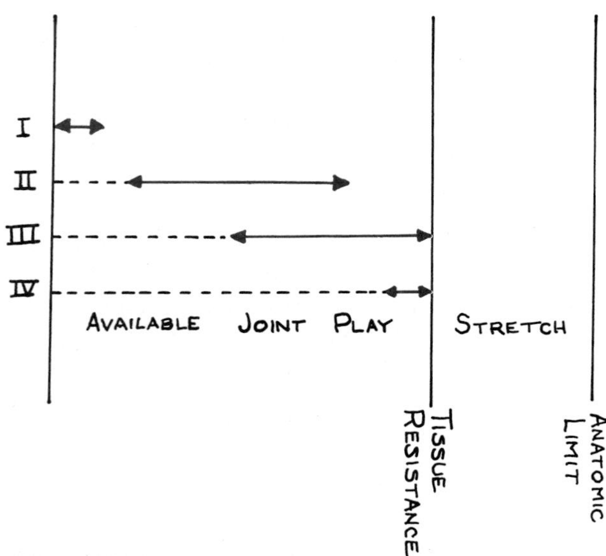

Figure 6–9 Diagrammatic representation of graded oscillation techniques. (Adapted from Maitland[9])

- ***Grade II.*** Large-amplitude rhythmic oscillations are performed within the range, not reaching the limit.
- ***Grade III.*** Large-amplitude rhythmic oscillations are performed up to the limit of the available motion and are stressed into the tissue resistance.
- ***Grade IV.*** Small-amplitude rhythmic oscillations are performed at the limit of the available motion and stressed into the tissue resistance.
- ***Grade V.*** A small-amplitude, high-velocity thrust technique is performed to snap adhesions at the limit of the available motion. Thrust techniques used for this purpose require advanced training and are beyond the scope of this book.

Uses

- Grades I and II are primarily used for treating joints limited by pain. The oscillations may have an inhibitory effect on perception of painful stimuli by repetitively stimulating mechanoreceptors that block nociceptive pathways at the spinal cord or brain stem levels.[16,24] These nonstretch motions help move synovial fluid to improve nutrition to the cartilage.
- Grades III and IV are primarily used as stretching maneuvers.

Techniques

The oscillations may be performed using physiologic (osteokinematic) motions or joint-play (arthrokinematic) techniques.

Sustained Translatory Joint-Play Techniques (Fig. 6–10)

Dosages

- ***Grade I (loosen).*** Small-amplitude distraction is applied where no stress is placed on the capsule. It equalizes cohesive forces, muscle tension, and atmospheric pressure acting on the joint.
- ***Grade II (tighten).*** Enough distraction or glide is applied to tighten the tissues around the joint. Kaltenborn[6] calls this "taking up the slack."
- ***Grade III (stretch).*** A distraction or glide is applied with an amplitude large enough to place a stretch on the joint capsule and on surrounding periarticular structures.

Uses

- Grade I distraction is used with all gliding motions and may be used for relief of pain.
- Grade II distraction is used for the initial treatment to determine how sensitive the joint is. Once joint reaction is known, the dosage of treatment is either increased or decreased accordingly.
- Gentle grade II distraction applied intermittently may be used to inhibit pain. Grade II glides may be used to maintain joint play when ROM is not allowed.
- Grade III joint distraction or glides are used to stretch the joint structures and, thus, increase joint play.

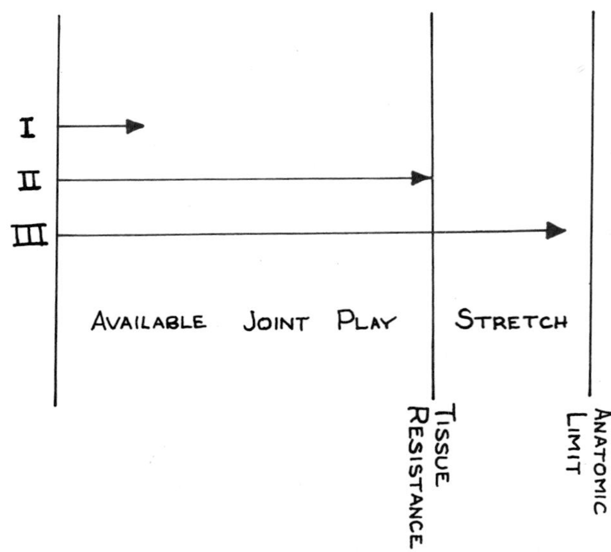

Figure 6–10 Diagrammatic representation of sustained translatory joint-play techniques. (Adapted from Kaltenborn[6])

Techniques

This grading system describes only joint-play techniques that separate (distract) or glide (slide) the joint surfaces.

Comparison

When using either grading system, dosages I and II are low intensity and so do not cause a stretch force on the joint capsule or surrounding tissue, although, by definition, sustained grade II techniques take up the slack of the tissues whereas grade II oscillation techniques stay within the slack. Grades III and IV oscillations and grade III sustained stretch techniques are similar in intensity in that they all are applied with a stretch force at the limit of motion. The differences are related to the rhythm or speed of repetition of the stretch force.

- For clarity and consistency, when referring to dosages in this text:
  - The notation *graded oscillations* means: use the dosages as described in the section on graded oscillation techniques.
  - The notation *sustained grade* means: use the dosages as described in the section on sustained translatory joint-play techniques.
- The choice of using oscillating or sustained techniques depends on the patient's response.
  - When dealing with managing pain, either grade I or II oscillation techniques or slow intermittent grade I or II sustained joint distraction techniques are recommended; the patient's response dictates the intensity and frequency of the joint-play technique.
  - When dealing with loss of joint play and thus decreased functional range, sustained techniques applied in a cyclic manner are recommended; the longer the stretch force can be maintained, the greater the creep and plastic deformation of the connective tissue.
  - When attempting to maintain available range by using joint-play techniques, either grade II oscillating or sustained grade II techniques can be used.

Positioning and Stabilization

- The patient and the extremity to be treated should be positioned so that the patient can relax. To relax the muscles crossing the joint, techniques of inhibition (see Chapter 5) may be appropriately used prior to or between joint mobilization techniques.
- Examination of joint play and the first treatment are initially performed in the resting position for that joint so that the greatest capsule laxity is possible. In some cases, the position to use is the one in which the joint is least painful. With progression of treatment, the joint is positioned at or near the end of the available range prior to application of the mobilization force. This places the restricting tissue in its most lengthened position where the stretch force can be more specific.
- Firmly and comfortably stabilize one joint partner, usually the proximal bone. A belt, one of the therapist's hands, or an assistant holding the part, may provide stabilization. Appropriate stabilization prevents unwanted stress to surrounding tissues and joints and makes the stretch force more specific and effective.

Treatment Force and Direction of Movement

- The treatment force (either gentle or strong) is applied as close to the opposing joint surface as possible. The larger the contact surface is, the more comfortable the procedure will be. For example, instead of forcing with your thumb, use the flat surface of your hand.
- The direction of movement during treatment is either parallel to or perpendicular to the treatment plane. *Treatment plane* is described by Kaltenborn[8] as a plane perpendicular to a line running from the axis of rotation to the middle of the concave articular surface. the plane is in the concave partner so its position is determined by the position of the concave bone (Fig. 6–11).
- Joint traction techniques are applied perpendicular to the treatment plane. The entire bone is moved so that the joint surfaces are separated.
- Gliding techniques are applied parallel to the treatment plane.
  - Glide in the direction in which the slide would normally occur for the desired motion. Direction of sliding is easily determined by using the convex-concave rule (earlier in this chapter). If the surface of the moving bony partner is convex, the treatment glide should be opposite to the direction in which the bone swings. If the surface of the moving bony partner is concave, the treatment glide should be in the same direction (see Figs. 6–5*A* and *B*).
  - The entire bone is moved so that there is gliding of one joint surface on the other. The bone should not be used as a lever; it should have no arcing

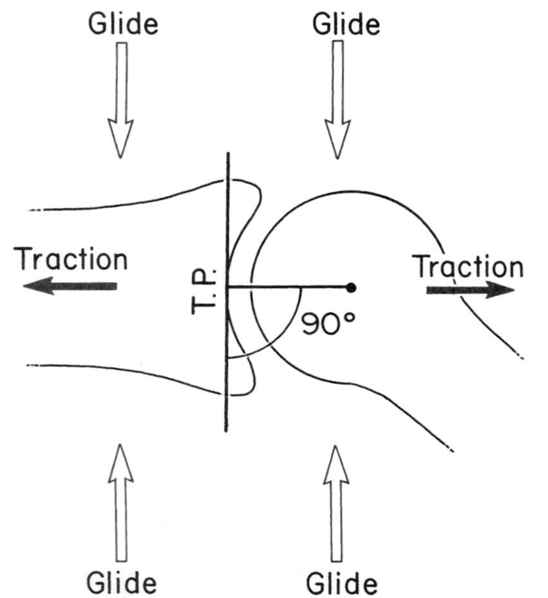

Figure 6–11 Treatment plane (T.P.) is at right angles to a line drawn from the axis of rotation to the center of the concave articulating surface and lies in the concave surface. Joint traction is applied perpendicular and glides are applied parallel to the treatment plane.

motion (swing) that would cause rolling and thus compression of the joint surfaces.

Initiation and Progression of Treatment (Fig. 6–12)

1. The initial treatment is the same whether treating to decrease pain or to increase joint play. The purpose is to determine joint reactivity before proceeding. Use a sustained grade II distraction of the joint surfaces with the joint held in resting position or the position of greatest relaxation.[6] Note the immediate joint response relative to irritability and range.
2. The next day, evaluate joint response, or have the patient report the response at the next visit.
   - If there is increased pain and sensitivity, reduce the amplitude of treatment to grade I oscillations.
   - If the joint is the same or better, perform either of the following: (1) Repeat the same maneuver if the goal of treatment is to maintain joint play. (2) Progress the maneuver to sustained grade III traction or glides if the goal of treatment is to increase joint play.
3. To progress the stretch technique, move the bone to the end of the available ROM, then apply the sustained grade III distraction or glide techniques. Advanced progressions include prepositioning the bone at the end of the available range and rotating it prior to applying grade III distraction or glide techniques. The direction of the rotation will be dictated by the joint mechanics. For example, laterally rotate the humerus as abduction is progressed; medially rotate the tibia as knee flexion is progressed.
4. Hints:
   - Warm the tissue around the joint prior to stretching. Modalities, massage, or gentle muscle contractions will increase the circulation and warm the tissues.
   - Muscle relaxation techniques and oscillation techniques may inhibit muscle guarding and should be alternated with the stretching techniques, if necessary.
   - When using grade III gliding techniques, a grade I distraction should be used with it. A grade II or III distraction should not be used with a grade III glide to avoid excessive trauma to the joint.
   - If gliding in the restricted direction is too painful, begin gliding mobilizations in the painless direction. Progress to gliding in the restricted direction when mobility improves a little and it is not painful.
   - When applying stretching techniques, move the bony partner through the available range of joint play first, that is, "take up the slack." When tissue resistance is felt, apply the stretch force against the restriction.
   - Incorporate MWM techniques (described later in this chapter) as part of the total approach to treatment.
5. To maintain joint play by using gliding techniques when range of motion techniques are contraindicated or not possible for a period of time, use sustained grade II or grade II oscillation techniques.

Speed, Rhythm, and Duration of Movements

Oscillations

- Grades I and IV are usually rapid oscillations, like manual vibrations.
- Grades II and III are smooth, regular oscillations at 2 or 3 per second for 1 to 2 minutes.

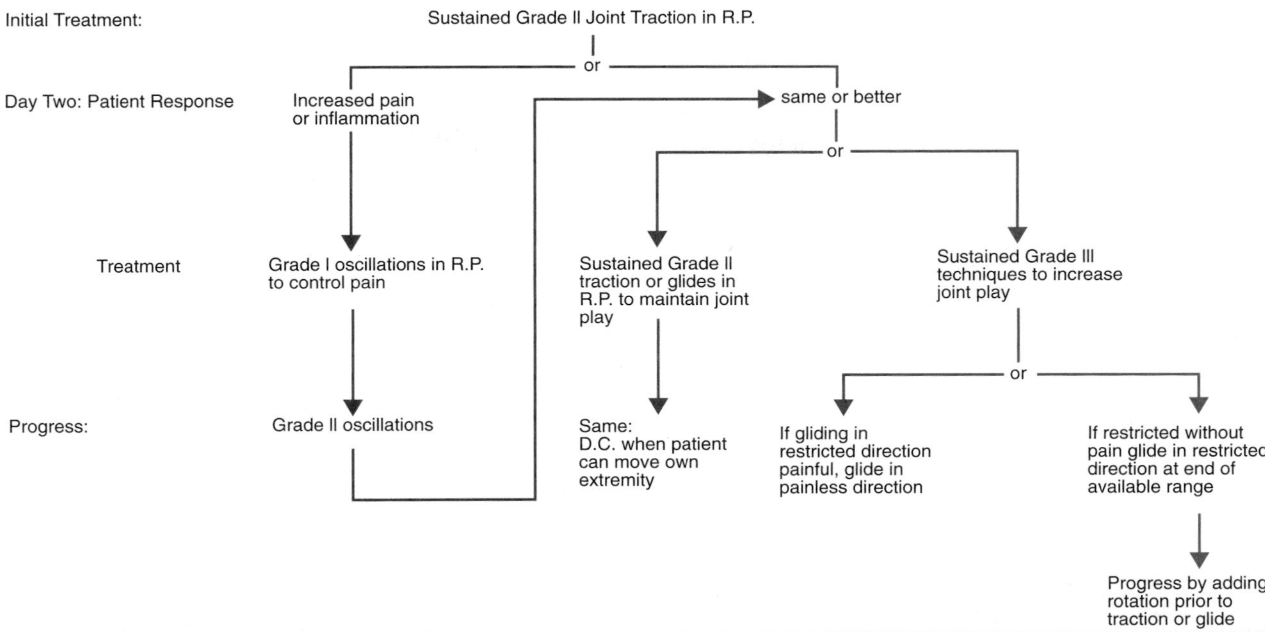

Figure 6–12 Initiation and progression of treatment.

- Vary the speed of oscillations for different effects such as low amplitude and high speed to inhibit pain or slow speed to relax muscle guarding.

Sustained

- For painful joints, apply intermittent distraction for 7 to 10 seconds with a few seconds of rest in between for several cycles. Note response and either repeat or discontinue.
- For restricted joints, apply a minimum of a 6-second stretch force, followed by partial release (to grade I or II), then repeat with slow, intermittent stretches at 3- to 4-second intervals.

Patient Response

- Stretching maneuvers usually cause soreness. Perform the maneuvers on alternate days to allow soreness to decrease and tissue healing to occur between stretching sessions. The patient should perform ROM into any newly gained range during this time. If there is increased pain after 24 hours, the dosage (amplitude) or duration of treatment was too vigorous. Decrease the dosage or duration until the pain is under control.
- The patient's joint and ROM should be reassessed after treatment and again before the next treatment. Alterations in treatment are dictated by the joint response.

Total Program

Mobilization techniques are one part of a total treatment program when there is decreased function. If muscles or connective tissues are also limiting motion, inhibition and passive stretching techniques

Box 6–1 Suggested Sequence of Treatment to Gain and Reinforce Functional Mobility

1. Warm the tissues
2. Relax muscles
   - Hold-relax inhibition technique
   - Grade I or II oscillation techniques
3. Joint mobilization stretches
   - Position and dosage for level of tissue tolerance
4. Passive stretch periarticular tissues
5. Patient actively uses new range
   - Reciprocal inhibition
   - Active ROM
   - Functional activities
6. Maintain new range; patient instruction
   - Self-stretching
   - Automobilization
   - Active, resistive ROM
   - Functional activities using the new range

are alternated with joint mobilization in the same treatment session. Therapy should also include appropriate ROM, strengthening, and functional exercises so that the client learns effective control and use of the gained mobility (Box 6–1).

▶ Mobilization with Movement, Principles and Procedures

Brian Mulligan's concept of Mobilization with Movement (MWM) is the natural continuance of the progression in the development of manual therapy from active self-stretching exercises, to therapist-applied passive physiological movement, to passive accessory mobilization techniques.[11] Mobilization with movement is the concurrent application of a pain-free accessory mobilization with active and/or passive physiological movement.[12] Passive end range overpressure or stretching is then applied without pain as a barrier. These techniques are applicable when:

- No contraindication for manual therapy exists (described earlier in this chapter).
- A full orthopedic scanning examination has been completed and evaluation of the results indicate local musculoskeletal pathology.[2]
- A specific biomechanical analysis reveals localized loss of movement and/or pain associated with function.[9]
- No pain is produced during or immediately after application of the technique.[10]

Principles of MWM in Clinical Practice

- One or more *comparable signs* are identified during the examination.[9] A comparable sign is a positive test sign that can be repeated after a therapeutic maneuver to determine the effectiveness of the maneuver. For example, a comparable sign may include loss of joint play movement, loss of ROM, or pain associated with movement during specific functional activities such as lateral elbow pain with resisted wrist extension, painful restriction of ankle dorsiflexion, or pain with overhead reaching.
- A passive joint mobilization is applied as described in the previous section following the principles of Kaltenborn.[6] This accessory glide or distraction performed parallel or perpendicular to the treatment plane must be pain-free.[12]
- Utilizing knowledge of joint anatomy and mechanics, a sense of tissue tension, and sound clinical reasoning, the therapist investigates various combinations of parallel or perpendicular accessory glides to find the pain-free direction and grade of accessory movement. This may be a glide, spin, distraction or combination of movement.
- While the therapist sustains the pain-free accessory mobilization, the patient is requested to perform the comparable sign. The comparable sign should now be significantly improved, i.e., there should be increased ROM and the motion should *be free of the original pain.*[12]
- The therapist must continuously monitor the patient's reaction to ensure no pain is produced. Failure to improve the comparable sign would indicate that the therapist has not found the correct direction of accessory mobilization, grade of movement or that the technique is not indicated.
- The previously restricted and/or painful motion or activity is repeated 6 to 10 times by the patient while the therapist continues to maintain the appropriate accessory mobilization. Further gains are expected with repetition during a treatment session particularly when *pain-free* passive overpressure is applied to achieve end-range loading.

Pain Is Always the Guide

Successful MWM techniques should render the comparable sign painless while significantly improving function during the application of the technique. Self-treatment is often possible using MWM principles with sports type adhesive tape and/or the patient providing the mobilization component of the MWM concurrent with the active physiologic movement.[5] Having restored articular function with MWMs, the therapist progresses the client through the ensuing rehabilitation sequences of the recovery of muscular power, endurance, and neural control. Sustained improvements are necessary to justify ongoing intervention.

Theoretical Framework

Mulligan postulates a positional fault model to explain the results gained through his concept. Alternately, inappropriate joint tracking mechanisms due to an altered instantaneous axis of rotation and neurophysiologic response models have also been considered.[5,10,11,13] Early research into this approach confirms its benefits; however, the mechanism through which it affects the musculoskeletal system has yet to be fully determined.[7,15,18,21] For further details of the application of the Mulligan Concept as it applies to the spine and extremities, refer to *Manual Therapy, "NAGS," "SNAGS," "MWMs,"* etc.[12]

Techniques

Techniques applicable to the extremity joints are described throughout this text in the treatment sections for various conditions (see Chapters 9 through 14).

▶ Peripheral Joint Mobilization Techniques

The following are suggested joint distraction and gliding techniques for use by entry level therapists and those attempting to gain a foundation in joint mobilization. A variety of adaptations can be made from these techniques. The distraction and glide techniques should be applied with respect to the dosage, frequency, progression, precautions, and procedures as described in the previous sections.

Note: Terms such as proximal hand, distal hand, lateral hand, or other descriptive terms indicate that the therapist should use the hand that is more proximal, distal, or lateral to the patient or the patient's extremity.

Shoulder Girdle Complex (Fig. 6–13)

Glenohumeral (GH) Joint

The concave glenoid fossa receives the convex humeral head.

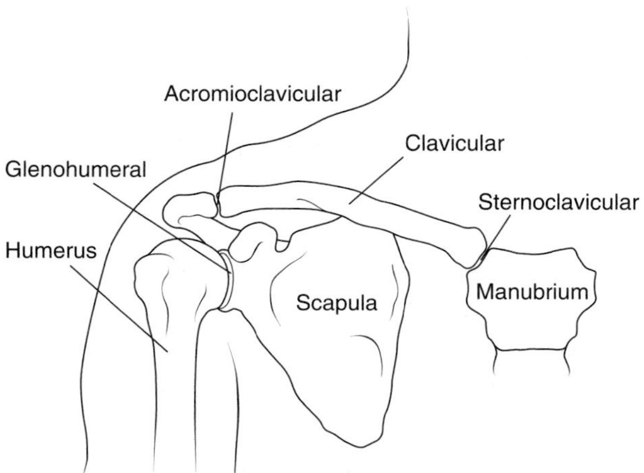

Figure 6–13 Bones and joints of the shoulder girdle complex.

Resting Position
Shoulder is abducted 55 degrees, horizontally adducted 30 degrees, and rotated so that the forearm is in the horizontal plane.

Treatment Plane
In the glenoid fossa and moves with the scapula.

Stabilization
Fixate the scapula with a belt or have an assistant help.

GH Joint Traction/Distraction (Fig. 6–14)

Indications
Testing; initial treatment (sustained grade II); pain control (grade I or II oscillations); general mobility (sustained grade III).

Patient Position
Supine, with arm in resting position; support the forearm between your trunk and elbow.

Hand Placement
- Use the hand nearer the part being treated (for example, left hand if treating the patient's left shoulder), and place it in the patient's axilla with your thumb just distal to the joint margin anteriorly and fingers posteriorly.
- Your other hand supports the humerus from the lateral surface.

Mobilizing Force
With the hand in the axilla, move the humerus laterally.

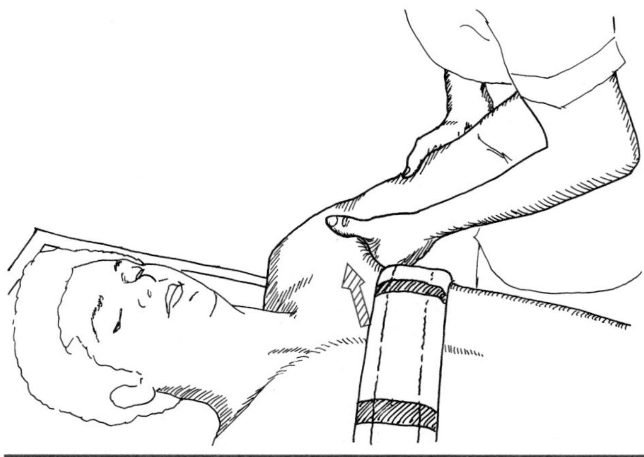

Figure 6–14 Joint traction; glenohumeral joint.

Note: The entire arm moves in a translatoric motion away from the plane of the glenoid fossa. Distractions may be performed with the humerus in any position (see Figs. 6–17, 6–19, and 9–8). You must be aware of the amount of scapular rotation and adjust the distraction force against the humerus so it is perpendicular to the plane of the glenoid fossa.

GH Caudal Glide (Fig. 6–15)

Indications
To increase abduction (sustained grade III); to reposition humeral head if superiorly positioned.

Patient Position
Same as with distraction.

Hand Placement
- Place one hand in the patient's axilla to provide the grade I distraction.
- The web space of your other hand is placed just distal to the acromion process.

Mobilizing Force
With the superiorly placed hand, glide the humerus in an inferior direction.

GH Caudal Glide: Alternate

Hand Placement
Same as with distraction (see Fig. 6–14).

Mobilizing Force
Comes from the hand around the arm, pulling caudally as you shift your body weight inferiorly.

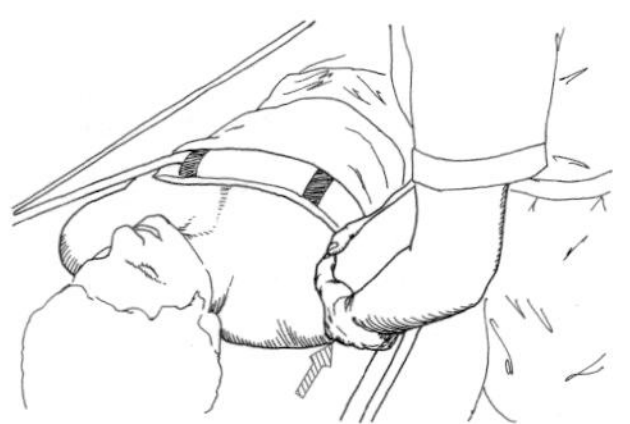

Figure 6–15 Caudal glide; glenohumeral joint.

Note: This glide is also called long-axis traction.

GH Caudal Glide Progression (Fig. 6–16*A*)

Indication
To increase abduction when range approaches 90 degrees.

Patient Position
- Supine, with the arm abducted to the end of its available range.
- External rotation of the humerus should be added to the end-range position as the arm approaches and goes beyond 90 degrees.

Therapist Position and Hand Placement
- Stand facing the patient's feet, and stabilize the patient's arm against your trunk with the hand farthest from the patient. Slight lateral motion of your trunk will provide the grade I distraction.
- Place the web space of your other hand just distal to the acromion process on the proximal humerus.

Mobilizing Force
With the hand on the proximal humerus, glide the humerus in an inferior direction.

Alternate Position
Sitting (Fig. 6–16*B*).

GH Elevation Progression (Fig. 6–17*A*)

Indication
To increase elevation beyond 90 degrees of abduction.

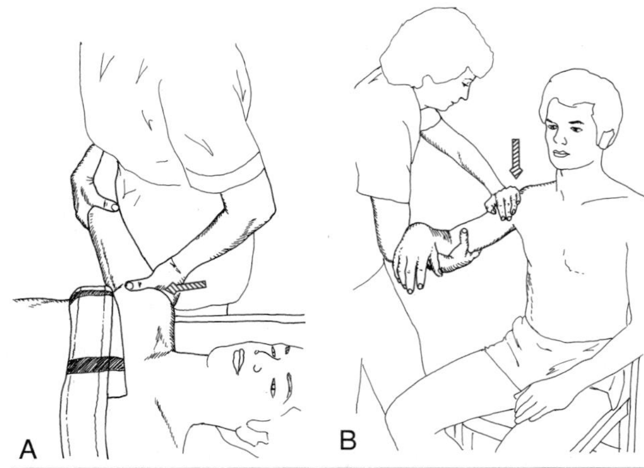

Figure 6–16 Caudal glide with the shoulder near 90 degrees, *(A)* supine and *(B)* sitting.

Patient Position

Supine, with the arm abducted and elevated to the end of its available range. The humerus is then externally rotated to its limit.

Therapist Position and Hand Placement

- Same as caudal glide progression.
- Adjust your body position so that the hand applying the mobilizing force is aligned with the treatment plane.
- With the hand grasping the elbow, apply a grade I distraction force.

Mobilizing Force

- With the hand on the proximal humerus, glide the humerus in a progressively anterior direction against the inferior folds of the capsule in the axilla.
- The direction of force with respect to the patient's body will depend on the amount of upward rotation and protraction of the scapula.

Alternate Position

Sitting (Fig. 6–17*B*).

GH Posterior Glide (Fig. 6–18)

Indications

To increase flexion; to increase internal rotation.

Patient Position

Supine, with the arm in resting position.

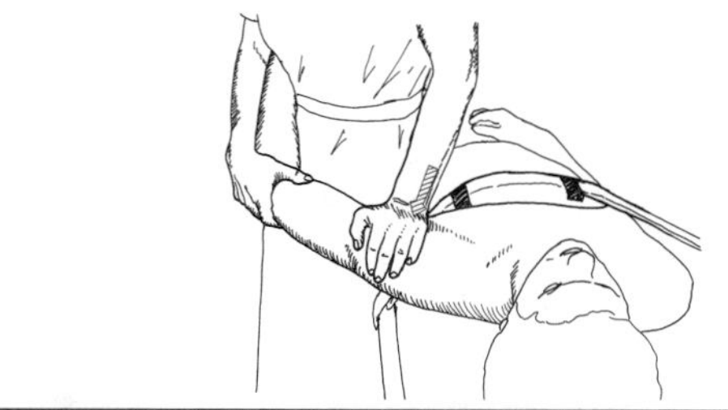

Figure 6–18 Posterior glide; glenohumeral joint.

Therapist Position and Hand Placement

- Stand with your back to the patient, between the patient's trunk and arm.
- Support the arm against your trunk, grasping the distal humerus with your lateral hand. This position provides grade I distraction to the joint.
- Place the lateral border of your top hand just distal to the anterior margin of the joint, with your fingers pointing superiorly. This hand gives the mobilizing force.

Mobilizing Force

Glide the humeral head posteriorly by moving the entire arm as you bend your knees.

GH Posterior Glide Progression (Fig. 6–19)

Indications

To increase posterior gliding when flexion approaches 90 degrees; to increase horizontal adduction.

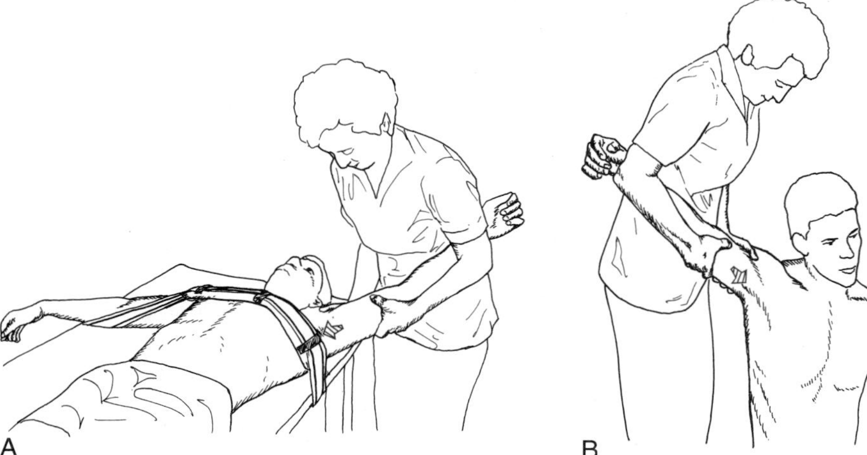

Figure 6–17 Elevation progression; glenohumeral joint *(A)* supine and *(B)* sitting. Used when the range is greater than 90 degrees. Note the externally rotated position of the humerus.

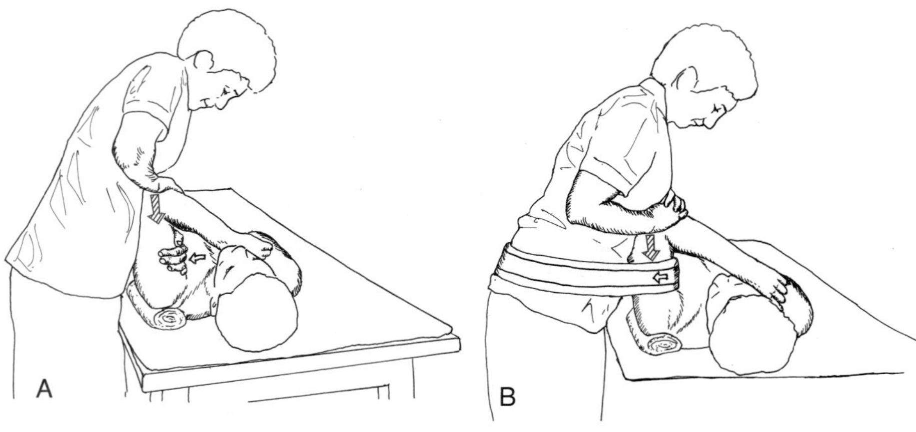

Figure 6–19 Posterior glide progression; glenohumeral joint. *(A)* Using one hand or *(B)* using a belt to give a grade 1 distraction force.

Patient Position
Supine, with arm flexed to 90 degrees, internally rotated, with elbow flexed. The arm may also be placed in horizontal adduction.

Hand Placement
- Place padding under the scapula for stabilization.
- Place one hand across the proximal surface of the humerus to apply a grade I distraction.
- Place your other hand over the patient's elbow.
- A belt placed around your pelvis and the patient's humerus may be used to apply the distraction force.

Mobilizing Force
Glide the humerus posteriorly by pushing down at the elbow through the long axis of the humerus.

GH Anterior Glide (Fig. 6–20)

Indications
To increase extension; to increase external rotation.

Patient Position
Prone, with arm in resting position over the edge of the treatment table, supported on your thigh. Stabilize the acromion with padding.

Therapist Position and Hand Placement
- Stand facing the top of the table with the leg closer to the table in a forward stride position.
- Support the patient's arm against your thigh with your outside hand; the arm positioned on your thigh provides a grade I distraction.
- Place the ulnar border of your other hand just distal to the posterior angle of the acromion process, with your fingers pointing superiorly; this hand gives the mobilizing force.

Mobilizing Force
Glide the humeral head in an anterior and slightly medial direction. Bend both knees so the entire arm moves anteriorly.

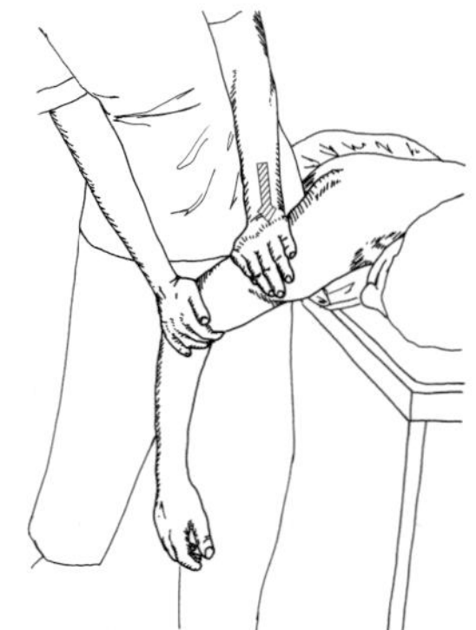

Figure 6–20 Anterior glide; glenohumeral joint.

Precaution: Do not lift the arm at the elbow and thereby cause an angulation of the humerus: such angulation could lead to an anterior subluxation or dislocation of the humeral head.

GH Anterior Glide Progression

Indication
To increase external rotation.

Precaution: Do not place the shoulder in 90 degrees abduction and then progress to externally rotating the arm while applying an anterior glide. Such a technique may lead to anterior subluxation of the humeral head.

Techniques
- Use a distraction progression of the humerus. Begin with the shoulder in resting position, externally rotate the humerus, then apply a grade III distraction perpendicular to the plane of the glenoid fossa (see Fig. 8–7).
- Use elevation progression (see Fig. 6–17) because external rotation is incorporated into that technique.

Note: To gain full elevation of the humerus, the accessory and component motions of clavicular elevation and rotation, scapular rotation, and external rotation of the humerus as well as adequate joint play anteriorly and inferiorly are necessary. The clavicular and scapular mobilizations are described in the following sections.

Acromioclavicular Joint: Anterior Glide (Fig. 6–21)

Indication
To increase mobility of the joint.

Stabilization
Fixate the scapula at the acromion process.

Patient Position
Sitting or prone.

Hand Placement
- With the patient sitting, stand behind the patient and stabilize the acromion process with the fingers of your lateral hand.
- The thumb of your other hand is placed posteriorly on the clavicle, just medial to the joint space.

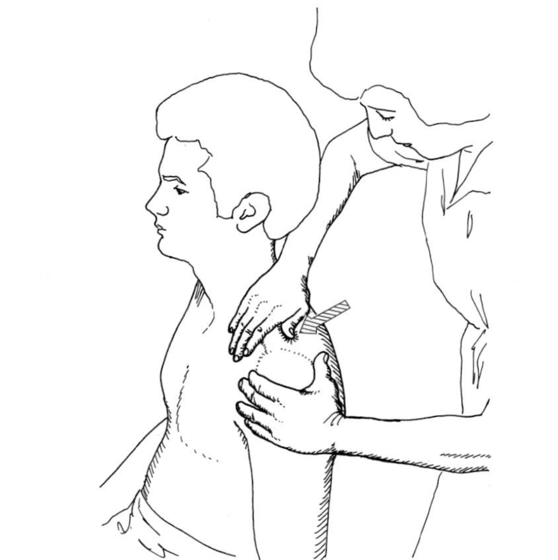

Figure 6–21 Anterior glide; acromioclavicular joint.

- With the patient prone, stabilize the acromion with a towel roll under the shoulder.

Mobilizing Force
Your thumb pushes the clavicle anteriorly.

Sternoclavicular (SC) Joint

The proximal articulating surface of the clavicle is convex superiorly/inferiorly and concave anteriorly/posteriorly.

Patient Position and Stabilization
Supine. The thorax provides stability to the sternum.

SC Posterior Glide (Fig. 6–22)

Indication
To increase retraction.

Hand Placement
- Place your thumb on the anterior surface of the proximal end of the clavicle.
- Flex your index finger and place the middle phalanx along the caudal surface of the clavicle to support the thumb.

Mobilizing Force
Push with your thumb in a posterior direction.

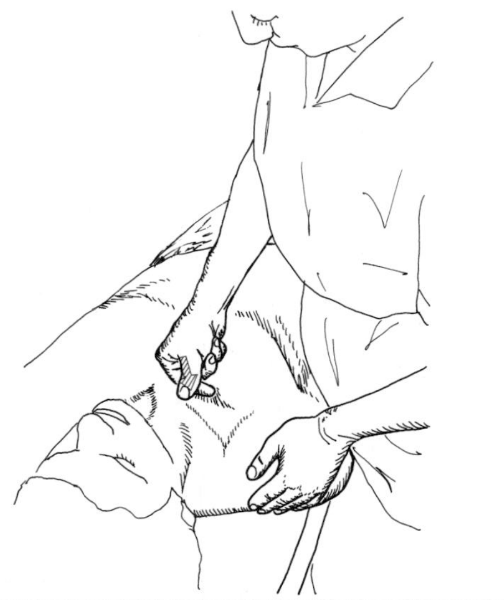

Figure 6–22 Posterior glide of the sternoclavicular joint; the same hand placement is used for superior glide.

SC Anterior Glide (Fig. 6–23)

Indication
To increase protraction.

Hand Placement
Your fingers are placed superiorly and thumb inferiorly around the clavicle.

Mobilizing Force
The fingers and thumb lift the clavicle anteriorly.

SC Inferior Glide (Fig. 6–23)

Indication
To increase elevation.

Hand Placement
Your fingers are placed superior to the clavicle.

Mobilizing Force
Your fingers pull the proximal clavicle caudally.

SC Superior Glide (see Fig. 6–22)

Indication
To increase depression.

Hand Placement
Flex the PIP joint of your index finger and place the radial border along the inferior aspect of the clavicle.

Mobilizing Force
Push the clavicle with your index finger in a superior direction.

Scapulothoracic Articulation

This is not a true joint, but the soft tissue is stretched to obtain normal shoulder girdle mobility (Fig. 6–24).

Indications
To increase scapular motions of elevation, depression, protraction, retraction, rotation, and winging. (Winging is an accessory motion that occurs when a person attempts to place the hand behind the back,

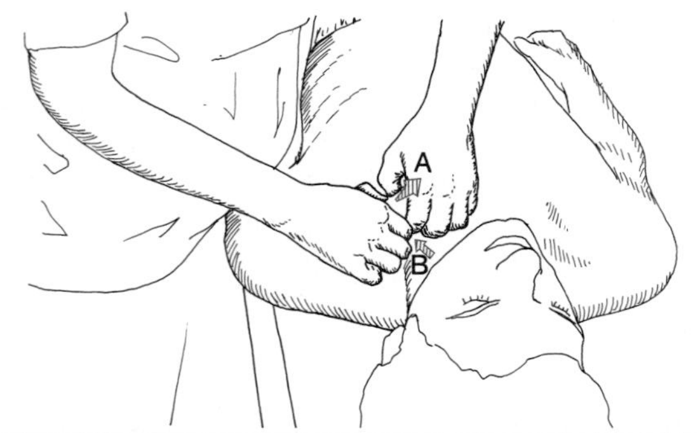

Figure 6–23 *(A)* Anterior glide of the sternoclavicular joint. *(B)* Same hand placement is used for inferior glide.

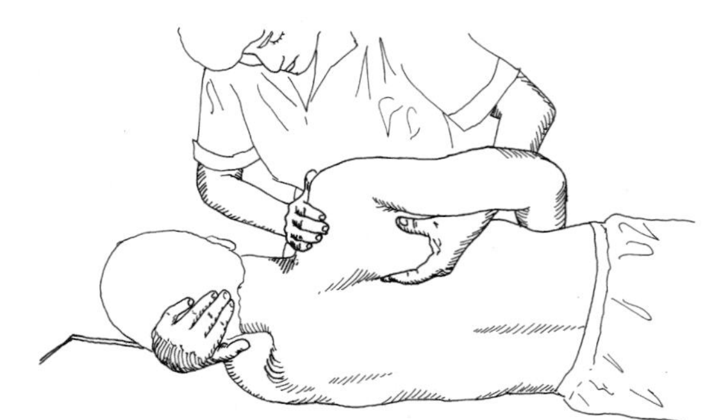

Figure 6–24 Scapulothoracic mobilization.

accompanying shoulder internal rotation and scapular downward rotation.)

Patient Position

- If there is little mobility, begin prone (see Fig. 2–6), and progress to side-lying, with the patient facing you.
- The patient's arm is draped over your inferior arm and allowed to hang so that the muscles are relaxed.

Hand Placement

- Your superior hand is placed across the acromion process to control the direction of motion.
- The fingers of your inferior hand scoop under the medial border and inferior angle of the scapula.

Mobilizing Force

The scapula is moved in the desired direction by lifting from the inferior angle or by pushing on the acromion process.

The Elbow and Forearm Complex (Fig. 6–25)

The Humeroulnar (HU) Articulation

The convex trochlea articulates with the concave olecranon fossa.

Resting Position

Elbow flexed 70 degrees, forearm supinated 10 degrees.

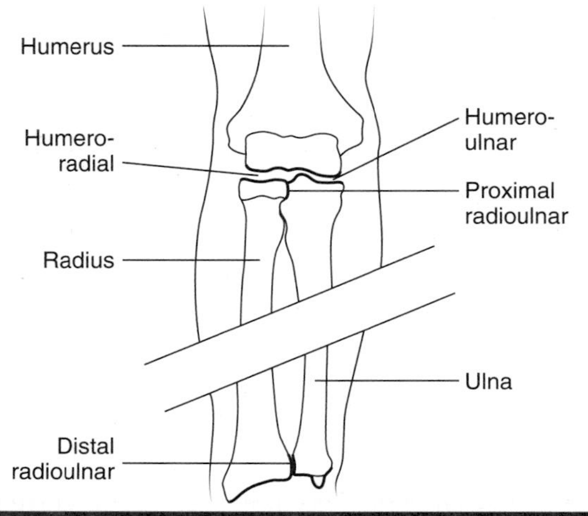

Figure 6–25 Bones and joints of the elbow complex.

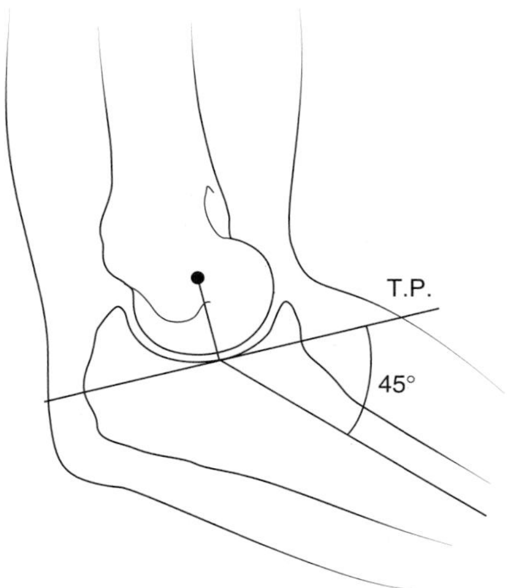

Figure 6–26 Lateral view of the humeroulnar joint, depicting the treatment plane (T.P.).

Treatment Plane

In the olecranon fossa, angled approximately 45 degrees from the long axis of the ulna (Fig. 6–26).

Stabilization

Fixate the humerus against the treatment table with a belt or use an assistant to hold it. The patient may roll on to his or her side and fixate the humerus with the contralateral hand if muscle relaxation can be maintained around the elbow joint being mobilized.

HU Joint Traction/Distraction (Fig. 6–27A)

Indications

Testing; initial treatment (sustained grade II); pain control (grade I or II oscillation); to increase flexion or extension.

Patient Position

Supine, elbow over the edge of the treatment table or supported with padding just proximal to the olecranon process. The wrist rests against your shoulder, allowing the elbow to be in resting position.

Hand Placement

Using your medial hand, place your fingers over the proximal ulna on the volar surface; reinforce it with your other hand.

Mobilizing Force

Force against the proximal ulna at a 45-degree angle to the shaft.

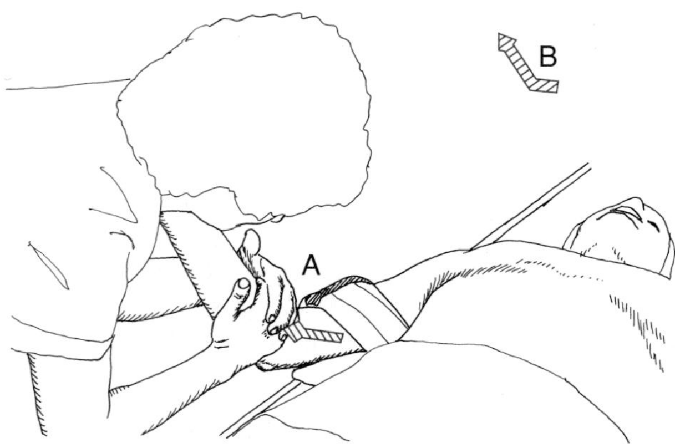

Figure 6–27 Joint traction. *(A)* Humeroulnar articulation. *(B)* Arrow indicating joint traction with distal glide.

HU Distraction Progression

Indications
To increase flexion or extension.

Patient Position
The elbow is positioned at the end of its available ROM before applying the distracting force.

Hand Placement
- Adjust your position to best apply the mobilization force and stabilize the humerus.
- When the elbow is near extension, stand and place the base of your hand against the proximal ulna.

Mobilizing Force
Always force against the ulna at a 45-degree angle, no matter at what angle the elbow is.

HU Distal Glide (Fig. 6–27*B*)

Indication
To increase flexion.

Patient Position and Hand Placement
Supine, elbow over the edge of the treatment table. Begin with the elbow in resting position. Progress by positioning it at the end range of flexion.

Mobilizing Force
Use a scooping motion in which distraction is applied to the joint first. Then pull along the long axis of the ulna (distal traction).

HU Radial Glide

Indication
To increase flexion.

Patient Position
- Side-lying with the shoulder laterally rotated and the humerus supported on the table.
- Begin with the elbow in resting position; progress to end of range flexion.

Hand Placement
The base of the proximal hand is just distal to the elbow; the distal hand supports the distal forearm.

Mobilizing Force
Force against the ulna in a radial direction.

HU Ulnar Glide

Indication
To increase extension.

Patient Position
- Same as with radial glide except a block or wedge is placed under the proximal forearm for stabilization (using distal stabilization).
- Initially, the elbow is placed in resting position and is progressed to end of range extension.

Mobilizing Force
Force against the distal humerus in a radial direction, causing the ulna to glide ulnarly.

The Humeroradial (HR) Articulation

The convex capitulum articulates with the concave radial head.

Resting Position
Elbow extended, forearm supinated to the end of the available range.

Treatment Plane
In the concave radial head perpendicular to the long axis of the radius.

Stabilization
Fixate the humerus with one of your hands.

HR Joint Traction/Distraction (Fig. 6–28)

Indications
To increase mobility of the radius; to correct a pushed elbow (proximal displacement of the radius).

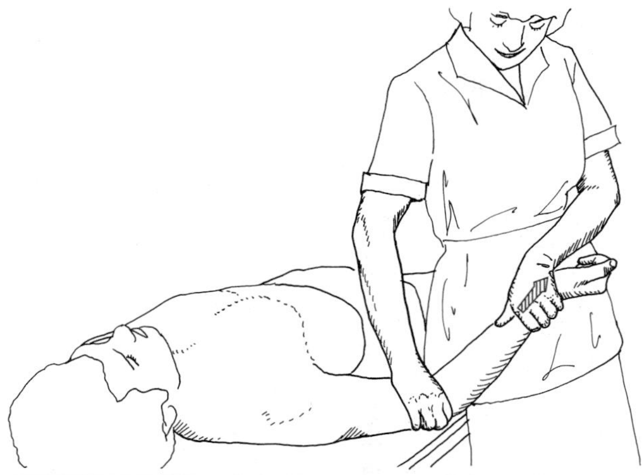

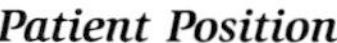

Figure 6–28 Joint traction; humeroradial articulation.

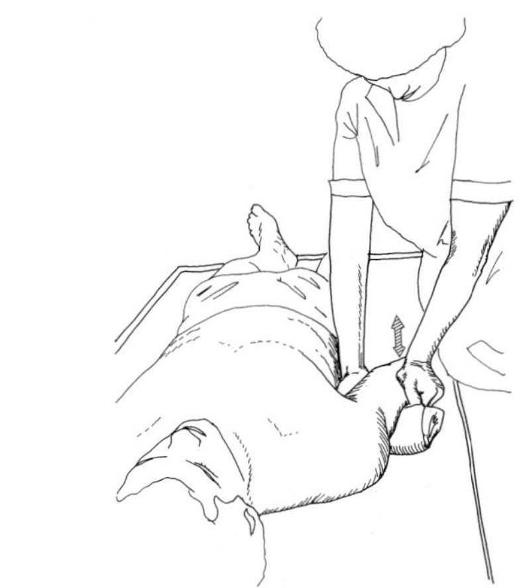

Figure 6–29 Dorsal and volar glide; humeroradial articulation.

Patient Position

Supine; or sitting, with the arm resting on the treatment table.

Therapist Position and Hand Placement

- Position yourself on the ulnar side of the patient's forearm.
- Stabilize the patient's humerus with your superior hand.
- Grasp around the distal radius with the fingers and thenar eminence of your inferior hand. Be sure your are not grasping around the distal ulna.

Mobilizing Force

Pull the radius distally (long-axis traction will cause joint traction).

HR Dorsal or Volar Glide (Fig. 6–29)

Indications

Dorsal glide head of the radius to increase elbow extension; volar glide, to increase flexion.

Patient Position

Supine, or sitting with the elbow extended and supinated to the end of the available range.

Hand Placement

- Stabilize the humerus with your hand that is on the medial side of the patient's arm.
- Place the palmar surface of your lateral hand on the volar aspect and your fingers on the dorsal aspect of the radial head.

Mobilizing Force

- Move the radial head dorsally with the palm of your hand or volarly with your fingers.
- If a stronger force is needed for the volar glide, realign your body, and push with the base of your hand against the dorsal surface in a volar direction.

HR Joint Compression (Fig. 6–30)

Indication

To reduce a pulled elbow subluxation.

Patient Position

Sitting or supine.

Hand Placement

- Using the same as that of the patient, place your thenar eminence against the patient's thenar eminence (locking thumbs).
- Fixate the humerus and proximal ulna against a firm object (treatment table or your other hand).

Mobilizing Force

Push along the long axis of the radius by putting pressure against the thenar eminence; simultaneously supinate the forearm.

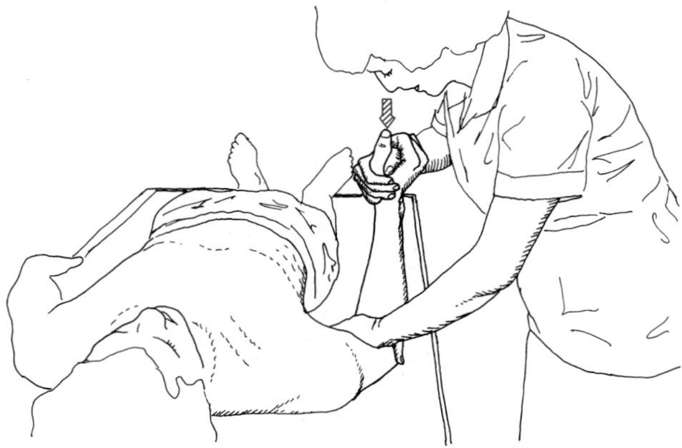

Figure 6–30 Joint compression; humeroradial articulation.

Note: To replace an acute subluxation, a quick motion (thrust) is used.

Proximal Radioulnar (RU) Joint (Fig. 6–31)

The convex rim of the radial head articulates with the concave radial notch on the ulna.

Resting Position
Elbow flexed 70 degrees, forearm supinated 35 degrees.

Treatment Plane
In the radial notch of the ulna, parallel to the long axis of the ulna.

Stabilization
Proximal ulna.

Indications
Dorsal glide, to increase pronation; volar glide, to increase supination.

Patient Position

- Sitting or supine, with the elbow and forearm in resting position.
- Progress by placing the forearm at the limit of the range of pronation prior to administering the dorsal glide, or at the limit of the range of supination prior to administering the volar glide.

Hand Placement

- Fixate the ulna with your medial hand around the medial aspect of the forearm.
- Place your other hand around the head of the radius with the fingers on the volar surface and the palm on the dorsal surface.

Mobilizing Force

- Force the radial head volarly by pushing with your palm or dorsally by pulling with your fingers.
- If a stronger force is needed for the dorsal glide, move around to the other side of the patient, switch hands, and push from the volar surface with the base of your hand against the radial head.

Distal Radioulnar Joint (Fig. 6–32)

The concave ulnar notch of the radius articulates with the convex head of the ulna.

Resting Position
Supinated 10 degrees.

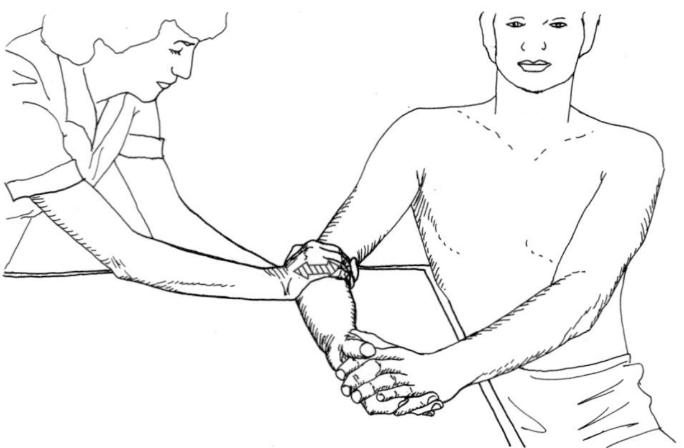

Figure 6–31 Dorsal-volar glide; proximal radioulnar joint.

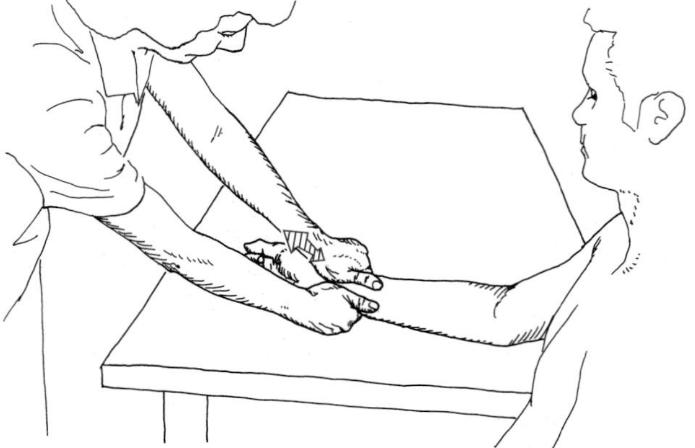

Figure 6–32 Dorsal-volar glide; distal radioulnar joint.

Treatment Plane
Articulating surface of the radius, parallel to the long axis of the radius.

Stabilization
Distal ulna.

Indications
Dorsal glide, to increase supination; volar glide to increase pronation.

Patient Position
Sitting, with arm on the treatment table; forearm in resting position.

Hand Placement
Stabilize the distal ulna by placing the fingers of one hand on the dorsal surface and the thenar eminence and thumb on the volar surface. Place your other hand in the same manner around the distal radius.

Mobilizing Force
Glide the distal radius dorsally or volarly parallel to the ulna.

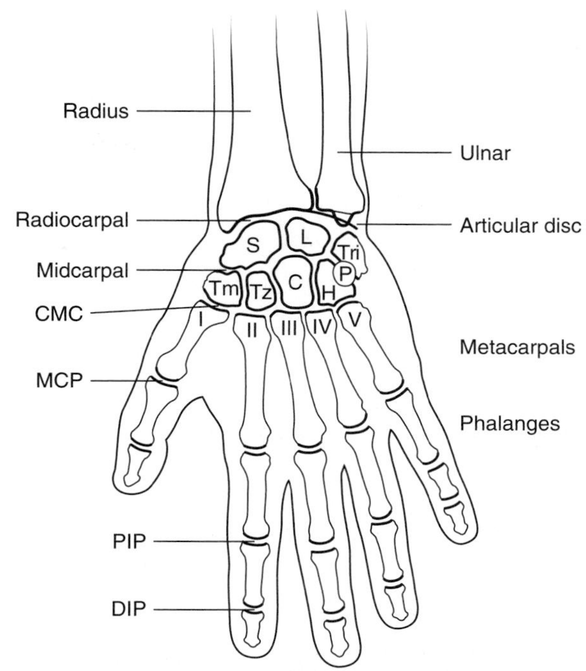

Figure 6–33 Bones and joints of the wrist and hand.

The Wrist Complex (Fig. 6–33)

Radiocarpal (RC) Joint

The concave distal radius articulates with the convex proximal row of carpals, which is composed of the scaphoid, lunate, and triquetrum.

Resting Position
Straight line through the radius and third metacarpal with slight ulnar deviation.

Treatment Plane
In the articulating surface of the radius perpendicular to the long axis of the radius.

Stabilization
Distal radius and ulna.

RC Joint Traction—Distraction (Fig. 6–34)

Indications
Testing; initial treatment; pain control; general mobility of the wrist.

Patient Position
Sitting, with forearm supported on the treatment table, wrist over the edge of the table.

Hand Placement
- With the hand closest to the patient, grasp around the styloid processes and fixate the radius and ulna against the table.
- Grasp around the distal row of carpals with your other hand.

Mobilizing Force
Pull in a distal direction with respect to the arm.

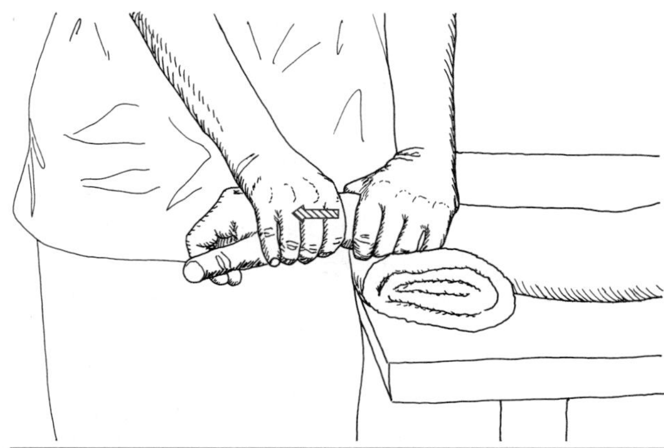

Figure 6–34 Joint traction; wrist joint.

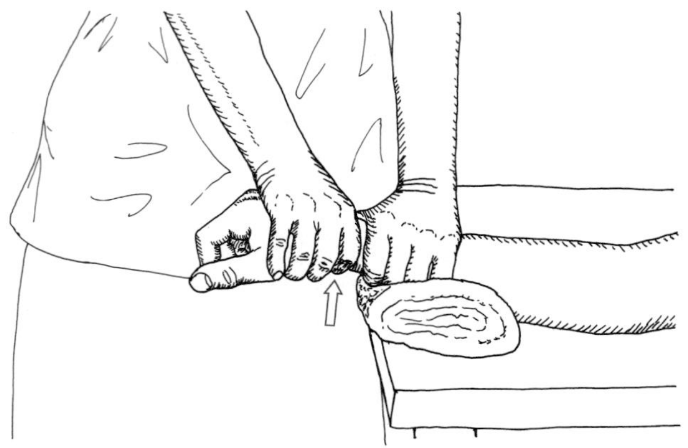

Figure 6–35 Dorsal glide; general mobilization of the wrist joint.

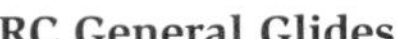

RC General Glides

Indications

Dorsal glide to increase flexion (Fig. 6–35); volar glide to increase extension (Fig. 6–36); radial glide to increase ulnar deviation; ulnar glide to increase radial deviation (Fig. 6–37).

Patient Position and Hand Placement

Same as with the distraction technique, except rotate the forearm when performing radial or ulnar glides for ease in accomplishing the technique.

Mobilizing Force

Comes from the hand around the distal row of carpals.

Progression

Progress by moving the wrist to the end of the available range and glide in the defined direction. Specific carpal gliding techniques described in the next sections are used to increase mobility at isolated articulations.

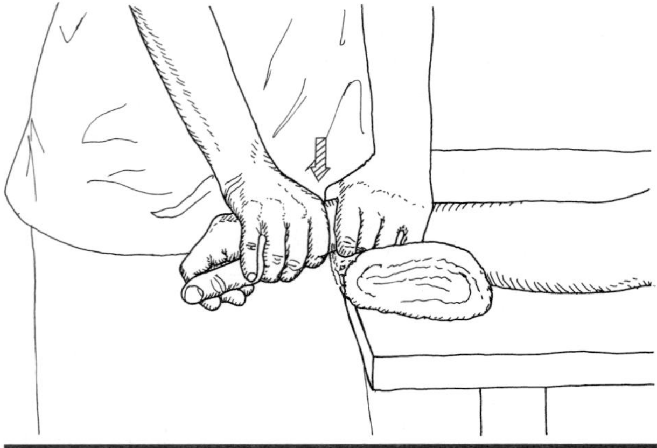

Figure 6–36 Volar glide; general mobilization of the wrist joint.

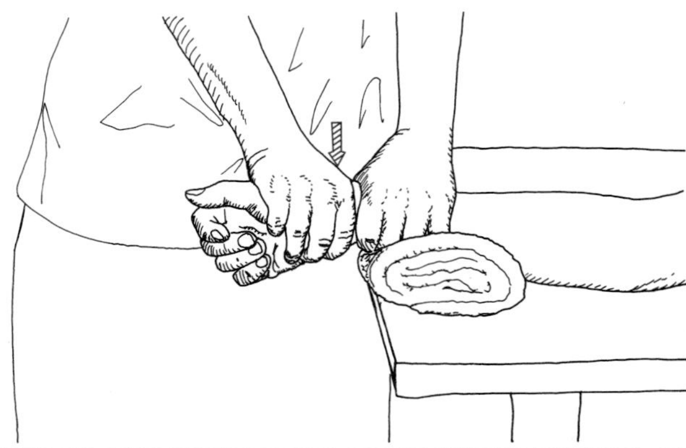

Figure 6–37 Ulnar glide; general mobilization of the wrist joint.

Specific Glides of the Carpals in the Proximal Row with the Radius and Ulna

Patient and Therapist Positions

- The patient sits.
- You stand and grasp the patient's hand so that the elbow hangs unsupported.
- The weight of the arm provides slight joint traction (grade I) so you then need only to apply the glides.

Hand Placement

Place your index fingers on the volar surface of the bone to be stabilized (see stabilization), the thumbs on the dorsal surface of the bone to be mobilized. The rest of your fingers hold the patient's hand so it is relaxed.

Stabilization

To increase flexion, the index fingers stabilize the distal bone (scaphoid or lunate) (Fig. 6–38). To increase extension, the index fingers stabilize the proximal bone (radius) (Fig. 6–39).

Mobilizing Force

- In each case, the force comes from the thumbs on the dorsal surface of the bone to be moved.
- Place one thumb on top of the other so that the force can be concentrated on a specific carpal.
- By mobilizing from the dorsal surface, pressure against the nerves, blood vessels, and tendons in the carpal tunnel and Guyon's canal is minimized

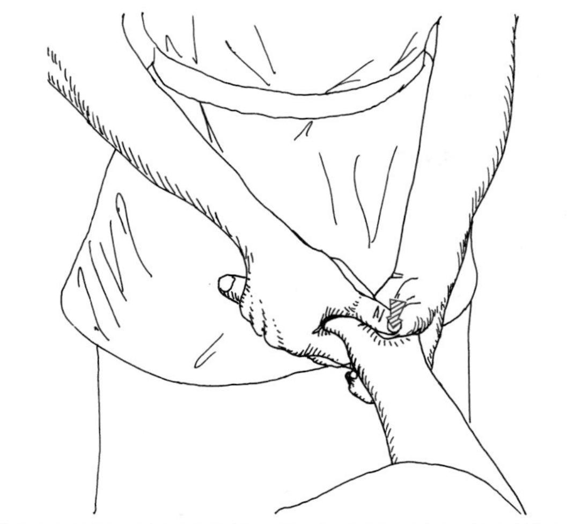

Figure 6–38 Stabilization of the distal bone; volar glide of the proximal bone; shown is stabilization of the scaphoid and lunate with the volar glide to the radius.

and a stronger mobilizing force can be used without pain.

Scaphoid-Radius and Lunate-Radius

In the scaphoid-radius, the scaphoid is convex, and the radius is concave. In the lunate-radius, the lunate is convex, and the radius is concave.

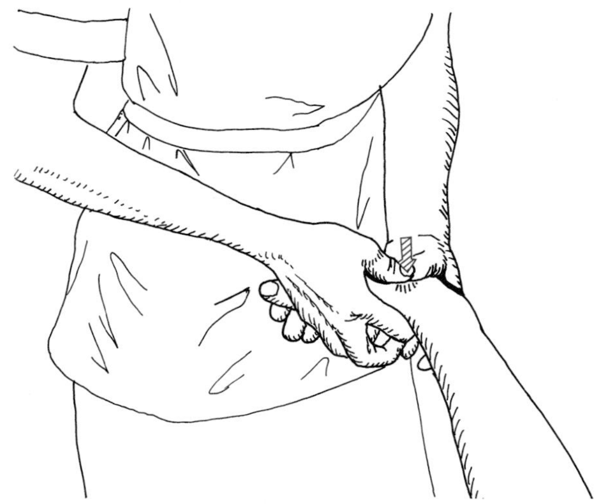

Figure 6–39 Stabilization of the proximal bone: volar guide of the distal bone; shown is stabilization of the radius with volar glide to the lunate.

Indications

To increase flexion, glide radius volarly on fixed scaphoid or glide radius volarly on fixed lunate (see Fig. 6–38). To increase extension, glide scaphoid volarly on fixed radius or glide lunate volarly on fixed radius (Fig. 6–39).

Ulnar-Meniscal Triquetral Articulation

Indications

To unlock the articular disk, which may block motions of the wrist or forearm, glide the ulna volarly on a fixed triquetrum.

Specific Glides of the Intercarpal Joints

Patient Position and Hand Placement

- The patient sits with the elbow unsupported as with the specific RC glides.
- You stand and grasp the patient's hand. The index fingers are on the volar surface, the thumbs on the dorsal surface, and the rest of the fingers hold the patient's hand.

Stabilization

In all cases, the stabilization is applied with the index fingers overlapped on the volar surface.

Mobilization Force

In all cases, the force comes from the overlapped thumbs on the dorsal surface.

Glides to Increase Extension

Stabilize the bone that has the concave articulating surface, and apply the mobilizing force against the dorsal surface of the bone with the convex articulating surface. The force is in a volar direction.

Examples

- To increase extension and radial deviation at the trapezium-trapezoid/scaphoid articulation, glide the scaphoid volarly with your thumbs while stabilizing the trapezium-trapezoid unit with your index fingers.
- To increase extension at the capitate/lunate articulation, glide the capitate volarly with your thumbs while stabilizing the lunate with your index fingers.

Glides to Increase Flexion

Stabilize the bone that has the convex articulating surface and apply the mobilizing force against the dorsal surface of the bone with the concave articulating surface. The force is in a volar direction.

Examples

- To increase flexion at the trapezium-trapezoid/ scaphoid articulation, glide the trapezium-trapezoid unit volarly with your thumbs while stabilizing the scaphoid with your index fingers.
- To increase flexion at the capitate/lunate articulation, glide the lunate volarly with your thumbs while stabilizing the capitate.

The Hand and Finger Joints

The Carpometacarpal (CMC) and Intermetacarpal (IMC) Joints of Digits II-V: Joint Traction (Fig. 6–40)

Indication

To increase mobility of the hand.

Stabilization and Hand Placement

Stabilize the respective carpal with thumb and index finger of one hand. With your other hand, grasp around the proximal portion of a metacarpal.

Mobilizing Force

Apply long-axis traction to the metacarpal to separate the joint surfaces.

CMC and IMC Volar Glide

Indication

To increase mobility of the arch of the hand.

Stabilization and Hand Placement

Stabilize the carpals with the thumb and index finger of one hand; place the thenar eminence of your other hand along the dorsal aspect of the metacarpals to provide the mobilization force.

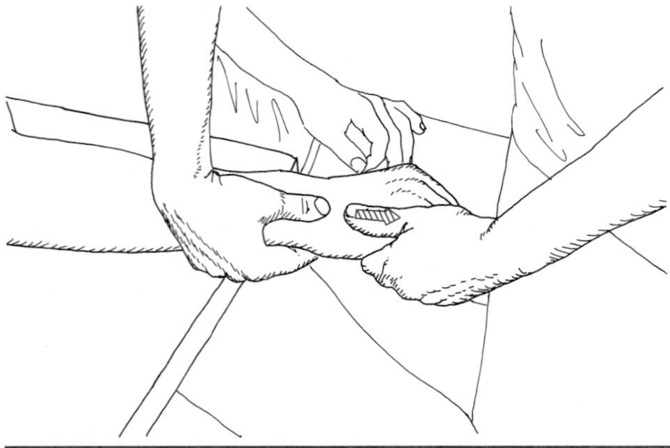

Figure 6–40 Joint traction; carpometacarpal joint.

Mobilizing Force

Glide the proximal portion of the metacarpal volar ward. See also the technique for cupping and flattening the arch of the hand described in Chapter 2.

The Carpometacarpal (CMC) Joint of the Thumb

This is a saddle joint. The trapezium is concave and the proximal metacarpal convex for abduction/ adduction. The trapezium is convex, and the proximal metacarpal is concave for flexion/extension.

Resting Position

Midway between flexion and extension and between abduction and adduction.

Stabilization

Fixate the trapezium with the hand that is closer to the patient.

Treatment Plane

In the trapezium, for abduction-adduction; in the proximal metacarpal, for flexion-extension.

CMC Joint Traction of the Thumb

Indications

Testing; initial treatment; pain control; general mobility.

Patient Position

Forearm and hand resting on the treatment table.

Hand Placement

- Fixate the trapezium with the hand that is closer to the patient.
- Grasp the patient's metacarpal by wrapping your fingers around it (similar to Fig. 6–41*A*).

Mobilizing Force

Apply long-axis traction to separate the joint surfaces.

CMC Glides of the Thumb (Fig. 6–41)

Indications

To increase flexion, ulnar glide; to increase extension, radial glide; to increase abduction, dorsal glide; to increase adduction, volar glide.

Patient Position and Hand Placement

- The trapezium is stabilized by grasping it directly or by wrapping your fingers around the distal row of carpals.
- Place the thenar eminence of your other hand against the base of the patient's first metacarpal on the side opposite the desired glide. For example, as pictured in Fig. 6–41*A*, the surface of the thenar eminence is on the radial side of the metacarpal to cause an ulnar glide.

Mobilizing Force

Comes from your thenar eminence against the base of the metacarpal. Adjust your body position to line up the force as illustrated in Figure 6–41*A* through *D*.

The Metacarpophalangeal (MP) and Interphalangeal (IP) Joints of the Fingers

In all cases, the distal end of the proximal articulating surface is convex, and the proximal end of the distal articulating surface is concave.

Note: Because all the articulating surfaces are the same for the digits, all techniques are applied in the same manner to each joint.

Resting Position

Slight flexion in all joints.

Treatment Plane

In the distal articulating surface.

Stabilization

Rest the forearm and hand on the treatment table; fixate the proximal articulating surface with the fingers of one hand.

MP and IP Joint Traction/Distraction (Fig. 6–42)

Indications

Testing; initial treatment; pain control; general mobility.

Hand Placement

Use your proximal hand to stabilize the proximal bone; wrap the fingers and thumb of your other hand around the distal bone close to the joint.

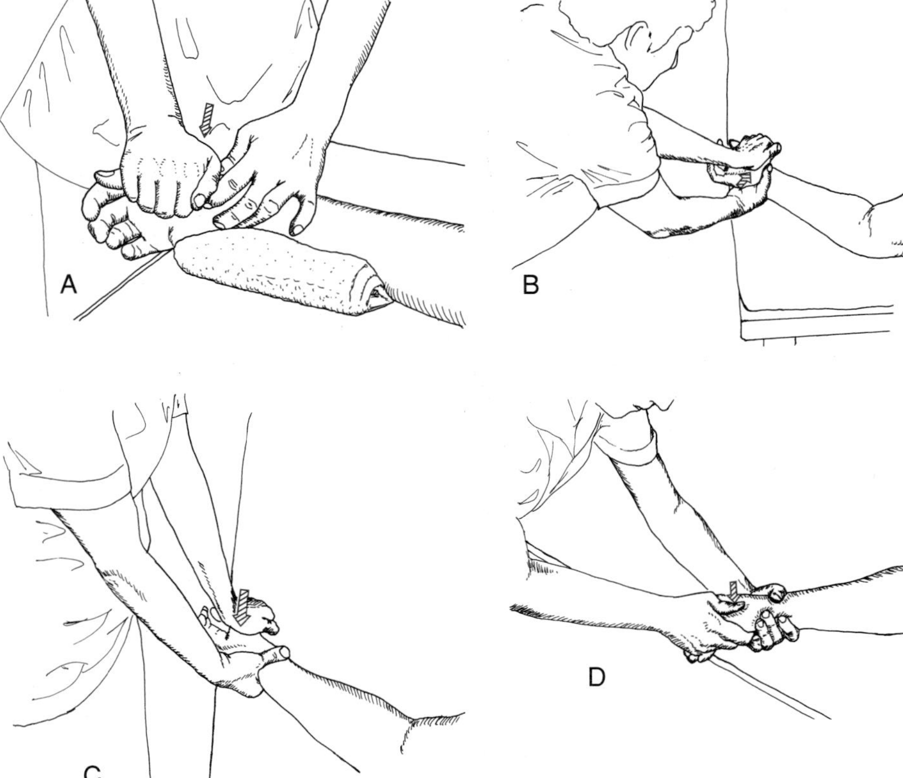

Figure 6–41 Carpometacarpal joint of the thumb. *(A)* Ulnar glide to increase flexion. *(B)* Radial glide to increase extension. *(C)* Dorsal glide to increase abduction. *(D)* Volar glide to increase adduction. Note that the thumb of the therapist is placed in the web space between the index and thumb of the patient's hand to apply a volar glide.

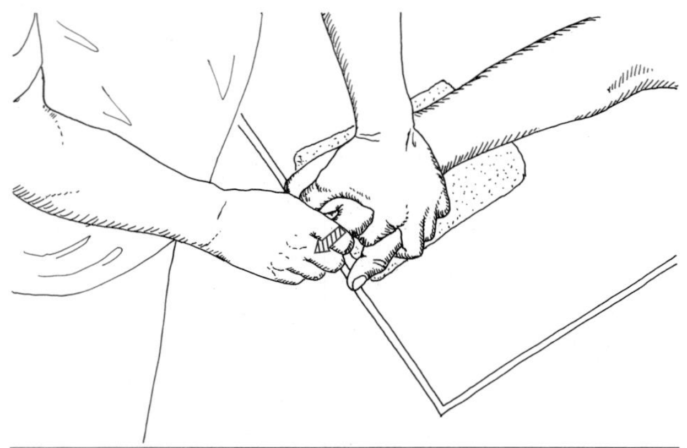

Figure 6–42 Joint traction of a metacarpophalangeal joint.

Mobilizing Force
Apply long-axis traction to separate the joint surface.

MP and IP Glides

Indications
To increase flexion, volar glide (Fig. 6–43); to increase extension, dorsal glide; to increase abduction or adduction, radial or ulnar glide (depending on finger).

Mobilizing Force
The glide force is applied by the thumb against the proximal end of the bone to be moved.

MP and IP Rotations (Fig. 6–44)

Indications
To increase final degrees of motion.

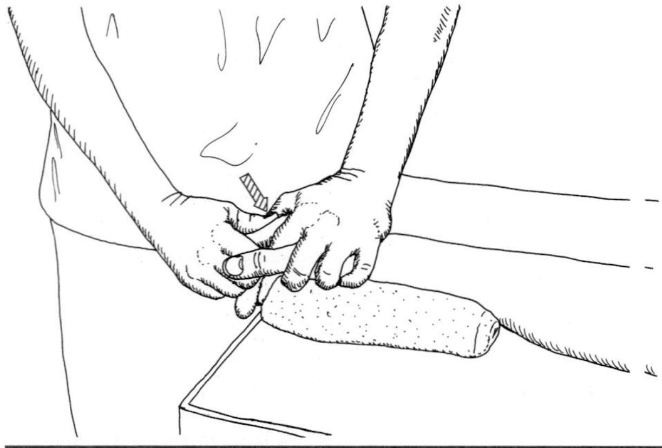

Figure 6–43 Volar glide of a metacarpophalangeal joint.

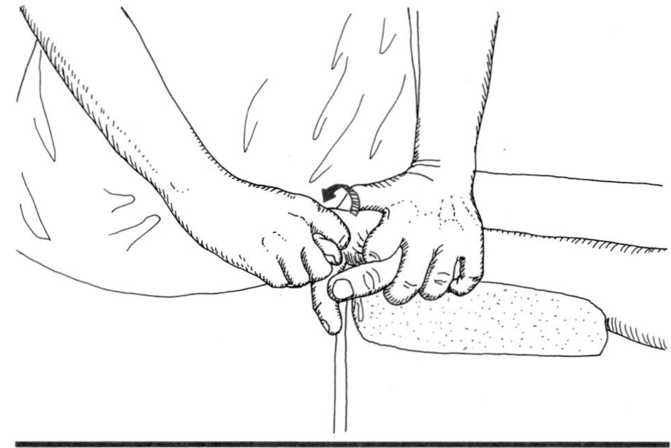

Figure 6–44 Rotation of a metacarpophalangeal joint.

Mobilizing Force
Initially, rotate the distal bone on the stabilized proximal bone, then apply a traction force.

The Hip Joint (Fig. 6–45)

The concave acetabulum receives the convex femoral head.

Resting Position
Hip flexion 30 degrees, abduction 30 degrees, and slight external rotation.

Stabilization
Fixate the pelvis to the treatment table with belts.

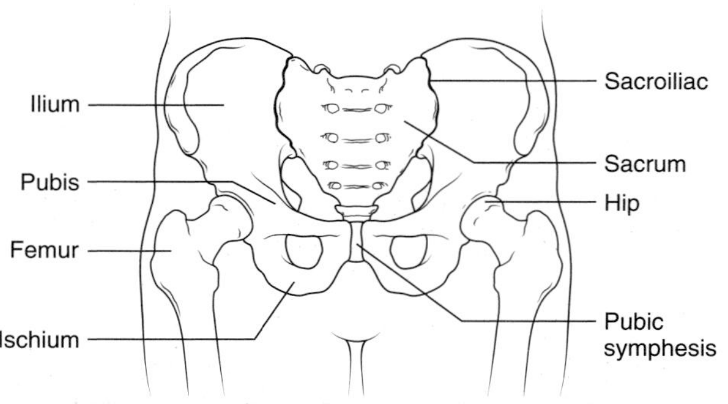

Figure 6–45 Bones and joints of the pelvis and hip.

Hip Distraction of the Weight-Bearing Surface—Caudal Glide (Fig. 6–46)

Note: Because of the deep configuration of this joint, traction applied perpendicular to the treatment plane causes a lateral glide of the superior, weight-bearing surface. To get separation of the weight-bearing surface, a caudal glide is used.

Indications
Testing; initial treatment; pain control; general mobility.

Patient Position
Supine, with hip in resting position and the knee extended.

Precaution: With knee dysfunction, this position should not be used; see alternate position following.

Therapist Position and Hand Placement
Stand at the end of the treatment table; place a belt around your trunk, then cross the belt over the patient's foot and around the ankle. Place your hands proximal to the malleoli, under the belt. The belt allows you to use your body weight to apply the mobilizing force.

Mobilizing Force
A long-axis traction is applied by pulling on the leg as you lean backward.

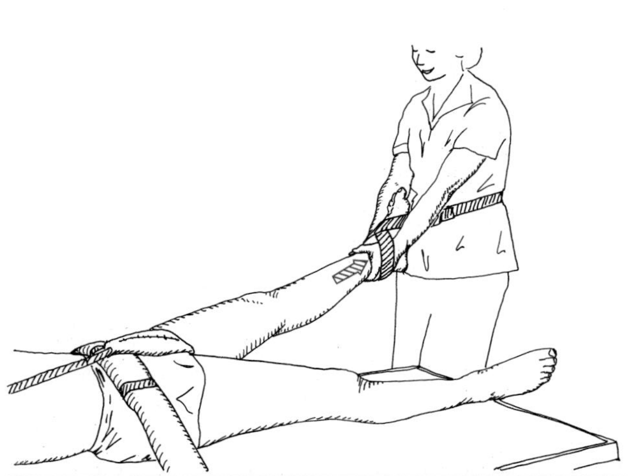

Figure 6–46 Distraction of the weight-bearing surface of the hip joint; caudal glide.

Alternate Position for Hip Caudal Glide

Indication
To apply distraction to the weight-bearing surface of the hip joint when there is knee dysfunction.

Patient Position
Supine, with the hip and knee flexed.

Therapist Position and Hand Placement
Wrap your hands around the epicondyles of the femur and distal thigh. Do not compress the patella.

Mobilizing Force
Comes from your hands and is applied in a caudal direction as you lean backward.

Hip Posterior Glide (Fig. 6–47)

Indications
To increase flexion; to increase internal rotation.

Patient Position
- Supine, with hips at the end of the table.
- The patient helps stabilize the pelvis and lumbar spine by flexing the opposite hip and holding the thigh against the chest with the hands.
- Initially, the hip to be mobilized is in resting position; progress to the end of the range.

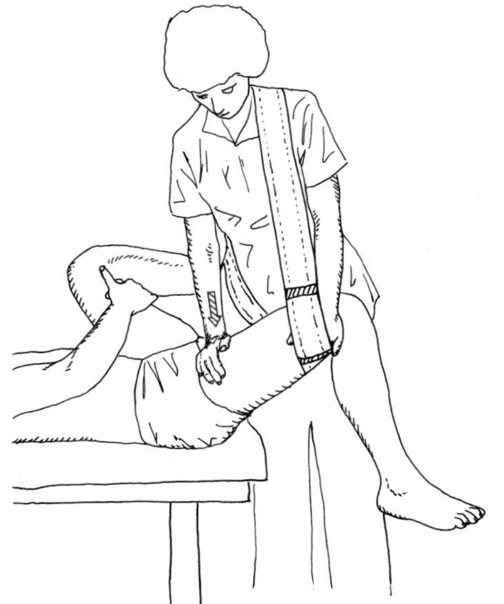

Figure 6–47 Posterior glide; hip joint.

Therapist Position and Hand Placement

Stand on the medial side of the patient's thigh. Place a belt around your shoulder and under the patient's thigh to help hold the weight of the lower extremity. Place your distal hand under the belt and distal thigh. Place your proximal hand on the anterior surface of the proximal thigh.

Mobilizing Force

Keep your elbows extended and flex your knees; apply the force through your proximal hand in a posterior direction.

Hip Anterior Glide (Fig. 6–48)

Indications

To increase extension; to increase external rotation.

Patient Position

Prone, with trunk resting on the table and hips over the edge. The opposite foot is on the floor.

Therapist Position and Hand Placement

- Stand on the medial side of the patient's thigh.
- Place a belt around your shoulder and the patient's thigh to help support the weight of the leg.
- With your distal hand, hold the patient's leg.
- Place your proximal hand posteriorly on the proximal thigh, just below the buttock.

Mobilizing Force

Keep your elbow extended and flex your knees; apply the force through your proximal hand in an anterior direction.

Alternate Position (Fig. 6–48B)

- Position patient side-lying with the thigh comfortably flexed and supported by pillows.
- Stand posterior to the patient and stabilize the pelvis across the anterior superior iliac spine with your cranial hand.
- Push against the posterior aspect of the greater trochanter in an anterior direction with your caudal hand.

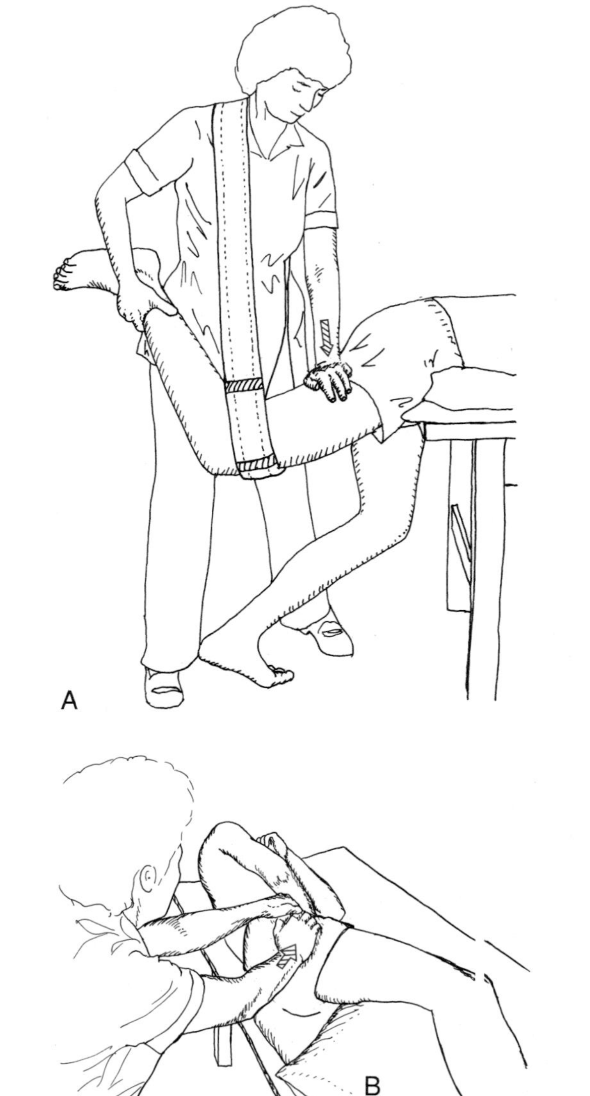

Figure 6–48 Anterior glide; hip joint (A) prone and (B) side-lying.

The Knee and Leg (Fig. 6–49)

The Tibiofemoral (TF) Articulation

The concave tibial plateaus articulate on the convex femoral condyles.

Resting Position

Flexion 25 degrees.

Treatment Plane

Along the surface of the tibial plateaus; therefore, it moves with the tibia as the knee angle changes.

Stabilization

In most cases, the femur is stabilized with a belt or by the table.

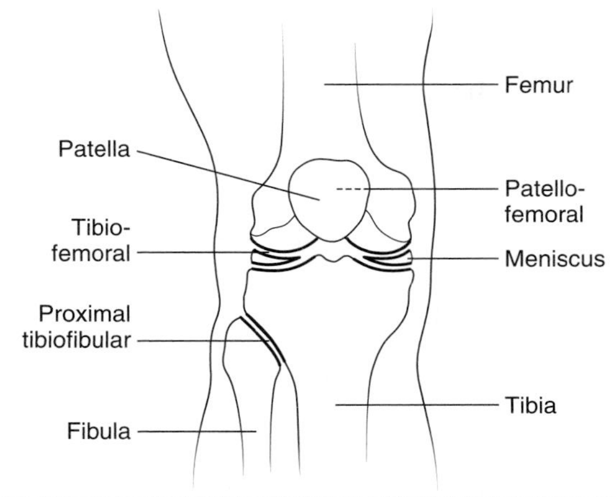

Figure 6–49 Bones and joints of the knee and leg.

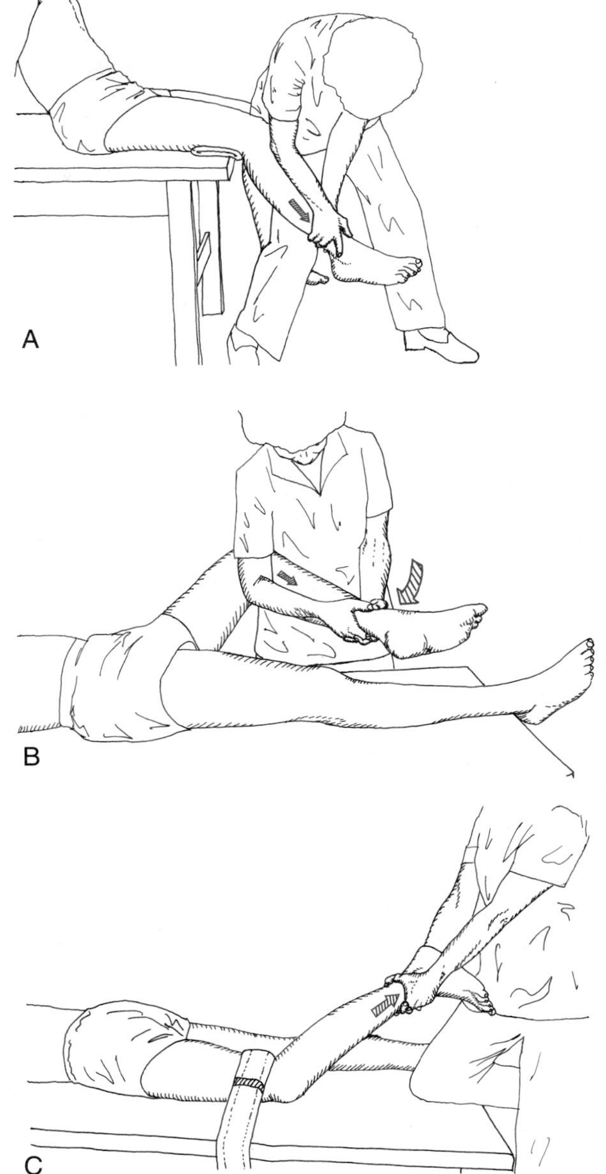

Figure 6–50 Traction of the knee joint *(A)* sitting, *(B)* supine, or *(C)* prone.

TF Joint Traction: Long-Axis Traction (Figs. 6–50A, *B*, and *C*)

Indications

Testing; initial treatment; pain control; general mobility.

Patient Position

- Sitting, supine, or prone, beginning with the knee in resting position.
- Progress to positioning the knee at the limit of the range of flexion or extension.
- Rotation of the tibia may be added prior to applying the traction force.

Hand Placement

Grasp around the distal leg, proximal to the malleoli with both hands.

Mobilizing Force

Pull on the long axis of the tibia to separate the joint surfaces.

TF Posterior Glide (Fig. 6–51)

Indications

Testing; to increase flexion.

Patient Position

Supine, with the foot resting on the table. The position for the drawer test can be used to mobilize the tibia either anteriorly or posteriorly, although no grade I distraction can be applied with the glides.

Therapist Position and Hand Placement

Sit on the table with your thigh fixating the patient's foot. With both hands, grasp around the tibia, fingers pointing posteriorly and thumbs anteriorly.

Mobilizing Force

Extend your elbows and lean your body weight forward; push the tibia posteriorly with your thumbs.

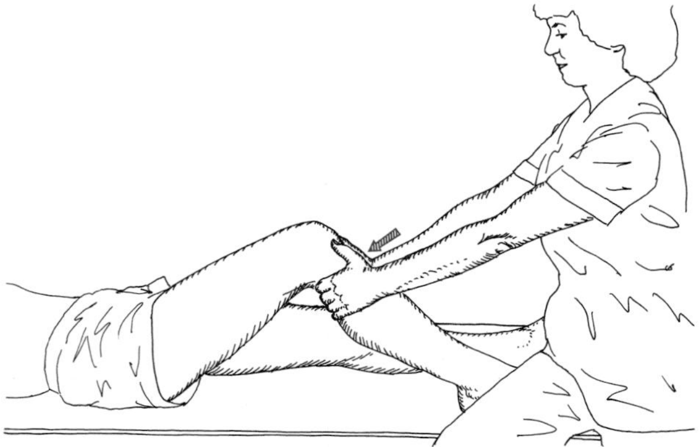

Figure 6–51 Posterior glide (drawer); knee joint.

TF Posterior Glide, Alternate Position, and Progression (Fig. 6–52)

Indication

To increase flexion.

Patient Position

- Sitting, with the knee flexed over the edge of the treatment table, beginning in resting position (Fig. 6–52*A*) and progressing to near 90 degrees with the tibia positioned in internal rotation (Fig. 6–52*B*).
- Once the knee flexes past 90 degrees, position the patient prone; place a small rolled towel proximal to the patella to minimize compression forces against the patella during the mobilization.

Therapist Position and Hand Placement

- When in resting position, stand on the medial side of the patient's leg. Hold the distal leg with your distal hand and place the palm of your proximal hand along the anterior border of the tibial plateaus.
- When near 90 degrees, sit on a low stool; stabilize the leg between your knees and place one hand on the anterior border of the tibial plateaus.
- When prone, stabilize the femur with one hand and place the other hand along the border of the tibial plateaus.

Mobilizing Force

- Extend your elbow and lean your body weight onto the tibia, gliding it posteriorly.
- When progressing with medial rotation of the tibia at the end of the range of flexion, the force is applied in a posterior direction against the medial side of the tibia.

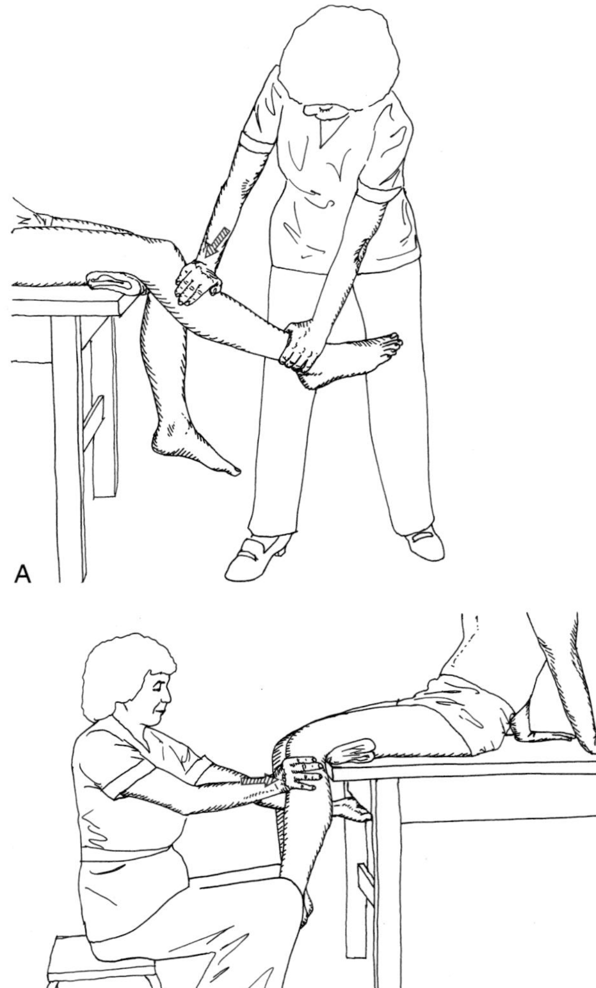

Figure 6–52 Posterior glide of the knee joint *(A)* in resting position and *(B)* near 90 degrees.

TF Anterior Glide (Fig. 6–53)

Indication

To increase extension.

Patient Position

- Prone, begin with the knee in resting position; progress to the end of the available range.
- The tibia may also be positioned in lateral rotation.
- Place a small pad under the distal femur to prevent patellar compression.

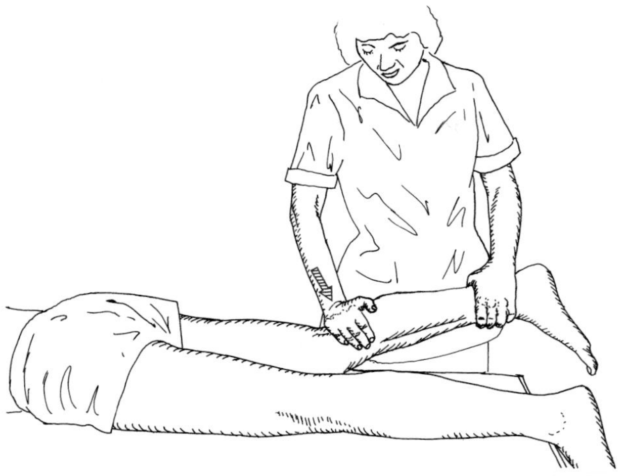

Figure 6–53 Anterior glide; knee joint.

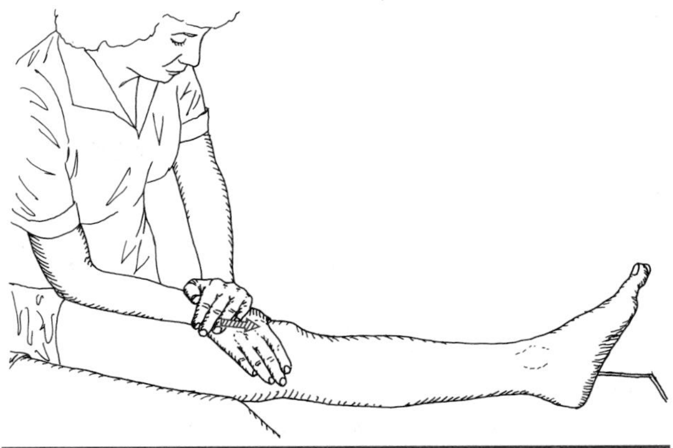

Figure 6–54 Distal glide; patellofemoral joint.

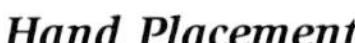

Hand Placement
Grasp the distal tibia with the hand that is closer to it, and place the palm of the proximal hand on the posterior aspect of the proximal tibia.

Mobilizing Force
Force with the hand on the proximal tibia in an anterior direction. The force may be directed to the lateral or to the medial tibial plateau to isolate one side of the joint.

Alternate Position

- If the client cannot be positioned prone, position supine with a fixation pad under the tibia.
- The mobilizing force is placed against the femur in a posterior direction.

Note: The drawer test position can also be used. The mobilizing force comes from the fingers on the posterior tibia as you lean backward (see Fig. 6–51).

Patellofemoral (PF) Joint, Distal Glide (Fig. 6–54)

Indication
To increase patellar mobility for knee flexion.

Patient Position
Supine, begin with knee extended; progress to positioning the knee at the end of the available range in flexion.

Hand Placement
Stand next to the patient's thigh, facing the patient's feet. Place the web space of the hand that is closer to the thigh around the superior border of the patella. Use the other hand for reinforcement.

Mobilizing Force
Glide the patella in a caudal direction, parallel to the femur.

Precaution: Do not compress the patella into the femoral condyles while performing this technique.

PF Medial-Lateral Glide (Fig. 6–55 and Fig. 13–3)

Indication
To increase patellar mobility.

Patient Position
Supine, with knee extended.

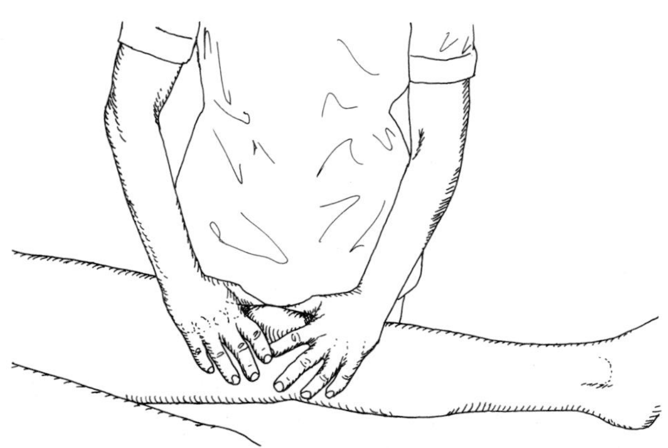

Figure 6–55 Medial-lateral glide of the patella.

Hand Placement
Place your fingers medially and thumbs laterally around the medial and lateral borders of the patella, respectively.

Mobilizing Force
Glide the patella in a medial or lateral direction, against the restriction.

Proximal Tibiofibular Articulation: Anterior (Ventral) Glide (Fig. 6–56)

Indications
To increase movement of the fibular head; to reposition a posteriorly positioned head.

Patient Position
- Side-lying, with the trunk and hips rotated partially toward prone.
- The top leg is flexed forward so that the knee and lower leg are resting on the table or supported on a pillow.

Therapist Position and Hand Placement
- Stand behind the patient, placing one of your hands under the tibia to stabilize it.
- Place the base of your other hand posterior to the head of the fibula, wrapping your fingers anteriorly.

Mobilizing Force
Comes from the heel of your hand against the posterior aspect of the fibular head, in an anterior-lateral direction.

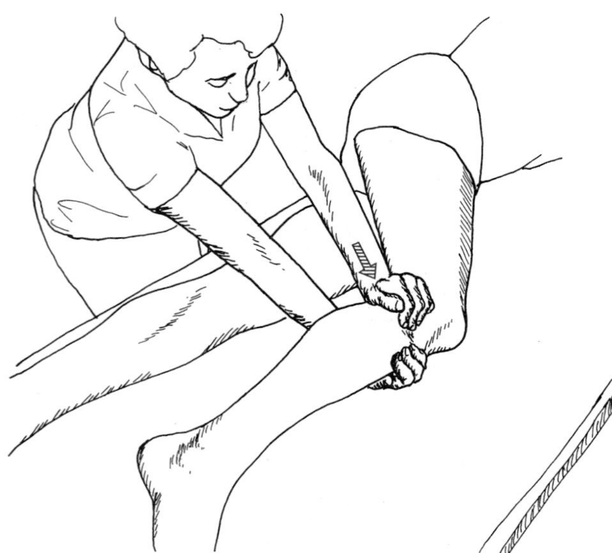

Figure 6–56 Anterior glide; fibular head.

Distal Tibiofibular Articulation: Anterior (Ventral) or Posterior (Dorsal) Glide (Fig. 6–57)

Indication
To increase mobility of the mortise when it is restricting ankle dorsiflexion.

Patient Position
Supine or prone.

Hand Placement
Working from the end of the table, place the fingers of the more medial hand under the tibia and the thumb over the tibia to stabilize it. Place the base of your other hand over the lateral malleolus, with the fingers underneath.

Mobilizing Force
Against the fibula in an anterior direction when prone and a posterior direction when supine.

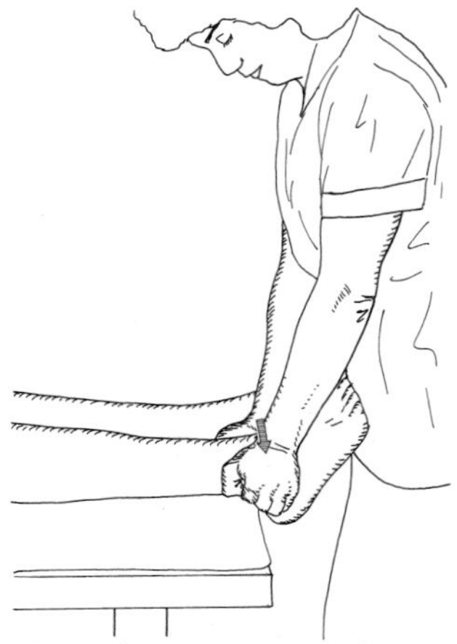

Figure 6–57 Posterior glide; distal tibiofibular articulation.

Ankle and Tarsal Joints (Fig. 6–58)

Talocrural (TC) Joint (Upper Ankle Joint)

Convex talus articulates with the concave mortise made up of the tibia and fibula.

Resting Position
Plantarflexion 10 degrees.

Treatment Plane
In the mortise, in an anterior-posterior direction with respect to the leg.

Stabilization
Tibia strapped or held against the table.

TC Joint Traction—Distraction (Fig. 6–59)

Indications
Testing; initial treatment; pain control; general mobility.

Patient Position
Supine, with the lower extremity extended. Begin with the ankle in resting position. Progress to the end of the available range of dorsiflexion or plantarflexion.

Therapist Position and Hand Placement

- Stand at the end of the table; wrap the fingers of both hands over the dorsum of the patient's foot, just distal to the mortise.
- Place your thumbs on the plantar surface of the foot to hold it in resting position.

Mobilization Force
Pull the foot away from the long axis of the leg in a distal direction by leaning backward.

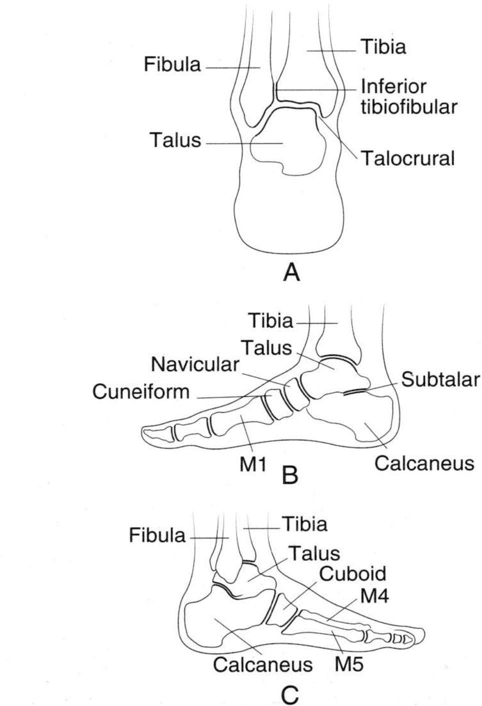

Figure 6–58 *(A)* Anterior view of the bones and joints of the lower leg and ankle. *(B)* Medial view. *(C)* Lateral view of the bones and joint relationships of the ankle and foot.

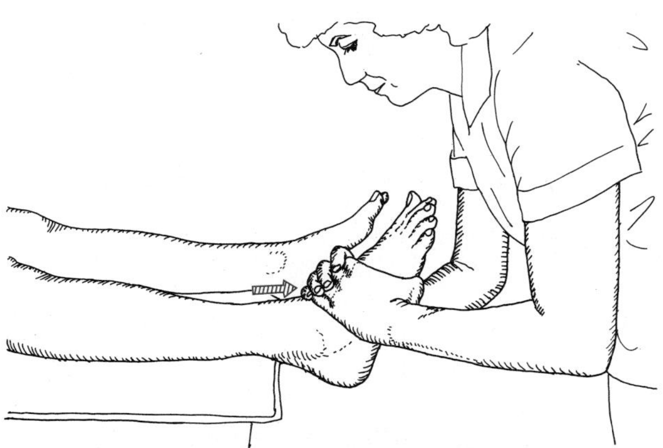

Figure 6–59 Joint traction; talocrural joint.

TC Dorsal (Posterior) Glide (Fig. 6–60)

Indication

To increase dorsiflexion.

Patient Position

Supine, with the leg supported on the table and the heel over the edge.

Therapist Position and Hand Placement

- Stand to the side of the patient.
- Stabilize the leg with your cranial hand or use a belt to secure the leg to the table.
- Place the palmar aspect of the web space of your other hand over the talus just distal to the mortise.
- Wrap your fingers and thumb around the foot to maintain the ankle in resting position. A grade I distraction force is applied in a caudal direction.

Mobilizing Force

Glide the talus posteriorly with respect to the tibia by pushing against the talus.

TC Ventral (Anterior) Glide (Fig. 6–61)

Indication

To increase plantarflexion.

Patient Position

Prone, with the foot over the edge of the table.

Therapist Position and Hand Placement

- Working from the end of the table, place your lateral hand across the dorsum of the foot to apply a grade I distraction.
- Place the web space of your other hand just distal to the mortise on the posterior aspect of the talus and calcaneus.

Mobilizing Force

Push against the calcaneus in an anterior direction (with respect to the tibia); this glides the talus anteriorly.

Alternate Position

- Patient is supine. Stabilize the distal leg anterior to the mortise with your proximal hand.
- The distal hand cups under the calcaneus.
- When you pull against the calcaneus in an anterior direction, the talus glides anteriorly.

Subtalar (ST) Joint (Talocalcaneal), Posterior Compartment

The calcaneus is convex, articulating with a concave talus in the posterior compartment.

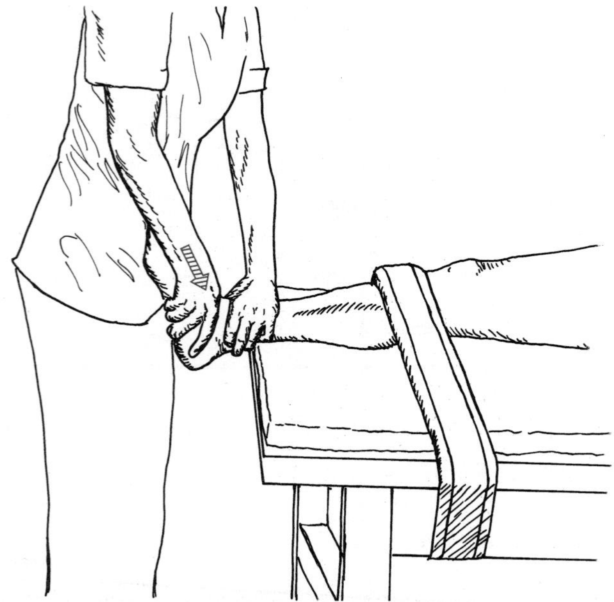

Figure 6–60 Posterior glide; talocrural joint.

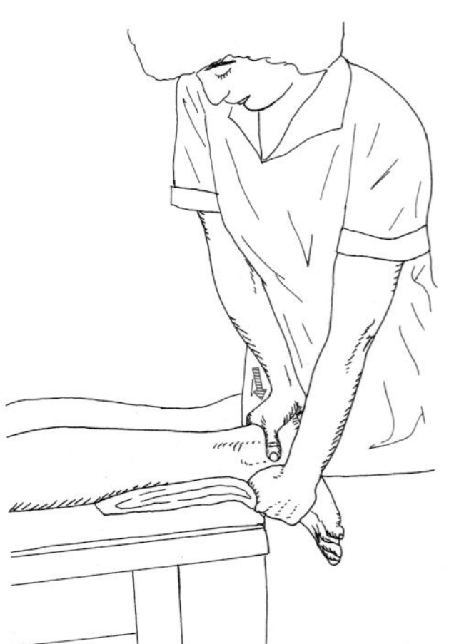

Figure 6–61 Anterior glide; talocrural joint.

Resting Position
Midway between inversion and eversion.

Treatment Plane
In the talus, parallel to the sole of the foot.

ST Joint Traction/Distraction (Fig. 6–62)

Indications
Testing; initial treatment; pain control; general mobility for inversion/eversion.

Patient and Therapist Positions
- The patient is placed in a supine position, with the leg supported on the table and heel over the edge.
- The hip is externally rotated so that the talocrural joint can be stabilized in dorsiflexion with pressure from your thigh against the plantar surface of the patient's forefoot.

Hand Placement
The distal hand grasps around the calcaneus from the posterior aspect of the foot. The other hand fixes the talus and malleoli against the table.

Mobilizing Force
Pull the calcaneus distally with respect to the long axis of the leg.

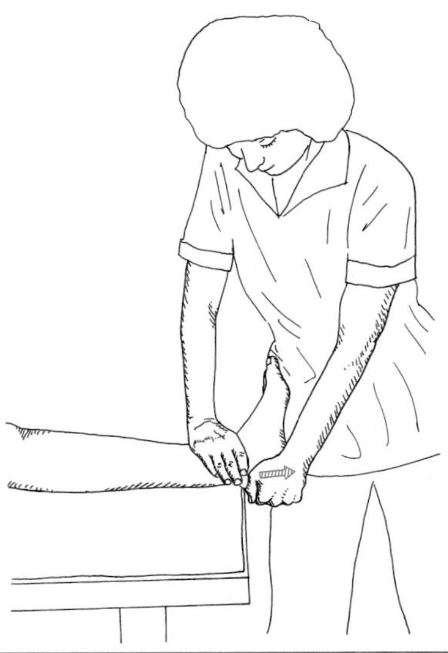

Figure 6–62 Joint traction; subtalar(talocalcaneal) joint.

ST Medial Glide or Lateral Glide (Fig. 6–63)

Indication
Medial glide to increase eversion; lateral glide to increase inversion.

Patient Position
Side-lying or prone, with the leg supported on the table or with a towel roll.

Therapist Position and Hand Placement
- Align your shoulder and arm parallel to the bottom of the foot.
- Stabilize the talus with your proximal hand.
- Place the base of the distal hand on the side of the

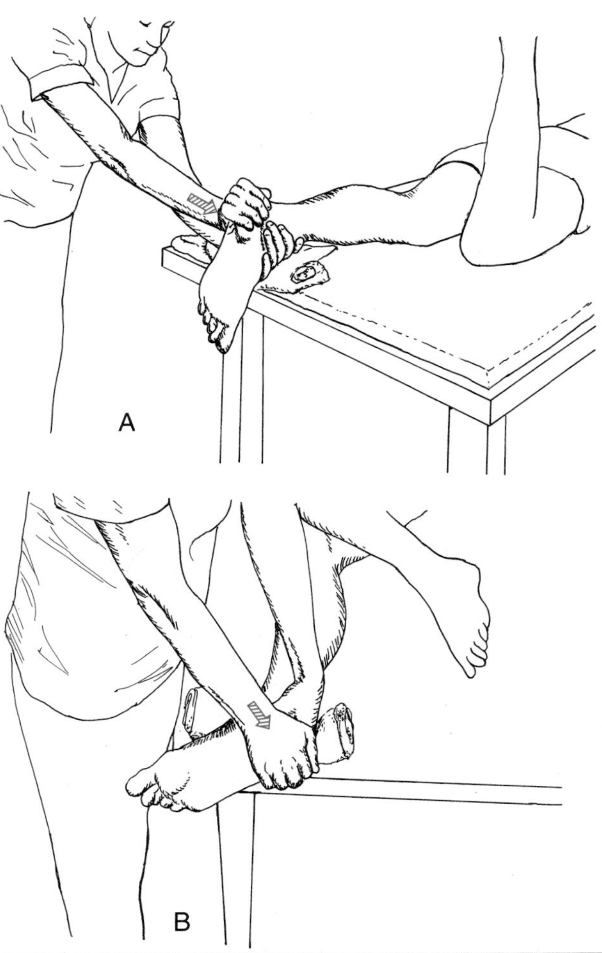

Figure 6–63 *(A)* Medial glide with patient prone to increase eversion. *(B)* Lateral glide with patient side-lying to increase inversion; subtalar joint.

calcaneus, medially to cause a lateral glide and laterally to cause a medial glide.
- Wrap the fingers around the plantar surface.

Mobilizing Force
Apply a grade I distraction force in a caudal direction, then push with the base of your hand against the side of the calcaneus parallel to the planter surface of the heel.

Alternate Position
Same as in the position for distraction, moving the calcaneus in the medial direction with the fingers, or a lateral direction with the base of the hand.

Intertarsal (IT) and Tarsometatarsal (TMT) Joints

When moving in a dorsal-plantar direction with respect to the foot, all of the articulating surfaces are concave and convex in the same direction. For example, the proximal articulating surface is convex and the distal articulating surface is concave. The technique for mobilizing each joint is the same. The hand placement is adjusted to stabilize the proximal bone partner so the distal bone partner can be moved.

IT and TMT Plantar Glide (Fig. 6–64)

Indication
To increase plantarflexion accessory motions (necessary for supination).

Patient Position
Supine, with hip and knee flexed; or sitting, with knee flexed over the edge of the table and heel resting on your lap.

Stabilization
Fixate the more proximal bone with your index finger on the plantar surface of the bone.

Hand Placement
- To mobilize the tarsal joints along the medial aspect of the foot, position yourself on the lateral side of the foot. Place the proximal hand on the dorsum of the foot with the fingers pointing medially, so that the index finger can be wrapped around and placed under the bone to be stabilized.
- Place your thenar eminence of the distal hand over the dorsal surface of the bone to be moved and wrap the fingers around the plantar surface.
- To mobilize the lateral tarsal joints, position yourself on the medial side of the foot, point your fingers laterally and position your hands around the bones as just described.

Mobilizing Force
Push the distal bone in a plantar direction from the dorsum of the foot.

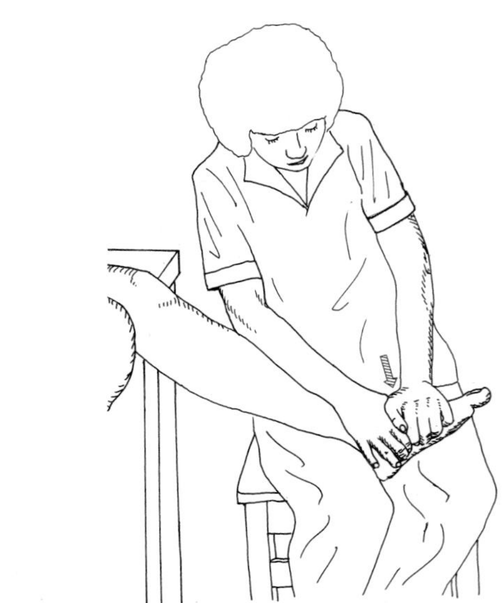

Figure 6–64 Plantar glide of a distal tarsal bone on a stabilized proximal bone; shown is the cuneiform bone on the navicular.

IT and TMT Dorsal Glide (Fig. 6–65)

Indication
To increase dorsal gliding accessory motion (necessary for pronation).

Patient Position
Prone, with knee flexed.

Stabilization
Fixate the more proximal bone.

Hand Placement

- To mobilize the lateral tarsal joints (for example, cuboid on calcaneus), wrap your fingers around the lateral side of the foot (as in Fig. 6–65).
- To mobilize the medial bones (for example, navicular on talus), wrap your fingers around the medial aspect of the foot.
- Place your second metacarpophalangeal joint against the bone to be moved.

Mobilizing Force
Push from the plantar surface in a dorsal direction.

Alternate Technique
Same as position and hand placement for plantar glides, except the distal bone is stabilized and the proximal bone is forced in a plantar direction. This is a relative motion of the distal bone moving in a dorsal direction.

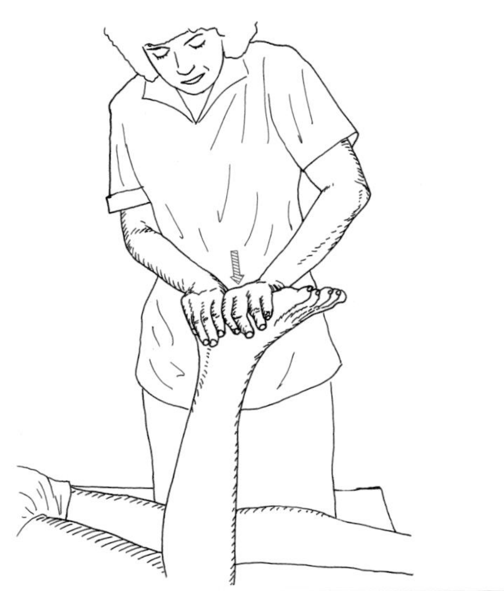

Figure 6–65 Dorsal gliding of a distal tarsal on a proximal tarsal; shown is the cuboid bone on the calcaneus.

Intermetarsal, Metatarsophalangeal, and Interphalangeal Joints

The intermetatarsal, metatarsophalangeal, and interphalangeal joints of the toes are stabilized and mobilized in the same manner as the fingers. In each case, the articulating surface of the proximal bone is convex, and the articulating surface of the distal bone is concave. It is easiest to stabilize the proximal bone and glide the surface of the distal bone either plantarward for flexion, dorsalward for extension, medially or laterally for adduction and abduction.

Independent Learning Activities

CRITICAL THINKING AND DISCUSSION

1. An individual is immobilized in a cast for 4 to 6 weeks following a fracture. In general, what structures will lose their elasticity, and what restrictions will you feel when testing range of motion, joint play, and flexibility?
2. Describe the normal arthrokinematic relationships for the extremity joints, and define the location of the treatment plane for each joint.
3. Using the information from number 1, define a specific fracture, such as a Colle's fracture of the distal forearm. Identify what techniques will be necessary to gain joint mobility and range of motion in the related joints such as the wrist, forearm and elbow joints, connective tissues, and muscles. Practice using each of the techniques.
4. Explain the rationale for use of passive joint techniques to treat patients with limitations because of pain and muscle guarding or to treat patients with restricted capsular or ligamentous tissue. What is the difference in the way the techniques are applied in each case?
5. Describe how joint mobilization techniques fit into the total plan of therapeutic intervention for patients with impaired joint mobility.
6. Explain the difference between passive joint mobilization techniques and mobilization with movement techniques.

LABORATORY PRACTICE

With a partner, practice mobilizing each joint in the upper and lower extremities.

Precaution: Do not practice on an individual with a hypermobile or unstable joint.

1. Begin with the joint in its resting position and apply distraction techniques at each intensity (sustained grade I, II, and III) to develop the feel for "very gentle," "taking up the slack," and "stretch." Do not apply a vigorous stretch to someone with a normal joint. Be sure to use appropriate stabilization.
2. With the joint in its resting position, practice all appropriate glides for that joint. Be sure to use a grade I distraction with each gliding technique. Vary the techniques between sustained and oscillation.
3. Practice progressing each technique by taking the joint to a point that you determine to be the "end of the range" and:
   - Apply a distraction technique with the extremity in that position.
   - Apply the appropriate glide at that range (be sure to apply a grade I distraction with each glide).
   - Add rotation (example external rotation for shoulder abduction) and then apply the appropriate glide.

REFERENCES

1. Akeson, WH, et al: Effects of immobilization on joints. Clin Orthop Rel Res 219:28, 1987.
2. Cyriax, J: Textbook of Orthopaedic Medicine, Vol I: The Diagnosis of Soft Tissue Lesions, ed 8. Bailliere and Tindall, London, 1982.
3. Donatelli, R, and Owens-Burkhart, H: Effects of immobilization on the extensibility of periarticular connective tissue. J Orthop Sports Phys Ther 3:67, 1981.
4. Enneking, WF, and Horowitz, M: The intra-articular effects of immobilization on the human knee. J Bone Joint Surg Am 54:978, 1972.
5. Exelby, L: Mobilizations with movement, a personal view. Physiotherapy 81(12):724, 1995.
6. Kaltenborn, FM: The Kaltenborn Method of Joint Examination and Treatment, Vol I: The Extremities, ed 5. Olaf Norlis Bokhandel, Oslo, 1999.
7. Kavanagh, J: Is there a positional fault at the inferior tibiofibular joint in patients with acute or chronic ankle sprains compared to normals? Manual Therapy 4(1):19, 1999.
8. Magee, DJ: Orthopedic Physical Assessment, ed 3. WB Saunders, Philadelphia, 1997.
9. Maitland, GD: Peripheral Manipulation, ed 3. Butterworth-Heinemann, Boston, 1991.

9a. McDavitt, S: Practice affairs corner; a revision for the *Guide to Physical Therapist Practice; Mobilization or manipulation? Yes! That is my final answer!* Orthop Phys Ther Practice 12 (4), 2000.15.

10. Meadows, J: Orthopedic differential diagnosis in physical therapy: A case study approach. McGraw-Hill, Toronto, 1999.
11. Miller, J: The Mulligan concept—the next step in the evolution of manual therapy. Orthopedic Division Review 2:9, 1999.
12. Mulligan, BR: Manual Therapy "NAGS", "SNAGS", "MWM'S: Etc., ed 4. Plane View Press, Wellington, 1999.
13. Mulligan, BR: Mobilizations with movement (MWM'S). Journal of Manual and Manipulative Therapy 1(4):154, 1993.
14. Norkin, C, and Levangie, P: Joint structure and function: A comprehensive analysis, ed 2. FA Davis, Philadelphia, 1992.
15. O'Brien, T, Vincenzino, B: A Study of the effects of Mulligan's mobilization with movement of lateral ankle pain using a case study design. Manual Therapy 3(2):78, 1998.
16. Paris, SV: Mobilization of the spine. Phys Ther 59:998, 1979.
17. Smith, LK, Weiss, EL, and Lehmkuhl, LD: Brunnstrom's Clinical Kinesiology, ed 5. FA Davis, Philadelphia, 1996.
18. Vincenzino, B, and Wright, A: Effects of a novel manipulative physiotherapy technique on tennis elbow: a single case study. Manual Therapy 1(1):30, 1995.
19. Warwick, R, and Williams, S (eds): Arthrology. In Gray's Anatomy, 35th British ed. WB Saunders, Philadelphia, 1973.
20. Wegener, L, Kisner, C, and Nichols, D: Static and dynamic balance responses in persons with bilateral knee osteoarthritis. J Orthop Sports Phys Ther 25:13, 1997.
21. Wilson, E. Mobilizations with movement and adverse neutral tension: an exploration of possible links. Manip Phys Therap 27(1):40, 1995.
22. Wyke, B: The neurology of joints. Ann R Coll Surg 41:25, 1967.
23. Wyke, B: Articular neurology: A review. Physiotherapy March: 94, 1972.
24. Wyke, B: Neurological aspects of pain for the physical therapy clinician. Physical Therapy Forum '82, Lecture, Columbus, 1982.

Chapter 7

Aquatic Exercise

Robert Schrepfer, MS, PT

OBJECTIVES

After studying this chapter the reader will be able to:

1. Define aquatic exercise.
2. Describe the basic goals of aquatic therapeutic exercise.
3. Explain precautions and contraindications to aquatic therapeutic exercises.
4. Describe the physical properties of water and hydromechanics.
5. Describe the clinical significance of the body's physiologic response to immersion.
6. Explain the impact of water temperature as it relates to aquatic therapeutic exercise.
7. Demonstrate correct stretching, strengthening and cardiovascular techniques in the aquatic environment.
8. Apply the principles of exercise unique to the aquatic environment to design an exercise program for patients with musculoskeletal conditions.

The use of water for healing purposes dates back several centuries. Near the end of the 19th century in Europe, and soon after in the United States, the use of an aquatic environment to facilitate exercise began to grow in popularity. In recent years, healthcare practitioners have increasingly utilized the aquatic medium to facilitate therapeutic exercises. The unique properties of the aquatic environment provide clinicians with treatment options that would otherwise be difficult or impossible to implement on land. Through the use of buoyant devices and varied depths of immersion the practitioner may position the patient supine, seated, kneeling, prone, side-lying, or vertically with any desired amount of weight bearing. Aquatic exercise has been successfully used for a wide variety of rehabilitation populations including pediatric, orthopedic, neurological, and cardiopulmonary patients.

Definition of Aquatic Exercise

Aquatic exercise refers to the use of multidepth immersion pools or tanks that facilitate the application of various established therapeutic interventions including stretching, strengthening, joint mobilization, balance and gait training, and endurance training.

Goals and Indications for Aquatic Exercise

The specific purpose of aquatic exercise is to facilitate functional recovery by providing an environment that augments a patient's and/or practitioner's ability to perform various therapeutic interventions. The specific goals include:

- Facilitate range of motion (ROM) exercise*
- Initiate resistance training[6,18,28,36,38,40]
- Facilitate weight-bearing activities[38,39]
- Enhance delivery of manual techniques[4,5,54]
- Provide three-dimensional access to the patient[5,51,54]
- Facilitate cardiovascular exercise†
- Initiate functional activity replication‡
- Minimize risk of injury or reinjury during rehabilitation[4,18,60,61]
- Enhance patient relaxation[4,41,42]

*See references 6, 18, 19, 28, 30, 32, 36, 38, 39, 40, 59.
†See references 3, 10, 12, 13, 15, 18, 21, 23, 33, 45, 47, 48, 50, 51, 58, 60.
‡See references 6, 8, 19, 28, 30, 40, 51, 56, 59, 62, 63.

Precautions and Contraindications to Aquatic Exericse

Although most patients will easily tolerate aquatic exercise, the practitioner must consider several physiologic and psychologic aspects of immersion that will affect the selection of an aquatic environment.

Precautions

Fear of Water

Fear of water can limit the effectiveness of any immersed activity. Fearful patients often experience increased symptoms during and after immersion because of muscle guarding, stress response, and improper form with exercise.[19,20] Often patients require an orientation period designed to provide instruction regarding the effects of immersion on balance, control of the immersed body, and proper use of flotation devices.[51]

Neurologic Disorders

Ataxic patients may experience increased difficulty controlling purposeful movements.[51] Patients with heat intolerant multiple sclerosis may fatigue with immersion in temperatures greater than 33°C.[51]

Seizures

Patients with controlled epilepsy require close monitoring during immersed treatment and must be compliant with medication prior to treatment.[51]

Cardiac Dysfunction

Patients with angina and abnormal blood pressure also require close monitoring. For patients with cardiac disease, low-intensity aquatic exercise may result in lower cardiac demand than similar land exercise. [35,44,47]

Small Open Wounds and Lines

Small, open wounds and tracheotomies may be covered by waterproof dressings. Patients with intravenous lines, Hickman lines, and other open lines will require proper clamping and fixation.[51]

Contraindications

- Incipient cardiac failure and unstable angina.
- Respiratory dysfunction; vital capacity of less than 1 liter.
- Severe peripheral vascular disease.
- Danger of bleeding or hemorrhage.
- Severe kidney disease: Patients will be unable to adjust to fluid loss during immersion.
- Open wounds, colostomy, and skin infections such as tinea pedis and ringworm.
- Uncontrolled bowel or bladder: Bowel accidents will require pool evacuation, chemical treatment, and possibly drainage.
- Water and airborne infections or diseases: Examples include influenza, gastrointestinal infections, typhoid, cholera, and poliomyelitis.
- Uncontrolled seizures: Uncontrolled seizures create a safety issue for both the clinician and patient if immediate removal from the pool is necessary.

Properties of Water

The unique properties of water and immersion have profound physiologic implications in the delivery of therapeutic exercise. To efficiently utilize aquatics, practitioners must possess a basic understanding of the clinical significance of the static and dynamic properties of water as they affect human immersion and exercise.

Physical Properties of Water

The properties provided by buoyancy,[4,8,19,37,51] hydrostatic pressure,[2,4,8,9,51] viscosity,[4,8,51] and surface tension[4,8,51] have a direct effect on the body in the aquatic environment.

Buoyancy (Fig. 7–1)

Definition. Buoyancy is the upward force that works opposite to gravity.

Properties. Archimedes' principle states that an immersed body experiences upward thrust equal to volume of liquid displaced.

Clinical significance

- Buoyancy provides the patient with relative weightlessness and joint unloading allowing performance of active motion with increased ease.
- Buoyancy allows the practitioner three-dimensional access to the patient.

Hydrostatic Pressure

Definition. Hydrostatic pressure is the pressure exerted on immersed objects.

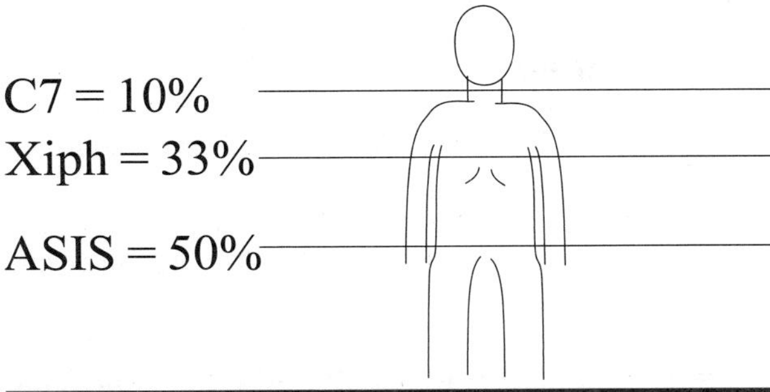

Figure 7–1 Percentage of weight bearing at various immersion depths.

Properties
- Pascal's law states that the pressure exerted by fluid on an immersed object is equal on all surfaces of the object.
- As the density of water and depth of immersion increase so does hydrostatic pressure.

Clinical significance
- Increased pressure reduces or limits effusion, assists venous return, induces bradycardia, and centralizes peripheral blood flow.
- The proportionality of depth and pressure allows patients to perform exercise more easily when closer to the surface.

Viscosity

Definition. Viscosity is friction occurring between molecules of liquid resulting in resistance to flow.

Properties. Resistance from viscosity is proportional to the velocity of movement through liquid.

Clinical significance
- Water's viscosity creates resistance with all active movements.
- A shorter lever arm results in increased resistance. During manual resistance exercises stabilizing an extremity proximally will require the patient to perform more work. Stabilizing an extremity distally will require the patient to perform less work.
- Increasing the surface area moving through water will increase resistance.

Surface Tension

Definition. The surface of a fluid acts as a membrane under tension. Surface tension is measured as force per unit length.

Properties
- The attraction of surface molecules is parallel to the surface.
- The resistive force of surface tension changes proportionally to the size of the object moving through the fluid surface.

Clinical significance
- An extremity that moves through the surface will perform more work than if kept under water.
- Using equipment at the surface of the water will increase the resistance.

Hydromechanics

Definition. Hydromechanics are the physical properties and characteristics of fluid in motion.[4,8,51]

Components of flow motion
- ***Laminar flow.*** Movement where all molecules move parallel to each other, typically slow movement.
- ***Turbulent flow.*** Movement where molecules do not move parallel to each other, typically faster movements.
- ***Drag.*** The cumulative effects of turbulence and fluid viscosity acting on an object in motion.

Clinical significance of drag
- As the speed of movement through water increases, resistance to motion will increase.
- Moving water past the patient will require the patient to work harder to maintain his/her position in pool.
- Application of equipment (glove/paddle/boot) will increase drag and resistance as the patient moves the extremity through water.

Thermodynamics

Water temperature will have an effect on the body and, therefore, performance in an aquatic environment.[4,7,8,51]

Specific Heat

Definition. Specific heat is the amount of heat (calories) required to raise the temperature of 1 gram of substance by 1°C.

Properties. Rate of temperature change is dependent upon mass and specific heat of the object.

Clinical significance

- Water retains heat 1000 times more than air.
- Differences in temperature between an immersed object and water will equilibrate with minimal change in temperature of the water.

Temperature Transfer

- Water conducts temperature 25 times faster than air.
- Heat transfer increases with velocity. A patient moving through the water will lose body temperature faster than an immersed patient at rest.

Center of Buoyancy (Fig. 7–2)

Center of buoyancy, rather than center of gravity, affects the body in an aquatic environment[4,8,51]

Definition. The center of buoyancy is the reference point of an immersed object upon which buoyant (vertical) forces of fluid predictably act.

Properties. Vertical forces that do not intersect the center of buoyancy create rotational motion.

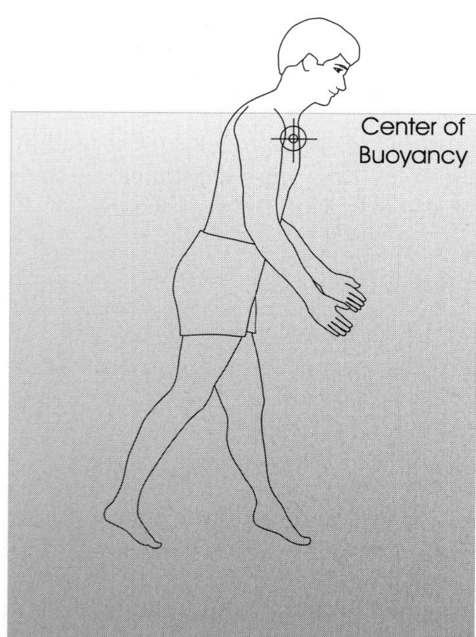

Figure 7–2 Center of buoyancy.

Clinical significance

- In the vertical position, the human center is located at the sternum.
- In the vertical position, posteriorly placed buoyancy devices will cause the patient to lean forward; anterior buoyancy will cause the patient to lean back.
- During unilateral manual resistance exercises the patient revolves around the practitioner in a circular motion.
- A patient with a unilateral lower extremity amputation will lean toward the residual limb side when in a vertical position.
- Patients bearing weight on the floor of the pool (i.e., sitting, kneeling, standing) will experience aspects of both the center of buoyancy and center of gravity.

▶ Aquatic Temperature and Therapeutic Exercise

A patient's impairments and the intervention goals will determine the water temperature selection. In general, utilize cooler temperatures for higher intensity exercise; utilize warmer temperatures for mobility and flexibility exercise and for muscle relaxation.[4,7,14,51] Ambient air temperature should be 3°C higher than water temperature for patient comfort. Incorrect water or ambient air temperature selection may adversely affect a patient's ability to tolerate or maintain immersed exercise.*

Temperature Regulation

- Temperature regulation during immersed exercise differs from land exercise because of alterations in temperature conduction and in the body's ability to dissipate heat.[4,8,19,37,51] With immersion there is less skin exposed to air resulting in less opportunity to dissipate heat through normal sweating mechanisms.
- Water conducts temperature 25 times faster than air,[11] more if the patient is moving through the water and molecules are forced past the patient.
- Patients will perceive small changes in water temperature more profoundly than small changes in air temperature.

*See references 3, 11, 16, 19, 22, 27, 28, 37, 54, 56.

- Over time, water temperature may penetrate to deeper tissues. Internal temperature changes are known to be inversely proportional to subcutaneous fat thickness.[11]
- Patients will be unable to maintain adequate core warmth during immersed exercise at temperatures less than 25°C.[11]
- Conversely, exercise at temperatures greater than 37°C may be harmful if prolonged or maintained at high intensities. Hot water immersion may increase the cardiovascular demands at rest and with exercise.[53]
- In waist-deep water exercise at 37°C, the thermal stimulus to increase heart rate overcomes the centralization of peripheral blood flow due to hydrostatic pressure.
- At temperatures greater than or equal to 37°C, cardiac output increases significantly at rest alone.[7,16]

Mobility and Functional Control Exercise

- Aquatic exercises including flexibility, strengthening, gait training, and relaxation may be performed in temperatures between 26°C and 33°C.[4,8,51]
- Therapeutic exercise performed in warm water (33°C) may be beneficial for patients with acute painful musculoskeletal injuries because of the effects of relaxation, elevated pain threshold, and decreased muscle spasm.[4,8,51]

Aerobic Conditioning

- Cardiovascular training and aerobic exercise should be performed in water temperatures between 26°C and 28°C. This range maximizes exercise efficiency, increases stroke volume, and decreases heart rate.[3,16,51,60]
- Intense aerobic training performed above 80% of a patient's maximum heart rate should take place in temperatures between 22°C and 26°C to minimize the risk of heat illness.[3,16,51,60]

▶ Special Equipment for Aquatic Exercise

A large variety of equipment exists for use with aquatic exercise. Aquatic equipment is used to provide buoyant support to the body or an extremity, challenge or assist balance, and generate resistance to movement. By adding or removing equipment, the practitioner can progress exercise intensity.

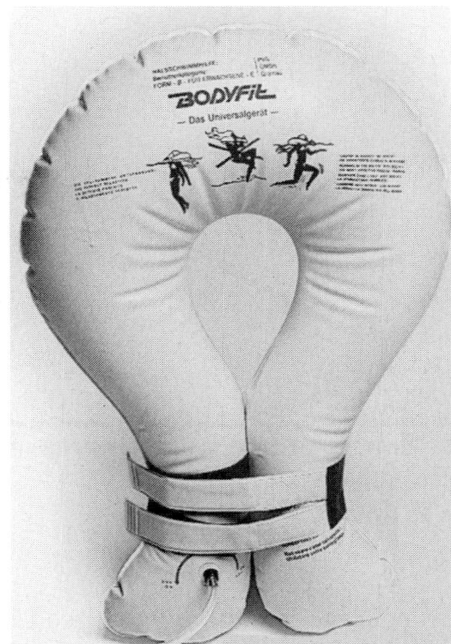

Figure 7–3 Cervical collar. (Courtesy of Rothhammer International Inc., San Luis Obispo, CA.)

Collars, Rings, Belts, and Vests

Equipment designed to assist with patient positioning by providing buoyancy assistance can be applied to the neck, extremities, or trunk. Inflatable cervical collars are used with the patient supine in order to

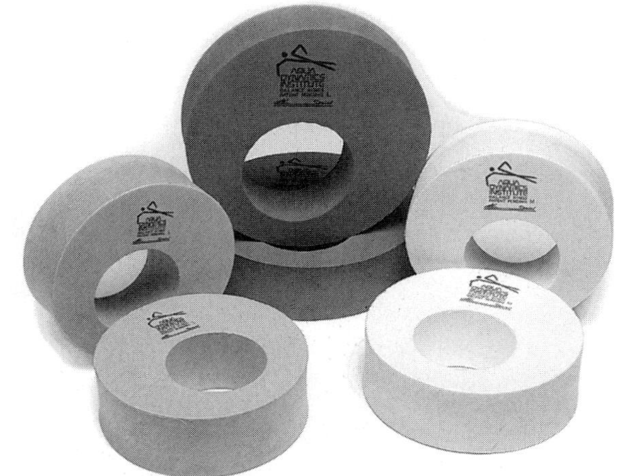

Figure 7–4 Flotation rings. (Courtesy of Rothhammer International Inc., San Luis Obispo, CA.)

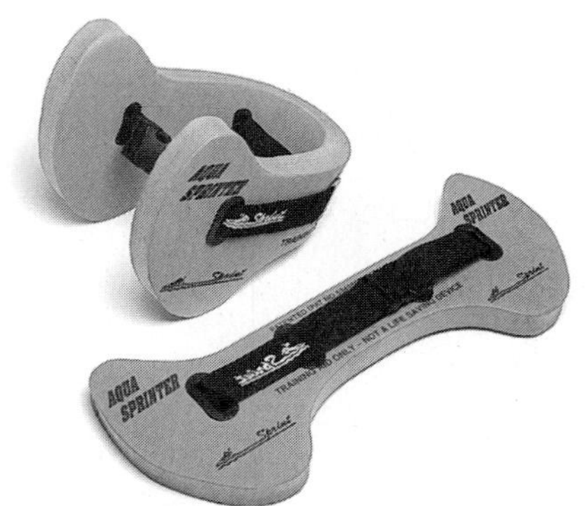

Figure 7–5 Buoyancy belts. (Courtesy of Rothhammer International Inc., San Luis Obispo, CA.)

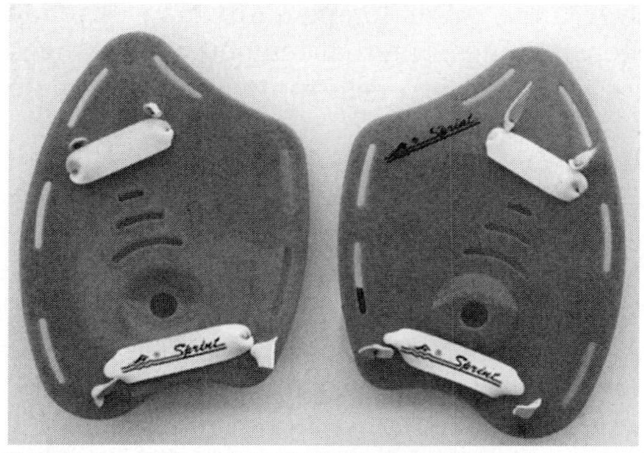

Figure 7–7 Hand paddles. (Courtesy of Rothhammer International Inc., San Luis Obispo, CA.)

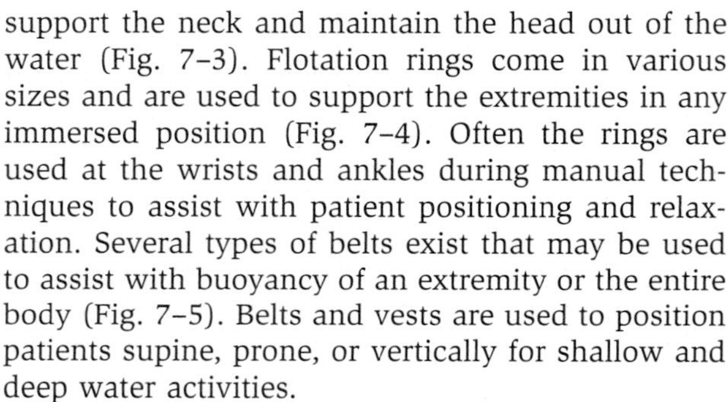

support the neck and maintain the head out of the water (Fig. 7–3). Flotation rings come in various sizes and are used to support the extremities in any immersed position (Fig. 7–4). Often the rings are used at the wrists and ankles during manual techniques to assist with patient positioning and relaxation. Several types of belts exist that may be used to assist with buoyancy of an extremity or the entire body (Fig. 7–5). Belts and vests are used to position patients supine, prone, or vertically for shallow and deep water activities.

Swim Bars

Buoyant dumbbells (swim bars) are available in short and long lengths. They are useful for supporting the upper body or trunk in upright positions and the lower extremities in the supine or prone positions (Fig 7–6). Patients can balance (seated or standing) on long swim bars in deep water to challenge balance, proprioception, and trunk strength.

Gloves, Hand Paddles, and Hydro-tone® Bells

Resistance to upper extremity movements is achieved by applying webbed gloves or progressively larger paddles to the hands (Fig 7–7). These devices are not buoyant and, therefore, only resist motion in the direction of movement. Hydro-tone® bells are large, slotted plastic devices that increase drag during upper extremity motions (Fig 7–8). The bells generate substantially more resistance than gloves or hand paddles.

Fins and Hydro-tone® Boots

The application of fins or boots to the feet during lower extremity motions generates resistance by in-

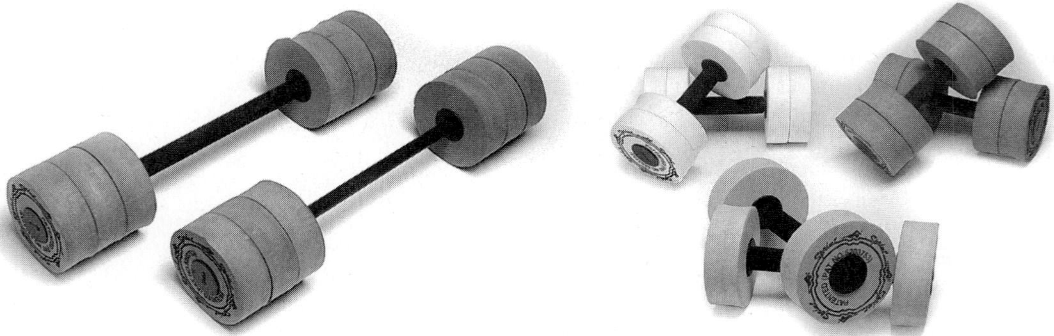

Figure 7–6 Swim bars. (Courtesy of Rothhammer International Inc., San Luis Obispo, CA.)

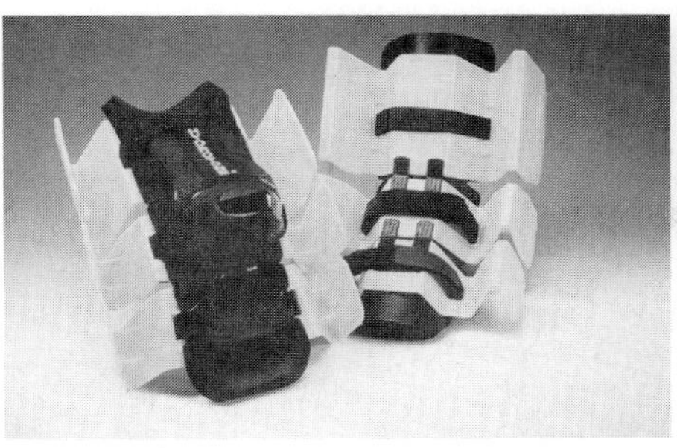

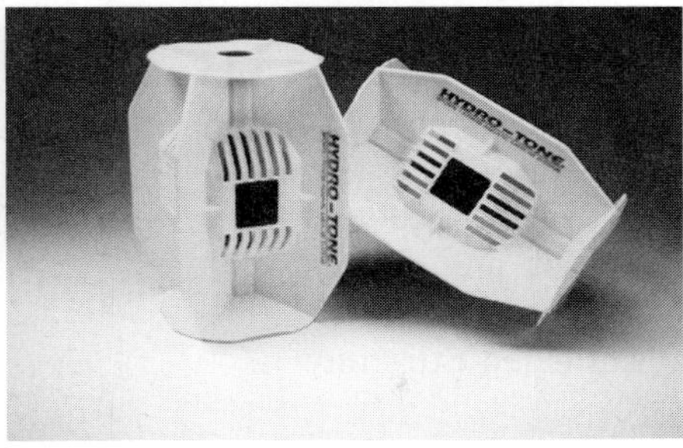

Figure 7–8 Hydro-tone boots and bells. (Courtesy of Rothhammer International Inc., San Luis Obispo, CA.)

creasing the surface area moving through the water. Fins are especially useful for challenging hip, knee, and ankle strength. Hydro-tone® boots are most effective during deep water walking and running (Fig 7–8).

Kickboards (Fig 7–9)

The shapes and styles of kickboards vary extensively among manufacturers. Nevertheless, kickboards remain a versatile and effective aquatic tool for augmenting any exercise program. Kickboards may be used to provide buoyancy in the prone or supine positions, held vertically to create resistance to walking patterns in shallow water, or used to challenge seated, kneeling, or standing balance in the deep water.

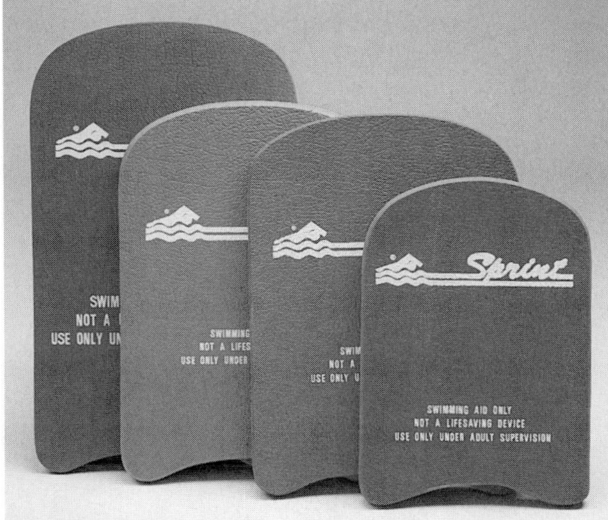

Figure 7–9 Kickboards. (Courtesy of Rothhammer International Inc., San Luis Obispo, CA.)

Stretching Exercises

Patients may tolerate immersed stretching exercises better than land stretching because of the effects of relaxation, soft tissue warming, and ease of positioning. However, buoyancy creates an inherently less stable environment than the land. Therefore, careful consideration is warranted when recommending aquatic stretching.

Manual Stretching Techniques

Manual stretching is typically performed with the patient supine in waist depth water with buoyancy devices at the neck, waist, and feet. Alternatively, the patient may be seated on steps. The buoyancy-supported supine position improves both access to the patient as well as control by the practitioner and position of the patient versus land techniques.

However, turbulence from wave activity can adversely affect both the patient and practitioner's ability to perform manual stretching. Difficulties may be experienced maintaining and perceiving the subtleties of end-range stretching and with scapular stabilization in the supine buoyancy-supported position. Anecdotal evidence indicates that careful consideration of all factors is warranted prior to initiating manual stretching in an aquatic environment.[5,54]

The manual stretching techniques described in this section are considered passive techniques, but may be adapted to utilize muscle inhibition techniques. The principles of stretching are the same as those discussed in Chapter 5.

The following terms will be used to describe the stretching techniques:

- ***Practitioner position.*** Describes the orientation of the practitioner to the patient.
- ***Patient position.*** Includes *buoyancy-assisted (BA)* seated or upright and *buoyancy-supported (BS)* supine positioning.

- ***Hand placement.*** The *fixed hand,* which stabilizes the patient, is typically the same (ipsilateral) hand as the patient's affected extremity, and it is positioned proximally on the affected extremity. The *movement hand,* which guides the patient's extremity through the desired motion and applies the stretch force, is typically the opposite (contralateral) hand as the patient's affected extremity and is positioned distally.
- ***Direction of movement.*** Describes the motion of the movement hand.

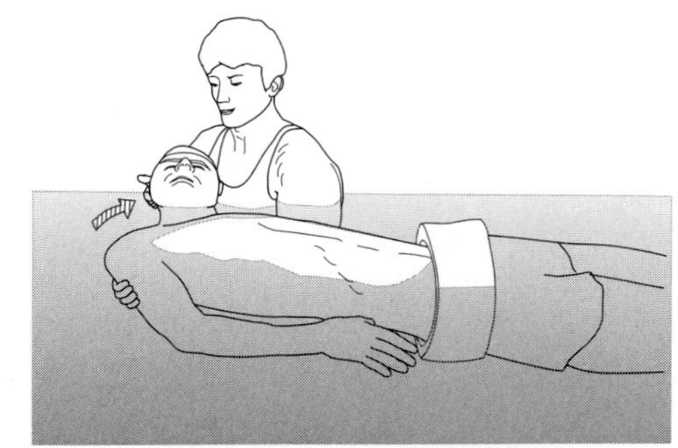

Figure 7–10 Hand placement and stabilization for stretching to increase cervical lateral flexion.

Cervical Spine: Flexion

Practioner Position
Stand at the patient's head facing caudalward.

Patient Position
BS supine without cervical collar.

Hand Placement
Cup the patient's head with your hands, the forearms supinated and thumbs placed laterally. Alternatively, place your hands in a pronated position with the thumbs at the occiput. This results in a more neutral wrist position at end range stretch.

Direction of Movement
As you flex the cervical spine, the patient will have a tendency to drift away from you if care is not taken to perform motion slowly.

Cervical Spine: Lateral Flexion (Fig. 7–10)

Practitioner Position
Stand at the side facing patient.

Patient Position
BS supine without cervical collar.

Hand Placement
Reach the fixed hand dorsally under the patient and grasp the contralateral arm; support the head with the movement hand.

Direction of Movement
Move the patient into lateral flexion and apply stretch force at desired intensity. This position prevents patient drift as the fixed hand stabilizes the patient against the practitioner.

Thoracic and Lumbar Spine: Lateral Flexion/ Side Bending (Fig 7–11)

Practitioner Position
Stand on the side opposite that to be stretched, facing cephalad with ipsilateral hips in contact (e.g., if stretching the left side of the trunk, the therapist's right hip is against patient's right hip).

Patient Position
BS supine, if tolerated. The patient's stretch side arm is abducted to end range to facilitate stretch.

Hand Placement
Grasp the patient's abducted arm with the fixed hand; alternately, grasp at the deltoid if patient's arm is not abducted. The movement hand is at the lateral aspect of the lower extremity of the side to be

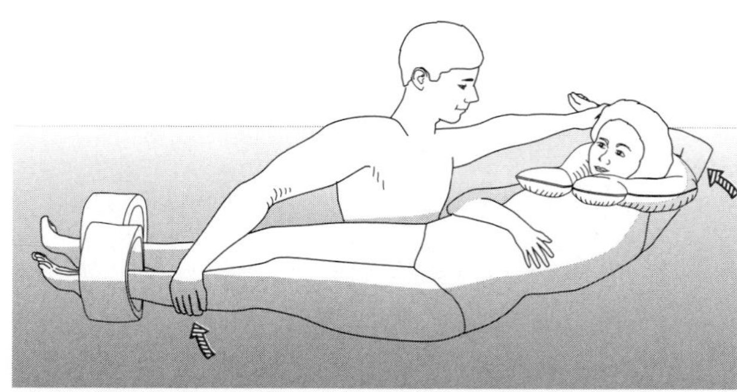

Figure 7–11 Hand placement and stabilization for stretching to increase lateral trunk flexion.

stretched (more distal placement improves leverage with stretch).

Direction of Movement
With the patient stabilized by your hip, pull the patient into lateral flexion. This technique allows for variability in positioning and hand placement to isolate distinct segments of the spine

Shoulder Flexion (Fig. 7–12)

Practitioner Position
Stand on the side to be stretched facing cephalad.

Patient Position
BS supine with the affected shoulder positioned in slight abduction.

Hand Placement
Grasp the buoyancy belt with the fixed hand; the movement hand is at the elbow of the affected extremity.

Direction of Movement
After positioning the arm in the desired degree of abduction, direct the arm into flexion and apply the stretch force with the movement hand.

Shoulder Abduction

Practitioner Position
Stand on the affected side facing cephalad with your hip in contact with the patient's hip.

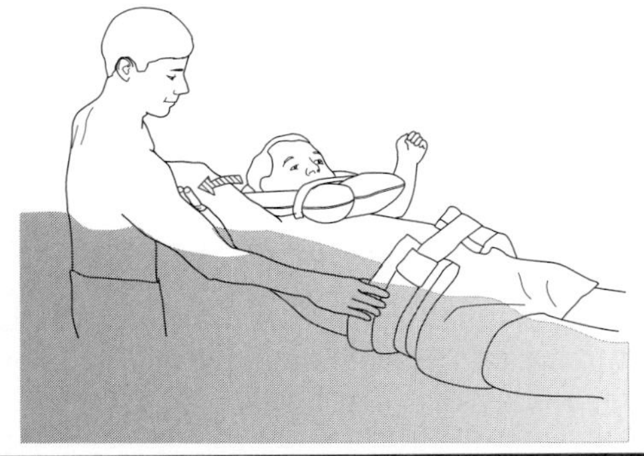

Figure 7–12 Hand placement and stabilization for stretching to increase shoulder flexion.

Patient Position
BS supine.

Hand Placement
Stabilize the scapula with the fixed hand; the movement hand grasps medially on the affected elbow joint.

Direction of Movement
Guide the arm into abduction and apply the stretch force. The hip contact provides additional stabilization as the stretch force is applied.

Shoulder External Rotation

Practitioner Position
Stand lateral to the affected extremity facing cephalad.

Patient Position
BS supine; position arm in desired degree of abduction with elbow flexed to 90 degrees.

Hand Placement
Grasp the medial side of the patient's elbow with the palmar aspect of the fixed hand while fingers hold laterally; grasp the midforearm with the movement hand.

Direction of Movement
Movement hand guides forearm dorsally to externally rotate shoulder and apply stretch force.

Shoulder Internal Rotation

Practitioner Position
Stand lateral to the patient's affected extremity facing caudal.

Patient Position
BS supine; position arm in desired degree of abduction with elbow flexed to 90 degrees.

Hand Placement
Stabilize the scapula with the dorsal aspect of the fixed hand entering from the axilla; the movement hand is at the distal forearm.

Direction of Movement
Direct the forearm palmarward and apply the stretch force. Use care to observe the glenohumeral joint to avoid a forward thrust and substitution.

Hip Extension

Practitioner Position
Kneel on one knee at the patient's affected side.

Patient Position
BS supine with the hip extended and the knee slightly flexed.

Hand Placement
Stabilize the patient's affected extremity by hooking the top of the foot with your ipsilateral thigh. Grasp the buoyancy belt with the movement hand and guide the motion with fixed hand on the knee.

Direction of Movement
Direct the patient caudally with the movement hand. To increase the stretch on the rectus femoris, lower the patient's knee in the water. Motion is performed slowly to limit spinal and pelvic substitution.

Hip External Rotation

Practitioner Position
Face the lateral aspect of the patient's thigh with your ipsilateral arm under the patient's flexed knee.

Patient Position
BS supine; hip flexed 70 degrees, and knee flexed 90 degrees.

Hand Placement
Grasp the buoyancy belt with the contralateral (fixed) hand while the ipsilateral (movement) hand grasps the thigh.

Direction of Movement
Externally rotate hip with the movement hand as patient's body lags through water to create stretch force.

Hip Internal Rotation

Practitioner Position
Face the lateral aspect of the involved thigh with the ipsilateral arm under the flexed knee.

Patient Position
BS supine, hip flexed 70 degrees, knee flexed 90 degrees.

Hand Placement
Stabilize the buoyancy belt with the contralateral (fixed) hand while grasping the thigh with the ipsilateral (movement) hand.

Direction of Movement
Internally rotate the hip as patient's body lags through water to create the stretch force.

Knee Extension with Patient on Steps

Practitioner Position
Half-kneel lateral to the affected knee with the ankle of the affected extremity resting on your thigh.

Patient Position
Semi-reclined on pool steps.

Hand Placement
Place one hand just proximal and one just distal to knee joint.

Direction of Movement
Extend the patient's knee.

Knee Flexion with Patient on Steps

Practitioner Position
Half-kneel lateral to the affected knee.

Patient Position
Semi-reclined on pool steps.

Hand Placement
Grasp the distal tibia with the ipsilateral hand; the contralateral hand stabilizes the lateral aspect of affected knee.

Direction of Movement
Apply the stretch force into flexion.

Knee Flexion with Patient Supine (Fig 7–13)

Practitioner Position
Half-kneel lateral to the affected knee with the dorsal aspect of the patient's foot hooked under the ipsilateral thigh.

Patient Position
BS supine, affected knee flexed.

Hand Placement
Place the ipsilateral (fixed) hand on distal tibia and the contralateral (movement) hand on buoyancy belt to pull body over fixed foot.

Direction of Movement
Pull the patient's body over the fixed foot creating the stretch to increase knee flexion. Lower the pa-

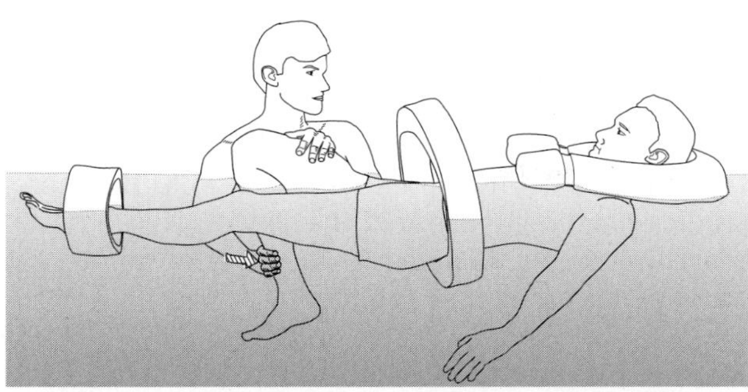

Figure 7–13 Hand placement and stabilization for stretching to increase knee flexion.

tient's knee into the water to extend the hip and increase the stretch on the rectus femoris. Perform the motion slowly to limit spinal and pelvic substitution.

Hamstrings Stretch

Practitioner Position
Face the patient and rest the patient's affected extremity on your ipsilateral shoulder.

Patient Position
BS supine, knee extended.

Hand Placement
Place both hands at distal thigh.

Direction of Movement
Start in the squatting position and gradually stand to flex the hip and apply the stretch force. Maintain knee extension by pulling the patient closer and increasing the stretch.

Self-Stretching with Aquatic Equipment

Often the intervention plan is to instruct the patient to perform independent stretching.* Self-stretching can be performed in either waist-depth or deep water. The patient frequently utilizes the edge of the pool for stabilization in both waist-depth and deep water.

Applying buoyancy devices may assist with stretching and increase the intensity of the aquatic stretch.[60] However, buoyancy devices are not required to achieve buoyancy-assisted stretching. That is, as buoyancy acts upon any submersed extremity, correct patient positioning will adequately produce a gentle stretch. The following guidelines describe the use of equipment for mechanical stretching; the descriptions apply similarly for use without buoyancy equipment. Providing verbal cueing and visual demonstration for patient positioning and form will aid in achieving the desired stretching effects.

Positioning for self-stretching of every body part is not described in this section. Typically, positioning for immersed self-stretches reflects traditional land positioning.

The following terms will be used to describe the self-stretching techniques.

- ***Patient position.*** Includes buoyancy-assisted (seated/upright), buoyancy-supported (supine), or vertical
- ***Buoyancy-assisted.*** Using the natural buoyancy of water to "float" the extremity toward the surface
- ***Equipment-assisted.*** Includes use of buoyancy devices attached or held distally on an extremity.

The following are some examples of self-stretching.

Shoulder Flexion and Abduction

Patient Position
Upright, neck level immersion.

Equipment
Small or large buoyant dumbbell or wrist strap.

Direction of Movement
Grasping buoyant device with affected extremity allows extremity to float to surface as buoyancy device provides the gentle stretch.

Hip Flexion (Fig. 7–14)

Patient Position
Upright, immersed to waist, or seated at edge of pool/on steps with hips immersed.

Equipment
Small buoyant dumbbell or ankle strap. For hip flexion with knee flexion, place strap/dumbbell proximal to the knee. For hip flexion with knee extension, (to stretch the hamstrings) place strap/dumbbell at the ankle.

Direction of Movement
Allow buoyancy device to float hip into flexion applying stretch to hip extensors or hamstrings.

Knee Extension

Patient Position
Seated on steps/edge of pool with knee in a position of comfort.

*See references 6, 29, 43, 46, 48, 49, 51, 57, 63.

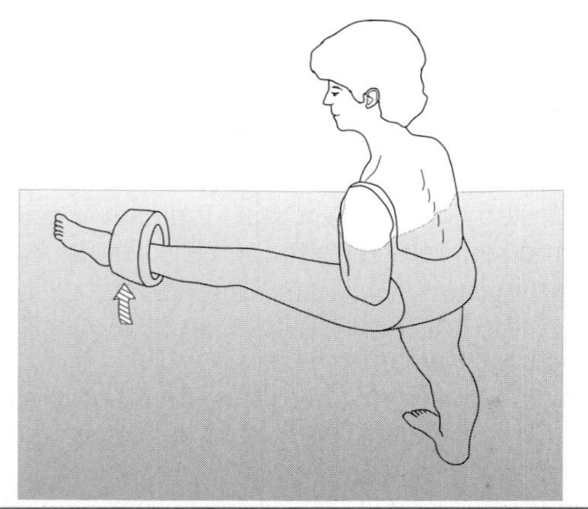

Figure 7–14 Self-stretching technique to increase hip flexion (stretch the hamstrings) using aquatic equipment.

Equipment
Small dumbbell or ankle strap.

Direction of Movement
Allow buoyancy device to extend knee toward the surface applying stretch to increase knee extension.

Knee Flexion

Patient Position
Stand immersed to waist with hip and knee in neutral position; increasing the amount of hip extension will increase the stretch on the two joint knee extensors.

Equipment
Small dumbbell or ankle strap.

Direction of Movement
Allow buoyancy device to flex knee toward surface applying stretch to knee extensors.

▶ Strengthening Exercises

By reducing joint compression, providing three-dimensional resistance, and dampening perceived pain, immersed strengthening exercises may be safely initiated earlier in the rehabilitation program than traditional land strengthening exercises.[4] Both manual and mechanical immersed strengthening exercises typically are done in waist-depth water. However, some mechanical strengthening exercises may also be performed in deep water. Frequently, immersion will alter the mechanics of active motion. For example, the vertical forces of buoyancy support the immersed upper extremity and alter the muscular demands on the shoulder girdle.[60] Furthermore, studies have demonstrated that lower extremity demand is inversely related to the level of immersion during closed-chain strengthening.[25]

Manual Resistance Exercises

Application of aquatic manual resistance exercises for the extremities typically occurs in a concentric, closed-chain fashion.[5,54] Manual aquatic resistance exercises are designed to fixate the distal segment of the extremity as the patient contracts the designated muscle group(s). The practitioner's hands provide primary fixation and guidance during contraction. As the patient contracts his or her muscles, the body moves over or away from the fixed distal segment (generally over the fixed segment for the lower extremity and away from the fixed segment for the upper extremity). The patient's movement through the viscous water generates resistance; the patient's body produces the drag forces. Verbal cueing by the practitioner is essential to direct the patient when to contract and when to relax, thereby synchronizing practitioner and patient.

Stabilization of the distal extremity segment is essential for maintaining proper form and isolating desired muscles. However, appropriate stabilization is not possible in the buoyancy-supported supine position for eccentric exercises or rhythmic stabilization of the extremities. The patient's body will have a tendency to tip and rotate in the water. In addition, the practitioner will have difficulty generating adequate resistance force, and the patient's body will move easily across the surface of the water with minimal drag producing inadequate counterforce to the practitioner's resistance. When supine, some motions including horizontal shoulder adduction and abduction should be avoided because of the difficulty the patient may have isolating proper muscle groups. Nevertheless, for many motions, the aquatic environment allows for closed-chain resistive training through virtually limitless planes of motion.

The following terms refer to manual resistance exercise in water:

- ***Practitioner position.*** Describes the orientation of the practitioner to the patient.

- ***Patient position.*** *Buoyancy-supported (BS)* in the supine position.
- ***Hand placement.*** The *guide hand* is generally the ipsilateral hand as the patient's affected extremity and typically is positioned more proximally. It directs the patient's body as muscles contract to move the body through the water. The *resistance hand* is generally the contralateral hand and typically is placed at the distal end of the contracting segment. More distal placement will increase overall resistance.
- ***Direction of movement.*** Describes the motion of the patient.

Shoulder Flexion/Extension (Fig. 7–15*A* and *B*)

Practitioner Position
Face caudal, lateral to the patient's affected shoulder.

Patient Position
BS supine; affected extremity flexed to 30 degrees.

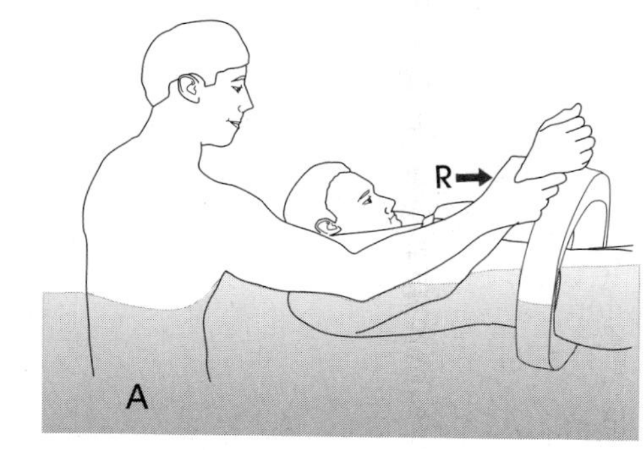

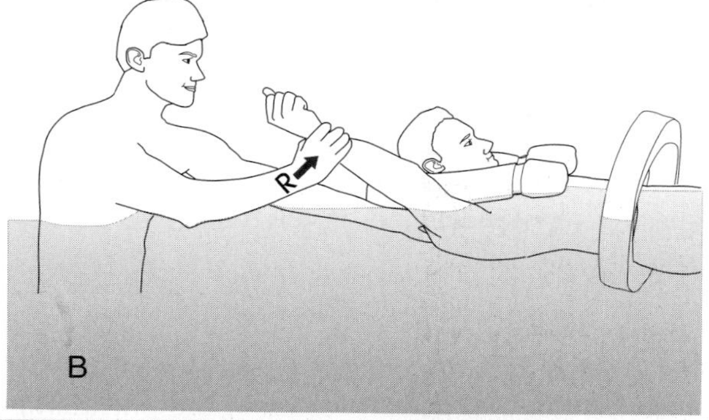

Figure 7–15 Manual resistance exercise for strengthening shoulder flexion, *(A)* start position, *(B)* end position.

Hand Placement
Place the palmar aspect of the guide hand at the patient's acromioclavicular joint. The resistance hand grasps the distal forearm. An alternative placement for the resistance hand may be the distal humerus; this placement will alter muscle recruitment.

Direction of Movement
Active shoulder flexion against the resistance hand causes the body to move away from the practitioner. Active shoulder extension from a flexed position causes the body to glide toward the practitioner.

Note: The patient must be able to actively flex through 120 degrees for proper resistance to be provided.

Shoulder Abduction

Practitioner Position
Face medially, lateral to the patient's affected extremity.

Patient Position
BS supine; affected extremity in neutral.

Hand Placement
Place the palmar aspect of guide hand at the proximal humerus as the thumb wraps anteriorly and the fingers wrap posteriorly. Place the resistance hand at the lateral aspect of distal humerus.

Direction of Movement
The practitioner determines the amount of external rotation and elbow flexion. Active abduction against the resistance hand will cause the body to glide away from the affected extremity and the practitioner.

Shoulder Internal/External Rotation (Fig. 7–16*A* and *B*)

Practitioner Position
Face medially on the lateral side of the patient's affected extremity.

Patient Position
BS supine; affected extremity's elbow flexed to 90 degrees with the shoulder in the desired amount of abduction and initial rotation.

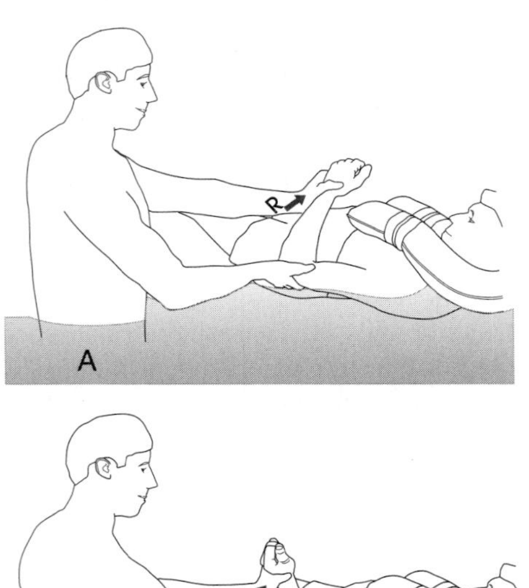

Figure 7–16 Manual resistance exercise for strengthening shoulder external rotation, *(A)* start position, and *(B)* end position.

Hand Placement
Place the palmar aspect of the guide hand at the lateral aspect of the elbow. The resistance hand grasps the palmar aspect of the distal forearm. An alternative method requires the practitioner to "switch" hands. The practitioner's ipsilateral hand becomes the guide hand and grasps the buoyancy belt laterally. The practitioner's contralateral hand becomes the resistance hand as described above. This approach allows for improved stabilization; however, the practitioner loses contact with the patient's elbow and must cue the patient to maintain the desired degree of shoulder abduction during the exercise.

Direction of Movement
Active internal rotation by the patient against the resistance hand will cause the body to glide toward the affected extremity; active external rotation will cause the body to glide away from the affected extremity.

Unilateral Diagonal Pattern D_1 Flexion/Extension of the Upper Extremity

Practitioner Position
Stand lateral to the patient's unaffected extremity and face medial and caudal.

Patient Position
BS supine; affected extremity internally rotated and pronated with slight forward flexion.

Hand Placement
Secure the medial and lateral epicondyles of distal humerus with the guide hand. Place the resistance hand on the dorsal surface of the distal forearm.

Direction of Movement
Prior to contraction, cue the patient to execute the specific joint motions expected within the diagonal patterns. Active contraction through the D_1 flexion pattern will cause the body to glide away from the practitioner. At the end position of D_1 secure the medial and lateral epicondyles of the distal humerus with the guide hand. The resistance hand will be on the palmar aspect of the distal forearm. From the flexed position the practitioner cues the patient to contract through the D_1 extension pattern.

Unilateral Diagonal D_2 Flexion/Extension of the Upper Extremity (Fig. 7–17*A* and *B*)

Practitioner Position
Stand lateral to the patient's affected shoulder, face medial and caudal.

Patient Position
BS supine; affected extremity adducted and internally rotated.

Hand Placement
Secure the medial and lateral epicondyles of the distal humerus with the guide hand. Wrap the palmar aspect of resistance hand on the dorsal wrist medial to the palmar surface.

Direction of Movement
Active movement through the D_2 flexion pattern will cause the body to glide away from the practitioner. From the fully flexed position, cue the patient to then move into the D_2 extension pattern. This will cause the body to glide toward the practitioner.

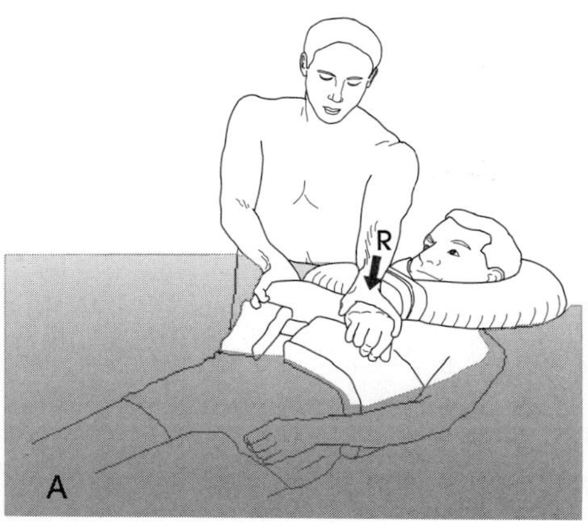

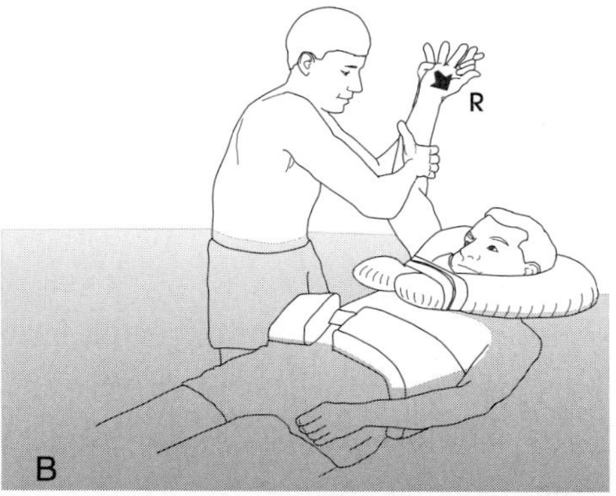

Figure 7–17 Manual resistance exercise for upper extremity unilateral diagonal D_2 flexion pattern, *(A)* start position, and *(B)* end position.

Bilateral Diagonal D_2 Flexion/Extension of the Upper Extremities (Fig. 7–18*A* and *B*)

Practitioner Position
Stand cephalad to patient, facing caudal.

Patient Position
BS supine; upper extremities adducted and internally rotated.

Hand Placement
Use both hands to provide resistance. Grasp the dorsal aspect of each of the patient's wrists, wrapping medially to the palmar surface.

Direction of Motion
Active contraction through the D_2 flexion pattern will cause the body to glide away from the practitioner. From the fully flexed position, cue the patient to contract through D_2 extension causing the patient to move toward the practitioner.

Hip Adduction

Practitioner Position
Stand lateral to patient's affected extremity and face medial.

Patient Position
BS supine; hip abducted.

Hand Placement
Place the guide hand on the buoyancy belt and the resistance hand on the patient's medial thigh.

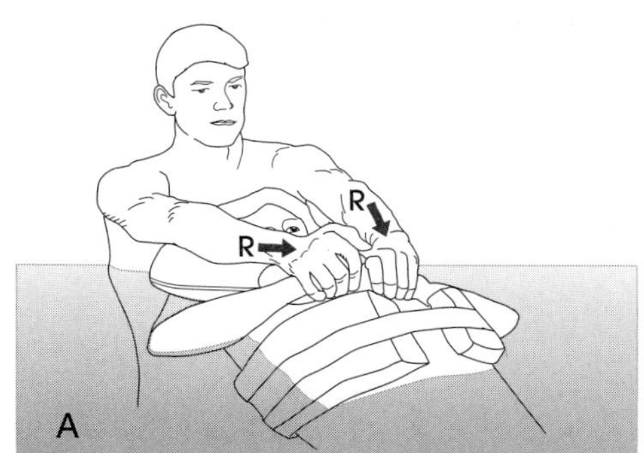

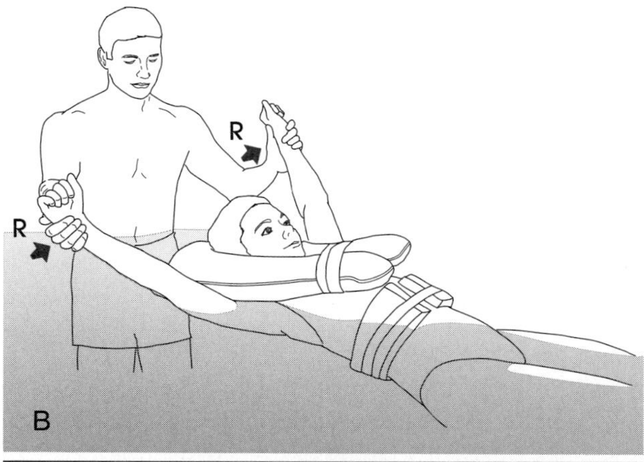

Figure 7–18 Manual resistance exercise for upper extremity bilateral diagonal D2 pattern, *(A)* start position, and *(B)* end position.

Direction of Movement
Active contraction of the hip adductors causes the affected leg to adduct as the contralateral leg and body glides toward affected leg and practitioner.

Hip Abduction (Fig. 7–19)

Practitioner Position
Stand lateral to patient's affected extremity, facing medially.

Patient Position
BS supine; hip adducted.

Hand Placement
Place the guide hand on the buoyancy belt or lateral thigh and the thumb and base of the resistance hand on the patient's lateral leg.

Direction of Movement
Active contraction of the hip abductors causes the affected leg to abduct as the contralateral leg and body glides away from affected leg and practitioner.

Hip Flexion with Knee Flexion (Fig. 7–20)

Practitioner Position
Stand at the side of the patient's affected extremity, facing cephalad.

Patient Position
BS supine.

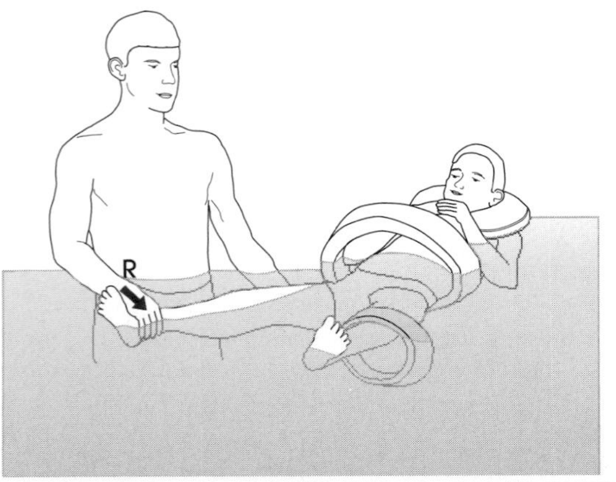

Figure 7–19 Manual resistance exercise for strengthening hip abduction with resistance applied to lateral aspect of the leg.

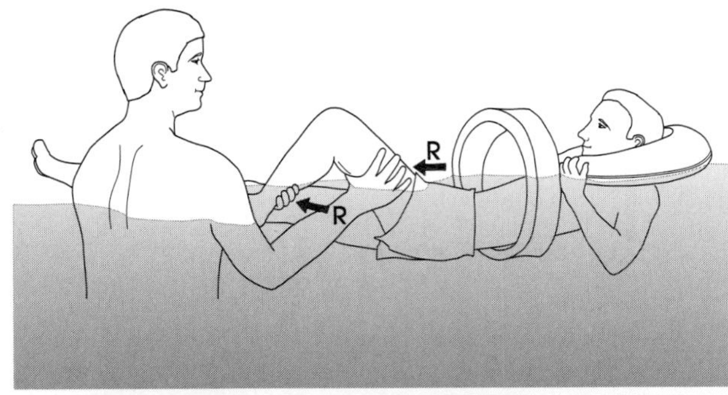

Figure 7–20 Manual resistance exercise for strengthening hip and knee flexion.

Hand Placement
Place the guide hand on the buoyancy belt or lateral hip. The resistance hand grasps proximal to the distal tibiofibular joint.

Direction of Movement
Active contraction of the hip and knee flexors will cause the patient's body to glide toward the practitioner and fixed distal extremity.

Hip Internal/External Rotation

Practitioner Position
Stand lateral to the patient's affected extremity, face medially.

Patient Position
BS supine; hip in neutral at 0 degrees extension with knee flexed to 90 degrees.

Hand Placement
Contact the distal thigh medially with the guide hand for resisted internal rotation and laterally for resisted external rotation. Place the resistance hand at the distal leg.

Direction of Movement
Active contraction of hip rotators (alternating between internal and external rotation) causes the patient's body to glide away from the distal fixed segment. **Caution:** Avoid this exercise for patients with possible medial or lateral knee joint instability.

Knee Extension

Practitioner Position
Stand at the patient's feet, facing cephalad.

Patient Position
BS supine.

Hand Placement
Place the guide hand at the patient's lateral thigh and the resistance hand on the dorsal aspect of the distal tibiofibular joint.

Direction of Movement
Active contraction of the quadriceps against the practitioner's resistance hand will direct the body away from the practitioner as the knee extends.

Ankle Motions

Practitioner Position
Stand lateral to the affected leg, facing caudal.

Patient Position
BS supine.

Hand Placement
The hand placement creates a short lever arm at the patient's ankle. As the patient moves through the resisted ankle motions the patient's entire body will move through the water producing a significant amount of drag and demand on the ankle complex.

Precaution: For patients with ligamentously unstable ankles or compromised ankle musculature, the practitioner should cue the patient to avoid maximal effort during contraction to avoid potential injury.

Ankle Dorsiflexion and Plantarflexion

Hand Placement
Place the guide hand on lateral aspect of the leg and the resistance hand over dorsal aspect of the foot to resist dorsiflexion, and on the plantar aspect to resist plantarflexion.

Direction of Movement
The body will move toward the practitioner during dorsiflexion and away from the practitioner during plantarflexion.

Ankle Inversion and Eversion

Hand Placement
Place the guide hand on lateral aspect of the lower leg during inversion and on the medial aspect of tibia during eversion. To resist inversion grasp the dorsal medial aspect of the foot, and to resist eversion, grasp the lateral foot.

Direction of Movement
During inversion the body will glide toward the practitioner, and during eversion the body will glide away from the practitioner.

Dynamic Trunk Stabilization

By applying concepts utilized for spinal stabilization exercises on land (see Chapters 15 and 16), the practitioner can challenge the dynamic control and strength of the trunk muscles in the aquatic environment. The BS supine position creates a unique perceptual environment for the patient.

Dynamic Trunk Stabilization—Frontal Plane (Fig. 7–21)

Practitioner Position
Hold the patient at the shoulders or feet.

Patient Position
Typically, the patient is placed in a supine position with buoyancy devices at the neck, waist, and legs.

Execution
Instruct the patient to identify his or her neutral spine position, perform a "drawing-in maneuver" (see Chapter 16), and maintain the spinal position (isometric abdominal contraction). Move the patient from side to side through the water; monitor and cue the patient to avoid lateral trunk flexion, an indication that the patient is no longer stabilizing the spine.

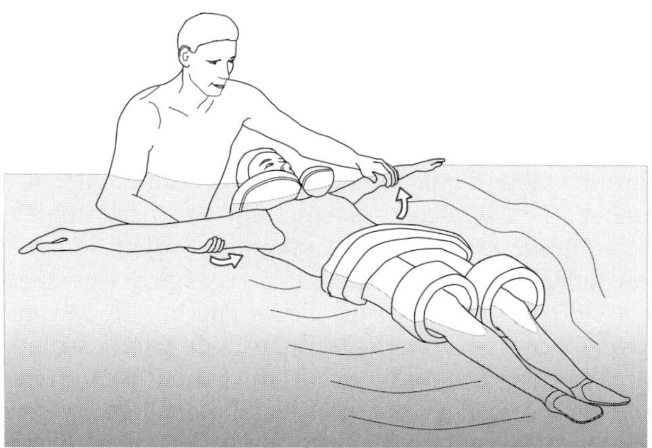

Figure 7–21 Isometric trunk stabilization exercise using side to side motions of the trunk.

Intensity

Moving the patient through the water faster will increase drag and exercise intensity. Holding the patient more distally will increase exercise intensity.

Dynamic Trunk Stabilization—Multidirectional

Practitioner Position

Stand at the shoulders or feet of the patient and grasp the patient's extremity to provide fixation as the patient contracts.

Patient Position

Typically, the patient is placed in a supine position with buoyancy devices at the neck, waist, and legs.

Execution

Instruct the patient to assume a neutral spine, perform the drawing-in maneuver, and "hold" the spine stable. Instruct the patient to perform either unilateral or bilateral resisted extremity patterns while maintaining a neutral spine and abdominal control. Monitor and cue the patient to avoid motion at the trunk, an indication that the patient is no longer stabilizing with the deep abdominal and spinal muscles. Upper extremity motions include shoulder flexion, abduction, and diagonal patterns. Lower extremity motions include hip and knee flexion and hip abduction and adduction.

Intensity

Unilateral patterns are more demanding than bilateral patterns. Increasing speed or duration will increase exercise intensity.

Independent Strengthening Exercises

Often patients perform immersed strengthening exercises independently. Because the resistance created during movement through water is speed dependent, patients are able to control the amount of work performed and demands imposed on contractile elements.[4,24,51] Typically, positioning and performance of equipment-assisted strengthening activities in water reflect that of traditional land exercise. However, the aquatic environment allows patients to assume many positions (supine, prone, side-lying, seated, and vertical). Attention to specific patient positioning allows the practitioner to utilize the buoyant properties of water and/or the buoyant and resistive properties of equipment that can either assist or resist patient movement.[31,34] Before initiating immersed strengthening activities, patients should be oriented to the effects of speed and surface area on resistance. Specific exercises for mechanical strengthening of every body part are not described. Only selected exercises are discussed and illustrated to reinforce major concepts and principles of application.

The following terms are used for equipment-assisted exercise.

- ***Buoyancy assisted (ba).*** Vertical movement directed parallel to vertical forces of buoyancy that assist motion (patient may use buoyant equipment to assist with motion).
- ***Buoyancy supported (bs).*** Horizontal movement with vertical forces of buoyancy eliminating or minimizing the need to support an extremity against gravity (patient may use buoyant equipment to assist with motion).
- ***Buoyancy resisted (br).*** Movement directed against or perpendicular to vertical forces of buoyancy creating drag (performed without equipment).
- ***Buoyancy super resisted (bsr).*** Use of equipment generates resistance by increasing the total surface area moving through water by creating greater drag. Increasing the speed of motion through water generates further drag.

Extremity Strengthening Exercises (Fig. 7–22*A* through *E*)

The most common aquatic upper and lower extremity strengthening exercises are outlined in Box 7–1.[1,31,34] Typically, patients are positioned standing immersed to shoulder level for upper extremity strengthening and to mid-trunk level for lower extremity strengthening. However, many exercises may be performed with the patient positioned vertically in deep water. The prone or supine position is useful when practitioners wish to progress patients or when patients require position-specific or sports-specific strengthening. Some exercises, most notably bilateral lower extremity diagonals, require the patient to be positioned supine, prone, or vertical in deep water.

Lumbar Spine Strengthening

Spinal stabilization may be performed in shallow, mid-depth, or deep water levels. Typically, patients are instructed to maintain a neutral spine with the drawing-in maneuver (see Chapter 16) while performing functional activities or moving the extremities. The patient's ability to stabilize the spine can

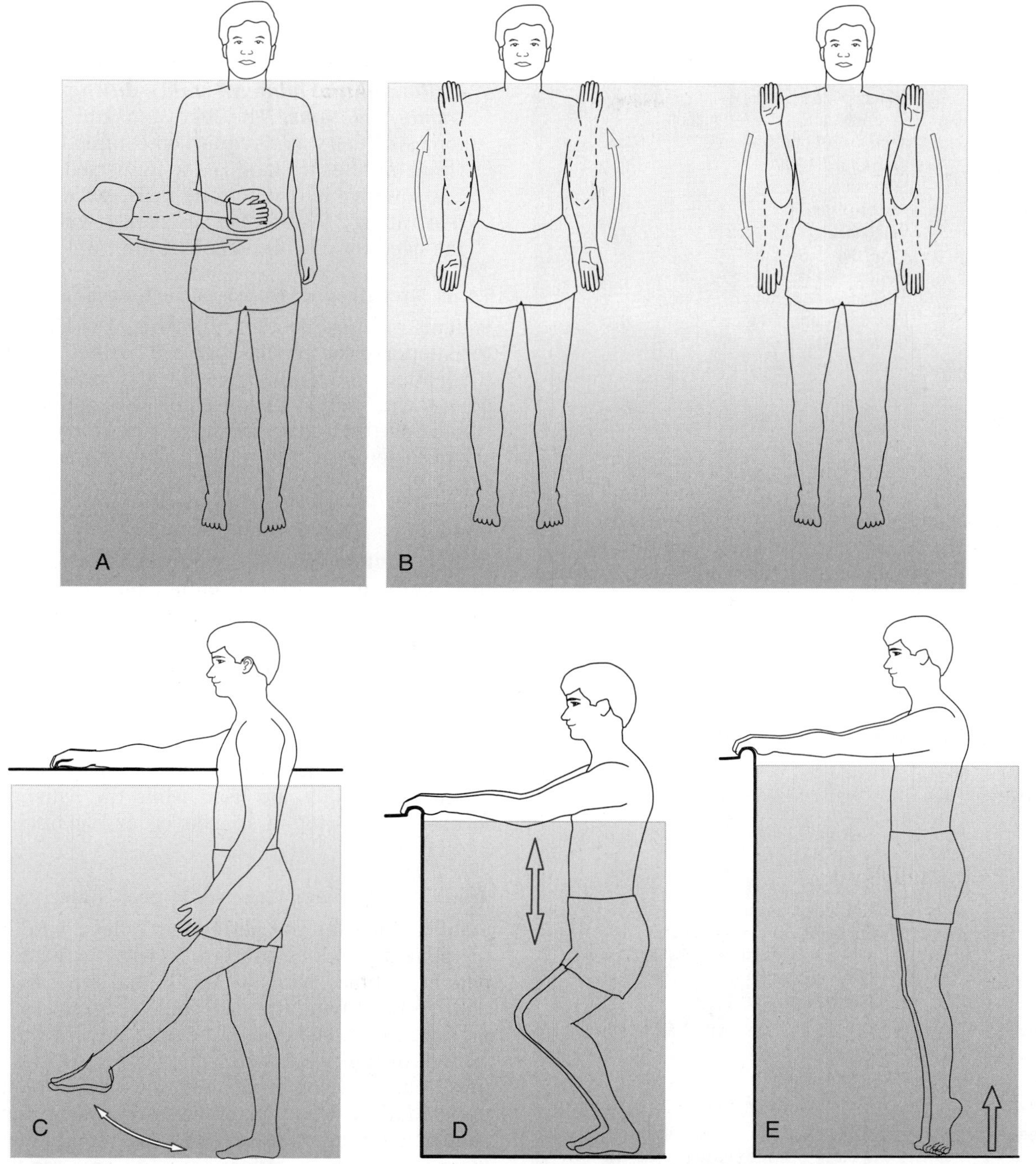

Figure 7–22 Mechanical resistance for strengthening *(A)* shoulder internal and external rotation, *(B)* elbow flexion and extension, *(C)* hip flexion and extension, *(D)* functional squatting, and *(E)* ankle plantarflexion. (Adapted from Bates and Hanson[6])

Box 7–1 Summary of Motions Used for Upper and Lower Strengthening Exercises

Shoulder	Flexion/extension Abduction/adduction Horizontal abduction/adduction Internal/external rotation Unilateral diagonals Bilateral diagonals
Elbow	Flexion/extension Diagonals Push/pull
Hip	Flexion/extension Abduction/adduction Internal/external rotation Unilateral diagonals Bilateral diagonals
Knee	Flexion/extension Diagonals

be challenged by increasing the duration of the activity, the speed or surface area moving through water, and by the addition of buoyant devices in the deep water. The exercises are summarized in Box 7–2.

Box 7–2 Summary of Lumbar Spine-Strengthening Exercises

Standing	Walking patterns: forward, backward, lateral, lunge walk, high stepping Unilateral/bilateral stance with upper extremity motions
Semi-reclined	Bicycling Hip abduction/adduction Flutter kick Bilateral lower extremity PNF patterns Unilateral/bilateral hip and knee flexion/extension
Supine	Bridging with long dumbbell placed at knees Swimming kicks
Prone	Swimming kicks
Deep water	Vertical stabilization exercises; abdominal bracing with arm and leg motions in the pike and iron-cross positions Seated on dumbbell; abdominal bracing and balance while performing unilateral or bilateral arm motions Standing on a kickboard or dumbbell; abdominal bracing and balance while performing bicycling motions and/or arm motions

Trunk Strengthening Exercises: Standing

- ***Walking patterns.*** Holding a kickboard vertically in the water will increase resistance.
- ***Unilateral and bilateral stance during upper extremity motions.*** The buoyant and turbulent forces of the water require co-contraction of the trunk muscles to stabilize the immersed body; using equipment (Hydro-tone bells, paddles, resistive tubing) to increase resistance will increase the need for co-contraction of the trunk muscles.

Trunk Strengthening Exercises: Semi-Reclined

Patients may use noodles, dumbbells, or kickboards for support. The practitioner can further challenge the patient by having him or her hold buoyant equipment, such as paddles, and having the patient stabilizing the trunk against the movement. A variety of lower extremity movements are suggested in Box 7–2.

Trunk Strengthening Exercises: Supine

In this position, various swimming kicks are used; instruct the patient to concentrate on the drawing-in maneuver and maintaining the neutral spine position while moving the legs. Bridging while maintaining a neutral spine can be done with a long dumbbell placed at the knees.

Trunk Strengthening Exercises: Prone

In the prone position, various swimming kicks, such as the flutter kick, are used while the patient performs the drawing-in maneuver and maintains a neutral spine.

Trunk Strengthening Exercises in Deep Water

Stabilization exercises performed in deep water with the patient positioned vertically typically require the patient to brace with the abdominal muscles. Emphasize identifying the neutral spine, activating the drawing-in maneuver, and holding the spine in the stable position while performing the various activities. Utilize any combination of unilateral or bilateral upper and/or lower extremity motions to further challenge the stabilization effort. Add equipment devices to the hands or legs for additional resistance and increased challenge when the patient can maintain good stabilization control. Variations include:

- Altering trunk positions such as the pike position or the iron-cross position.
- Sitting on a dumbbell and bicycling forward or backward or moving the upper extremities through any combination of motions.

- Standing on a kickboard or dumbbell and moving the upper extremities through various combinations of motions, first without then with equipment. Such standing activities typically induce obligatory abdominal bracing and challenges to balance.

Aerobic Conditioning

Aquatic exercise that emphasizes aerobic/cardiovascular conditioning can be an integral component of many rehabilitation programs. Aerobic/cardiovascular exercise typically takes place with the patient suspended vertically in deep water pools and the feet not touching the pool bottom. Alternative activities that may be performed in mid-level water, 4 to 6 feet in depth, include jogging, swimming strokes, immersed cycling, and immersed treadmill. Understanding the various treatment options, physiologic responses, monitoring methods, proper form, and equipment selection allows the clinician to use this form of exercise effectively and safely in a rehabilitation program.

Treatment Interventions

Deep water walking/running (Fig. 7–23). Deep water walking and running are the most common vertical deep water cardiovascular endurance exercises. Alternatives include cross-country motions and high-knee marching. Deep water cardiovascular training, which may be used as a precursor to midwater or land-based cardiovascular training, eliminates the effects of impact on the lower extremities and spine.

The patient can be tethered to the edge of the pool to perform deep water running in those pools with limited space. Some small tanks provide resistance jets for the patient to move against.

Midwater jogging/running (immersed treadmill running). Midwater aerobic exercise, which may be used as a precursor to land training, lessens the effects of impact on the spine and lower extremities. As a patient's tolerance to impact improves, mid-water jogging may be performed in progressively shallower depths to provide increased weight bearing and functional replication. In pools with limited space, tethering with resistive tubing can provide resistance.

Immersed equipment. Immersed equipment includes immersed cycling, treadmill, or upper body ergometer.

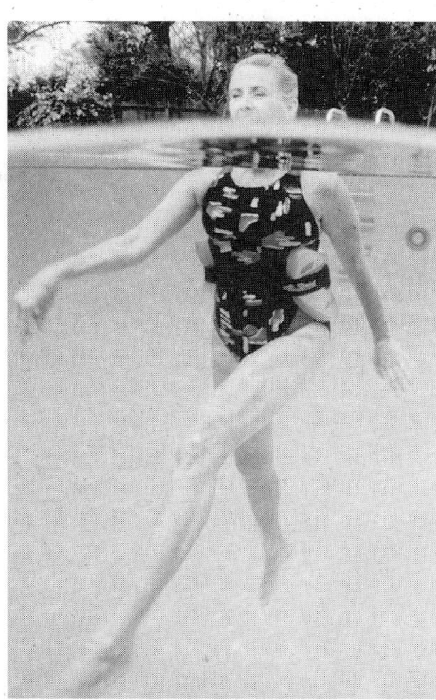

Figure 7–23 Deep water walking/jogging. (Courtesy of Rothhammer International Inc. San Luis Obispo, CA.)

Swimming strokes. For patients able to tolerate the positions necessary to perform various swim strokes (neck and shoulder ROM and prone, supine, or side-lying positions) swimming can be an excellent tool to train and improve cardiovascular fitness. Swimming may elicit significantly higher elevations of heart rate, blood pressure, and $\dot{V}O_{2\ max}$ than other aquatic activities. Swimming contributes the added benefit of hip and trunk strengthening for some patients with spinal conditions.

Precaution: Recommending swimming for poorly skilled swimmers with cardiac compromise may adversely challenge the patient's cardiovascular system.

Physiologic Response to Deep Water Walking/Running

Various physiologic responses to deep water walking and running have been reported.*

Cardiovascular Response

Patients without cardiovascular compromise may experience dampened elevation of heart rate, ventilation and $\dot{V}O_{2\ max}$ compared to similar land-based

*See references 3, 10, 12, 13, 15, 21, 27, 33, 55, 58.

exercise. During low-intensity exercise, cardiac patients may experience lower cardiovascular stresses.[22,23] As exercise intensity increases, cardiovascular stresses approach those of related exercise on land.[23,35]

Training Effect

Patients will experience carryover gains in $\dot{V}O_{2\ max}$ from aquatic to land conditions.[45] Additionally, aquatic cardiovascular training maintains leg strength and maximal oxygen consumption in healthy runners.[33,45,58,60]

Proper Form for Deep Water Running

Instruction for Beginners

Proper instruction is important to ensure correct form because many beginners will experience a significant learning curve.[8] Once immersed, the patient should maintain a neutral cervical spine and slightly forward flexed trunk with the arms at the sides. During running the hips should alternately flex to approximately 80 degrees with the knee extended and then extend to neutral as the knee flexes.

Accommodating Specific Patient Populations

For patients with positional pain associated with spinal conditions, a posterior buoyancy belt will help maintain a slightly forward flexed position while a flotation vest will help maintain a more erect posture and relatively extended spine. Patients with unilateral lower extremity amputations may have difficulty maintaining a vertical position. Placing the buoyancy belt laterally (on the contralateral side of the amputation) will allow the patient to remain vertical more easily.

Exercise Monitoring

Monitoring Intensity of Exercise

- ***Rate of perceived exertion.*** Because skill may affect technique, subjective numeric scales depicting perceived effort may inadequately identify the level of intensity for novice deep water runners. However, at both submaximal and maximal levels of exertion subjective numeric rating of effort appears to adequately correlate to heart rate during immersed exercise.[10,13,26,33]
- ***Heart rate.*** Because of the physiologic changes that occur with neck level immersion, various adjustments have been suggested in the literature to *lower* immersed maximum heart rate during near maximum cardiovascular exercise.[12,13,17,50,60] Suggested adjustments range from a decrease of between 7 and 20 beats per minute.[17,50,60] Immersed heart rate can be reliably monitored manually or with water-resistant electronic monitoring devices.

Monitoring Beginners

Care should be taken to regularly monitor the cardiovascular response of novice deep-water runners or of patients with known cardiac, pulmonary, or peripheral vascular disease. Novice deep-water runners may experience higher levels of perceived exertion and $\dot{V}O_{2\ max}$ compared to responses during similar land exercise.[26]

Equipment Selection

Deep Water Equipment

Selection of buoyancy devices should reflect the desired patient posture, comfort, and the projected intensity level. The most common buoyant device for deep water running is the flotation belt positioned posteriorly (see Fig. 7–5). Patients presenting with injuries or sensitivity of the trunk may require an alternative buoyant device; alternatives include vests, flotation dumbbells, or noodles. Providing the patient with smaller buoyant equipment (i.e., smaller belts, fewer noodles) will require the patient to work harder to maintain adequate buoyancy, thereby increasing the intensity of the activity. Fins and specially designed boots can be applied to the legs and feet to add resistance. Also, bells or buoyant dumbbells can be held in the hands to increase resistance (see Fig. 7–8).

Midwater Equipment

Specially designed socks can help eliminate the potential problem of skin breakdown on the feet during impact activities, such as running. Patients can run against forced current or tethered with elastic tubing for resistance. Using noodles around the waist or running while holding a kickboard will increase the amount of drag and resistance that the patient must move against.

Independent Learning Activities

CASE STUDIES

Postoperative Arthroscopic Knee Meniscectomy

Mike is a 54-year-old man who tore his right medial meniscus playing basketball. He is 2 weeks status postarthroscopic debridement of the torn piece of cartilage. Mike has returned to his desk job as a computer programmer but has a strong desire to return to his active workout schedule and weekend sports leagues. The surgeon has told Mike that he has no limitations except pain.

Past Medical History: Mike is healthy with no prior medical problems. He has never had an injury that made him miss more than a few days of sports participation.

Functional Status: Mike is ambulating without assistive devices, but he limps slightly because of a stiff knee. He is able to go up and down stairs but only one step at a time and has to lead with his left leg.

Musculoskeletal Status: Mike has only minimal swelling of the right knee. He rates his pain as a 1 out of 10 at rest and a 3 out of 10 with activity. His active knee ROM is 5 to 100 degrees. He has normal ROM in the remaining joints of the right leg. Mike is able to perform a straight leg raise and has a good quadriceps contraction. Manual muscle testing reveals 4/5 quadriceps strength, 4+/5 hamstring and gastrocsoleus strength. He has good patellofemoral joint mobility.

Physician Referral: The prescription that Mike's physician gives him states "Evaluate and treat right knee, S/P arthroscopic meniscal debridement; may utilize land and aquatic exercise for ROM and strength."

- Formalize a program to utilize the shallow water (4-ft depth) to start Mike with independent exercises for strength and flexibility.
- Describe what manual techniques you might be able to perform with Mike for strength or flexibility.
- As Mike progresses to full ROM and near-normal strength, how could you use aquatics to replicate the demands of basketball?
- What can Mike do in the pool to maintain his cardiovascular fitness while his knee heals?

Calf Tear

Cecily is a 30-year-old weather anchor who happens to be an elite marathon runner. Four days ago she was running up a hill and felt a "pulling" in her left calf, just distal to the knee. She decided to run in a 10K marathon the next day but had to quit after about 5K because of a sharp pain in her calf. The doctor has told her to use crutches and remain 25% weight bearing for the next 3 days. After that she can gradually begin to increase the weight she puts through the leg over the next week. The doctor has told Cecily that she should be full weight-bearing in 1 week and able to run in 3 weeks. Cecily is anxious to return to her intensive training schedule.

Past Medical History: Cecily is healthy with no prior medical problems. She has worn orthotic inserts in her shoes for "flat feet" for as long as she can remember. She says she has pulled her left calf several times during a running career that goes back to high school.

Functional Status: Cecily enters the facility ambulating with crutches. She is putting about 25% of her weight through her left foot. She is able to perform stairs without difficulty using the crutches and/or a railing.

Musculoskeletal Status: Cecily has a visible bruise at the medial head of the left gastrocnemius muscle belly. She is very tender to palpation there and has some swelling. She rates her pain at rest as a 1 out of 10 and her pain with activity as a 2 out of 10. Her ankle ROM is normal for all motions actively and passively with the exception of dorsiflexion. She dorsiflexes actively 5 degrees and passively 8 degrees. You grade her ankle strength as 5/5 except for plantarflexion, which you grade as a 4-/5; this may be limited due to pain. You also notice that her left hip flexors, quadriceps, and hamstrings are all tight.

Physician Referral: The prescription that Cecily's doctor gives her states "Aquatic therapy, evaluate and treat for left calf strain, gait training, ROM, strength. Progress to land as tolerated."

- Write up a program to address Cecily's dysfunctions and impairments utilizing the aquatic environment.
- At what depth of mid-water does Cecily need to be to gait train in the water and still maintain 25% weight bearing?
- Write up a program for the deep water to help Cecily maintain her high level of cardiovascular fitness.
- What equipment might be useful to assist her with independent stretching in the deep water and for cardiovascular training in the deep water?

Chronic Low Back Pain

Develop an aquatic program for a patient who has chronic low back pain and needs a comprehensive flexibility and strengthening program for the legs and trunk. The patient only has one visit approved by the insurance company. However, the patient has a pool in his or her back yard that gradually goes from 3 feet to 7 feet in depth. The 7-foot deep area is only 10 feet long and 5 feet wide. The patient has no other medical problems that will limit his or her performance of the aquatic program.

REFERENCES

1. Abidin, MR, et al: Hydrofitness devices for strengthening upper extremity muscles. J Burn Care Rehab 9:199, 1988.
2. Arborelius, M, Balldin, UI, et al: Hemodynamic changes in man during immersion with the head above water. Aerospace Med 43:592, 1972.
3. Avellini, BA, Shapiro, Y, and Pandolf, KB: Cardio-respiratory physical training in water and on land. Europ J Appl Physiol 50:255, 1983.
4. Babb, R, and Muntzer, E: Hydrotherapy: whirlpools to aquatic pools. In Michlovitz SL: Thermal Agents In Rehabilitation. FA Davis, Philadelphia, 1990.
5. Babb, R, and Simelson-Warr, A: Manual techniques of the lower extremities in aquatic physical therapy. J Aquatic Phys Ther 4(2):7, 1996.
6. Bates, A, and Hanson, N: Aquatic Exercise Therapy: A Comprehensive Approach to Use of Aquatic Exercise in Treatment of Orthopedic Injuries. Swystun and Swystun, British Columbia, Canada, 1992.
7. Bazett, HC, Maxfield, ME, and Blithe, MD: Effect of baths at different temperature on oxygen exchange and on the circulation. Am J Physiol 119:93, 1938.
8. Becker, BE, and Cole, AJ (eds): Comprehensive Aquatic Therapy. Butterworth-Heinemann, Mass, 1997.
9. Begin, R, Epstein, M, Sackner, MA, et al: Effects of water immersion to the neck on pulmonary circulation and tissue volume in man. J Appl Physiol 60:293, 1976.
10. Brennan, DK, Michaud, TJ, et al: Gains in aquarunning peak oxygen consumption after eight weeks of aquarun training (abstract). Med Sci Sports Exerc 24:S23, 1992.
11. Bullard, RW, and Rapp, GM: Problems of body heat loss in water immersion. Aerospace Med 41:1269, 1970.
12. Butts, NK, Tucker, M, and Greening, C: Physiologic responses to maximal treadmill and deep water running in men and women. Am J Sports Med 19:612, 1991.
13. Butts, NK, Tucker, M, and Smith, R: Maximal responses to treadmill and deep water running in high school female cross country runners. Res Q Exerc Sport 62:236, 1991.
14. Campion, M: Hydrotherapy: Principles and Management. Butterworth-Heinemann, England, 1997.
15. Cassady, SL, and Neilsen, DH: Cardiorespiratory responses to calisthenics performed with upper and lower extremities on land and in water at given cadences. Phys Ther 72:532, 1992.
16. Choukroun, ML, and Varene, P: Adjustments in oxygen transport during head-out immersion in water at different temperatures. J Appl Physiol 68:1475, 1990.
17. Christie, JL, et al: Cardiovascular regulation during head-out immersion exercise. J Appl Physiol 69:657, 1990.
18. Croce, P, and Gregg, JR: Keeping fit when injured. Clin Sports Med 10:181, 1991.
19. Duffield, MH, Skinner, AT, and Thompson, AM: Duffield's Exercise In Water. Bailliere Tindall, England, 1983.
20. Egan, S: Reduction of anxiety in aquaphobics. Can J Appl Sports Sci 6:68, 1981.
21. Evans, FW, Cureton, KJ, and Purvis, JW: Metabolic and circulatory responses to walking and jogging in water. Res Q Exerc Sport 49:442, 1987.
22. Fernhall, B, Congdon, K, and Manfredi, T: ECG response to water and land based exercise in patients with cardiovascular disease. J Cardiopulm Rehab 10:5, 1990.
23. Fernhall, B, Manfredi, TG, and Congdon, K: Prescribing water-based exercise from treadmill and arm ergometry in cardiac patients. Med Sci Sports Exerc 24:139, 1992.
24. Frey Law, LA, and Smidt, GL: Underwater forces produced by the Hydro-Tone bell. J Orthop Sports Phys Ther 23:267, 1996.
25. Fuller, RA, Dye, KK, Cook, NR, and Awbrey, BJ. The activity levels of the vastus medialis oblique muscle during a single leg squat on the land and at varied water depths. J Aquatic Phys Ther 7(1):13, 1999.
26. Gehring, M, Keller, B, and Brehm, B: Physiological responses to deep water running in competitive and non-competitive runners (abstract). Med Sci Sports Exerc 24:S23, 1992.
27. Gleim, GW, and Nicholas, JA: Metabolic costs and heart rate responses to treadmill walking in water at different depths and temperatures. Am J Sports Med 17:248, 1989.
28. Golland, A: Basic hydrotherapy. Physiotherapy 67(9):258, 1981.
29. Green, J, et al: Home exercises are as effective as outpatient hydrotherapy for osteoarthritis of the hip. Br J Rheumatol 32:812, 1993.
30. Hall, J, Skevington, SM, et al: A randomized and controlled trial of hydrotherapy in rheumatoid arthritis. Arth Care Res 9(3):206, 1996.
31. Harrison, RA: A quantitative approach to strengthening exercises in the hydrotherapy pool. Physiotherapy 65:60, 1980.
32. Harrison, RA: Tolerance of pool therapy by ankylosing spondylitis patients with low vital capacities. Physiotherapy 67:296, 1981.
33. Hertler, L, Provost-Craig, M, Sestili, D, Hove, A, and Fees, M: Water running and the maintenance of maximal oxygen consumption and leg strength in runners (abstract). Med Sci Sports Exerc 24:S23, 1992.
34. Hillman, MR, Matthews, L, and Pope, JM: The resistance to motion through water created with hydrotherapy table-tennis bats. Physiotherapy 73:570, 1987.
35. Johnson, BK, Adamcyk, J, Stromme, SG, and Tennoe, KO: Comparison of oxygen uptake and heart rate during exercises on land and in water. Phys Ther 57:3, 1977.
36. Kelsey, DD, and Tyson, E: A new method of training for the lower extremity using unloading. J Orthop Sports Phys Ther, 19(4):218, 1994.
37. Kolb, ME: Principles of underwater exercise. Phys Ther Rev 37:361, 1957.
38. Lawson, GE: An overview of aquatic rehabilitation therapy. Topics Clin Chiro 3(9):82, 1996.
39. Langridge, JC, and Phillips, D: Group hydrotherapy exercises for chronic low back pain sufferers. Physiotherapy 74:269, 1988.
40. LeFort SM, and Hannah, TE: Return to work following an aquafitness and muscle strengthening program for the low back injured. Arch Phys Med Rehabil 75:1247, 1994.
41. Levine, BA: Use of hydrotherapy in reduction of anxiety. Psychol Rep 55:226, 1984.
42. Mano, T, Iwase, S, Yamazaki, Y, and Saito, M: Sympathetic nervous adjustments in man to simulated weightlessness induced by water immersion. Sngyo Ika Daigaku Zasshi 7(suppl):215, 1985.
43. McGrath, AM, Johnson, AS, and Moeller, JM: The effects of hamstring stretching on land versus water (abstract). Phys Ther 73(6):S30, 1993.

44. McMurray, RG, Fieselman, CC, et al: Exercise hemodynamics in water and on land in patients with coronary artery disease. J Cardiopulm Rehabil 8:69, 1988.
45. Michaud, TL, Brennan, DK, et al: Aquarun training and changes in treadmill running maximal oxygen consumption (abstract). Med Sci Sports Exerc 24:S23, 1992.
46. Norton, CO, Shaha, S, and Stewart, L: Aquatic versus traditional therapy: contrasting effectiveness for acquisition rates (abstract). Phys Ther 73(6):S10, 1993.
47. Perk, J, Perk, L, and Boden, C: Cardiopulmonary adaptation of COPD patient to physical training on land and in water. Europ Resp J 9:248, 1996.
48. Prins, J, and Cutner, D: Aquatic therapies in the rehabilitation of athletic injuries. Clin Sports Med 18(2):447, 1999.
49. Revay, S, Dahlstrom, M, and Dalen, N: Water exercise versus instruction for self-training following a shoulder fracture. Int J Rehab Res 15, 1992.
50. Ritchie, SE, and Hopkins, WG: The intensity of exercise in deep-water running. Int J Sports Med 12:27, 1991.
51. Ruoti, RG, Morris, DM, and Cole, AJ: Aquatic Rehabilitation. Lippincott, Philadelphia, 1997.
52. Ruoti, RG, Troup, JT, and Berger, RA: The effects of non-swimming water exercise on older adults. J Orthop Sports Phys Ther 19(3):140, 1994.
53. Sagawas, S, et al: Water temperature and intensity of exercise in maintenance of thermal equilibrium. J Appl Physiol 65:2413, 1988.
54. Schrepfer, R, and Babb, R: Manual techniques of the shoulder in aquatic physical therapy. J Aquatic Phys Ther 6(1)11, 1998.
55. Sheldahl, LM, Clifford, PS, et al: Effects of head-out water immersion on response to exercise training. J Appl Physiol 60:1878, 1986.
56. Simmons, V, and Hansen, PD: Effectiveness of water exercise on postural mobility in the well elderly: an experimental study on balance enhancement. J Gerontol 51A:M233, 1996.
57. Speer, KP, Cavanaugh, JT, et al: A role for hydrotherapy in shoulder rehabilitation. Am J Sports Med 21(6):850,1993.
58. Svendenhag, J, and Seger, J: Running on land and in water: Comparative exercise physiology. Med Sci Sports Exerc 24:1155, 1992.
59. Templeton, MS, Booth, DL, and O'Kelly, WD: Effects of aquatic therapy on joint flexibility and functional ability in subjects with rheumatic disease. J Orthop Sports Phys Ther 6:376, 1996.
60. Thein, JM, and Brody, LT: Aquatic-based rehabilitation and training for the elite athlete. J Orthop Sports Phys Ther 27(1):32, 1998.
61. Tovin, BJ, Wolf, SL, et al: Comparison of the effects of exercise in water and on land on the rehabilitation of patients with intra-articular anterior cruciate ligament reconstructions. Phys Ther 74:710, 1994.
62. Whitlach, S, and Adema, R: Functional benefits of a structured hot water group exercise program. Activities, Adaptation, and Aging 20(3):75, 1996.
63. Woods, DA: Rehabilitation aquatics for low back injury: functional gains or pain reduction. Clin Kines 43:96, 1989.

Part II

Application of Therapeutic Exercise Techniques to Regions of the Body

Chapter 8

Principles of Treating Soft Tissue, Bony, and Postsurgical Conditions

OBJECTIVES

After studying this chapter, the reader will be able to:

1 Describe examples of soft tissue lesions.

2 Differentiate characteristics of soft tissue repair during each of the stages of inflammation and healing after injury or surgery.

3 Describe special considerations, impairment goals, and treatment plan for soft tissue lesions during each of the stages of recovery.

4 Describe general management strategies for impairments and functional limitations related to repetitive trauma syndromes.

5 Describe general management strategies for mobility impairments related to joint pathologies and fractures.

6 Apply guidelines for management of impairments and functional limitations to develop appropriately graded exercise programs for each stage of recovery after soft tissue and joint trauma.

7 Describe common surgical procedures used to manage musculoskeletal impairments associated with a variety of musculoskeletal disorders or conditions.

8 Design a preoperative patient education program for individuals planning to undergo surgery to the musculoskeletal system.

9 Apply appropriate guidelines for management to develop a postoperative exercise program for each of the three progressive phases of rehabilitation after musculoskeletal surgery.

The proper use of therapeutic exercise in the management of musculoskeletal disorders depends on identifying the structure involved, recognizing its stage of recovery, and determining the functional limitations or disabilities. Examination of the involved region is an important prerequisite for identifying the anatomic structure or structures that are causing the impairments and limiting function and also for determining whether the tissue is in the acute, subacute, or chronic stage of recovery. This chapter and subsequent chapters in this section have been written with the assumption that the reader has a background in examination, evaluation, and program planning to be able to assess impairments and develop functional goals. Utilizing the principles presented in this chapter, the reader should be able to design therapeutic exercise programs that meet the goals and choose techniques for intervention that are at an appropriate intensity for the stage of healing, disease process, or phase of postsurgical recovery. Subsequent chapters in this section expand on these principles for each joint region.

▶ Soft Tissue Lesions

Examples of Soft Tissue Lesions

- ***Strain.*** Overstretching, overexertion, overuse of soft tissue. Tends to be less severe than a sprain. Occurs from slight trauma or unaccustomed repeated trauma of a minor degree.[16] This term is frequently used to refer specifically to some degree of disruption of the musculotendinous unit.[34]
- ***Sprain.*** Severe stress, stretch, or tear of soft tissues, such as joint capsule, ligament, tendon, or muscle. This term is frequently used to refer specifically to injury of a ligament and is graded

as first- (mild), second- (moderate), or third- (severe) degree sprains.[34]

- ***Subluxation.*** An incomplete or partial dislocation that often involves secondary trauma to surrounding soft tissue.
- ***Dislocation.*** Displacement of a part, usually the bony partners within a joint, leading to soft tissue damage, inflammation, pain, and muscle spasm.
- ***Muscle/tendon rupture or tear.*** If a rupture or tear is partial, pain is experienced in the region of the breach when the muscle is stretched or when it contracts against resistance. If a rupture or tear is complete, the muscle does not pull against the injury, so stretching or contraction of the muscle does not cause pain.[20]
- ***Tendinous lesions.*** **Tenosynovitis** is an inflammation of the synovial membrane covering a tendon. **Tendinitis** is an inflammation of a tendon; there may be resulting scarring or calcium deposits. **Tenovaginitis** is inflammation with thickening of a tendon sheath. **Tendinosis** is a degeneration of the tendon from repetitive microtrauma.
- ***Synovitis.*** Inflammation of a synovial membrane; an excess of normal synovial fluid within a joint or tendon sheath from trauma or disease.[71]
- ***Hemarthrosis.*** Bleeding into a joint, usually from severe trauma.[71]
- ***Ganglion.*** Ballooning of the wall of a joint capsule or tendon sheath. Ganglia may arise after trauma, and they sometimes occur with rheumatoid arthritis.
- ***Bursitis.*** Inflammation of a bursa.
- ***Contusion.*** Bruising from a direct blow, resulting in capillary rupture, bleeding, edema, and an inflammatory response.
- ***Overuse syndromes, cumulative trauma disorders, repetitive strain injury.*** Repeated, submaximal overload and/or frictional wear to a muscle or tendon resulting in inflammation and pain.

Clinical Conditions Resulting from Trauma or Pathology

In many conditions involving soft tissue, the primary pathology is difficult to define, or the tissue has healed with limitations, resulting in a secondary loss of function. The following are examples of clinical manifestations resulting from a variety of causes, including those listed under the previous section:

- ***Dysfunction.*** Loss of normal function of a tissue or region. The dysfunction may be caused by adaptive shortening of the soft tissues, adhesions, muscle weakness, or any condition resulting in loss of normal mobility.
- ***Joint dysfunction.*** Mechanical loss of normal joint play in synovial joints; commonly causes loss of function and pain. Precipitating factors may be trauma, immobilization, disuse, aging, or a serious pathologic condition.[69]
- ***Contractures.*** Adaptive shortening of skin, fascia, muscle, or joint capsule that prevents normal mobility or flexibility of that structure.
- ***Adhesions.*** Abnormal adherence of collagen fibers to surrounding structures during immobilization, after trauma, or as a complication of surgery, which restricts normal elasticity and gliding of the structures involved.
- ***Reflex muscle guarding.*** The prolonged contraction of a muscle in response to a painful stimulus. The primary pain-causing lesion may be in nearby or underlying tissue or from a referred pain source. When not referred, the contracting muscle functionally splints the injured tissue against movement. Guarding ceases when the painful stimulus is relieved.
- ***Intrinsic muscle spasm.*** The prolonged contraction of a muscle in response to the local circulatory and metabolic changes that occur when a muscle is in a continued state of contraction. Pain is a result of the altered circulatory and metabolic environment, so the muscle contraction becomes self-perpetuating regardless of whether the primary lesion that caused the initial guarding is still irritable (Fig. 8–1). Spasm may also be a response of muscle to viral infection, cold, prolonged periods of immobilization, emotional tension, or direct trauma to muscle.[69]
- ***Muscle weakness.*** A decrease in the strength of contraction of muscle. Muscle weakness may be the result of a systemic, chemical, or local lesion of a nerve of the central or peripheral nervous system or the myoneural junction. It may also be the result of a direct insult to the muscle or may simply be due to inactivity.

Severity of Tissue Injury

- ***Grade 1 (first-degree).*** Mild pain at the time of injury or within the first 24 hours. Mild swelling, local tenderness, and pain occur when the tissue is stressed.[34,35]

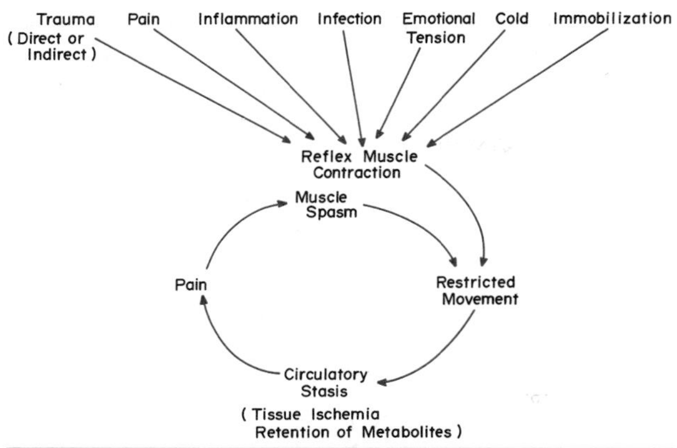

Figure 8–1 Schematic of the self-perpetuating cycle of muscle spasm.

- ***Grade 2 (second-degree).*** Moderate pain that requires stopping the activity. Stress and palpation of the tissue greatly increase the pain. When the injury is to ligaments, some of the fibers are torn, resulting in some increased joint mobility.[34,35]
- ***Grade 3 (third-degree).*** Near-complete or complete tear or avulsion of the tissue (tendon or ligament) with severe pain. Stress to the tissue is usually painless; palpation may reveal the defect. A torn ligament results in instability of the joint.[34,35]

Irritability of Tissue: Stages of Inflammation and Repair

After any insult to connective tissue, whether it is from mechanical injury (including surgery) or chemical irritant, the vascular and cellular response is similar (Table 8–1). Tissue irritability, or sensitivity, is the result of these responses and is usually divided into three stages of inflammation and repair with the following clinical signs and symptoms.

Acute Stage (Inflammatory Reaction)

The signs of inflammation are present; they are swelling, redness, heat, pain at rest, and loss of function. When testing the range of motion (ROM), movement is painful and the patient usually guards against the motion before completion of the range is possible (Fig. 8–2*A*). The pain and impaired movement are from the altered chemical state that irritates the nerve endings, increased tissue tension from edema or joint effusion, and muscle guarding, which is the body's way of immobilizing a painful area. This stage usually lasts 4 to 6 days unless the insult is perpetuated.

Table 8–1 Characteristics and Clinical Signs of the Stages of Inflammation, Repair, and Maturation of Tissue

Acute Stage: Inflammatory Reaction	Subacute Stage: Repair and Healing	Chronic Stage: Maturation and Remodeling
Characteristics		
Vascular changes	Removal of noxious stimuli	Maturation of connective tissue
Exudation of cells and chemicals	Growth of capillary beds into area	Contracture of scar tissue
Clot formation	Collagen formation	Remodeling of scar
Phagocytosis, neutralization of irritants	Granulation tissue	Collagen aligns to stress
Early fibroblastic activity	Very fragile, easily injured tissue	
Clinical Signs		
Inflammation	Decreasing inflammation	Absence of inflammation
Pain before tissue resistance	Pain synchronous with tissue resistance	Pain after tissue resistance
Physical Therapy Intervention		
PROTECTION PHASE Control effects of inflammation Modalities Selective rest/ immobilization Promote early healing and prevent deleterious effects of rest Passive movement, massage, and muscle setting with caution	CONTROLLED-MOTION PHASE Promote healing; develop mobile scar Nondestructive active, resistive, open- and closed-chain stabilization, and muscular endurance exercises, carefully progressed in intensity and range	RETURN-TO-FUNCTION PHASE Increase strength and alignment of scar; develop functional independence Progressive stretching, strengthening, endurance training, functional exercises, and specificity drills

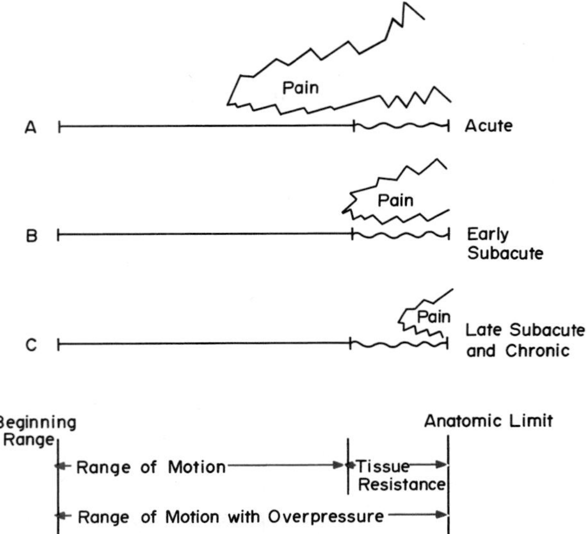

Figure 8–2 Pain experienced with ROM when involved tissue is in the *(A)* acute stage, *(B)* early subacute stage, and *(C)* late subacute or chronic stage.

Subacute Stage (Repair and Healing)

The signs of inflammation progressively decrease and eventually are absent. When testing ROM, the patient may experience pain synchronous with encountering tissue resistance at the end of the available ROM (Fig. 8–2*B*). Pain occurs only when the newly developing tissue is stressed beyond its tolerance or when tight tissue is stressed. Muscles may test weak, and function will be limited as a result of the weakened tissue. This stage usually lasts 10 to 17 days (14–21 days after the onset of injury), but may last up to 6 weeks in some tissues with limited circulation, such as tendons.[22]

Chronic Stage (Maturation and Remodeling)

There are no signs of inflammation. There may be contractures or adhesions that limit range, and there may be muscle weakness limiting normal function. Connective tissue continues to strengthen and remodel during this stage. A stretch pain may be felt when testing tight structures at the end of their available range (Fig. 8–2*C*). Function may be limited by muscle weakness, poor endurance, or poor neuromuscular control. This stage may last 6 months to 1 year depending on the tissue involved and amount of tissue damage.

Chronic Inflammation (Overuse Syndrome)

This is a state of prolonged inflammation. There are symptoms of increased pain, swelling, and muscle guarding that last more than several hours after activity. There are increased feelings of stiffness after rest, loss of ROM 24 hours after activity, and progressively greater stiffness of the tissue as long as the irritation persists.

Chronic Pain Syndrome

This is a state that persists longer than 6 months. It includes pain that cannot be linked to a source of irritation or inflammation and functional limitations and disability that include physical, emotional, and psychosocial parameters.

▶ Management During The Acute Stage

Tissue Response—Inflammation

This stage involves cellular, vascular, and chemical responses within the tissue. During the first 48 hours after insult to soft tissue, vascular changes predominate. Exudation of cells and solutes from the blood vessels takes place, and clot formation occurs. Within this period, neutralization of the chemical irritants or noxious stimuli, phagocytosis (cleaning up of dead tissue), early fibroblastic activity, and formation of new capillary beds begin. These physiological processes serve as a protective mechanism as well as a stimulus for subsequent healing and repair.[12] Usually this stage lasts 4 to 6 days unless the insult is perpetuated.

Management Guidelines—The Protection Phase

The therapist's role during this phase of intervention is to control the effects of the inflammation, facilitate wound healing, and maintain normal function in unaffected tissues and body regions. The following information is summarized in Box 8–1.

Patient Education

Inform the patient about the expected duration of symptoms (4–6 days), what he or she can do during this stage, any precautions or contraindications, and what to expect when the symptoms lessen. Patients need reassurance that the acute symptoms are usually short-lived, and need to learn what is safe to do during this stage of healing.

Protection of the Injured Tissue

To minimize musculoskeletal pain and promote healing, protection of the part affected by the in-

Box 8–1 Management Guidelines—Acute Stage/Protection Phase

Impairments:
- Inflammation, pain, edema, muscle spasm
- Impaired movement
- Joint effusion (if the joint is injured or if there is arthritis)
- Decreased use of associated areas

Plan of Care	Intervention (up to 1 week postinjury)
1. Educate the patient.	1. Inform patient of anticipated recovery time and how to protect the part while maintaining appropriate functional activities.
2. Control pain, edema, spasm.	2. Cold, compression, elevation, massage (48 hours). Immobilize the part (rest, splint, tape, cast). Avoid positions of stress to the part. Gentle (grade I) joint oscillations with joint in pain-free position.
3. Maintain soft tissue and joint integrity and mobility.	3. Appropriate dosage of passive movements within limit of pain, specific to structure involved. Appropriate dosage of intermittent muscle setting or electrical stimulation.
4. Reduce joint swelling if symptoms are present.	4. May require medical intervention if swelling is rapid (blood). Provide protection (splint, cast).
5. Maintain integrity and function of associated areas.	5. Active-assistive, free, resistive, and/or modified aerobic exercises, depending on proximity to associated areas and effect on the primary lesion. Adaptive or assistive devices as needed to protect the part during functional activities.

Precautions: The proper dosage of rest and movement must be used during the inflammatory stage. Signs of too much movement are increased pain or increased inflammation.

Contraindications: Stretching and resistance exercises should not be performed at the site of the inflamed tissue.[71]

flammatory process is necessary during the first 24 to 48 hours. This is usually provided by rest (splint, tape, cast), cold (ice), compression, and elevation. Depending on the type and severity of injury, manual methods of pain and edema control, such as massage and gentle (grade I) joint oscillations, may be beneficial. Depending on the part involved, protection with assistive devices for ambulation may be required.

Prevention of Adverse Effects of Immobility

Complete or continuous immobilization should be avoided whenever possible as it can lead to the adherence of developing fibrils to surrounding tissue, weakening of connective tissue, and changes in articular cartilage.[20,57,58,70]

The *long-term goal of treatment* is the formation of a strong, mobile scar at the site of the lesion so that there is complete and painless restoration of function. Initially, the network of fibril formation is random. It acquires an organized arrangement according to the mechanical forces acting on the tissue. To influence the development of an organized scar, begin treatment during the acute stage, when tolerated, with carefully controlled *passive movements.*

Tissue-specific movement. These movements should be specific to the structure involved to prevent abnormal adherence of the developing fibrils to surrounding tissue and thus avoid future disruption of the scar. Tissue-specific techniques are described below.

Intensity. The intensity (dosage) of movement should be gentle enough so that the fibrils are not detached from the site of healing. Too much movement too soon will be painful and will reinjure the tissue. The dosage of passive movement depends on the severity of the lesion. Some patients tolerate no movement during the first 24 to 48 hours; others tolerate only a few degrees of gentle passive movement. Continuous passive movement (CPM; see Chapter 2) has been useful immediately after various types of surgery to joints; intra-articular, metaphyseal, and diaphyseal fractures; surgical release of extra-articular contractures and adhesions; as well as other selected conditions.[57,58] Any movement tolerated at this stage is beneficial, but it must *not* increase the inflammation or pain. Active movement is usually *contraindicated* at the site of an active pathological process unless it is a chronic disease, such as rheumatoid arthritis.

General movement. Active movement is appropriate in neighboring regions to maintain integrity in uninjured tissue as well as to aid in circulation and lymphatic flow.

Specific Interventions and Dosages

Precaution: If the movement increases pain or inflammation, it is either of too great a dosage or it should not be done. Extreme care must be used with movement at this stage.

Passive range of motion (PROM). PROM within the limit of pain is valuable for maintaining mobility in joint, ligaments, tendons, and muscles as well as improving fluid dynamics and maintaining nutrition within the joints.[57,58] Initially, the range will probably be very small.[70] Stretching at this stage is contraindicated. Any motion gained from the PROM techniques is because of decreased pain, swelling, and muscle guarding.

Low-dosage joint mobilization techniques. Grade I or II distraction and glide techniques have the benefit of improving fluid dynamics within the joint to maintain cartilage health. These techniques may also reflexively inhibit or gate the perception of pain. Low-dosage joint mobilizations are beneficial with joint pathologies as well as any other connective tissue injury that affects joint motion during the acute stage.

Muscle setting. Gentle isometric muscle contractions performed intermittently and at a very low intensity so as not to cause pain or joint compression have several purposes. The pumping action of the contracting muscle assists the circulation and, therefore, fluid dynamics. If there is muscle damage or injury, the setting techniques are done with the muscle in the shortened position to help maintain mobility of the actin-myosin filaments without stressing the breached tissue. If there is joint injury, the position during the setting techniques is dictated by pain; usually the resting position for the joint is most comfortable. If tolerated, the intermittent setting techniques are performed in several positions.

Massage. Massage serves the purpose of moving fluid, and if applied cautiously and gently to injured tissue, may assist in preventing adhesions. Tendinous lesions are treated with a gentle dosage applied transverse to the fibers to smooth roughened surfaces or to maintain mobility of the tendon within its sheath. When applied, the tendon is kept taut. When treating muscle lesions, the muscle is usually kept in its shortened position in order not to separate the healing breach.[20]

Interventions for Associated Areas

During the protection phase, maintain as normal a physiological state as possible in related areas of the body. Include techniques to maintain or improve:

Range of motion. These techniques may be done actively or passively, depending on the proximity to and the effect on the injured tissue.

Muscle strength. Resistance may be applied at an appropriate dosage to muscles not directly related to the injured tissue to prepare the patient for use of assistive devices, such as crutches or a walker, and to improve functional activities.

Functional activities. Supportive or adaptive devices may be necessary depending on area of injury and expected functional activities.

Circulation. It will be helped by doing the functional activities as well as by using supportive elastic wraps, by elevating the part, and by using appropriate massage and muscle-setting techniques.

▶ Management During The Subacute Stage

Tissue Response—Repair and Healing

During the 2nd to 4th day after tissue injury, the inflammation will begin to decrease. Resolution of the clot and repair of the injured site begins. This usually lasts an additional 10 to 17 days (14–21 days after the onset of injury), but may last up to 6 weeks.

The synthesis and deposition of collagen characterize this stage. Noxious stimuli are removed, and growth of capillary beds into the area takes place. Fibroblastic activity, collagen formation, and granulation tissue development increase. Fibroblasts are in tremendous number by the 4th day after injury and continue in large number until about the 21st day.[64] The fibroblasts produce new collagen. The immature collagen replaces the exudate that originally formed the clot. In addition, myofibroblastic activity begins about day 5, causing scar shrinkage (contraction).[64] Wound closure in muscle and skin usually takes 5 to 8 days; in tendons and ligaments, 3 to 6 weeks.[22]

During this stage, the immature connective tissue that is produced is thin and unorganized. It is very fragile and easily injured if overstressed, yet proper growth and alignment can be stimulated by appropriate tensile loading in the line of normal stresses for that tissue. At the same time, adherence to surrounding tissues can be minimized.[19]

Management Guidelines—The Controlled Motion Phase

The therapist's role during this stage is critical. The patient feels much better because the pain is no longer constant, and active movement can begin. It is easy to begin too much movement too soon or be tempted to approach intervention cautiously and not progress rapidly enough. Understanding the healing process and tissue response to stresses underlies the critical decisions that are made throughout this phase of intervention. The key is to initiate and progress *nondestructive* exercises and activities, i.e., exercises and activities that are within the tolerance of the healing tissues to respond to without reinjury and inflammation. The following information is summarized in Box 8–2.

Patient Education

Inform the patient about what to expect at this stage, the time frame for healing, and what signs and symptoms indicate that he or she is pushing beyond tissue tolerance. Encourage him or her to return to normal activities that do not exacerbate symptoms, but caution against returning to recreational, sport, or work-related activities that will be detrimental to

Box 8–2 Management Guidelines—Subacute Stage/Controlled Motion Phase

Impairments:

- Pain when end of available ROM is reached
- Decreasing soft tissue edema
- Decreasing joint effusion (if joints are involved)
- Developing soft tissue, muscle, and/or joint contractures
- Developing muscle weakness from reduced usage
- Decreased functional use of the part and associated areas

Plan of Care	Intervention (up to 3 weeks postinjury)
1. Educate the patient.	1. Inform patient of anticipated healing time and importance of following guidelines. Teach home exercises and encourage functional activities consistent with plan; monitor and modify as patient progresses.
2. Promote healing of injured tissues.	2. Monitor response of tissue to exercise progression; decrease intensity if inflammation increases. Protect healing tissue with assistive devices, splints, tape, or wrap; progressively increase amount of time the joint is free to move each day and decrease use of assistive device as strength in supporting muscles increases.
3. Restore soft tissue, muscle, and/or joint mobility.	3. Progress from passive to active-assistive to active ROM within limits of pain. Gradually increase mobility of scar, specific to structure involved. Progressively increase mobility of related structures if they are tight; use techniques specific to tight structure.
4. Develop neuromuscular control, muscle endurance, and strength in involved and related muscles.	4. Initially, progress multiple-angle isometric exercises within patient's tolerance; begin cautiously with mild resistance. Initiate AROM and protected closed-chain stabilization exercises. As ROM, joint play, and healing improve, progress isotonic exercises with increased repetitions. Emphasize control and proper mechanics. Progress resistance later in this stage.
5. Maintain integrity and function of associated areas.	5. Apply progressive strengthening and stabilizing exercises, monitoring effect on the primary lesion. Resume low-intensity functional activities involving the healing tissue that do not exacerbate the symptoms.

Precautions: The signs of inflammation or joint swelling normally decrease early in this stage. Some discomfort will occur as the activity level is progressed, but it should not last longer than a couple of hours. Signs of too much motion or activity are resting pain, fatigue, increased weakness, and spasm.[71]

the healing process. Teach the patient a home exercise program, and help the patient adapt work and recreational activities that are consistent with intervention strategies so that he or she becomes an active participant in the recovery process.

Management of Pain and Inflammation

Pain and inflammation decrease as healing progresses. Criteria for initiation of active exercises and stretching in the early subacute stage include decreased swelling, pain that is no longer constant, and pain that is not exacerbated with motion in the available range.

Monitor activities and exercises. As new exercises are introduced or as the intensity of exercises is progressed, monitor the patient response, so that if symptoms warrant, the intensity of exercise can be modified.

Precaution: The new tissue being developed is fragile and easily interrupted. The patient often feels good and returns to normal activity too soon, causing an exacerbation of symptoms. Exercises progressed too vigorously or functional activities begun too early can be injurious to the fragile, newly developing tissue and, therefore, may delay recovery by perpetuating the inflammatory response.[64,71] However, if movement is not progressed, the new tissue adheres to surrounding structures and will become a source of pain and limited tissue mobility.

Initiation of Active Exercises

Because of the restricted use of the injured region, there will be muscle weakness even in the absence of muscle pathology. The subacute phase is a transition period during which *active* exercises within the pain-free range of the injured tissue can begin and be progressed to muscular endurance and strengthening exercises with care, keeping within the tolerance of the healing tissues (nondestructive motion). If activity is kept within a safe intensity and frequency, symptoms of pain and swelling will progressively decrease each day. Patient response is the best guide to how quickly or vigorously to progress. Clinically, if signs of inflammation increase or the ROM progressively decreases, then the intensity of the exercise and activity must decrease because a chronic inflammation has developed and a retracting scar will become more limiting.[8,9,41]

Multiple-angle, submaximal isometric exercises. Submaximal isometric exercises are used in the early subacute stage to initiate control and strengthening of the muscles in the involved region in a nonstressful manner. They may also help the patient become aware of using the correct muscles. The intensity and angles for resistance are determined by the absence of pain.

- To initiate isometric exercise in an injured, healing muscle, place it in the shortened or relaxed position so that the new scar is not pulled from the breached site.[19,64]
- To initiate isometric exercises when there is joint pathology, the resting position for the joint may be the most comfortable position. The intensity of contraction should be kept below the perception of pain.

Active range of motion (AROM) exercises. AROM activities in pain-free ranges are used to develop control of the motion. Initially isolated, single plane motions are used. Emphasize control of the motion using light-resistive, concentric exercises of involved muscle and muscles needed for proper joint mechanics. Use of combined motions or diagonal patterns may facilitate contraction of the desired muscles, but care must be taken not to use patterns of motion dominated by stronger muscles with the weaker muscles not effectively participating at this early stage. Do not stress beyond the ability of the involved or weakened muscles to participate in the motion.

Muscular endurance. Exercises for muscle endurance are emphasized in the subacute phase because slow-twitch muscle fibers are the first to atrophy when there is joint swelling, trauma, or immobilization. Initially, only active ROM is used with emphasis on control. Later in the healing phase low-intensity, high-repetition exercise using light resistance is used rather than high-intensity resistance. The therapist must be certain that the patient is using correct motor patterns without substitution and is informed of the importance of stopping the exercise or activity when the involved muscle fatigues or involved tissue develops symptoms. For example, if the patient is doing shoulder flexion or abduction activities, substitution with scapular elevation should be avoided; or if the patient is doing leg-lift exercises, proper stabilization of the pelvis and the spine is important to assure safety and correct motor learning.

Protected closed-chain exercises. Partial weight bearing within the tolerance of the healing tissues may be used early to load the region in a controlled manner and stimulate stabilizing co-contractions in the muscles. Reinforcement from the therapist helps develop awareness of appropriate muscle contractions as well as helps develop control while the patient shifts his or her weight in a side-to-side or anterior-to-posterior motion. As tolerated by the patient, progress by increasing the amplitude of movement or by decreasing the amount of support or protection. Resistance is added to progress strength in the stabilizing muscles.

Precaution: Eccentric and heavy-resistance exercises (such as PRE) may cause added trauma to muscle and are not used in the early subacute stage after muscle injury when the weak tensile quality of the healing tissue could be jeopardized.[47] For nonmuscular injuries, eccentrics may not reinjure the part, but the resistance should be limited to a low intensity at this stage to avoid delayed-onset muscle soreness. (This is in contrast to using eccentrics to facilitate and strengthen weak muscles when there has been no injury to take advantage of greater tension development with less energy in eccentric contractions, which is described in Chapter 3).

Initiation and Progression of Stretching

Restricted motion during the acute stage and adherence of the developing scar usually cause decreased flexibility in the healing tissue as well as related structures in the region. To increase mobility and stimulate proper alignment of the developing scar, initiate stretching techniques that are specific to the tissues involved. More than one technique may have to be used to regain the ROM.

Warm the tissues. Use modalities or active ROM to increase the tissue temperature and relax the muscles for ease in stretching.

Inhibition techniques. Muscles that are not relaxed interfere with joint mobilization and passive stretching of inert tissue. If necessary, utilize hold-relax techniques first to be able to take the tissues to the end of their available range.

Joint mobilization. If there is decreased joint play restricting range, it is important to begin stretching with joint mobilization techniques. Use grade III sustained or grade III and IV oscillation techniques to restore some of the joint slide prior to physiologic stretching so as to minimize excessive compression of vulnerable cartilage. Joint distraction and gliding techniques are applied to stretch restricting capsular tissue (see Chapter 6 for principles and techniques of joint mobilization).

Stretching techniques. Use of passive stretching techniques, self-stretching, and prolonged mechanical stretching are used to increase the extensibility of inert connective tissue, which permeates every structure in the body. These techniques are interspersed with neuromuscular inhibition techniques to relax and elongate the muscles crossing the joints (see Chapter 5 for principles and techniques of stretching).

Massage. Various types of massage can be used for their soft tissue mobilizing effects. For example, cross-fiber friction massage is used to mobilize ligaments and incision sites so they move freely across the joint. Cross-fiber massage is also used at the site of muscle scar tissue or tendon adhesions to gain mobility of the scar tissue. The intensity and duration of the technique is progressively increased as the tissue responds.

Use of the new range. The patient must use the new range to maintain any extensibility gained with the stretching maneuvers as well as to develop control of the new range. Teach home exercises that include light resistance using the agonist in the new range as well as self-stretching techniques. Also help the patient incorporate the new range into his or her daily activities.

Correction of Contributing Factors

Continue to maintain or develop as normal a physiologic and functional state as possible in related areas of the body. Correct postural stability problems or muscle length and strength imbalances that could have contributed to the problem. Resume low-intensity functional activities as the patient tolerates without exacerbating symptoms. Continue to reassess the patient's progress and understanding of the controlled activities.

▶ Management During The Chronic Stage

Tissue Response—Maturation and Remodeling

Scar retraction from activity of the myofibroblasts is usually complete by the 21st day and the scar stops increasing in size, so that from day 21 to day 60 there is a predominance of fibroblasts that are easily remodeled.[64] The process of maturation begins in the late subacute stage and continues for several months. The maturation and remodeling of the scar tissue occurs as collagen fibers become thicker and reorient in response to stresses placed on the connective tissue. Remodeling time is influenced by factors that affect density and activity level of the fibroblasts including amount of time immobilized, stress placed on the tissue, location of the lesion, and vascular supply.

Maturation of Tissue

The primary differences in the state of the healing tissue between the late subacute and chronic stages are the improvement in quality (orientation and tensile strength) of the collagen and the reduction in size of the wound during the chronic stages. The quantity of collagen stabilizes; there is a balance between the synthesis and degradation. Depending on the size of the structure or degree of injury or pathology, healing, with progressively increasing tensile quality in the injured tissue, may continue for 12 to 18 months.[22,48,64]

Remodeling of Tissue

Because of the way immature collagen molecules are held together (hydrogen bonding) and adhere to surrounding tissue, they can be easily remodeled with gentle and persistent treatment. This is possible for up to 10 weeks. If not properly stressed, the fibers adhere to surrounding tissue and form a restricting scar. As the structure of collagen changes to covalent bonding and thickens, it becomes stronger and resistant to remodeling. At 14 weeks, the scar tissue is unresponsive to remodeling. Consequently an old scar has a poor response to stretch.[19] Treatment under these conditions requires either adaptive lengthening in the tissue surrounding the scar or surgical release.

Management Guidelines—Return to Function Phase

The therapist's role during this phase is to design a progression of exercises that safely stress the maturing connective tissue both in terms of flexibility and strength so that the patient can return to his or her functional and work-related activities. Individuals returning to high-intensity activities require more intense exercises to prepare the tissues to withstand the stresses and train the neuromuscular system to respond to the demands of the activity.

Because remodeling of the maturing collagen occurs in response to the stresses placed on it, it is important to use controlled forces that duplicate normal stresses on the tissue. Maximum strength of the collagen will develop in the direction of the imposed forces. Pain that the patient now experiences arises only when stress is placed on restrictive contractures or adhesions, or when there is soreness from increased stress of resistive exercise. To avoid chronic or recurring pain, the contractures need to be stretched or the adhesions need to be broken up and mobilized. Excessive or abnormal stresses will lead to reinjury and chronic inflammation, which can be detrimental to the return of function. The following information is summarized in Box 8–4.

Patient Education

Unless there is restrictive scar tissue requiring manual techniques for intervention, the patient becomes more responsible for carrying out the exercises in the plan of treatment. Instruct the patient in biomechanically safe progressions of resistance and self-stretching and how to self-monitor for detrimental effects and signs of excessive stress (Box 8–3). Establish guidelines for what must be attained to safely return to recreational, sport, or work-related activities. Re-examine and evaluate the patient's progress and modify the exercises as progress is noted or if problems develop. Recommend modifications in living, work, or sport activities if they are contributing to the patient's impairments and preventing return to desired activities.

Considerations for Progression of Exercises

Free joint play within a useful (or functional) ROM is necessary to avoid joint trauma. If joint play is restricted, joint mobilizing techniques should be used. These stretching techniques can be vigorous as long as no signs of increased irritation result.

Box 8–3 Signs of Excessive Stress with Exercise or Activities

- Exercise or activity soreness that does not decrease after 4 hours and is not resolved after 24 hours
- Exercise or activity pain that comes on earlier or is increased over the previous session
- Progressively increased feelings of stiffness and decreased ROM over several exercise sessions
- Swelling, redness, and warmth in the healing tissue
- Progressive weakness over several exercise sessions
- Decreased functional usage of the involved part

Exercise progressions may cause some temporary soreness that may last 4 hours, but if the above signs and symptoms occur, the activity, exercise, or stretching maneuvers are too stressful and should be modified or reduced in intensity.

Joint motion without adequate muscle support will cause trauma to that joint, or faulty neuromuscular patterns will be used as functional activities are attempted. Zohn and Mennell[71] recommend that the criterion for strength should be a muscle test grade of 4 on a 5-point scale in lower extremity musculature before discontinuing use of supportive or assistive devices for ambulation.

- To increase strength when there is a loss of joint play, use multiple-angle isometric exercises.
- Once joint play within the available ROM is restored, use resistive dynamic exercises within the available range. This does not imply that normal ROM needs to be present before initiating dynamic exercises but that joint play, within the available range, should be present (see Chapter 6 for information on joint play).

In summary, both joint dynamics and muscle strength and flexibility should be balanced as the injured part is progressed to functional exercises.[71]

Progression of Stretching

Stretching of any restricting contractures or adhesions should be specific to the tissue involved using manual techniques such as joint mobilization, myofascial massage, neuromuscular inhibition techniques, and passive stretching in addition to instruction in self-stretching (see Chapters 5 and 6). At this stage, progress the intensity and duration of the stretching maneuvers as long as no signs of increased irritation persist beyond 24 hours.

Box 8–4 Management Guidelines—Chronic Stage/Return to Function Phase

Impairments:

Soft tissue and/or joint contractures and adhesions that limit normal ROM or joint play
Decreased muscle performance: weakness, poor endurance, poor neuromuscular control
Decreased functional usage of the involved part
Inability to function normally in an expected activity

Plan of Care	Interventions (>3 weeks postinjury)
1. Educate the patient.	1. Instruct patient in safe progressions of exercises and stretching. Monitor understanding and compliance. Teach ways to avoid reinjuring the part. Teach safe body mechanics. Provide ergonomic counseling.
2. Increase soft tissue, muscle and/or joint mobility.	2. Stretching techniques specific to tight tissue: • Joint and selected ligaments (joint mobilization). • Ligaments, tendons and soft tissue adhesions (cross-fiber massage). • Muscles (neuromuscular inhibition, passive stretch, massage, and flexibility exercises).
3. Improve neuromuscular control, strength, muscle endurance.	3. Progress exercises: • Submaximal to maximal resistance. • Specificity of exercise using resisted concentric and eccentric, open- and closed-chain. • Single plane to multiplane motions. • Simple to complex motions, emphasizing movements that simulate functional activities. • Controlled proximal stability, superimpose distal motion. • Safe biomechanics. • Increase time at slow speed; progress complexity and time; progress speed and time.
4. Improve cardiovascular endurance.	4. Progress aerobic exercises using safe activities.
5. Progress functional activities.	5. Continue using supportive and/or assistive devices until the ROM is functional with joint play, and strength in supporting muscles is adequate. Progress functional training with simulated activities from protected and controlled to unprotected and variable. Continue progressive strengthening exercises and advanced training activities until the muscles are strong enough and able to respond to the required functional demands.

Precautions: There should be no signs of inflammation. Some discomfort will occur as the activity level is progressed, but it should not last longer than a couple of hours. Signs that activities are progressing too quickly or with too great a dosage are joint swelling, pain that lasts longer than 4 hours or that requires medication for relief, a decrease in strength, or fatiguing more easily.[71]

Progression of Muscle Performance Exercises: Developing Neuromuscular Control, Strength, and Endurance

As the patient's tissues heal, not only does treatment progress to stimulate proper maturation and remodeling in the healing tissue, but also emphasis is placed on controlled progressive exercises designed to prepare the patient to meet the functional outcomes.

- If the patient is not using some of the muscles because of inhibition, weakness, or dominance of substitute patterns, isolate the desired muscle action or use unidirectional motions to develop awareness of muscle activity and control of the movement.
- Progress exercises from isolated, unidirectional, simple movements to complex patterns and multidirectional movements requiring coordination with all muscles functioning for the desired activity.[68]
- Progress strengthening exercises to simulate specific demands including both closed- and open-chain (weight-bearing and nonweight-bearing), and both eccentric and concentric contractions.
- Progress trunk stabilization, postural control, and balance exercises and coordinate with extremity motions for effective total body movement patterns.[68]
- Teach safe body mechanics and have the patient practice activities that replicate his or her work environment.
- Often overlooked but of importance in preventing injury associated with fatigue is developing muscular endurance in the prime mover muscles and stabilizing muscles as well as cardiovascular endurance.

Return to High-Demand Activities

Patients who must return to activities with greater-than-normal demand such as is required in sports participation and heavy work settings are progressed further to more intense exercises including plyometrics, agility training, and skill development. Develop exercise drills that simulate the work[30] or sport[8,68] activities using a controlled environment with specific, progressive resistance and plyometric drills. As the patient demonstrates capabilities, increase the repetitions and speed of the movement. Progress by changing the environment and introducing surprise and uncontrolled events into the activity.[6,68]

The importance of proper education to teach a safe progression of exercises and how to avoid damaging stresses cannot be overemphasized. To return to the activity that caused the injury prior to regaining functional pain-free motion, strength, endurance, and skill to match the demands of the task will probably result in recurring injury and pain.

Cumulative Trauma—Chronic Recurring Pain

Tissue Response—Chronic Inflammation

When connective tissue is injured, it goes through a healing process of repair. This was described in the preceding sections. However, in connective tissue that is repetitively stressed beyond its ability to repair itself, the inflammatory process is perpetuated. Proliferation of fibroblasts with increased collagen production and degradation of mature collagen leads to a predominance of new, immature collagen. This has an overall weakening effect on the tissue. In addition, myofibroblastic activity continues, which may lead to progressive limitation of motion.[64] Efforts to stretch the inflamed tissue perpetuate the irritation and progressive limitation.

Etiology of Chronic Inflammation Leading to Prolonged or Recurring Pain

Overuse, cumulative trauma, repetitive strain. These are terms descriptive of the repetitive nature of the precipitating event.[26] Repetitive microtrauma or repeated strain overload over time results in structural weakening, or fatigue breakdown of connective tissue with collagen fiber cross-link breakdown and inflammation. Initially, the inflammatory response from the microtrauma is subthreshold but eventually builds to the point of perceived pain and resulting dysfunction.

Trauma. Trauma that is followed by superimposed repetitive trauma results in a condition that never completely heals. This may be the result of too early return to high-demand functional activities before proper healing of the original injury has occurred. The continued reinjury leads to the symptoms of chronic inflammation and dysfunction.

Reinjury of an "old scar." Scar tissue is not as compliant as surrounding, undamaged tissue. If the scar adheres to the surrounding tissues or is not properly aligned to the stresses imposed on the tissue, there is an alteration in the force transmission and energy absorption. This region becomes more susceptible to injury with stresses that normal, healthy tissue could sustain.

Contractures or poor mobility. Faulty postural habits or prolonged immobility may lead to connective tissue contractures that became stressed with repeated or vigorous activity.

Contributing Factors

By nature of the condition, there is usually some factor that perpetuates the problem. Not only should the tissue at fault and its stage of pathology be identified, but the *mechanical cause* of the repetitive trauma needs to be defined. Evaluate for faulty mechanics or faulty habits that may be sustaining the irritation. Possibilities include:

- ***Imbalances between the length and strength of the muscles*** around the joint, leading to faulty mechanics of joint motion or abnormal forces through the muscles.
- ***Rapid or excessive repeated eccentric demand*** placed on muscles not prepared to withstand the load, leading to tissue failure, particularly at the musculotendinous region.[47]
- ***Muscle weakness*** or inability to respond to excessive strength demands that results in muscle fatigue with decreased contractility and shock-absorbing capabilities and increased stress to supporting tissues.[47]
- ***Bone malalignment or weak structural support*** that causes faulty joint mechanics of force transmission through the joints (poor joint stability as in a flat foot).[50]
- ***Change in the usual intensity or demands*** of an activity such as an increase or change in an exercise or a training routine or change in job demands.[47]
- ***Returning to an activity too soon after an injury*** when the muscle-tendon unit is weakened and not ready for the stress of the activity.[27]
- ***Sustained awkward postures or motions*** placing parts of the body at a mechanical disadvantage that lead to postural fatigue or injury.
- ***Environmental factors*** such as a work station not ergonomically designed for the individual, excessive cold, continued vibration, or inappropriate weight-bearing surface (for standing, walking, or running), which may contribute to any of the previous factors.
- ***Age-related factors*** such that a person attempts activities that could be done when younger but tissues are no longer in condition to withstand the sustained stress.[53]
- ***Training errors,*** such as using improper methods, intensity, amount, equipment, or condition of the participant, which lead to abnormal stresses.[50]
- ***A combination of several contributing factors*** are frequently seen that cause the symptoms.

Management Guidelines—Chronic Inflammation

When the patient has symptoms and signs of chronic inflammation, it is imperative that treatment begins by controlling the inflammation—in other words, treat as an acute condition. Once the inflammation is under control, treatment progresses to dealing with the impairments and functional limitations. Management guidelines are summarized in Box 8–5.

Chronic Inflammation—Acute Stage

When the inflammatory response is perpetuated because of continued tissue irritation, the inflammation must be controlled to avoid the negative effects of continued tissue breakdown and excessive scar formation.

- Besides the use of modalities and rest of the part, it is imperative to identify and modify the mechanism of chronic irritation with appropriate biomechanical counseling. This will require cooperation from the patient. Describe to the patient how the tissue reacts and breaks down under the continued inflammation, and explain the strategy of intervention. Using illustrations such as what happens when a person repeatedly hits a thumbnail with a hammer or repeatedly scrapes a skin area before it heals helps the patient visualize the repeated trauma occurring in the musculoskeletal problem and understand the need to quit "hitting the sore."
- Initially, allow only nonstressful activities.
- Initiate exercises at *nonstressful* intensities in the involved tissues, as with any acute lesion, and at appropriate corrective intensities in related regions without stressing the involved tissues.

Subacute and Chronic Stages of Healing Following Chronic Inflammation

Once the constant pain from the chronic inflammation has decreased, progress the patient through an exercise program with controlled stresses until the

Box 8–5 Management Guidelines—Chronic Inflammation/Cumulative Trauma Syndromes

Impairments:

Pain in the involved tissue of varying degrees:[53]

- Only after doing repetitive activities
- When doing repetitive activities as well as after
- When attempting to do activities; completion of demands prevented
- Continued and unremitting

Soft tissue, muscle, and/or joint contractures or adhesions that limit normal ROM or joint play
Muscle weakness and poor muscular endurance in postural or stabilizing muscles as well as primary muscle at fault
Imbalance in length and strength between antagonistic muscles; biomechanical dysfunction
Decreased functional use of the region
Faulty position or movement pattern perpetuating the problem

Plan of Care	Interventions During Chronic Inflammation
1. Educate the patient.	1. Counsel as to cause of chronic irritation and need to avoid stressing the part while inflamed. Adapt the environment to decrease tissue stress. Home exercise program to reinforce therapeutic interventions.
2. Promote healing; decrease pain and inflammation.	2. Cold, compression, massage. Rest to the part (stop mechanical stress, splint, tape, cast).
3. Maintain integrity and mobility of involved tissue.	3. Nonstressful passive movement, massage, and muscle setting within limits of pain.
4. Develop support in related regions.	4. Posture training. Stabilization exercises.

Plan of Care	Interventions—Controlled Motion and Return to Function Phases
1. Educate the patient.	1. Ergonomic counseling in ways to prevent recurrence. Home instruction in safe progression of stretching and strengthening exercises. Instruction on signs of too much stress (see Box 8-3).
2. Develop strong, mobile scar.	2. Friction massage. Soft tissue mobilization.
3. Develop a balance in length and strength of the muscles.	3. Correct cause of faulty muscle and joint mechanics with appropriately graded stretching and strengthening exercises.
4. Progress functional independence.	4. Train muscles to function according to demand; provide alternatives or support if it cannot. Train coordination and timing. Develop endurance.
5. Analyze job/activity.	5. Adapt home, work, sport environment/tools.

Precaution: If there is progressive loss of range of motion as the result of stretching, do not continue to stretch. Re-evaluate the condition and determine if there is still a chronic inflammation with contracting scar or if there is protective muscle guarding. Emphasize stabilizing the part and training in safe adaptive patterns of motion.

connective tissue in the involved region has developed the ability to withstand the stresses imposed by the functional activities.

- Locally, if there is a chronic, contracted scar that limits range or continually becomes irritated with microruptures, mobilize the scar within the tissue with friction massage, soft tissue manipulation, or stretching techniques.
  - If inflammation occurs from the stretching maneuvers, treat it as an acute injury.
  - Because chronic inflammation can lead to proliferation of scar tissue and contraction of the scar, progressive loss of range is a warning sign that the intensity of stretching is too vigorous.
  - Muscle guarding could be a sign that the body is attempting to protect the part from excessive motion. In this case the emphasis is on developing stabilization of the part and training in safe adaptive patterns of motion.
- Identify the cause of the faulty muscle and joint mechanics. Strengthening and stabilization exercises, in conjunction with working or recreational adaptations, are necessary to minimize the irritating patterns of motion.

- Because chronic irritation problems frequently result from inability to sustain repetitive activities, muscle endurance is an appropriate component of the muscle re-education program. Consider endurance in the postural stabilizers as well as in the prime movers of the desired functional activity.
- As when treating patients in the chronic stage of healing, progress exercises to develop functional independence. The exercises become specific to the demand and include timing, coordination, and skill. Work-conditioning and work-hardening programs may be used to prepare the person for return to work; training in sports-specific exercises is important in returning an individual to sports.

Note: Specific overuse syndromes are covered in detail in the respective chapters associated with the involved region.

▶ Arthritis—Arthrosis

Arthritis is inflammation of a joint. There are many types of arthritis, both inflammatory and noninflammatory that affect joints and other connective tissues in the body. The most common types treated by therapists are rheumatoid arthritis and osteoarthritis. **Arthrosis** is limitation of a joint without inflammation. Unless the cause of the joint problems is known, such as recent trauma or immobility, medical intervention is necessary to diagnose and manage osteoarthritis and systemic diseases, such as rheumatoid arthritis and lupus erythematosis. Traumatic arthritis may require aspiration if there is bloody effusion.

Clinical Signs and Symptoms

Mobility Impairments

The patient usually presents with signs typical of joint involvement that include a characteristic pattern of limitation (called a capsular pattern), usually a firm end feel (unless acute, then the end feel may be guarded), decreased and possibly painful joint play, and joint swelling (effusion).[33] Additional signs may be present depending on the specific disease process (Table 8–2). Arthrosis may be present if the individual is recovering from a fracture or other problem requiring immobilization. There will be limited joint play along with other connective tissue and muscular contractures limiting ROM.

Muscle Impairments

Examination of the patient by the therapist should include identifying any mechanical imbalances in flexibility and strength in supporting muscles. This is important because poor muscle support allows the joint to be more susceptible to trauma; conversely,

Table 8–2 Comparison of Osteoarthritis and Rheumatoid Arthritis[3,28,59,61,62]

Characteristics	Osteoarthritis	Rheumatoid Arthritis
Age of onset	Usually after age of 40	Usually begins between 15 and 50
Progression	Usually develops slowly over many years in response to mechanical stress	May develop suddenly, within weeks or months
Manifestations	Cartilage degradation, altered joint architecture, osteophyte formation	Inflammatory synovitis and irreversible structural damage to cartilage and bone
Joint involvement	Affects a few joints; typically –DIP, PIP, 1st CMC of hands –Cervical and lumbar spine –Hips, knees, 1st MTP of feet	Usually affects many joints, usually bilateral; typically –MCP and PIP of hands, wrists, elbows, shoulders –Cervical spine –MTP, talonavicular and ankle
Joint signs and symptoms	Morning stiffness (usually less than 30 min), increased joint pain with weight-bearing and strenuous activity	Redness, warmth, swelling, and prolonged morning stiffness; increased joint pain with activity
Systemic signs and symptoms	None	General feeling of sickness and fatigue, weight loss and fever; may develop rheumatoid nodules, may have ocular, respiratory, hematological, and cardiac symptoms

good muscle support will help protect an arthritic joint. Any asymmetry of muscle pull may be a deforming force, and if it cannot be corrected with exercises, splinting or bracing may be necessary to prevent progressive deformity. Stabilizing muscles are often inhibited when there are swollen or restricted joints; strength returns with decreased swelling and increased joint mobility, so it is important to protect the joints when swollen and the muscles are weak.

Balance Impairments

Patients may develop balance deficits because of impaired sensory input from joint mechanoreceptors and altered muscle spindle input. This is particularly a problem with weight-bearing joints.[67]

Functional Limitations

Limitations in daily activities, work demands, and social activities may be minimally to significantly restrictive. Adaptive and assistive devices may be used by the patient to improve function or help prevent possible deforming forces. A variety of classification systems and functional instruments have been developed for use in clinical studies as well as routine practice to measure patient function and outcomes in response to interventions.[27]

Rheumatoid Arthritis (RA)

RA is a chronic, inflammatory, systemic disease affecting the connective tissue. The onset and progression vary from mild joint symptoms with aching and stiffness to abrupt swelling, stiffness, and progressive deformity.[3,12,38,52] The criteria for classification of RA are summarized in Table 8–3.

Characteristics of Rheumatoid Arthritis (RA)

- There are usually periods of exacerbation (flare) and remission.[12,38]
- Joints are characteristically involved with early inflammatory changes in the synovial membrane, peripheral portions of the articular cartilage, and subchondral marrow spaces. In response, granulation tissue (pannus) forms, covers, and erodes the articular cartilage, bone and ligaments within the joint capsule. Adhesions may form, restricting joint mobility. With progression of the disease, cancellous bone becomes exposed. Fibrosis or ossific ankylosis may eventually result, causing deformity and disability.[3,52]
- Inflammatory changes also occur in tendon sheaths (tenosynovitis), and if subjected to a lot of friction, the tendons may fray or rupture.

Table 8–3 Criteria for Diagnosis of Rheumatoid Arthritis[5]

1. Morning stiffness in and around the joints, lasting at least 1 hour before maximal improvement
2. At least 3 joint areas simultaneously have soft tissue swelling or fluid observed by a physician
3. Swelling in the wrist, MCP, or PIP joints
4. Symmetric arthritis (bilateral involvement of PIPs, MCPs, or MTPs may occur without absolute symmetry)
5. Rheumatoid nodules
6. Serum rheumatoid factor
7. Radiographic changes including erosions or periarticular osteopenia in hand and/or wrist joints

Note: RA is defined by the presence of at least 4 of these 7 criteria. #1–4 must have been present for at least 6 weeks.

- Extra-articular pathological changes sometimes occur; these include rheumatoid nodules, atrophy and fibrosis of muscles, and mild cardiac changes.

Signs and Symptoms During Periods of Exacerbation

- With synovial inflammation, there is effusion and swelling of the joints, which cause aching and limited motion. Joint stiffness is prominent in the morning. Usually there is pain on motion, and a slight increase in temperature can be detected over the joints. The pain and stiffness worsen after strenuous activity.
- Onset is usually in the smaller joints of the hands and feet, most commonly in the proximal interphalangeal joints. Usually symptoms are bilateral.
- With progression, the joints become deformed and may ankylose or subluxate.
- Pain is often felt in adjoining muscles; eventually muscle atrophy and weakness occur. Asymmetry in muscle strength and alterations in line of pull of muscles and tendons add to the deforming forces.
- The person often experiences nonspecific symptoms such as fatigue, low-grade fever, loss of appetite and weight, malaise, and fatigue.

Management Guidelines—Active Inflammatory Period of RA

Management guidelines for treating patients with RA are as follows.

- Because periods of exacerbation may last several months to greater than a year, initiate education

Box 8–6 Principles of Joint Protection[37,51]

- Monitor activities and stop when discomfort or fatigue begins to develop.
- Use frequent but short episodes of exercise (3–5 sessions per day) rather than one long session.
- Alternate activities to avoid fatigue.
- Decrease level of activities or omit provoking activities if joint pain develops and persists for more than 1 hour after activity.
- Maintain a functional level of joint ROM and muscular strength and endurance.
- Balance work and rest to avoid muscular and total body fatigue.
- Increase rest during flares of the disease.
- Avoid deforming positions.
- Avoid prolonged static positioning; change positions during the day every 20–30 minutes.
- Use stronger and larger muscles and joints during activities whenever possible.
- Use appropriate adaptive equipment.

in the overall treatment plan, safe activity, and joint protection (Box 8–6) as soon as possible.[49]

- If medication controls the swelling and secondary pain, active exercises that encourages as much ROM as possible are progressed carefully (not stretching). Also encourage performance of ADLs with appropriate modification to protect the joints. If necessary, use splints and assistive devices.
- Secondary effects of steroidal medications may include osteoporosis and ligamentous laxity, so exercises should not cause excessive stress to bones or joints.
- The type and intensity of exercise varies depending on the symptoms. It is imperative to involve the patient in the management so that he or she learns how to conserve energy and how to avoid potential deforming stresses during activities and when exercising.

  A recent study[65] using patients with medically controlled active RA documented improved function, decreased number of clinically active joints, improved muscle strength, and improved rate of diminished disease activity in patients in a carefully controlled intensive exercise program compared with patients in a conservative ROM and isometric exercise program. The intensive exercises included isokinetic resistance to the knees at 70% maximum voluntary contraction and angular velocity at 60 degrees/second, isometric exercises at 70% maximum voluntary contraction, bicycling at 60% age-predicted maximum for 15 minutes as well as ROM exercises. All exercises were adjusted to pain tolerance of the individual when needed. The primary conclusion of this study was that there is no evidence that patients with active disease should be prevented from vigorous exercise as long as fatigue and pain are respected. The study did not look at erosion and cartilage damage.
- Instruct the patient to respect fatigue and, when tired, to rest to minimize undue stress to all the body systems. Because inflamed joints are easily damaged, and rest is encouraged to protect the joints, teach the patient how to rest the joints in nondeforming positions and to intersperse the rest with ROM.
- Stretching techniques should not be performed across swollen joints. The limited motion when there is effusion is from the excessive fluid in the joint space. To force motion on the distended capsule will overstretch it with subsequent hypermobility (or subluxation) when the swelling abates. It may also increase the irritability of the joint and prolong the joint reaction.
- Therapeutic exercises cannot positively alter the pathological process of RA, but if administered carefully, they can help prevent, retard, or correct the mechanical limitations and deforming forces that occur, especially in the early stages of the disease, and, therefore, help maintain function.

Guidelines are summarized in Box 8–7.

Management Guidelines—Subacute and Chronic Stages of RA

- As the intensity of pain, joint swelling, morning stiffness and systemic effects diminish the disease is considered subacute. Often medications will decrease the acute symptoms so that the patient can function as if subacute. The chronic stage is between exacerbations. This may be very short in duration, or it may last for many years.
- The treatment approach is the same as with any subacute and chronic musculoskeletal disorder, except appropriate precautions must be taken because the pathologic changes from the disease process make the parts more susceptible to damage. Nonimpact or low-impact conditioning exercises such as swimming and bicycling, performed within the tolerance of the individual with arthritis, improve aerobic capacity and physical activity and decrease depression and anxiety.[46] Group activities such as water aerobics also provide social support in conjunction with the activity.

Box 8–7 Management Guidelines—Rheumatoid Arthritis/Active Disease Period

Impairments:
- Tenderness and warmth over the involved joints with joint swelling
- Muscle guarding and pain on motion
- Joint stiffness and limited motion
- Muscle weakness and atrophy
- Potential deformity and ankylosis from the degenerative process and asymmetric muscle pull
- Fatigue, malaise, sleep disorders
- Restricted ADLs and IADLs

Plan of Care	Interventions
1. Educate the patient.	1. Inform the patient on importance of rest, joint protection, energy conservation, and performance of ROM. Teach home exercise program and activity modifications that conserve energy and minimize stress to vulnerable joints.
2. Relieve pain and muscle guarding and promote relaxation.	2. Modalities. Gentle massage. Immobilize in splint. Relaxation techniques.
3. Minimize joint stiffness and maintain available motion.	3. Passive or active-assistive ROM within limits of pain, gradual progression as tolerated. Gentle joint techniques using grade I or II oscillations.
4. Minimize muscle atrophy.	4. Gentle isometrics in pain-free positions, progression to ROM when tolerated.
5. Prevent deformity and protect the joint structures.	5. Use of supportive and assistive equipment for all pathologically active joints. Good bed positioning while resting. Avoidance of activities that stress the joints.

Precautions: Respect fatigue and increased pain; do not overstress osteoporotic bone or lax ligaments.

Contraindications: Do not stretch swollen joints or apply heavy resistance exercise that cause joint stress.

Precautions: The joint capsule, ligaments, and tendons may be structurally weakened by the rheumatic process (also as a result of using steroids), so the dosage of stretching techniques used to counter any contractures or adhesions must be carefully graded.

Contraindications: Vigorous stretching or manipulative techniques.

Osteoarthritis (OA)

Characteristics of Osteoarthritis or Degenerative Joint Disease (DJD)

- OA is a chronic degenerative disorder primarily affecting the articular cartilage of synovial joints, with eventual bony remodeling and overgrowth at the margins of the joints (spurs and lipping). There is also a progression of synovial and capsular thickening and joint effusion. With degeneration, there may be capsular laxity as a result of bone remodeling and capsule distention, resulting in hypermobility or instability in some ranges. With pain and decreased willingness to move, contractures eventually develop in portions of the capsule and overlying muscle, so that as the disease progresses, motion becomes more limited.[23,28,63]
- Causes may be from mechanical injury to the joint, from either a major stress or repeated minor stresses, or due to poor movement of synovial fluid when the joint is immobilized. Rapid destruction of articular cartilage occurs with immobilization, because the cartilage is not being bathed by moving synovial fluid and is thus deprived of its nutritional supply.
- OA is also genetically related especially in the hands and hips, and to some degree, in the knees.[23] Other risk factors that show a direct relationship to OA are obesity, weakness of the quadriceps muscles, joint impact or sports with repetitive impact and twisting (such as soccer, baseball pitching and football), and occupational activities such as jobs requiring kneeling and squatting with heavy lifting.[23]

- The cartilage loses its ability to withstand stress; it splits and thins out. Eventually the bone becomes exposed. There is increased density of the bone along the joint line, with cystic bone loss and osteoporosis in the adjacent metaphysis. In the early stages, the joint is usually asymptomatic because the cartilage is avascular and aneural.

Signs, Symptoms, and Management Guidelines in OA

Management guidelines are summarized in Box 8–8.

- Pain usually occurs because of compressive stresses on or excessive activity of the involved joint and is relieved with rest. In the late stages of the disease, pain is often present at rest. The pain is probably from secondary involvement of subchondral bone, synovium, and the joint capsule. In the spine, if bony growth encroaches on the nerve root, there may be radicular pain.
- Usually there are brief periods of stiffness in the morning or after periods of rest due to gelling of the involved joints after periods of inactivity.[1] Movement relieves the stiffness.
- Affected joints may become enlarged. Heberden's nodes (enlargement of the distal interphalangeal joint of the fingers) and Bouchard's nodes (enlargement of the proximal interphalangeal joints) are common.
- Most commonly involved are weight-bearing joints (hips and knees), the cervical and lumbar spine, and the distal interphalangeal joints of the fingers and carpometacarpal joint of the thumb.
- Crepitation or loose bodies may occur within the joint.
- Stiffness occurs with inactivity, but increased pain occurs with excessive mechanical stress or activity. Therefore, moderation of activity and correction of the biomechanical stresses can prevent, retard, or correct the mechanical limitations. It is important to instruct the patient to maintain a balance between activity and rest.

Box 8–8 Management Guidelines: Osteoarthritis

Impairments:

- Pain with mechanical stress or excessive activity
- Pain at rest in the advanced stages
- Stiffness after inactivity
- Limitation of motion
- Muscle weakness
- Decreased proprioception and balance
- Functional limitations in ADLs and IADLs

Plan of Care	Intervention
1. Educate the patient.	1. Teach about deforming forces and prevention. Teach home exercise program to reinforce interventions and minimize symptoms.
2. Decrease effects of stiffness.	2. Active ROM. Joint-play mobilization techniques.
3. Decrease pain from mechanical stress and prevent deforming forces.	3. Splinting and/or assistive equipment to minimize stress or to correct faulty biomechanics, strengthen supporting muscles. Alternate activity with periods of rest.
4. Increase ROM.	4. Stretch muscle, joint, or soft tissue restrictions with specific techniques.
5. Improve neuromuscular control, strength, and muscle endurance.	5. Low-intensity resistance exercises and muscle repetitions.
6. Improve balance.	6. Balance training activities.
7. Improve physical conditioning.	7. Nonimpact or low-impact aerobic exercise.

Precautions: When strengthening supporting muscles, increased pain in the joint during or following resistive exercises probably means that too great a weight is being used or stress is being placed at an inappropriate part of the ROM. Analyze the joint mechanics and at what point during the range the greatest compressive forces are occurring. Maximum resistance exercise should not be performed through that ROM.

- With progression of the disease, the bony remodeling, swelling, and contractures alter the transmission of forces through the joint, which further perpetuates the deforming forces and creates joint deformity. Functional activities become more difficult and adaptive or assistive devices, such as a raised toilet seat, cane, or walker may need to be used to maintain function.
- Progressive weakening in the muscle occurs either from inactivity or from inhibition of the neuronal pools. Weak muscles may add to the joint dysfunction.[1]
- Impairment of joint position sense may occur.[67]
- A recent literature review[24] summarized factors that put an individual with OA at risk for disability. They include pain, depression, muscle weakness, and poor aerobic capacity.
- In addition to medical interventions, patient education and exercises to improve strength and endurance are important in treatment. Use of assistive devices and shock-absorbing footwear may decrease stresses in OA of the knees.[24]

Fractures—Post-Traumatic Immobilization

Reduction, alignment, and immobilization for healing of a fracture are medical procedures and are not discussed in this text.

Tissue Response and Management Guidelines—Period of Immobilization

Management guidelines are summarized in Box 8–9.

Local Tissue Response

With immobilization, there is connective tissue weakening, articular cartilage degeneration, muscle atrophy, and contracture development as well as sluggish circulation.[19,40] In addition, because of the fracture there is also soft tissue injury with bleeding and scar formation. Because immobilization is necessary for bone healing, the soft tissue scar cannot become organized along lines of stress as it develops. Early nondestructive motion, within the tolerance of the fracture site, is ideal but usually not feasible unless there is some type of internal fixation to stabilize the fracture site. Structures in the related area should be kept in a state as near to normal as possible by using appropriate exercises without jeopardizing alignment of the fracture site while it is healing.

Immobilization in Bed

If bed rest or immobilization in bed is required, as with skeletal traction, secondary physiologic changes will occur systematically throughout the body. General exercises for the uninvolved portions of the body can minimize these problems.

Functional Adaptations

If there is a lower extremity fracture, alternate modes of ambulation need to be taught to the patient who is allowed out of bed, such as use of crutches or walker. The choice of device and gait pattern will depend on the fracture site, the type of immobilization, and the functional capabilities of the patient. Consultation with the patient's physi-

Box 8–9 Management Guidelines—Postfracture/Period of Immobilization

Impairments:

Initially, inflammation and swelling
In the immobilized area, progressive muscle atrophy, contracture formation, cartilage degeneration, and decreased circulation
Potential overall body weakening if confined to bed
Functional limitations imposed by the fracture site and method of immobilization used

Plan of Care	Intervention
1. Educate the patient.	1. Teach functional adaptations. Teach safe ambulation, bed mobility.
2. Decrease effects of inflammation during acute period.	2. Ice, elevation.
3. Decrease effects of immobilization.	3. Intermittent muscle setting. Active ROM to joints above and below immobilized region.
4. If patient is confined to bed, maintain strength and ROM in major muscle groups.	4. Resistive exercises to major muscle groups not immobilized, especially in preparation for future ambulation.

cian is necessary to determine the amount of weight bearing allowed.

The Postimmobilization Period

Signs and Symptoms

- There will be decreased ROM, joint play, and muscle flexibility. Muscle atrophy with weakness and poor muscle endurance, and pain in the structures that have been immobilized occur.
- Initially, the patient will experience pain as movement begins, but it should progressively decrease as joint movement, muscle strength, and ROM improve.
- If there was soft tissue damage at the time of fracture, an inelastic scar will also restrict tissue mobility in the region of the scar.

Management Guidelines—Postimmobilization

Management guidelines are summarized in Box 8–10.

Determine bone healing. Consult with the referring physician to determine if there is clinical or radiological healing. Until the fracture site is radiologically healed, use care any time stress is placed across the fracture site such as when applying resistance, a stretch force, or during weight-bearing activities. Once radiologically healed, the bone has normal structural integrity and can withstand normal stress.

Examine the patient. Determine the degree of ROMs lost, the strength available, the tissues that are in dysfunction, and the functional limitations. Usually all of the joint and periarticular tissues are affected in the region that was immobilized.

Joint mobilization. Joint mobilization techniques are very effective for regaining lost joint play without traumatizing the articular cartilage or stressing the fracture site.[33] Begin with gentle stretches (grades III and IV) and progress the intensity as joint reaction becomes predictable.

Neuromuscular inhibition. Hold-relax and agonist-contraction techniques may be used early in the postimmobilization period, but use caution with the intensity of contraction, and do not apply the resistive force beyond the fracture site.

Self-stretching and passive stretching. These techniques may not be appropriate early in the postimmobilization period due to the use of the long bony lever in the application of the force across the fracture site. Once the bone is healed, these techniques may be used if needed.

Box 8–10 Management Guidelines—Postfracture/Postimmobilization

Impairments:
- Pain with movement, which progressively decreases
- Decreased ROM
- Decreased joint play
- Scar tissue adhesions
- Decreased strength and endurance

Plan of Care	Interventions
1. Educate the patient.	1. Inform patient of limitations until fracture site is radiologically healed. Teach home exercises that reinforce interventions.
2. Provide protection until radiologically healed.	2. Use partial weight bearing in lower extremity and nonstressful activities in the upper extremity.
3. Initiate active exercises.	3. Active ROM, gentle multiangle isometrics.
4. Increase joint and soft tissue mobility.	4. Initiate joint play stretching techniques (using grades III and IV) with the force applied proximal to the healing fracture site. For muscle stretching, apply the force proximal to the healing fracture site until radiologically healed.
5. Increase strength and muscle endurance.	5. As the ROM increases and the bone heals, initiate resistive and repetitive exercises.
6. Improve cardiorespiratory fitness.	6. Initiate safe aerobic exercises that do not stress the fracture site until it is healed.

Precautions: No stretch or resistive forces distal to the fracture site until the bone is radiologically healed. No excessive joint compression or shear for several weeks after the period of immobilization. Use protected weight bearing until the site is radiologically healed.

Activities. Initiate activities carefully in order not to traumatize the weakened structures, including muscle, cartilage, bone, and connective tissue. Partial weight bearing will need to be continued for several weeks after a lower extremity fracture until the fracture site is completely healed and able to tolerate full weight bearing.

Muscle performance: Strengthening and muscle endurance. Use caution with resisted exercises during the first couple of weeks, not only because the bone cannot tolerate the stress but neither can the cartilage tolerate excessive compressive forces after periods of immobilization. Begin with light isometrics; then as joint play and ROM improves, progress to light resistance. The resistive force should be applied proximal to the fracture site until the bone is healed.

Scar tissue mobilization. If there is scar tissue, begin mobilization techniques to the scar. Choice of technique will depend on the tissue involved.

▶ Surgery

An array of injuries, diseases, and disorders of the musculoskeletal system that affect muscles, fascia, tendons, ligaments, cartilage, joint capsules, or bones and subsequently cause impairments and functional limitations of the upper or lower extremities or the spine often must be managed through surgical intervention coupled with pre- and postoperative rehabilitation. Surgery may be indicated if one or more impairments limit a person's ability to function. Indications for common musculoskeletal surgeries are listed in Box 8–11.[7,12,13,43,55,58,60,66]

Surgical procedures, in part, include releases, transfers, or reattachments of muscle-tendon units, decompression of painful structures, removal or repair of cartilage, reconstruction of ligaments, and debridement, stabilization, realignment, or replacement of joint.

A well-planned program of patient education, therapeutic exercise, and carefully progressed functional activities are integral components of care of the surgical patient. Appropriate rehabilitative management takes into consideration many factors, any of which will play a part in determining the components and progression of the rehabilitation program. These factors are noted in Box 8–12.

Each of these factors also influences the postoperative functional outcomes for the patient and the ultimate success of the surgical procedure. To design a safe and effective rehabilitation program for the surgical patient, a therapist must understand the indications and rationale for a particular surgical procedure, must become familiar with the procedure itself, must be aware of special precautions related to the surgery, and must communicate effectively with the patient and surgeon.

This section provides an overview of considerations for preoperative management and general guidelines for postoperative management during progressive phases of rehabilitation. In addition, this section concludes with a brief description of selected surgeries for the management of musculoskeletal conditions of the upper and lower extremities and the factors and potential complications that can interfere with the achievement of optimal functional outcomes after surgery. Descriptions of surgical procedures for specific injuries or disorders of the extremities are included in Chapters 9–14. In these chapters, specific guidelines for postoperative management are based on the application of principles of tissue healing and exercise management rather than adherence to specific protocols. These principles can be applied by the therapist when designing

Box 8–11 Indications for Surgery for Musculoskeletal Disorders of the Extremities and Spine

- Incapacitating pain at rest or with functional activities
- Marked limitation of active or passive motion
- Gross instability of a joint or bony segment
- Joint deformity or abnormal joint alignment
- Chronic joint swelling
- Failed conservative (nonsurgical) or previous surgical management
- Significant loss of function as the result of any of the preceding factors

Box 8–12 Factors that Influence the Components, Progression, and Outcomes of a Postoperative Rehabilitation Program

- Extent of tissue pathology or damage
  - Size or severity of the lesion
- Type and unique characteristics of the surgical procedure
- Stage of healing of involved tissues
- Characteristics of types of tissues involved
  - Response to immobilization and remobilization
- Integrity of structures adjacent to involved tissues
- Patient's general health and use of medications
- Patient's needs, expectations, and level of motivation
- Philosophy of the surgeon

exercise interventions for patients undergoing current surgical procedures and can also be applied as a basis of rehabilitation in the future as surgical techniques continue to change and evolve.

Guidelines for Preoperative Management

Preoperative contact with a patient is advisable. Of course, this is possible only with preplanned, elective surgery. A preoperative visit helps the therapist begin to establish rapport with a new patient and alleviate some of the patient's anxiety about the scheduled surgery and early postoperative days. This visit also enables the therapist to perform a thorough examination to document the patient's impairments and functional status prior to surgery.[42,56] The preoperative evaluation provides a basis to determine the patient's needs, goals, and expected functional outcomes.

Patient education can also be initiated preoperatively, either during an individual instruction session with the patient or in a group setting with patients planning to undergo similar surgeries. For example, some acute care facilities provide preoperative group instruction by team members from several disciplines, such as nursing, physical therapy, or occupational therapy, for patients scheduled for joint replacement surgery.[21,32,36] Preoperative instruction gives the patient an opportunity to become familiar with wound care, any special precautions that must be followed after surgery, or the use of assistive or supportive equipment such as crutches, a splint, or a sling.[42,56] Of equal importance, it enables the patient to practice and learn early postoperative exercises without being hampered by postoperative pain or the side effects of pain medication, such as disorientation and drowsiness.[42,56] For those patients scheduled for outpatient surgery, preoperative instruction allows the patient to be safe at home during the early postoperative days and to begin a home exercise program the day after surgery and then follow up with the therapist a week or so after surgery.

Examination and Evaluation

- Determine the patient's preoperative level of functional independence or functional limitation and the level of function he or she expects after surgery. Measure the patient's perceived level of disability.
- Determine the primary impairments such as the amount and type of joint pain, swelling, or crepitation the patient is experiencing.
- Measure the active and passive ROM of the involved joint or extremity.
- Check the ROM of all other joints.
- Grade the strength of the affected extremity.
- Estimate the functional strength of the unaffected joints or extremities as a basis for postoperative ambulation, transfers, and activities of daily living (ADL).
- Evaluate the gait characteristics, type of assistive devices, and degree of weight bearing used during ambulation. Note any inequalities in leg lengths.

Components of Preoperative Patient Education

- Explain the general plan of care the patient can expect during the postoperative period.
- Advise the patient of any precautions or contraindications to movement or weight bearing that must be followed postoperatively.
- Teach the patient any exercises that will be started in the very early postoperative period. These often include:
  - Deep-breathing and coughing exercises.
  - Active ankle exercises, if possible, to prevent venous stasis.
  - Gentle muscle-setting exercises of immobilized joints.
- Teach the patient safe and efficient bed mobility.
- Teach use of any assistive devices, such as crutches or canes, that may be needed after surgery.
- Explain or reinforce care of the incision for optimal wound healing.

Guidelines for Postoperative Management

After surgery and throughout a postoperative rehabilitation program a number of primary and secondary impairments must be addressed that can have an impact on the success of the surgical procedure and the functional outcomes for the patient. In addition to impairments, such as pain, limitation of motion, or loss of strength, potential complications after surgery (Box 8–13) can also affect outcomes.[7,31,58,60,66]

As with any other individually designed rehabilitation program, the postoperative goals and the plan of care, including therapeutic exercise interventions, change throughout the postoperative course. For example, early on, after surgery, the emphasis of management focuses on minimizing pain, preventing postoperative complications, which include secondary impairments, and retaining a safe level of functional mobility while protecting the surgical site.

Box 8–13 Potential Postoperative Complications

- Increased risk of pneumonia or atelectasis
- Local or systemic infection
- Deep vein thrombosis or pulmonary embolism
- Delayed wound healing
- Muscle function deficits secondary to tourniquet compression and resulting ischemia
- Delayed healing of repaired soft tissue or bone
- Subluxation or dislocation of joint surfaces or implants
- Adhesions and contractures of soft tissues and joints
- Loosening of joint implants secondary to periprosthetic osteolysis
- Failure, loosening, or displacement of internal fixation devices

Later, as the patient recovers from surgery, interventions are directed toward improving strength, stability, muscular and cardiorespiratory endurance, and balance and returning a patient to an optimal level of functional capabilities.

Without disregarding the fact that each patient's recovery after surgery is unique, postoperative rehabilitation can be divided into three general phases: (1) the very early phase when maximum protection of acutely involved tissues is paramount; (2) the intermediate phase when only moderate protection is necessary and progressive levels of stress can be placed on healing tissues; and (3) the final phase when only minimum protection is required, and the patient can gradually return to most or all functional activities. These phases of postoperative rehabilitation are based on the stages of healing of involved soft tissue and bone, the characteristics of the surgical procedure and, of course, the individual qualities, needs, and abilities of each patient. Therefore, the timeframe for each phase of rehabilitation varies from one procedure to another and from one patient to another. For example, after an arthroscopic meniscectomy or synovectomy, the maximum protection phase, during which movement of the involved area is restricted to passive or assisted motion within a protected range, may extend for only 1 day postoperatively. After a complex tendon repair in the hand, maximum protection may be required for several weeks.

Because surgical intervention usually occurs with the more serious injuries, severe deformities or late-stage joint diseases, the progression of exercises may be more gradual and the return to a full functional activity level may take more time for postoperative patients than for patients who do not require surgery. On the other hand, surgical intervention after some soft tissue or bony injuries actually allows earlier movement or weight bearing than would have been allowable with nonoperative management. Therefore, each patient's readiness to progress from one phase of postoperative rehabilitation to the next must be judged on an individual basis. Although many published protocols include estimated time frames for each phase of postoperative rehabilitation, these time periods must be viewed only as general guidelines. Progression from one phase to the next should not be based solely on time but also on the patient's attainment of predetermined criteria, such as the absence of pain or inflammation or the achievement of a particular level of strength or motion.

Given the relatively few number of justifiable visits available for postoperative rehabilitation, it is highly unlikely for a therapist to directly treat a patient through all three phases of postoperative rehabilitation. Therefore, the key to successful postoperative outcomes is effective self-management that includes a home program of selected interventions, in particular, a progression of exercises that have been carefully taught and periodically monitored by the therapist during each phase of rehabilitation. The following guidelines, summarized in Box 8–14, highlight the key components of management during the three phases of postoperative rehabilitation.

Overview of Common Orthopedic Surgical Procedures and Guidelines for Postoperative Management

Surgical management of musculoskeletal conditions encompasses many different procedures and combinations of procedures that can involve a variety of tissues and structures including muscles, tendons, fascia, joint capsules, cartilage, ligaments, nerves, and bones. The surgical methods can be divided into several broad categories: *repair, release, resection, realignment, reconstruction, replacement, and fusion.*[43,57] Some specific examples of procedures that employ these methods are listed in Table 8–4.

It is the purpose of this section to provide a brief description of some of the more common orthopedic procedures and associated postoperative management. As previously mentioned, postoperative management of specific surgical procedures for various regions of the upper or lower extremities are found in Chapters 9 through 14.

Note: In these general descriptions of various orthopedic procedures, the duration of immobilization and the initiation, progression, and intensity of exercise may vary according to differences in surgical techniques and the philosophy of the surgeon. A patient's health status, age, and use of medications will also affect the rate of healing and subsequent progression in a postoperative exercise program.

Open, Arthroscopic and Arthroscopically Assisted Procedures

An open surgical procedure involves an incision of adequate length and depth through superficial and deep layers of skin, fascia, muscles, and joint cap-

Box 8–14 Management Guidelines—Postoperative Rehabilitation

Impairments:

- Postoperative pain because of disruption of soft tissue
- Postoperative swelling
- Potential circulatory and pulmonary complications
- Joint stiffness or limitation of motion because of injury to soft tissue and necessary postoperative immobilization
- Muscle atrophy because of immobilization
- Loss of strength for functional activities
- Limitation of weight bearing
- Potential loss of strength and mobility in unoperated joints

Maximum Protection Phase

Plan of Care	Interventions
1. Educate the patient in preparation for self-management.	1. Instruction in safe positioning and limb movements and special postoperative precautions or contraindications.
2. Decrease postoperative pain, muscle guarding, or spasm.	2. Relaxation exercises. Use of modalities such as transcutaneous nerve stimulation (TNS), cold, or heat. Continuous passive motion (CPM) during the early postoperative period.
3. Prevent wound infection.	3. Instruction or review of proper cleaning and dressing the incision.
4. Minimize postoperative swelling.	4. Elevation of the operated extremity. Active muscle pumping exercises at the distal joints. Use of compression garment. Gentle distal-to-proximal massage.[69]
5. Prevent circulatory and pulmonary complications such as deep vein thrombosis, pulmonary embolus, or pneumonia.	5. Active exercises to distal musculature. Deep-breathing and coughing exercises.
6. Prevent unnecessary, residual joint stiffness, or soft tissue contractures.	6. CPM or passive or active-assistive ROM initiated in the immediate postoperative period.
7. Minimize muscle atrophy across immobilized joints.	7. Muscle-setting exercises.
8. Maintain motion and strength in areas above and below the operative site.	8. Active and resistive ROM exercises to unoperated areas.
9. Maintain functional mobility while protecting the operative site.	9. Adaptive equipment and assistive devices.

Moderate Protection/Controlled Motion Phase

Plan of Care	Interventions
1. Educate the patient.	1. Teach the patient to monitor the effects of the exercise program and make adjustments if swelling or pain increases.
2. Gradually restore soft tissue and joint mobility.	2. Active-assistive or active ROM within limits of pain. Joint mobilization procedures.
3. Establish a mobile scar.	3. Gentle massage across and around the maturing scar.
4. Strengthen involved muscles and improve joint stability.	4. Multiple-angle isometrics against increasing resistance. Alternating isometrics and rhythmic stabilization procedures. Dynamic exercise against light resistance in open- and closed-chain positions. Light functional activities with operated limb.

cont'd on page 310

Box 8–14 Management Guidelines—Postoperative Rehabilitation *(continued)*

Minimum Protection/Return to Function Phase

Plan of Care	Interventions
1. Continue patient education.	1. Emphasize gradual but progressive incorporation of improved muscle performance, mobility, and balance into functional activities.
2. Prevent reinjury or postoperative complications.	2. Reinforce self-monitoring and review the signs and symptoms of excessive use; identify unsafe activities.
3. Restore full joint and soft tissue mobility, if possible.	3. Joint stretching (mobilization) and self-stretching techniques.
4. Maximize muscle performance, dynamic stability, and neuromuscular control.	4. Progressive strengthening exercises using higher loads and speeds and combined movement patterns. Integrate movements and positions into exercises that simulate functional activities.
5. Restore balance and coordinated movement.	5. Progressive balance and coordination training.
6. Acquire or relearn specific motor skills.	6. Apply principles of motor learning (appropriate practice and feedback during task-specific training).

Precautions: In addition to the precautions already addressed that relate to the stages of tissue repair and healing, there are several additional precautions that are of particular importance to the postsurgical patient.

- Avoid positions, movements, or weight bearing that could compromise the integrity of the surgical repair.
- Keep the wound clean to avoid postoperative infection. Monitor for wound drainage and signs of systemic or local infection, such as elevated temperature.
- Avoid vigorous/high-intensity stretching or resistance exercises with soft tissues, such as muscles, tendons, or joint capsules that have been repaired or reattached for at least 6 weeks to ensure adequate healing and stability.
- Modify level and selection of physical activities, if necessary, to prevent premature wear and tear of repaired or reconstructed soft tissues and joints.

sule so that the operative field can be fully visualized by the surgeon during the procedure.[39,58,60] The term **arthrotomy** is used to describe an open procedure in which the joint capsule is incised and joint structures are exposed. Open approaches are necessary for surgeries, such as joint replacement, arthrodesis, and internal fixation of fractures, and for some soft tissue repairs and reconstruction, such as muscle or tendon ruptures. There is extensive disturbance of soft tissues during an open procedure that requires a lengthy period of rehabilitation while soft tissues heal.

Arthroscopy is used as a diagnostic tool and as a means of treating a variety of intra-articular disorders.[4,41,44] Arthroscopic procedures are usually performed on an outpatient basis and under local anesthesia.

An arthroscopy involves several very small incisions (punctures) in the skin, muscle, and joint capsule for insertion of an endoscope into the joint for

Table 8–4 General Methods and Examples of Musculoskeletal Surgeries

Surgical Methods	Examples of Procedures
• Repair	• Tenorrhaphy, tendon repair; meniscus or ligament repair; articular cartilage repair by implantation
• Release or decompression	• Myotomy, tenotomy, fasciotomy; capsulotomy; tenolysis; muscle-tendon lengthening; retinacular release; arthroscopic subacromial decompression
• Resection or removal	• Synovectomy, meniscectomy, capsulectomy; debridement and lavage; laminectomy; excision of soft tissue or bony neoplasms
• Realignment or stabilization	• Tendon transfer, tenodesis; extensor mechanism realignment; capsulorrhaphy, capsular shift; osteotomy
• Reconstruction or replacement	• Tenoplasty; capsulolabral reconstruction; ligamentous reconstruction; chondroplasty; arthroplasty
• Fusion or fixation for bony union	• Arthrodesis; open reduction with internal fixation

visualization of the interior of the joint by means of a camera. The small incisions are called *portals.* Miniature, motorized surgical tools are inserted through the portals and used to repair soft tissues within or around the joint, remove loose bodies, or debride the joint surfaces. Arthroscopic techniques are most commonly used at the shoulder and knee.[4,39] Procedures include ligament and tendon repairs or reconstruction, debridement of joints, meniscectomy, and synovectomy.[4,41,44] Because the incisions for the portals are so small, there is minimal disturbance of soft tissues during arthroscopic procedures. Therefore, rehabilitation *usually* but not always can proceed more quickly than after an open procedure. An arthroscopically assisted procedure uses arthroscopy for a portion of the procedure, but also necessitates an open surgical field for selected aspects of the operative procedure.[4,39,41] This sometimes is referred to as a "mini-open" procedure.

Repair, Reattachment, Reconstruction, or Transfer of Soft Tissues

Surgical repair, reattachment, or reconstruction of soft tissues may be employed after a severe injury of a muscle, tendon, or ligament. Transfer of a muscle-tendon unit may be indicated to improve the stability of an unstable joint or prevent deformity and improve neuromuscular control in patients with neuropathic or myopathic disorders.[2,34,43,58] Although there are a multitude of surgeries that fall into this category, in all instances the therapist must consider the effects of immobilization and remobilization and the characteristics of healing of the types of tissues involved when designing a postoperative exercise program.[34]

Repair of a muscle. A complete tear or rupture of a muscle is unusual, but it may occur if a muscle that is already in a state of contraction takes a direct blow or is forcibly stretched.[2,6,17]

Procedure

Immediate surgical repair of a severe tear or even a complete rupture of a muscle is uncommon because inflammation affects the texture of muscle tissue making it difficult to hold sutures in place. A patient can achieve a more satisfactory outcome with a late repair (approximately 48–72 hours after injury) after acute symptoms have decreased. The muscle is reopposed, sutured, and immobilized so that the muscle is in a *shortened* position.[2,43,58]

Exercise

- Muscle-setting exercise of the sutured muscle may be initiated immediately after surgery.
- When the immobilization is removed, active ROM emphasizing controlled motion may be started to regain joint motion and prevent contractures.
- Weight bearing is partially restricted until the patient achieves a functional level of strength and flexibility.
- Low-intensity, high-repetition exercises are progressed very gradually and should not elicit pain.
- Vigorous stretching or return to a full level of activity are contraindicated until soft tissue healing is complete—as long as 6 to 8 weeks postoperatively.

Repair of a tendon. A tendon usually ruptures from severe trauma in a young person or with a sudden, unusual motion in an elderly person with a history of chronic impingement and progressive deterioration of the tendon.[9] Tendons usually rupture at musculotendinous or tendo-osseous junctions.[47] Common sites of acute rupture are the bicipital tendon at the shoulder or the Achilles tendon.[2]

In patients with chronic tenosynovitis of the hand and wrist, the extensor tendons often erode over time and may eventually rupture along the dorsum of the hand.[7,10] The superficial tendons of the hand and foot are also vulnerable to injuries that could require surgical repair. For example, the flexor tendons of the fingers are commonly severed as the result of a deep laceration to the palm of the hand.

Procedure

The tendon is sutured, and the muscle and tendon are put in a shortened position, as with a complete tear of a muscle. A longer immobilization period may be required for a repaired tendon than for a repaired muscle, because the vascular supply to tendons is poor.

Exercise

- Muscle setting is begun immediately after surgery to prevent adhesions of the tendon to the sheath or surrounding tissues and to promote alignment of healing tissue. If it is possible to remove the immobilization for brief periods of exercise, passive motion within a protected range also may be permissible within a few days after surgery.[10]
- Controlled active ROM is initiated after the repaired tendon has had several weeks to heal.

- After an upper or lower extremity tendon repair, weight bearing may be restricted, and after an upper extremity repair, heavy lifting activities are often contraindicated for as long as 6 to 8 weeks.
- Vigorous stretching and high-intensity resistance exercise may be initiated after about 8 weeks, when healing of the tendon has occurred.

Repair or reconstruction of ligaments. When ligaments cannot be approximated for healing through closed reduction, surgical repair is indicated. Reconstruction of a ligament with tissue taken from a donor site may also be necessary. The knee and ankle joints are commonly affected.

Procedure

The torn ligament is repaired or reconstructed, and the joint is immobilized in a position that places limited tension on the sutured ligament.[4] Immobilization is required postoperatively, but the duration varies with the site and severity of injury and the type of repair or reconstruction employed.[4,13,17,58]

Exercise

Rehabilitation after ligament surgery emphasizes early but protected motion and progressive strengthening and weight bearing to consistently but safely load the healing tissues. How quickly the rehabilitation program is progressed depends on many factors such as the type of repair or reconstruction that has been done. For example, an anterior cruciate ligament (ACL) reconstruction utilizing a patellar tendon graft and bone to bone fixation can be progressed more rapidly than a soft tissue stabilization procedure, involving a transfer of the iliotibial band or hamstrings.[2,4,6,17] The rate of progression also depends on the site of the repair or reconstruction. For example, support should be worn and weight bearing restricted for an extended period of time if the repair is at a potentially unstable joint and until muscle power can adequately protect the joint.

Generally, postoperative rehabilitation after ligamentous surgery is a long process. For patients wishing to return to high-intensity sports after knee ligament surgery for example, it may take at least 6 months to a year of rehabilitation.[6]

Tendon transfer or realignment. The transfer or realignment of a muscle-tendon unit alters the line of pull of a muscle. This may be indicated, for example, to improve the stability of an unstable shoulder joint or to stabilize a chronically dislocating patella. Although a realignment procedure slightly alters the line of pull of the muscle, it does not change the *action* of the muscle-tendon unit. For instance, after an extensor mechanism realignment, the quadriceps remains an extensor of the knee.

A tendon transfer from one bony surface to another is often indicated for a patient with a significant neurological deficit to prevent deformity and improve functional control. In this type of procedure, not only is the line of pull of the muscle-tendon unit altered, the *action* of the muscle is also changed. For example, transfer of the distal attachment of the flexor carpi ulnaris to the extensor surface of the wrist can prevent a wrist flexion deformity and improve active wrist extension for functional grasp in a child with cerebral palsy.[58]

Procedures

In both tendon transfer or realignment procedures, usually the distal attachment of the muscle-tendon unit is removed from its bony insertion and reattached to a different bone, to a different location on the same bone, or to adjacent soft tissues.[43,58] The muscle-tendon unit is then immobilized in a shortened position for a period of time.

Exercise

- As with a tendon repair, early muscle setting and protected motion are important to maintain tendon gliding. Resisted movements are progressed very carefully and gradually to protect the reattached tendon.
- If the purpose of the transfer was to change the function of the muscle, biofeedback and electrical muscle stimulation are often used to help a patient learn to control the new action of the transferred muscle-tendon unit.[58]

Soft Tissue Release, Lengthening, or Decompression Procedures

Soft tissues may be incised or sectioned to improve ROM, prevent or minimize progressive deformity, or relieve pain. Procedures include *myotomy, tenotomy,* or *fasciotomy.*[14,43,58]

A surgical release of soft tissues may be appropriate in young patients with severe arthritis and resulting contractures in whom joint replacement is not advisable or as a preliminary procedure in adults prior to joint replacement.[7,60] Releases are also performed in patients with myopathic and neuropathic diseases, such as cerebral palsy and muscular dystrophy, to improve functional mobility.[58] Some form of splinting or bracing in the corrected position in conjunction with exercise is always used postoperatively to maintain the gained ROM. A release of soft tissues to achieve decompression of tissues and relieve pain may be indicated for a person with an impingement or compartmental syndrome, such as a shoulder impingement or carpal tunnel syndrome.[4,13,43]

Procedures

In a release or lengthening of a shortened muscle group, a portion of the muscle-tendon unit is surgically sectioned and fibrotic tissues are incised. A tendon can also be partially incised to allow greater extensibility. The incised structures are then immobilized in a *lengthened* position except during exercise.[43,58] In decompression procedures, fasciae that are causing pressure on muscles, tendons, or nerves may either be released or removed. Some decompression procedures, for example at the shoulder, also involve removal of osteophytes or alteration of bony structures that are creating excessive pressure on soft tissues.

Exercise

- CPM and/or active-assistive ROM is usually initiated several days after surgery. This is followed by active ROM through the gained ranges as soft-tissue healing progresses.[14,58]
- Strengthening of the antagonists of the lengthened muscle should also be started early to maintain active control of movement within the newly gained range.

Synovectomy

Procedure

Removal of the synovium (lining of the joint) in patients with chronic joint inflammation can be done arthroscopically or by an arthrotomy.[60] It is occasionally performed in patients who have rheumatoid arthritis with chronic proliferative synovitis but with minimal articular changes. It is indicated if medical management has failed to alleviate joint inflammation for 4 to 6 months. Synovectomy is most commonly performed on the knee, elbow, wrist, and metacarpophalangeal joints.[7,10,70] Although synovium tends to regenerate, resection of the inflamed synovium temporarily relieves pain and joint swelling and is thought to protect articular cartilage or tendons from enzymatic damage.[7,15,70]

A compression dressing is applied at the time of surgery and worn for a brief period of time. The operated extremity is elevated to reduce edema.

Exercise

- During the brief period of immobilization postoperatively, setting exercises of the muscles that surround the affected joint are begun.
- CPM or active-assistive exercises are initiated as soon as the immobilization can be removed. Exercises quickly progress to active ROM.
- Full weight bearing or lifting heavy objects is restricted for 6 to 8 weeks.
- Progression of the rehabilitation program is based on the patient's response to exercise as well as the overall response to medication for the primary inflammatory disease. Every effort should be made to avoid excessive exercise or activity that could increase joint pain or swelling.[60,70]

Osteotomy

Procedure

The surgical cutting and realignment of bone is undertaken in cases of severe arthritis to correct joint deformity and reduce pain. It is most often performed in osteoarthritis of the knee or hip.[15] Osteotomy of the hip is also appropriate for young patients with severe hip pain secondary to hip problems such as Legg-Calvé-Perthes disease or congenital dislocation of the hip.[43] In some instances, an osteotomy is employed to improve ambulation and prevent eventual joint deterioration by correcting angular or rotational deformities of the lower extremities associated with neurological deficits, such as cerebral palsy or traumatic brain injury.[58] Osteotomy is also necessary for surgical shortening or lengthening of bone to correct a severe leg length discrepancy.

An osteotomy realigns bone and redistributes loads placed on joint surfaces. If articular degeneration has led to joint pain and swelling, an osteotomy reduces these symptoms and may also stimulate the development of fibrocartilage in the unloaded compartment of the joint.[7,15,18,55] A successful osteotomy delays the need for a total joint replacement in young, active patients or very obese patients who will most likely require a revision arthroplasty sooner than the average patient with degenerative arthritis.

Immobilization

Either the osteotomy site is immobilized with internal fixation, which allows early joint motion and protected weight bearing, or the involved bones and adjacent joints are placed in a cast until bony healing occurs, which may take as long as 8 to 12 weeks.[7,18,55]

Exercise

- During immobilization in a cast, the patient should be encouraged to actively move the joints above and below the site of the osteotomy to prevent joint stiffness and undue weakness.
- When motion and weight bearing are allowed or when the cast is removed, active-assistive, active, and mild resistive exercise may be started to restore joint ROM and strength (see discussion of the chronic stage of soft tissue healing earlier in this chapter).
- If chronic stiffness persists because of the long-term immobilization, joint mobilization and soft tissue stretching will be necessary.

Arthrodesis

Procedure

Surgical fusion of bony surfaces of a joint with internal fixation, such as with pins, nails, plates, and bone grafts, is most frequently indicated in cases of severe joint pain and instability in which mobility of the joint is a lesser concern.[11,43,55,58] It is commonly performed at the spine, wrist, thumb, and ankle. Arthrodesis of the extremity joints is also reserved for patients with significant weakness of muscles surrounding a joint as the result of neurological abnormalities, such as a peripheral neuropathy of the ankle or a severe brachial plexus injury. In addition, it may be the only salvage procedure available for a patient with a failed total joint arthroplasty who is not a candidate for a revision arthroplasty. Optimal positions for arthrodesis are listed in Table 8–5. Optimal position is somewhat dependent on the functional needs or goals of the patient and may vary slightly in some joints, such as the elbow and ankle. For example, the optimal position for elbow fusion in the dominant upper extremity is usually between 70 and 90 degrees. However, in the nondominant limb, the elbow must be in more extension for assistive activities.[11] For a woman, the optimal position for arthrodesis of the ankle might be in slightly greater plantarflexion than for a man to allow a woman to wear shoes with a slightly higher heel height.[58]

Table 8–5 Optimal Positions for Arthrodesis

Joint	Position
Shoulder	15–30 degrees of abduction and flexion and 45 degrees of internal rotation: a position so that the hand can reach the mouth
Elbow	Dominant upper extremity: 70–90 degrees of flexion and midposition of the forearm; nondominant limb: more extension for assisting during tasks
Wrist	Slight extension
MCP of the thumb	20 degrees of flexion
Hip	10–15 degrees of flexion to allow ambulation and comfortable sitting
Ankle	
Tibiotalar joint	Neutral (90 degrees) or slight equinus for women who wear low heels
Subtalar joint	Neutral so there is no varus or valgus
Spine	Neutral so normal lordosis or kyphosis is maintained

Immobilization

The joint is immobilized with bone grafts and some type of internal or external fixation device in the desired position for maximum function for 6 to 12 weeks to ensure bony fusion.

Exercise

- Because no movement will be possible in the fused joint, ROM and strength must be maintained above and below the operated joint.
- Weight bearing is restricted until there is evidence of bony healing.

Arthroplasty

Any reconstructive joint procedure, with or without joint implant, designed to relieve pain and/or restore joint motion is generally referred to as an arthroplasty of which there are several types.

Procedures

Abrasion arthroplasty. This procedure, also known as *abrasion chondroplasty,* is used to promote healing of chondral lesions. It involves abrasion of an articular surface with an arthroscopic burr or drill to stimulate local fibrocartilage ingrowth.[13] In the past the procedure was often performed for chondral lesions of the patella. Although rehabilitation after this procedure is quite protracted, the benefits appear to be short-lived because the fibrocartilage replacement tissue is not as strong as hyaline cartilage and, therefore, deteriorates steadily.[13]

Excision arthroplasty. This procedure involves removal of periarticular bone from one or both articular surfaces. A space is left where fibrotic (scar) tissue is allowed to be laid down during the healing process. This is sometimes called *resectional arthroplasty.*[7,43,55,58,66] This procedure may be performed in a variety of joints such as the hip, elbow, wrist, and foot to reduce pain and increase joint motion. Disadvantages of these procedures are:

- Possible joint instability.
- A poor cosmetic result because of shortening of the operated extremity.
- Persistent muscular imbalance and weakness.

Excision arthroplasty, although an old procedure, is still appropriate in selected cases.

Excision arthroplasty with implant. After removal of the articular surface, an artificial implant is fixed in place to help in the remodeling of a new joint. This is sometimes called *implant resection arthroplasty.*[58,66] The implant usually is made of a flexible silicone material and becomes encapsulated by fibrous tissue as the joint reforms.

Interpositional arthroplasty. Débridement of the joint is performed initially, and a foreign material is placed between (interposed) the two joint surfaces. A variety of materials may be used to cover the joint surface such as fascia, Silastic material, or metal.

Some examples of interpositional arthroplasties are Smith-Petersen cup arthroplasty of the hip (rarely performed now, with the advent of the total hip replacement), condylar replacement of the knee, and humeral replacement of the shoulder.

Total joint replacement arthroplasty. This procedure is a common operative option to relieve pain and improve function in patients with severe joint destruction associated with late-stage arthritis.[7,58] It involves removal of both affected joint surfaces and replacement with artificial joint components.[7,42,43,55,66]

Prosthetic replacements for almost every joint of the extremities have been developed and refined. A more complete description of those implants will be reviewed joint by joint in Chapters 9 through 14. Overall, total joint replacement arthroplasty has been most successful in the large joints, such as the hip and knee, rather than in the smaller joints of the foot and hand.[7,55]

The materials, designs, and methods of fixation used in total joint arthroplasty are noted in Box 8–15. In almost all designs, one articular surface is metal and the other is plastic. Designs range from unconstrained (resurfacing) joint components that have no inherent stability to semiconstrained and fully constrained (articulated) implants that provide stability to an unstable joint. Choice of fixation is based, in part, on the anticipated loads that will be placed on the prosthetic implants over an extended period of time. Cemented fixation eventually tends to deteriorate over time at the bone-cement interface resulting in loosening of the implant and pain.[7,58,66] Therefore, cemented fixation is used primarily for older or sedentary patients who are unlikely to place high stresses on the implants. Bio-ingrowth fixation is less likely to deteriorate over time and appears to be a better choice for younger, more active patients.

Despite the positive functional outcomes of total joint replacement, not every patient with advanced joint disease is a candidate for this procedure. Contraindications to total joint arthroplasty are noted in

Box 8–15 Materials, Design, and Fixation Used in Total Joint Arthroplasty

Implant Materials

- ***Rigid.*** Inert metal (cobalt-chrome alloy, titanium alloy, or ceramic)
- ***Semirigid.*** Plastic (high-density polymers such as polyethylene)

Implant Designs

- Unconstrained (resurfacing)—no inherent stability
- Semiconstrained
- Fully constrained (articulated)—inherent stability

Methods of Fixation

- Cemented
  - Acrylic cement (methyl methacrylate)
- Uncemented
  - Biological fixation (microscopic ingrowth of bone into a porous-coated prosthesis
  - Press fit (tight fit between bone and implant)
  - Screws, bolts, or nails
- Hybrid
  - Uncemented component for one joint surface and cemented component for opposing joint surface.

Box 8–16.[7,43,55,58,66] Although opinions vary as to which of these are absolute versus relative contraindications, there is general agreement that infection is of the utmost concern.

Exercise

Postoperative management, which includes therapeutic exercise interventions, for various forms of arthroplasty of major joints of the extremities are described in detail in Chapters 9 through 14.

Articular Cartilage Implantation

Procedure

This procedure, also referred to as *autologous chondrocyte implantation,* is designed to repair focal, full thickness defects of hyaline cartilage and prevent progressive deterioration of joint cartilage leading to osteoarthritis.[14,25,45] The procedure is a relatively new alternative to abrasion arthroplasty. It has been used most often for patients with articular defects of the femoral condyles or patella.[14] The procedure occurs in two stages. First, healthy articular cartilage is harvested arthroscopically from the patient, cultured for several weeks, and processed in a laboratory to increase the volume of healthy tissue. The second phase is the implantation phase. This phase sometimes is combined with another necessary procedure, such as an extensor mechanism realignment or ligamentous reconstruction. After the chondral defect sites are debrided and covered with a periosteal patch, the autologous chondrocytes are injected into the articular defect.

Exercise

Rehabilitation after articular cartilage implantation is a slow and arduous process.[14,25,45] Exercise is an important aspect of postoperative management at each stage of rehabilitation. Early passive motion and protected weight bearing are essential to promote the maturation and maintain the health of the implanted chondrocytes. A knee immobilizer is worn during functional activities for approximately 6 weeks. Full weight bearing is allowable by 8 to 9 weeks. A well-controlled program of progressive exercises continues for 6 months to a year to achieve optimal functional outcomes.

Box 8–16 Contraindications to Total Joint Arthroplasty

- Active infection in the joint
- Chronic osteomyelitis
- Systemic infection
- Substantial loss of bone or malignant tumors that prohibit adequate implant fixation
- Significant paralysis of muscles surrounding the joint
- Neuropathic joint
- Inadequate patient motivation

Independent Learning Activities

CRITICAL THINKING AND DISCUSSION

1. Your patient has experienced an injury to a muscle; describe the symptoms that he or she will experience during each stage of inflammation and repair, and describe the principles of exercise intervention that should be used during each stage. Once you have identified the principles, choose a commonly injured muscle, such as the hamstrings, and describe the symptoms, test results, goals treatment plan, and actual interventions that you would use for each stage of intervention.
2. Do the same activity as in #1 except use a ligamentous injury, such as strain of the humeroulnar ligament or anterior talofibular ligament.
3. Describe the mechanism of injury for common overuse syndromes, such as lateral epicondylitis or shin splints, and explain the differences between such an injury and an acute-traumatic injury.
4. Describe the benefits of nondestructive, controlled motion to injured or surgically traumatized tissue. What is nondestructive motion? How do you know if too much motion has occurred during the acute and early subacute stages of healing, or when treating an overuse syndrome?
5. Your patient sustained a traumatic knee joint injury in an automobile accident; there is joint effusion, limited ROM, and decreased joint play 2 days after the accident. The patient guards against motion as you approach the end of the available range. Identify the principles of treatment, the goals, and plan of care for this patient. Describe and practice specific therapeutic techniques that you would use for intervention, and

describe how you would progress the techniques through the stages of healing.

6. An individual sustained a fracture 6 weeks ago, and the limb was just removed from the cast. How will treatment differ from that of other traumatic conditions 6 weeks postinjury? Describe what precautions you will follow and why they are important.

7. Differentiate among the following types of soft tissue or bony surgeries primarily used in the management of arthritis: arthrodesis, arthroplasty, osteotomy, and synovectomy. Briefly describe each surgery and compare and contrast postoperative management with respect to the use of exercise.

8. Discuss the similarities and differences of postoperative management of the following soft-tissue surgeries: tendon repair, tendon transfer, ligament reconstruction, tenotomy or myotomy, and decompression procedures.

REFERENCES

1. American College of Rheumatology Subcommittee on Osteoarthritis Guidelines: Recommendations for the medical management of osteoarthritis of the hip and knee: 2000 update. Arthritis Rheum 43(9):1905, 2000.
2. Anderson, MK, Hall, SJ: Fundamentals of sports injury management. Williams & Wilkins, Baltimore, 1997.
3. Anderson, RJ: Rheumatoid arthritis: Clinical and laboratory features. In Klippel, JH, (ed): Primer on the Rheumatic Diseases, ed 11. Arthritis Foundation, Atlanta, 1997, p 161.
4. Andrews, JR, Timmerman, LA (eds): Diagnostic and operative arthroscopy. WB Saunders, Philadelphia, 1997.
5. Arnett, FC, Edworthy, SM, Bloch, DA, et al: The American Rheumatism Association 1987 revised criteria for the classification of rheumatoid arthritis. Arthritis Rheum 31:315, 1988.
6. Arnheim, DD, and Prentice, WE: Principles of Athletic Training, ed 3. McGraw-Hill, Boston, 1997.
7. Ballard, WT, and Buckwalter, JA: Operative treatment of rheumatic disease. In Klippel, JH, (ed): Primer on the Rheumatic Diseases (ed 11). Arthritis Foundation, Atlanta, 1997, p 443.
8. Bandy, WD: Functional rehabilitation of the athlete. Orthop Phys Ther Clin North Am 1:269, 1992.
9. Barrick, EF: Orthopedic trauma. In Kauffman, TL (ed): Geriatric Rehabilitation Manual. Churchill Livingstone, New York, 1999.
10. Batts Shanku, CD: Rheumatoid arthritis. In Hansen, RA and Atchison, B (eds): Conditions in Occupational Therapy, ed 2. Lippincott Williams & Wilkins, Baltimore, 2000.
11. Beckenbaugh, RD: Arthrodesis. In Morrey, BF (ed): The Elbow and Its Disorders. WB Saunders, Philadelphia, 2000, p 751.
12. Boissonnault, WG: Joint and muscle disorders. In Goodman, CC and Boissonnault, WG: Pathology: implications for the physical therapist. WB Saunders Co, Philadelphia, 1998, p 660.
13. Brinker, M, and Miller, M: Fundamentals of Orthopedics. WB Saunders, Philadelphia, 1999.
14. Brittberg, M, et al: Treatment of deep cartilage defects in the knee with autologous chondrocyte transplantation. N Engl J Med 331:889, 1994.
15. Buckwalter, JA, and Lohmander, S: Operative treatment of osteoarthritis. J Bone Joint Surg 76A:1405, 1994.
16. Cailliet, R: Soft tissue pain and disability, ed 2. FA Davis, Philadelphia, 1988.
17. Canavan, PK: Rehabilitation in Sports Medicine: A Comprehensive Guide. Appleton and Lange, Stamford, CT, 1998.
18. Coventry, MB, Ilstrup, DM, and Wallrichs, SL: Proximal tibial osteotomy: a critical long-term study of eighty-seven cases. J Bone Joint Surg 75A:196, 1993.
19. Cummings, GS, and Tillman, LJ: Remodeling of dense connective tissue in normal adult tissues. In Currier, DP, and Nelson, RM (eds): Dynamics of Human Biologic Tissues. FA Davis, Philadelphia, 1992, p 45.
20. Cyriax, J: Textbook of Orthopaedic Medicine, Vol 1. Diagnosis of Soft Tissue Lesions, ed 8. Bailliere and Tindall, London, 1982.
21. D'Lima, DD, et al: The effect of preoperative exercise on total knee replacement outcomes. Clin Orthop Rel Res 326:174, 1996.
22. Enwemeka, CS: Connective tissue plasticity: ultrastructural, biomechanical, and morphometric effects of physical factors on intact and regenerating tendons. J Orthop Sports Phys Ther 14(5):198, 1991.
23. Felson, DT, Lawrence, RC, Dieppe, PA, et al: Osteoarthritis: new insights. Part 1: the disease and its risk factors. Ann Internal Med 133(8):635, 2000.
24. Felson, DT, Lawrence, RC, Hockberg, MC, et al: Osteoarthritis: new insights. Part 2: treatment approaches. Ann Internal Med 133 (9):726, 2000.
25. Gillogly, SD, Voight, M, and Blackburn, T: Treatment of articular cartilage defects of the knee with autologous chondrocyte implantation. J Orthop Sports Phys Ther 28(4):241, 1998.
26. Guidotti, TL: Occupational repetitive strain injury. Am Fam Physician 45:585, 1992.
27. Hawley, DJ: Health status assessment. In Wegener, ST (ed): Clinical Care in the Rheumatic Diseases. American College of Rheumatology, Atlanta, 1996.
28. Hockberg, MC: Osteoarthritis: clinical features and treatment. In Klippel, JH, (ed): Primer on the Rheumatic Diseases, ed 11. Arthritis Foundation, Atlanta, 1997, p 218.
29. Irrgang, JJ, and Pezzullo, D: Rehabilitation following surgical procedures to address articular cartilage lesions in the knee. J Orthop Sports Phys Ther 28 (4):232, 1998.
30. Isernhagen, SJ: Exercise technologies for work rehabilitation programs. Orthop Phys Ther Clin North Am 1:361, 1992.
31. Jacobson, MD, et al: Muscle function deficits after tourniquet ischemia. Am J Sports Med 22(3):372, 1994.

32. Jones, RE, and Blackburn, WD: Joint replacement surgery preoperative management. Bull Rheum Dis 47(4):5, 1998.
33. Kaltenborn, F: Manual Mobilization of the Extremity Joints: The Kaltenborn Method of Joint Examination and Treatment, Vol I. The Extremities, ed 5. Olaf Norlis Bokhandel Norway, 1999.
34. Keene, J, and Malone, TR: Ligament and muscle-tendon unit injuries. In Malone, TR, McPoil, Nitz, AJ GJ (eds): Orthopaedic and Sports Physical Therapy, ed 3. CV Mosby, St Louis, 1997, p 135.
35. Kellet, J: Acute soft tissue injuries: A review of the literature. Med Sci Sports Exerc 18:489, 1986.
36. King, L: Case study: physical therapy management of hip osteoarthritis prior to total hip arthroplasty. J Orthop Sports Phys Ther 26(1):35, 1997.
37. Leonard, JB: Joint protection for inflammatory disorders. In Lichtman, DM and Alexander, AH (eds): The Wrist and Its Disorders, ed 2. WB Saunders, Philadelphia, 1997, p 1377.
38. Margolis, S, and Flynn, JA: Arthritis: The Johns Hopkins White Papers. The Johns Hopkins Medical Institutions, Baltimore, Maryland, 2000.
39. Matsen, FA, et al: Glenohumeral arthritis and its management. In Rockwood, CA and Matsen, FA (eds): The Shoulder, Vol 2, ed 2. WB Saunders, Philadelphia, 1998, p 841.
40. McDonough, A: Effect of immobilization and exercise on articular cartilage: A review of literature. J Orthop Sports Phys Ther 3:2, 1981.
41. McGinty, JB (ed): Operative Arthroscopy. Lippincott-Raven Publishers, Philadelphia, 1996.
42. Melvin, JL, and Gall, V: Surgical rehabilitation for arthritis: achieving optimal results. In Melvin, JL and Gall, V (eds): Rheumatologic Rehabilitation Series, Vol 5: Surgical Rehabilitation. American Occupational Therapy Assoc., Bethesda MD, 1999.
43. Mercier, LR: Practical Orthopedics, ed 4. Mosby, St. Louis, 1995.
44. Metcalf, RW: Arthroscopy. In Sledge, CB, et al (eds): Arthritis Surgery. WB Saunders, Philadelphia, 1994.
45. Minas, T, and Nehrer, S: Current concepts in the treatment of articular cartilage defects. Orthopedics 20:525, 1997.
46. Minor, MA, et al: Efficacy of physical conditioning exercise in patients with rheumatoid arthritis and osteoarthritis. Arthritis Rheum 32:1396, 1989.
47. Noonan, TJ, and Garrett, WE: Injuries at the myotendinous junction. Clin Sports Med 11:783, 1992.
48. Noyes, FR, Keller, CS, et al: Advances in understanding of knee ligament injury, repair and rehabilitation Med Sci Sports Exerc 16:427, 1984.
49. Paget, SA: Rheumatoid arthritis: treatment. In Klippel, JH, (ed): Primer on the Rheumatic Diseases, ed 11. Arthritis Foundation, Atlanta, 1997, p 168.
50. Pease, BJ: Biomechanical assessment of the lower extremity. J Orthop Phys Ther Clin North Am 3:291, 1994.
51. Phillips, CA: Therapist's management of patients with RA. In Lichtman, DM and Alexander, AH (eds): The Wrist and Its Disorders, ed 2. WB Saunders, Philadelphia, 1997, p 1345.
52. Pincus, T: Rheumatoid arthritis. In Wegener, ST (ed): Clinical Care in the Rheumatic Diseases. American College of Rheumatology, Atlanta, 1996, p 147.
53. Puffer, JC, and Zachazewski, JE: Management of overuse injuries. Am Fam Physician 38:225, 1988.
54. Rand, JA, et al: A comparison of cemented vs cementless porous-coated anatomic total knee arthroplasty. In Rand, JA (ed): Total Arthroplasty of the Knee. Aspen, Rockville, MD, 1987.
55. Richterman, I, and Keenan, MA: Surgical Interventions. In Walker, JM and Helewa, A: Physical Therapy in Arthritis. WB Saunders Co, Philadelphia, 1996.
56. Roach, JA, Tremblay, LM, and Bowers, DL: A preoperative assessment and education program: implementation and outcomes. Patient Education Counseling 25:83, 1995.
57. Salter, RB: Continuous Passive Motion, A Biological Concept. Williams & Wilkins, Baltimore, 1993.
58. Salter, RB: Textbook of Disorders and Injuries of the Musculoskeletal System, ed 3. Williams & Wilkins, Baltimore, MD, 1999.
59. Simon, LS: Arthritis: New agents herald more effective symptom management. Geriatrics 54(6):37, 1999.
60. Sledge, CB: Introduction to surgical management. In Sledge, CB, et al (eds): Arthritis Surgery. WB Saunders, Philadelphia, 1994.
61. The Arthritis Foundation's Guide to Good Living with Osteoarthritis. Arthritis Foundation, Atlanta, 2000.
62. The Arthritis Foundation's Guide to Good Living with Rheumatoid Arthritis. Arthritis Foundation, Atlanta, 2000.
63. Threlkeld, JA, and Currier, DP: Osteoarthritis: Effects on synovial joint tissues. Phys Ther 68:346, 1988.
64. Tillman, LJ, and Cummings, GS: Biologic Mechanisms of Connective Tissue Mutability. In Currier, DP and Nelson, RM (eds): Dynamics of Human Biologic Tissues. FA Davis, Philadelphia, 1992, p 1.
65. van den Ende, CH, Breedveld, FC, le Cessie, S, et al: Effect of intensive exercise on patients with active rheumatoid arthritis: a randomised clinical trial. Ann Rheum Dis 59 (8):615, 2000.
66. Waugh, T: Arthroplasty rehabilitation. In Gouldgold, J (ed): Rehabilitation Medicine. CV Mosby, St Louis, 1988.
67. Wegener, L, Kisner, C, and Nichols, D: Static and dynamic balance responses in persons with bilateral knee osteoarthritis. J Orthop Sports Phys Ther 25:13, 1997.
68. Wilk, KE, and Arrigo, C: An integrated approach to upper extremity exercises. J Orthop Phys Ther Clin North Am 1:337, 1992.
69. Woolf, CJ: Generation of acute pain: Central mechanisms. Br Med Bull 47:523, 1991.
70. Wynn Parry, CB, and Stanley, JK: Synovectomy of the hand. Br J Rheumatol 32:1089, 1993.
71. Zohn, D, and Mennell, J: Musculoskeletal pain: Principles of physical diagnosis and physical treatment. Little, Brown & Company, Boston, 1976.

Chapter 9

The Shoulder and Shoulder Girdle

OBJECTIVES

After studying this chapter, the reader will be able to:

1 Identify important aspects of shoulder girdle structure and function for review.

2 Establish a therapeutic exercise program to manage soft tissue and joint lesions in the shoulder girdle region related to stages of recovery after an inflammatory insult to the tissues.

3 Establish a therapeutic exercise program to manage common musculoskeletal lesions, recognizing unique circumstances for their management.

4 Discuss the background of, indications for, and outcomes of common surgical procedures for soft tissue and joint pathology of the shoulder.

5 Explain the goals and appropriate interventions for postoperative management of shoulder and shoulder girdle dysfunction.

6 Establish a postoperative intervention program that includes therapeutic exercise for management of common surgical procedures.

The design of the shoulder girdle allows for mobility of the upper extremity. As a result, the hand can be placed almost anywhere within a sphere of movement, being limited primarily by the length of the arm and the space taken up by the body. The combined mechanics of its joints and muscles provide for and control the mobility. When establishing a therapeutic exercise program for impaired function of the shoulder region, as with any other region of the body, the unique anatomic and kinesiologic features must be taken into consideration as well as the state of pathology and functional limitations imposed by the impairments. The first section of this chapter briefly reviews anatomic and kinesiologic information on the shoulder complex. The following sections then describe common problems and guidelines for conservative and postsurgical management. The last three sections describe exercise techniques commonly used to meet the goals of treatment during the stages of tissue healing and phases of rehabilitation.

▶ Review of the Structure and Function of the Shoulder and Shoulder Girdle

Bony Parts: Proximal Humerus, Scapula, and Clavicle (see Fig. 6–13)

The shoulder girdle has only one bony attachment to the axial skeleton. The clavicle articulates with the sternum via the small sternoclavicular joint. As a result, considerable mobility is allowed in the upper extremity. Stability is provided by an intricate balance between the scapular and glenohumeral muscles and the structures of the joints in the shoulder girdle.

Synovial Joints

Glenohumeral (GH) joint

Characteristics

This joint is an incongruous, ball-and-socket (spheroidal) triaxial joint with a lax joint capsule. It is supported by the tendons of the rotator cuff and the glenohumeral (superior, middle, and inferior) and coracohumeral ligaments. The concave bony partner, the glenoid fossa, is located on the superior-lateral margin of the scapula. It faces anteriorly, laterally, and upward, which provides some stability to the joint. A fibrocartilagenous lip, the glenoid labrum, deepens the fossa for greater congruity and serves as the attachment site for the capsule. The convex bony partner is the head of the humerus. Only a small portion of the head comes in contact with the fossa at any one time, allowing for considerable humeral movement and potential instability.[127]

Arthrokinematics

According to the convex-concave theory of joint motion (see Chapter 6), with motions of the humerus (physiologic motions), the convex head rolls in the same direction and slides in the opposite direction in the glenoid fossa (Box 9–1). Of interest, and apparent contradiction of this theory, one study reported that through the midrange of the arc of passive motion there is minimal displacement of the humeral head. However, beyond midrange the overall displacement of the head is anterior with shoulder flexion and posterior with shoulder extension in normal joints.[66] This cadaveric study demonstrated that the integrity of the capsular ligamentous system influenced the displacement, and that both hyper- and hypomobility of the capsule changed the overall displacement of the humeral head with passive range of motion. In another study, Howel et al,[79] using radiographs, measured humeral head displacement in normal and unstable shoulders. These investigators reported posterior displacement of the humeral head during end-range horizontal abduction with the humerus at 90 degrees and in full external rotation in normal subjects, yet anterior displacement in subjects with anterior instability. These studies support the importance of joint mobility testing to examine restricted accessory motions to determine if interventions with joint mobilization techniques should be used and the direction of the mobilization force rather than just using the convex-concave rule to determine direction of mobilizations.

Stability

Static and dynamic restraints provide joint stability (Table 9–1).[32,44,150,183,187]

The structural relationship of the bony anatomy, ligaments, and glenoid labrum and the adhesive and cohesive forces within the joint provide static stability. The tendons of the rotator cuff blend with the ligaments and glenoid labrum at the sites of attachment so that when the muscles contract, they provide dynamic stability by tightening the static restraints. The coordinated response of the muscles of the cuff and tension in the ligaments provide varying degrees of support depending on the position and motion of the humerus.[143,150,172] In addition, the long head of the biceps and long head of the triceps brachii reinforce the capsule with their attachments and provide superior and inferior shoulder joint support respectively when functioning with elbow motions.[92] The long head of the biceps in particular stabilizes against humeral elevation[92] and contributes to anterior stability of the glenohumeral joint by resisting torsional forces when the shoulder is abducted and externally rotated.[14,143] Neuromuscular control, including movement awareness and motor response, underlies coordination of the dynamic restraints.[183,187]

Acromioclavicular (AC) Joint

Characteristics

This joint is a plane, triaxial joint, which may or may not have a disk. The weak capsule is reinforced by the superior and inferior acromioclavicular ligaments. The convex bony partner is a facet on the lateral end of the clavicle. The concave bony partner is a facet on the acromion of the scapula.

Arthrokinematics

With motions of the scapula, the acromial surface slides in the same direction in which the scapula moves, because the surface is concave. Motions affecting this joint include upward rotation (the

Box 9–1 Summary of Joint Arthrokinematics of the GH Joint

Physiologic Motion of Humerus	Roll	Slide	Translation*
Flexion	Anterior	Posterior	Anterior†
Horizontal adduction	Anterior	Posterior	Anterior†
Internal rotation	Anterior	Posterior	Anterior†
Extension	Posterior	Anterior	Posterior†
Horizontal abduction	Posterior	Anterior	Posterior‡
External rotation	Posterior	Anterior	Posterior†
Abduction	Superior	Inferior	

*Joints with normal capsular integrity

†Cadaveric study with passive humeral motion[66]

‡Radiographic study with arm abducted to 90 degrees and positioned in external rotation[79]

Table 9–1 Static and Dynamic Stabilizers of the Scapula and Glenohumeral Joint

Description	Static Stabilizers	Dynamic Stabilizers
Scapula		
Weight of upper extremity creates downward rotation and forward tipping moment on the scapula	Cohesive forces of subscapular bursa	Upper trapezius and serratus anterior, middle trapezius and rhomboids
Glenohumeral Joint		
In dependent position: if scapula is in normal alignment, weight of arm creates an adduction moment on the humerus	Superior capsule and suprahumeral ligament are taut Adhesive and cohesive forces of synovial fluid and negative joint pressure hold surfaces together Glenoid labrum deepens fossa and improves congruency	Rotator cuff, deltoid, and long head of biceps brachii
When the humerus is elevating and the scapula is rotating upward	Tension placed on static restraints by the rotator cuff Glenohumeral ligaments provide stability against forward, upward, and inferior translation of humeral head	Rotator cuff and deltoid; elbow action brings in two-joint muscle support: • Long head of biceps stabilizes against humeral elevation • Long head of triceps stabilizes against inferior translation

scapula turns so that the glenoid fossa rotates upward), downward rotation, winging of the vertebral border, and tipping of the inferior angle.

Stability
The acromioclavicular ligaments are supported by the strong coracoclavicular ligament. No muscles directly cross this joint for dynamic support.

Sternoclavicular (SC) Joint

Characteristics
This joint is an incongruent, triaxial, saddle-shaped joint with a disk. The joint is supported by the anterior and posterior sternoclavicular ligaments and the interclavicular and costoclavicular ligaments. The medial end of the clavicle is convex superior to inferior and concave anterior to posterior. The joint disk attaches to the upper end. The superior-lateral portion of the manubrium and first costal cartilage is concave superior to inferior and convex anterior to posterior.

Arthrokinematics
The motions of the clavicle occur as a result of the scapular motions of elevation, depression, protraction (abduction), and retraction (adduction) (Box 9–2). Rotation of the clavicle occurs as an accessory motion when the humerus is elevated above the horizontal position and the scapula upwardly rotates; it cannot occur as an isolated voluntary motion.

Stability
The ligaments crossing the joint provide static stability. There are no muscles crossing the joint for dynamic stability.[42]

Functional Articulations

Scapulothoracic Articulation

Motions of the Scapula
Normally there is considerable soft tissue flexibility, allowing the scapula to slide along the thorax and participate in all upper extremity motions. Motions of the scapula are:

- Elevation, depression, protraction (abduction), and retraction (adduction), seen with clavicular motions at the SC joint. They are also component motions when the humerus moves.
- Upward and downward rotation, seen with clavicular motions at the SC joint and rotation at the AC joint, occurs concurrently with motions of the

Box 9–2 Summary of Arthrokinematics of the SC Joint

Physiologic Motion of Clavicle	Roll	Slide
Protraction	Anterior	Anterior
Retraction	Posterior	Posterior
Elevation	Superior	Inferior
Depression	Inferior	Superior

humerus. Upward rotation of the scapula is a necessary component motion for full range of motion (ROM) of flexion and abduction of the humerus.

- Winging of the medial border and tipping of the inferior angle, seen with motion at the AC joint concurrently with motions of the humerus. Tipping of the scapula is necessary to reach the hand behind the back in conjunction with internal rotation and extension of the humerus. Winging is an accessory motion with horizontal adduction of the humerus.

Scapular Stability

In the dependent position, the scapula is stabilized primarily through a balance of forces. The weight of the arm creates a downward rotation, abduction, and forward tipping moment on the scapula. The downward rotation is balanced by the dynamic support of the upper trapezius and serratus anterior. The forward tipping and abduction is balanced by the dynamic support of the rhomboids and middle trapezius.[94,151] (See Table 9–1.)

With active arm motions the muscles of the scapula function in synchrony to stabilize and control the position of the scapula so that the scapulohumeral muscles can maintain a good length-tension relationship as they function to stabilize and move the humerus. Without the positional control of the scapula, the efficiency of the humeral muscles decreases. The upper and lower trapezius with the serratus anterior upwardly rotate the scapula whenever the arm abducts or flexes, and the serratus anterior abducts (protracts) the scapula on the thorax to align the scapula during flexion or pushing activities. During arm extension or during pulling activities, the rhomboids function to downwardly rotate and adduct (retract) the scapula in synchrony with the latissimus dorsi, teres major, and rotator cuff muscles. These stabilizing muscles also eccentrically control acceleration motions of the scapula in the opposite directions.[128]

With a faulty scapular posture from muscle imbalances, muscle length and strength imbalances also occur in the humeral muscles, altering the mechanics of the glenohumeral joint. A forward tilt of the scapula is associated with a tight pectoralis minor muscle and possibly a weak serratus anterior or trapezius. This scapular posture changes the posture of the humerus in the glenoid, assuming a relatively abducted and internally rotated position. This results in shortened glenohumeral internal rotators and stretched or weakened lateral rotators.

Suprahumeral Space

The coracoacromial arch, composed of the acromion and coracoacromial ligament, overlies the subacromial/subdeltoid bursa, the supraspinatus tendon, and a portion of the muscle.[94]

These structures allow for and participate in normal shoulder function. Compromise of this space from faulty muscle function, faulty joint mechanics, injury to the soft tissue in this region, or structural anomalies of the acromion lead to impingement syndromes.[28,31] After a rotator cuff tear, the bursa may communicate with the glenohumeral joint cavity.[44]

Shoulder Girdle Function

Scapulohumeral Rhythm

- Motion of the scapula, synchronous with motions of the humerus, allows for 150 to 180 degrees of shoulder ROM into flexion or abduction with elevation. The ratio has considerable variation among individuals but is commonly accepted to be 2:1 (2 degrees of glenohumeral motion to 1 degree of scapular rotation) overall motion. During the setting phase (0–30 degrees abduction, 0–60 degrees flexion), motion is primarily at the glenohumeral joint, whereas the scapula seeks a stable position. During the midrange, the scapula has greater motion, approaching a 1:1 ratio with the humerus; later in the range, the glenohumeral joint again dominates the motion.[41,94,157]
- The synchronous motion of the scapula allows the muscles moving the humerus to maintain an effective length-tension relationship throughout the activity and helps maintain congruency between the humeral head and fossa while decreasing shear forces.[41,94,157]
- Muscles causing the upward rotation of the scapula are the upper and lower trapezius and serratus anterior. Weakness or complete paralysis of these muscles results in the scapula being rotated downward by the contracting deltoid and supraspinatus as abduction or flexion is attempted. These two muscles then reach active insufficiency, and functional elevation of the arm cannot be reached, even though there may be normal passive ROM and normal strength in the shoulder abductor and flexor muscles.[157]

Clavicular Elevation and Rotation with Humeral Motion

- Initially, with upward rotation of the scapula, 30 degrees of elevation of the clavicle occurs at the

SC joint. Then, as the coracoclavicular ligament becomes taut, the clavicle rotates 38 to 50 degrees about its longitudinal axis, which elevates its acromial end (because it is crank-shaped). This motion allows the scapula to rotate an additional 30 degrees at the AC joint.

- Loss of any of these functional components will decrease the amount of scapular rotation and, thus, the ROM of the upper extremity.

External Rotation of the Humerus with Full Elevation Through Abduction

- During abduction of the arm in the frontal plane, for the greater tubercle of the humerus to clear the coracoacromial arch, the humerus must externally rotate as it is elevated above the horizontal.
- Weak or inadequate external rotation will result in impingement of the soft tissues in the suprahumeral space, causing pain, inflammation, and eventually loss of function.

Internal Rotation of the Humerus with Full Elevation Through Flexion

- Medial rotation begins around 50 degrees of passive shoulder flexion when all structures are intact.[129] With full range of shoulder flexion and elevation, the humerus medially rotates 90 degrees, and the medial epicondyle faces anteriorly.[21,22,129]
- As the arm elevates above the horizontal position in the sagittal plane, the anterior capsule and ligaments become taut, causing the humerus to rotate medially. The bony configuration of the posterior aspect of the glenoid fossa contributes to the inward rotation motion of the humerus as the shoulder flexes.[157] Most of the shoulder flexor muscles are also medial rotators of the humerus.[157]
- The infraspinatus and teres minor stabilize the humeral head against the inward rotating forces, helping to maintain alignment and stability of the head in the fossa. Weakness in these muscles may contribute to excessive anterior translation and instability.[32]

Elevation of the Humerus Through the Plane of the Scapula—Scaption

- The plane of the scapula is described as 30 degrees anterior to the frontal plane. Motion of the humerus in this plane is popularly called **scaption**[171,182] or scapular plane abduction.[41]
- In this range, there is less tension on the capsule and greater elevation is possible than with pure frontal or sagittal plane elevation. Neither internal nor external rotation of the humerus is necessary to prevent greater tubercle impingement in elevation through scaption.[41,171] Many functional activities occur with the shoulder oriented in this plane.

Deltoid-Short Rotator Cuff and Supraspinatus Mechanisms

- The majority of the force of the deltoid muscle causes upward translation of the humerus; if unopposed, it leads to impingement of the soft tissues within the suprahumeral space between the humeral head and the coracoacromial arch.
- The combined effect of the short rotator muscles (infraspinatus, teres minor, and subscapularis) causes a stabilizing compression and a downward translation of the humerus in the glenoid.
- The combined actions of the deltoid and short rotators result in a balance of forces that abduct the humerus and control the humeral head.
- The supraspinatus muscle has a significant stabilizing, compressive, and slight upward translation effect on the humerus; these effects, combined with the effect of gravity, lead to abduction of the arm.
- Interruption of function leading to fatigue or poor coordination of any of these muscles can cause microtrauma and eventual dysfunction in the shoulder region.

Referred Pain: Common Sources of Pain in the Shoulder Region

Cervical Spine

- Vertebral joints between C-3 and C-4 or between C-4 and C-5
- Nerve roots C-4 or C-5

Referred Pain from Related Tissues

- Dermatome C-4 is over the trapezius to the tip of the shoulder.
- Dermatome C-5 is over the deltoid region and lateral arm.
- Diaphragm: pain perceived in the upper trapezius region.
- Heart: pain perceived in the axilla and left pectoral region.
- Gallbladder irritation: pain perceived at the tip of shoulder and posterior scapular region.

Nerve Injury: Common Sites in the Shoulder Girdle

Brachial Plexus in the Thoracic Outlet

Common sites for compression are the scalene triangle, costoclavicular space and under the coracoid process, and pectoralis minor muscle.[96]

Suprascapular Nerve in the Suprascapular Notch

This injury occurs from direct compression or from nerve stretch, such as when carrying a heavy bookbag over the shoulder.

Radial Nerve in the Axilla

Compression occurs from continual pressure, such as when leaning on axillary crutches.

▶ Joint Hypomobility: Nonoperative Management

Glenohumeral (GH) Joint

Related Diagnoses and Etiology of Symptoms

Rheumatoid arthritis and osteoarthritis. These disorders follow the clinical picture described in Chapter 8.

Traumatic arthritis. This disorder occurs in response to a fall or blow to the shoulder or to microtrauma from faulty mechanics or overuse.

Postimmobilization arthritis or stiff shoulder. This disorder occurs as a result of lack of movement or secondary effects from conditions, such as heart disease, stroke, or diabetes mellitus.

Idiopathic frozen shoulder. This disorder, which is also called *adhesive capsulitis* or *periarthritis,* is characterized by the development of dense adhesions and capsular restrictions, especially in the dependent fold of the capsule, rather than arthritic changes in the cartilage and bone, as seen with rheumatoid arthritis or osteoarthritis. The insidious onset usually occurs between the ages of 40 and 60 years, without a known cause (primary frozen shoulder), although problems already mentioned, in which there is a period of pain and/or restricted motion, such as with rheumatoid arthritis, osteoarthritis, trauma, or immobilization, may lead to a frozen shoulder (secondary frozen shoulder). In primary frozen shoulder, the pathogenesis may be from a provoking chronic inflammation in musculotendinous or synovial tissue such as the rotator cuff, biceps tendon, or joint capsule that results in formation of capsular thickening and adhesions, particularly in the folds of the inferior capsule.[42,63,117,120] Consistent with this is a faulty posture and muscle imbalance predisposing the suprahumeral space to impingement and overuse syndromes.[1]

Clinical Signs and Symptoms

Acute joint problems. Pain and muscle guarding limit motion, usually external rotation and abduction. Pain is frequently experienced radiating below the elbow and may disturb sleep.

Subacute joint problems. Capsular tightness begins to develop. Limited motion is detected, consistent with a capsular pattern. Usually external rotation and abduction are most limited, and internal rotation and flexion are least limited. Often, the patient will feel pain as the end of the limited range is reached. Joint-play testing will also reveal limited joint play. If the patient can be treated as the acute condition begins to subside by gradually increasing shoulder motion and activity, the complication of joint and soft tissue contractures can usually be minimized.[117,112]

Chronic joint problems. Progressive restriction of the glenohumeral joint capsule magnifies the signs of limited motion in a capsular pattern and decreased joint play. There is significant loss of function with an inability to reach overhead, outward, or behind the back. Aching is usually localized to the deltoid region.

Idiopathic frozen shoulder. This clinical entity follows a classic pattern.*

- ***"Freezing."*** Characterized by intense pain even at rest and limitation of motion by 2 to 3 weeks after onset. These acute symptoms may last 10 to 36 weeks.
- ***"Frozen."*** Characterized by pain only with movement, significant adhesions, and limited glenohumeral motions with substitute motions in the scapula. Atrophy of the deltoid, rotator cuff, biceps, and triceps brachii muscles occurs. This stage lasts 4 to 12 months.
- ***"Thawing."*** Characterized by no pain and no synovitis but significant capsular restrictions from

*See references 42, 60, 63, 117, 120, 145, 175.

adhesions. This stage lasts 2 to 24 months or longer. Some patients never regain normal ROM. Spontaneous recovery occurs on the average of 2 years from onset.[60,63] Inappropriately aggressive therapy at the wrong time may prolong the symptoms.[18] Treatment guidelines are the same as acute for the freezing stage, and subacute and chronic for the frozen and thawing stages, respectively.

Common Impairments

- Night pain and disturbed sleep during acute flares
- Pain on motion and often at rest during acute flares
- Decreased joint play and ROM, usually limiting external rotation and abduction with some limitation of internal rotation and elevation in flexion
- Possible faulty postural compensations with protracted and anteriorly tipped scapula, rounded shoulders, and elevated and protected shoulder
- Decreased arm swing during gait
- General muscle weakness and poor endurance in the glenohumeral muscles with overuse of the scapular muscles leading to pain in the trapezius and posterior cervical muscles
- Guarded shoulder motions with substitute scapular motions

Common Functional Limitations/Disabilities

- Inability to reach overhead, behind head, out to the side and behind back; thus, having difficulty with dressing (such as putting on a jacket or coat or women fastening undergarments behind their back), with reaching hand into back pocket of pants (to retrieve wallet), with reaching out a car window (to use an ATM machine) with self-grooming (such as combing hair, brushing teeth, washing face), and with bringing eating utensils to the mouth
- Difficulty lifting weighted objects, such as dishes into a cupboard
- Limited ability to sustain repetitive activities

GH Joint Management: Protection Phase

See guidelines for management in Chapter 8 and Box 8–1.

Control Pain, Edema, and Muscle Guarding

- The joint may be immobilized in a sling to provide rest and minimize pain.
- Initiate intermittent periods of controlled motion and gentle joint oscillation techniques as soon as the patient tolerates movement to minimize adhesion formation.

Maintain Soft Tissue and Joint Integrity and Mobility

- ***Passive range of motion (PROM)*** in all ranges of pain-free motion (see Chapter 2). As pain decreases, progress to active ROM with or without assistance using activities such as rolling a small ball or sliding a rag on a smooth table top in flexion, abduction, and circular motions. Initiate use of an overhead pulley. Be sure the patient is taught proper mechanics and avoids faulty patterns such as scapular elevation or a slumped posture.
- ***Passive joint traction and glides,*** with the joint placed in a pain-free position (see Chapter 6). Begin with grade I; progress to grade II as symptoms subside.
- ***Pendulum (Codman's) exercises*** are techniques that use the effects of gravity to distract the humerus from the glenoid fossa.[31,36] They help relieve pain through gentle traction and oscillating movements (grade II) and provide early motion of joint structures and synovial fluid. No weight is used during this phase of treatment (see Figure 9–10).

Precaution: If there is increased pain or irritability in the joint after use of these techniques, either the dosage was too strong or the techniques should not be used at this time.

Contraindication: Stretching (grade III) techniques. If there are mechanical restrictions causing limited motion, appropriate stretching can be initiated only *after* the inflammation subsides.

- ***Gentle muscle setting*** to all muscle groups of the shoulder. Also include scapular and elbow muscles because of their close association with the shoulder. Instruct the patient to gently contract a group of muscles while you apply slight resistance—just enough to stimulate a muscle contraction. It should not provoke pain. The emphasis is on rhythmic contracting and relaxing of the muscles to help stimulate blood flow and prevent circulatory stasis.

Maintain Integrity and Function of Associated Areas

- Educate the patient in the importance of keeping the joints distal to the injured site as active and mobile as possible. Teach the patient or family member to perform ROM exercises of the elbow, forearm, wrist, and fingers several times each day while the shoulder is immobilized. If tolerated, active or gentle resistive ROM is preferred to passive for a greater effect on circulation and muscle integrity.

- Reflex sympathetic dystrophy (sympathetically maintained pain) is a potential complication after shoulder injury or immobility; give special attention to the hand with additional exercises, such as having the patient repetitively squeeze a ball or other soft object.
- If edema is noted in the hand, instruct the patient to elevate the hand, whenever possible, above the level of the heart.

Note: Conditions in which there is potentially a prolonged acute/inflammatory stage such as with rheumatoid arthritis and during the freezing stage of idiopathic frozen shoulder, it is critical to teach the patient active-assistive exercises to maintain muscle integrity and as much mobility as possible without exacerbating the symptoms.

GH Joint Management: Controlled Motion Phase

Follow the guidelines as described in Chapter 8, Box 8–2 emphasizing joint mobility, neuromuscular control, and instructions to the patient for self-care.

Note: For normal shoulder joint mechanics, there must be good scapular posture and control, and the humerus must be able to externally rotate. To avoid suprahumeral impingement, do not stretch above 90 degrees until there is adequate glenohumeral external rotation. With a traumatic injury that involves the AC or SC joints, these joints tend to become hypermobile with improper stretching. Care should be taken to provide stabilization to the scapula and clavicle so as not to stretch these joints when mobilizing the glenohumeral joint.

Control Pain, Edema, and Joint Effusion

- Carefully monitor increasing activities. If the joint was splinted, progressively increase the amount of time that the shoulder is free to move each day.
- ***Range of motion.*** Begin with active ROM up to the point of pain, including all shoulder and scapular motions. Use self-assistive ROM techniques, such as the overhead pulleys, wand exercises, or hand slides on a table.

Precaution: With increased pain or decreased motion, the activity may be too intense or the patient may be using faulty mechanics. Reassess the technique and modify it if faulty joint mechanics exist.

Progressively Increase Soft Tissue and/or Joint Mobility

- ***Passive joint mobilization techniques.*** Progress to stretch grades (grade III sustained or grade III and IV oscillation) using techniques that focus on the restricting capsular tissue at the end of the available ROM[86,122] (see Table 9–1 and Figs. 6–15 through 6–20 in Chapter 6).
  - Use a grade I distraction with all gliding techniques.
  - If the joint is highly irritable and gliding in the direction of restriction is not tolerated, glide in the opposite direction. As pain and irritability decrease, begin to glide in the direction of restriction.[86]
  - Advanced progressions in the shoulder include prepositioning the humerus at the end of the ROM, rotating the humerus then either applying a grade III distraction or a grade III glide to stretch the restrictive capsular tissue or adhesions (see Figs. 6–17, 6–20, and 9–8).
  - Pendulum exercises can also be used for joint stretching by adding a cuff weight to the wrist or a weight to the hand to cause a grade III joint distraction force (see Fig. 9–10). To direct the stretch force to the glenohumeral joint, stabilize the scapula against the thorax manually or with a belt.

Precaution: Vigorous stretching should not be undertaken until the chronic stage of healing.

- ***Self-mobilization techniques.*** Teach the patient the following techniques for a home program:
  - ***Caudal glide.*** Patient position and procedure: Sitting on a firm surface and grasping the fingers under the edge. He or she then leans the trunk away from the stabilized arm (Fig. 9–1).
  - ***Anterior glide.*** Patient position and procedure: Sitting with both arms behind or lying supine supported on a solid surface. He or she then leans the body weight between the arms (Fig. 9–2).
  - ***Posterior glide.*** Patient position and procedure: Prone, propped up on both elbows. The body weight shifts downward between the arms (Fig. 9–3).

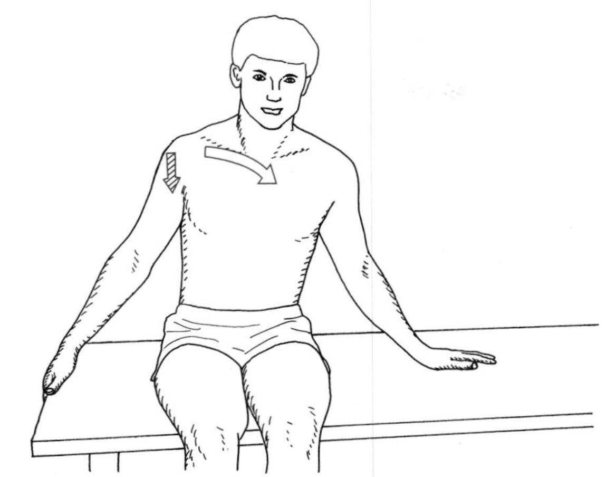

Figure 9–1 Self-mobilization; caudal glide of the humerus occurs as the person leans away from the fixed arm.

- ***Manual stretching.*** Cautiously initiate manual stretching techniques to restricting tissue.
- ***Self-stretching exercises.*** As the joint reaction becomes predictable and the patient begins to tolerate stretching, teach self-stretching using techniques in which the body is moved in relation to the stabilized arm (see Figs. 9–13 through 9–17).[46]

Inhibit Muscle Spasm and Correct Faulty Mechanics

Muscle spasm may lead to a faulty deltoid-rotator cuff mechanism and scapulohumeral rhythm when the patient attempts abduction (Fig. 9–4). The head of the humerus may be held in a cranial position within the joint, making it difficult and/or painful to abduct the shoulder because the greater tuberosity impinges on the coracoacromial arch. In this case, repositioning the head of the humerus with a caudal

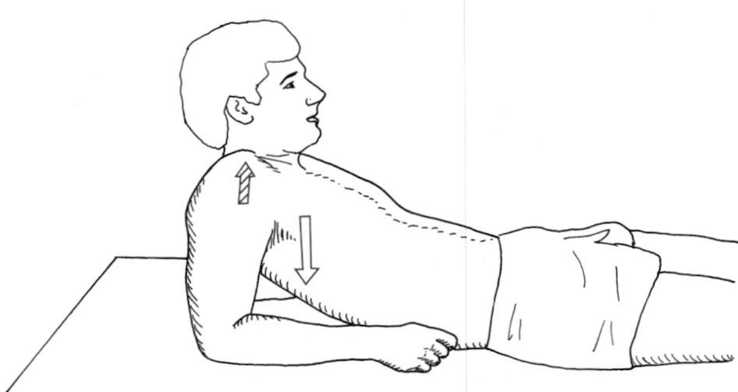

Figure 9–2 Self-mobilization; anterior glide of the humerus occurs as the person leans between the fixed arms.

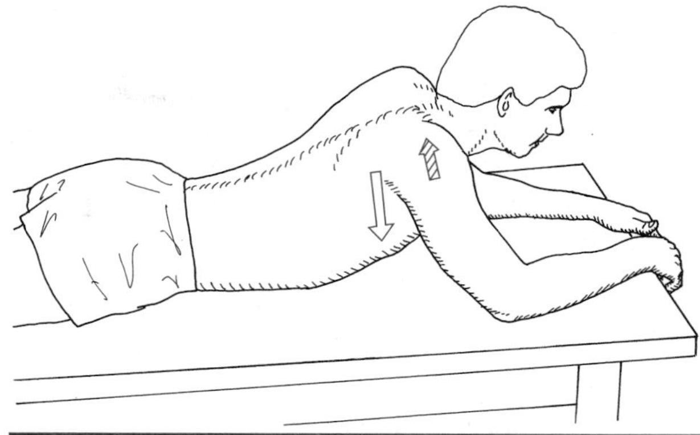

Figure 9–3 Self-mobilization; posterior glide of the humerus occurs as the person shifts his weight downward between the fixed arms.

glide is necessary before proceeding with any other form of shoulder exercise. The patient also needs to learn to avoid “hiking the shoulder” when abducting or flexing the arm. The following techniques may address these problems and faulty mechanics. See also mobilization with movement techniques in the next section.

- Gentle joint oscillation techniques will help decrease the muscle spasm (grade I or II).
- Sustained caudal glide joint techniques will help reposition the humeral head in the glenoid fossa.
- Protected weight bearing, such as leaning hands against a wall or on a table, stimulates co-contraction of the rotator cuff and scapular stabilizing muscles. If tolerated, gentle rocking

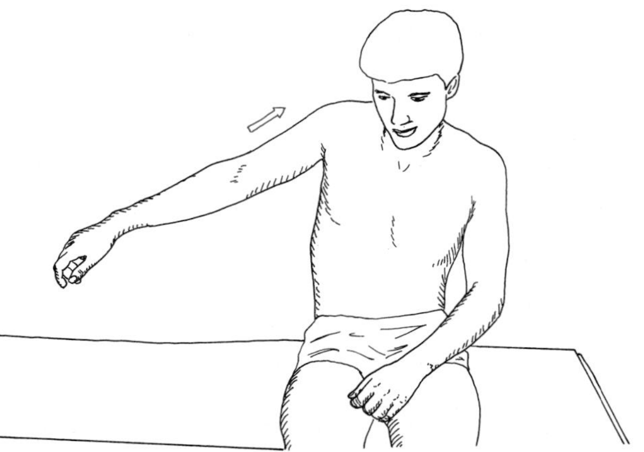

Figure 9–4 Poor mechanics with patient hiking the shoulder while trying to abduct the shoulder, thus elevating rather than depressing the humeral head.

forward/backward and side to side requires the muscles to begin controlling motion. Because weight bearing causes joint compression, the benefits of intermittent compression stimulates synovial fluid motion; progress within the tolerance of the joint.

- Training the external rotators of the shoulder will help to depress the humeral head as the arm abducts. Teach the patient active and progress to resistive external rotation exercises (see Fig. 9–36).

Improve Joint Tracking

Mobilization with movement (MWM) techniques may assist with retraining muscle function for proper tracking of the humeral head.[110]

- ***Shoulder MWM for painful restriction of shoulder external rotation*** (Fig. 9–5). Patient position and procedure: Supine lying with folded towel under scapula; the elbow is near the side and flexed to 90 degrees. A cane is held in both hands.
  - Stand on the opposite side of the bed facing the patient, and reach across the patient's torso to cup the anteromedial aspect of the head of the humerus with reinforced hands. Apply a pain-free graded posterolateral glide of the humeral head on the glenoid. Instruct the patient to use the cane to push the affected arm into the previously restricted range of external rotation.
  - Sustain the movement for 10 seconds and repeat in sets of 5 to 10. It is important to maintain the elbow near the side of the trunk and ensure no pain is experienced during the procedure. Adjust the grade and direction of the glide as needed to achieve pain-free function.
- ***Shoulder MWM for painful restriction of internal rotation*** and inability to reach hand behind back (Fig. 9–6). Patient position and procedure: Standing with a towel draped over the unaffected upper trapezius and affected hand at current range of maximum pain-free position behind back. The hand on the affected side grasps the towel behind the back.
  - Stand facing the patient's affected side. Place the hand closest to patient's back high up in the axilla with the palm facing outward to stabilize the scapula with an upward and inward pressure. With the hand closest to the patient's abdomen hook the thumb in the cubital fossa and grasp the lower humerus to provide an inferior glide. Your abdomen is in contact with the patient's elbow to provide an adduction force to the arm.
  - Have the patient pull on the towel with the unaffected hand to draw the affected hand up the back while the mobilization force is being applied in an inferior direction.
  - Ensure no pain is experienced during the procedure. Adjust grade and direction of glide as

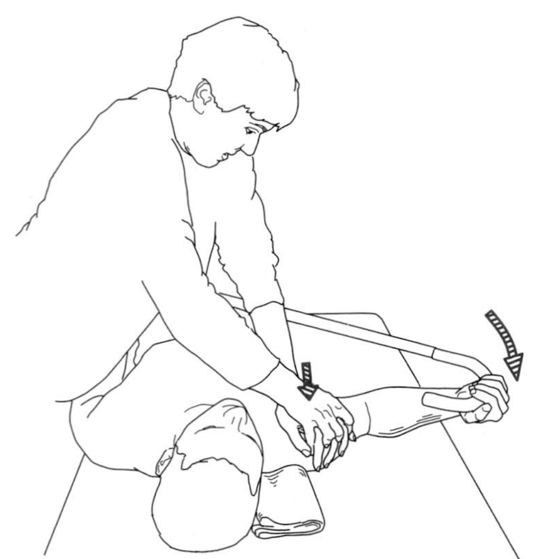

Figure 9–5 MWM to improve external rotation. A posterolateral glide is applied to the humeral head while the patient pushes the arm into the end-range of external rotation with a cane.

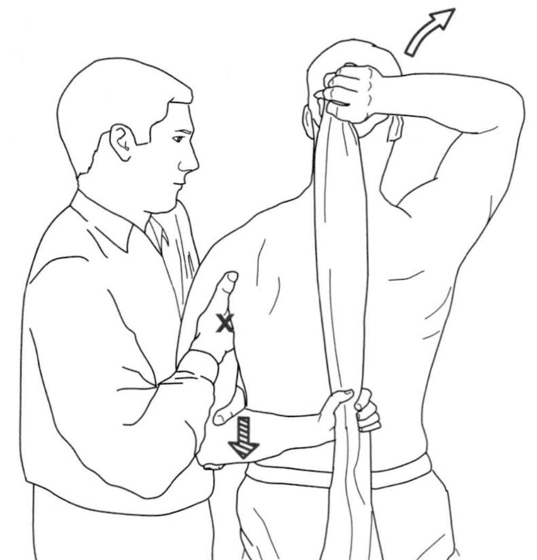

Figure 9–6 MWM to improve internal rotation. An inferior glide is applied to the humerus while the patient pulls the hand up the back with a towel.

needed to achieve pain-free function. Maximal glide should be applied to achieve end-range loading.

- ***Shoulder MWM for painful arc or impingement signs.*** MWM active elevation technique may be appropriate; see description with Figure 9–7*A* and *B*.

Progressively Increase Strength

- Determine any faulty postures or shoulder girdle mechanics that the patient displays when moving the upper extremity in various functional patterns.
- Initiate stabilization exercises to the scapular and glenohumeral musculature in open- and closed-chain as described later in this chapter.
- Exercises to manage faulty spinal posture are described in Chapter 16. Initiate dynamic strengthening, utilizing light resistance, with emphasis on developing control in weak musculature. As the patient develops control, progress the resistance. Strengthening exercises and progressions are described in the final section of this chapter.
- Once proper mechanics are restored, the patient should perform active ROM of all shoulder motions daily and return to functional activities to the extent tolerated.

GH Joint Management—Return to Function Phase

Progressively Increase Flexibility and Strength

- Progress stretching and strengthening exercises as the joint tissue tolerates. The patient should be actively involved in self-stretching and strengthening by this time so that emphasis during treatment is on correct mechanics, safe progressions, and exercise strategies for return to function.
- If capsular tissue is still restricting ROM apply vigorous manual stretching and joint mobilization techniques. Vermeulen et al.[174] reported good outcomes for increased ROM, decreased pain, and improved function in seven subjects with adhesive capsulitis utilizing intensive end-range mobilization and muscle relaxation techniques twice a week for 3 months. The improved function continued in six of the seven subjects 9 months after cessation of treatment.

Prepare for Functional Demands

If the patient is involved in repetitive heavy lifting, pushing, pulling, carrying or reaching, when joint range and strength allow, exercises are progressed to replicate these demands. See the last section of this chapter for suggestions.

Management Postmanipulation Under Anesthesia

Occasionally, no progress is made, and the physician chooses to perform manipulation under anesthesia. Following this procedure, there is an inflammatory reaction and the joint is treated as an acute lesion. Begin joint-play and passive ROM techniques while the patient is still in the recovery room. Surgical intervention with incision of the dependent capsular fold may be used if the adhesions are not broken with the manipulation. Postoperative treatment is the same with the following considerations.[120]

- Keep the arm elevated overhead in abduction and external rotation during the inflammatory reaction stage; treatment principles progress as with any joint lesion.
- Begin therapeutic exercise the same day while the patient is still in the recovery room, with emphasis on internal and external rotation in the 90-degree (or higher) abducted position.
- Use joint mobilization procedures, particularly a caudal glide, to prevent re-adherence of the inferior capsular fold.
- When sleeping, the patient may be required to position the arm abducted for up to 3 weeks post-manipulation.[120]

Joint Lesions: Acromioclavicular (AC) and Sternoclavicular (SC) Joints

Related Diagnoses and Etiology of Symptoms

Overuse syndromes. Overuse syndromes of the AC joint are frequently arthritic or post-traumatic conditions. The causes may be from repeated stressful movement of the joint with the arm at waist level, such as with grinding, packing assembly, and construction work,[64] or repeated diagonal extension, adduction, and internal rotation motions, as with spiking a volleyball or serving in tennis.

Subluxations or dislocations. Subluxations or dislocations of either joint are usually caused by falling against the shoulder or against an outstretched arm. In the AC joint, the distal end of the clavicle displaces posteriorly and superiorly on the acromion; the ligaments supporting the AC joint may rupture.[119] Clavicular fractures may result from the fall.[119] After trauma and associated overstretching of the capsules and ligaments of either joint, hypermobility is usually permanent because there is no muscle support to restrict movement.

Hypomobility. Decreased clavicular mobility may occur with sustained faulty postures involving clavicular and scapular depression or retraction. Complications from this may contribute to a thoracic outlet syndrome (TOS) with a compromise of space for the neuromuscular bundle as it courses between the clavicle and first rib (described later in this chapter).

Common Impairments

- Pain localized to the involved joint or ligament
- Painful arc with shoulder elevation
- Pain with shoulder horizontal adduction or abduction
- Hypermobility in the joints if trauma or overuse is involved
- Hypomobility in the joints if sustained posture or immobility is involved
- Neurological or vascular symptoms if TOS is present

Common Functional Limitations/Disabilities

- Limited ability to sustain repeated loaded movements related to forward/backward motions of the arm, such as with grinding, packing, assembly, and construction work.[64]
- Inability to reach overhead without pain.
- Inability to effectively serve at tennis or spike a volley ball.
- See also limitations/disabilities from TOS if present.

Nonoperative Management of AC or SC Joint Strain or Hypermobility

- Rest the joint by putting the arm in a sling to support the weight of the arm.
- Cross-fiber massage to the capsule or ligaments.
- ROM to the shoulder and grade II traction and glides to the glenohumeral joint to prevent glenohumeral restriction.
- Teach the patient how to apply cross-fiber massage if joint symptoms occur after excessive activity.

Nonoperative Management of AC or SC Joint Hypomobility

Joint mobilization techniques are used to increase joint mobility (see Figs. 6–21 through 6–23).

Surgery for Clavicular Problems and Postoperative Management

Surgical resection of the distal clavicle is sometimes used when AC joint pain is unrelenting and causes disability.[64] For example, an arthroscopic or open resection of the distal clavicle, as a component of a subacromial decompression procedure, is sometimes indicated for patients with primary shoulder impingement syndrome.[125,133] Grade III instabilities, in which the clavicle has been acutely or chronically dislocated on the acromion, may be surgically reduced and stabilized with a variety of techniques.[119] Techniques for management of acute dislocations include primary stabilization of the AC joint with Kirschner wires, Steinman pins, screws, or most recently bioabsorbable tacks. A muscle-tendon transfer, that includes the tip of the coracoid process and the attached tendons of the coracobrachialis and short head of the biceps to the undersurface of the clavicle[125] or resection of the distal clavicle with coracoacromial ligament reconstruction also can be performed.[119] Based on a small body of evidence in the literature, it appears the best results are achieved with primary AC and coracoclavicular stabilization procedures. Chronic AC dislocations, which are usually associated with degenerative changes of the AC joint, are most often managed with distal clavicle resection coupled with coracoclavicular stabilization.[125,141]

Although most SC dislocations are managed nonoperatively, an acute posterior dislocation of the SC joint that cannot be successfully reduced with a closed maneuver or an SC joint that dislocates recurrently are managed surgically. Surgical reduction of a traumatic anterior dislocation is not recommended.[140] Surgical options for posterior SC dislocations include open reduction with repair of the stabilizing ligaments or resection of a portion of the medial clavicle and fixation of the remaining clavicle to the first rib or sternum with a soft tissue graft.[140,190]

Postoperative management usually involves immobilization in a sling or strapping. Exercise intervention should be directed at functional recovery as the signs of healing allow. No specific muscles cross the AC and SC joints, so scapular and glenohumeral strength is developed to provide indirect control.

▶ Glenohumeral Joint Surgery and Postoperative Management

Surgical intervention and postoperative rehabilitation for severe glenohumeral joint arthritis are often indicated to achieve the following goals: (1) relieve pain, (2) correct deformity, (3) improve mobility or stability, and (4) restore or improve functional use of the upper extremity. The most common forms of surgical intervention used to treat severe arthritis of the shoulder and restore upper extremity function are either *glenohumeral joint arthroplasty* (total shoulder replacement), or hemiarthroplasty of the shoulder. In rare situations, arthrodesis (surgical ankylosis) of the glenohumeral joint is used as an alternative or salvage procedure.

Glenohumeral Arthroplasty

Indications for Surgery

The following impairments are widely accepted indications for glenohumeral arthroplasty.*

- Incapacitating pain (at rest or with motion) and severe glenohumeral joint destruction associated with advanced arthritis (OA, RA, or traumatic arthritis) or osteonecrosis of the head of the humerus as the result of a fracture of the anatomic neck of the humerus or long-term use of steroids for systemic disease
- Severe loss of upper extremity strength and control secondary to pain
- Inability to perform functional tasks with the involved upper extremity
- Decreased ROM

Procedures

Background: Selection of Procedure and Implant Design

Since the pioneering work of Neer in the 1960s[116] several procedures and many types of prosthetic implants for the shoulder joint have been developed. A *total shoulder replacement* (TSR) *arthroplasty* is composed of a high-density polyethylene (plastic) glenoid component (some with metal backing) and a modular humeral component made of an inert metal. The glenoid component is usually cemented in place although biological or screw fixation has also been used. The humeral stem component is fit tightly (a press fit) into the intramedullary canal of the humerus for fixation but may need to be cemented in place in patients with severe osteoporosis.† A *hemiarthroplasty* involves only the replacement of the head and neck of the humerus with a metal stemmed prosthesis.[39,54,103,149]

*See references 6, 12, 13, 39, 103, 114, 116, 149, 163, 164.

†See references 13, 102, 103, 112, 114, 163, 188.

The designs of total shoulder replacements, ranging from *unconstrained* to *constrained,* provide varying amounts of mobility and stability of the GH joint. The unconstrained design, also referred to as a *resurfacing* replacement, provides the greatest freedom of movement but is indicated only when the rotator cuff and deltoid mechanisms are intact or can be adequately repaired to provide dynamic stability to the glenohumeral joint.[47,55,103,114,116,149] *Semiconstrained* and *constrained* replacements have more stability built into their designs but are indicated only when the rotator cuff functions insufficiently.[47,55,103,112,114] Loosening or excessive wear of the polyethylene glenoid component are the most common long-term complications after TSR.[37,38,103] Although loosening of the humeral component can occur, the major concern after hemiarthroplasty is premature wear of the articular cartilage of the glenoid fossa.[37,38,103]

Controversy exists over the specific criteria for selection of TSR versus hemiarthroplasty, but in general, it depends on the etiology and severity of the joint deterioration and soft tissue dysfunction.[6,103,112] Patients with primary OA usually have loss or thinning or the articular cartilage of the head of the humerus and the posterior portion of the glenoid fossa,[54,103,149] but the rotator cuff is intact in approximately 90% of these patients.[135] Selection of a resurfacing TSR usually yields the best results for shoulders with these characteristics. As many as 30 to 40% of patients with advanced RA of the glenohumeral joint have rotator cuff insufficiency, and many have bony erosion of the glenoid.[164] These characteristics lend themselves well to a TSR with bone grafting at the glenoid to improve prosthetic fixation and a repair of the rotator cuff. If an effective cuff repair cannot be achieved, then a more constrained design of TSR is selected by some surgeons.[103,149,164]

A hemiarthroplasty is often used when the articular surface and underlying bone of the head of the humerus have deteriorated but the glenoid fossa is reasonably intact.[103] (This is referred to as osteonecrosis of the head of the humerus.) Patients with severe pain and loss of function as the result of massive, irreparable cuff tears may also be candidates for hemiarthroplasty.[54] Some surgeons prefer a hemiarthroplasty to a TSR for patients with RA in whom joint destruction is coupled with longstanding cuff insufficiency or contractures that cannot be resolved effectively. (This is often referred to as *cuff tear arthropathy.*)[103] These problems may lead to superior migration of the head of the humerus within the glenoid fossa. If the glenoid is resurfaced under these conditions, the superior migration creates an incongruous articulation that accentuates the risk of loosening and premature wear of the glenoid implant.[164] These examples underscore the complexity of the clinical decision-making process involved in choice of operative procedure and prosthetic design.

Operative Procedures

The patient is placed in a semireclining position. The procedure involves an anterior approach with a deltopectoral incision that extends from the AC joint to the deltoid insertion. The pectoralis major is released, an anterior capsulotomy is performed, the GH joint is dislocated, a humeral osteotomy is performed, and the head of the humerus is removed. Deltoid reflection usually is not required. The glenoid fossa is also débrided.*

Concomitant procedures that may be performed include:

- Repair of a deficient rotator cuff
- Anterior acromioplasty for a history of impingement syndrome
- Subscapularis lengthening for a significant internal rotation contracture
- Bone graft of the glenoid if bone stock is insufficient for fixation of the glenoid implant

After implantation of the prosthetic components and repair of soft tissues, the shoulder is passively moved through all planes of motion to visually evaluate the stability of the prosthetic joint and the integrity of the repaired soft tissues. This determines the anatomic ROM possible and how aggressive the postoperative program can be.[103,112]

Postoperative Management

Note: The guidelines for TSR and hemiarthroplasty are similar. Effective patient education and close communication among the surgeon, therapist, and patient are the basis of successful outcomes.

Special Considerations

Integrity of the rotator cuff. Patients with an intact rotator cuff mechanism prior to shoulder arthroplasty are most likely to achieve significant functional improvements postoperatively.[103,112,149] Coexisting rotator cuff deficiency that cannot be adequately repaired by a concomitant procedure necessitates a more cautious postoperative treatment plan that emphasizes joint stability over functional mobility.[54,103]

Posture concerns. Since many patients undergoing shoulder arthroplasty are elderly, the postural changes associated with aging (increased thoracic kyphosis and scapular protraction) cause malalignment (excessive downward rotation) of the glenoid fossa, which predisposes the patient to shoulder impingement and pain during shoulder motions. For these patients, it is particularly important to emphasize an erect sitting or standing posture for joint stability during elevation of the arm and to incorporate spinal extension and scapular retraction exercises into the postoperative program.

Immobilization and Postoperative Positioning

At the close of the surgical procedure the operated arm is placed in some type of shoulder immobilizer, usually a sling and swathe or Velpeau dressing, to protect reattached and repaired soft tissues.[6,103,164] Positioning is detailed in Box 9–3.

Initially the immobilizer is removed only for exercise and bathing. The patient is weaned from the immobilizer during the day as quickly as possible to prevent postoperative stiffness. The immobilizer is worn during sleep for approximately 6 weeks to pro-

Box 9–3 Positioning After Shoulder Arthroplasty: Maximum Protection Phase

Supine

- Arm immobilized in sling-swathe dressing
  - Elbow flexed to 90 degrees
  - Forearm and hand resting on abdomen
- Arm at patient's side in slight abduction and supported on a folded blanket or pillow
  - Forward flexion (10–20 degrees) and internal rotation of the shoulder
- Head of bed elevated about 30 degrees

Sitting

- Arm supported in sling or resting in the above position on a pillow in the patient's lap

With Tenuous Rotator Cuff Repair

- Shoulder positioned in abduction splint or airplane splint for an extended period of time

*See references 6, 13, 54, 103, 112, 114, 149, 163.

tect incised and reattached tissues until they are reasonably well healed.[24,27,47,83,102,108,164]

Exercise

The guidelines for progression of exercises during each phase of rehabilitation set forth in this section are drawn from several published protocols, none of which has been shown to be more effective than another.*

Note: The guidelines in this section are for patients *without* rotator cuff deficiency. Modifications in guidelines are noted throughout this section for patients with a tenuous rotator cuff mechanism.

Precaution: Remember, pain relief is the primary goal of shoulder arthroplasty, with improvement in functional mobility a secondary goal. Although improvements in surgical techniques and implant technology now allow an accelerated progression of postoperative rehabilitation, it is still important to proceed judiciously during each phase of rehabilitation to avoid excessive muscle fatigue or irritation of healing soft tissues.

Since almost all published protocols for shoulder arthroplasty are time-based, few criteria for advancing a patient from one phase of rehabilitation to the next are reported in the literature. Specific criteria for progression should be established by close communication between the therapist and the surgeon and individualized for each patient.

Exercise: Maximum Protection Phase

This phase of rehabilitation, which emphasizes pain control protected motion and prevention of atrophy, may extend from 2 to 3 weeks or, if the patient has a tenuous rotator cuff, as long as 6 weeks.

■ ***Maintain mobility of adjacent joints.***

- While the shoulder is immobilized, encourage the patient to keep the shoulder, neck, and upper trunk musculature as relaxed as possible. Use gentle massage to these areas, and have the patient perform active movements of the neck and scapula to maintain normal motion and minimize muscle guarding and spasm.
- Active ROM of the hand, wrist, and elbow when the arm can be removed from the sling.

■ ***Regain shoulder mobility.***

- Initiate passive or therapist-assisted shoulder motions within a protected range and with the patient lying supine begun the day after surgery or no later than 48 hours postoperatively. Emphasize forward elevation of the arm in the plane of the scapula for patient comfort. Perform abduction and limited internal and external rotation within a protected range with the elbow flexed and the arm on a folded towel slightly away from the side of the trunk. In addition, some surgeons prescribe the immediate use of a CPM unit for passive elevation of the arm.
- Self-assisted shoulder ROM performed in supine. Incorporate reaching movements (to the nose, forehead, or over the head as comfort allows) to simulate functional movements. Initially, teach the patient to assist with the sound hand and later with a wand or dowel rod.
- Pendulum exercises without a hand-held weight and with the elbow flexed (for a shorter moment arm). Encourage the patient to periodically remove the sling and gently swing the arm during ambulation.
- Active-assistive shoulder ROM in sitting or standing with a wand, by performing "gear shift" exercises (see Fig. 9–11) or use of an overhead rope-pulley system to lessen the weight of the arm. Add horizontal abduction and adduction to ROM exercises. Remind the patient to maintain an erect trunk when performing assisted shoulder motions while seated or standing. Incorporate "shoulder rolls" by elevating, adducting, and then relaxing the scapulae to reinforce an erect posture of the trunk.

■ ***Minimize muscle atrophy.***

- Gentle muscle-setting of shoulder musculature with the elbow flexed. Teach these exercises in preparation for discharge (usually 3–4 days postoperatively) by having the patient practice isometrically contracting the muscles of the sound shoulder. Postpone setting exercises of the operated shoulder until about 7 days postoperatively in the home exercise program.
- Scapular stabilization exercises in nonweight-bearing positions. Target the serratus anterior and trapezius muscles.

Precautions: Precautions for the maximum protection phase are noted in Box 9–4. A patient's understanding of these precautions is of the utmost importance during this phase of rehabilitation.

*See references 24, 27, 47, 83, 91, 102, 108, 164.

Box 9–4 Precautions for Maximum Protection Phase of Rehabilitation After Shoulder Arthroplasty

Exercise

- Begin exercises gradually and within a protected ROM.
  - Implement short but frequent exercise sessions (four to five per day).
  - Keep repetitions low and intensity gentle.
- Progress exercises more slowly in patients with a severely damaged and repaired rotator cuff mechanism.
  - After a repair of the supraspinatus or deltoid mechanism, avoid active antigravity abduction until the patient can initiate the movement without first shrugging the shoulder.
  - If the subscapularis has been repaired or divided for lengthening, perform external rotation with the arm at the side and *only to neutral.*
- During passive or assisted shoulder rotation with the patient lying supine, position the humerus slightly anterior to the midline of the body (by placing the arm on a folded towel) to avoid excessive stress to the anterior capsule and suture line.
- In sitting or standing, avoid excessive thoracic kyphosis during overhead reaching exercises. Emphasize spinal extension and scapular retraction.
- If an overhead rope-pulley system is used for assisted elevation of the arm, initially *have the patient face the doorway and pulley apparatus* so that shoulder elevation only occurs within a protected range.

ADL

- Avoid weight bearing on the operated extremity, such as pushing with the arm during transfers or when moving in bed, especially the first week after surgery.
- Avoid lifting heavy objects.
- Support the arm in a sling during extended periods of standing or walking.
- Wear the sling while sleeping.

Exercise: Moderate Protection/Controlled Motion Phase

This phase of rehabilitation places an emphasis on moving toward active (unassisted) control of the shoulder while continuing to increase shoulder mobility.[24,27,83,91,108,164] If the rotator cuff is intact, these exercises in this phase may begin as easily as 2 to 3 weeks postoperatively; if the cuff repair is tenuous, these exercises sometimes are not initiated for at least 6 weeks after surgery.

- ***Re-establish mobility and control of shoulder motions.***
  - Transition from assisted to active ROM in all anatomic and diagonal planes of motion.
  - Wall-climbing exercises, emphasizing overhead reaching.
  - Addition of wand exercises behind the back to emphasize shoulder extension and internal rotation as well as scapular winging and tipping (necessary for reaching behind the back).
  - Use of active ROM in dressing and grooming.
- ***Improve strength, endurance and stability of the shoulder girdle.***
  - Scapular stabilization (alternating isometrics and rhythmic stabilization) exercises in a variety of positions combined with minimal to moderate weight bearing; light weight bearing during functional activities.
  - Continuation of isometric exercise of shoulder musculature against gradually increasing resistance at multiple points in the ROM.
  - Dynamic strengthening of the scapula and shoulder musculature (from 0–90 degrees) using light weights or elastic resistance. Begin in the supine position to support and stabilize the scapula. Progress to the sitting position.
  - Upper extremity ergometry with the UBE or a portable reciprocal exerciser on a table. Emphasize progressive repetitions to increase muscular endurance.

Exercise: Minimum Protection/Return to Functional Activity Phase

The final phase of rehabilitation after shoulder arthroplasty usually begins no earlier than 6 weeks postoperatively (with an intact rotator cuff) or considerably later if the rotator cuff mechanism is deficient.[91,103,112]

To advance to this phase of rehabilitation the following criteria should be met: (1) pain-free, active shoulder ROM through functional ranges and (2) greater than a Fair (3/5) grade of strength of shoulder musculature. To return to use of the involved arm for light ADL and modified recreational activities, 85% active ROM and a muscle strength grade of at least Good (4/5) should be achieved.[108] There is a continued effort to restore functional ROM during this final phase of rehabilitation. It is useful for the therapist to recheck the patient and possibly modify the exercise program during this phase. For optimal results, the home exercise program may need to be continued for at least 6 months to a year.

- ***Continue to improve mobility.***
  - End-range, therapist-assisted, or self-stretching
  - Grade III joint mobilization and self-mobilization, if appropriate[24,27,108]

- ***Continue to improve strength, stability, and endurance of the shoulder.***
  - Low-load, high-repetition PRE of shoulder musculature in anatomic and diagonal planes and in patterns of movement that replicate functional tasks throughout the available ROM. Position the patient in gravity-resisted positions.
  - Increased weight bearing through the upper extremity during functional activities.
  - Use of the involved upper extremity for light lifting, carrying, pushing, or pulling activities against increasing loads.
  - Use of the involved upper extremity for modified recreational or sport-related activities.

Outcomes

Almost all patients report a total relief of a substantial decrease in shoulder pain, as well as an improvement in functional use of the arm.[6,13,91,102,112,114] If the rotator cuff and deltoid muscles are functioning well, a patient can expect to regain active ROM necessary for most functional activities within a year after surgery. Overall, patients with OA show greater improvement in ROM (forward flexion) than patients with RA. Both groups report similar improvement in pain relief and functional status.* It is usually necessary to modify activities of daily living as well as work-related and recreational activities after shoulder arthroplasty. Heavy lifting and high-impact activities should be avoided to minimize the potential for postoperative wear and tear or loosening of the prosthetic components.[27,39,108,164]

Arthrodesis of the Shoulder

Indications for Surgery

The following are generally accepted indications for arthrodesis of the glenohumeral joint.[12,39,103,138,180]

- Incapacitating pain
- Gross instability of the GH joint
- Complete paralysis of the deltoid and rotator cuff muscles
- Severe joint destruction from infection
- Failed shoulder arthroplasty in a young, active patient who is not a candidate for revision arthroplasty
- Good compensatory scapular motion and strength of the serratus anterior and trapezius muscles

Procedure

The GH joint is fused with pins and bone grafts in a position of 15 to 30 degrees of flexion and abduction and up to 30 to 45 degrees of internal rotation so that the hand can reach the middle of the body or mouth.[103,138,139,164,180] The shoulder is immobilized in a shoulder spica cast or a thoracobrachial (airplane) orthosis that extends across the elbow joint. The immobilizer is worn for 3 to 5 months.

Postoperative Management

Place emphasis on maintaining mobility of peripheral joints. While the shoulder and elbow are immobilized, have the patient focus on maintaining mobility in the wrist and hand. If an orthosis with a hinged elbow joint is used, begin elbow flexion and extension when permissible, often as early as the day after surgery. After the immobilization device may be removed for exercise, begin active scapulothoracic ROM. Strengthen scapulothoracic musculature to maximize control and stability of the scapula.

Outcomes

A patient may expect to achieve 90 to 130 degrees of active elevation of the arm because of scapulothoracic mobility.[103,138,180] After bony and soft tissue healing is complete, the shoulder is stable and pain free for activities that require strength or weight bearing at the shoulder. Patients are able to bring the hand to the mouth, behind the head, and to the hip.[138,164,180] Over time, excessive stress may be placed on the AC joint, resulting in AC joint hypermobility and pain.[138,139,164]

▶ Painful Shoulder Syndromes: Rotator Cuff Disease, Impingement Syndromes, and Shoulder Instabilities

Mechanical compression and irritation of the soft tissues (rotator cuff and subacromial bursa) in the suprahumeral space is called **impingement syndrome** and is the most common cause of shoulder pain.[98] Impingement is generally classified as primary or secondary.

Primary impingement is the result of intrinsic or extrinsic factors that encroach against the tissues in

*See references 39, 54, 102, 103, 114, 116, 149.

the subacromial space. Structural encroachment includes structural variations in the acromion,[56,142] hypertrophic degenerative changes of the AC joint, or other trophic changes in the coracoacromial arch or humeral head, which decrease the suprahumeral space. Extrinsic factors that result in decreased suprahumeral space and repetitive trauma to the soft tissues during elevation of the arm include posterior capsular tightness, poor neuromuscular control of the rotator cuff or scapular muscles, faulty scapulothoracic posture or a partial or complete tear of the tissues in the suprahumeral space (either from traumatic or degenerative situations).[70,97,98,113,155] Neer described three pathologic stages of impingement which demonstrate the potentially progressive nature of the pathology over time.[113] These are outlined in Box 9–5.

Secondary impingement is used to describe symptoms from faulty mechanics that occur from hypermobility or instability of the GH joint with increased translation of the humeral head. The instability may be unidirectional or multidirectional. Unidirectional instability usually occurs from trauma and results in partial tearing of some of the supporting ligaments or glenoid labrum, but may also occur from lax capsular tissues. The trauma may occur in an anterior, posterior, or inferior direction. Physiologically lax connective tissue of the capsule may also lead to multidirectional instability. The hypermobility can cause other problems besides impingement such as subluxation, dislocation or rotator cuff tendinitis, which with repetitive microtrauma can lead to degenerative changes including bone spurs, tendon rupture, or capsular restrictions and frozen shoulder. Jobe has developed a classification system incorporating the progression of impingement and instability in the overhead athlete based on progressive microtrauma.[84] These are outlined in Box 9–5.

Symptoms from impingement, whether from primary causes or secondary instability, are usually brought on with excessive or repetitive overhead activities that load the shoulder joint, particularly in the midrange. Other types of musculotendinous strains that occur in the shoulder region may occur from overuse or trauma, such as in the anterior pectoral region from racket sports or in the long head of triceps and serratus anterior from impact trauma such as holding on to a steering wheel in an automobile accident.

Box 9–5 Categories of Painful Shoulder Syndromes

Impingement syndromes and other painful shoulder conditions have varying etiological factors and, therefore, can be categorized several ways.

Based on Degree or Stage of Pathology of the Rotator Cuff (Neer's Classification of Rotator Cuff Disease)[113]

- **Stage I.** Edema, hemorrhage (patient usually less than 25 years of age)
- **Stage II.** Tendinitis/bursitis and fibrosis (patient usually 25–40 years of age)
- **Stage III.** Bone spurs and tendon rupture (patient usually over 40 years of age)

Based on Impaired Tissue[42]

- Supraspinatus tendinitis
- Infraspinatus tendinitis
- Bicipital tendinitis
- Subdeltoid (subacromial) bursitis
- Other musculotendinous strains (specific to type of injury or trauma)
  - Anterior—from overuse with racket sports (pectoralis minor, subscapularis, coracobrachialis, short head of biceps strain)
  - Inferior—from motor vehicle trauma (long head of triceps, serratus anterior strain)

Based on Mechanical Disruption and Direction of Instability or Subluxation

- Multidirectional instability from lax capsule with or without impingement
- Unidirectional instability (anterior, posterior, or inferior) with or without impingement
  - Traumatic injury with tears of capsule and/or labrum
  - Insidious (atraumatic) onset from repetitive microtrauma
  - Inherent laxity

Based on Progressive Microtrauma (Jobe's classification)[84]

- **Group 1.** Pure impingement (usually in an older recreational athlete with partial undersurface rotator cuff tear and subacromial bursitis)
- **Group 2.** Impingement associated with labral and/or capsular injury, instability, and secondary impingement
- **Group 3.** Hyperelastic soft tissues resulting in anterior or multidirectional instability and impingement (usually attenuated but intact labrum, undersurface rotator cuff tear)
- **Group 4.** Anterior instability without associated impingement (result of trauma, results in partial or complete dislocation)

Based on Degree and Frequency

- Instability → subluxation → dislocation
- Acute, recurrent, fixed

Related Diagnoses and Etiology of Symptoms

The cause of impingement is multifactoral, involving both structural and mechanical impairments. Impingement syndrome is often used as the diagnosis when patient signs and symptoms are related to pain with overhead reaching, a painful arc midrange, and positive impingement tests. Other test results may more specifically identify the tissue involved, faulty mechanics associated with the condition, or degree of instability or injury.

Primary Impingement—Rotator Cuff Disease

Primary impingement is believed to occur as a result of mechanical wear of the rotator cuff against the anteroinferior one-third of the acromion in the suprahumeral space during elevation activities of the humerus. Structural variants, in the acromion and coracoacromial arch, may be the cause of primary impingement[77] and often have to be dealt with surgically. Other factors that influence the amount of suprahumeral space and may contribute to impingement include posture, muscle imbalances, and joint restrictions are dealt with using therapeutic exercise interventions. Neer[113] identified impingement lesions of the rotator cuff and long head of the biceps in three progressive stages:

Stage I. Edema and hemorrhage: Typically occurs in patients who are below the age of 25 years.

Stage II. Fibrosis and tendinitis (the bursa may also become fibrotic and thickened): Seen typically in patients between 25 and 40 years of age.

Stage III. Bone spurs, rotator cuff tears, and biceps rupture: Typically seen in persons over 40 years of age.

Other authors have identified chronic inflammation, possibly from repetitive microtraumas in the joint region, as a stimulus for the development of frozen shoulder.[63,117,120]

Tendinitis/Bursitis—Impaired Musculotendinous Tissues

Neer has identified tendinitis/bursitis as a stage II impingement syndrome. The following describe specific diagnoses and presenting signs and symptoms.

Supraspinatus tendinitis. The lesion is usually near the musculotendinous junction and results in a painful arc with overhead reaching. Pain occurs with the impingement test (forced humeral elevation in the plane of the scapula while the scapula is passively stabilized so that the greater tuberosity impacts against the acromion;[70,113] or with the arm in internal rotation while flexing the humerus).[70] There is pain on palpation of the tendon just inferior to the anterior aspect of the acromion when the patient's hand is placed behind the back. It is difficult to differentiate partial tears from subdeltoid bursitis because of the anatomic proximity.

Infraspinatus tendinitis. The lesion is usually near the musculotendinous junction and results in a painful arc with overhead or forward motions. It may present as a deceleration (eccentric) injury from overload during repetitive or forceful throwing activities. Pain occurs on palpation of the tendon just inferior to the posterior corner of the acromion when the patient horizontally adducts and laterally rotates the humerus.

Bicipital tendinitis. The lesion involves the long tendon in the bicipital groove beneath or just distal to the transverse humeral ligament. Swelling in the bony groove is restrictive and compounds and perpetuates the problem. Pain occurs with resistance to the forearm in a supinated position while the shoulder is flexing (Speed's sign) and on palpation of the bicipital groove.[99] A rupture or dislocation of this humeral depressor may escalate impingement of tissues in the suprahumeral space.[113,121]

Bursitis (subdeltoid or subacromial). When acute, symptoms are the same as supraspinatus tendinitis. Once the inflammation is under control, there are no symptoms with resistance.

Other musculotendinous problems. The following are examples of other musculotendinous problems in the shoulder region.

- The pectoralis minor, short head of the biceps, and coracobrachialis are subject to microtrauma, particularly in racket sports requiring a controlled backward then a rapid forward swinging of the arm, as are the scapular stabilizers as they function to control forward motion of the scapula.[95]
- The long head of the triceps and scapular stabilizers are often injured in motor vehicle accidents as the driver holds firmly to the steering wheel on impact.
- A fall on an outstretched hand or against the shoulder may also cause trauma to the scapular stabilizers, which, if not properly healed, will continue to cause symptoms whenever using the arm or when maintaining a shoulder posture.
- Injury, overuse, or repetitive trauma can occur in any muscle being subjected to stress.[124] Pain will occur when the involved muscle is placed on a

stretch or when contracting against resistance. Palpation of the site of the lesion will cause the familiar pain.

Secondary Impingement—Shoulder Instability/Subluxation

Multidirectional instability. Some individuals have physiologically lax connective tissue causing excessive mobility in the joints of the body. In the GH joint, the humeral head translates to a greater degree than normal in all directions.[127,148,168] Many individuals, particularly those involved in overhead throwing or lifting activities, have some inherent laxity or develop laxity of the capsule and instability from continually subjecting the joint to stretch forces.[56,84] With strong rotator cuff muscles a hypermobile joint is satisfactorily supported, but once they fatigue, poor humeral head stabilization leads to faulty humeral mechanics, trauma, and inflammation to the suprahumeral tissues.[84,109] This trauma is magnified with the rapidity of control demanded in the overhead throwing action.[56] Similarly, in individuals with poor rotator cuff muscle strength and function, the ligaments become stressed with repetitive use and hypermobility, and impingement results. With instability, the impingement of tissue in the suprahumeral space is the secondary effect.[56]

Unidirectional instability with or without impingement (anterior, posterior or inferior). Unidirectional instability may be the result of physiologically lax connective tissue but is usually the result of trauma and usually involves rotator cuff tears. The tears can be classified as acute, chronic, degenerative, or partial- or full-thickness tears. Often there is damage to the glenoid labrum and tearing of some of the supporting ligaments.

Traumatic tears or paralysis. Partial-thickness tears or full avulsion of the greater tubercle may occur in the elderly as the result of a fall on an outstretched arm.[118] In young patients, trauma is usually associated with capsular injury, with or without labrum injury, resulting in instability. Dislocation of the humerus may occur with ensuing instability. The instability can lead to progressive degeneration and eventually tears in the supporting structures. Tears are associated with pain and most commonly weakness of shoulder abduction and external rotation.

- *Anterior instability* usually occurs with force against the arm when it is in an abducted and externally rotated position and frequently involves detachment of the anterior capsule and glenoid labrum (Bankart lesion). There may also be a fractured piece or flattening of the anterior lip of the glenoid.[65] Positive signs include apprehension, load and shift, and anterior drawer tests.[99,186]
- *Posterior instability* results from a forceful thrust against a forward flexed humerus or fall on an outstretched arm. There is a positive posterior drawer sign.[99,186]
- *Inferior instability* results from rotator cuff weakness/paralysis and is frequently seen in patients with hemiplegia.[61] It is also prevalent in patients with multidirectional instability. This is detected with a positive sulcus sign.[99,186]

Insidious (atraumatic) onset. Neer has identified rotator cuff tears as a stage III impingement syndrome, a condition that typically occurs in persons over the age of 40 after repetitive microtrauma to the rotator cuff or long head of the biceps.[113] With aging, the distal portion of the supraspinatus tendon is particularly vulnerable to impingement or stress from overuse strain. With degenerative changes, calcification and eventual tendon rupture may occur.[56,126] Chronic ischemia caused by tension on the tendon and decreased healing in the elderly are possible explanations, although Neer states that, in his experience, 95% of tears are initiated by impingement wear rather than by impaired circulation or trauma.[113]

Common Impairments

Various impairments have been reported to be common in impingement syndromes; it is not known if they are the cause or effect of the faulty mechanics.[32,97,98,128,178] A thorough examination of the cervical spine and shoulder girdle is necessary to differentiate signs and symptoms related to primary and secondary impingements or other causes of shoulder pain.[23,85,99]

Postural Malalignment and Muscle Imbalances: Increased Thoracic Kyphosis with Accompanying Forward Head, Abducted, and Forward Tipped Scapula

Faulty upper quadrant posture leads to an imbalance in the length and strength of the scapular and glenohumeral musculature and decreases the effectiveness of the dynamic and passive stabilizing structures of the GH joint.[187] Typically with increased thoracic kyphosis, the scapula is protracted and tipped forward, and the GH joint is in an internally rotated posture. With this posture, the pectoralis minor, levator scapulae, and shoulder internal rotators are tight, and the lateral rotators of the shoulder and upward rotators of the scapula test weak and have poor muscular endurance. There is no longer the stabilizing tension on the superior joint capsule and coracohumeral ligament or compressive forces from the rotator cuff muscles. Therefore, the effect of gravity tends to cause an inferior force on the humerus.

When reaching overhead there is faulty scapular and humeral mechanics resulting in faulty alignment of the scapula and altered function in the muscles controlling the scapula and glenohumeral joint. Ludewig and Cook[97] documented delayed upward rotation of the scapula during the 31- to 60-degrees range of humeral elevation, incomplete backward tipping of the scapula, and excessive scapular elevation in individuals with impingement. This mechanical alteration may contribute to decreased clearance under the anterior acromion. Overuse of the upper trapezius with scapular elevation may be a compensation for the weak posterior tipping action of the serratus anterior[97] and points to the importance of re-establishing control and balance in strength in this muscle along with flexibility in the pectoralis minor.

Decreased Thoracic ROM

Thoracic extension is a component motion that is needed for full overhead reaching; incomplete thoracic extension will decrease the functional range of humeral elevation.

Rotator Cuff Overuse and Fatigue

If the rotator cuff musculature or long head of the biceps fatigue from overuse, they no longer provide the dynamic stabilizing, compressive and translational forces that support the joint and control the normal joint mechanics. This is thought to be a precipitating factor in secondary impingement syndromes when there is capsular laxity and increased need for muscular stability.[131] The tissues in the subacromial space may then become impinged from faulty mechanics. There is also a relationship between muscle fatigue and joint position sense in the shoulder that may play a roll in impaired performance in repetitive overhead activities.[33]

Muscle Weakness Secondary to Neuropathy

Muscle weakness may be related to nerve involvement. Long thoracic nerve palsy has been identified as a cause of faulty scapular mechanics from serratus anterior muscle weakness leading to impingement in the suprahumeral region.[151]

Hypomobile Posterior GH Joint Capsule

Tightness in the posterior joint capsule compromises the normal arthrokinematics and increases forces on the head of the humerus against the anterior capsule. Harryman et al[66] has demonstrated increased anterior translation in the humeral head when there is a tight posterior capsule.

Summary of Common Impairments with Rotator Cuff Disease and Impingement Syndromes

Note: Some, all, or none of these may be present.

- Pain at the musculotendinous junction of the involved muscle with palpation, with resisted muscle contraction, and when stretched
- Positive impingement sign (forced internal rotation at 90 degrees of flexion) and painful arc
- Faulty posture: Thoracic kyphosis, forward head, and forward (anterior) tipped scapula with decreased thoracic mobility
- Muscle imbalances: Hypomobile pectoralis major and minor, levator scapulae, and internal rotators of GH joint; weak serratus anterior and lateral rotators
- Hypomobile posterior GH joint capsule
- Faulty kinematics with humeral elevation: decreased posterior tipping of scapula related to weak serratus anterior; scapular elevation and overuse of upper trapezius; and uncoordinated scapulohumeral rhythm
- With a complete rotator cuff tear, inability to abduct the humerus against gravity
- When acute, pain referred to the C-5 and C-6 reference zones

Common Functional Limitations/Disabilities

- When acute, pain may interfere with sleep, particularly when rolling onto the involved shoulder.
- Pain with overhead reaching, pushing, or pulling.
- Difficulty with lifting loads.
- Inability to sustain repetitive shoulder activities

(such as reaching, lifting, throwing, pushing, pulling, or swinging the arm).
- Difficulty with dressing, particularly putting a shirt on overhead.

Nonoperative Management: Painful Shoulder Syndromes (Without Dislocation)

Note: Even though symptoms may be "chronic" or recurring, if there is inflammation, the initial treatment priority is to get the inflammation under control.

Management: Protection Phase

Control Inflammation and Promote Healing

- Use modalities and low-intensity cross-fiber massage to the site of the lesion. While applying the modalities position the extremity to maximally expose the involved region.[43,45]
- Support the arm in a sling for rest.

Patient Education

The environment and habits that provoke the symptoms must be modified or avoided completely during this stage.[43]

Maintain Integrity and Mobility of the Soft Tissues

- Initiate early motion with passive, active-assistive, or self-assisted ROM.
- Apply multiple-angle muscle setting and protected stabilization exercises. Of particular importance in the shoulder is to stimulate the stabilizing function of the rotator cuff, biceps brachii, and scapular muscles at an intensity tolerated by the patient.
- Use caution with exercises in this stage to avoid the impingement positions, which are often in the midrange of abduction or end-range position when the involved muscle is on a stretch.

Control Pain and Maintain Joint Integrity

Use pendulum exercises without weights to cause pain-inhibiting grade II joint distraction and oscillation motions (see Fig. 9–10).

Develop Support in Related Regions

- Teach the patient postural awareness and correction techniques.
- Initiate training of scapular and thoracic posture using shoulder strapping or scapular taping, tactile cues, and use of mirrors for reinforcement. Repetitive practice of correct posture is necessary throughout the day.
- Forward head posture is often related to forward shoulder posture (see Chapter 15 for additional suggestions if this dysfunction is present).

Management: Controlled Motion Phase

Once the acute symptoms are under control, the main emphasis becomes use of the involved region with progressive, nondestructive movement and proper mechanics while the tissues heal. The components of the desired functions are analyzed and initiated in a controlled exercise program.[44,45,87,182,183] If there is a functional laxity in the joint, the intervention is directed toward learning neuromuscular control of and developing strength in the stabilizing muscles of both the scapula and glenohumeral joint.[29,87,90,150,171] If there is restricted mobility that prevents normal mechanics or interferes with function, mobilization of the restricted tissue is performed. Exercise techniques and progressions are described later in this chapter.

Patient Education

Patient adherence with the program and avoidance of irritating the healing tissue are necessary. The home exercise program is progressed as the patient learns safe and effective execution of each exercise.

Develop a Strong, Mobile Scar

- Position the tissue on a stretch if it is a tendon or in the shortened position if it is in the muscle belly and apply cross-fiber or friction massage to the tolerance of the patient.
- Follow this with an isometric contraction of the muscle in several positions of the range and at an intensity that does not cause pain.
- Teach the patient how to self-administer the massage and isometric techniques.

Improve Postural Awareness

Continue to reinforce proper postural habits. Every time an exercise is performed, make the patient aware of scapular and cervical posture with tactile and verbal reinforcement such as touching the scapular adductors and chin and reminding the patient to "pull the shoulders back" and "lift the head" while doing the shoulder exercises.

Modify Joint Tracking

Mobilization with movement (MWM) may be useful to modify joint tracking and reinforce full movement when there is painful restriction of shoulder elevation because of a painful arc or impingement[110] (see Chapter 6 for description of principles).

- ***Posterolateral glide with active elevation*** (Fig 9–7*A*)
  - Patient position and procedure: Sitting with the arm by the side and head in neutral retraction. Stand on the side opposite the affected arm and reach across the patient's torso to stabilize the scapula with the palm of one hand. The other hand is placed over the anteromedial aspect of the head of the humerus.
  - Apply a graded posterolateral glide of the humeral head on the glenoid. Request that the patient perform the previously painful elevation. Maintain the posterolateral glide mobilization throughout both elevation and return to neutral. Ensure no pain is experienced during the procedure. Adjust the grade and direction of the glide as needed to achieve pain-free function.
  - Add resistance in the form of elastic resistance or a cuff weight to load the muscle.
- ***Self-treatment.*** A mobilization belt provides the posterolateral glide while the patient actively elevates the affected limb against progressive resistance to end range (Fig. 9–7*B*).

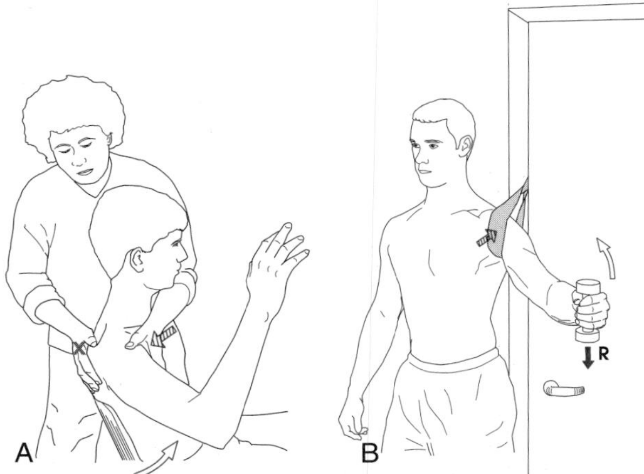

Figure 9–7 MWM to modify joint tracking and improve active elevation. A posterolateral glide is applied to the humeral head *(A)* manually, or *(B)* with a belt for self-treatment, while the patient actively elevates the humerus. A weight is used to strengthen the muscles through the pain-free range.

Develop Balance in Length and Strength of Shoulder Girdle Muscles

Design a program that specifically addresses the patient's limitations. Typical interventions in the shoulder girdle include but are not limited to:

- ***Stretch shortened muscles.*** These typically include the pectoralis major, pectoralis minor, latissimus dorsi and teres major, subscapularis, and levator scapulae.
- ***Strengthen and train the scapular stabilizers.*** These typically include the serratus anterior and lower trapezius for posterior tipping and upward rotation and the middle trapezius and rhomboids for scapular retraction. It is important that the patient learns to avoid scapular elevation when raising the arm. Therefore, practice scapular depression when abducting and flexing the humerus.
- ***Strengthen and train the rotator cuff muscles,*** especially the shoulder lateral rotators.

Develop Co-Contraction, Stabilization, and Endurance in the Muscles of the Scapula and Shoulder

- Isolate the scapular muscles in open-chain positions (side-lying, sitting, supine) and apply alternating isometric resistance to protraction/retraction, elevation/depression, and upward/downward rotation so the patient learns to stabilize the scapula against the outside forces (see Fig. 9–25).
- Combine scapular and glenohumeral patterns with the humerus in various positions of flexion, abduction, and rotation and apply alternating isometric resistance while the patient holds against the changing directions of the resistance force (see Fig 9–29).
- Closed-chain stabilization is performed with the patient's hands fixated against a wall, a table, or the floor (quadruped position) while the therapist provides a graded, alternating isometric resistance or rhythmic stabilization. Observe for abnormal scapular winging. If it occurs the scapular stabilizers are not strong enough for the demand; so the position should be changed to reduce the amount of body weight (see Fig 9–30).
- Increased muscular endurance by increasing the amount of time the individual holds the pattern against the alternating resistance. The limit is reached when any one of the muscles in the pattern can no longer maintain the desired hold. The goal at this phase should be stabilization for approximately 3 minutes.

Progress Shoulder Function

As the patient develops strength in the weakened muscles, develop a balance in strength of all shoulder and scapular muscles within the range and tolerance of each muscle. Increase coordination between scapular and arm motions; dynamically load the upper extremity within tolerance of the synergy with submaximal resistance. Improve muscular endurance and develop control from 1 to 3 minutes.

Management: Return to Function Phase

As soon as the patient has developed control of posture and the basic components of the desired activities without exacerbating the symptoms, initiate specificity of training toward the desired functional outcome.

Increase Muscular Endurance

Increase repetitive loading of defined patterns from 3 to 5 minutes.

Develop Quick Motor Responses to Imposed Stresses

- Increase the speed at which the stabilization exercises are applied.
- Initiate plyometric training in both open- and closed-chain patterns if power is needed.

Develop Function

Progress to specificity of training; emphasize timing and sequencing of events.

- Progress eccentric training to maximum load.
- Simulate desired functional activities, first under controlled conditions, then under progressively challenged situations using acceleration/deceleration drills.
- Assess the total-body function while doing a desired activity and modify any component that causes faulty patterning.

Educate the Patient

Inform the patient of the time frames for healing and any exercises and activities that can be done. Instruct the patient on how to progress the program when discharged as well as how to prevent recurrences. Suggestions are summarized in Box 9–6.

Box 9–6 Patient Instructions to Prevent Recurrences of Shoulder Pain

- Prior to exercise or work, massage the involved tendon or muscle; follow with isometric resistance and then with full ROM and stretching of the muscle.
- Take breaks from the activity if repetitive in nature. If possible, alternate the stressful, provoking activity with other activities or patterns of motion.
- Maintain good postural alignment; adapt seating or work station to minimize stress. If sport-related, seek coaching in proper techniques or adapt equipment for safe mechanics.
- Prior to initiating a new activity or returning to an activity not conditioned for, begin a strengthening and training program.

Impingement Syndromes: Surgical and Postoperative Management

Indications for Surgery

The following are generally accepted indications for surgical management of impingement syndromes.*

- Insufficient subacromial joint space leading to pain during overhead activities as the result of primary impingement of soft tissues at the anterior edge and undersurface of the acromion.
- Stage II (Neer classification) impingement with nonreversible fibrosis or bony alterations (degenerative spurring) of the subacromial compartment.
- Intact or minor tears of the rotator cuff; calcific deposits in the cuff tendons; symptomatic subacromial crepitus.
- Unsuccessful conservative (nonoperative) management for 3 to 6 months or as long as a year.

Procedures

Impingement syndromes of the shoulder are managed by a variety of surgical methods known as *subacromial decompression* procedures or *anterior acromioplasty.*[1,50,68,133,147] An arthroscopic subacromial decompression involves removal of a portion of the anterior acromion (arthroscopic acromioplasty) and debridement of the undersurface of the acromion through several portal sites.[1,4,50,68,133] The inferior aspect of the remaining portion of the acromion is often beveled to provide adequate gliding space for the inflamed tendons.[142] In an arthroscopic approach, the deltoid is left intact.

An open procedure involves an arthrotomy through an anterolateral incision at the lateral border of the acromion. The anterior and lateral origins of the deltoid are detached from the acromion and later repaired before closure.[71,112,115,132] In open and arthroscopic approaches, the coracoacromial ligament is released. In both approaches sometimes the distal clavicle is also resected.[1,68]

Postoperative Management

The position and duration of immobilization of the shoulder and initiation and progression of exercise

*See references 4, 50, 68, 71, 115, 132, 133, 142, 147.

vary with the surgical approach. Rehabilitation after arthroscopic acromoplasty is quite rapid, primarily because the deltoid is left intact. Since the arthroscopic approach is used far more frequently for surgical management of primary impingement syndrome than an open acromoplasty, *the postoperative guidelines and the progression of exercises outlined in this section are appropriate after arthroscopic subacromial decompression.* If arthroscopic decompression is combined with a mini-open (arthroscopically assisted) repair of the rotator cuff, many of the same exercises are appropriate but in a slower progression. With an open acromioplasty, which is frequently used in combination with a traditional open rotator cuff repair, as noted previously, the deltoid must be detached and then repaired. Accordingly, the progression of exercises, discussed later in this chapter for open rotator cuff repair, is advisable.

Regardless of the type of procedure selected, close communication among the patient, therapist, and surgeon is necessary throughout all phases of postoperative rehabilitation. Effective patient education is the basis of early self-management by the patient and positive functional outcomes.

Immobilization

The shoulder is usually positioned in adduction and internal rotation, and the forearm is supported in a sling with the elbow flexed to 90 degrees. The sling is removed for exercise the day after surgery but otherwise is worn for several days for comfort.[50,162,185]

Exercise: Maximum Protection Phase

The goals and interventions for exercise in this phase of rehabilitation, which usually extends from 1 to 2 weeks postoperatively, are consistent with the guidelines for nonoperative management of acute impingement syndrome outlined previously in this chapter. *Emphasis is placed on immediate but pain-free assisted movement.*[50,83,162,185] Use of modalities and prescribed anti-inflammatory medication is indicated to control inflammation and pain.

■ ***Control pain.***

- Cervical spine active ROM and shoulder relaxation exercises

■ ***Prevent or correct postural malalignment.***

- Active exercises of the scapula with emphasis on retraction
- Posture awareness training, placing emphasis on an erect trunk (avoiding excessive thoracic kyphosis) during exercises and ADL

■ ***Prevent loss of mobility of all joints and muscles in the involved upper extremity.***

- CPM from 0 to 90 degrees of shoulder flexion initiated in the recovery room or the day after surgery, predicated on the philosophy of the surgeon.[104] It is used for only 48 hours postoperatively for patients undergoing inpatient surgery.
- Active ROM of the elbow, wrist, and hand through full ranges.
- Active-assistive shoulder ROM begun on the first postoperative day, emphasizing shoulder flexion, scaption, abduction, and horizontal abduction and adduction within pain-free ranges. Start in the supine position to provide additional stability to the scapula against the thorax using therapist-assisted, short-arc motion, progressing to full-arc ROM; then transition to self-assisted ROM with the uninvolved hand and finally with a wand. Progress to assisted elevation of the arm in the seated position.
- Active-assistive external and internal rotation with a wand, first in supine and later while seated. Keep the elbow flexed to 90 degrees and the arm slightly flexed and abducted during assisted rotation.
- Gear-shift exercises in sitting.
- Pendulum exercises for pain control and mobility.
- Assisted shoulder extension in a standing position with a wand held behind the back.
- Assisted scaption above the level of the shoulder with a rope-pulley system through a pain-free range.
- Transition to active-free (unassisted) ROM of the shoulder by 10 days to 2 weeks postoperatively.

■ ***Prevent atrophy and improve strength, stability, and endurance of the shoulder girdle musculature.***

- *Pain-free,* low-intensity, multiple-angle isometrics of GH musculature against minimal resistance. Begin isometrics a few days to a week postoperatively. Lightly resist with the uninvolved upper extremity. Focus on increasing repetitions more than resistance.[97,151]
- Alternating isometric and rhythmic stabilization exercises for scapulothoracic muscles with the involved arm supported by the therapist. Target the serratus anterior and trapezius muscles.

Exercise: Moderate Protection/Controlled Motion Phase

Rehabilitation proceeds very rapidly after arthroscopic subacromial decompression. Controlled active motion is emphasized while moderate protection of the shoulder is maintained by only performing pain-free movements. This phase of rehabilitation usually begins by 2 weeks postoperatively.

Criteria to advance to this phase include pain-free active elevation of the arm well above the level of the shoulder and at least Fair (3/5) muscle testing grade of shoulder musculature.[83,184,185] The priorities during this phase are to restore full ROM, strengthen key muscle groups, and begin to use the involved arm for light functional activities.[45,83,88,89,162,185]

- ***Restore and maintain full, pain-free passive mobility of the shoulder.***
  - Joint mobilization, emphasizing posterior and caudal glides of the humerus and scapulothoracic mobility.
  - Gentle stretching of range-limiting muscles that could restrict sufficient upward rotation of the scapula and rotation of the humerus necessary for full elevation of the arm overhead, specifically the levator scapulae, rhomboids, middle trapezius, latissimus dorsi, and pectoralis major and minor. Remember, shortening of these muscles contributes to impingement of soft tissues during overhead movements of the arm.
  - Self-stretching (cross-chest stretch) of the posterior deltoid and posterior capsule of the GH joint, which is usually tight in stage II and stage III impingement. A tight posterior capsule causes excessive anterior translation and superior migration of the head of the humerus in the glenoid, which, in turn, causes impingement of soft tissues during overhead reach.[66,104]
  - Active shoulder motions, incorporating the gained ROM into exercises and functional movement patterns during ADL.
- ***Continue to improve strength, stability, endurance and control of scapulothoracic and GH muscles.***
  - Stabilization exercises against greater resistance and in weight-bearing postures.[88,89] Use a Bodyblade® in various positions of the shoulder.
  - Upper extremity ergometry. Initiate in a standing position rather than while seated to avoid an impingement arc.[88,89]
  - Dynamic exercises of isolated shoulder muscles against low levels of resistance (1–5 lb) and gradually increasing repetitions. Use manual or mechanical resistance. Once again, begin shoulder elevation in the supine position to stabilize the scapula against the thorax; progress to sitting. Target the upward rotators of the scapulothoracic joint (serratus anterior, the upper and lower trapezius) and the rotator cuff muscles,[154] as well as the latissimus dorsi, teres major, and biceps brachii, which act as humeral head depressors and, therefore, oppose superior translation during active elevation of the arm. Initially perform resisted motions of the humerus below the level of the shoulder; later progress to overhead exercises if motions remain pain-free.

Note: If winging of the scapula occurs with progressive resistance or weight bearing, provide manual support or decrease the imposed loads. Emphasize isolated strengthening or the serratus anterior and trapezius muscles.

- Use the involved arm for light functional activities.

Exercise: Minimum Protection/ Return to Function Phase

The final phase of rehabilitation usually begins by 6 weeks postoperatively at which time soft tissues are reasonably well healed and require minimum protection. Criteria to progress to this phase is full, pain-free, active ROM of the shoulder, 70 to 75% strength of shoulder musculature compared with the sound shoulder, and a negative impingement test.[83,185] Criteria to return to full activity, which usually occurs by 8 to 12 weeks postoperatively, depends primarily on desired functional outcomes and the potential demands and stresses that will be placed on the shoulder. A patient wishing to return to competitive sports will require a more demanding progression of advanced exercises than a sedentary individual.[68,83] Include the following goals, exercises, and activities in the final phase of rehabilitation.[83,89,162,184,185]

- Progress exercises to include advanced activities, such as more rapid motions and directional changes.
  - Isokinetic exercises.
  - Kinesthetic/proprioceptive training, using rapid, alternating resistance with rhythmic stabilization.
  - Plyometric training.[181]
- Simulate functional activities in drills and then gradually return to actual work or sports-related functional activities. Refer to detailed, sports-specific protocols in the literature to return to

such sports as golf, volleyball, throwing sports, and tennis. Modify functional activities, if necessary, to prevent recurrence of impingement.

Note: Exercises for the final phase of nonoperative rehabilitation of impingement syndrome, cuff tears, and instabilities discussed earlier in this chapter are also appropriate in the final stage of postoperative rehabilitation.

Outcomes

There appears to be no significant difference in the *long-term* results (pain-free ROM and return to desired functional activities) after either open or arthroscopic surgery for primary impingement syndrome with or without associated rotator cuff disease.[50] Based on the results of numerous outcome studies of open and arthroscopic procedures, between 85 and 95% of patients report good to excellent results 1 to 2.5 years postoperatively.[2,184,185] In general, patients reporting the least satisfaction with their function after surgery are those involved in high-demand athletic activities, involving overhead throwing and those with work-related injury receiving workers' compensation.[104] Follow-up studies have documented several advantages of an arthroscopic over comparable open surgical management of impingement syndrome. They are: less postoperative pain; earlier restoration of full ROM and strength; earlier return to work, often as early as 1 week postoperatively; less cost (shorter hospital stay or outpatient surgery); and a more favorable cosmetic result.[1,68,104]

Rotator Cuff Tears: Surgical and Postoperative Management

Indications for Surgery

- Partial-thickness or full-thickness tears of the rotator cuff tendons as the result of repetitive microtrauma and chronic impingement, which lead to irreversible degenerative changes in soft tissues. Some patients with stage II and most with stage III lesions, who continue to be symptomatic and have functional limitations after 6 months to a year of nonoperative treatment, are candidates for surgery.*
- Acute, traumatic rupture (frank, full-thickness tears) of the rotator cuff tendons, often combined with avulsion of the greater tuberosity, labral damage, or acute dislocation of the GH joint in individuals with no known history of cuff injury. Full-thickness, traumatic tears occur most often in young, active adults.

Procedures

Depending on the severity and location of the tear of the rotator cuff tendons, the extent of associated lesions, the quality of the torn tissues as well as other considerations, there are several operative options. *Partial-thickness cuff tears,* if managed surgically after failed nonoperative treatment, are usually debrided arthroscopically along the margins of the tear rather than repaired. Debridement is often combined with subacrominal decompression.[2,8,105,161,169]

Repair is indicated for most *full-thickness cuff tears* after a trial of nonoperative management or sometimes immediately after an acute injury. Options for repair now include *arthroscopic cuff repair, mini-open (arthroscopically assisted) repair,* or a traditional *open repair.* Concomitant subacromial decompression is usually indicated particularly with chronic cuff disease. Capsular tightening or reconstruction may also be performed if unidirectional or multidirectional instability of the GH joint is present. The three approaches involve the following:

- In an arthroscopic repair, only a few small incisions are made for portal sites.[4,29,57,105,161,164]
- In a mini-open approach, an anterolateral incision is made at the acromion and is extended distally along the fibers of the deltoid muscle. The deltoid is then longitudinally split for several centimeters to allow visualization of the cuff tear. The proximal insertion of the deltoid remains intact.[8,57,68,105,134,169,170]
- In an open repair, a deltopectoral approach is used. An anterolateral incision begins at the inferior aspect of the lateral portion of the clavicle and extends inferiorly and obliquely to the lateral aspect of the acromion. The proximal insertion of the deltoid must be detached and reflected for exposure of the rotator cuff. After the cuff repair is complete, the deltoid is reattached to the acromion.†

Small to medium cuff tears (<1–3 cm) are usually managed with an arthroscopic or mini-open repair. Large tears (3–5 cm) are usually repaired with an open procedure or less frequently with a mini-open

*See references 2, 4, 8, 15, 68, 72, 74, 105, 134, 136, 155, 168.

†See references 15, 72, 74, 93, 105, 136, 164, 169.

procedure. Massive tears (>5 cm) are almost exclusively repaired with an open procedure and sometimes require transposition of other adjacent soft tissues to reinforce the repair. In massive cuff tears, other structures, such as the biceps tendon, may also have to be repaired.[105] In addition to the size and location of the cuff tear and the presence of associated injury, other factors influence the surgeon's selection of surgical approach and types of procedure and fixation used. They include the amount of retraction present in the torn tendons, the quality of the bone and remaining cuff tendons, and, of course, the training and previous experience of the surgeon.[105,164] The cuff repair involves either a *tendon-to-tendon repair* or, more commonly, a *tendon advancement* and reattachment to bone. Fixation is accomplished with either direct nonabsorbable or absorbable sutures, percutaneous tacks, or staples.[57,68,105,164,169]

Postoperative Management

After surgical repair of a rotator cuff tear, there are numerous factors that can determine the position and duration of immobilization, the selection and application of exercises, and the rate of progression of each patient's postoperative rehabilitation program. These factors and their potential impact are summarized in Table 9–2.

It should be apparent that many of these factors may also affect postoperative outcomes. There is little consensus of opinion reported in the literature or practiced in the clinical setting as to how and to what extend each of these factors, singularly or collectively, have an impact on the decisions made about a patient's postoperative rehabilitation program by the surgeon and the therapist.* Hence, published guidelines and protocols for postopera-

*See references 8, 25, 49, 83, 111, 133, 134, 184.

Table 9–2 Factors that Influence Progression of Rehabilitation After Repair of the Rotator Cuff

Factors	Potential Impact on Rehabilitation
• Onset of injury	• Chronic impingement and atraumatic cuff deficiency → slower progression than after acute traumatic injury.
• Size and location of the tear	• Larger tears with more structures involved and probability of more extensive surgery → slower progression.
• Associated pathologies such as GH instability or fracture	• Associated pathologies often lengthen the period of immobilization → slower progression of exercises or the need for additional precautions.
• Preoperative strength and mobility of the shoulder	• Pre-existing weakness and atrophy of the dynamic stabilizers or limited passive and active mobility of the shoulder → slower postoperative progression.
• Patient's general health	• Patient in poor health; history of smoking; history of inflammatory disease → slower progression.
• History of steroid injections or previous, failed cuff surgery	• Compromised bone and tendon tissue quality, which affects the security of the repair (fixation) → slower progression.
• Preinjury level of activity of postoperative goals	• Higher level goals require a more extended and advanced postoperative training program because of a higher risk of reinjury.
• Age of patient	• Older patient who has an insidious (chronic) onset and may have articular changes → slower progression.
• Type of approach	• Traditional open approach (with deltoid detachment and repair) → slightly slower progression than after an arthroscopic or arthroscopically assisted (mini-open/deltoid splitting) repair.
• Type of repair	• Tendon to tendon → slower progression than tendon to bone.
• Mobility (no excessive tension on the repaired tendon when arm at side) and integrity of the repair	• If mobility is inadequate → longer duration of exercise within a protected ROM during early rehabilitation.
• Patient's compliance with the program	• Lack of compliance (doing too much or too little) can affect outcome.
• Philosophy, skill, and training of the surgeon	• All have an impact that could → either slower or more accelerated progression.

tive management of rotator cuff tears are diverse and sometimes contradictory. For example, many authors point out that if the deltoid is detached during the surgery, as is necessary in an open repair, deltoid strengthening should be postponed for approximately 6 weeks postoperatively until the repaired deltoid has healed.[49,83,105] Yet another author suggests that rehabilitation should proceed similarly whether or not deltoid detachment was required.[68]

As with postoperative protocols for so many other musculoskeletal pathologies of the shoulder or other joints, no one single protocol has been shown to be the most appropriate or effective for all patients who have undergone the same type of surgery for rotator cuff repair. The many variables summarized in Table 9–2 highlight the complexity of rotator cuff rehabilitation and why an exercise program based on a comprehensive examination and ongoing re-examination of the patient's response to intervention is so important. For instance, the preinjury strength of shoulder musculature will influence postoperative management. A young, active patient who sustains an acute tear most likely will have had a strong rotator cuff mechanism prior to injury, whereas an elderly patient with a history of chronic impingement often will exhibit preoperative weakness and atrophy. These two patients need to be managed differently during their rehabilitation. In addition, intraoperative observations by the surgeon, for example, of the quality of bone and remaining tendons or the mobility of the repair, will also influence the rate of progression of exercises postoperatively. These examples underscore the need for development of individualized rehabilitation programs or at least modification of pre-existing protocols for each patient through close communication between the therapist and the surgeon.

It is the purpose of this section to highlight and compare *general* guidelines and precautions for each phase of postoperative management of a *full-thickness* cuff tear after a mini-open repair (with deltoid splitting) and an open repair (with deltoid detachment and repair). To date, very limited information on postoperative management after arthroscopic repair is available.[58] The progression of exercises after an arthroscopic repair appears to be essentially comparable to or slightly more accelerated than after a mini-open (arthroscopically assisted) repair. Therefore, in this section, there is no significant distinction made between postoperative management after these two approaches to cuff repair.

Note: Remember, repair of most cuff tears, particularly when associated with chronic impingement, also includes subacromial decompression. The same treatment principles and types of upper extremity exercises, such as assisted ROM, stabilization and strengthening exercises, stretching, and advanced activities already discussed and outlined for management after subacromial decompression for impingement syndrome, are also applicable and appropriate after a cuff repair with an arthroscopic, mini-open, or open approach. The key differences are that the rate of progression must proceed more gradually and additional precautions must be taken with open approaches. The progression of rehabilitation after debridement of a partial-thickness tear is comparable to postoperative management after subacromial decompression.

Immobilization

There are many inter-related factors that influence a surgeon's decision about the position and duration of immobilization of the operated shoulder after rotator cuff repair. Most of these factors were summarized in Table 9–2. Two of those factors, the type of surgical approach (mini-open or open) and the size of the tear, in part, determine whether the patient's operated upper extremity is supported in a sling (shoulder adducted, internally rotated, and elbow flexed to 90 degrees) or in an abduction orthosis (shoulder abducted 45 to 65 degrees, internally rotated and elbow flexed).

The rationale for initially immobilizing the operated shoulder in abduction is based on two principles. (1) In the abducted position, the repaired cuff, as well as the reattached deltoid in an open approach, are held in a relaxed position, which reduces the possibility of reflexive muscle contractions that could disrupt the repairs. (2) Supporting the arm in abduction rather than adduction reduces tension on the tendons and, therefore, may improve blood flow to the repaired tendon(s). Table 9–3 summarizes the diversity of opinions found in the literature on how the size of the tear and the type of surgical approach influence surgeons' decisions on postoperative immobilization after cuff repair.[49,68,83,105,179]

Exercise

Early self-management by the patient through effective patient education is emphasized in each phase

Table 9–3 Relationships of Type and Duration of Immobilization to the Size of the Rotator Cuff Tear and Surgical Approach*

Mini-Open (Arthroscopically Assisted/Deltoid Splitting) Approach			
Size of Tear	Small (<1 cm)	Medium to Large (>1–5 cm)	Massive (>5 cm)
Type and Duration	Sling or abduction splint 1–2 weeks; removal for exercise the day of surgery or 1 day postop	Sling or abduction orthosis 3–6 weeks; removal for exercise 1–2 days postop	Sling or abduction orthosis 4–8 weeks; removal for exercise 1–3 days postop
Open Approach			
Size of Tear	Small (<1 cm)	Medium and Large (>1–5 cm)	Massive (>5 cm)
Type and Duration	Sling, sling and swathe, or abduction orthosis up to 6 weeks, depending on tissue quality; removal for exercise 1 day postop	Sling, sling and swathe, or abduction orthosis for 6 weeks depending on tissue quality; removal for exercise 2–3 days postop	Abduction orthosis for 6–8 weeks; removal of splint as early as 1 day postop; in some instances, orthosis is worn continually for 1 week before removal for exercise

*Age of the patient, onset of the injury, and quality of repaired tissue also influence position and duration of immobilization.

of postoperative rehabilitation. General ***precautions*** for exercise after either a mini-open or open procedure are addressed in Box 9–7 for each of the phases of rehabilitation. Note that the rate of progression is consistently more gradual after an open repair than after a mini-open repair.

Exercise: Maximum Protection Phase

The important priorities in this initial phase of rehabilitation are the protection of the repaired tissues and prevention of the adverse effects of immobilization. Therefore, in almost all situations the immobilization is removed for brief sessions of passive or assisted ROM within a limited (protected) range as soon as possible after surgery (see Table 9–3). The maximum protection phase extends for as little as 3 weeks after a mini-open repair or as long as 6 to 8 weeks after an open repair. The following goals and selected interventions combined with the appropriate use of pain medication may be initiated during the maximum protection phase.*

- ***Control pain.***
  - Cervical spine ROM and shoulder relaxation exercises
  - Grade I oscillations on the GH joint
- ***Prevent or correct postural malalignment,*** especially excessive thoracic kyphosis. Exercises for posture training are described in Chapter 16.

*See references 8, 25, 49, 83, 105, 133, 134, 184.

- ***Prevent loss of mobility in the involved upper extremity.***
  - CPM from 0 to 90 degrees of shoulder flexion initiated in the recovery room or the day after surgery and continued for 48 hours. Use is based on the surgeon's philosophy.[105]
  - Assisted ROM of the elbow and active ROM of the wrist and hand.
  - Active movements of the scapula.
- Passive ROM of the shoulder within safe and pain-free ranges when the immobilization can be removed for exercise. In the supine position, include elevation in the scapular plane and external rotation. After a mini-open procedure progress to self-assisted motions by 1[184] to 3 weeks,[49] but much more gradually after an open procedure.
  - Pendulum exercises.
- ***Develop control of scapulothoracic musculature.*** (appropriate after open and mini-open procedures). Use submaximal isometrics to isolated scapular muscles.[97]

Precaution: During this period of maximum protection provide support to the arm during scapular motions and avoid weight bearing on the operated arm to avoid excessive tension in repaired GH musculature.[83,184]

- ***Prevent inhibition and atrophy of GH musculature,*** especially the rotator cuff. Low-intensity

Box 9–7 Precautions for Exercise After Repair of a Full-Thickness Rotator Cuff Tear (Open or Mini-Open Procedure)

- Perform passive or assisted shoulder ROM within *safe and pain-free ranges* based on the surgeon's intraoperative observation of the mobility and strength of the repair and the patient's comfort level during exercise.
- Initially perform passive and active-assistive shoulder ROM in the supine position to maintain stability of the scapula on the thorax.
- See that the humerus is positioned slightly anterior to the frontal plane of the body and in slight abduction to minimize anterior translation of the humeral head and the potential for impingement.
  - In the supine position while at rest or during passive or assisted shoulder rotation exercises, support the humerus on a folded towel.
  - When initiating assisted shoulder extension, perform the exercise in prone (arm over the edge of the bed) from 90 degrees to just short of neutral. Later progress to exercises behind the back.
- When beginning isometric resistance to scapulothoracic musculature, be sure to support the arm to avoid excessive tension in repaired GH musculature.
- After an open repair, postpone isometric resistance exercises to the shoulder for at least 6 weeks unless advised otherwise.
- Avoid vigorous passive stretching, the use of contract-relax procedures or grade III joint mobilizations for at least 6 and often for 12 weeks postoperatively to give time for the repaired tendon(s) to heal and become strong.
- Delay dynamic strengthening after a mini-open procedure for a minimum of 8 weeks (for small, strong repair) and after an open procedure until 3 months postoperatively.
- Restore strength in the rotator cuff, especially the supraspinatus and infraspinatus muscles, before dynamically strengthening the shoulder flexors and abductors.
- Avoid weight bearing on the involved arm for approximately 6 weeks, particularly after an open procedure.
- Wait until about 6 weeks after a mini-open and 12 weeks after an open repair before using the operated arm for light functional activities.
- After an open repair, avoid use of the involved arm for *resisted* functional activities (pushing, pulling, lifting, carrying heavy loads) for 4 to 12 *months* postoperatively.

muscle setting exercises that are not provocative to healing cuff tendons against minimal resistance, as early as 1–3 weeks postoperatively.[49,184] This is *only recommended after a mini-open procedure and only if the repair is strong.* Even gentle isometrics are *not* recommended for 6 weeks after an open repair.

Note: Recommendations for the safest position of the shoulder in which to begin isometric training of the GH musculature after cuff repair are inconsistent. One suggestion is to start in a position that creates minimum tension on the repaired cuff tendons (shoulder internally rotated and flexed and abducted to about 45 to 65 degrees and elbow flexed).[49] Another opinion recommends placing the shoulder in 100 to 110 degrees of flexion and 10 to 20 degrees of horizontal abduction. In this position the deltoid creates a compression force on the head of the humerus into the glenoid fossa, thus diminishing the superior sheer forces generated by the deltoid than when the arm is in less flexion.[184] As the strength of the cuff muscles improves in the later phases of rehabilitation, the isometric activities can be performed with the arm positioned in less shoulder flexion.

Exercise: Moderate Protection/Controlled Motion Phase

Criteria to advance to this phase are approximately 120 to 145 degrees of pain-free, assisted elevation and 60 degrees of rotation of the involved arm.[8,83] The focus of this phase of rehabilitation after both mini-open and open repairs is to achieve near-normal ROM by means of continued assisted ROM, transition to active ROM, and initiation of limited strengthening exercises so that the operated arm can be used for selected functional activities. This phase *begins* no earlier than 4 to 6 weeks and often as late as 6 to 12 weeks depending on the strength and mobility of the repaired cuff.[8,25,49,105,133,134,184] The following goals and interventions are appropriate during this phase of rehabilitation.

- ***Restore near-normal, nonpainful, passive mobility of the shoulder.***
  - Continuation of self-assisted ROM with an end-range hold by means of wand or pulley exercises, in single plane and combined (diagonal) patterns.
- Mobilization of the incision site if well-healed.

Precaution: The use of passive stretching and grade III joint mobilizations, if initiated during this phase of rehabilitation, must be done very cautiously. Vigorous stretching is not routinely considered safe for about 3 to 4 months, that is, until after the repaired tendons have healed and have become reasonably strong.[105,184]

- ***Increase strength, stability, and endurance and restore dynamic control of the shoulder musculature.***
  - Transition to active ROM of the shoulder through gradually increasing ranges
  - Isometric and dynamic strengthening to key scapulothoracic stabilizers

- Submaximal multiple-angle isometrics against very gradually increasing resistance to rotator cuff and other GH musculature[49]
- Dynamic strengthening and endurance training of the GH musculature against light resistance, begun at about 8 to 12 weeks[105,133,134]
- Use of the involved upper extremity for *light* (no-load or low-load) functional activities at 6 weeks after a mini-open repair and delayed until 12 weeks after an open repair

Note: Since weakness and atrophy of the supraspinatus and infraspinatus muscles were probably present prior to injury, strengthen the rotator cuff before dynamically strengthening the shoulder abductors and flexors.

Precaution: Dynamic strengthening in this phase is only appropriate after a mini-open repair, not an open repair.

Exercise: Minimum Protection/ Return to Function Phase

Criteria to move into the final phase of rehabilitation and gradually return to unrestricted activities include full, pain-free ROM, progressive improvement of shoulder strength and a stable GH joint.[83] This phase usually begins no earlier than 3 to 4 months postoperatively for patients with strong repairs but as late as 4 to 5 months for tenuous repairs.[49,83,184] If full ROM has not been restored with active-assistive and active exercises, passive stretching of the GH musculature and joint mobilization is now typically initiated. Advanced strengthening activities dominate this phase of rehabilitation. Patients may not be allowed to return to full activities for 6 months or possibly 1 year postoperatively depending on the patient's level of comfort, strength, and flexibility as well as the demands of the desired activities.

The goals and interventions in this final phase of rehabilitation are consistent with those previously discussed for late-stage nonoperative management of cuff disorders and for the final phase of rehabilitation after subacromial decompression. However, the progression of activities is more gradual and the time frame for adhering to precautions is extended after mini-open and open repairs.

Outcomes

Because the etiology and severity of rotator cuff tears are so diverse, the results of rotator cuff repair are also variable. Both mini-open (arthroscopically assisted) and traditional open repairs result in comparably favorable functional outcomes and pain relief with small to medium size tears (<3 cm).[9,68,105] Patients who have undergone a mini-open repair return to functional activities earlier (about a month earlier in one study) than those who have had an open repair.[9] This outcome may be skewed by the fact that mini-open repairs are performed more often in younger patients with less severe tears. During postoperative rehabilitation, although gains in strength continue to occur for a year, the most substantial gains are seen in the first 6 months. In most cases, patients achieve 80% strength in the operated shoulder (compared to noninvolved shoulder) at 6 months and 90% at 1 year.[144] Early follow-up of patients who have undergone arthroscopic repair is promising and appears to yield similar results.[58,161] In addition, immediate postoperative pain is significantly less, and the cosmetic outcome is more favorable with an arthroscopic repair.[58,161]

Repairs of acute tears in young patients are more successful than repairs of chronic cuff impingement and insufficiency in elderly patients (over age 65 years).[64] Other factors that are directly related to more favorable cuff repair outcomes are smaller size tears and fewer associated impairments and pathologies, such as a biceps tendon tear or joint instability.[105] There is inconsistent evidence whether there is a direct relationship between the integrity of the repair and functional outcomes.[67]

Shoulder Dislocations

Related Diagnoses and Mechanisms of Injury

Traumatic Anterior Shoulder Dislocation

There is complete separation of the articular surfaces of the glenohumeral joint caused by direct or indirect forces applied to the shoulder.[127] Anterior dislocation most frequently occurs when there is a blow to the humerus while it is in a position of external rotation and abduction. Stability normally is provided by the subscapularis, glenohumeral ligament, and long head of the biceps when in that position.[92,143,172] Poor integrity of any of these structures can predispose the joint to dislocation, or a significant blow to the arm may damage them along with the attachment of the anterior capsule and glenoid labrum (Bankart lesion). When dislocated, the humeral head usually rests in the subcoracoid region, rarely subclavicular or intrathoracic. Traumatic anterior dislocation is usually associated with a complete rupture of the rotator cuff. Neurologic or vascular injuries may occur during dislocations.[65] The axillary nerve is most commonly injured, but the brachial plexus or one of the peripheral nerves could be stretched or compressed.

Traumatic Posterior Shoulder Dislocation

This injury is less common. Most posterior dislocations are subacromial, although subglenoid or subspinous posterior dislocations may occur. The mechanism of injury is usually a force applied to the humerus that combines flexion, adduction, and internal rotation, such as a fall on an outstretched arm.[152] The person will complain of symptoms when doing activities such as push-ups, bench press, or follow-through on a golf swing.[65]

Recurrent Dislocation

With significant ligamentous and capsule laxity, unidirectional or multidirectional recurrent subluxations or dislocations may occur with any movement that reproduces the abduction and external rotation forces or the flexion, adduction, and internal rotation forces, causing significant pain and functional limitation. Some individuals can voluntarily dislocate the shoulder anteriorly or posteriorly without apprehension and with minimal discomfort.[127,152] The group in which the rate of recurrence after first traumatic dislocation is highest is the younger population (<30 years). Because they are more active and place greater demands on the shoulder, longer immobilization (>3 weeks) is advocated after dislocation than in the less than 30-year-old patient. Shorter immobilization (1–2 weeks) is advocated for older patients.[104,107]

Common Impairments

- After an acute traumatic injury, symptoms from tissue damage include pain and muscle guarding from bleeding and inflammation.
- When a dislocation is associated with a complete rotator cuff tear, there is an inability to abduct the humerus against gravity, except the range provided by the scapulothoracic muscles.
- Asymmetric joint restrictions/hypermobilities. In an anterior instability, the posterior capsule may be tight; in a posterior instability, the anterior capsule may be tight. After healing, there may be adhesions.
- With recurrent dislocations, the individual can dislocate the shoulder at will, or the shoulder may just dislocate when doing specific activities. Instabilities, as described previously in this chapter, are present.

Common Functional Limitations/Disabilities

- With rotator cuff rupture, inability to reach or lift objects to the level of horizontal, thus interfering with all activities using humeral elevation
- Possibility of recurrence when replicating the dislocating action
- With anterior dislocation, restricted ability in sports activities such as pitching, swimming, serving (tennis, volleyball), spiking (volleyball)
- Restricted ability, particularly when overhead or horizontal abduction movements are required in dressing, such as putting on a shirt or jacket, and with self-grooming, such as combing the back of the hair
- Discomfort or pain when sleeping on the involved side in some cases
- With posterior dislocation, restricted ability in sports activities such as follow-through in pitching and golf; restricted ability in pushing activities, such as pushing open a heavy door or pushing one's self up out of a chair or out of a swimming pool

Nonoperative Management: Dislocations

Management: Protection Phase After Closed Reduction of Anterior Dislocation

Note: Reduction manipulations should be undertaken only by someone specially trained in the maneuver because of the vulnerability of the brachial plexus and axillary blood vessels.

Protect the Healing Tissue

- After acute anterior dislocation in a young patient, the arm is immobilized for 3 to 4 weeks in a sling, which is removed only for exercise. During the first week, the patient's arm may be continuously immobilized because of pain and muscle guarding.
- An older, less active patient (over 40 years of age) may require immobilization for only 2 weeks.

- The position of dislocation must be avoided when exercising, when dressing, or doing other daily activities

Promote Tissue Health

Use protected ROM, intermittent muscle setting of the rotator cuff, deltoid, and biceps brachii muscles, and grade II joint techniques.

Precautions: In order not to disrupt healing of the capsule and other damaged tissues after anterior dislocation, ROM into external rotation is performed with the elbow at the patient's side, with the shoulder flexed in the sagittal plane, and with the shoulder in the resting position (in the plane of the scapula, abducted 55 degrees and 30 to 45 degrees anterior to the frontal plane), but not in the 90-degree abducted position. The forearm is moved from in front of the trunk (maximal internal rotation) to 0 or possibly 10 to 15 degrees external rotation. Extension beyond 0 degrees is contraindicated.

- Intermittent muscle setting of the rotator cuff, deltoid, and biceps brachii muscles
- Grade II joint techniques: Maintain joint play by using sustained grade II distraction or gentle grade II oscillations with the glenohumeral joint at the side or in the resting position (see Fig. 6–13).

Management: Controlled Motion Phase After Closed Reduction of Anterior Dislocation

Provide Protection

The patient continues to wear the sling for 3 weeks, then increases the time the sling is off; the sling is used when the shoulder is tired or if protection is needed.

Increase Shoulder Mobility

- Begin mobilization techniques using all appropriate glides except the anterior glide. The anterior glide is ***contraindicated*** even though external rotation is necessary for functional elevation of the humerus. To safely stretch for external rotation, place the shoulder in the resting position (abducted 55 degrees and horizontally adducted 30 degrees), then externally rotate it to the limit of its range, and then apply a grade III distraction force perpendicular to the treatment plane in the glenoid fossa (Fig. 9–8).
- Passively stretch the posterior joint structures with horizontal adduction self-stretching techniques.

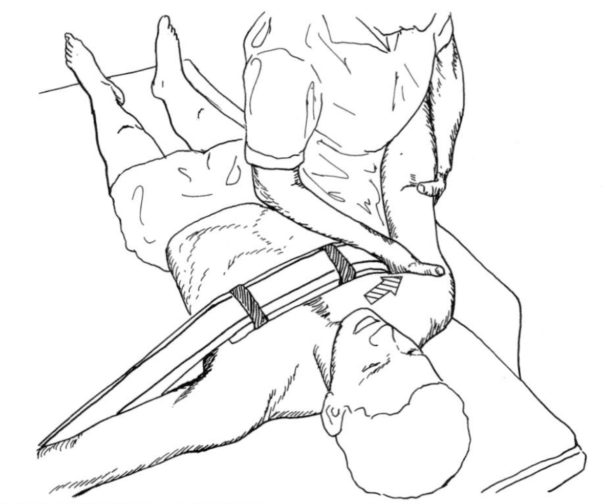

Figure 9–8 Mobilizing to increase external rotation when an anterior glide is contraindicated. Place the shoulder in resting position, externally rotate it, then apply a grade III distraction force.

Increase Stability and Strength of Rotator Cuff and Scapular Muscles

Both the internal and external rotators need to be strengthened as healing occurs.[26] The internal rotators and adductors must be strong to support the anterior capsule. The external rotators must be strong to stabilize the humeral head against anterior translating forces and to participate in the deltoid-rotator cuff force couple when abducting and laterally rotating the humerus. Scapular stability is important for normal shoulder function.

- Begin with *isometric resistance* exercises with the joint positioned at the side and progress to various pain-free positions within the available ranges.
- Initiate closed-chain, partial weight-bearing, and stabilization exercises.
- Progress to *dynamic resistance,* limiting external rotation to 50 degrees and avoiding the position of dislocation.
- At 3 weeks, begin supervised *isokinetic resistance* for internal rotation and adduction at speeds 180 degrees per second or higher.[7] Position the patient standing with the arm at the side or in slight flexion and elbow flexed 90 degrees. The patient performs internal rotation beginning at the zero

position with the hand pointing anteriorly and moving across the front of the body. Progress to positioning the shoulder at 90 degrees flexion, then perform the exercise from zero to full internal rotation. Do not position in 90 degrees abduction.

- By 5 weeks, all shoulder motions are incorporated into exercises on isokinetic or other mechanical equipment except in the position of 90 degrees abduction with external rotation.

Return to Function Phase After Anterior Shoulder Dislocation

Restore Functional Control

- Develop a balance in strength of all shoulder and scapular muscles.
- Develop coordination between scapular and arm motions.
- Develop endurance for each exercise as previously described for shoulder instabilities.
- As stability improves, progress eccentric training to maximum load, increase speed and control, and progress to simulating desired functional patterns for activity.

Return to Maximum Function

- Help the patient learn to recognize signs of fatigue and impingement and stay within the tolerance of the tissues.
- The patient can return to normal activities when there is no muscle imbalance, when good coordination of skill is present, and when the apprehension test is negative. Full rehabilitation takes 2 1/2 to 4 months.[7]

Management After Posterior Dislocation of the Shoulder with Closed Reduction

The management approach is the same as anterior dislocation with the exception of avoiding the position of flexion with adduction and internal rotation during the acute and healing phases.

Protect the Part

The arm is immobilized. A sling may be uncomfortable because of the adducted and internally rotated position, particularly if the sling elevates the humerus so the head translates in a superior and posterior direction. The patient may be more comfortable with the arm hanging freely in a dependent position while kept immobile.

Increase Limited Ranges

Begin joint mobilization techniques using all appropriate glides except the posterior glide. Posterior glide is ***contraindicated.*** If adhesions develop, preventing internal rotation, mobility can safely be regained by placing the shoulder in the resting position (abducted 55 degrees and horizontally adducted 30 degrees), internally rotating it to the limit of its range, and then applying a grade III distraction force perpendicular to the treatment plane in the glenoid fossa (same as Fig. 9–8 but with the arm internally rotated).

Glenohumeral Joint Instabilities: Surgical and Postoperative Management

Indications for Surgery

The following are common indications for surgical stabilization of the GH joint.[76,104,106,107,165,179]

- Recurrent episodes of GH joint dislocation or subluxation, which impairs functional activities
- Unidirectional or multidirectional instability during active shoulder movements that causes apprehension of placing the arm in positions of potential dislocation and, hence, compromises use of the arm for functional activities
- Instability-related impingement (secondary impingement syndrome) of the shoulder
- Significant inherent joint laxity resulting in recurrent instability
- High probability of subsequent episodes of instability after an acute dislocation in young patients involved in high-risk (overhead), work-related or sport activities
- Dislocations associated with significant cuff tears
- Failure to resolve the instability and restore function with nonoperative management

Procedures

Procedures designed to improve stability and prevent recurrent instability, while maintaining near-normal rotation of the GH joint, are performed today using either an arthroscopic or open approach. An open stabilization is done if an open reduction is required or if extensive damage to surrounding structures has also occurred.[104,106,133,165] These procedures, which are designed to balance stabilization of the anterior, posterior, or inferior portions of the capsule with retention of functional mobility, can be organized into several categories.

- ***Capsulorrhaphy*** is a tightening of the capsule *(capsular shift)* to reduce capsular redundancy and overall capsule volume by incising, overlapping (imbrication) and then suturing, tacking, or stapling the lax or overstretched portion of the capsule.* A capsular shift procedure is tailored to the direction(s) of instability: anterior, inferior, posterior, or multidirectional (anteroinferior or posteroinferior). For example, if a patient has recurrent anterior instability, an anterior capsular shift is performed. The anterior portion of the capsule is incised, tightened by imbrication, and resutured. This can be done using an arthroscopic or open approach.† Posterior capsulorrhaphy, a far less common procedure, is briefly described at the conclusion of this section.
- ***Electrothermally assisted capsulorrhaphy (ETAC)*** is an arthroscopic procedure that uses thermal energy (radio frequency thermal-delivery or nonablative laser) to shrink and tighten loose capsuloligamentous structures. The procedure (also referred to as a *thermal-assisted capsular shift*) can be done alone or in combination with other arthroscopic procedures, such as debridement of a partial rotator cuff tear or subacromial decompression.[48,53,106,167,173] It has been shown in animal and human cadaveric studies that thermal energy initially makes collagen fibrils more extensible, but as the collagen tissue of the capsuloligamentous structures heals, it shortens or "shrinks," thus causing a decrease in capsular laxity.[75,153] If one or more of the glenohumeral ligaments is detached or if rotator cuff lesions are detected that could be contributing to the instability, they are repaired arthroscopically prior to ETAC.
- ***Bankart reconstruction*** is an open or arthroscopic repair of a Bankart lesion (a detachment of the capsulolabral complex from the anterior rim of the glenoid), which commonly occurs during traumatic anterior dislocation. An anterior capsulolabral reconstruction involves reattachment of the labrum to the surface of the glenoid lip with bioabsorable tacks, direct sutures, or suture anchors.‡ This is sometimes combined with a capsular shift if capsular laxity is present. In an open repair, access to the lesion and capsule is through the subscapularis tendon (which must then be repaired) or through the rotator cuff interval, which allows the subscapularis to remain intact.[3,104,106] In an arthroscopic repair, multiple portal sites are used. Generally, more secure fixation is achieved with an open repair than with an arthroscopic repair.
- ***Soft tissue transfers.*** Open transfer and realignment of the subscapularis tendon *(Putti-Platt or Magnuson-Stack procedures)* to stabilize the anterior capsule is rarely done today, as they have resulted in poor functional outcomes because of significant loss of external rotation.[104,107,136]
- ***Bony procedures.*** Open transfer of the tip of the coracoid process to the anterior glenoid rim (with the short head of the biceps and the coracobrachialis still attached) to form a bony block *(Bristow procedure)* is only of interest from an historical perspective to understand how the management of recurrent anterior dislocation has evolved.[104,107] As with procedures involving transfer of the subscapularis, the Bristow procedure also resulted in a significant loss of external rotation.
- ***Repair of a SLAP lesion.*** A tear of the proximal attachment of the biceps and the superior labrum is classified as a SLAP (superior labrum anteroposterior) lesion.[133,165] Some SLAP lesions are associated with recurrent anterior glenohumeral instability. The lesion is debrided arthroscopically, and the torn portion of the superior labrum and biceps anchor are reattached with tacks or suture anchors. A concomitant anterior stabilization is also performed if instability is present.
- ***Posterior capsulorrhaphy (posterior or posteroinferior capsular shift).*** Recurrent, involuntary posterior or posteroinferior instabilities, if treated surgically, are managed with an open or arthroscopic stabilization procedure to tighten the capsule if the capsule is lax.§ In addition, plication and advancement of the infraspinatus to reinforce the posterior capsule may also be necessary. Shoulders without an effective posterior glenoid can be surgically managed with labral reconstruction or, occasionally, with a glenoid osteotomy. In these procedures, a posterior incision is made, the deltoid is split, and the infraspinatus, teres minor, and posterior capsule are incised.[137,166] In some instances of a traumatic mul-

*See references 3, 16, 62, 81, 104, 106, 107, 189.
†See references 3, 34, 35, 62, 81, 107, 127, 189.
‡See references 3, 5, 34, 35, 59, 81, 104, 133, 146.
§See references 17, 73, 76, 104, 106, 137, 165, 166.

tidirectional instability, an anterior approach is used even if the predominant instability appears to be posterior.[104,137]

- ***In summary,*** GH stabilization procedures may be performed with an open or arthroscopic approach for correction of unidirectional or multidirectional instabilities. Associated procedures such as a repair of the rotator cuff may also be required.

Postoperative Management

General Considerations

As with rehabilitation after repair of rotator cuff tears, guidelines for postoperative management of recurrent instability of the GH joint are based on many factors. The factors that can influence the composition and progression of a postoperative program are summarized in Table 9–4. Additional factors, such as philosophy and training of the surgeon and several patient-related variables (general health, medications, preinjury functional status and postoperative goals, education, and compliance), and their potential impact have already been discussed in Table 9–2 are common to postoperative rehabilitation after rotator cuff repair and GH stabilization. As such, no additional discussion of these common factors and their influence is included in this section on postoperative management of instabilities.

The guidelines in this section address *general* principles of management across the three broad phases of postoperative rehabilitation after a variety of surgical stabilization and reconstruction procedures for recurrent, unidirectional, or multidirectional glenohumeral instabilities. These general guidelines cannot begin to address the many variations of postoperative management of shoulder instabilities that therapists encounter. Many detailed protocols or case-based descriptions of rehabilitation of different patient populations, specific types of instabilities or associated labral lesions, and different stabilization or reconstructive surgeries have been documented extensively in the literature.* These protocols can be used to complement the general guidelines in this section that apply to postoperative rehabilitation of the more common types of surgical stabilization procedures.

In many instances traumatic and atraumatic instabilities of the shoulder are coupled with lesions (tears) of the rotator cuff tendons. For example, it is

*See references 25, 48, 83, 88, 89, 106, 123, 173, 184.

Table 9–4 Factors that Influence the Rehabilitation Program After Surgery for Recurrent Instability of the GH Joint

Factors	Potential Impact on Rehabilitation
• Onset of instability	• Capsular redundancy and greater risk of recurrent dislocation is more often associated with atraumatic instability, which requires more conservative postoperative rehabilitation than stabilization of recurrent instability of traumatic origin.[104]
• Severity of associated lesions	• The more severe the underlying pathology, the slower the progression of rehabilitation.
• Previous failure of a surgical stabilization procedure	• Slower progression after previous failed surgery.
• Direction of instability	• Stabilization of anterior instability: more rapid advancement than after stabilization of posterior or multidirectional instabilities.[137]
• Type of surgical approach	• Open stabilization or reconstruction: more rapid advancement than after arthroscopic procedures because of more secure methods of tissue fixation.[184]
• Type of procedure	• Thermally assisted capsulorrhaphy: slower progression than open capsular tightening.[48,173] • Bony reconstruction: slower progression than after soft tissue reconstruction.
• Patient variables –tissue integrity –preoperative status of dynamic stabilizers –generalized joint laxity	• The progression of postoperative rehabilitation is conservative for the inactive patient with multidirectional atraumatic instability who has generalized joint laxity and poor preoperative strength of the dynamic stabilizers.

estimated that the incidence of a tear of the rotator cuff tendons in the older patient (over 40 years of age) who experiences an anterior dislocation is at least 85%.[88] Consequently, many patients who undergo surgery for recurrent instability of the shoulder will also require a repair of the rotator cuff. Therefore, the postoperative guidelines after rotator cuff repair already outlined in this chapter must also be considered when treating a patient after a surgical stabilization of the GH joint.

Always keep in mind that regardless of the type of instability or associated pathology or choice of surgical procedure, the focus of rehabilitation must always be to *prevent recurrence of shoulder instability* while restoring an adequate level of strength and mobility to meet the patient's functional needs.

Immobilization

Position. The position in which the patient's shoulder is immobilized after surgery is determined by the *direction(s) of instability* prior to surgery. After surgical reconstruction for recurrent *anterior or anteroinferior* instability, the shoulder is immobilized in a sling or splint in adduction (or slight abduction) and internal rotation (forearm across the abdomen) with the arm slightly anterior to the frontal plane of the body.[81,104] After surgery for *posterior or posteroinferior* instability the upper extremity is immobilized and supported in an orthosis in the "handshake" position (neutral rotation, 20–30 degrees of abduction and sometimes slight extension of the shoulder).[51,104,137]

Duration. The duration of immobilization, that is, the period of time before use of the immobilizer is completely discontinued, is determined by the surgeon and ranges from 1 to 3 weeks to as long as 6 to 8 weeks. Continuous immobilization of the operated shoulder (before shoulder ROM can be initiated) is usually maintained for only a day to a few days or up to 1 to 2 weeks unless a bony procedure has been performed. These time frames are dependent upon many of the same factors, summarized in Table 9–4, that influence all aspects of postoperative rehabilitation. For example, the duration of immobilization is usually shorter for an elderly patient than for a young patient because the elderly patient is more likely to develop postoperative shoulder stiffness than the younger patient.[104] Posterior or multidirectional instabilities usually require a longer period of immobilization than an anterior instability to minimize the risk of recurrence.[104,137,166] With recurrent posterior instability the shoulder may be continuously immobilized and ROM delayed for up to 6 weeks postoperatively.[88] The more extensive the soft tissue or bony reconstruction, the longer the immobilization.

Exercise

The decisions of when the arm may be temporarily removed from the immobilizer to begin shoulder exercises and to what extent specific shoulder motions are either permissible or contraindicated are also based on many of the factors summarized in Table 9–4. As with postoperative management of other surgical procedures, close communication between therapist and surgeon and careful patient education are both imperative for optimal postoperative outcomes.

The overall goal of postoperative exercise is to develop strength and stability as well as mobility of the shoulder consistent with functional needs while preventing recurrence of the instability. Specific goals and interventions for each phase of rehabilitation are essentially the same as those already outlined for postoperative management of primary impingement of the shoulder and rotator cuff tears and nonoperative management of recurrent instabilities. Therefore, it is appropriate to include the same variations of exercises in a postoperative program after surgical stabilization of the shoulder while implementing special precautions for specific surgeries. Precautions, particularly during the early weeks of rehabilitation after different types of stabilization procedures, are noted in Box 9–8.

Exercise: Maximum Protection Phase

Protection of the capsule that has been tightened or of reinforced and repaired structures, such as the labrum, is necessary for about 6 weeks. The goals and exercises for the maximum protection phase are summarized in the following section. Some additional precautions are also noted. Use of prescribed medications and modalities for pain control are indicated during this phase of rehabilitation.

- ***Control pain.***
  - Active ROM of the cervical spine and shoulder relaxation exercises.
  - Grade I and II joint mobilizations avoiding motions in the direction of the preoperative instability.
- ***Prevent or correct postural malalignment,*** especially excessive thoracic kyphosis. Emphasize spinal extension and scapular retraction.

Box 9–8 Summary of Precautions During Early Rehabilitation After Surgical Stabilization of the GH Joint

Anterior Stabilization Procedure

- Limit elevation of the arm to 90 to 100 degrees during the initial phase of rehabilitation.
- Limit *ER, horizontal abduction,* and *extension* during maximum protection phase (up to 6 weeks postoperatively). Recommendations for initial limitation of ER vary from 0 degrees (no ER past neutral),[104] 15 to 20 degrees,[83] and up to 40 degrees[123] depending on the type of pathology, surgical procedure, and intraoperative evaluation of shoulder stability. Progress these motions cautiously.
- Avoid positioning and activities that place stress on the anterior aspect of the capsule for about 4 to 6 weeks.
  - Avoid functional activities that require ER, especially if combined with horizontal abduction during early rehabilitation as when reaching to put on a coat or shirt.
  - Avoid upper extremity weight bearing particularly if the shoulder is extended as when pushing up from the armrests of a chair.

Repair of Bankart Lesion

- Progress rehabilitation more cautiously after an arthroscopic repair than after an open repair.[184]
- Avoid resisted IR for approximately 4 weeks, particularly after arthroscopic reconstruction, to avoid rupture of the subscapularis.[59]

Posterior Stabilization Procedure

- Limit elevation of the arm to 90 degrees during early rehabilitation.
- Limit IR to neutral or 15 to 20 degrees and horizontal adduction during maximum protection phase (up to 6 weeks postoperatively).
- Restrict upper extremity weight bearing, particularly when the shoulder is flexed, to avoid stress to the posterior aspect of the capsule, for example, during closed-chain scapulothoracic and GH stabilization exercises and functional activities for at least 6 weeks postoperatively.

Thermally Assisted Capsular Tightening

- Postpone initiation of ROM of the shoulder for approximately 10 days to 2 weeks, because collagen in the thermally treated capsuloligamentous structures is initially more extensible (more vulnerable to stretch) until it heals.[106,173]

Bony Reconstruction

- Delay passive or assisted ROM for 6 to 8 weeks to allow bony healing.

- ***Prevent loss of mobility in the involved upper extremity*** while protecting the tightened or reconstructed capsule.
  - Active ROM of the elbow, forearm, wrist, and fingers the day after surgery.
  - Active scapulothoracic movements.
  - While seated, remove the sling (if permissible) and rest the forearm on a table with the shoulder positioned in slight flexion and abduction and neutral rotation.
  - Self-assisted ROM, wand exercises, and nonweighted pendulum exercises for the GH joint, initially *within protected ranges,* but gradually to near-normal ROM by 6 to 8 weeks, except for external rotation after an anterior stabilization and internal rotation after a posterior stabilization procedure. Begin shoulder rotation with the arm in a slightly abducted and flexed position.[88,184]

Note: Shoulder motion is begun when temporary removal of the immobilizer is permitted. This may be as soon as the day after surgery for selected patients who have had an anterior stabilization procedure,[83] but more often is begun 1–2 weeks postoperatively.[88,123] Remember, ROM is delayed for a longer period of time after a thermally assisted stabilization[48,53,173] or a posterior stabilization procedure.[51,88,137] Generally, motion can be progressed slightly more rapidly after an open stabilization than after an arthroscopic stabilization because stabilization of the capsule tends to be more secure by direct suturing in an open procedure than by bioabsorbable tacks in an arthroscopic procedure.[184]

- ***Develop control and strength of scapulothoracic, elbow, wrist, and hand musculature.***
  - Isometric and dynamic strengthening exercises

Precaution: Initially strengthen the scapular stabilizing muscles in an open-chain to avoid the need for weight bearing on the operated upper extremity. When weight-bearing activities are initiated, be cautious about the position of the operated shoulder to avoid undue stress to the vulnerable portion of the capsule for about 6 weeks postoperatively.

- ***Prevent inhibition and atrophy of GH musculature.***
  - Multiple angle muscle-setting exercises (very gentle isometrics) of GH musculature as early as the first week or by 3 to 4 weeks postoperatively after some procedures.[83]

Precaution: Be particularly cautious with musculature that has been torn or surgically detached, incised, or advanced and then repaired. Resistance to the subscapularis, which is longitudinally split during an anterior approach, may need to be delayed as long as 6 weeks.[59,123]

  - Use of the operated arm for *unresisted, nonweight-bearing, waist-level* functional activities by 2 to 4 weeks postoperatively.

- Possible initiation of dynamic exercises against *light* resistance below shoulder level at 4 to 6 weeks. Emphasize the GH stabilizers. During internal and external rotation position the arm at the side, slightly anterior to the frontal plane or in the plane of the scapula.

Note: In some cases dynamic exercises against light resistance are often delayed until 6 to 8 weeks when only moderate protection is necessary.

Exercise: Moderate Protection/Controlled Motion Phase

This phase of rehabilitation begins between 6 and 8 weeks postoperatively and continues until approximately 12 to 16 weeks. The focus is on achievement of normal active (unassisted) ROM of the shoulder, continued development of strength and endurance of scapulothoracic and GH musculature, and progressive use of the upper extremity through greater ranges of motion for functional activities. Goals and interventions include the following as well as those activities already suggested for nonoperative management.[25,83,106,123,184]

- ***Restore full, pain-free ROM of the shoulder*** by 8 to 12 weeks except in motions limited by the specifics of the surgery.
  - Continuation of active ROM.
  - Stretching and grade III mobilizations in positions that do not provoke instability. After an anterior stabilization procedure for chronic (atraumatic) anterior instability, pay particular attention to increasing horizontal adduction, as the posterior structures are often tight preoperatively and continue to be tight postoperatively.
- ***Continue to increase strength, endurance, stability, and control of shoulder musculature*** through available ROM.
  - Progression of dynamic strengthening to overhead positions if strength of dynamic stabilizers is adequate.

Precautions: *After a posterior stabilization* do not initially begin dynamic strengthening of the external rotators from full internal rotation. *After anterior stabilization,* do not initiate dynamic strengthening of the internal rotators from full external rotation, particularly in the 90-degree abducted position. When strengthening the shoulder extensors, *do not extend the arm posterior to the frontal plane.* Therefore, strengthen the extensors in prone with the arm over the side of the table or standing and leaning forward with the hips flexed to approximately 90 degrees. Use the same precaution when strengthening the horizontal abductors and adductors. In addition, maintain the shoulder in neutral rotation during horizontal abduction and adduction.

  - Upper extremity ergometry with a portable reciprocal exerciser on a table or with the UBE® for muscular endurance. Include forward and backward motions.
  - Progressive upper extremity weight bearing during strengthening and stabilization exercises.
  - Dynamic strengthening in diagonal and simulated functional movement patterns.

Exercise: Minimum Protection/ Return to Function Phase

Criteria to progress to this final phase of rehabilitation and the focus of exercise are similar to criteria already discussed for rehabilitation after rotator cuff repair. This phase usually begins as early as 10 to 12 weeks postoperatively or as late as 16 to 18 weeks, depending on individual characteristics of the patient and the surgical procedure. Participation in desired work-related and sports activities often takes up to 6 months postoperatively.

Precautions: Some patients may have permanent restrictions placed on functional activities that involve high-risk movements and that could potentially cause recurrence of the instability. After some anterior stabilization procedures, full ER in 90 degrees of abduction may not be advisable or possible.

Outcomes

A successful postoperative outcome involves regaining the ability to participate in desired functional activities without a recurrence of instability of the GH joint. Follow-up studies measure subjective and objective outcomes such as restoration of ROM and strength, rate of recurrence of pain, apprehension or instability, ability to participate in desired activities, and general patient satisfaction. Rates of recurrent instability (dislocation, subluxation, and/or apprehension) and patient satisfaction vary substantially from study to study. For example, reported rates of recurrent instability after anterior stabilization procedures range from 0 to 30%.[104]

Although results of surgery and postoperative rehabilitation are usually reported for specific pathologies, patient populations, and surgical stabilization procedures and are determined by means of a variety of outcome measures, a few generalizations can be made.

- Surgical stabilization of a recurrent unidirectional anterior instability yields better results than stabilization of posterior or multidirectional instabilities.[17,104,137,189]
- Recurrent instability of traumatic origin responds more favorably to surgical management than atraumatic instabilities.[17,104] In addition, the rate of recurrence of anterior instability over 5 years after repair of a Bankart lesion is as low as 1%.[104]
- Rate of recurrence of instability is substantially higher in young patients (younger than 20–30 years of age) or patients who return to high-demand, competitive overhead sports than elderly patients (older than 40–50 years of age).[104,106,133]
- The rate of recurrence of instability is also higher after an arthroscopic stabilization than after an open stabilization, most likely because of a higher rate of problems with arthroscopic fixation techniques than open fixation techniques. The rate of recurrence of posterior instability after arthroscopic stabilization has been reported to be particularly high, up to 30 to 40%.[166]
- After some anterior stabilization procedures, full ER or horizontal abduction is sometimes not advisable or possible.[88] Likewise, some posterior stabilization procedures permanently limit full IR and, to some degree, overhead elevation of the arm.[104]
- Although the rate of progression early on in a rehabilitation program is slightly more rapid after open stabilization procedures than after comparable arthroscopic procedures (because fixation is more secure in open procedures), the period of time required to return to full physical activity is comparable.[88,104]
- Early follow-up of patients who have undergone thermally assisted anterior stabilization is encouraging,[53,106] but long-term outcomes are not yet available.

Thoracic Outlet Syndrome

The thoracic outlet is the region along the pathway of the brachial plexus from just distal to the nerve roots exiting the intervertebral foramen to the lower border of the axilla. The outlet is bordered medially by the scalenus anterior, medius, and posterior and first rib; posteriorly by the upper trapezius and scapula; anteriorly by the clavicle, coracoid, pectoralis minor, and deltopectoral fascia; and laterally by the axilla. The plexus enters the outlet between the scalenus anterior and medius; the subclavian artery runs posterior to the scalenus anterior; and the subclavian vein runs anterior to the scalenus anterior. The blood vessels join the brachial plexus and course together under the clavicle, over the first rib, and under the coracoid process posterior to the pectoralis minor. Vascular and/or neurologic symptoms that are not consistent with nerve root or peripheral nerve dermatome and myotome patterns should lead the therapist to suspect thoracic outlet problems.[96]

Related Diagnoses

Thoracic outlet syndrome (TOS) encompasses many diagnoses that involve upper extremity neurological and vascular symptoms including pain, paresthesia, numbness, weakness, discoloration, swelling, ulceration, gangrene, and in some cases, Raynaud's phenomenon. Diagnoses that have been used to describe TOS include cervical rib, scalenus anticus syndrome, costoclavicular syndrome, subcoracoid-pectoralis minor syndrome, droopy shoulder syndrome, and hyperabduction syndrome.*

Etiology of Symptoms

Walsh[177] has identified three causative factors that could be interrelated or exist separately: compressive neuropathy, faulty posture, and entrapment.

Compressive Neuropathy

Compression of the neurovascular structures can occur if there is a decrease in the size of the area through which the brachial plexus and subclavian vessels pass. Compression can occur from muscle hypertrophy in the scalenes or pectoralis minor, anatomic anomalies such as cervical rib or fractured clavicle, adaptive shortening of fascia, or a space-occupying lesion.

Faulty Posture

Changes in posture, particularly forward head with increased thoracic kyphosis, protracted scapulae,

*See references 40, 52, 130, 156, 159, 160, 177.

and forward shoulders narrow the spaces through which the neurovascular structures pass. Specifically, adaptive shortening of the scaleni and pectoralis minor muscles can potentially compress the neurovascular tissues or can cause repetitive trauma and adhesions with overuse.

Entrapment of the Neural Tissue from Scar Tissue or Pressure

Entrapment affects the ability of nerve tissue of the brachial plexus to tolerate tension as it courses through the various tissues in the thoracic outlet.

Location of Compression or Entrapment and Tests of Provocation

There are three primary sites for compression or entrapment of the neurovascular structures.

Interscalene Triangle, Bordered by the Scalenus Anterior and Medius Muscles and First Rib

If these muscles are hypertrophied, tight, or have anatomic variations they may compress the proximal portion of the brachial plexus and subclavian artery. Inflammation from overuse can lead to adhesions preventing normal mobility of the neural tissues with head and arm movements.

Symptoms from dysfunction in this area are reproduced with Adson's maneuver, which stretches the scalene muscles and places tension on the nerves. If the artery is compressed, there will also be a decreased pulse.[99] Palpation of the scalene muscles may also provoke symptoms.

Costoclavicular Space Between the Clavicle Superiorly and the First Rib Inferiorly

Compression of the neurovascular bundle can occur between the clavicle and first rib especially if the clavicle is depressed for periods of time as occurs when carrying a heavy suitcase or shoulder bag or with a faulty, slouched posture. A fractured clavicle or anomalies in the region can also lead to symptoms. An elevated first rib, which can occur with a first rib subluxation, or with upper thoracic breathing (as with asthma or chronic emphysema) will also narrow the costoclavicular space.

Symptoms caused by a depressed clavicle are reproduced when the shoulders are retracted and depressed as with the Military Brace Test.[99] If, when in this posture, a patient is asked to take in a breath and symptoms are reproduced, the rib elevation is causing the symptoms.

Axillary Interval Between the Anterior Deltopectoral Fascia, the Pectoralis Minor, and the Coracoid Process

Compression or restricted movement of the neurovascular structures may occur in this region if the pectoralis minor is tight from a faulty posture with the scapula tipped forward or from repetitive overuse.

Holding the arms in an elevated position places a stretch on the lower branches of the brachial plexus and blood vessels. If there is poor neurovascular mobility and tension is placed on the brachial plexus, a patient will have reproduction of symptoms when the arm is abducted. In addition, if the person does repetitive opening and closing of the hand and there is increased ischemic pain (Roos test),[99] there is vascular compromise. Palpation pressure against the pectoralis minor will reproduce the neurological symptoms if the muscle is tight.

Restricted Nerve Mobility

Restricted mobility of nerve roots or portions of the brachial plexus from scar tissue adhesion secondary to trauma and inflammation may cause symptoms when tension is placed on the nerves. The Halstead test[99] elongates portions of the brachial plexus and may obliterate the radial pulse, thus reproducing TOS symptoms. This test is similar to the upper limb tension test for the median nerve[30] and, therefore, may indicate restricted nerve gliding or tension.

Summary of Contributing Factors

There is a wide latitude of motion in the various joints of the shoulder complex that may result in compression or impingement of the nerves or vessels.

- ***Postural variations,*** such as a forward head or round shoulders, lead to associated muscle tightness in the scalene, levator, subscapularis, and pectoralis minor muscles and a depressed clavicle.
- ***Respiratory patterns*** that continually use the action of the scalene muscles to elevate the upper ribs lead to hypertrophy of these muscles. Also, the elevated upper ribs decrease the space under the clavicle.
- ***Congenital factors*** such as an accessory rib, a long transverse process of the C-7 vertebra, or other anomalies in the region can reduce the space for the vessels. A traumatic or arteriosclerotic insult can also lead to TOS symptoms.
- ***Traumatic injuries*** such as clavicular fracture or subacromial dislocations of the humeral head can

injure the plexus and vessels, leading to TOS symptoms.

- ***Hypertrophy or scarring*** in the pectoralis minor muscles can lead to TOS symptoms.
- ***Injuries*** that result in inflammation, scar tissue formation, and adhesions can restrict nerve tissue mobility when tension is placed on the nerve. This may occur anywhere from the intervertebral foramina at the spine to the distalmost portion of the peripheral nerve. There will be nerve tension signs from restricted mobility.

Common Impairments

- Intermittent brachial plexus and vascular symptoms of pain, paresthesia, numbness, weakness, discoloration, and swelling.
- Muscle length-strength imbalances in the shoulder girdle with tightness in anterior and medial structures and weakness in posterior and lateral structures.
- Faulty postural awareness in the upper quarter.
- Poor endurance in the postural muscles.
- Shallow respiratory pattern, characterized by upper thoracic breathing.
- Poor clavicular and anterior rib mobility.
- Nerve tension symptoms when the brachial plexus is placed on a stretch.

Common Functional Limitations/Disabilities

- Sleep disturbances that could be from excessive pillow thickness or arm posture.
- Inability to carry briefcase, suitcase, purse with shoulder strap, or other weighted objects on the involved side.
- Inability to maintain prolonged overhead reaching position.
- Inability to do sustained desk work, cradling a telephone receiver between head and involved shoulder, and driving a car.

Nonoperative Management

If the symptoms demonstrate that there is inflammation, treatment is first directed at eliminating the provoking mechanism and to control the inflammation. The primary emphasis of management is to decrease the mechanical pressure by increasing mobility of tissues in the thoracic outlet region, preventing recurrence of the compression loads by correcting the postural alignment, and developing endurance to maintain the correct posture.[10,177]

Patient Education

Teach the patient how to modify or eliminate provoking postures and activities, as well as introducing a home exercise program. Emphasize the importance of compliance to reduce the stresses on the nerve or vascular structures.

Mobilize Restricted Nerve Tissue

Use nerve mobilization maneuvers if nerve tension tests are positive. These are described in Chapter 15.

Increase Flexibility in Tight Structures

Use manual and self-stretching techniques. Common problems include but are not limited to the scalene, levator scapulae, pectoralis minor, pectoralis major, anterior portion of the intercostals and short suboccipital muscles, and to the sternoclavicular joint.

Train Weak Muscles

Develop a program to develop strength, endurance, and postural awareness. Common weaknesses include but are not limited to scapular adductors and upward rotators, shoulder lateral rotators, short anterior throat cervical flexor muscles, and thoracic extensors. Techniques for cervical exercises and posture correction are discussed in Chapter 16.

Correct a Faulty Respiratory Pattern and Elevated Upper Ribs

Teach diaphragmatic breathing patterns and relaxation exercises to relax the upper thorax (see Chapter 19).

Progress to Functional Independence

Determine activities that provoke the symptoms, and involve the patient in adapting the environment and faulty habits to minimize the stress.

▶ Reflex Sympathetic Dystrophy

Related Diagnoses and Symptoms

Reflex sympathetic dystrophy (RSD) is classified as a subcategory of the diagnosis Complex Regional Pain Syndrome (CRPS type I).[176] Common synonyms of

RSD include shoulder-hand syndrome, Sudeck's atrophy, sympathetically mediated pain syndrome, reflex neurovascular dystrophy, traumatic angiospasm or vasospasm, and sympathetically maintained pain (SMP).[31,158,176]

Etiology and Symptoms

The underlying mechanism that stimulates onset of this condition is unclear. It develops in association with a persistent painful lesion such as a painful shoulder after a cardiovascular accident or myocardial infarction, cervical osteoarthritis, trauma such as a fracture or sprain, or after cardiac catheterization. The condition can last for months or years, but spontaneous recovery often occurs in 18 to 24 months. Three stages are identified.

Stage I: Reversible stage. This stage of vasodilation lasts 3 weeks to 6 months. Pain is the predominant feature, usually out of proportion to the severity of the injury. There is hyperhidrosis, warmth, erythema, rapid nail growth, and edema in the hand.

Stage II: Dystrophic or vasoconstriction stage. This stage lasts 3 to 6 months. It is characterized by sympathetic hyperactivity, burning pain, and hyperesthesia exacerbated by cold weather. There is mottling and coldness, brittle nails, and osteoporosis.

Stage III: Atrophic stage. This stage is characterized by pain either decreasing or becoming worse and by severe osteoporosis. Muscle wasting and contractures may occur.

Common Impairments

- Pain or hyperesthesia at the shoulder, wrist, or hand out of proportion to the injury.
- Limitation of motion develops. Typically, the shoulder develops limitation in a capsular pattern with most restriction in lateral rotation and abduction. In the wrist and hand, the most common restrictions are limited wrist extension and metacarpophalangeal and proximal interphalangeal flexion.
- Edema of the hand and wrist secondary to circulatory impairment of the venous and lymphatic systems, which, in turn, precipitates stiffness in the hand.
- Vasomotor instability.
- Trophic changes in the skin.

As the condition progresses, pain subsides but limitation of motion persists. The skin becomes cyanotic and shiny, intrinsic muscles of the hand atrophy, subcutaneous tissue in the fingers and palmar fascia thicken, nail changes occur, and osteoporosis develops.

Management

This is a progressive disorder unless vigorous intervention is used. The best intervention is prevention when it is recognized that development of RSD is a possibility, such as when there has been trauma to the shoulder. It requires that the therapist motivate the patient to safely move the entire upper extremity, minimize edema and vascular stasis with elevation and hand activity, and be alert to the development of adverse symptomology.

Medical intervention is a necessity to manage this syndrome. The physician may choose to block the sympathetic stimuli with sympatholytic drugs, local anesthetic blocks, stellate ganglion blocks, or upper thoracic sympathectomy, or may use oral steroids or intramuscular medication. This is done in conjunction with therapeutic exercise to interrupt the sympathetic response and manage impairments and functional limitations.

Educate the Patient

Emphasize the importance of following the program of increased activity.

Increase ROM of the Shoulder and Hand

Use techniques specific to the limiting structures and work within the pain-free range. Do not stretch when painful, or the symptoms may be exacerbated.

Facilitate Active Muscle Contractions

Use both dynamic and isometric exercise and controlled closed-chain activities for neuromuscular control as well as afferent fiber stimulation.

Relieve Pain

Use modalities such as ultrasound, vibration, transcutaneous electrical nerve stimulation (TENS), or ice.

Control Edema

Apply intermittent pneumatic compression and massage. Elevate and use elastic compression when not receiving the pneumatic compression treatment.

Desensitize the Area

Utilize desensitization techniques for brief periods five times per day, such as having the patient work with various textures, tap or vibrate over the sensitive area. The patient is instructed to wear a protective glove during activities of daily living.

► Exercise Techniques for Management During Acute and Early Subacute Stages of Tissue Healing (Protection and Early Controlled Motion Phases of Intervention)

During the *protection* and *early controlled motion* phases of intervention, when inflammation is present or just beginning to resolve and the healing tissues should not be stressed, some early motion may be utilized to inhibit pain and muscle guarding and help prevent deleterious effects of complete immobilization. This section describes and summarizes techniques that may be used for these purposes. During the acute and early subacute stages, when motion in the shoulder itself is limited to allow tissues to begin to heal, it is also valuable to treat associated areas such as the cervical and thoracic spine, the scapulae, and the remainder of the upper extremity (elbow, wrist, and hand) to begin correcting faulty posture, relieve stresses to the shoulder girdle, and prevent fluid stasis in the extremity.

General guidelines for management during the acute stage are described in Chapter 8, and specific precautions for various pathologies and surgical interventions in the shoulder are identified throughout the previous sections of this chapter. Early motion is usually passive (PROM) and applied within the pain-free range. When tolerated, active-assistive range of motion (A-AROM) is utilized.

Early Motion of the Glenohumeral Joint

Manual PROM and A-AROM techniques are described in detail in Chapter 2. This section expands on self-assisted exercises.

Wand Exercises

Several wand exercises are described in Chapter 2. Additional suggestions include:

- Initiate A-AROM using a cane, wand, or T-bar in the supine position to provide stabilization and control of the scapula during the protection and early controlled motion phases. Motions usually included are flexion, abduction, flexion in the plane of the scapula (scaption), and rotation (Fig. 9–9*A*).
- If it is necessary to relieve stress on the anterior capsule, such as following surgical repair of the capsule or labrum, place a folded towel under the humerus to position the humerus anterior to the midline of the body when the patient performs internal or external rotation (Fig. 9–9*B*).
- When treating a shoulder impingement (primary or secondary), have the patient grasp the wand with the forearm supinated when flexing and abducting to emphasize external rotation.

Ball Rolling or Dusting a Table Top

Patient position and procedure: Sitting with the arm resting on a table and hand placed on a 6- to 8-inch ball or towel and the shoulder in the plane of the scapula. Have the patient initiate gentle circular motions of the shoulder by moving the trunk forward, backward, and to the side allowing the hand to roll the ball or "dust the table." As pain subsides, have

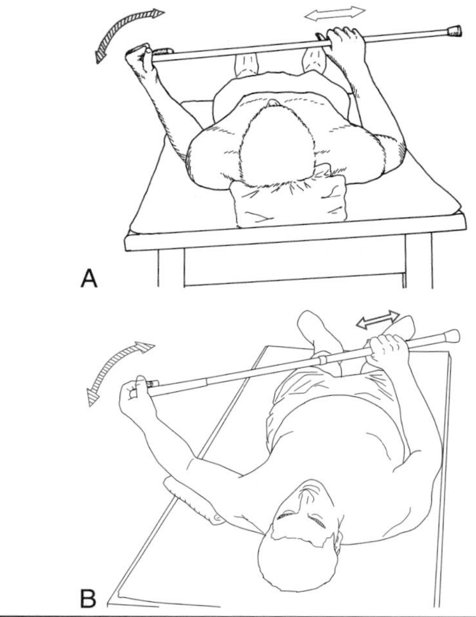

Figure 9–9 Self-assisted shoulder rotation using a cane *(A)* with the arm at the side and *(B)* in scaption. To relieve stress on the anterior capsule, elevate the distal humerus with a folded towel.

the patient use the shoulder muscles to actively move the ball or cloth through greater ROMs.

Pendulum (Codman's) Exercises

Patient position and procedure: Standing, with the trunk flexed at the hips about 90 degrees. The arm hangs loosely downward in a position between 60 and 90 degrees flexion or scaption (Fig. 9–10).

- A pendulum or swinging motion of the arm is initiated by having the patient move the trunk slightly back and forth. Motions of flexion, extension, and horizontal abduction, adduction, and circumduction can be done.[36] Increase the arc of motion as tolerated. This technique should not cause pain.
- If patients cannot balance themselves leaning over, have them hold on to a solid object or lie prone on a table.
- If the patient experiences back pain from bending over, use the prone position.
- Adding a weight to the hand or using wrist cuffs causes a greater distraction force on the glenohumeral joint. Weights should be used only when joint stretching maneuvers are indicated late in the subacute and chronic stages—and then only if the scapula is stabilized by the therapist or a belt is placed around the thorax and scapula, so that the stretch force is directed to the joint, not the soft tissue of the scapulothoracic region.

Precautions: Some patients may get dizzy when standing upright after being bent over; if so, have them sit and rest. With increased pain or decreased ROM, the technique may be an inappropriate choice. Pendulum exercises are also inappropriate for a patient with peripheral edema.

"Gear Shift" Exercises

Patient position: Sitting with the involved arm at the side, holding a cane or wand with the tip resting on the floor to support the weight of the arm. Instruct the patient to move the pole forward and back, diagonally, or laterally and medially in a motion similar to shifting gears in a car with a floor shift (Fig. 9–11).

"Table Dusting" or "Wall Washing"

Patient position: Standing with hand placed on a table or against a wall (on a towel or ball). Instruct the patient to perform clockwise and counterclockwise circular motions with the hand moving on the table or wall or rolling the ball. Progress this activity by having the patient reach upward and outward as far as tolerated without causing symptoms.

Early Motion of the Scapula

Passive and A-AROM of the scapula are described in Chapter 2. In the acute phase, the side-lying position

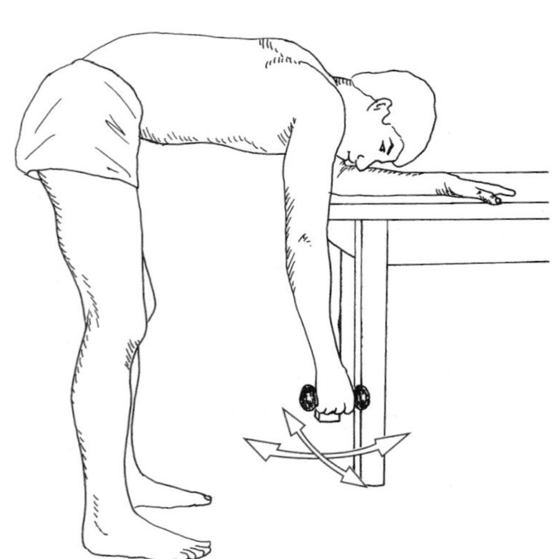

Figure 9–10 Pendulum exercises. For gentle distraction, no weight is used. Use of a weight causes a grade III (stretching) distraction force.

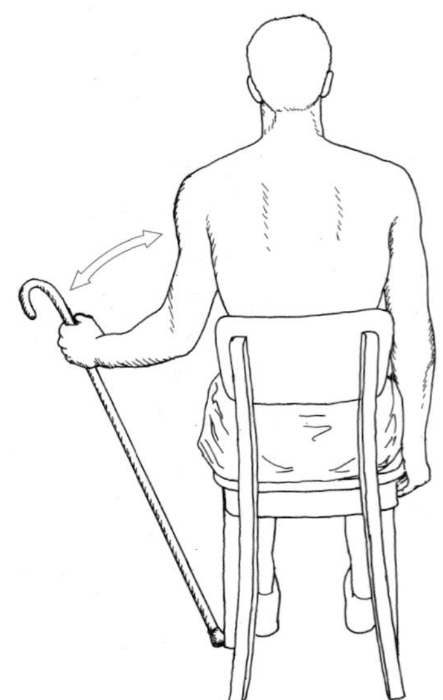

Figure 9–11 Gear shift exercise. Self-assisted shoulder rotation using a cane. Flexion/extension and diagonal patterns can also be done.

is usually more comfortable than prone-lying. If the patient can perform active scapular elevation/depression and protraction/retraction, use the sitting position.

Early Neuromuscular Control

Frequently, the muscles of the rotator cuff are inhibited after trauma or surgery.[182] Initiate the following to stimulate activation and develop control in key muscles as soon as the patient tolerates.

Multiple-Angle Muscle Setting

Begin gentle multiple-angle muscle-setting exercises of the rotators internal and external in pain-free positions of humeral flexion or scaption. Activate the scapular and rest of the glenohumeral muscles with gentle muscle-setting techniques in positions that do not exacerbate symptoms.

Closed-Chain or Protected Weight Bearing

Have the patient lean onto his or her hands or elbows and gently move from side to side. This helps to seat the humeral head in the glenoid fossa and stimulate muscle action.

▶ Exercise Techniques to Increase Flexibility and Range of Motion

To regain neuromuscular control and function in the shoulder girdle, it may be necessary to increase flexibility in restricted muscles and fascia so that proper shoulder girdle alignment and functional ranges are possible. Techniques to stretch tight joints in the shoulder girdle were discussed earlier in this chapter. Principles of inhibition and passive stretching were presented in Chapter 5. Specific manual and self-stretching techniques are described in this section.

Self-Stretching Techniques

Teach the patient a low-intensity prolonged stretch. Emphasize the importance of not bouncing at the end of the range.

To Increase Horizontal Flexion/Adduction—Cross-Chest Stretch

Patient position and procedure: Sitting or standing. Teach the patient to horizontally adduct the tight shoulder by placing the arm across the chest and then apply a sustained overpressure to the adducted arm by pulling the arm toward the chest being careful not to rotate the trunk (Fig. 9–12).

Note: This stretch is used when treating impingement syndromes to increase mobility in the structures of the posterior GH joint.

To Increase Flexion and Elevation of the Arm

Patient position and procedure: Sitting with the involved side next to the table, forearm resting along the table edge and elbow slightly flexed (Fig. 9–13*A*). Have the patient slide the forearm forward along the table while bending from the waist. Eventually the head should be level with the shoulder (Fig. 9–13*B*).

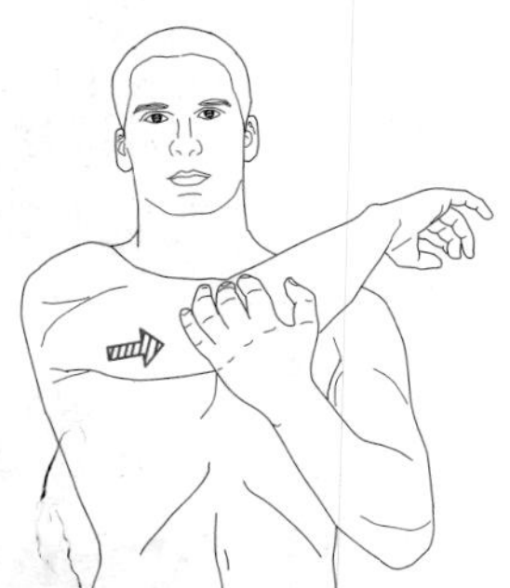

Figure 9–12 Self-stretching to increase horizontal adduction.

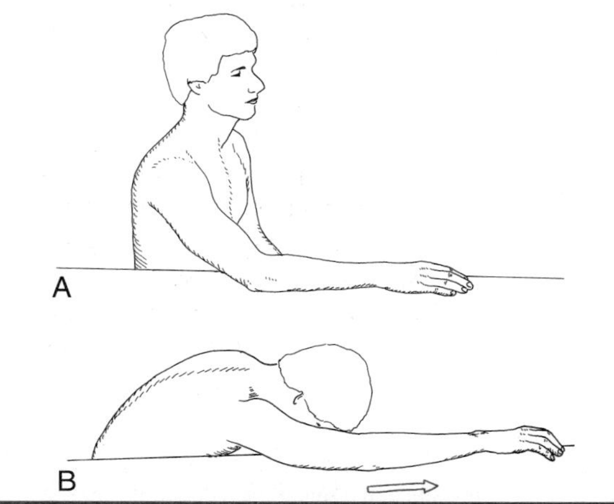

Figure 9–13 *(A)* Beginning and *(B)* end positions for self-stretching to increase shoulder flexion with elevation.

To Increase External (Lateral) Rotation

- Patient position and procedure: Standing and facing a doorframe with the palm of the hand against the edge of the frame and elbow flexed 90 degrees. While keeping the arm against the side or in slight abduction (held in abduction with a folded towel or small pillow under the axilla) have the patient turn away from the fixed hand (Fig. 9–14*A*).
- Patient position and procedure: Sitting with his or her side next to a table with the forearm resting on the table and elbow flexed to 90 degrees. Have the patient bend from the waist, bringing the head and shoulder level with the table (Fig. 9–14*B*).

Precaution: Avoid this stretch position if there is anterior GH instability.

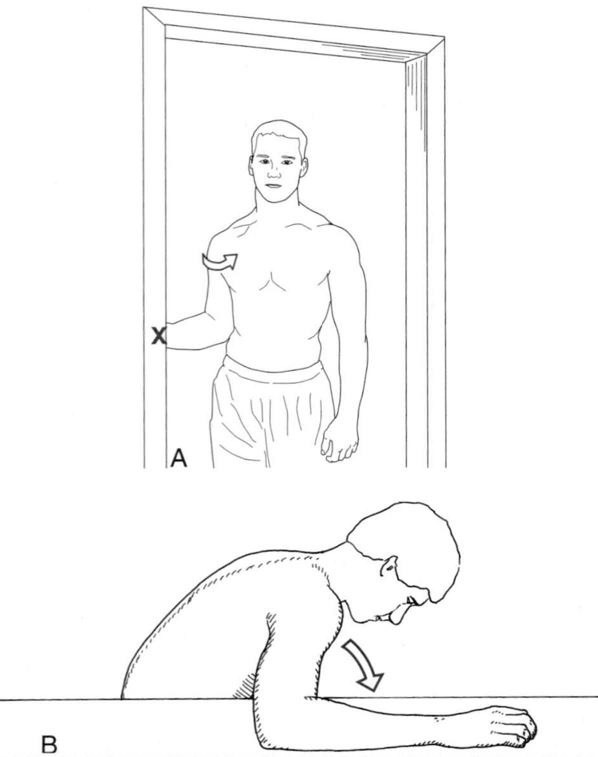

Figure 9–14 Self-stretching to increase lateral rotation of the shoulder *(A)* with the arm at the side using a doorframe and *(B)* with the arm in scaption, using a table to stabilize the forearm.

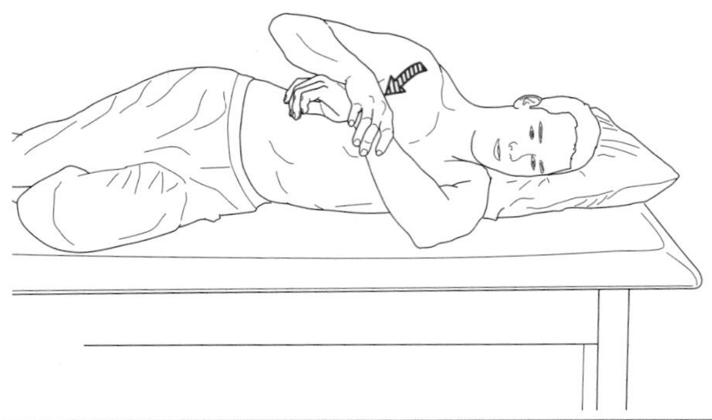

Figure 9–15 Self-stretching to increase internal rotation of the shoulder using a table to stabilize the humerus.

To Increase Internal Rotation

- Patient position and procedure: Standing facing a doorframe with the elbow flexed to 90 degrees and the back of the hand against the frame. Have the patient turn his or her trunk toward the fixed hand.
- Patient position and procedure: Side-lying on the affected side, with the shoulder and elbow each flexed to 90 degrees and arm internally rotated to end position. Have the patient then push the forearm toward the table with the opposite hand (Fig. 9–15).

To Increase Abduction and Elevation of the Arm

- Patient position and procedure: Sitting with the side next to a table, the forearm resting with palm up (supinated) on the table and pointing toward the opposite side of the table (Fig 9–16*A*). Have the patient slide his or her arm across the table as the head is brought down toward the arm and the thorax moves away from the table (Fig. 9–16*B*).
- Patient position and procedure: Same as above with a folded towel or belt placed across the proximal humerus and held in the opposite hand. Have the patient pull downward on the towel to cause a caudal slide of the humeral head when in the end-range stretch position of abduction.

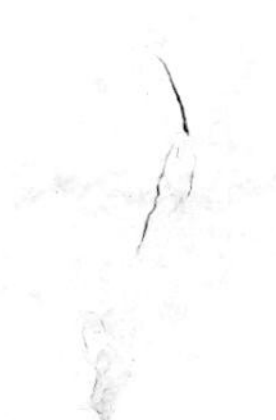

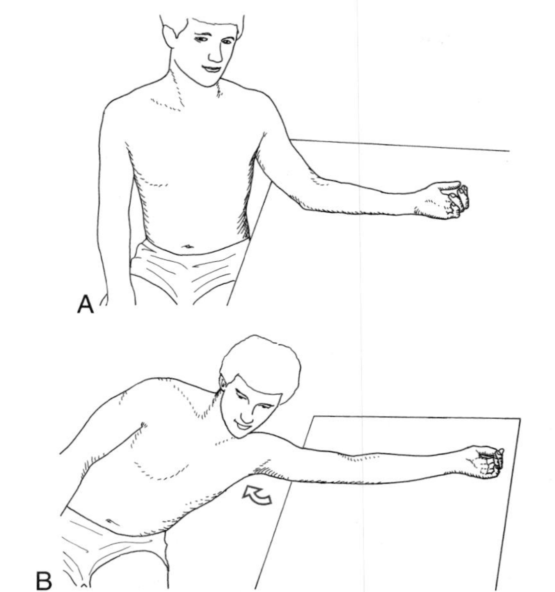

Figure 9–16 *(A)* Beginning and *(B)* end positions for self-stretching to increase shoulder abduction with elevation.

To Increase Extension of the Arm

Patient position and procedure: Standing with the back to the table, both hands grasping the edge with the fingers facing forward (Fig. 9–17*A*). Have the patient begin to squat while letting the elbows flex (Fig. 9–17*B*).

Precaution: If a patient is prone to anterior subluxation or dislocation, this stretching technique should not be done.

To Increase Internal Rotation, Extension and Scapular Tipping (Towel or Wand Stretch)

Patient position and procedure: Sitting or standing. Instruct the patient to hold each end of a towel (or wand) with one arm overhead and the arm to be stretched behind the lower back, and then pull up on the towel with the overhead hand (see Fig. 9–3).

Precaution: If a patient has anterior or multidirectional GH joint instability, or has had recent anterior stabilization surgery to correct a dislocated shoulder, this exercise should not be done because it forces the head of the humerus against the anterior capsule.

Note: This stretch is used to increase the ability to reach behind the back. It is a generalized stretch that does not isolate specific tight tissues. Before using it, each component of the motion should be stretched so that no one component becomes the "weak link" in the chain.

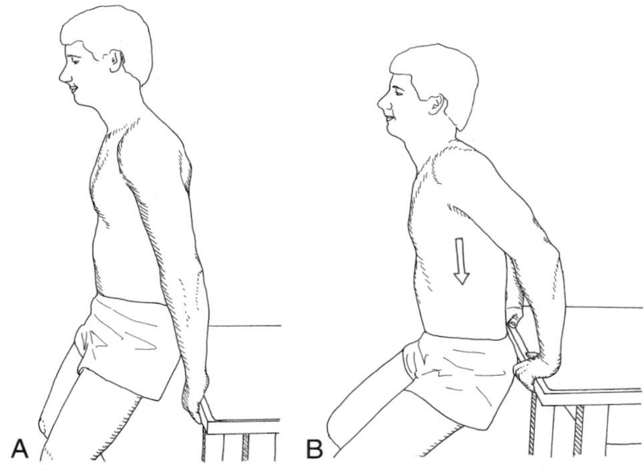

Figure 9–17 *(A)* Beginning and *(B)* end positions for self-stretching to increase shoulder extension.

Manual and Self-Stretching Exercises for Specific Muscles

General manual stretching techniques to increase ROM were described and illustrated in Chapter 5. Specific multijoint muscles that affect alignment of the shoulder girdle that were not presented in Chapter 5 are presented in this section along with self-stretching techniques of these muscles.

To Stretch the *Latissimus Dorsi* Muscle

Manual Stretch

Patient position and procedure: Supine, with hips and knees flexed so the pelvis is stabilized in a posterior pelvic tilt. Provide additional stabilization to the pelvis with one hand, if necessary; with the other hand grasp the distal humerus and flex, laterally rotate, and partially abduct it to the end of the available range. Instruct the patient to contract into extension, adduction, and medial rotation while providing resistance for a hold-relax maneuver. During the relaxation phase, elongate the muscle.

Self-Stretch—Supine

Patient position and procedure: Hook-lying with the pelvis stabilized in a posterior pelvic tilt and the arms flexed, laterally rotated, and slightly abducted overhead as far as possible (thumbs pointing toward floor). Allow gravity to provide the stretch force. Instruct the patient to not allow the back to arch.

Self-Stretch—Standing

Patient position and procedure: Standing with back to a wall and feet forward enough to allow the hips and knees to partially flex and flatten the low back against the wall, and the arms in a "hold-up" position (abducted 90 degrees and laterally rotated 90 degrees if possible). Tell the patient to slide the back of the hands up the wall as far as possible without allowing the back to arch.

Note: This exercise is also used to strengthen the lower trapezius and serratus anterior as they upwardly rotate and depress the scapulae during humeral abduction.

To Stretch the *Pectoralis Major* Muscles

Manual Stretch

Patient position and procedure: Sitting on a treatment table or mat, with the hands behind the head. Kneel behind the patient and grasp the patient's elbows (Fig. 9–18). Have the patient breathe in as he or she brings the elbows out to the side (horizontal abduction and scapular adduction). Hold the elbows at this end-point as the patient breathes out. No forceful stretch is needed against the elbows, because the rib cage is elongating the proximal attachment of the pectoralis major muscles bilaterally. As the patient repeats the inhalation, again move the elbows up and out to the end of the available range, and hold as the patient breathes out. Repeat only three times in succession to avoid hyperventilation.

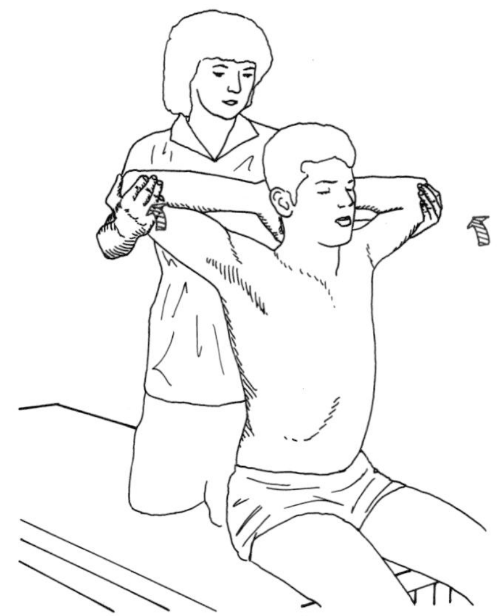

Figure 9–18 Active stretching of the pectoralis major muscle. The therapist holds the elbow at the end-point as the patient breathes out.

Note: Hyperventilation should not occur, because the breathing is slow and comfortable. If the patient does become dizzy, allow him or her to rest, then reinstruct for proper technique. Be sure the patient maintains the head and neck in the neutral position, not forward.

Corner Stretch

Patient position and procedure: Standing, facing a corner or open door, with the arms in a reverse T or a V against the wall (Fig. 9–19*A* and *B*). Have the patient lean the entire body forward from the ankles (knees slightly bent). The degree of stretch can be adjusted by the amount of forward movement.

Wand Exercises for Self-Stretch

Patient position and procedure: sitting or standing and grasping the wand with the forearms pronated and elbows flexed 90 degrees. Have the patient then elevate the shoulders and bring the wand behind the head and shoulders (Fig. 9–20). The scapulae are adducted and the elbows are brought out to the side. Combine with breathing by having the patient inhale as he or she brings the wand into position behind the shoulders, then exhale while holding this stretched position.

To Stretch the *Pectoralis Minor* Muscle

Patient position and procedure: sitting, place one hand posterior on the scapula and the other hand anterior on the shoulder, just above the coracoid process (Fig. 9–21). As the patient breathes in, tip the scapula posteriorly by pressing up and back against the coracoid process while pressing downward against the inferior angle of the scapula, and then hold it at the end-position while the patient breathes out. Repeat, readjusting the end-position with each inhalation, and stabilizing as the patient exhales.

To Stretch the *Levator Scapulae* Muscle

Note: The muscle attaches to the superior angle of the scapula and causes it to rotate downward and elevate; it also attaches to the transverse processes of the upper cervical vertebrae and causes them to backward bend and rotate to the ipsilateral side. Because the muscle is attached to two movable structures, both ends must be stabilized opposite to the pull of the muscle.

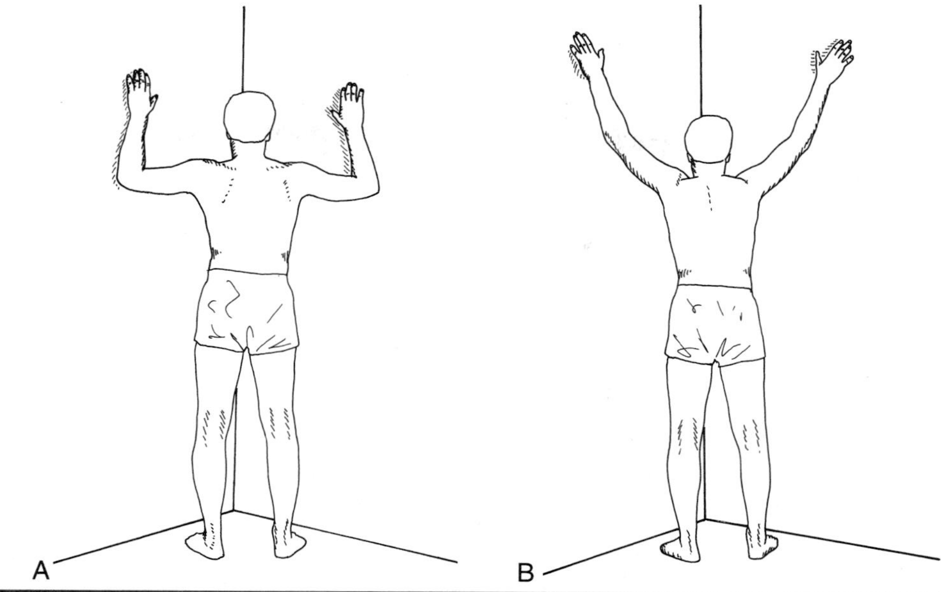

Figure 9–19 Self-stretching the pectoralis major muscle with the arms in a reverse T to stretch *(A)* the clavicular portion, and in a V to stretch *(B)* the sternal portion.

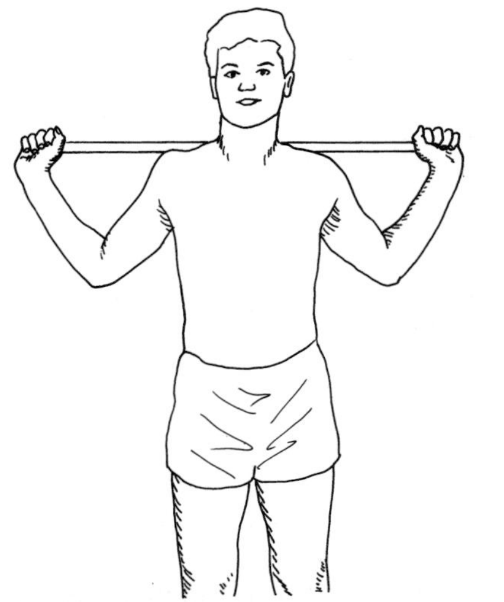

Figure 9–20 Wand exercises to stretch the pectoralis major muscle.

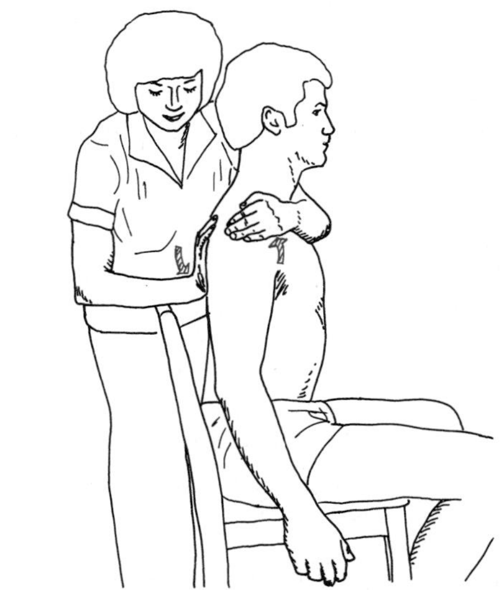

Figure 9–21 Active stretching of the pectoralis minor muscle. The therapist holds the scapular and coracoid process at the end-point as the patient breathes out.

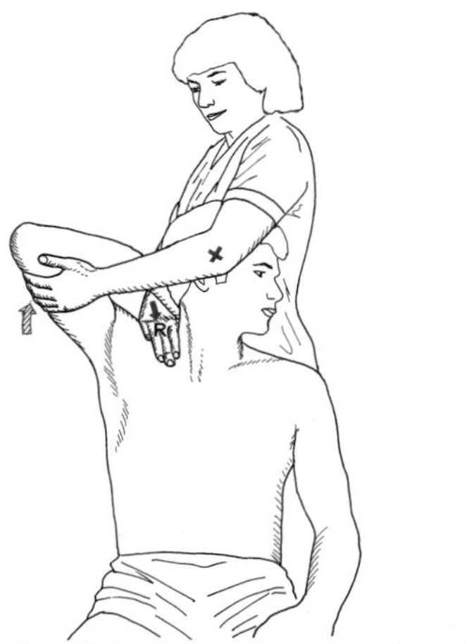

Figure 9–22 Active stretching of the levator scapulae muscle. The therapist stabilizes the head and scapula as the patient breathes in, contracting the muscle against the resistance. As the patient relaxes, the rib cage and scapula depress, which stretches the muscle.

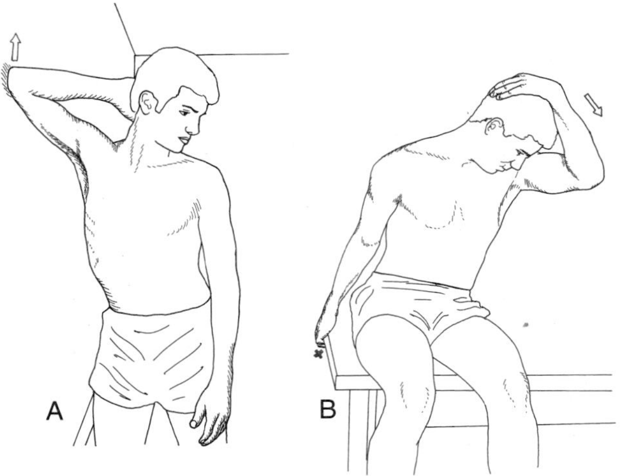

Figure 9–23 Self-stretching the levator scapulae muscle. *(A)* Using upward rotation of the scapula and *(B)* using depression of the scapula.

Manual Stretch

Patient position and procedure: sitting with the head rotated opposite to side of tightness (looking away from the tight side) and forward bent until a slight pull is felt in the posterolateral aspect of the neck (in the levator muscle). The arm on the side of tightness is abducted and the hand is placed behind the head to help stabilize it in the rotated position. Stand behind the patient and stabilize his or her head with one arm, and place the other hand (same side as tight muscle) over the superior angle of the scapula (Fig. 9–22). With the muscle now in its stretched position, have the patient breathe in, then out. Hold the shoulder and scapula down to maintain the stretch as the patient breathes in again (he or she contracts the muscle against the resistance of the fixating hand). To increase the stretch, press down against the superior angle of the scapula. This is not a forceful stretch but a gentle hold-relax maneuver. Do not stretch the muscle by forcing rotation on the head and neck.

Self-Stretch

Patient position and procedure: Standing with the head side bent and rotated away from the tight side and bent elbow against a wall. The other hand can be placed across the forehead to stabilize the rotated head. Instruct the patient to slide the elbow up the wall as he or she takes in a breath, then hold the position while exhaling (Fig. 9–23*A*).

Self-Stretch

Patient position and procedure: Sitting with head side bent and rotated away from the tight side. To stabilize the scapula, have the patient reach down and back with the hand on the side of tightness and hold on to the seat of the chair. The other hand is placed on the head to gently pull it forward and to the side in an oblique direction opposite the line of pull of the tight muscle (Fig. 9–23*B*).

▶ Exercises to Develop and Improve Muscle Performance and Functional Control

Developing control of the scapula and glenohumeral joint musculature is fundamental to correcting faulty shoulder mechanics and for improving strength, muscle endurance, power, and performance of functional activities. During observation of scapular alignment and movement, if excessive tipping, winging, or poorly coordinated scapulohumeral rhythm during humeral elevation is identified, it is important to correct these faulty mechanics with properly chosen exercises. Poor stabilization and control of GH rotation and translation during humeral elevation likewise requires concentration on training the rotator cuff musculature. When designing an exercise program, the intensity and type of exercises must not exceed the capability of the healing tissues whether the cause of the impaired control is nerve injury, disuse, traumatic insult, overuse, instability, or surgery.

Box 9–9 Summary of Exercise Progressions for the Shoulder

- Develop awareness and control of weak or disused muscles.
- If weak, begin with minimal resistance, multiangle isometrics and active-assistive ROM, open- and closed-chain (pain-free ranges).
- Develop postural stability of scapula and glenohumeral joint with stabilization exercises in both open- and closed-chain.
- Provide just enough resistance and repetitions to challenge the muscles.
- Do not allow substitution with stronger muscles.
- When stabilizing control develops in the scapula and GH muscles, progress to dynamic exercises.
- First strengthen weak motions and weak muscles so that substitute actions do not dominate; emphasize scapular and rotator cuff muscle control in open- and closed-chain.
- Develop muscle endurance and control.
- Progress to patterns of motion and train muscle groups to function in a coordinated sequence of control and motion.
- Use simple functional activities.
- Progress to more complex and challenging activities.

The exercises described in the following sections begin at the simplest or least stressful level and progress to a more difficult level for each type of exercise. They also progress from uniplanar or isolated muscle activity to more complex and functional patterns. Initially, choose exercises that help the patient focus on utilizing correct muscles to counteract the identified impairments; then increase the challenge by utilizing patterns of exercises that will prepare the musculature to respond to functional demands.* No matter what the level of exercise, it is important to challenge patients at intensities they can meet so they can safely progress to more intense levels. Chapter 3 describes principles and techniques of resistance exercises; it is important that the reader understands and applies these principles, as well as the principles of tissue healing described in Chapter 8, and precautions for various pathologies as presented in this chapter before teaching exercises to patients. This section describes shoulder exercises; see also Chapter 16 for correction of cervical and thoracic postural problems that might underlie faulty shoulder girdle mechanics. Improvement of muscle performance is multifactoral; Box 9–9 summarizes a method of progressing an individual toward functional recovery.

Isometric Exercises

Isometric exercises are applied along a continuum of very gentle, to maximum contraction, and they are applied at varying muscle lengths and joint angles. Choice of the intensity, muscle length, or joint angle and number or repetitions is based on strength, stage of recovery after injury or surgery, and/or pathomechanics of the region.

Scapular Motions

Patient position and procedure: Side-lying, prone-lying, or sitting, with the arm supported if necessary. Resist elevation, depression, protraction, or retraction with pressure directly on the scapula in the direction opposite the motion (Fig. 9–24).

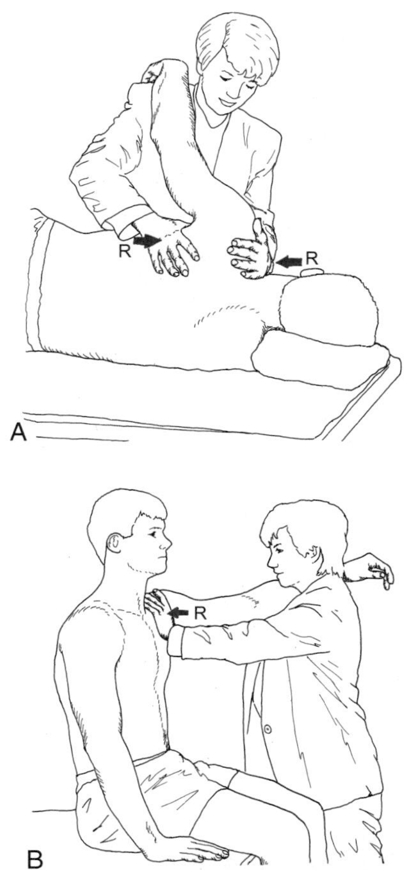

Figure 9–24 Isometric or dynamic manual resistance to scapular motions. *(A)* Resistance to elevation/depression. *(B)* Resistance to protraction/retraction. Direct the patient to reach across the therapist's shoulder to protract the scapula while the therapist resists against the coracoid and acromion process; the other hand is placed behind the scapula to resist retraction.

*See references 11, 20, 28, 44, 45, 82, 88, 90, 95, 101, 150, 171, 182.

Depression (lower trapezius). Activation of the lower trapezius is emphasized when there is forward tipping and delayed upward rotation often seen with impingement syndromes. Apply resistance against the inferior angle of the scapula (Fig. 9–24*A*).

Protraction (serratus anterior). Activation of the serratus anterior is emphasized when there is scapular winging or when there is delayed or incomplete upward rotation of the scapula with GH elevation. Apply resistance against the axillary border of the scapula or coracoid process, or indirectly against the humerus positioned in the plane of the scapula (Fig. 9–24*B*).

Retraction (rhomboids and trapezius). Activation of the rhomboids and trapezius muscle groups is emphasized when there the scapular posture is protracted (abducted). Apply resistance against the medial border of the scapula.

Multiple-Angle Isometrics to the GH Muscles

Patient position and procedure: Supine, sitting, or standing. During the protection and early motion phases of treatment when the tissue has symptoms of inflammation, use the supine position to provide scapular and trunk stability and manual resistance for the best control of position and intensity of resistance. If pain from joint compression occurs, apply a slight distractive force to the GH joint as the resistance is given.

Internal and external rotation. Position the humerus at the patient's side, in slight flexion, slight abduction, or scaption (plane of the scapula), and with the elbow flexed 90 degrees. Apply resistance against the forearm as if turning a crank (see Fig. 3–12*A*).

Abduction. Maintain the humerus neutral to rotation and resist abduction at 0, 30, 45, and 60 degrees. If there are no contraindications to motion above 90 degrees, preposition the humerus in external rotation before elevating the humerus and resisting above 90 degrees abduction.

Scaption. Position midway between flexion and abduction and resist at various ranges such as 30 and 60 degrees in the plane of the scapula (Fig. 9–25).

Extension. Position the humerus at the side or in various positions of flexion and apply resistance against the humerus.

Adduction. Position the humerus between 15 and 30 degrees abduction and apply resistance.

Elbow flexion with the forearm supinated. Position the humerus at the side and neutral to rotation. Apply resistance to the forearm, causing tension in the long head of the biceps (see Fig. 3–14). Change the position of shoulder rotation and repeat the isometric resistance to elbow flexion.

Self-Applied Multiple-Angle Isometrics

Teach the patient how to independently apply isometric resistance using positions and intensities consistent with therapeutic goals. The patient can use the opposite hand (Fig. 9–26) or a stationary object such as a wall or door frame (Fig. 9–27).

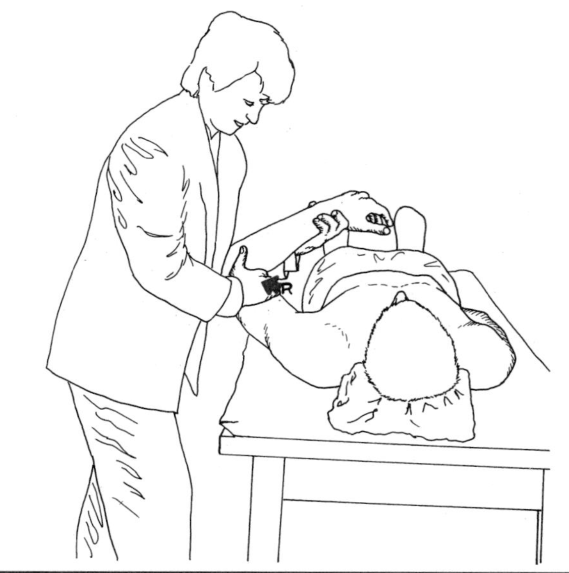

Figure 9–25 Isometric resistance in scaption. The shoulder is positioned between 30 and 60 degrees of scaption, and controlled manual resistance is applied against the humerus.

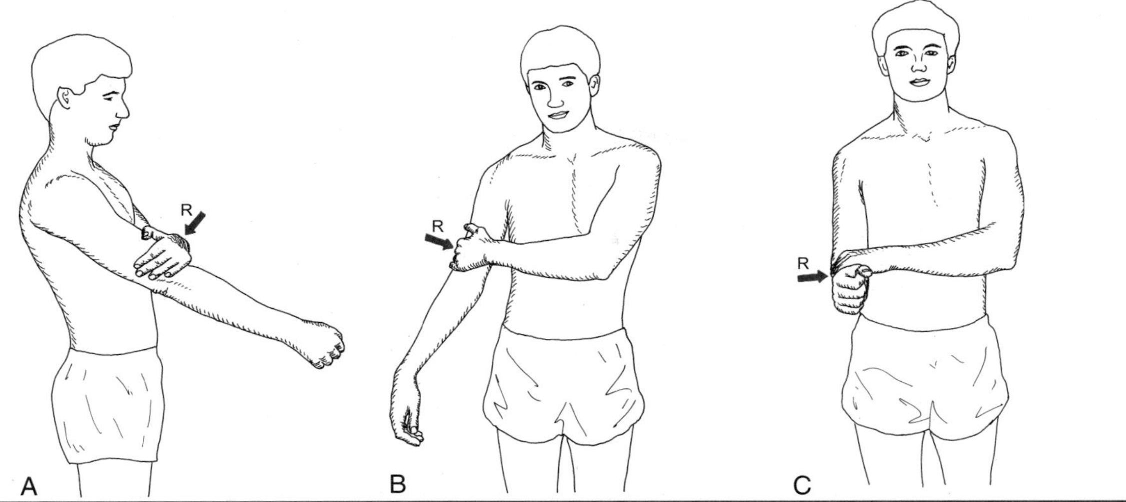

Figure 9–26 Self-resistance for isometric *(A)* shoulder flexion, *(B)* abduction, and *(C)* rotation.

Stabilization Exercises

The application of alternating isometrics and rhythmic stabilization techniques (described in Chapter 3) is designed to develop strength and stability of proximal muscle groups in response to shifting loads. The shoulder girdle functions in both open- and closed-chain activities, and therefore, the muscles should be trained to respond to both situations. Initially, apply the alternating resistance slowly and command the patient to "hold" against the resistance. At the beginning of training it may also be necessary to tell the patient which way you are going to push to help the patient focus on the contracting muscles and alternating forces. As the patient learns to respond by contracting the proper muscles and stabilizing the joints, increase the rapidity of the shifting resistance and also decrease the verbal warning so that the muscles learn to respond accordingly.

Begin training the scapular muscles so that when the muscles of the GH joint need to contract they will have a stable base (scapular stability).

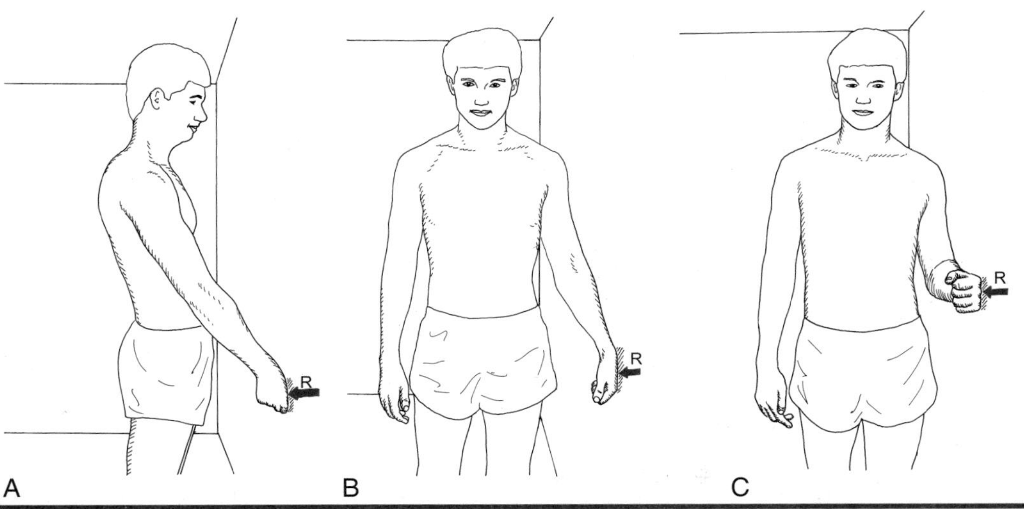

Figure 9–27 Using a wall to provide resistance for isometric *(A)* shoulder flexion, *(B)* abduction, or *(C)* rotation.

Open-Chain Stabilization Exercises for the Scapular Muscles

Begin with the patient side-lying, with the affected extremity up. Drape the forearm of the involved extremity over your shoulder. The degree of shoulder flexion, scaption, or abduction can be controlled by your stance and the relative position of the patient. Progress the patient to sitting with his or her arm draped over your shoulder; apply resistance to all scapular motions in the same manner as described previously.

Scapular elevation/depression. Place your top hand superiorly and the other hand inferiorly around the scapula to provide manual resistance (see Fig. 9–24*A*).

Scapular protraction/depression. Place your top hand along medial border and the other around the coracoid process to provide resistance (see Fig. 9–24*B*).

Scapular upward and downward rotation. Place one hand around the inferior angle and the other hand around the acromion and coracoid process to provide resistance.

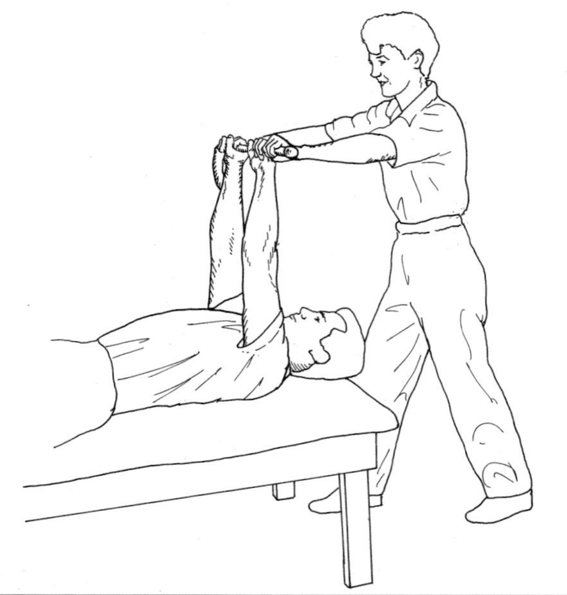

Figure 9–28 Stabilization exercises. The patient stabilizes with the shoulder girdle musculature (isometrically) against the resistance imposed by the therapist. Flexion/extension, abduction/adduction, and rotation resistance is applied in a rhythmic sequence.

Open-Chain Stabilization Exercises for the Shoulder Girdle

Patient position and procedure: Supine holding a rod or ball with elbows extended and shoulders flexed to 90 degrees. Stand at the patient's head and grasp the rod; instruct the patient to hold against or match the resistance you provide. Push, pull, and rotate the rod in various directions (Fig. 9–28). Resistance can also be applied directly against the arm or forearm.

- If too much assistance is being given by the normal extremity, apply the stabilization technique to just the involved extremity.
- As the patient gains control, progress to sitting and then standing, and have the patient hold the arm in various positions as the alternating resistance is applied. Observe the scapula to be sure there is good stabilization. If not, return to the exercises described above or decrease the intensity of resistance. Progress these exercises to functional patterns as strength and control improves.

Closed-Chain (Weight-Bearing) Stabilization Exercises

Weight bearing activates contraction of stabilizing muscles in proximal joints and may be a stimulus for improving fluid dynamics of the articular cartilage as described in Chapter 6. Early in the controlled motion phase of treatment (subacute stage), if the healing tissues tolerate, it may be beneficial to initiate protected weight-bearing stabilization exercises. The amount and intensity of weight bearing and resistance is progressed as tissues heal.

Note: If scapular winging is observed when the patient is weight bearing, do not progress these exercises until there is enough strength to stabilize the scapula against the rib cage.

Scapular stabilization. Patient position and procedure: Side-lying on uninvolved side. Both the elbow and shoulder of the involved arm are flexed to 90 degrees with the hand placed on the table and bearing some weight. Resist the scapular motions of elevation/depression and retraction directly against the scapula; resist protraction by pushing against the elbow.

Protected weight bearing. Patient position and procedure: Sitting with forearms resting on thighs or a table, or standing with arms resting on a table. Apply a gentle resistance force against the shoulders and ask the patient to match the resistance and "hold." Alternate from side to side and forward.

Closed-chain stabilization progressions. Patient position and procedure: Standing with shoulder at 90 degrees and one or both hands leaning against a wall or on a ball (Fig. 9–29). Additional, more advanced progressions include having the patient in the all-4s or quadruped position with hands on the floor, on a rocker or wobble board, or on a ball. The ball provides an unstable surface and requires greater neuromuscular control and balance reactions. Each of the positions can also be done with the patient supporting his or her weight on only the involved upper extremity. Apply alternating resistance against the patient's shoulders or trunk and ask him or her to "hold" against the force. Pressing forward against the trunk will increase the effect of the body weight and require the serratus anterior to stabilize more strongly against the additional force. As already noted, if the scapula wings, the resistance is too strong and should be reduced.

Closed-Chain (Weight-Bearing) Dynamic Stabilization

Dynamic stabilization requires the stabilizing muscles to maintain control of the scapula and GH joint while moving the body weight over the fixed extremity or extremities.

- Patient position and procedure: Standing with shoulders flexed 90 degrees and hands supported against a wall, leaning hands on a table, or quadruped (all 4s) position. Instruct the patient to shift his or her body weight from one extremity to the other (rock back and forth). Apply resistance against the shoulders (see Fig. 9–29).
- Progress by having the patient alternately lift one extremity, then the other, so that one extremity bears the body weight and stabilizes against the shifting load. Apply manual resistance to the shoulders or strap a weight around each wrist.
- When the muscles are able to control and stabilize, progress to using unstable surfaces (such as a rocker board, BAPS board, or ball). Suggestions for more vigorous closed-chain activities are described in the following section.

Dynamic Strengthening—Open- and Closed-Chain

It is imperative that the proximal stabilizing muscles of the thorax, neck, and scapula function properly before initiating dynamic strengthening of the muscles that move the glenohumeral joint through the ROM to avoid faulty mechanics. Strengthening exercises can be done in both open- and closed-chains. Progress exercises with repetitions and resistance that are within the mechanical limits of the involved tissues.

Initially utilize light resistance with multiple repetitions to develop dynamic control and muscular endurance. As control develops, progress to combined patterns of motion and training for muscle groups to function in a coordinated sequence. Begin

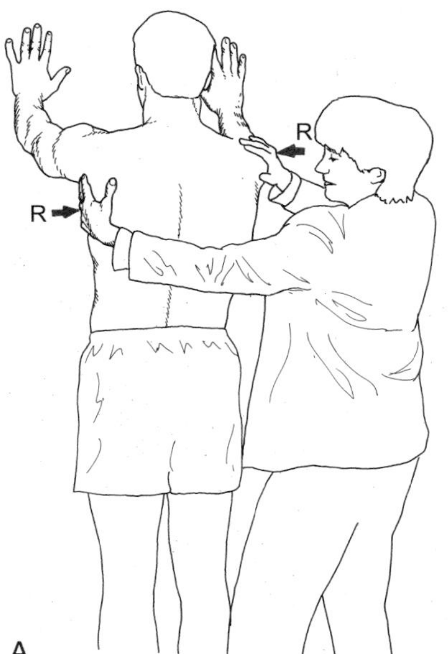

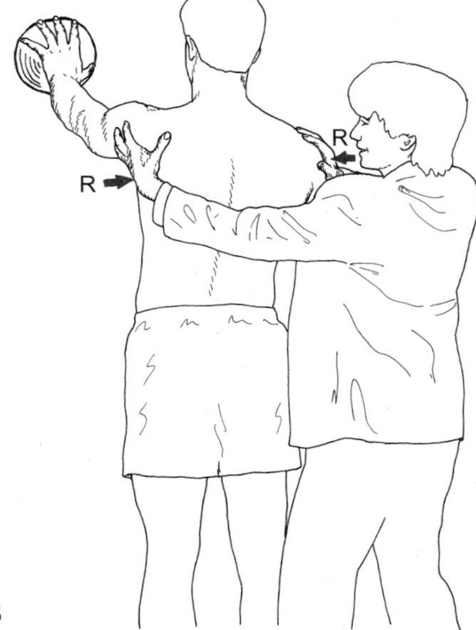

Figure 9–29 Closed-chain scapular and glenohumeral stabilization exercises. *(A)* Bilateral support in a minimal weight-bearing position with both hands against a wall. *(B)* Unilateral support on a less stable surface (ball). The therapist applies alternating resistance while the patient stabilizes against the resistance or the therapist applies resistance as the patient moves from side to side.

with simple functional activities and then more complex and challenging activities. Both muscular endurance and strength are necessary for postural and dynamic control of activities.

Scapular Retraction (Rhomboids and Middle Trapezius)

These exercises are designed to isolate scapular retraction; once the patient is able to retract the scapula against resistance, combine patterns with the GH joint to progress strength and functional patterns as described in the next sections.

- Patient position and procedure: Prone, sitting and standing. Instruct the patient to clasp the hands together behind the low back. This activity should cause scapular adduction. Draw attention to the adducted scapulae, and have the patient hold the adducted position of the scapulae while the arms are lowered to the sides. Have the patient repeat the activity without arm motion.
- Patient position and procedure: Prone with the arm over the edge of the table in a dependent position and a weight in the hand. Instruct the patient to pinch the scapulae together (Fig. 9–30). Progress this exercise to prone rowing and horizontal abduction against gravity described below.
- Patient position and procedure: Sitting or standing with the shoulder flexed to 90 degrees and elbows extended. Have the patient grasp each end of an elastic band or tubing that has been secured at shoulder level or a two-handled pulley that is at shoulder level, and pinch the scapulae together by pulling against the resistance.

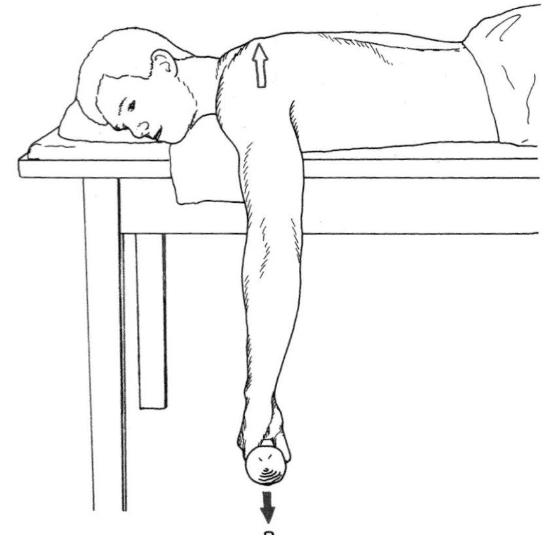

Figure 9–30 Scapular retraction against handheld resistance in the prone position.

Scapular Retraction Combined with Shoulder Horizontal Abduction/Extension (Rhomboids, Middle Trapezius, and Posterior Deltoid)

Prone and Sitting

Patient position and procedure: Prone with shoulders abducted 90 degrees, elbows flexed and forearms pointed vertically toward the floor. Instruct the patient to perform horizontal abduction with scapular retraction. This exercise can also be done with the elbows extended for greater resistance (Fig. 9–31). Progress this exercise by adding weights and then by having the patient perform the rowing motion standing or sitting in front of a length of elastic resistance that has been secured at shoulder level.

Corner Press-Outs

Patient position and procedure: Standing with his or her back toward a corner, shoulders are abducted 90 degrees, and elbows are flexed. Instruct the patient to press the elbows into the walls and push the body weight away from the corner (Fig. 9–32).

Scapular Retraction and Shoulder Horizontal Abduction Combined with External Rotation (Rhomboids, Trapezius, Posterior Deltoid, Infraspinatus, and Teres Minor)

- Patient position and procedure: Prone with shoulders abducted 90 degrees and externally rotated 90 degrees (90–90 position). The elbows can be flexed 90 degrees (easier position) or extended (more difficult position). Instruct the patient to lift

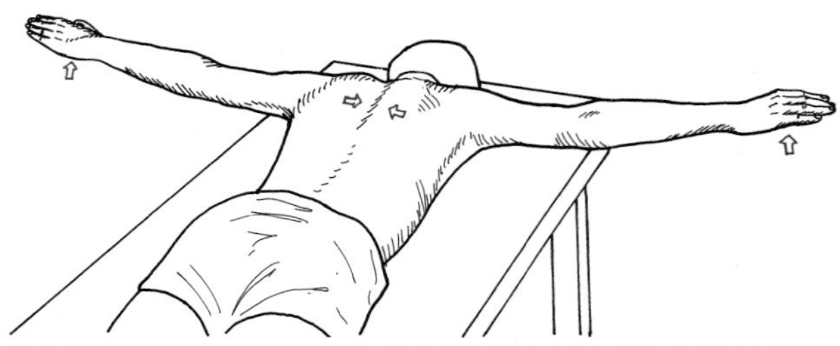

Figure 9–31 Horizontal abduction and scapular adduction exercises, with the arms positioned for maximal resistance from gravity. To progress the exercise further, weights can be placed in the patient's hands.

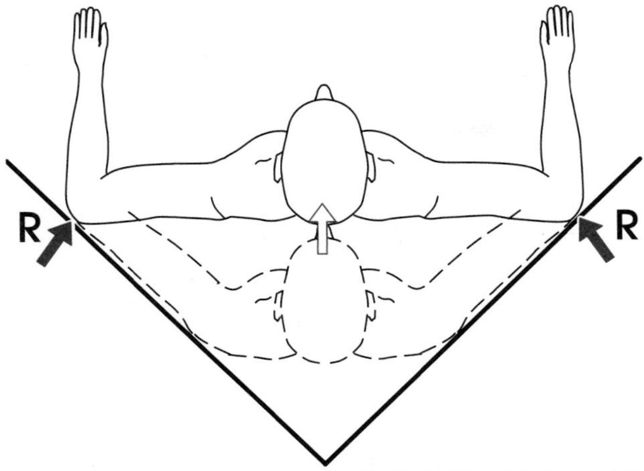

Figure 9–32 Corner press-outs to strengthen scapular retraction and shoulder horizontal abduction (view looking from above).

the arm a few degrees off the table. To do this correctly the scapulae must simultaneously adduct.

Note: Greater ROM can be used if these exercises are done on a narrow bench so that the arm can begin in a horizontally adducted position.

- Patient position and procedure: Sitting or standing with shoulders in the 90–90 position. Secure the middle of a piece of elastic resistance in front of the patient slightly above the shoulders, and have the patient grasp each end of the resistance. Then have the patient pull the hands and elbows back while simultaneously adducting the scapulae (Fig. 9–33).

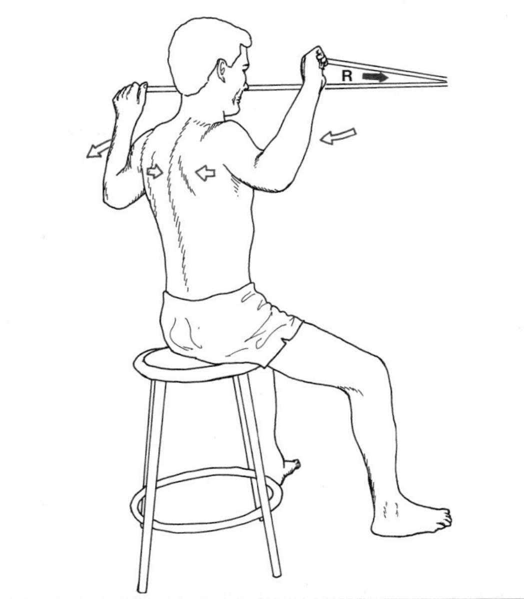

Figure 9–33 Combined scapular adduction with shoulder horizontal abduction and lateral rotation against resistance.

Scapular Protraction (Serratus Anterior)

- Patient position and procedure: Sitting or standing with shoulder flexed around 90 degrees and elbow extended. Secure a piece of elastic resistance behind the patient at shoulder level (or use a pulley system). Instruct the patient to "push" outward against the resistance without rotating the body (Fig. 9–34).
- Patient position and procedure: Supine with the arm flexed 90 degrees and slightly abducted, and the elbow extended. Place a light weight in the hand if resistance is tolerated, and have the patient "push" the weight upward without rotating the body.
- ***Push-ups with a "plus."*** Patient position and procedure: Standing with arms against a wall, leaning on a table or lying prone. Have the patient place his or her hands directly in front or slightly to the side of his or her shoulders and push the trunk up (or away from the wall); once full GH range is reached, instruct the patient to "give an

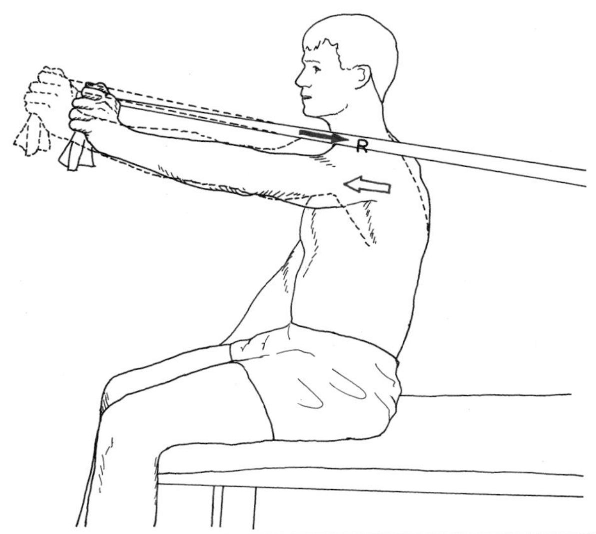

Figure 9–34 Scapular protraction; pushing against elastic resistance.

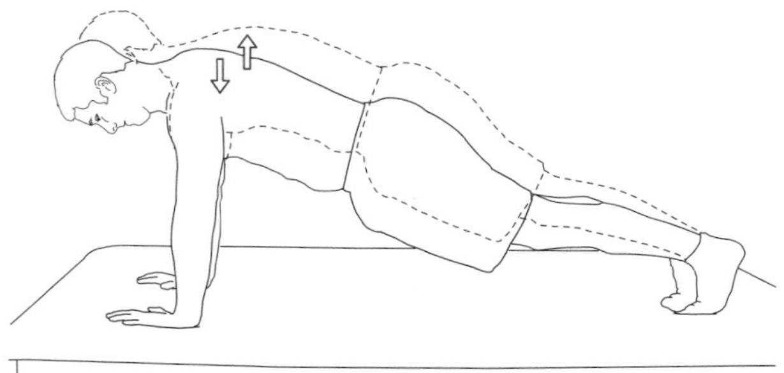

Figure 9–35 Push-ups with a "plus" to strengthen scapular protraction.

extra push" to protract the scapulae. Progress the wall push-ups to table push-ups then, prone push-ups with knees as a fulcrum, and finally prone-lying push-ups, lifting full body weight (Fig. 9–35). Add weight around the trunk if the patient is able to tolerate greater resistance.

Shoulder External Rotation (Infraspinatus and Teres Minor)

Position the arm at the patient's side or in various positions of abduction, scaption, or flexion. Flex the elbow to 90 degrees and apply the resistive force through the hand at right angles to the forearm. Be sure the patient rotates the humerus and does not extend the elbow.

- Patient position and procedure: Sitting or standing, using elastic resistance or wall pulley in front of the body at elbow level. Instruct the patient to grasp the elastic material or the pulley handle and rotate his or her arm outward (Fig. 9–36*A*).
- Patient position and procedure: Side-lying on normal side with involved shoulder upright and arm resting on the side of the thorax with a rolled towel under the axilla. Have the patient use a handheld weight, weight cuff, or elastic resistance and rotate the arm through the desired ROM.
- Patient position and procedure: Prone on a treatment table, upper arm resting on the table with shoulder at 90 degrees if possible, elbow flexed with forearm over the edge of the table. Lift the weight as far as possible by rotating the shoulder, not extending the elbow (Fig. 9–36*B*). It has been reported[20] that the activation of the infraspinatus and teres minor is maximized with this exercise.
- Patient position and procedure: Sitting with elbow flexed 90 degrees and supported on a table so the shoulder is in the resting position (scaption). The patient lifts the weight from the table by rotating the shoulder (Fig. 9–36*C*).

Shoulder Internal Rotation (Subscapularis)

Position the arm at the patient's side or in various positions of flexion, scaption, or abduction. The elbow is flexed to 90 degrees and the resistive force is held in the hand.

- Patient position and procedure: Side-lying on involved side with the arm forward in partial flex-

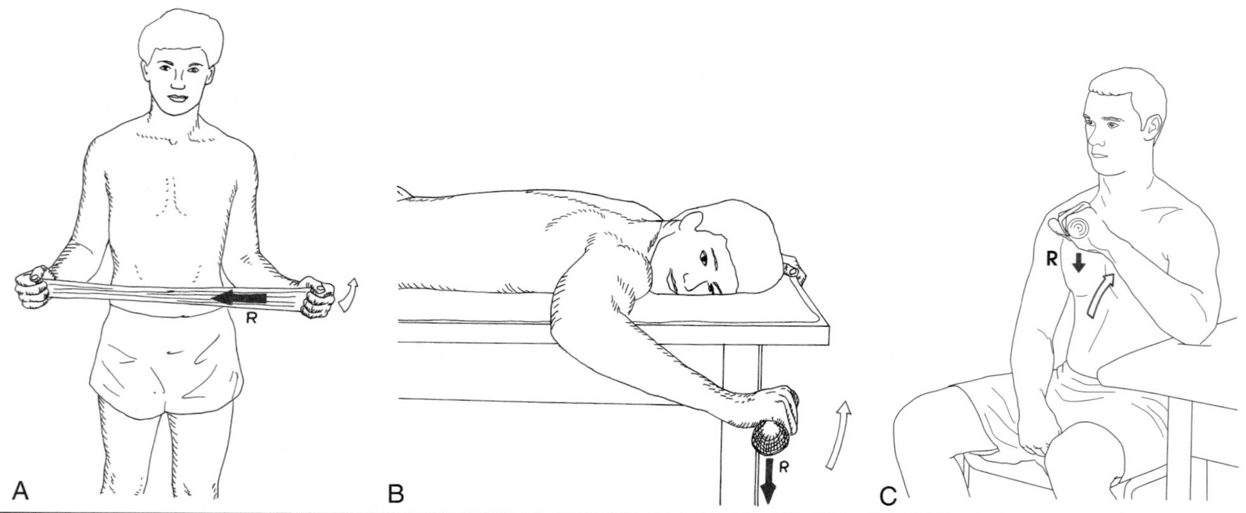

Figure 9–36 Strengthening external rotation with *(A)* the arm at the side using elastic resistance *(B)* prone with the arm at 90 degrees using a free weight, and *(C)* sitting with the shoulder in scaption using a free weight.

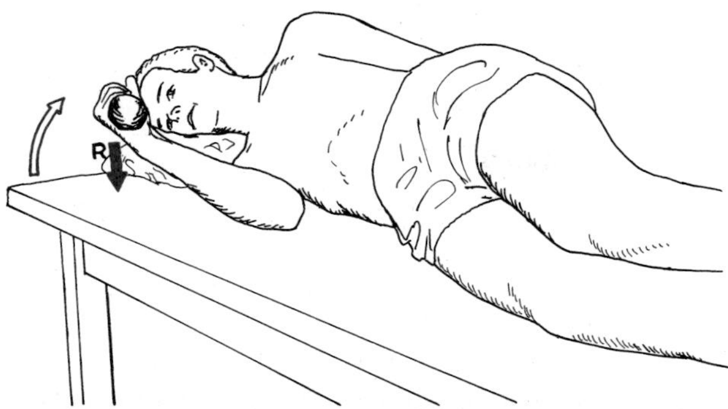

Figure 9–37 Resisted internal rotation of the shoulder using a handheld weight. To resist external rotation, place the weight in the patient's upper hand.

ion. Have the patient lift the weight upward off the table into internal rotation (Fig. 9–37).

- Patient position and procedure: Sitting or standing using an elastic material or pulley system with the line of force out to the side and at the level of the elbow. Have the patient pull across the front of the trunk into internal rotation.

Shoulder Abduction and Scaption (Deltoid and Supraspinatus)

Abduction exercises are classically done with the humerus moving in the frontal plane. It is commonly accepted that most functional activities occur with the humerus 30 to 45 degrees forward to the frontal plane where the arc of motion is more in line with the glenoid fossa of the scapula; this motion is called scaption. Many abduction exercises can be adapted to be performed in scaption.

Precaution: Teach the patient that whenever the shoulder elevates beyond 90 degrees, it must externally rotate to avoid impingement of the greater tubercle against the acromion.

"Military Press"

Patient position and procedure: Sitting, arm at the side in external rotation with elbow flexed and forearm supinated (thumb pointing posteriorly). Have the patient lift the weight straight up overhead (Fig. 9–38).

Abduction Against Gravity

- Patient position and procedure: Sitting or standing with a weight in hand. Have the patient abduct the arm to 90 degrees, then laterally rotate

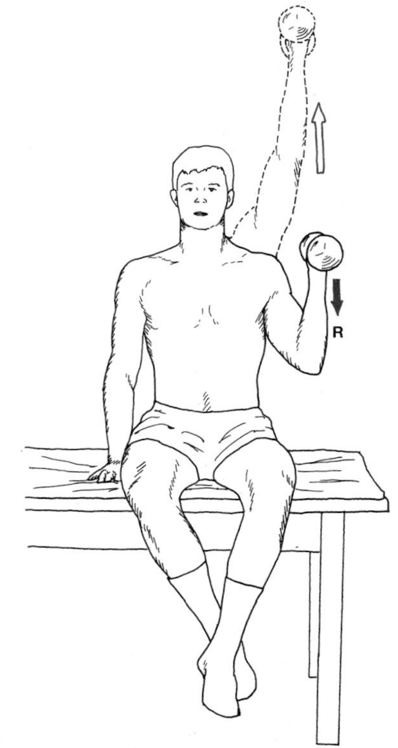

Figure 9–38 Military press-up. Beginning with the arm at the side in external rotation with elbow flexed and forearm supinated (thumb pointing posteriorward), the weight is lifted overhead.

and elevate the arm through the rest of the range. This same motion can be performed with elastic resistance secured under the patient's foot, but be cautious in that the greater the elastic stretch, the greater the resistance. The patient may not be able to complete the ROM because of the increased resistance at the end of the range.

- Patient position and procedure: Side-lying with involved arm uppermost. Have the patient lift a weight up to 90 degrees. The greatest effect of the resistance is at the beginning of the range. At 90 degrees, all of the force is through the long axis of the bone.

Full Can and Empty Can

Patient position and procedure: Standing with the humerus either externally rotated (full can) or internally rotated (empty can). Have the patient raise the arm away from the side in the plane of the scapula, halfway between abduction and flexion (Fig. 9–39). Performing scaption with the humerus in various positions of rotation has the value of emphasizing

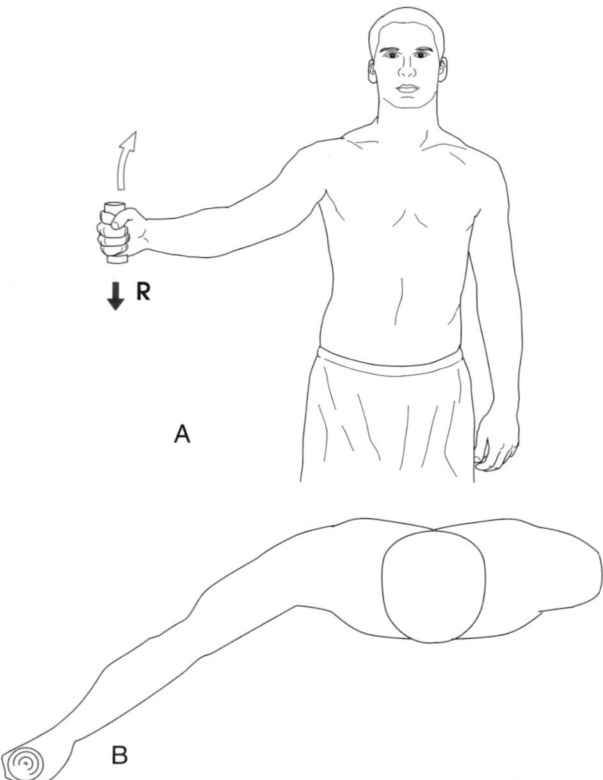

Figure 9–39 Abduction in the plane of the scapula (scaption). This is called the "full can" exercise because the shoulder is held in external rotation as if lifting a full can: *(A)* front view, *(B)* top view. If the shoulder is held in internal rotation it is called "empty can."

each of the rotatory muscles of the cuff in their synergy with the supraspinatus and deltoid muscles.[99] Resistance is applied with a handheld weight or from elastic resistance secured under the patient's foot.

Note: Recent EMG studies have confirmed that no one exercise isolates the action of the supraspinatus muscle from the other rotator cuff or deltoid muscles.[100,171] The supraspinatus muscle is effectively activated in both the "empty can"[82,182] and "full can" exercises.[80,100,171] It also contracts strongly with the military press[171] and horizontal abduction with external rotation exercises.[20,100,191] These findings give the therapist several choices of exercises for strengthening the supraspinatus. Several authors[45,78,80] as well as the authors of this text have suggested the "empty can" exercise (scaption with internal rotation of the humerus) should not be used in shoulder rehabilitation because it cause impingement of the suprahumeral tissues, especially as the arm approaches and elevates above 90 degrees. The "full can" position (scaption with external rotation) does not cause impingement.[45,80]

Shoulder Flexion (Anterior Deltoid Rotator Cuff and Serratus Anterior)

Patient position and procedure: Sitting, standing, or supine. If a free weight is used when supine, the greatest resistive force is at the beginning of the range; during standing, the greatest resistive force is when the shoulder is flexed 90 degrees. An elastic resistive force also can be used if secured under the patient's foot or solid object.

Shoulder Adduction (Pectoralis Major, Teres Major, and Latissimus Dorsi)

Patient position and procedure: Sitting or standing with the arm abducted. Have the patient pull down against a pulley force or elastic resistance tied overhead. The greatest resistance will be when the line of the resistive force is at right angles to the patient's arm.

Shoulder Horizontal Adduction (Anterior Deltoid, Coracobrachialis, and Pectoralis Major)

Patient position and procedure: Supine, begin with one or both arms out to the side in horizontal abduction. Have the patient bring the arms forward into horizontal adduction until the arm or arms are vertical.

Shoulder Extension (Posterior Deltoid Latissimus Dorsi and Rhomboids)

- Patient position and procedure: Prone with the arm over the side of the table in 90 degrees flexion. Have the patient lift the weight and extend the shoulder. Simultaneous elbow flexion while extending the shoulder is easiest (shortest lever arm); maintaining elbow extension while extending the shoulder is more difficult (longer lever arm).
- Patient position and procedure: Sitting or standing with the arm flexed; a pulley or elastic resistance is secured overhead. Have the patient pull down against the resistance into extension.

Scapular Depression (Lower Trapezius and Lower Serratus Anterior)

Shoulder Rolls

- Patient position and procedure: Sitting or standing. Ask the patient to roll the shoulders forward, up, and then around to the back so that the scapulae are resting in the retracted and depressed position. Instruct the patient to do this frequently throughout the day as part of a posture correction activity (see Chapter 16).

- Patient position and procedure: Sitting with elbow flexed. Provide manual resistance in an upward direction under the patient's elbow, and ask him or her to push down into your hands. Caudal gliding of the humeral head may also occur (Fig. 9–40*A*).

Closed-Chain Scapular Push-Ups (Scapular Depression and Humeral Adduction)

Patient position and procedure: Sitting or standing with both hands on blocks, on the armrests of a chair, or on parallel bars. Have the patient push down on the hands and lift the body (Fig. 9–40*B*).

Scapular Upward Rotation with Depression (Lower Trapezius and Serratus Anterior)

This motion cannot be isolated. The upward rotation action of the lower trapezius and serratus anterior require strengthening in coordination with humeral elevation. As noted elsewhere in this chapter, a patient may substitute with scapular elevation, primarily using the upper trapezius, so this exercise draws attention to maintaining the scapula in depression while upwardly rotating.

- ***"Superman" motion.*** Patient position and procedure: Prone, with humerus elevated overhead (if possible). Ask the patient to barely lift the arm off the table.
- Alternate position and procedure: Sitting or standing if the patient has a tight shoulder and cannot do the "superman motion" lying prone. Secure elastic resistance overhead and instruct the patient to move the shoulder into greater flexion with scapular depression. The scapular depression is most important; it may be necessary to use tactile cues on the lower trapezius to help the patient focus on the scapular depression, not scapular elevation (Fig. 9–40*C*).

Note: This is not a rowing motion; nor should trunk extension occur.

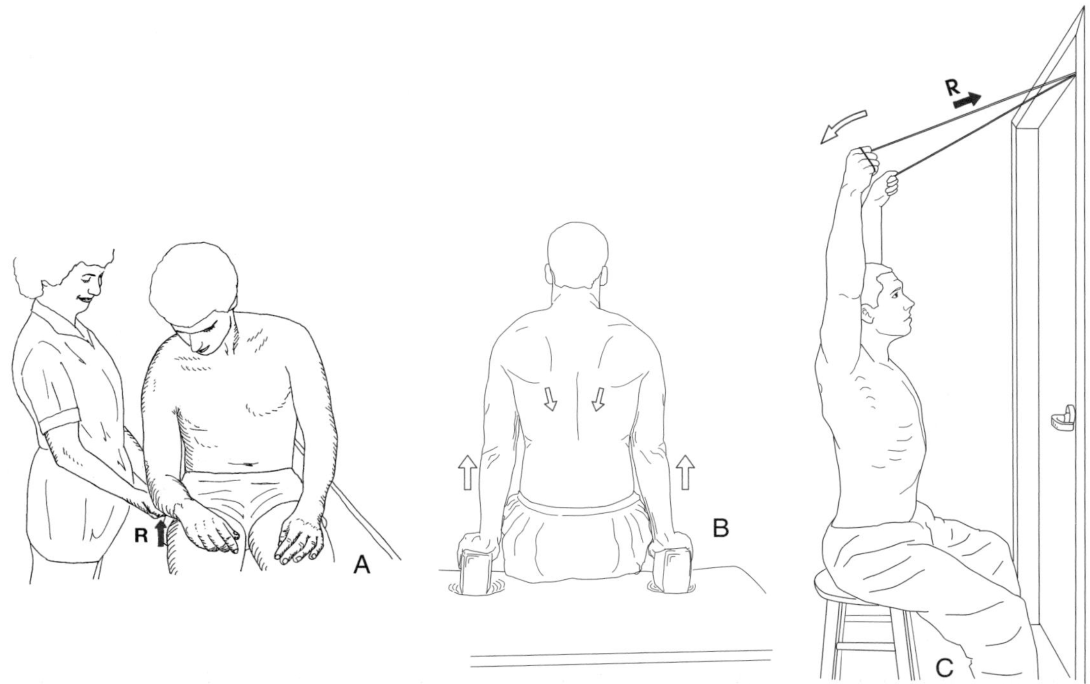

Figure 9–40 Exercises that emphasize the lower trapezius: *(A)* shoulder girdle depression against manual resistance, *(B)* closed-chain shoulder girdle depression using body weight for resistance, and *(C)* scapular depression with upward rotation of the scapula against elastic resistance.

- Patient position and procedure: Standing with back to the wall, heels away from the wall enough to be able to comfortably do a posterior pelvic tilt and maintain the back flat against the wall. Begin with arms slightly abducted and externally rotated and elbows flexed 90 degrees (back of hands should be against the wall). Instruct the patient to slide the hands and arms up the wall (abduction) as far as possible while maintaining the back flat against the wall.

Elbow Flexion (Biceps Brachii)

Biceps Curls

Patient position: Sitting or standing. Have the patient flex the elbow with a handheld weight while keeping the forearm supinated and the arm at the side or with the shoulder moving into slight extension (see Fig. 10–7).

Note: Since the biceps brachii is a two-joint muscle, the long head not only serves to flex the elbow as its primary function, it also assists the rotator cuff muscles by acting as an additional dynamic stabilizer of the GH joint by approximating the humeral head against the glenoid fossa and by depressing the head of the humerus as the arm elevates and the scapula upwardly rotates.[94] As such, the biceps brachii must be strengthened in a shoulder rehabilitation program.

PNF (Diagonal) Patterns

Note: PNF patterns as described in Chapter 3 utilize the entire upper extremity or address specific regions, such as the scapula. Apply resistance manually to emphasize specific muscles within the pattern by adjusting hand placement and resistance. Teach the patient exercises utilizing PNF patterns with weights or elastic resistance.

D_1 Flexion Pattern

Patient position and procedure: Standing. The arm begins in extension, internal rotation and slight abduction. Have the patient bring the arm into flexion, adduction, and external rotation while holding a weight or pulling against elastic resistance that is secured under the foot.

D_2 Flexion Pattern

Patient position and procedure: Standing. The arm begins in extension, internal rotation, and slight adduction. Have the patient bring the arm into flexion, abduction, and external rotation while holding a weight or pulling against elastic resistance (Fig. 9–41).

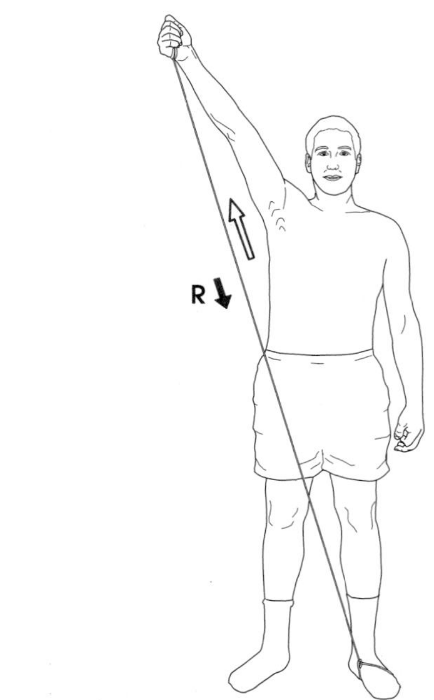

Figure 9–41 Elastic resistance to the D_2 flexion pattern, emphasizing shoulder flexion, abduction, and external rotation using elastic resistance.

D_1 Extension Pattern

Patient position and procedure: Supine, standing, or sitting. The arm begins in flexion, adduction, and external rotation. Have the patient pull against elastic resistance that is secured above the head or against an overhead cable attached to a weighted pulley system with a combined extension, abduction, and internal rotation motion.

D_2 Extension Pattern

Patient position: Supine, standing, or sitting. The arm begins in flexion, abduction, and external rotation. Have the patient pull against elastic resistance that is secured above the head with a combined extension, adduction, and internal rotation.

Isokinetic Training

Principles of isokinetic training are discussed in Chapter 3. Early in the exercise program have the patient use a submaximal effort at slow speeds. As tissues heal, have the patient perform maximum effort concentric and eccentric exercises at medium to high speeds. Simulate functional patterns of movement if the equipment setup allows.

Resisted Exercises Using Functional Patterns of Motion with Equipment

There are a variety of exercise devices that can be used or modified to use for shoulder girdle strengthening that require coordination between the stabilizing and dynamic functions of the scapula and humerus. Some are considered closed-chain in that the proximal segments move over the stabilized extremity, or there is pressure through the extremity causing approximation of the GH joint surfaces. The exercises may be used to accomplish several goals, such as improving strength, power, endurance (muscular and/or cardiovascular/pulmonary), balance, coordination, and skill.

Handwalking on a Treadmill

Patient position and procedure: Kneeling at the end of a treadmill. The surface can be moving forward or backward. Have the patient "walk" with his or her hands while bearing weight through the shoulders.

ProFitter™

Patient position and procedure: Kneeling with one or both hands on the movable platform. The hands slide the platform from side to side. Change the position of the unit to obtain different angles of motion (Fig. 9–42).

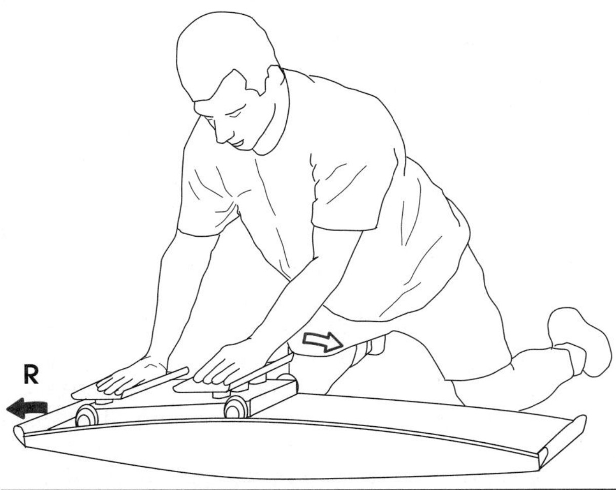

Figure 9–42 Advanced closed-chain exercise to resist the upper extremity using a ProFitter™ to provide an unstable, moving surface.

Stepping Machine

Patient position and procedure: Kneeling with each hand on a step of the unit. The upper extremities do the climbing. Encourage the patient to use scapular protraction/retraction rather than elbow flexion/extension.

Rowing Machine

Patient position and procedure: Long-sitting. Follow the instructions provided by the manufacturer if a commercial unit is used. Elastic resistance or cable system on a pulley can be used to simulate a commercial rowing machine. Have the patient secure the elastic resistance under the feet or around a solid object, grasp the ends of the resistance, and pull backward in a rowing action with the arms. Also have the patient long sit facing a cable system with the pulley at ground level. If there is just one cable, secure a bar to the cable, and have the patient pull the bar toward his or her trunk in a rowing action.

Lawnmower Pull

Patient position and procedure: Standing with hips partially flexed and holding onto a table or chair for balance with the hand of the sound upper extremity. Have the patient reach diagonally across the midline and grasp a piece of elastic resistance that is secured under the foot of the sound side or attached to the floor. Then have the patient pull upward on the resistance as if starting a lawnmower. This may also be simulated with a free weight (see Fig. 10–14).

Upper Body Ergometry

Patient position and procedure: Sitting or standing in front of an ergometer with hands on the handles. Determine arc of motion, and direction (forward or backward), speed, and time. This machine may be used for general warm-up, ROM, strengthening, or endurance training. Since tight or overused anterior structures and weak or underused posterior structures tend to be the pattern with shoulder impairments, place emphasis on backward (retro) motions of the ergometer.

Advanced Closed-Chain Stabilization and Balance Activities

Patient position and procedure: Quadruped on the floor with hands on an unstable surface such as BAPS board, rocker board, wobble board, foam roll, or 8- to 10-inch ball. Or have the patient assume a quadruped position with knees on a mat and hands on a large gym ball on the floor next to the mat. A variety of activities can then be done. For example, have the patient perform the following activities.

- Maintain a balanced posture as resistance is applied to the shoulders or trunk to disturb balance.
- Shift body weight from one hand to the other using an alternating protraction/retraction motion of the scapulae.
- Alternately flex each upper extremity so that only one hand is balanced on the unstable surface.
- Perform push-ups and push-ups with a plus on the unstable surface.
- Increase speed of the above activities.

Functional Activities

As soon as the patient develops control of scapular and humeral motions and the basic components of the desired activities without exacerbating the symptoms, initiate specificity of training toward the desired functional outcome by progressing the strengthening exercises to maximum resistance concentrically and eccentrically. Use the actual patterns and type of contraction required in the desired outcome and progress to the desired speed first in a controlled manner, then with less control.

An individual who has a sedentary lifestyle may require postural adaptations and ergonomic analysis of his or her home environment or work station to change repetitive stress whereas an athlete or industrial worker may require high-intensity exercises that develop endurance, power, and skill. Functional exercises may begin simply by instructing the patient to unload a dishwasher and place the dishes on a low shelf using correct shoulder mechanics or washing windows using small circular motions. Body mechanics are incorporated into lifting, pushing, or pulling activities (Fig. 9–43). If catching and throwing or swinging a bat or golf club are necessary, total body patterns are practiced with the upper extremity exercises. Creativity in adapting exercises to meet progressive upper extremity challenges is a must. Basic principles to progress the patient during the return to function phase of therapy follow.

Endurance Training

Muscle and cardiovascular/pulmonary endurance is important for general health as well as to function throughout a workday. Utilize repetitive loading of each exercise from 3 to 5 minutes using patterns of motion that simulate work or functional activities. Principles of conditioning are discussed in Chapter

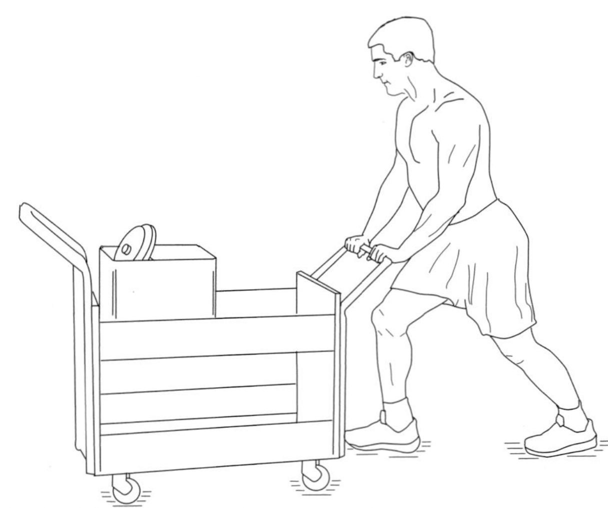

Figure 9–43 Functional exercise incorporating body mechanics

4. Have the patient maintain his or her target heart rate for 20 minutes with repetitive exercises.

Eccentric Training

Eccentric exercises are high-intensity exercises and may be used for specific training. Because eccentric contractions tolerate greater resistance than concentric, when loading resistance for eccentric training, the patient is taught to assist the arm to the end of the shortened range of the muscles to be stressed; then the muscles control the return motion. This can be performed with elastic resistance, pulleys, or free weights first in single-plane motions and then progressed to simulated functional patterns.

Plyometric Training

Initiate *stretch-shortening drills* in safe, controlled patterns with light resistance; then progress speed and resistance as tolerated.

Example. The therapist tosses a weighted ball such as a Plyoball® for the patient to reach for and catch and then immediately toss back using the reciprocal pattern (Fig. 9–44). Progress to total body patterns including step and throw and overhead pass activities. Spring-loaded rebounders or elastic tubing is commercially available so the patient can do the activity independently once the drills are learned.[181–183]

Total Body Training

Increase *speed* with superimposed stresses to tolerance while simulating the desired activity. Assess

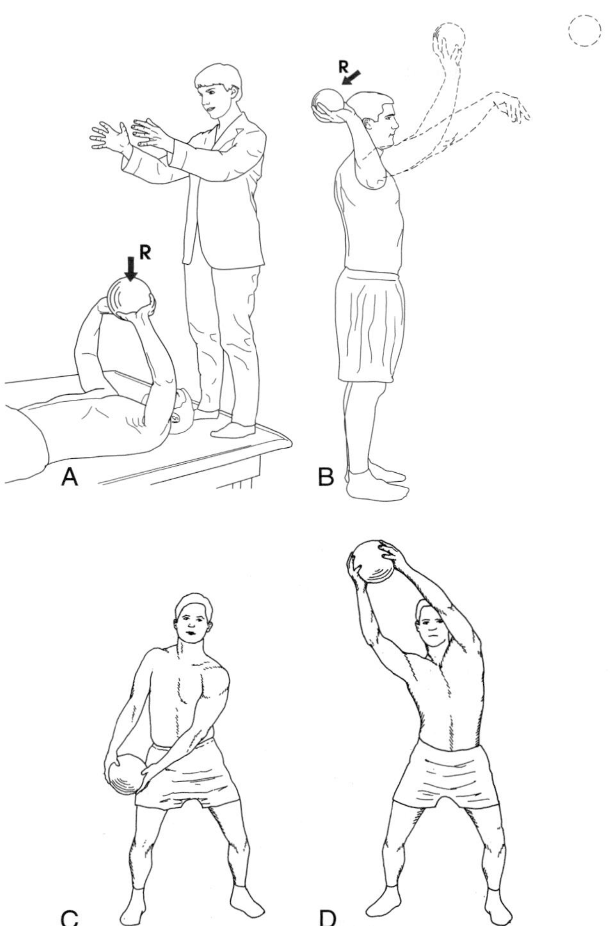

Figure 9–44 Plyometric activities catching and throwing a weighted ball *(A)* in a stable supine position, *(B)* in a standing position, *(C)* in a diagonal extension pattern, and *(D)* in a diagonal flexion pattern

the total-body function while the desired activity is being carried out. Develop timing and sequencing of events that are consistent with the functional activity.

Independent Learning Activities

CRITICAL THINKING AND DISCUSSION

1. Describe the functions and inter-relationships of the scapulothoracic and glenohumeral musculature as dynamic stabilizers of the shoulder.
2. Which structures can restrict normal upward rotation of the scapula, and how does inadequate passive or active upward rotation of the scapula adversely affect elevation of the arm?
3. How does sitting or standing in a slumped posture (excessive thoracic kyphosis and forward head) with scapular abduction versus an erect posture with scapular adduction alter ROM of the shoulder?
4. Which mechanisms and structures could be sources of pain in primary impingement syndrome?
5. How are impingement and instability related to each other in secondary impingement syndrome?
6. A patient experienced a traumatic shoulder injury, falling down five cement steps 2 weeks ago. She now has a capsular pattern, decreased joint play, and muscle guarding with passive glenohumeral motions. She does not actively use the extremity because of pain. You observe edema in the hand. What potential complications could develop if left untreated? Design an exercise program for this patient at her present level of involvement. What would you teach the patient about her symptoms, impairments, and parameters for recovery?
7. An individual with a history of diabetes has developed a frozen shoulder. She has had shoulder discomfort for several months, but she did not seek treatment until 1 week ago when she was unable to wash or fix her hair with her left hand. Identify your intervention plan and instructions for this patient.
8. A new patient describes experiencing episodes of numbness and tingling in the hand with occasional periods of "puffiness." She reports it is particularly annoying because it happens whenever she carries her briefcase or heavy purse with a shoulder strap. She also experiences pain at night and wakes up with her hand "having fallen asleep." What shoulder girdle problems could cause these symptoms? What is the probable cause of the symptoms? Create a scenario of objective findings, identify impairment and functional goals, and a plan of intervention. What precautions are related to nerve pathologies?
9. In the early and middle stages of a rehabilitation program, what types of functional activities (ADL, work-related, or sport-related) should initially be avoided or modified for patients with a history of recurrent anterior dislocation of the GH joint? With recurrent posterior dislocation of the GH joint?

10. What criteria should patients with each of the following shoulder diagnoses meet before progressing to *overhead* exercises and functional activities: primary impingement syndrome; anterior GH instability; frozen shoulder; S/P rotator cuff repair?

LABORATORY PRACTICE

1. With your partner, review and practice key tests and measurements that you might need to do to determine what is causing shoulder pain and/or diminished upper extremity function. What do each of those tests indicate?
2. Mobilize the scapula with manual techniques.
3. Mobilize the glenohumeral joint capsule with manual techniques.
4. Teach your partner a series of self-mobilization techniques for the GH joint capsule.
5. Using appropriate stabilization manually stretch all major muscle groups of the shoulder.
6. Teach your partner effective self-stretching techniques for each of these muscle groups.
7. Practice a sequence of exercises to strengthen the muscles of the scapula using manual resistance (applied by the therapist). Use open-chain and closed-chain positions.
8. Teach your partner a progressive sequence of strengthening exercises that he or she could do in a home exercise program to develop stability and dynamic control of the scapula.
9. Teach your partner a progressive sequence of strengthening exercises that he or she could do in a home exercise program to develop strength, stability, and endurance of the GH muscles. Have your patient perform each exercise for a specified number of repetitions and at a specified level of resistance. Correct any faulty postures or motions as your partner executes each exercise. Watch for and teach your partner signs of fatigue and poor exercise technique.
10. Develop a series of functional activities to complement the self-stretching and self-strengthening exercise you have taught your partner.

CASE STUDIES

1. A patient referral states: evaluate and treat shoulder pain S/P MVI. The patient describes shoulder pain whenever reaching overhead. She is a nurse and finds symptoms worsen whenever placing solutions on an IV pole, a frequent activity for her. She was the driver of the car in a head-on collision. Examination reveals painful resisted scapular protraction, elbow extension, and shoulder extension with pain on palpation of the long head of the triceps near its insertion on the inferior glenoid, and pain in the serratus anterior in the axilla. Other impairments include weak rhomboids and lower trapezius muscles (4-/5).
   - Explain why these muscles would be injured in this type of accident.
   - Explain why this patient's job would perpetuate these symptoms.
   - Outline a treatment plan to manage the acute symptoms and initiate a therapeutic exercise program.
   - Identify a measurable functional outcome goal and interventions you would use to reach the goal.
   - As the patient's symptoms subside, how would you progress her exercise program?
2. Your patient describes pain whenever reaching overhead. He likes to play volleyball in a weekend league, but otherwise has a sedentary lifestyle. On examination, you observe moderate atrophy in the infraspinous fossa, protracted scapula, and a thoracic kyphosis with forward head. You have him assume the quadruped position in anticipation of instruction in closed-chain rhythmic stabilization and scapular protraction exercises and note significant winging of the scapula.
   - Describe what muscles probably test weak with these observations.
   - How would you change the quadruped exercise to develop control and strength in the involved muscles at a safe resistance level?
   - Based on your assumptions of muscle involvement, develop an intervention plan for this patient that includes a home exercise program. Indicate parameters (frequency, repetitions), positions, safety, and progressions.
3. You have received a referral to "evaluate and treat" a 62-year-old patient who had a total shoulder arthroplasty for osteoarthritis 2 weeks ago. The patient has been wearing a sling to support and protect the operated shoulder but has been allowed to remove the sling only for daily pendulum exercises and active ROM of the elbow, wrist, and hand.

- Prior to initiating your examination and developing an exercise program, what additional information would you like to find out from the surgeon?
- What information will you want to gather from the patient?
- What examination procedures would you wish to perform during the patient's initial visit?
- The patient's insurance, most likely, will initially approve 6 visits. Develop, implement, and teach and then progress a series of exercises over a period of 6 visits with the patient.

4. Six months ago your patient underwent surgery for repair of a Bankart lesion and stabilization of the anterior capsule (capsular shift) after a traumatic anterior dislocation of the GH joint. The patient now has full ROM and 90% strength in the shoulder after a program of rehabilitation. Your patient wants to return to recreational sports, such as tennis, softball, and volleyball but is apprehensive that the shoulder will dislocate during these activities. Design an advanced rehabilitation program to gradually return the patient to the desired recreational activities.

REFERENCES

1. Altchek, DW, et al: Arthroscopic acromioplasty: Technique and results. J Bone Joint Surg 72A:1198, 1990.
2. Andrews, JR, Brousard, TS, and Carson, WG: Arthroscopy of the shoulder in the management of partial tears of the rotator cuff: A preliminary report. Arthroscopy 1:117, 1985.
3. Andrews, JR, and Satterwhite, YE: Anatomic capsular shift. J Orthop Tech 1:151, 1993.
4. Andrews, JR, and Angelo, RL: Shoulder arthroscopy for the throwing athlete. In Paulos, LE, and Tibone, JE (eds): Operative Technique in Shoulder Surgery. Aspen, Gaithersburg, MD, 1991.
5. Arciero, RA, et al: Arthroscopic Bankart repair versus nonoperative treatment for acute, initial anterior shoulder dislocation. Am J Sports Med 22:589, 1994.
6. Arntz, CT, and Jackins, S: Prosthetic replacement of the shoulder for the treatment of defects in the rotator cuff and the surface of the glenohumeral joint. J Bone Joint Surg Am 75:485–491, 1993.
7. Aronen, JG, and Regan, K: Decreasing the incidence of recurrence of first-time anterior dislocations with rehabilitation. Am J Sports Med 12:283, 1984.
8. Arroyo, JS, and Flatow, EL: Management of rotator cuff disease: Intact and repairable cuff. In Iannotti, JP, and Williams, GR (eds): Disorders of the Shoulder: Diagnosis and Management. Lippincott Williams & Wilkins, Philadelphia, 1999, p 31.
9. Baker, CL, and Liu, SH: Comparison of open and arthroscopically-assisted rotator cuff repair. Am J Sports Med, 23:99, 1995.
10. Baker, CL, and Liu, SH: Neurovascular injuries to the shoulder. J Orthop Sports Phys Ther 18:361, 1993.
11. Ballantyne, BT, et al: Electromyographic activity of selected shoulder muscles in commonly used therapeutic exercises. Phys Ther 73:668, 1993.
12. Ballard, WT, and Buckwalter, JA: Operative treatment of rheumatic disease. In Klippel, JH (ed): Primer on the Rheumatic Diseases, ed 11. Arthritis Foundation, Atlanta, 1997, p 443.
13. Barrett, WP, and Frankin, JL: Total shoulder arthroplasty. J Bone Joint Surg Am 69:866–872, 1987.
14. Bassett, RW, et al: Glenohumeral muscle force and movement mechanics in a position of shoulder instability. J Biomech 23:405, 1990.
15. Bigliani, LV, et al: Repair of rotator cuff tears in tennis players. Am J Sports Med 20(2):112–117, 1992.
16. Bigliani, LV, et al: Inferior capsular shift procedure for anterior-inferior shoulder instability in athletes. Am J Sports Med 22:578, 1994.
17. Bigliani, LV, et al: Shift of the posteroinferior aspect of the capsule for recurrent posterior glenohumeral instability. J Bone Joint Surg 77A:1011, 1995.
18. Binder, AI, et al: Frozen shoulder: A long-term prospective study. Ann Rheum Dis 43:361, 1984.
19. Black, KP, et al: In vitro evaluation of shoulder external rotation after a Bankart reconstruction. Am J Sports Med 25:449, 1997.
20. Blackburn, TA, et al: EMG analysis of posterior rotator cuff exercises. Athletic Training 25:40, 1990.
21. Blakely, RL, and Palmer, ML: Analysis of rotation accompanying shoulder flexion. Phys Ther 64:1214, 1984.
22. Blakely, RL, and Palmer, ML: Analysis of shoulder rotation accompanying a proprioceptive neuromuscular facilitation approach. Phys Ther 66:1224, 1986.
23. Boublik, M, and Hawkins, RJ: Clinical examination of the shoulder complex. J Orthop Sports Phys Ther 18:379, 1993.
24. Brems, JJ: Rehabilitation following total shoulder arthroplasty. Clin Ortho Rel Res 307:70, 1994.
25. Brewster, C, and Schwar, DRM: Rehabilitation of the shoulder following rotator cuff injury or surgery. J Orthop Sports Phys Ther 18:422, 1993.
26. Brostrom, LA, et al: The effect of shoulder muscle training in patients with recurrent shoulder dislocations. Scand J Rehabil Med 24:11, 1992.
27. Brown, DD, and Friedman, RJ: Postoperative rehabilitation following total shoulder arthroplasty. Orthop Clin North Am 29:535, 1998.
28. Brunet, ME, Haddad, RJ, and Porche, EB: Rotator cuff impingement syndrome in sports. Physician Sports Med 10:87, 1982.
29. Burkhead, WZ, and Rockwood, CA: Treatment of instability of the shoulder with an exercise program. J Bone Joint Surg Am 74:890, 1992.
30. Butler, DS: Mobilization of the Nervous System. Churchill Livingstone, New York, 1991.
31. Cailliet, R: Shoulder Pain, ed 3. FA Davis, Philadelphia, 1991.

32. Cain, PR, et al: Anterior stability of the glenohumeral joint. Am J Sports Med 15:144, 1987.
33. Carpenter, JE, Blasier, RB, and Pellizzon, GG: The effects of muscle fatigue on shoulder joint position sense. Am J Sports Med 26:262, 1998.
34. Cash, JD: Recent advances and perspectives on arthroscopic stabilization of the shoulder. Clin Sports Med 10(4):871–886, 1991.
35. Caspari, RB: Arthroscopic reconstruction for anterior shoulder instability. In Paulos, LE, and Tibone, JE (eds): Operative Techniques in Shoulder Surgery. Aspen, Gaithersburg, MD, 1991.
36. Codman, EA: The Shoulder. Thomas Todd Company, Boston, 1934.
37. Cofield, RH, Chang, W, and Sperling, JW: Complications of shoulder arthroplasty. In Iannotti, JP, and Williams, GR (eds): Disorders of the Shoulder: Diagnosis and Management. Lippincott Williams & Wilkins, Philadelphia, 1999, p 571.
38. Cofield, RH: Results and complications of shoulder arthroplasty. In Morrey, B (ed): Reconstructive Surgery of the Joints. Churchill Livingstone, New York, 1996.
39. Cofield, RH: The shoulder. In Kelley, WN, Harris, ED, Ruddy, S, and Sledge, CB (eds): Textbook of Rheumatology, WB Saunders, Philadelphia, 1997.
40. Cuetter, AC, and Bartoszek, DM: The thoracic outlet syndrome: Controversies, overdiagnosis, overtreatment, and recommendations for management. Muscle Nerve 12:410, 1989.
41. Culhan, E, and Peat, M: Functional anatomy of the shoulder complex. J Orthop Sports Phys Ther 18:342, 1993.
42. Cyriax, J: Textbook of Orthopaedic Medicine, Vol. 1. Diagnosis of Soft Tissue Lesions, ed 8. Bailliere Tindall, London, 1982.
43. Cyriax, J: Textbook of Orthopaedic Medicine, Vol. 2. Treatment by Manipulation, Massage and Injection, ed 10. Bailliere Tindall, London, 1980.
44. Davies, GJ, and Dickoff-Hoffman, S: Neuromuscular testing and rehabilitation of the shoulder complex. J Orthop Sports Phys Ther 18:449, 1993.
45. Davies, GJ, and Durall, C: "Typical" rotator cuff impingement syndrome: it's not always typical. PT Magazine 8:58, 2000.
46. Dontigny, R: Passive shoulder exercises. Phys Ther 50:1707, 1970.
47. Edmonds, A: Shoulder arthroplasty. In Clark, GL, et al (eds): Hand Rehabilitation. Churchill Livingstone, New York, 1998, p 267.
48. Ellenbecker, TS, and Mattalino, AJ: Glenohumeral joint range of motion and rotator cuff strength following arthroscopic anterior stabilization with thermal capsulorraphy. J Orthop Sports Phys Ther 29:160, 1999.
49. Ellenbecker, TS: Etiology and evaluation of rotator cuff pathology and rehabilitation. In Donatelli, RA (ed): Physical Therapy of the Shoulder. Churchill Livingstone, Philadelphia, 1997, p 279.
50. Ellman, H: Arthroscopic subacromial decompression. In Welsh, RP, and Shephard, RJ (eds): Current Therapy in Sports Medicine, Vol 2. BC Decker, Toronto, 1990.
51. Engle, RP, and Canner, GC: Posterior shoulder instability: Approach to rehabilitation. J Orthop Sports Phys Ther 10(12):70–78, 1989.
52. Fahey, VA: Thoracic outlet syndrome. J Cardiovasc Nurs 1:12, 1987.
53. Fanton, G, and Thabit, G: Orthopedic uses of arthroscopy and lasers. Orthopedic knowledge. Update Sports Medicine, AAOS, 1994.
54. Fenlin, JM, and Friedman, B: Shoulder arthroplasty: massive cuff deficiency. In Iannotti, JP, and Williams, GR (eds): Disorders of the Shoulder: Diagnosis and Management. Lippincott Williams & Wilkins, Philadelphia, 1999, p 559.
55. Friedman, RJ: Biomechanics of total shoulder arthroplasty. In Friedman, RJ (ed): Arthroplasty of the Shoulder. Thieme Medical, New York, 1994, p 27.
56. Fu, FH, Harner, CD, and Klein, AH: Shoulder impingement syndrome: a critical review. Clin Orthop 269:162, 1991.
57. Gartsman, GM, and Hammerman, SM: Full-thickness tears: arthroscopic repair. Orthop Clin North Am 28:83, 1997.
58. Gartsman, GM, Khan, M, and Hammerman, SM: Arthroscopic repair of fullthickness tears of the rotator cuff. J Bone Joint Surg, 80A:832, 1998.
59. Greis, PE, Dean, M, and Hawkins, RJ: Subscapularis tendon disruption after Bankart reconstruction for anterior instability. J Shoulder Elbow Surg 5:219, 1996.
60. Grey, RG: The natural history of idiopathic frozen shoulder. J Bone Joint Surg Am 60:564, 1978.
61. Griffin, JW: Hemiplegic shoulder pain. Phys Ther 66:1884, 1986.
62. Gross, RM: Arthroscopic shoulder capsulorrhaphy: Does it work? Am J Sports Med 17:495, 1989.
63. Grubbs, N: Frozen shoulder syndrome: A review of literature. J Orthop Sports Phys Ther 18:479, 1993.
64. Guidotti, TL: Occupational repetitive strain injury. Am Fam Physician 45:585, 1992.
65. Haig, SV: Shoulder Pathophysiology Rehabilitation and Treatment. Aspen Publishers Inc, Gaithersburg, Maryland, 1996.
66. Harryman, DT, et al: Translation of the humeral head on the glenoid with passive glenohumeral motion. J Bone Joint Surg 72A:1334, 1990.
67. Harryman, DT II, et al: Reports of the rotator cuff: Correlation of functional results with integrity of the cuff. J Bone Joint Surg, 73A:982, 1991.
68. Hartzog, CW, Savoie, FH, and Field, LD: Arthroscopic acromioplasty and arthroscopic distal clavicle resection, mini-open rotator cuff repair: Indications, techniques, and outcome. In Iannotti, JP (ed): The Rotator Cuff: Current Concepts and Complex Problems. American Academy of Orthopedic Surgeons, Rosemont, IL, 1998, p 25.
69. Hattrup, SJ: Rotator cuff repair: relevance of patient age. J Shoulder Elbow Surg 4:95, 1995.
70. Hawkins, RJ, and Abrams, JS: Impingement syndrome in the absence of rotator cuff tear (stages 1 and 2). Orthop Clin North Am 18:373, 1987.
71. Hawkins, RJ, et al: Acromioplasty for impingement with an intact rotator cuff. J Bone Joint Surg Br 70 (5):795–797, 1988.
72. Hawkins, RJ, and Kunkel, SS: Rotator cuff tears. In: Welsh, RP, and Shepherd, RJ (eds): Current Therapy in Sports Medicine, Vol 2. BC Decker, Toronto, 1990.
73. Hawkins, RJ, Koppert, G, and Johnston, G: Recurrent posterior instability (subluxation) of the shoulder. J Bone Joint Surg Am 66:169, 1984.

74. Hawkins, RJ, Misamore, GW, and Hobeika, PE: Surgery for full-thickness rotator cuff tears. J Bone Joint Surg Am 67:1349, 1985.
75. Hayashi, K, Markel, M, et al: The effect of nonablative laser energy on joint capsular properties: an in vitro mechanical study using a rabbit model. Am J Sports Med 23: 482, 1995.
76. Hernandez, A, and Drez, D: Operative treatment of posterior shoulder dislocation by posterior glenoidplasty, capsulorrhapy and infraspinatus advancement. Am J Sports Med 14:187, 1986.
77. Ho, CP: Applied MRI anatomy of the shoulder. J Orthop Sports Phys Ther 18:351, 1993.
78. Horrigan, JM, et al: Magnetic resonance imaging evaluation of muscle usage associated with three exercises for rotator cuff rehabilitation. Med Sci Sports Exerc 31:1361, 1999.
79. Howell, SM, Galinet, BJ, et al: Normal and abnormal mechanics of the glenohumeral joint in the horizontal plane. J Bone Joint Surg 70A:227, 1988.
80. Itoi, E, et al: Which is more useful, the "full can test" or the "empty can test," in detecting the torn supraspinatus tendon? Am J Sports Med 27:65, 1999.
81. Jobe, FW, Giangarra, CE, et al: Anterior capsulolabral reconstruction of the shoulder in athletes in overhead sports. Am J Sports Med 19:428, 1991.
82. Jobe, FW, and Moynes, DR: Delineation of diagnostic criteria and a rehabilitation program for rotator cuff injuries. Am J Sports Med 10:336, 1982.
83. Jobe, FW, Schwab, DM, Wilk, KE, and Andrews, JR: Rehabilitation of the shoulder. In Brotzman, SB (ed): Clinical Orthopedic Rehabilitation. CV Mosby, St. Louis, 1996, p 97.
84. Jobe, FW, and Pink, M: Classification and treatment of shoulder dysfunction in the overhead athlete. J Orthop Sports Phys Ther 18:427, 1993.
85. Johanson, MA, and Gonzalez-King, BZ: Differential Soft Tissue Diagnosis, p 57. In Donatelli, RA: Physical Therapy of the Shoulder, ed 3. Churchill Livingstone, New York, 1997, p 57.
86. Kaltenborn, F: Manual Mobilization of the Joints; The Kaltenborn Method of Joint Examination and Treatment. Vol 1: The Extremities, ed 5. Olaf Norlis Bokhandel, Oslo, 1999.
87. Kamkar, A, Irrgang, JJ, and Whitney, SI: Nonoperative management of secondary shoulder impingement syndrome. J Orthop Sports Phys Ther 17(5):212–224, 1993.
88. Kelley, MJ, and Leggin, BG: Shoulder rehabilitation. In Iannotti, JP, and Williams, GR (eds): Disorders of the Shoulder: Diagnosis and Management. Lippincott Williams & Wilkins, Philadelphia, 1999, p 979.
89. Kelley, MJ: Case studies. In Kelley, MJ, and Clark, WA: Orthopedic Therapy of the Shoulder, JB Lippincott, Philadelphia, 1995, p 424.
90. Kennedy, K: Rehabilitation of the unstable shoulder. Sportsmedicine Performance and Research Center, WB Saunders, 1993.
91. Kosmahl, EM: The shoulder. In Kauffman, TL (ed): Geriatric Rehabilitation Manual. Churchill Livingstone, New York, 1999, p 99.
92. Kumar, VP, Satku, K, and Balasubramaniam, P: The role of the long head of the biceps brachii in the stabilization in the head of the humerus. Clin Orthop 244:172, 1989.
93. Kunkel, SS, and Hawkins, RJ: Open repair of the rotator cuff. In Andrews, JR, and Wilk, KE (eds): The Athlete's Shoulder. Churchill Livingstone, New York, 1994.
94. Levangie, PK, and Norkin CC: Joint Structure and Function: A Comprehensive Analysis, ed 3. FA Davis, Philadelphia, 2001.
95. Litchfield, R, et al: Rehabilitation for the overhead athlete. J Orthop Sports Phys Ther 18:433, 1993.
96. Lord, J, and Rosati, JM: Thoracic outlet syndromes, Vol 23. CIBA Pharmaceutical Co, Summit, NJ, 1971.
97. Ludewig, PM, and Cook, TC: Alterations in shoulder kinematics and associated muscle activity in people with symptoms of shoulder impingement. Phys Ther 80:276, 2000.
98. Lukasiewics, AC, McClure, P, et al: Comparison of 3-dimensional scapular position and orientation between subjects with and without shoulder impingement. J Orthop Sports Phys Ther 29:574, 1999.
99. Magee, DJ: Orthopedic Physical Assessment, ed 3. WB Saunders, Philadelphia, 1997.
100. Malanga, GA, et al: EMG analysis of shoulder positioning in testing and strengthening the supraspinatus. Med Sci Sports Exerc 28:661, 1996.
101. Malone, TR: Principles of rehabilitation and prehabilitation. Sports Injury Management 1:42, 1988.
102. Matsen, FA: Early effectiveness of shoulder arthroplasty for patients who have primary degenerative disease. J Bone Joint Surg, 78A:260, 1996.
103. Matsen, FA, et al: Glenohumeral arthritis and its management. In Rockwood, CA, and Matsen, FA (eds): The Shoulder, Vol 2, ed 2. WB Saunders, Philadelphia, 1998, p 841.
104. Matsen, FA, et al: Glenohumeral instability. In Rockwood, CA, and Matsen, FA (eds): The Shoulder, Vol 2, ed 2. WB Saunders, Philadelphia, 1998, p 611.
105. Matsen, FA, Arntz, CT, and Lippitt, SB: Rotator cuff. In Rockwood, CA, and Matsen, FA (eds): The Shoulder, Vol 2, ed 2. WB Saunders, Philadelphia, 1998, p 755.
106. Mattalino, AJ: Instabilities. In Donatelli, RA (ed): Physical Therapy of the Shoulder, ed 3. Churchill Livingstone, Philadelphia, 1997, p 421.
107. Matthews, LS, and Pavlovich, LJ: Anterior and anteroinferior instability: diagnosis and management. In Iannotti, JP, and Williams, GR (eds): Disorders of the Shoulder. Lippincott Williams & Wilkins, Philadelphia, 1999, p 251.
108. McCluskey, GM, and Uhl, T: Total shoulder replacement. In Donatelli, RA (ed): Physical Therapy of the Shoulder, ed 3. Churchill Livingstone, Philadelphia, 1997, p 459.
109. Meister, K, and Andrews, JR: Classification and treatment of rotator cuff injuries in the overhand athlete. J Orthop Sports Phys Ther 18:413, 1993.
110. Mulligan, BR: Manual Therapy "NAGS", "SNAGS", "MWM's": etc, ed 4. Plane View Press, Wellington, 1999.
111. Murphy, MS: Rotator cuff repairs. In Clark, GL, et al (eds): Hand Rehabilitation, ed 2. Churchill Livingstone, New York, 1998, p 187.
112. Neer, CS: Surgery in the shoulder. In Kelly, WH, Harris, ED, Ruddy, S, and Sledge, CB (eds): Surgery in Arthritis. WB Saunders, Philadelphia, 1994, p 754.
113. Neer, CS: Impingement lesions. Clin Orthop 173:70, 1983.
114. Neer, CS: Shoulder Reconstruction. WB Saunders, Philadelphia, 1990.
115. Neer, CS: Anterior acromioplasty for the chronic impingement syndrome in the shoulder. A preliminary report. J Bone Joint Surg Am 54:41, 1972.
116. Neer, CS: Replacement arthroplasty for glenohumeral osteoarthritis. J Bone Joint Surg Am 56:1, 1974.

117. Nevaiser, RJ, and Nevaiser, TJ: The frozen shoulder: Diagnosis and management. Clin Orthop 223:59, 1987.
118. Nevaiser, RJ: Ruptures of the rotator cuff. Orthop Clin North Am 18:387, 1987.
119. Nevaiser, RJ: Injuries to the clavicle and acromioclavicular joint. Orthop Clin North Am 18:433, 1987.
120. Nevaiser, TJ: Adhesive capsulitis. Orthrop Clin North Am 18:439, 1987.
121. Nevaiser, TJ: The role of the biceps tendon in the impingement syndrome. Orthop Clin North Am 18:383, 1987.
122. Nicholson, GG: The effects of passive joint mobilization on pain and hypomobility associated with adhesive capsulitis of the shoulder. J Orthop Sports Phys Ther 6:238, 1985.
123. Nixon, RT, and Lindenfeld, TN: Early rehabilitation after a modified inferior capsular shift procedure for multidirectional instability of the shoulder. Orthopedics 21:441, 1998.
124. Noonan, TJ, and Garrett, WE: Injuries at the myotendinous junction. Clin Sports Med 11:783, 1992.
125. Nuber, GW, and Bowen, MK: Disorders of the acromioclavicular joint: pathophysiology, diagnosis and management. In Iannotti, JP, and Williams, GR (eds): Disorders of the Shoulder. Lippincott Williams & Wilkins, Philadelphia, 1999, p 739.
126. O'Brien, M: Functional anatomy and physiology of tendons. Clin Sports Med 11:505, 1992.
127. O'Brien, SJ, Warren, RF, and Schwartz, E: Anterior shoulder instability. Orthop Clin North Am 18:385, 1987.
128. Paine, RM, and Voight, M: The role of the scapula. J Orthop Sports Phys Ther 18:386, 1993.
129. Palmer, ML, and Blakely, RL: Documentation of medial rotation accompanying shoulder flexion: A case report. Phys Ther 66:55, 1986.
130. Pang, D, and Wessel, HB: Thoracic outlet syndrome. Neurosurgery 22:105, 1988.
131. Payne, LZ, Deng, XH, et al: The combined dynamic and static contributions to subacromial impingement: a biomechanical analysis. Am J Sports Med 25:801, 1997.
132. Penny, JW, and Welsh, MB: Shoulder impingement syndromes in athletes and their surgical management. Am J Sports Med 9:11, 1981.
133. Peterson, CA, Altchek, DW, and Warren, RE: Shoulder arthroscopy. In Rockwood, CA, and Matsen, FA (eds): The Shoulder, Vol 1, ed 2. WB Saunders, Philadelphhia, 1998, 290.
134. Pollock, RG, and Flatow, LL: Full-thickness tears: mini-open repair. Orthop Clin North Am, 28:169, 1997.
135. Post, M, and Grinblat, E: Preoperative clinical evaluation. In Friedman, RJ (ed): Arthroplasty of the Shoulder, Theime Medical, New York, 1994, p 41.
136. Post, M, Morrey, BE, and Hawkins, RJ (eds): Surgery of the Shoulder. Mosby Year-Book, St Louis, 1990.
137. Ramsey, ML, and Klimkiewicz, JJ: Posterior instability: diagnosis and management. In Iannotti, JP, and Williams, GR (eds): Disorders of the Shoulder: Diagnosis and Management. Lippincott Williams & Wilkins, Philadelphia, 1999, p 295.
138. Richards, RR: Redefining indications for and problems of shoulder arthrodesis. In Warner, JJP, Iannotti, JB, and Gerber, C (eds): Complex and Revision Problems in Shoulder Surgery. Lippincott-Raven, Philadelphia, 1997.
139. Richards, RR: Glenohumeral arthrodesis. In Iannotti, JP, and Williams, GR (eds): Disorders of the Shoulder: Diagnosis and Management. Lippincott Williams & Wilkins, Philadelphia, 1999, p 501.
140. Rockwood, CA, and Wirth, MA: Disorders of the sternoclavicular joint. In Rockwood, CA, and Matsen, FA (eds): The Shoulder, Vol 1, ed 2. WB Saunders, Philadelphia, 1998, p 555.
141. Rockwood, CA, Williams, GR, and Young, DC: Disorders of the acromioclavicular joint. In Rockwood, CA, and Matsen, FA (eds): The Shoulder, Vol 1, ed 2. WB Saunders, Philadelphia, 1998, p 483.
142. Rockwood, CA, and Lyons, FR: Shoulder impingement syndrome: Diagnosis, radiographic evaluation, and treatment with a modified Neer acromioplasty. J Bone Joint Surg Am 75:409, 1993.
143. Rodosky, MW, and Harner, CD: The role of the long head of the biceps muscle and superior glenoid labrum in anterior stability of the shoulder. Am J Sports Med 22:121, 1994.
144. Rokito, AS, et al: Strength after surgical repair of the rotator cuff. J Shoulder Elbow Surg 5:12, 1996.
145. Rose, BS: Frozen shoulder. N Z Med J 98(792):1039, 1985.
146. Rowe, CR: Anterior glenohumeral subluxation/dislocation: The Bankart procedure. In Welsh, RP, and Shephard, RJ (eds): Current Therapy in Sports Medicine, Vol 2. BC Decker, Toronto, 1990.
147. Roye, RP, Grana, WA, and Yates, CK: Arthroscopic subacromial decompression: two- to seven-year follow-up. Arthroscopy 11:301, 1995.
148. Schenk, T, and Brems, JJ. Multidirectional instability of the shoulder: pathophysiology, diagnosis, and management. J Am Acad Orthop Surg 6:65, 1998.
149. Schenk, T, and Iannotti, IP: Prosthetic arthroplasty for glenohumeral arthritis with an intact or repairable rotator cuff: Indications, techniques and results. In Iannotti, JP, and Williams, GR (eds): Disorders of the Shoulder: Diagnosis and Management. Lippincott Williams & Wilkins, Philadelphia, 1999, p 521.
150. Schieb, JS: Diagnosis and rehabilitation of the shoulder impingement syndrome in the overhand and throwing athlete. Rheum Dis Clin North Am, 16:971, 1990.
151. Schmitt, L, and Snyder-Mackler, L: Role of scapular stabilizers in etiology and treatment of impingement syndrome. J Orthop Sports Phys Ther 29:31, 1999.
152. Schwartz, E, et al: Posterior shoulder instability. Orthop Clin North Am 18:409, 1987.
153. Selecky, MT, Vangsness, CT, et al: The effects of laser-induced collagen shortening on the biomechanical properties of the inferior glenohumeral ligament complex. Am J Sports Med 27:168, 1999.
154. Sharkey, NA, and Marder, RA: The rotator cuff opposes superior translation of the humeral head. Am J Sports Med 23:270, 1995.
155. Simon, ER, and Hill, JA: Rotator cuff Injuries: An update. J Orthop Sports Phys Ther 10(10):394–398, 1989.
156. Smith, K: The thoracic outlet syndrome: A protocol of treatment. J Orthop Sports Phys Ther 1:89, 1979.
157. Smith, LK, Weiss, EL, and Lehmkuhl, LD: Brunnstrom's Clinical Kinesiology, ed 5. FA Davis Company, Philadelphia, 1996.
158. Stanton-Hicks, M, et al: Reflex sympathetic dystrophy: changing concepts and taxonomy. Pain 63:127, 1995.

159. Sucher, BM: Thoracic outlet syndrome: A myofascial variant: Part 1. Pathology and diagnosis. J Am Osteopath Assoc 90:686, 1990.
160. Sucher, BM: Thoracic outlet syndrome: A myofascial variant: Part 2. Treatment, J Am Osteopath Assoc 90:810, 1990.
161. Tauro, JL: Arthroscopic rotator cuff repair: An analysis of technique and results of 2- and 3-year follow-up. Arthroscopy 14:45, 1998.
162. Thein, LA, and Greenfield, BH: Impingement syndrome and impingement-related instability. In Donatelli, RA (ed): Physical Therapy of the Shoulder, ed 3. Churchill Livingstone, New York, 1997, p 229.
163. Thomas, BJ, and Amstuts, HC: Shoulder arthroplasty for rheumatoid arthritis. Clin Orthop 269:125, 1991.
164. Thornhill, TS, Gall, V, Vermetle, S, and Griffen, F: Shoulder surgery and rehabilitation. In Melvin, I, and Gall, V (eds): Rheumatologic Rehabilitation Series, Vol 5: Surgical Rehabilitation. American Occupational Therapy Association, Bethesda, MD, 1999, p 37.
165. Tibone, JE, and McMahon, PJ: Biomechanics and pathologic lesions in the overhead athlete. In Iannotti, JP, and Williams, GR (eds): Disorders of the Shoulder: Diagnosis and Management. Lippincott Williams & Wilkins, Philadelphia, 1999, p 233.
166. Tibone, JE, and Bradley, JP: The treatment of posterior subluxation in athletes. Clin Orthop 291:124, 1993.
167. Tibone, JE, et al: Glenohumeral joint translation after arthroscopic, nonablative thermal capsuloplasty with a laser. Am J Sports Med 26: 495, 1998.
168. Tibone, JE, et al: Surgical treatment of tears of the rotator cuff in athletes. J Bone Joint Surg Am 68:887, 1986.
169. Ticker, JB, and Warner, JJJP: Rotator cuff tears: principles of tendon repair. In Iannotti, JP (ed): The Rotator Cuff: Current Concepts and Complex Problems. American Academy of Orthopedic Surgeons, Rosemont, IL, 1998, p 17.
170. Timmerman, LA, Andrews, JR, and Wilk, KE: Mini-open repair of the rotator cuff. In Wilk, KE, and Andrews, JR (eds): The Athlete's Shoulder, Churchill-Livingstone, New York, 1994.
171. Townsend, H, et al: Electromyographic analysis of the glenohumeral muscles during a baseball rehabilitation program. Am J Sports Med 19:264, 1991.
172. Turkel, SJ, et al: Stabilizing Mechanisms Preventing Anterior Dislocation of the Glenohumeral Joint. J Bone Joint Surg Am 61:1208, 1981.
173. Tyler, TF, Calabrese, GJ, Parker, RD, and Nicholas, SJ: Electrothermally-assisted capsulorrhaphy (E.T.A.C.): A new surgical method for glenohumeral instability and its rehabilitation considerations. J Orthop and Sports Phys Ther 30:390, 2000.
174. Vermeulen, HM, Obermann, WR, et al: End-range mobilization techniques in adhesive capsulitis of the shoulder joint: a multiple-subject case report. Phys Ther 80:1204, 2000.
175. Wadsworth, CT: Frozen shoulder. Phys Ther 66:1878, 1986.
176. Walker, SM, and Cousins, MJ: Complex regional pain syndromes: including "reflex sympathetic dystrophy" and "causalgia". Anaesth Intensive Care 25 :113, 1997.
177. Walsh, MT: Therapist management of thoracic outlet syndrome. J Hand Ther April-June:131, 1994.
178. Warner, JP, Micheili, LJ, et al: Scapulothoracic motion in normal shoulders and shoulders with glenohumeral instability and impingement syndrome: a study using Moire's topographic analysis. Clin Orthop 285:191, 1992.
179. Warner, JP: Treatment options for anterior instability: Open vs. arthroscopic. Operative Tech Orthop 5:233, 1995.
180. Wilde, AH, Brems, JJ, and Bounphrey, FRS: Arthrodesis of the Shoulder: Current indications and operative technique. Orthop Clin North Am 18:463–472, 1987.
181. Wilk, KE, et al: Stretch-shortening drills for the upper extremities: Theory and clinical application. J Orthop Sports Phys Ther 17(5):225–239, 1993.
182. Wilk, KE, and Arrigo, C: An integrated approach to upper extremity exercises. Orthop Phys Ther Clin North Am 1:337, 1992.
183. Wilk, KE, and Arrigo, C: Current concepts in the rehabilitation of the athletic shoulder. J Orthop Sports Phys Ther 18:365, 1993.
184. Wilk, KE: The shoulder. In Malone, TR, McPoil, TG, and Nitz, AJ (eds): Orthopedic and Sports Physical Therapy, ed 3, CV Mosby, St. Louis, 1997, p 401.
185. Wilk, KE, and Andrews, JR: Rehabilitation following arthroscopic subacromial decompression. Orthopedics 16:349, 1993.
186. Wilk, KE, Andrews, JR, and Arrigo, CA: The physical examination of the glenohumeral joint: emphasis on the stabilizing structures. J Orthop Sports Phys Ther 25:380, 1997.
187. Wilk, KE, Arrigo, CA, and Andrews, JR: Current concepts: the stabilizing structures of the glenohumeral joint. J Orthop Sports Phys Ther 24:364, 1997.
188. Williams, GR, and Iannotti, JP: Biomechanics of the glenohumeral joint: Influence on shoulder arthroplasty. In Iannotti, JP, and Williams, GR (eds): Disorders of the Shoulder: Diagnosis and Management. Lippincott Williams & Wilkins, Philadelphia, 1999, p 471.
189. Wirth, MA, Blatter, G, and Rockwood, CA: The capsular imbrication procedure for recurrent anterior instability of the shoulder. J Bone Joint Surg 78A:246, 1996.
190. Wirth, MA, and Rockwood, CA: Disorders of the sternoclavicular joint: pathophysiology, diagnosis, and management. In Iannotti, JP, and Williams, GR (eds): Disorders of the Shoulder: Diagnosis and Management. Lippincott Williams & Wilkins, Philadelphia, 1999, p 763.
191. Worrell, TW, et al: An analysis of supraspinatus EMG activity and shoulder isometric force development. Med Sci Sports Exerc 24:744, 1992.

Chapter 10

The Elbow and Forearm Complex

OBJECTIVES

After studying this chapter, the reader will be able to:

1 Identify important aspects of elbow and forearm structure and function for review.
2 Establish a therapeutic exercise program to manage soft tissue and joint lesions in the elbow and forearm region related to stages of recovery after an inflammatory insult to the tissues, recognizing unique circumstances for their management.
3 Discuss the background of, indications for, and outcomes of common surgical procedures for soft tissue and joint pathology at the elbow.
4 Explain the goals and appropriate interventions for postoperative management of elbow dysfunction.
5 Establish a postoperative intervention program that includes therapeutic exercise for management of common surgical procedures for the elbow.

A freely mobile but strong and stable elbow complex is required for normal upper extremity function. The design of the elbow and forearm adds to the mobility of the hand in space by shortening and lengthening the upper extremity and by rotating the forearm. The muscles provide control and stability to the region as the hand is used for various activities from eating, dressing and grooming; pushing, pulling, turning, lifting, throwing, catching, and reaching for objects; to coordinated use of equipment, tools, and machines.[23,32,36,49,60] Most activities of daily living require a 100 degree arc of flexion and extension at the elbow, specifically between 30 and 130 degrees, as well as 100 degrees of forearm rotation, equally divided between pronation and supination.[49,50]

Injury or disease of bony, articular, or soft tissue structures of the elbow and forearm can cause pain and compromised mobility, strength, stability, and functional use of the upper extremity. Loss of active or passive elbow flexion interferes with grooming and eating, whereas loss of elbow extension restricts a person's ability to push up from a chair or reach out for objects. In general, loss of terminal flexion of the elbow contributes to greater limitation of function than loss of terminal extension.[49]

The anatomic and kinesiologic relationships of the elbow and forearm are outlined in the first section of this chapter. Chapter 8 presents information on principles of management; the reader should be familiar with that material before proceeding with establishing a therapeutic exercise program to improve function of the elbow and forearm.

► Review of the Structure and Function of the Elbow and Forearm

Bony Parts: Distal Humerus, Radius, and Ulna (see Fig. 6–25)

The distal end of the humerus has two articular surfaces, the trochlea, which articulates with the ulna and the capitulum, which articulates with the head of the radius. Flexion and extension occur between these two joint surfaces. The radius also articulates with the radial notch on the ulna and is called the proximal radioulnar joint. This joint participates in pronation and supination along with the distal radioulnar joint. The capsule of the elbow encloses the humeroulnar, humeroradial, and proximal radioulnar articulations. The distal radioulnar joint is structurally separate from the elbow complex even though its function is directly related to the proximal radioulnar joint.[31]

Elbow Joint Characteristics and Arthrokinematics

The elbow is a compound joint with a lax joint capsule, supported by two major ligaments: the medial (ulnar) and lateral (radial) collateral, which provide medial and lateral stability, respectively.[9,28,32,60]

Humeroulnar (HU) Articulation

- This is a modified hinge joint. The medially placed hourglass-shaped trochlea at the distal end of the humerus is convex. It faces anteriorly and downward 45 degrees from the shaft of the humerus. The concave trochlear fossa, on the proximal ulna, faces upward and anteriorly 45 degrees from the ulna (see Fig. 6–26).
- The primary motion is flexion and extension; the concave fossa slides in the same direction in which the ulna moves, so that with elbow flexion, the fossa slides around the trochlea in an anterior and distal direction. With elbow extension, the fossa slides in a posterior and proximal direction (Box 10–1).
- There is also slight medial and lateral sliding of the ulna, allowing for full elbow ROM; it results in a valgus angulation of the joint with elbow extension and a varus angulation with elbow flexion. When the bone moves in a medial/lateral direction, the trochlear ridge provides a convex surface, and the trochlear groove provides a concave surface, so with varus the ulna slides in a lateral direction and with valgus the ulna slides in a medial direction (Box 10–1).

Humeroradial (HR) Articulation

- This is a hinge-pivot joint. The laterally placed, spherical capitulum at the distal end of the humerus is convex. The concave bony partner, the head of the radius, is at the proximal end of the radius.
- As the elbow flexes and extends, the concave radial head slides in the same direction as the bone motion so that with elbow flexion the concave head slides anteriorly, and with elbow extension it slides posteriorly (Box 10–1). With pronation and supination of the forearm, the radial head spins on the capitulum.

Ligaments of the Elbow

Medial (ulnar) collateral ligament. This ligament consists of bundles of fibers that may be differentiated into anterior, posterior, and transverse positions. Various portions of the ligament are taut in different ranges of motion (ROMs) providing medial support to the elbow against valgus stresses. The ligament also keeps the joint surfaces in approximation.[60]

Lateral (radial) collateral ligament. This fan-shaped ligament on the lateral surface of the elbow provides stability against varus forces and prevents posterior translation of the radial head.

Box 10–1 Summary of Joint Arthrokinematics of the Elbow and Forearm Joints

Physiologic Motion	Roll	Slide
Humeroulnar articulation	Motion of ulnar joint surface	
Flexion	Anterior	Distal/anterior
Extension	Posterior	Proximal/posterior
Humeroradial articulation	Motion of radial joint surface	
Flexion	Anterior	Anterior
Extension	Posterior	Posterior
Forearm varus	Motion of proximal forearm	
	Medial	Lateral
Forearm valgus	Motion of proximal forearm	
	Lateral	Medial
Proximal radiounlar joint	Motion of rim of radial head	
Pronation	Anterior	Posterior (dorsal)
Supination	Posterior	Anterior (volar)
Distal radioulnar joint	Motion of distal radial joint surface	
Pronation	Anterior	Anterior
Supination	Posterior	Posterior

Forearm Joint Characteristics and Arthrokinematics

Both the proximal and distal radioulnar joints are uniaxial pivot joints that function together to produce pronation and supination (rotation) of the forearm.[9,28,32,60]

Proximal (Superior) Radioulnar (RU) Articulation

- It is within the capsule of the elbow joint but is a distinct articulation.
- The convex rim of the radial head articulates with the concave radial notch on the ulna and the annular ligament. This ligament encircles the rim of the radial head and stabilizes it against the ulna. As the forearm rotates into pronation and supination, the convex rim of the radial head slides opposite the bone motion, so that with pronation the head slides posteriorly (dorsal ward) on the radial notch and with supination it slides anteriorly (volarward). It also slides in the annular ligament and the proximal surface spins on the capitulum.

Distal (Inferior) Radioulnar Articulation

- The distal RU joint is an anatomically separate joint at the distal end of the radius and ulna.
- The concave ulnar notch on the distal radius articulates with the convex notch on the head of the ulna. As the forearm rotates, the concave radius slides in the same direction as the physiologic motion. It slides anterior (volar) with pronation and posterior (dorsal) with supination (Box 10–1).

Muscle Function at the Elbow and Forearm

Elbow Flexor Muscles

Brachialis. The brachialis is a one-joint muscle that inserts close to the axis of motion on the ulna, so it is unaffected by the position of the forearm or the shoulder; it participates in all flexion activities of the elbow.[9,32,60]

Biceps brachii. The biceps is a two-joint muscle that crosses both the shoulder and elbow and inserts close to the axis of motion on the radius, so it also acts as a supinator of the forearm. It functions most effectively as a flexor of the elbow between 80 and 100 degrees of flexion. For optimal length-tension relationship, the shoulder extends to lengthen the muscle when it contracts forcefully for elbow and forearm function.[9,32,60]

Brachioradialis. With its insertion a great distance from the elbow on the distal radius, the brachioradialis mainly functions to provide stability to the joint, but it also participates as the speed of flexion motion increases and a load is applied with the forearm from midsupination to full pronation.[9,32,60]

Elbow Extensor Muscles

Triceps brachii. The long head crosses both the shoulder and elbow; the other two heads are uniaxial. The long head functions most effectively as an elbow extensor if the shoulder simultaneously flexes; this maintains an optimal length-tension relationship in the muscle.[32,60]

Anconeus. This muscle stabilizes the elbow during supination and pronation and assists in elbow extension.[32,60]

Forearm Supinator Muscles

Supinator. The proximal attachment of the supinator at the annular and lateral collateral ligaments may function to stabilize the lateral aspect of the elbow. Its effectiveness as a supinator is not affected by the elbow position as is the biceps brachii.[62]

Biceps brachii. The biceps muscle acts as a supinator if the elbow simultaneously flexes, or if resistance is given to supination when the elbow is in extension.[5]

Brachioradialis. The brachioradialis contributes to pronation and supination only as an accessory muscle when resistance is provided to the motion.[5] It cannot function alone as a rotator or stabilizer of the forearm joints when other forearm muscles are paralyzed.[60]

Forearm Pronator Muscles

Pronator teres. This muscle pronates as well as stabilizes the proximal radioulnar joint and helps approximate the humeroradial articulation.[32]

Pronator quadratus. The pronator quadratus is a one-joint muscle and is active during all pronation activities.

Wrist and Hand Muscles

Many muscles that act on the wrist and hand are attached on the distal portion (epicondyles) of the humerus. This allows for movement of the fingers and wrist, whether the forearm is in pronation or supination. The muscles provide stability to the elbow but contribute little to motion at the elbow. The position of the elbow will affect the length-tension relationship of the muscles during their actions on the wrist and hand.[32]

Wrist Flexor Muscles

Originating on the medial epicondyle are the flexor carpi radialis, flexor carpi ulnaris, palmaris longus, and flexor digitorum superficialis and profundus.

Wrist Extensor Muscles

Originating on the lateral epicondyle are the extensor carpi radialis longus and brevis, extensor carpi ulnaris, and extensor digitorum.

Major Nerves Subject to Pressure and Trauma Around the Elbow

Ulnar Nerve

The nerve is superficial to the olecranon fossa, posterior to the medial epicondyle, and covered by a fibrous sheath, which forms the cubital tunnel; it then passes between the heads of the flexor carpi ulnaris. Pressure or injury to the nerve at these sites will cause sensory changes in the cutaneous distribution of the nerve (ulnar border of the hand, little finger, and ulnar half of the ring finger), with progressive weakness in the muscles innervated distal to the site of injury (flexor carpi ulnaris, ulnar half of the flexor digitorum profundus, hypothenar eminence, interossei, lumbricals III and IV, flexor pollicis brevis, and adductor pollicis).[29]

Radial Nerve

The nerve pierces the lateral muscular septum anterior to the lateral epicondyle and passes under the origin of the extensor carpi radialis brevis and then divides.[29] The deep branch may become entrapped as it passes under the edge of the extensor carpi radialis brevis and the fibrous slit in the supinator, causing progressive weakness in the wrist and finger extensor and supinator muscles (except the extensor carpi radialis longus, which is innervated proximal to the bifurcation). The deep branch may also be injured with a radial head fracture. The superficial radial nerve may receive direct trauma that causes sensory changes in the lateral aspect of the forearm to the anatomic snuffbox, and the radial side of the dorsum of the wrist and hand and radial three and one-half digits.

Median Nerve

The nerve courses deep in the cubital fossa, medial to the tendon of the biceps and brachial artery, then progresses between the ulnar and humeral heads of the pronator teres and dips under the flexor digitorum profundus muscle. Entrapment may occur between the heads of the pronator muscle, causing sensory changes duplicating carpal tunnel syndrome (palmar aspect of the thumb, index, middle, and half of the ring finger, and dorsal aspect of distal phalanges of index and ring fingers). Motor changes include the pronator teres, wrist flexors, extrinsic finger flexors, and the intrinsic thenar and lumbricals I and II.[29] (Carpal tunnel syndrome involves just the intrinsic muscles of the thenar eminence and lumbricals I and II; see Chapter 11.)

Joint Hypomobility: Nonoperative Management

Related Diagnoses and Etiology of Symptoms

Pathologies such as rheumatoid arthritis (RA), juvenile rheumatoid arthritis (JRA), and degenerative joint disease (DJD) as well as acute joint reactions after trauma, dislocations, or fractures affect this joint complex. Postimmobilization contractures and adhesions develop in the joint capsule and surrounding tissues any time the joint is immobilized in a cast or splint. This typically occurs after dislocations and fractures of the humerus, radius, or ulna.

Common Impairments

Acute stage. When symptoms are acute, joint effusion, muscle guarding, and pain restrict elbow flexion and extension, and there is usually pain at rest. If pronation and/or supination are restricted after an acute injury, other conditions such as fracture, subluxation, or dislocation may be present.[13] These require medical intervention.

Subacute and chronic stages. A capsular pattern usually exists in the subacute or chronic stages. Elbow flexion is more restricted than extension. There is a firm end-feel and decreased joint play. In longstanding arthritis at the elbow, pronation and supination also become restricted with a firm end-feel and decreased joint play in the proximal RU joint.[13] Arthritis in the distal RU joint results in pain on overpressure.

Common Functional Limitations/Disabilities

- Difficulty turning a doorknob or key in the ignition
- Difficulty or pain with pushing and pulling activities, such as opening and closing doors
- Restricted hand-to-mouth activities for eating and drinking and hand-to-head activities for personal grooming and using a telephone
- Difficulty or pain with pushing self up from a chair
- Inability to carry objects with a straight arm
- Limited reach

Joint Management: Protection Phase

See guidelines for management in Chapter 8, Box 8–1.

Patient Education

- Inform the patient of anticipated length of acute symptoms and teach methods of joint protection and how to modify ADL activities. For example, avoid activities that involve lifting or pushing off with the involved upper extremity.
- Avoid excessive fatigue by performing exercises frequently during the day but limiting the number of repetitions during each bout (set) of exercises.

Reduce Effects of Inflammation or Synovial Effusion and Protect the Area

- Immobilization in a sling provides rest to the part, but complete immobilization can lead to joint hypomobility, contractures, and limited motion, so frequent periods of controlled movement within a pain-free range should be performed.

Note: Often the elbow is immobilized in 90 degrees flexion. The position of relative extension (20–30 degrees of flexion) is used to prevent or treat ulnar neuropathy by preventing positions that could aggravate the ulnar nerve already at risk in the cubital tunnel because of joint swelling. The somewhat extended position, as well as use of a posterior splint bubbled out around the cubital tunnel, deepens the cubital tunnel, thus reducing pressure on the ulnar nerve.[7]

- Gentle grade I or II distraction and oscillation techniques in the resting position may inhibit pain and move synovial fluid for nutrition in the involved joints (see Chapter 6 for techniques).

Maintain Soft Tissue and Joint Mobility

- Passive or active-assistive ROM within limits of pain; include flexion/extension and pronation/supination.
- Multiple-angle muscle setting of elbow flexors, extensors, pronators, and supinators, and to wrist flexors and extensors in pain-free positions.

Maintain Integrity and Function of Related Areas

- Shoulder, wrist, and hand ROM and activities should be encouraged within the tolerance of the individual.
- If edema develops in the hand, the arm should be elevated whenever possible and distal-to-proximal massage techniques applied.

Joint Management: Controlled Motion Phase

If joint hypomobility exists, ROM is increased by utilizing joint mobilization techniques as well as passive stretching and muscle inhibition techniques following the principles described in Chapters 5 and 6. There are several important precautions if the joint restrictions are related to trauma. ***Precautions after trauma:*** (1) If the brachialis muscle is injured, ossification of the injured tissue is a potential complication, and stretching is contraindicated. (2) After healing of fractures in the forearm, malunion is not unusual, preventing full range of pronation or supination. A bony block end-feel or an abnormal appearance of the forearm should alert the therapist to the cause of this impairment. X-ray films are helpful in verifying the problem. No amount of stretching or mobilizing will change the patient's range. Indiscriminate stretching may lead to hypermobility of related joints, which could cause additional trauma and pain.

Progressively Increase Soft Tissue and Joint Mobility

Precaution: Initiate stretching cautiously, and note joint and tissue response. Vigorous stretching should not be undertaken until the chronic stage of healing.

- ***Passive joint mobilization techniques.*** Determine which of the articulations in the elbow complex have reduced joint play and apply grade III sustained or grade IV oscillation techniques. See Figures 6–27 through 6–32 and their descriptions in Chapter 6. Progress each technique by positioning the joint at the end of its available range before applying the mobilization technique.

Note: To progress joint mobility in the terminal ranges of flexion and extension it may be necessary to emphasize the accessory motions of varus and valgus, respectively. This is accomplished with medial and lateral gliding techniques or with a varus or valgus physiologic stretch at the elbow.

- ***Mobilization to reduce a "pushed elbow."*** Proximal subluxation of the radius may occur from falling on an outstretched hand.[70] The radial head is pushed proximally in the annular ligament and impinges against the capitulum. This sometimes accompanies a fracture of the distal radius (Colles' fracture) or scaphoid and is not identified as an impairment until after healing of the fracture and removal of the cast. It is often overlooked because there is considerable soft tissue and joint restriction caused by the period of immobilization. Bilateral palpation of the joint spaces will reveal the decreased space on the involved side. There may be limited flexion or extension of the elbow, limited wrist flexion, and limited pronation.
  - ***Technique.*** If acute (and no fracture), apply a distal traction to the radius to reposition the radial head. If chronic, repetitive stretching with sustained grade III distal traction to the radius will be necessary (see Fig. 6–28) in addition to the soft tissue stretching and strengthening techniques needed for increasing motion.
- ***Manipulation to reduce a "pulled elbow."*** Distal subluxation of the radius is usually seen as an acute injury in children and is sometimes labeled "tennis elbow" when it occurs in adults.[70] It occurs as a result of a forceful pull on the hand such as would occur when a child jerks away from a parent or caregiver, or a person trying to pick up a heavy object with a jerking motion on a handle. The force causes the radius to move distalward, and the head of the radius is unable to slide proximally in the annular ligament. The person usually holds the forearm in pronation; there is limited supination.
  - ***Technique.*** Apply a quick compressive manipulation with supination to the radius (see Fig. 6–30) to reposition the head. If it is an initial injury, there may be soft tissue trauma from the injury, which is treated with cold and compression.
- ***Manual and self-stretching.*** Stretch any periarticular tissues that are restricting mobility. Manual stretching and inhibition techniques are described in Chapter 5.
- Teach the patient self-stretching maneuvers followed by active exercise that utilize the new range. Suggestions are provided later in this chapter.

Improve Joint Tracking of the Elbow

A mobilization with movement (MWM) technique of a lateral glide combined with the active movement of flexion or extension and pain-free passive overpressure may improve articular surface tracking by allowing the muscles to move the joint in a pain-free manner.[51] (Refer to principles of MWM in Chapter 6.)

Technique. Patient position: Supine with elbow either flexed or extended to end of available range. Secure a mobilization belt around the proximal forearm and your hips. Stabilize the distal humerus at the olecranon process with one hand, and support the forearm with the other. Apply a gentle lateral glide to the proximal ulna with the belt by moving your hips. Have the patient produce an active elbow flexion or extension movement and apply a passive overpressure stretch at the end of the range (Fig. 10–1). This should not elicit any pain.

Progressively Increase Strength and Functional Activities

Initiate active and light resistance exercises in open- and closed-chain to develop control, muscular endurance, and strength in the muscles of the elbow and forearm. Exercises are described later in this chapter. Progress the patient toward return to functional activities. Include the shoulder girdle, wrist, and hand in the exercise program since their flexibility and strength will have an influence on the recovery of elbow function.

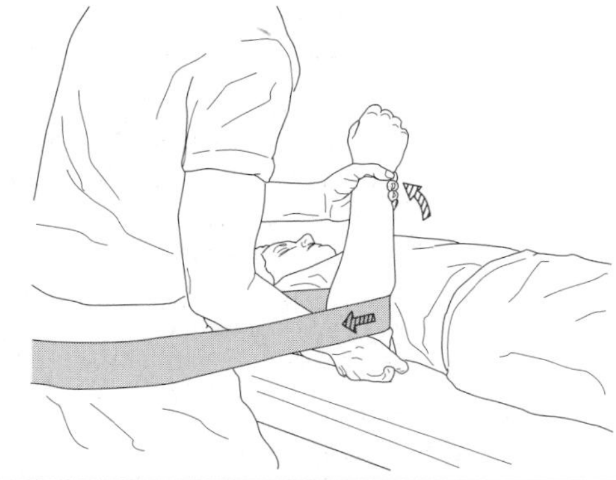

Figure 10–1 MWM to improve elbow flexion. A lateral glide is applied to the proximal ulna while the patient actively flexes, followed by a passive end range stretch.

Joint Management: Return to Function Phase

Stretching and Strengthening Exercises

Progress self-stretching and strengthening exercises as the joint tissue tolerates. Teach the patient safe progressions and exercise strategies that promote return to function.

Manual and Joint Mobilization Techniques

If restrictions remain, vigorous manual techniques are used.

Prepare for Functional Demands

The elbow and forearm are involved in pushing, pulling, lifting, carrying, and gripping activities. Develop exercises that replicate the repetitions and demands of daily tasks to prepare the joint and muscles for the tasks. Chronic arthritic conditions may require modification of high-load activities to minimize deforming stresses.

▶ Joint Surgery and Postoperative Management

Surgical intervention is often necessary after a variety of fractures or dislocations that affect the joints of the elbow and surrounding soft tissues. These injuries may require open reduction, internal fixation, or arthroscopic or open excision of bone fragments. In adults, the most common fracture in the elbow region is a fracture of the head and neck of the radius. This injury usually occurs when a person falls on an outstretched hand, causing a posterior dislocation and fracture of the radial head.[43] If the proximal radius is displaced and the radial head is comminuted, either open reduction with internal fixation or *radial head excision (resection)* with or without implant is usually indicated.[38,43] It has been suggested that rigid internal fixation (screws or plate fixation) of radial head fractures is indicated in the young, active adult, whereas excision of the radial head is more appropriate for the low-demand patient or if the fracture is severely comminuted and fixation is not possible.[24] Radial head fractures are relatively uncommon in children. When they do occur, closed reduction is preferred.[61]

Other indications for extra-articular or intra-articular surgery are long-standing RA, JRA, and post-traumatic DJD associated with synovial proliferation and destruction of articular surfaces of the elbow joints, which results in pain, limitation of motion, and impairment of upper extremity function. In early-stage rheumatoid arthritis in which synovial proliferation is present but joint surfaces are still in good condition, *open* or *arthroscopic synovectomy* is the procedure of choice for relief of pain if medications have not controlled the disease.[4,26,31] Late-stage arthritis may need to be treated surgically by *resection of the radial head* with or without joint implant and concurrent synovectomy,[63] *interpositional* or *total elbow arthroplasty,* or in rare instances, by *arthrodesis* of the elbow.[4,11,17a,41,46] Table 10–1 summarizes how the severity of joint and soft tissue involvement influences the choice of surgical procedure.[12,17a]

The goals of surgery and postoperative rehabilitation of the elbow joint complex[12,48,67] can include (1) relief of pain, (2) restoration of bony alignment and joint stability, and (3) sufficient strength and ROM to allow functional use of the elbow and upper extremity. Procedures done to relieve pain and improve elbow stability tend to be more successful than procedures done solely to increase ROM. Heterotopic

Table 10–1 Severity of Elbow Joint Disease and Selection of Surgical Procedure

Severity of Joint Disease	Selection of Surgical Procedure
Mild synovitis: joint surfaces normal or minimally deteriorated; osteoporosis	Nonoperative/medical management
Moderate synovitis; some loss of articular cartilage; narrowing of joint space but joint contour maintained	Arthroscopic synovectomy or resection of the radial head with synovectomy
Moderate to severe synovitis; loss of articular cartilage; loss of joint space; intact collateral ligaments	Resurfacing total elbow arthroplasty or, possibly, in a growing child, an interpositional arthroplasty
Severe synovitis; destruction of articular cartilage; complete loss of joint space (bone-to-bone articulation); significant joint instability; bone loss; ankylosis	Semiconstrained total elbow arthroplasty

bone formation, which leads to joint stiffness, is often a complication of elbow fractures, dislocations, and elbow joint surgery.[42] Therefore, the single goal of improving ROM is rarely an indication for surgery.[12,38,41]

Excision of the Radial Head

Indications for Surgery

- Severe comminuted fractures of the distal humerus,[10] or fracture-dislocations of the head of the radius that cannot be reconstructed and held in place with internal fixation.[38,43]
- Chronic synovitis and mild deterioration of the articular surfaces associated with arthritis of the humeroradial and proximal radioulnar joints resulting in joint pain at rest or with motion, possible subluxation of the head of the radius, and significant loss of upper extremity function.[4,12,17a,63]

Note: Excision of the radial head is contraindicated in the growing child.[61]

Procedure

A lateral triceps-sparing incision at the elbow and forearm is made (arthrotomy); the radial head is resected at the level of the annular ligament.[43,63]

For the patient with synovitis, a concomitant synovectomy is also done.[63] The head of the radius may or may not be replaced with a prosthetic implant to enhance stability at the elbow. The use of a prosthetic implant is indicated when there is clinical instability of the elbow as the result of disruption of the supporting ligaments.[17a,43,63] Implants were originally made of silicone (Silastic material), but this material has been associated with fatigue failure and adverse biological reactions, specifically, inflammatory arthrosis (synovitis) of the humeroulnar joint.[64] Other materials, such as cobalt-chrome, titanium, ceramics, and ultra-high molecular weight polyethylene are currently being used and investigated.[21,43] The optimal implant has yet to be designed and fabricated. If the elbow is unstable, ligamentous structures are repaired. To prevent injury to the ulnar nerve or if symptoms of compression are present, an ulnar nerve transposition is also performed.

Postoperative Management

Immobilization

The elbow is immobilized in a well-padded posterior splint for maximum protection in a position of 90 degrees of flexion and midposition of the forearm for 1 to 3 days after surgery.[43,63] The arm is elevated for comfort and to prevent or minimize edema distally. The splint is removed for exercise but is replaced after exercise and worn at night for several weeks.[37] If the stability of the elbow is tenuous and the surgery involved a prosthetic implant, ROM exercises may need to be delayed for a week and then initiated with the patient's arm in a hinged splint.

Exercise: Maximum Protection Phase

During the first 7 to 10 days postoperatively, include the following goals and interventions.

- ***Maintain mobility of unoperated joints.*** Active ROM exercises to the shoulder, wrist, and hand immediately after surgery.
- ***Maintain mobility of the elbow.*** Remove the splint several times daily to begin passive or active-assisted ROM within the pain-free ranges as soon as possible after surgery. Continuous passive motion (CPM) may also be used while the patient is hospitalized, usually for 3 to 5 days. Teach the patient self-assisted and active ROM for the home exercise program.
- ***Minimize muscle atrophy.*** Submaximal, pain-free, multiple-angle setting exercises of elbow musculature.

Exercise: Moderate and Minimum Protection Phases

By 10 to 14 days postoperatively the staples along the incision are removed if wound closure is satisfactory. The following goals and interventions are added to the rehabilitation program to improve functional mobility and strength.

Note: These activities often continue for 6 to 12 months postoperatively.[37] The rate of progression of the rehabilitation program depends on the extent of damage to soft tissues from injury or chronic inflammation, the necessity for repair of supporting structures (especially ligaments) of the elbow complex and, of course, the patient's response to treatment.[37] A resting splint is worn at night for an extended period of time to protect healing tissues.

- ***Increase ROM,*** particularly if contractures were noted preoperatively.
  - Gentle (low-intensity) manual stretching using inhibitory elongation techniques.
  - Low-load dynamic splinting or alternating use of static splints in maximum flexion and extension.

- Grades I and II joint mobilization techniques initially, followed by Grade III mobilizations after 6 weeks when the joint capsule is well healed.

Contraindication: Do not perform valgus/varus stretches in terminal extension/flexion, particularly if the radial head was not replaced with a prosthetic implant or if the integrity of the supporting ligaments and stability of joints are in question.

- ***Improve functional strength and muscular endurance.***
  - Use of the operated upper extremity for *light* ADL.

Precaution: Avoid using the involved upper extremity for moving or holding heavy objects.

- Low-load resistance exercises (maximum 1–2 lb), emphasizing high repetitions.

Note: Some surgeons and therapists prefer to improve strength and endurance solely through ADL, that is, without the use of specific resistance exercises.[37,43]

Outcomes

Excision of the radial head for a severely displaced and comminuted fracture or chronic arthritis yields pain-free motion (flexion/extension and pronation/supination) within functional ranges. If pre-existing contractures exist, ROM may not necessarily improve postoperatively.[31,41,43] Some patients also develop a slight increase (about 5–10 degrees) in valgus laxity of the elbow without complaints of instability during functional activities if the ulnar collateral ligament is intact. There may also be slight proximal migration of the radius that may or may not be associated with wrist pain.[43] Early postoperative results of excision arthroplasty with and without implant are similar with regard to relief of pain and functional motion. Patients with preoperative instability necessitating an implant and those with a tenuous repair of ligamentous structures have poorer results than those with a stable elbow.

Most long-term studies of excision with prosthetic implant have evaluated components made of silicone, which, as previously mentioned, are associated with material fatigue or inflammatory responses and lead to premature failure. In patients with chronic arthritis, synovitis eventually recurs necessitating another synovectomy or a total elbow arthroplasty.[63] Regardless of the underlying pathology, patients who have undergone excision of the radial head with or without prosthetic implant, should permanently refrain from high-demand, work-related or recreational activities.[37]

Total Elbow Arthroplasty

Indications for Surgery

- Severe joint pain and articular destruction of the humeroulnar and humeroradial joints, resulting in loss of functional use of the upper extremity.[12,17a,54,67] Underlying conditions include RA, JRA, post-traumatic arthritis, or osteoarthritis.[11,12,19,47,58]
- Gross instability of the elbow.[12,25,55]
- Acute comminuted fractures[10] and nonunion fractures[48] of the distal humerus.
- Failed resection of the radial head.[57]
- Marked limitation of motion at the elbow, particularly in patients with bilateral ankylosis of the elbow.[12,67]
- Bone stock loss from trauma or tumors.[67]

Procedure

General Background

The complex structural relationships among the humeroulnar (HU), humeroradial (HR), and proximal radioulnar (RU) joints have made total elbow arthroplasty a challenging task. Incremental improvements in design, fixation, and surgical technique, since the first cemented replacement of the elbow in 1972,[14] have contributed to increasingly predictable and successful outcomes. Early designs were *hinged, fully constrained* metal-to-metal humeral and ulnar implants that allowed only flexion and extension of the elbow joint. These designs made no allowances for normal varus and valgus and rotational movements, and hence, the implants rapidly loosened at the bone-cement interface. Metal fatigue at the linkage of the prosthesis and dislocation of the prosthetic joint were also common complications. Contemporary total elbow replacements now use either *semiconstrained* or *unconstrained (resurfacing)* designs that provide 5 to 10 degrees of varus and valgus and a small degree of rotation.[17,17a,33,44,56] A stemmed titanium humeral component that has a cobalt-chrome alloy articulating surface interfaces with a high-density polyethylene articulating surface of a stemmed ulnar component. Some designs also include a replacement of the head of the radius.

Semiconstrained designs, which are loosely hinged, have some degree of inherent stability;[15,20,44,58] unconstrained designs do not and therefore require integrity of the collateral ligaments for stability.[19,33,34] If significant preoperative joint instability is permanent, semiconstrained designs, some with an extra-articular anterior flange to enhance stability, are appropriate. Ultimately, the design selected by the surgeon is based on the etiology and extent of joint destruction, the degree of joint instability, the quality of the bone stock, the functional needs of the patient, and the training and experience of the surgeon.

Currently, prosthetic components are cemented in place with acrylic cement. Some designs also have a porous-coated extramedullary flange for osseous ingrowth.[40] To date, cementless fixation has not yet been developed for total elbow arthroplasty.[12] Despite improvements in fixation, loosening of the implants at the bone-cement interface continues to be the most common cause of failure of this procedure.

Overview of the Procedure

A longitudinal incision is made at the posterior aspect of the elbow. The distal attachment of the triceps is either reflected and detached *(triceps-reflecting approach)* or split and retracted along the midline *(triceps-sparing approach)*;[44] the ulnar nerve is identified and temporarily displaced or transposed to protect it; necessary ligaments are released; and the posterior aspect of the capsule is incised and retracted. The triceps-reflecting approach tends to give a greater area of exposure of the joint surfaces during the procedure.

Small portions of the distal humerus and proximal ulna are resected. Depending on the status of the radial head, the integrity of the collateral ligaments, and the design of the prosthesis, the head of the radius may or may not be resected. Then the intramedullary canals of the humerus and ulna and possibly the radius are prepared, and the components are inserted and cemented in place. The collateral ligaments are repaired, if indicated, based on the design of the prosthesis; the capsule and triceps mechanism are repaired.[33,41,44,56,67,68]

Postoperative Management

Immobilization

Immediately after surgery, a soft compression dressing and posterior or anterior splint are applied to immobilize the elbow in a position selected by the surgeon that may vary from almost full extension to 70 or 80 degrees of flexion and a neutral position of the forearm.[17a,33,37,67] If symptoms of ulnar neuropathy are present, the elbow is held in relative extension to alleviate pressure in the cubital tunnel.

The period of continuous immobilization after surgery, which is kept as short as possible to avoid stiffness, also varies widely, ranging from 1 to 2 days to a week or more. This time period depends on the design of the prosthesis, the type of surgical approach, the integrity of ligamentous structures, wound healing as well as intraoperative observations by the surgeon. In general, unconstrained (resurfacing) designs, which have no inherent stability, require a longer period of immobilization than semiconstrained designs. Even after it is permissible to remove the splint for exercise or self-care, the patient is encouraged to continue to wear the splint at night for protection for up to 6 weeks.

Exercise

The focus of rehabilitation after total elbow arthroplasty is to achieve pain-free ROM as well as strength and stability of the upper extremity sufficient for functional activities. The rate of progression of an exercise program is usually slower after a triceps-reflecting approach than after a triceps-splitting (triceps-sparing) approach.[37] Exercises must also be more controlled and guarded after an unconstrained replacement than after a semiconstrained replacement which has some degree of stability built into the design. Patients with significant preoperative instability of the elbow or tenuous ligament repairs, initially might need to wear a hinged splint during exercise that allows only flexion and extension and restricts rotation of the forearm. These factors and others that influence the progression of postoperative rehabilitation are summarized in Table 10–2.

Specific precautions for exercise and functional use of the operated upper extremity are noted throughout the following phases of rehabilitation. Adherence to these precautions ensures more positive outcomes and lessens the likelihood of short- or long-term postoperative complications related to exercise and use of the operated arm for functional activities. These complications include aseptic (biomechanical) loosening of the prosthesis over time, triceps insufficiency or avulsion, or joint instability and dislocation.[12,17a,33,45]

Table 10–2 Factors that Influence the Progression of Exercise After Total Elbow Arthroplasty

Factors	Impact on Rehabilitation
• Design of prosthesis: semiconstrained vs. unconstrained	• Earlier motion (CPM or exercise) and earlier use of the operated upper extremity for light ADL with semiconstrained replacement; more protected, controlled motion and use with unconstrained replacement
• Surgical approach: triceps-splitting (sparing) vs. triceps-reflecting	• Earlier antigravity extension and low-load resistance during exercise and ADL with triceps-splitting approach
• Pre- and postoperative status of supporting ligaments of the elbow	• Earlier and less protected motion during exercise, less protected use during ADL and less time in splint during the day and at night if ligaments are intact preoperatively or have undergone an effective repair
• Wound healing	• Delayed end-range flexion or extended immobilization of the elbow in an extension splint if healing of the posterior incision is tenuous
• Ulnar neuropathy	• May require extended immobilization in an extension splint or delay of exercises to regain elbow flexion

Exercise: Maximum Protection Phase

During the first 7 to 10 days after surgery, the arm is routinely elevated to prevent or minimize edema. Application of cold is also appropriate. Initially include the following goals and interventions during the maximum protection phase of rehabilitation when the elbow must remain immobilized and later when the splint may be temporarily removed for exercise.[6,12,15,37]

- ***Minimize edema in the hand and maintain mobility of the shoulder, wrist, hand.*** Active ROM of these regions in the immediate postoperative period
- ***Regain motion of the elbow and forearm.***
  - Active-assistive or active flexion and extension of the elbow with the forearm in midposition and within pain-free ranges.
  - Active-assistive or active pronation and supination with the elbow in a comfortably flexed position.
  - Self-assisted ROM in preparation for discharge, usually within 2 to 5 days postoperatively.

Precautions

- If a triceps-reflecting approach was used, perform elbow flexion/extension in a seated or standing rather than supine position to avoid antigravity extension, which could cause excessive stress to the reattached triceps mechanism.[12,37]
- If elbow stability is questionable after an unconstrained replacement, postpone rotation of the forearm, particularly supination past neutral, because this places stress on a lateral ligament repair.

- ***Minimize atrophy of elbow and forearm musculature.***
  - Gentle, pain-free muscle-setting exercises while the elbow is in the splint and later, multiple-angle setting exercises when the splint can be removed.

Precaution: If the triceps was reflected and reattached, postpone isometric contractions of the triceps for several weeks.[37]

Exercise: Moderate and Minimum Protection Phases

From 7 to 10 days through 4 to 6 weeks postoperatively during the moderate protection/controlled motion phase, the focus of rehabilitation is to increase ROM of the elbow and begin to use the operated arm for functional activities. After 6 weeks soft tissue healing is fairly complete and only minimum protection is required. Strength usually continues to improve up to 6 to 12 months postoperatively by cautious use of the operated arm for functional activities.

The following goals and interventions are added during the moderate protection and minimum protection phases of rehabilitation.

- ***Increase ROM of the elbow.***
  - Low-intensity manual self-stretching using inhibitory elongation procedures
  - Low-load dynamic splinting[8] or alternating use of static splints fabricated in maximum but comfortable extensions and flexion

Precautions: Initially emphasize end-range extension before end-range flexion to protect the posterior capsule and the triceps mechanism. If symptoms of cubital tunnel syndrome are present (aching along the medial forearm and hand, paresthesia, or hyperesthesia), avoid prolonged or repeated end-range positioning or stretching to increase elbow flexion.[2,7]

It is the opinion of the authors that use of joint mobilization techniques to increase ROM of the elbow or forearm is inappropriate after total elbow arthroplasty, particularly with semiconstrained (linked) implants or if the stability of the elbow is questionable. If selected as a stretching technique, it should be implemented only after specific consultation with the surgeon to determine appropriateness. It is a more prudent choice to forego full motion than to jeopardize the stability of the joint.

- ***Improve functional strength and endurance of the operated extremity.*** As soon as 1 week postoperatively with a triceps-sparring approach and semiconstrained prosthesis but later with a triceps-reflecting approach or unconstrained replacement begin the following:
  - Use of the operated extremity for *light* ADL (< 1 lb of resistance).
  - Low-load (1 lb or light-grade) elastic resistance exercises. Add low-load, closed-chain activities, such as wall push-ups after 6 weeks when the triceps mechanism and posterior capsule have healed.

Precautions

- Postpone resisted elbow extension for 6 weeks (or as long as 12 weeks) if a triceps-reflecting approach was used.
- When strengthening the shoulder, apply resistance above the elbow to eliminate stresses across the elbow joint.
- Avoid pushing up from a chair, using crutches or a cane, and moving or carrying objects with the operated extremity for 6 weeks.
- Limit repetitive lifting to 1 lb for the first 3 months; 2 lb for the first 6 months; and no more than 5 lb thereafter.[33,37,46,47] Consequently, high-load PRE is inappropriate after total elbow arthroplasty.[6,12,15,37]

Outcomes

Relief of pain is the most consistent outcome after total elbow arthroplasty occurring in more than 85 to 95% of patients.[11,17a,19,33,41,55,67] Follow-up studies of patients who have undergone total elbow arthroplasty indicate an overall high rate of patient satisfaction, with up to 90% of patients reporting "good" or "excellent" results.[10,19,33,55] Improvement in ROM is less consistent or significant. Most gains in ROM are usually seen within 6 to 12 weeks but may continue up to 6 months postoperatively. Patients with preoperative contractures associated with, for example, late-stage post-traumatic,[46] rheumatoid[17a,19] or juvenile arthritis,[11] tend to regain some motion but usually continue to have limited motion postoperatively. Patients with little active movement of the elbow because of preoperative instability have exhibited marked improvement of active motion postoperatively.[25,55] In general, ROM tends to improve more significantly after semiconstrained replacements than after unconstrained replacements. This difference may be related to more accelerated rehabilitation after semiconstrained than after unconstrained procedures.[19]

For the best long-term results a patient must be selective in the type of work-related or recreational activities performed. Over the lifetime of the prosthesis, patients must restrict repetitive lifting to 2 to 5 lb and a single lift to 10 lb to minimize the stresses on the joint replacement. High-impact or high-demand recreational activities, such as racquet or throwing sports, are not advisable.[37,41] The most common long-term complications that often require revision arthroplasty are infection, loosening of the prosthesis at the bone-cement interface, and instability of the prosthetic joint.[20,45] The incidence of these problems has steadily decreased since the 1970s. The frequency of aseptic (biomechanical) loosening after total elbow arthroplasty is still slightly higher than in other major joints (hip, knee, shoulder) replacements but has decreased as prosthetic design, methods of fixation, and surgical technique have improved. The incidence of radiologic loosening is consistently higher than clinical loosening (where the patient becomes symptomatic). The rate of clinical loosening of contemporary implants over a 5-year period has been reported to range from 2 to 6%.[20,45]

▶ Myositis Ossificans

Etiology of Symptoms

The terms *myositis ossificans* and *heterotopic* or *ectopic bone formation* are often used interchangeably to describe the formation of bone in atypical locations of the body. Some authorities[23,38,42] use the term myositis ossificans to denote only ossification of muscle. More often, the term is used generally to characterize heterotopic bone formation in muscle-tendon unit, capsule, or ligamentous structures. In this text, the terms myositis ossificans and heterotopic bone formation are used synonymously.

Although not a common phenomenon, the sites most frequently involved are the elbow region and thigh. In the elbow, heterotopic bone formation most often develops in the brachialis muscle or joint capsule as the result of trauma, such as a comminuted fracture of the radial head, a fracture-dislocation (supracondylar or radial head fracture) of the elbow, or a tear of the brachialis tendon.[13,23,42,43] Patients with neurological impairments, specifically traumatic brain injury or spinal cord injury, as well as patients with burns to the extremities are also prone to develop this complication.[42] It may also develop as the result of aggressive stretching of the elbow flexors after injury and a period of immobilization.[13]

Myositis ossificans is distinguished from traumatic arthritis of the humeroulnar joint in that passive extension is more limited than flexion, resisted elbow flexion causes pain, flexion is limited and painful when the inflamed muscle is pinched between the humerus and ulna, and resisted flexion in midrange causes pain in the brachialis muscle. Palpation of the distal brachialis muscle is tender.[13,23] After the acute inflammatory period, heterotopic bone formation is laid down in muscle, between, not within, individual muscle fibers or around the joint capsule within a 2- to 4-week period of time. This makes the muscle extremely firm to touch. Although this condition can permanently restrict elbow motion, in most cases, the heterotopic bone to a large extent is reabsorbed over several months, and motion usually returns to near normal.[38]

Management

Massage, passive stretching, and resistive exercise are contraindicated if the brachialis muscle is implicated after trauma. The elbow should be kept at rest in a splint, which should be removed only periodically during the day for active, pain-free ROM. Rest should continue until the bony mass matures and then resorbs. Surgical excision of heterotopic bone from muscle or a total elbow arthroplasty, if the capsule is also involved, is necessary only in rare instances.[38,42]

▶ Overuse Syndromes: Repetitive Trauma Syndromes

Related Diagnoses

Lateral Epicondylitis (Tennis Elbow)

There is pain in the common wrist extensor tendons along the lateral epicondyle and radiohumeral joint with gripping activities. Activities such as the backhand stroke in tennis, requiring firm wrist stability, or pulling weeds in a garden, which requires repeated wrist extension, can inflame the musculotendinous unit and cause symptoms. The highest incidence is in the musculotendinous junction of the extensor carpi radialis brevis.[13,16,23,53] Symptoms also occur when the annular ligament is stressed.

Note: Pulled elbow, pushed elbow, rotated elbow, radial head fracture, pinched synovial fringe, meniscal lock, radial tunnel syndrome, tendinosis,[30] and periosteal bruise are also possible sources of pain at the elbow and are sometimes erroneously called tennis elbow.[35,70]

Medial Epicondylitis (Golfer's Elbow)

This involves the common flexor/pronator tendon at the tenoperiosteal junction near the medial epicondyle and is associated with repetitive movements into wrist flexion such as swinging a golf club, pitching a ball, or work-related grasping, shuffling papers, and lifting heavy objects. Concomitant ulnar neuropathy is often an associated finding.[18,23]

Other

Overuse can occur in any muscle in the elbow region including the flexors and extensors of the elbow.

Etiology of Symptoms

- With epicondylitis the most common cause is excessive repetitive use or eccentric strain of the wrist or forearm muscles. The result is microdamage and partial tears, usually near the musculotendinous junction when the strain exceeds the strength of the tissues and when the demand exceeds the repair process. With continued irritation, chronic inflammation develops.

- Inflammation of the periosteum may develop with formation of granulation tissue and adhesions.[53]
- Recurring problems are seen because the resulting immobile or immature scar is redamaged when returning to activities before there is sufficient healing or mobility in the surrounding tissue.
- Causes of problems anterior or posterior to the elbow are frequently from excessive extension or flexion strain in sporting activities.[3]

Common Impairments

- Gradually increasing pain in the elbow region after excessive activity of the wrist and hand.
- Pain when the involved muscle is stretched or when it contracts against resistance.
- Decreased muscle strength and endurance for the demand.
- Decreased grip strength, limited by pain.
- Tenderness with palpation at the site of inflammation, such as over the lateral or medial epicondyle, head of the radius, or within the muscle belly.

Common Functional Limitations/Disabilities

- Inability to participate in provoking activities, such as racket sports, throwing, or golf.
- Difficulty with repetitive forearm/wrist tasks, such as sorting or assembling small parts, gripping activities, using a hammer, turning a screwdriver, shuffling papers, or playing a percussion instrument.

Nonoperative Management of Overuse Syndromes: Protection Phase

Control Pain, Edema, or Spasm

- Rest the muscles in a splint. If the extensor muscles are involved, immobilize the wrist in a cock-up splint, while keeping the elbow free to move.
- Instruct the patient to not perform any aggravating activities, such as strong or repetitive gripping activities.
- Utilize cryotherapy to help control edema and swelling.

Maintain Soft Tissue and Joint Mobility

- Remove the splint several times a day and perform nonstressful motion. Apply gentle multiple-angle setting techniques to the involved muscle followed by pain-free ROM.
  - ***Technique for wrist extensor muscles.*** Patient position and procedure: Sitting with the elbow flexed, forearm pronated and resting on a table, and the wrist in extension. Begin with gentle isometric contractions with the wrist extensors in the shortened position. Resist wrist extension, hold the contraction to the count of 6, relax and repeat several times, then move the wrist toward flexion and repeat the isometric resistance. Do not move into the painful range nor provide resistance that causes a painful contraction.

    When full wrist flexion is obtained without pain in the lateral epicondyle region, progress by placing the elbow in greater degrees of extension and repeat the isometric resistance sequence to the wrist extensors. Progress until gentle resistance can be applied to the wrist extensors in the position of elbow extension and wrist flexion. It may take several weeks to reach this position.
  - ***Technique for wrist flexor muscles.*** Patient position: Sitting with the elbow flexed, forearm resting on a table, and the wrist in flexion. Begin with gentle isometric contractions with the wrist flexors in the shortened position. Resist wrist flexion, hold the contraction to the count of 6, relax and repeat several times, then move the wrist toward extension and repeat the isometric resistance. Do not move into the painful range or provide resistance that causes a painful contraction.

    When full wrist extension is obtained without pain in the medial epicondyle region progress by placing the elbow in greater degrees of extension and supination and repeat the isometric resistance sequence to the wrist flexors. As stated above, it may take several weeks to reach the full range of elbow extension, forearm supination, and wrist extension and be able to tolerate gentle resistance.
- Apply gentle cross-fiber massage within tolerance at the site of the lesion.
- Teach the patient to self-administer the submaximal isometric and cross-fiber massage techniques in a home exercise program.

Maintain Integrity in Upper Extremity Function

- Perform active ROM in all other elbow, forearm, and wrist motions to maintain integrity of the rest of the upper extremity.

- Perform resistive shoulder and scapular ROM with the resistance applied proximal to the elbow.

Nonoperative Management: Controlled Motion and Return to Function Phases

Note: If there is chronic inflammation, treat the inflammation first as was described.

Gradually Increase the Flexibility of the Muscle and Create a Mobile Scar

- ***Inhibition and passive stretching.*** Use agonist-contraction, hold-relax, and passive stretching techniques, elongating the tight muscle to the end of its range. Application of the techniques have previously been described in Chapter 5. Use an intensity of muscle contraction and stretch that causes a stretching sensation but not increased pain. For both the wrist flexors and wrist extensors, the elbow must be extended. Then to stretch the wrist extensors, pronate the forearm, flex and ulnarly deviate the wrist, and flex the fingers. To stretch the wrist flexors supinate the forearm, extend and radially deviate the wrist, and extend the fingers. (See techniques later in this chapter.)
- ***Self-stretching techniques.*** Instruct the patient to stretch the involved muscle. A patient may use a wall (see Fig. 10–5) and slide his or her hand along the wall until a stretch force is experienced, or the opposite hand is used to apply the stretch force. The stretch positions are the same as described above.
- ***Cross-fiber (friction) massage.*** Palpate to localize the scar, then apply pressure and cross-fiber massage. Increase the intensity of massage as the inflammation decreases.

Restore Normal Joint Tracking of the Radiohumeral Joint

Mobilization with movement (MWM) techniques are proposed to restore normal tracking of the radius on the capitulum so that strengthening the forearm muscles can be done without painful symptoms.[51] Several researchers have reported decreased pain and increased grip strength during or shortly after MWM at the elbow.[39,65,66] One researcher observed decreased shoulder rotation in patients with lateral epicondylalgia and demonstrated significant improvement in shoulder range after MWM at the elbow. He proposed the mechanism was mediated neurophysiologically.[1] Refer to Chapter 6 for principles of application. The following techniques are used if the patient experiences pain when making a fist or with resisted wrist extension.

- Patient position and procedure: Supine with the forearm pronated. Place a mobilization belt around the patient's proximal forearm and across your shoulders and stabilize the distal humerus with one hand. Apply a lateral glide to the forearm through the belt and then have the patient do repeated wrist extension against manual resistance applied by your other hand (Fig. 10–2*A*).
- An alternative method is to apply the lateral glide force against the proximal forearm with your distal hand and have the patient do repeated gripping by squeezing a ball or inflatable bulb (Fig. 10–2*B*). Both the lateral glide force and the muscle contraction must be pain-free.
- ***Self-mobilization.*** Have the patient stand with the humerus of the involved elbow stabilized against a doorframe and the forearm in the opening. Have the patient apply a lateral glide force against the proximal forearm with the contralateral hand. The patient then does repetitive gripping or squeezing against a resistive force such as a pneumatic bulb or squeezable ball (Fig. 10–2*C*).

Strengthen the Muscle and Improve Muscular Endurance

- Progress the isometric exercises in various pain-free positions. When there is no pain through the ROM, progress to concentric resistance at an appropriate dosage.
- Strengthen the forearm and wrist muscles using free weights and elastic resistance. Initially use low-intensity resistance with multiple repetitions of the involved muscle. Progress the resistance to strengthen the muscles in preparation for functional demands.
- As strength improves progress to eccentric resistance.

Progress to Functional Training and Conditioning

Include strength, cardiovascular and muscle endurance, power, and flexibility exercises in the upper quarter with controlled loading of forces. Of equal importance is patient education. This should include advice and techniques on prevention, recognition of provoking factors, and identification of warning symptoms. The patient should be taught how to re-

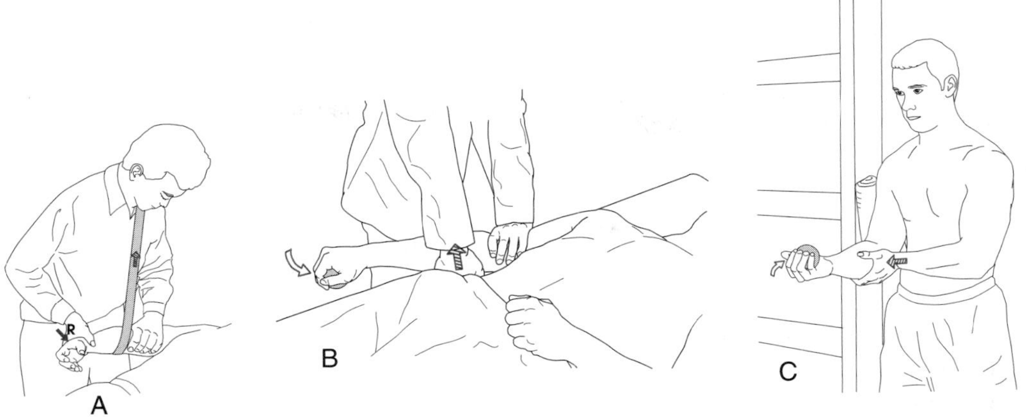

Figure 10–2 MWM for lateral epicondylitis; lateral glide is applied to the proximal forearm *(A)* with resistance added to wrist extension, *(B)* with patient squeezing a ball to bring in the wrist extensors, and *(C)* self-treatment.

duce the overload forces that caused the problem and be retrained in proper techniques.[16,23,29,52]

- Instruct the patient to apply friction massage and to stretch the involved muscle prior to using it.
- Begin strength and power training sessions with warm-up exercises that include general flexibility exercises for the shoulder, elbow, wrist, and trunk.
- Increase repetitions in the defined pattern progressing from 1 to 5 minutes to develop muscular endurance.
- Attain general strengthening and conditioning of any unused or underused part of the extremity or trunk before returning to the stressful activity.
- Include exercises simulating the desired activity. Progress from slow, controlled motions to high speeds with low resistance to improve timing (see Fig. 10–17).
- As strength improves, add plyometric exercises to the program if the patient's goals include returning to sport activities or occupational activities that require elbow and forearm power. Suggestions include
  - Bounce a tennis ball on a short-handled racket, progress to a long-handled racket.
  - Rapid eccentric/concentric elbow and forearm motions with an elastic resistance.
  - Rapid chest passes or overhead passes using a weighted plyometric ball.
- Assess the patient's technique and advise him or her on how to modify it before returning to the stressful activity. (This may require taking tennis lessons to correct improper tennis techniques.) If equipment is used (as in tennis or with a hammer), it should also be analyzed and modified to reduce stress.[16,23,52,53]

Exercise Techniques to Increase Flexibility and Range of Motion

Prior to initiating a muscle stretching program, be sure the joint capsule is not restricting motion. Techniques to increase joint play in the elbow and forearm joints were discussed earlier in this chapter with reference to joint mobilization techniques.

The description of principles and techniques for applying inhibition and passive stretching techniques are presented in Chapter 5. In addition to the general techniques described there, specific manual, mechanical, and self-stretching techniques are described in this section. When teaching the patient self-stretching, emphasize the importance of maintaining a low-intensity, prolonged stretch and not bouncing at the end of the range.

Manual, Mechanical, and Self-Stretching Techniques

To Increase Elbow Extension

Note: Of the three muscles that flex the elbow, only one, the biceps brachii, crosses two joints—the elbow and the shoulder. Therefore, techniques to fully elongate the biceps brachii must be done with the shoulder extended.

Mechanical Stretch—Mild Flexion Contracture
Patient position and procedure: Supine with the arm supported on the treatment table and a folded towel under the distal humerus as a fulcrum. Place a cuff weight around the distal forearm. Position the forearm in pronation, midposition and supination to affect each of the flexor muscles. Have the patient stabilize the proximal humerus with the other hand, or place a sandbag or belt across the proximal humerus to stabilize it. Instruct the patient to maintain the stretch for an extended period of time.[69]

Mechanical Stretch—Dynamic Splinting
Apply a low-intensity, long-duration mechanical stretch force with a dynamic splint to reduce a long-standing elbow flexion contracture by affecting the soft tissue properties of creep and stress-relaxation.[8,22]

Manual Stretch—Biceps Brachii
Patient position and procedure: Prone with the elbow in end-range but comfortable extension and forearm in pronation. Stabilize the scapula and passively extend the shoulder.

Mechanical Stretch—Biceps Brachii (Fig. 10–3A)
Patient position and procedure: Supine with a cuff weight around the distal forearm. The elbow is in extension and the forearm is in pronation. Have the patient stabilize the proximal humerus with the opposite hand and then place the arm over the side of the table; allow the elbow and shoulder to extend as far as possible and sustain the stretch position for an extended period of time.

Self-Stretch—Biceps Brachii (Fig 10–3B)
The patient can also self-stretch the biceps brachii (without the pronation component). Have the patient stand at the side of a table, grasp the end of the table and walk forward, causing shoulder extension with elbow extension.

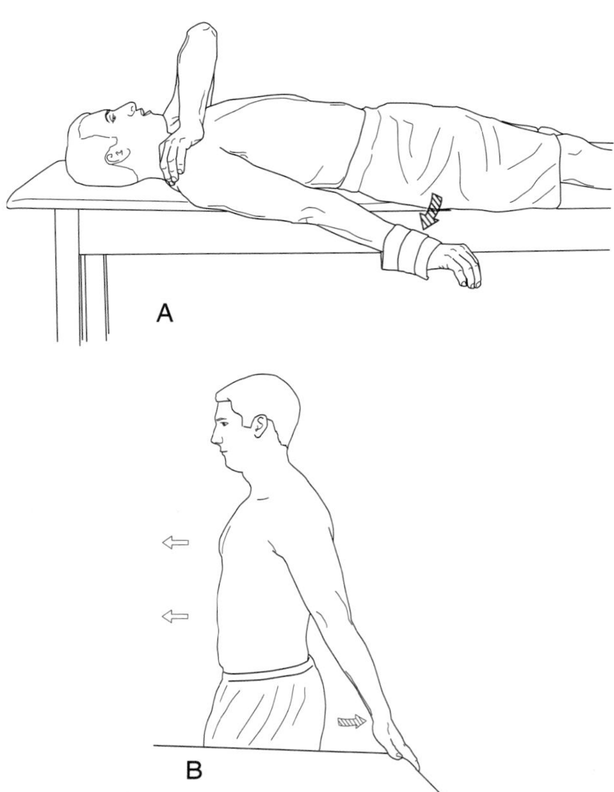

Figure 10–3 Self-stretching the biceps brachii musculotendinous unit includes stretching the long head across the shoulder joint *(A)* supine and *(B)* standing.

To Increase Elbow Flexion

Self-Stretch—Mild Extension Contracture
- Patient position and procedure: Prone lying and propped up on elbows with forearms resting on the exercise mat. Have the patient lower the chest as far as elbow flexion allows and maintain the position as long as tolerated.
- Patient position and procedure: Sitting with elbow flexed as far as possible. Have the patient press against the distal forearm with the opposite hand to provide the stretch force into flexion.

Self-Stretch Long Head of Triceps (Fig. 10–4)
Patient position: Sitting or standing. Have the patient flex the elbow and shoulder as far as possible. The other hand can either push on the forearm to flex the elbow, or push the shoulder into more flexion. Hold the stretch position as long as tolerated.

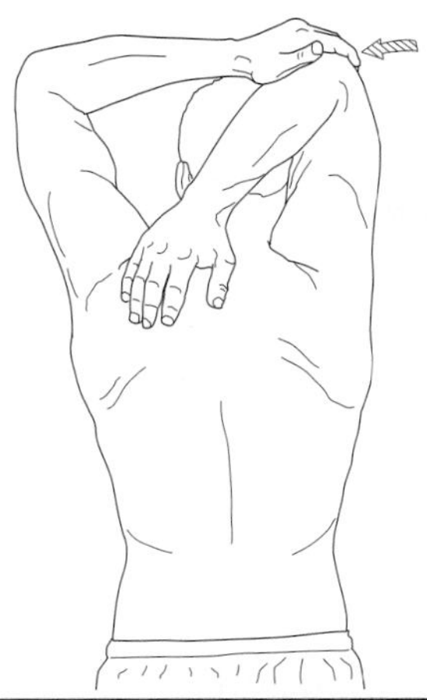
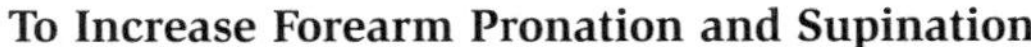

Figure 10–4 Self-stretching the triceps brachii musculotendinous unit includes stretching the long head across the shoulder joint.

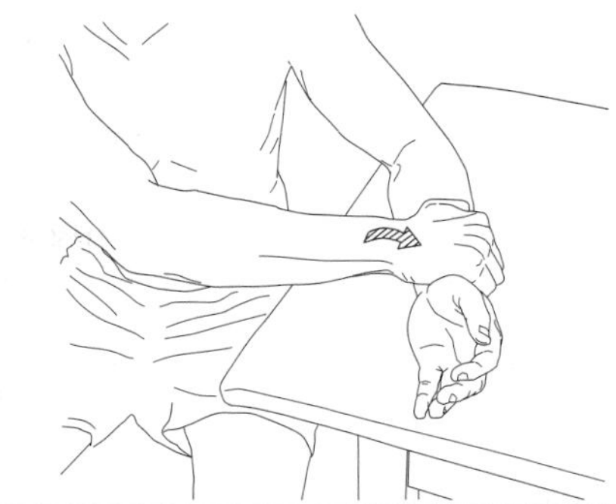

Figure 10–5 Self-stretching the forearm into supination. It is important that the stretch force is against the radium, not the hand.

To Increase Forearm Pronation and Supination

Patient position: Sitting with the elbow flexed to 90 degrees and the elbow resting on a padded table or stabilized against the side of the trunk.

Self-Stretch to Increase Pronation
Have the patient grasp the dorsal surface of the involved forearm so that the heel of the uninvolved hand is against the radius just proximal to the wrist and so that the fingers wrap around the ulna. Then have the patient pronate the forearm and sustain the stretch as long as tolerated. The force is applied against the radius so there is no trauma to the wrist.

Self-Stretch to Increase Supination (Fig. 10–5)
Have the patient place the heel of the uninvolved hand against the volar aspect of the involved radius just proximal to the wrist, supinate the forearm, and sustain the stretch as long as tolerated.

Self-Stretching Techniques: Muscles of the Medial and Lateral Epicondyles

To Stretch the Wrist Extensor Muscles (from the Lateral Epicondyle)

- Patient position and procedure: Sitting or standing with the elbow extended and forearm pronated. While holding this position have the patient ulnarly deviate the wrist and flex the wrist and fingers; then apply a gentle stretch force against the dorsum of the hand. The patient should feel a stretching sensation along the lateral epicondyle or proximal forearm.
- Patient position: Standing with elbow extended, forearm pronated, and back of the hand against a wall (fingers pointing down). Have the patient then slide the back of the hand up the wall[59] (Fig. 10–6). For additional stretch have the patient actively flex the fingers.

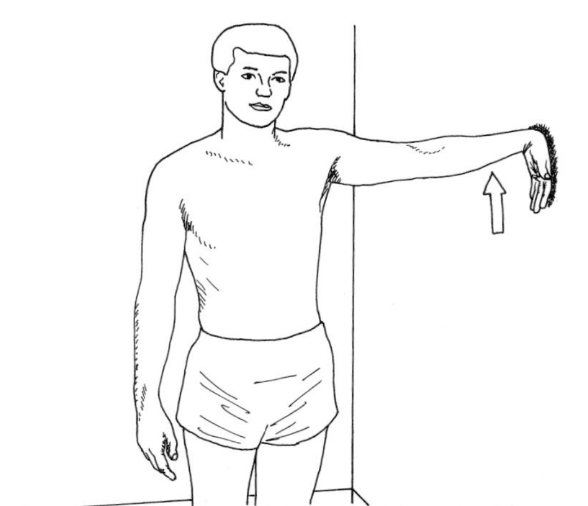

Figure 10–6 Self-stretching of the muscles of the lateral epicondyle.

To Stretch the Wrist Flexor Muscles (from the Medial Epicondyle)

- Patient position and procedure: Sitting or standing with the elbow extended and forearm supinated. While holding this position have the patient radially deviate and extend the wrist and apply a gentle stretch force with the other hand against the palm of the hand. A stretch sensation should be felt along the medial epicondyle or proximal forearm.
- Patient position and procedure: Standing with the elbow extended and forearm supinated. Have the patient place the palm of the hand against a wall, fingers pointing down, and then move the hand up the wall until a stretch sensation is felt in the wrist flexor muscles.[59]

Exercises to Develop and Improve Muscle Performance and Functional Control

In addition to the conditions already described in this chapter, imbalances in length and strength of muscles crossing the elbow and forearm can result from a variety of causes such as nerve injury or after surgery, trauma, disuse, or immobilization. Selection of appropriate exercises to develop neuromuscular control, increase strength, and improve endurance for return to functional activities can be made from the following exercises as well as the techniques described in Chapter 3. For patients with elbow impairments, exercises of the joints above (shoulder) and below (wrist and hand) should also be incorporated into the therapeutic program to prevent complications and restore proper function in the entire upper quarter. The general principles of managing acute soft tissue lesion are discussed in Chapter 8. The exercises described in this section are for use during the controlled motion and return to function phases of intervention when tissues are in the subacute and chronic stages of healing and require only moderate to minimum protection.

Isometric Exercises

Multiple-Angle Isometric Exercises

Use manual or mechanical resistance throughout the available ROM of elbow flexion and extension and forearm rotation. Isolate key musculature. Apply resistance at the distal forearm, not at the hand, to avoid forces across the wrist joints.

Angle-Specific Training

During isometric exercises emphasize joint positions that simulate use of the elbow for anticipated functional activities. For example, to simulate carrying large boxes close to the chest, strengthen the elbow flexors in a 70- to 90-degree position with the forearm in midposition.

Endurance

Emphasize holding objects for extended periods of time to increase muscular endurance.

Alternating Isometrics and Rhythmic Stabilization—Open- and Closed-Chain

Open-Chain

- Use alternating isometric contractions by means of manual resistance between antagonists at multiple angles of elbow flexion/extension and forearm pronation/ supination. Stabilize the humerus and apply the resistance against the forearm.
- Once the patient has learned to respond to the resistance at various elbow and forearm positions and at varying speeds of alternation, progress to alternating isometrics using the total upper extremity as described in the Chapter 9.

Closed-Chain

Patient positions include standing with hands on a wall or on a table, in the quadruped position, or in the prone push-up position (with knees as fulcrum, or toes as fulcrum). Have the patient hold the desired elbow position and apply alternating isometrics and rhythmic stabilization by means of manual resistance against the shoulders and trunk.

Dynamic Strengthening and Endurance

Many muscles that cross the elbow joint are multijoint muscles, such as the biceps, long head of the triceps, and wrist flexors and extensors. It is particularly important to consider the position of the shoulder and forearm during resistance training at the elbow.[60]

Dynamic strengthening and endurance activities for the *prime movers* of the elbow, forearm, and wrist using manual or mechanical resistance are noted in this section. Combined patterns of motion during open- and closed-chain activities are described in the next section. A comprehensive rehabilitation program after an elbow injury or surgery must also include exercises for the adjacent shoulder and hand, as well as general conditioning for the entire body.

Elbow Flexion (Biceps Brachii, Brachialis, Brachioradialis)

Curls

- Patient position and procedure: Sitting or standing, with the humerus at the side of the chest (arm perpendicular to the floor). Have the patient hold a weight or grasp a piece of elastic resistance material (secured under the foot or to the floor), and flex and extend the elbow. This strengthens the elbow flexors concentrically and eccentrically throughout the available ROM to simulate functional lifting and lowering. Perform this motion with the forearm supinated, pronated, and in midposition.
- Patient position: Supine or prone with the humerus supported on the treatment table. When the patient is supine, the resistive force from a free weight or gravity will have greater effect on the muscles near end-range extension and have little to no effect as the elbow reaches 90 degrees. To provide resistance with the patient prone with the forearm over the side of the bed, a pulley system or elastic resistance is necessary to provide resistance to the elbow flexors.
- Patient position: Standing or sitting while holding a weight with the forearm supinated. Have the patient extend the shoulder as the elbow flexes (Fig. 10–7). This combined motion elongates the biceps brachii over the shoulder as the muscle is shortening to move the elbow, and thus most efficiently maintains optimal length for development of maximum tension in the *biceps*. This combined motion develops control for carrying objects at the side.

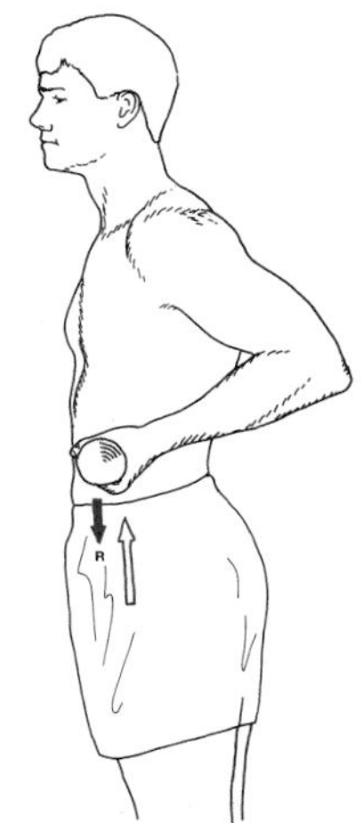

Figure 10–7 Resisting elbow flexion with emphasis on the biceps brachii. The shoulder extends as the elbow flexes with the forearm in supination. This combined action lengthens the proximal portion of the musculotendinous unit across the shoulder while it contracts to move the elbow, thus maintaining a more optimal length-tension relationship through a greater ROM.

Elbow Extension (Triceps, Anconeus)

- Patient position and procedure: Prone, humerus abducted to 90 degrees and supported on a rolled towel on a treatment table. Have the patient extend the elbow while holding a weight or pulling against elastic resistance.

Note: This position strengthens the elbow extensors from only 90 degrees of flexion to terminal extension.

- Patient position and procedure: Supine with the shoulder flexed 90 degrees, holding a weight in the hand. Have the patient begin with the elbow flexed and the weight either at the ipsilateral or contralateral shoulder (external or internal rotation of the shoulder); then extend and flex the elbow (lift and lower the weight) to strengthen the elbow extensors concentrically and eccentrically. To help maintain the shoulder in a stable position, have the patient stabilize the humerus in the 90-degree position with the opposite hand.

Long Head of Triceps with Elbow Extension

Patient position and procedure: Sitting or standing with the arm held overhead (shoulder flexed) and elbow flexed so that the weight is near the shoulder (Fig. 10–8). Have the patient lift the weight overhead and then lower the weight for a concentric and eccentric contraction.

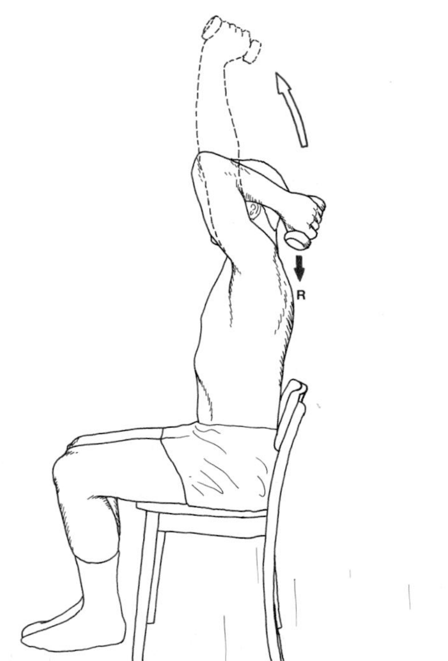

Figure 10–8 Resisting elbow extension, beginning with the long head of the triceps brachii on a stretch.

Precaution: Only perform this exercise if the patient has sufficient control of the shoulder.

Pronation (Pronator Teres and Quadratus) and Supination (Supinator and Biceps)

Patient position: Sitting or standing with the elbow flexed to 90 degrees.

- ***Free weights.*** When using a free weight to strengthen the pronators and supinators, the weight must be placed to one side or the other of the hand (Fig. 10–9). If a person holds a dumbbell with weight equal on each side of the hand, one side of the weight will be assistive while the other will be resistive, in essence cancelling out the resistive force. Note also the position of the thumb in each exercise so that it is not lifting the bar. The weight can also be turned through a downward arc by placing the resistance on the ulnar side of the hand.
- ***Elastic resistance.*** Patient position: Same as above. Have the patient grasp one end of the elastic resistance with the normal hand, or secure it by standing on it. Have the patient grasp the other end with the involved extremity and turn the forearm against the resistance. For greater resistance, secure the end of the resistance around the end of a short rod and have the patient pull against the resistance force.
- Patient position: Standing facing a doorknob with the arm kept at the side and the elbow flexed to 90 degrees to avoid substituting with shoulder rotation. Have the patient turn the knob.

Wrist Flexion (Muscles of the Medial Epicondyle) and Extension (Muscles of the Lateral Epicondyle)

- ***Free weights.*** Patient position and procedure: Sitting with forearm resting on a table and hand over the edge of the table holding a small weight. When the forearm is pronated, resistance is against the wrist extensors (Fig. 10–10); when supinated, the resis-tance is against the wrist flexors. Elastic resistance can be applied by securing a loop of material under the patient's foot and holding the other end in the hand.
- ***Wrist roller.*** Patient position and procedure: Sitting or standing with the elbows flexed or extended and the forearms pronated or supinated. Tie a 2- to 4-foot cord to the middle of a short rod; secure a weight to the other end of the cord. Have the patient hold each end of the rod and with an alternating wrist action, turn the rod causing the cord to wind around the rod and elevate the weight. The weight is then lowered with a reverse motion (Fig. 10–11).

Functional Patterns—Open- and Closed-Chain Strengthening Exercises

Note: Since the elbow primarily functions during activities that also involve the shoulder and hand, use combined patterns that strengthen the entire upper extremity. Be careful that substitute motions do not occur to compensate for a weak link in the chain. Include exercises to progressively improve strength, power, and endurance. Isokinetic exercises may also be used to address specific patterns of motion.

Diagonal Patterns

PNF patterns against manual or mechanical resistance. Use unilateral or bilateral diagonal (PNF) patterns as described in Chapter 3. Use manual resistance, free weights, elastic resistance, a weight-pulley system, or an isokinetic dynamometer to provide the resistance as the patient moves through the diagonal patterns; gradually increase resistance, speed (if appropriate with the choice of equipment), and repetitions.

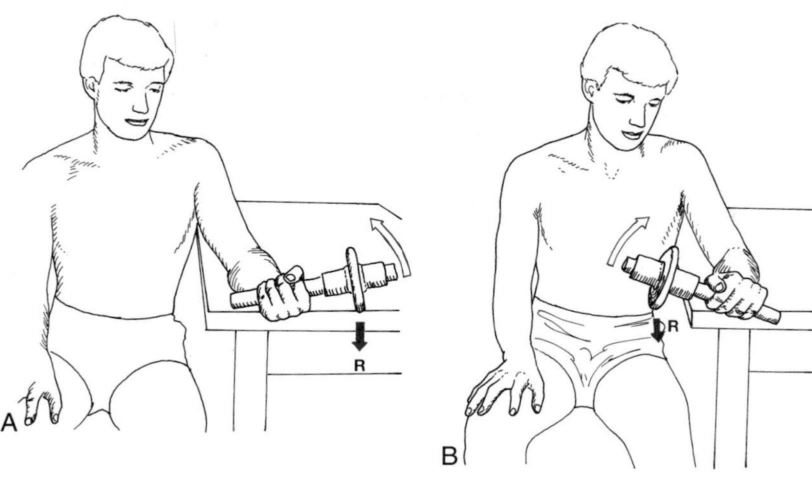

Figure 10–9 Mechanical resistance exercise using a small bar with asymmetrically placed weights for strengthening *(A)* forearm pronators and *(B)* supinators. The bar can also be rotated through a downward arc to affect the other half of the range for each muscle by placing the weight on the ulnar side of the hand.

Combined Pulling Motions

Elbow flexors are used in pulling, lifting, and carrying activities in open- and closed-chain. These upper extremity actions also require strength in the scapular retractors, shoulder extensors, and wrist and hand musculature. Many of the exercises that were described for the shoulder in Chapter 9 also involve resisted elbow flexion and, therefore, can be used to strengthen muscle groups during pulling motions.

Additional suggestions include:

- Bilateral pull-ups against elastic resistance (Fig. 10–12)
- Closed-chain chin-ups or modified pull-ups on an overhead bar (Fig. 10–13)

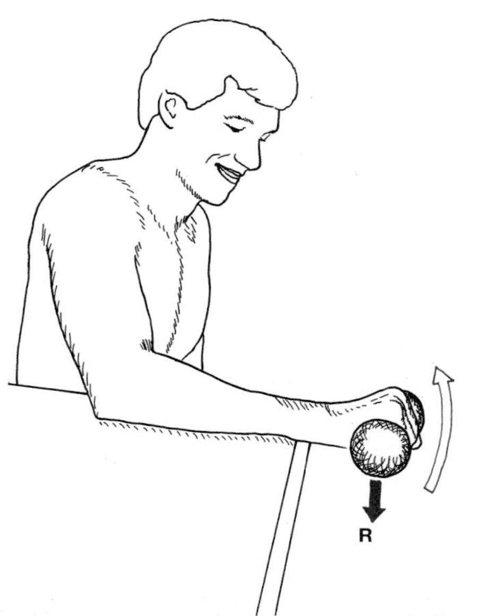

Figure 10–10 Mechanical resistance exercise using a handheld weight for strengthening the muscles of the lateral epicondyle (wrist extensors).

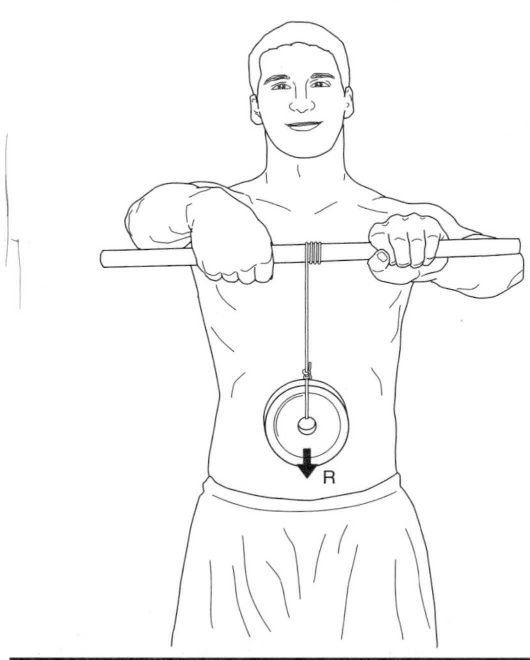

Figure 10–11 Wrist roller exercise to strengthen grip and develop muscles of the lateral epicondyle. This exercise requires stabilization in the shoulder girdle and elbow muscles. The elbows may be flexed or the forearms supinated to emphasize the elbow flexors or muscles of the medial epicondyle, respectively.

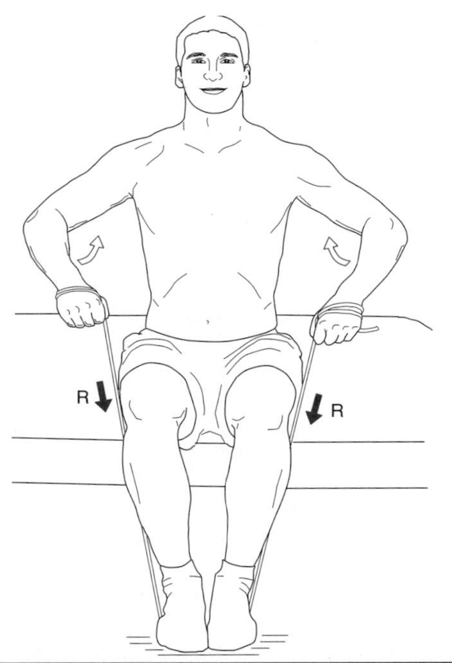

Figure 10–12 Bilateral pull-ups against elastic resistance.

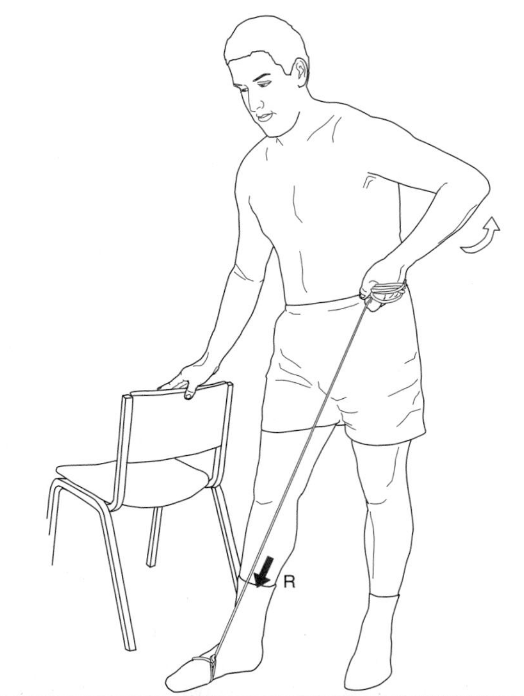

Figure 10–14 Simulation of a "lawn mower pull" for functional strengthening of the upper extremity.

- Bilateral or unilateral rowing motions, such as using a rowing machine or simulating starting a lawn mower (Fig. 10–14)
- Pulling a variety of weighted objects with one or both arms, emphasizing elbow flexion and proper body mechanics.

Combined Pushing Motions

The triceps are involved in pushing motions. Pushing also involves variations of shoulder flexion and scapular protraction or depression so that muscles controlling these motions are functioning with the triceps. Many of the exercises described in Chapter 9 for the shoulder also involve resisted elbow extension and may be used to strengthen muscles groups used in pushing patterns.

- Military press (see Fig. 9–38)
- Bench press
- Upper extremity ergometry (see Fig. 3–47)

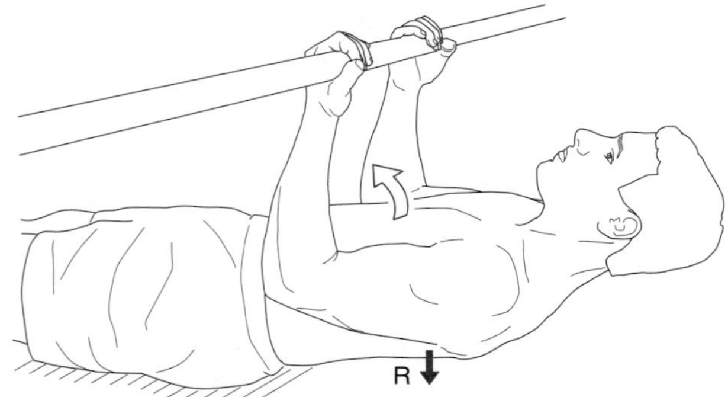

Figure 10–13 Closed-chain modified chin-ups using top half of body weight for resistance to strengthen the elbow flexors. This exercise may be performed in a bed with an overhead trapeze.

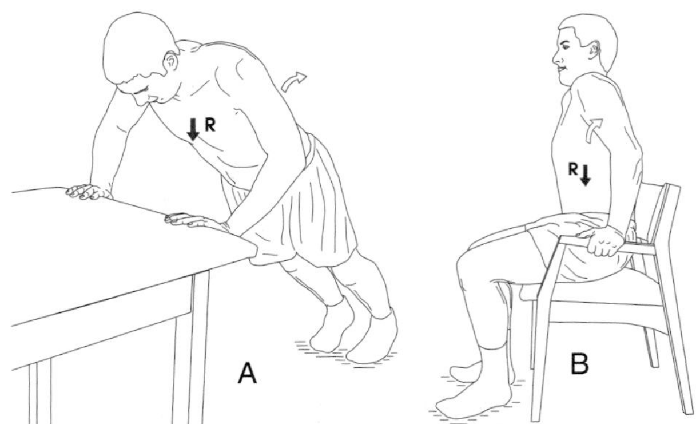

Figure 10–15 Closed-chain strengthening of the triceps. *(A)* Modified push-ups and *(B)* seated push-ups.

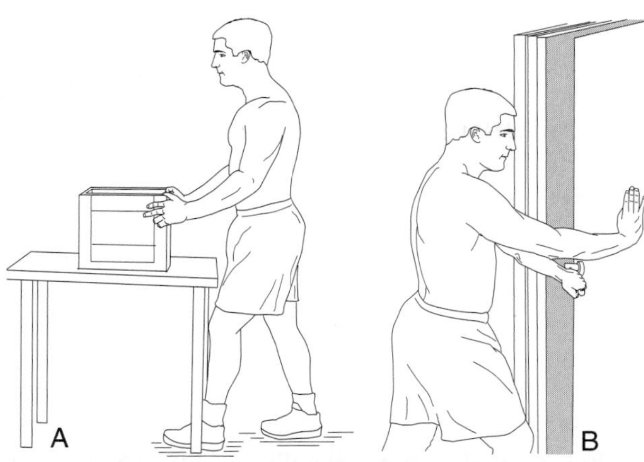

Figure 10–16 Strengthening the triceps with pushing activities: *(A)* pushing weighted objects across a table; *(B)* depressing a door handle and pushing open a door.

- Wall push-ups, semiprone, or prone push-ups (Fig. 10–15*A*)
- Push-ups from a chair or in the parallel bars. (Fig. 10–15*B*)
- Stairmaster; with hands on the "steps." Emphasize elbow extension.
- Pushing a variety of weighted objects with one or both arms using dynamic elbow extension (Fig. 10–16).

Stretch-Shortening Drills (Plyometrics)

Suggestions for increasing power using plyometric exercises include:

- Instruct the patient using rapid reversal between eccentric and concentric resistance using elastic resistance.
- Use a weighted plyometric ball and have the patient catch then quickly throw it back. Emphasize elbow motions with overhead passes, chest passes, and lateral passes.
- Have the patient bounce a tennis ball on a racket with the forearm pronated, and with it supinated.

Simulated Tasks and Activities

Determine the component motions of the patient's desired functional activities as well as occupational or recreational tasks. Have the patient simulate these motions as well as practice the entire task. Activities could involve lifting, lowering, carrying, pushing, pulling, twisting, turning, catching, throwing, or swinging. For example, if the patient is recovering from repetitive trauma to the muscles of the lateral epicondyle ("tennis elbow"), have the patient practice the various strokes using a wall pulley (Fig. 10–17). Impose controlled forces to challenge the patient by increasing the time or repetitions, speed, or resistance.[69]

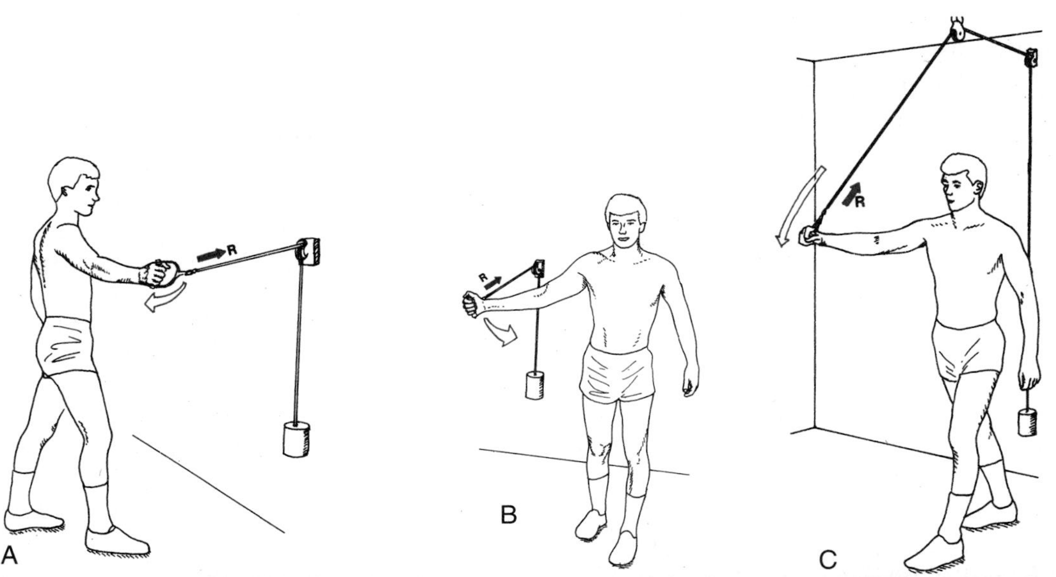

Figure 10–17 Mechanical resistance exercise using wall pulleys to simulate tennis swings. *(A)* Backhand stroke. *(B)* Forehand stroke. *(C)* Serve.

Independent Learning Activities

CRITICAL THINKING AND DISCUSSION

1. Differentiate between the etiology, signs, and symptoms and management of lateral and medial epicondylitis. Note similarities and differences.
2. Develop, compare, and contrast the postoperative management after two different types of total elbow arthroplasty: (1) a semiconstrained implant/triceps-reflecting approach and (2) a resurfacing implant/triceps-splitting approach.
3. The goal is to increase muscle performance and function in the elbow flexors that are currently functioning at a 3/5 strength level and endurance of four repetitions. Identify exercises that could be used at each increment of strength, including exercises for strength, endurance, power, control, stability, and function. Identify parameters for progression of each exercise and any precautions.
4. Do the same sequence of analysis and identification to increase muscle performance and function of the elbow extensors.
5. Analyze the following household, occupational, or sports-related activities. Identify the components and sequence of motions related to each of these motor tasks; pay particular attention to elbow and forearm motions in theses tasks. Design a sequence of upper extremity exercises and simulated activities that could be incorporated into a late-stage rehabilitation program to prepare a patient to return to the desired task after an elbow injury.
   - housecleaning
   - gardening
   - grocery store stocking
   - carpentry
   - volleyball
   - tennis
   - throwing sports

LABORATORY PRACTICE

1. Apply mobilization techniques on a laboratory partner to increase the following elbow and forearm motions: mid- and end-range elbow flexion; mid- and end- range elbow extension; forearm pronation and supination (proximal and distal articulations).
2. Demonstrate passive stretching and hold-relax techniques to elongate the following muscles that cross the elbow: brachialis, brachioradialis; biceps; long head of the triceps; extensor communis digitorum; flexor carpi ulnaris; flexor carpi radialis.
3. Using the following pieces of resistance equipment demonstrate at least two different methods (setups) to strengthen the elbow flexors/ extensors and forearm rotators: free weights, weight-pulley system, and elastic resistance. Then demonstrate a progressive sequence of resistance exercise to strengthen the same muscle groups using self-resistance (body weight or manual resistance).

CASE STUDIES

1. Describe the mechanical problem causing the impairments in the elbow and forearm in the following scenario and what techniques could be used for intervention. A patient is referred to you 4 weeks after S/P fracture of the distal radius and immobilization in a cast following a fall on an outstretched hand. She has limited elbow, forearm, and wrist motions. On palpation you note a decreased space between the lateral aspect of the head of the radius and capitellum as well as decreased joint play at all articulations of the elbow, forearm, and wrist.
2. A 15-year-old patient with a 5-year history of polyarticular JRA just had an open synovectomy and excision of the head of the radius with implant for late-stage joint disease of the elbow. Prior to surgery the patient had severe pain in the elbow region, lacked full elbow flexion/extension and forearm rotation and had very limited use of the arm for functional activities. CPM was implemented during the patient's hospitalization (3 days). On the day prior to discharge the patient was referred to physical therapy for a home program. Design an exercise program for this teenager. Prioritize and describe each exercise you want the patient to do for the first week at home. Outline a program of exercises for later use in the rehabilitation process. The patient plans to return to school within a week of discharge from the hospital. Indicate whether you will recommend outpatient therapy; if so, indicate frequency and duration; justify the need for this recommendation.

REFERENCES

1. Abbott, JH, Patla, CE, and Jensen, RH: Manual therapy to the elbow affects shoulder range of motion in subjects with lateral epicondylalgia. In Singer, KP (ed): Proceedings of the 7th Scientific Conference of the IFOMT, Perth, Australia, Nov 6–10, 2000, p 11.
2. Aiello, B: Ulnar nerve compression. In Clark, GL, et al (eds): Hand Rehabilitation, ed. 2. Churchill Livingstone, New York, 1998, p 213.
3. Andrews, JR, and Whiteside, JA: Common elbow problems in the athlete. J Orthop Sports Phys Ther 17:289, 1993.
4. Ballard, WT, and Buckwalter, JA: Operative treatment of rheumatic disease. In Klippel, JH (ed): Primer on the Rheumatic Diseases, ed. 11. Arthritis Foundation, Atlanta, 1997, p 443.
5. Basmajian, JV: Muscles Alive: Their Functions Revealed by Electromyography, ed 4. Williams & Wilkins, Baltimore, 1979.
6. Bentley, JA: Physiotherapy following joint replacements. In Downie, PA: Cash's Textbook of Orthopedics and Rheumatology for Physiotherapists. JB Lippincott, Philadelphia, 1984.
7. Blackmore, SM, and Hotchkiss, RN: Therapist's management of ulnar neuropathy at the elbow. In Hunter, JM, Mackin, EJ, and Callahan, AD (eds): Rehabilitation of the Hand: Surgery and Therapy, ed. 4. Mosby-Year Book, Inc., St. Louis, 1995, p 665.
8. Bonutti, PM, et al: Static progressive stretch to re-establish elbow range of motion. Clin Orthop Rel Res 303:128, 1984.
9. Bowling, RW, and Rockar, PA: The elbow complex. In Malone, TR, McPoil, TM, and Niyz, AJ (eds): Orthopedic and Sports Physical Therapy, ed 2. CV Mosby, St Louis, 1997, p 379.
10. Cobb, TK, and Morrey, BF: Total elbow arthroplasty as primary treatment for distal humeral fractures in elderly patients. J Bone Joint Surg 79A:826, 1997.
11. Connor, PM, and Morrey BF: Total elbow arthroplasty in patients who have juvenile rheumatoid arthritis. J Bone Joint Surg 80A:678, 1998.
12. Cooney, WP: Elbow arthroplasty: historical perspective and current concepts. In Morrey, BF (ed): The Elbow and Its Disorders, ed 3. WB Saunders, Philadelphia, 2000, p 581.
13. Cyriax, J: Textbook of Orthopaedic Medicine, Vol. 1. Diagnosis of Soft Tissue Lesions, ed 8. Bailliere Tindall, London, 1982.
14. Dee, R: Total replacement arthroplasty of the elbow for rheumatoid arthritis. J Bone Joint Surg 54B:88, 1972.
15. Edmonds, A: Elbow arthroplasty. In Clark, GL, et al (eds): Hand Rehabilitation, ed 2. Churchill Livingstone, New York, 1998, p 287.
16. Ellenbecker, TS, and Mattalino, A: The Elbow in Sport—Injury, Treatment and Rehabilitation. Human Kinetics Publishers, Champaign IL, 1997.
17. Ewald, FC, et al: Capitellocondylar total elbow replacement in rheumatoid arthritis: Long-term results. J Bone Joint Surg 75A:498, 1993.

17a. Ferlic, DC: Rheumatoid arthritis in the elbow. In Green, DP, Hotchkiss, RM, and Peterson, WC (eds): Green's Operative Hand Surgery, Vol 2, ed 4. Churchill Livingstone, New York 1999, p 1740.

18. Gebel, GT, and Morrey, BF: Operative treatment of medial epicondylitis. Influence of concomitant ulna neuropathy at the elbow. J Bone Joint Surg (Am) 77:1065, 1995.
19. Gill, DR, and Morrey, BF: The Coonrad-Morrey total elbow arthroplasty in patients who have rheumatoid arthritis: A 10 to 15 year follow-up study. J Bone Joint Surg 80A:1327, 1998.
20. Gschwend, N, Simmen BR, and Matejovsky, Z: Late complications in elbow arthroplasty. J Shoulder Elbow Surg 5:86, 1996.
21. Gupta, GG, Lucas, G, and Hahn DL: Biomechanical and computer analysis of radial head prostheses. J Shoulder Elbow Surg 6:37, 1997.
22. Hepburn, G, and Crivelli, K: Use of elbow dynasplint for reduction of elbow flexion contractures: A case study. J Orthop Sports Phys Ther 5:259, 1984.
23. Hertling, D, and Kessler, RM: Management of Common Musculoskeletal Disorders, Physical Therapy Principles and Methods (ed 3). Lippincott Williams & Wilkins, Philadelphia, 1996.
24. Hotchkiss, RN: Displaced fractures of the radial head: internal fixation or excisions? J Am Acad Orthop Surg 5:1, 1997.
25. Inglis, AE, Inglis AE Jr, Friggie, MM, and Asnis, L: Total elbow arthroplasty for flail and unstable elbows. J Shoulder Elbow Surg 6:29, 1997.
26. Jerosch, J, Schroder, M, and Schneider, T: Good and relative indications for elbow arthroscopy: A retrospective study on 103 patients. Arch Orthop Trauma Surg 117:246, 1998.
27. Jobe, FW, and Ciccotti, MG: Lateral and medial epicondylitis of the elbow. J Am Acad Orthop Surg 2:1, 1994.
28. Kapadji, IA, and Kandel, MJ: The Physiology of the Joints, Vol. I. ed 5. Churchill-Livingstone, Edinburgh, 1997.
29. Kopell, H, and Thompson, W: Peripheral Entrapment Neuropathies, ed 2. Robert E Krieger, Huntington, NY, 1976.
30. Kraushaar, BS, and Nirschl, RP: Tendinosis of the elbow (tennis elbow). Clinical features and findings of histological, immunohistochemical and electron microscopy studies. J Bone Joint Surg (Am) 81(2):259, 1999.
31. Lee, BP, and Morrey BF: Synovectomy of the elbow. In Morrey, BF (ed): The Elbow and Its Disorders, ed 3. WB Saunders, Philadelphia, 2000, p 708.
32. Levangie, P, and Norkin, C: Joint Structure and Function: A Comprehensive Analysis, ed 3. FA Davis, Philadelphia, 2001.
33. Linscheid, RL: Resurfacing elbow replacement arthroplasty: Rationale, technique and results. In Morrey, BF (ed): The Elbow and Its Disorders, ed 3. WB Saunders, Philadelphia, 2000, p 602.
34. Lowe, LW, et al: The development of an unconstrained elbow arthroplasty: A clinical review. J Bone Joint Surg Br 66:243, 1984.
35. Lutz, FR: Radial tunnel syndrome: An etiology of chronic lateral elbow pain. J Orthop Sports Phys Ther 14:14, 1991.
36. Magee, DJ: Orthopedic Physical Assessment, ed 3. WB Saunders, Philadelphia, 1997.
37. Manning-Kloos, S, and Nestor, BJ: Elbow surgery and rehabilitation. In Melvin, J and Gall, V (eds): Rheumatologic Rehabilitation Series, Vol. 5: Surgical Rehabilitation. American Occup Ther Assoc, Bethesda MD, 1999, p 13.
38. Mercier, LR: Practical Orthropedics, ed 4. CV Mosby Publishers, St. Louis, 1995.

39. Miller, J: Mulligan concept—management of "tennis elbow." Orthop Div Rev May/June: 45, 2000.
40. Morrey, BF, and Kavanagh, BF: Cementless joint replacement: Current status and future. Bull Rheum Dis 37:1, 1987.
41. Morrey, BF: Surgery of the elbow. In Sledge, CB, et al (eds): Arthritis Surgery. WB Saunders, Philadelphia, 1994.
42. Morrey, BF: Ectopic ossificans about the elbow. In Morrey, BF (ed): The Elbow and Its Disorders, ed 3. WB Saunders, Philadelphia, 2000, p 437.
43. Morrey BF: Radial head fracture. In Morrey BF (ed): The Elbow and Its Disorders, ed 3. WB Saunders, Philadelphia, 2000, p 341.
44. Morrey, BF: Semiconstrained elbow replacement arthroplasty: rationale and surgical technique. In Moorey, BF (ed): The Elbow and Its Disorders, ed 3. WB Saunders, Philadelphia, 2000, p 617.
45. Morrey, BF: Complications of elbow replacement surgery. In Morrey, BF (ed): The Elbow and Its Disorders, ed 3. WB Saunders, Philadelphia, 2000, p 667.
46. Morrey, BF, Adams, RA, and Bryan, RS: Total replacement for post-traumatic arthritis of the elbow. J Bone Joint Surg 73B:607, 1991.
47. Morrey, BF, and Adams, RA: Semiconstrained total elbow arthroplasty for rheumatoid arthritis. J Bone Joint Surg 74A:479, 1992.
48. Morrey, BF, and Adams, RA: Semiconstrained elbow for distal humeral nonunion. J Bone Joint Surg 77B:67, 1995.
49. Morrey, BF, and An, K: Functional evaluation of the elbow. In Morrey, BF (ed): The Elbow and Its Disorders, ed 3. WB Saunders, Philadelphia, 2000, p 74.
50. Morrey, BE, et al: A biomechanical study of normal functional elbow motion. J Bone Joint Surg 63A:87, 1981.
51. Mulligan, BR: Manual Therapy "NAGS", "SNAGS", "MWM'S" etc. (ed 4). Plane View Press, Wellington, 1999.
52. Nerschl, R, and Sobel, J: Conservative treatment of tennis elbow. Phys Sportsmed 9.6:43, 1981.
53. Noteboom, T, et al: Tennis elbow: A review. J Orthop Sports Phys Ther 19:357, 1994.
54. Pritchard, RW: Semiconstrained elbow prosthesis: A clinical review of five years' experience. Orthop Rev 8:33, 1979.
55. Ramsey, ML, Adams, RA, and Morrey, BF: Instability of the elbow treated with semiconstrained total elbow arthroplasty. J Bone Joint Surg 81A:38, 1999.
56. Risung, F: The Norway elbow replacement: design, technique and results after nine years. J Bone Joint Surg 79B:394, 1997.
57. Schemitsch, EH, Ewald, FC, and Thornhill, TS: Results of total elbow arthroplasty after excision of the radial head and synovectomy in patients who had rheumatoid arthritis. J Bone Joint Surg 78A:1541, 1996.
58. Schneeberger, AG, Adams, R, and Morrey, BF: Semiconstrained total elbow replacement for the treatment of posttraumatic osteoarthrosis. J Bone Joint Surg 79A:1211, 1997.
59. Sheon, R, Moskowitz, R, and Goldberg, V: Soft tissue rheumatic pain: recognition, management, prevention. Lea & Febiger, Philadelphia, 1982.
60. Smith, LK, Weiss, EL, and Lehmkuhl, LD: Brunnstrom's Clinical Kinesiology, ed 5. FA Davis, Philadelphia, 1996.
61. Stans, AA, and Wedge, JH: Fractures of the neck of the radius in children. In Morrey, BF (ed): The Elbow and Its Disorders, ed 3. WB Saunders, Philadelphia, 2000, pp 236.
62. Stroyan, M, and Wilk, KE: The functional anatomy of the elbow complex. J Orthop Sports Phys Ther 17:179, 1993.
63. Summers, GD, Talor, AR, and Wobley, M: Elbow synovectomy and excision of the radial head in rheumatoid arthritis: a short term palliative procedure. J Rheumatol 15:566, 1988.
64. Vander-Wilde, RS, et al: Inflammatory arthrosis of the ulnohumeral joint after failed silicone radial head implant. J Bone Joint Surg 76B:78, 1994.
65. Vicenzino, B, Buratowski, S, and Wright, A: Preliminary study of the initial hypoalgesic effect of a mobilisation with movement treatment for lateral epicondylalgia. In Singer, KP (ed): Proceedings of the 7th Scientific Conference of the IFOMT. Perth, Australia, Nov 6, 2000, p 460.
66. Vicenzino, B, and Wright, A: Effects of a novel manipulative physiotherapy technique on tennis elbow: a single case study. Manual Therapy 1:30, 1995.
67. Waugh, T: Arthroplasty rehabilitation. In Goodgold, J (ed): Rehabilitation Medicine. CV Mosby, St Louis, 1988.
68. Weiland, AJ, et al: Capitellocondylar total elbow replacement. J Bone Joint Surg Am 71:217, 1989.
69. Wilk, KE, Arrigo, C, and Andrews, JR: Rehabilitation of the elbow in the throwing athlete. J Orthop Sports Phys Ther 17:305, 1993.
70. Zohn, D, and Mennell, J: Musculoskeletal Pain: Principles of Physical Diagnosis and Physical Treatment. Little, Brown, Boston, 1976.

Chapter 11

The Wrist and Hand

OBJECTIVES

After studying this chapter, the reader will be able to:

1. Identify important aspects of wrist and hand structure and function for review.
2. Integrate presenting signs and symptoms of common wrist and hand impairments with goals for intervention.
3. Recognize unique structural and functional relationships in the wrist and hand that require special precautions when establishing and teaching therapeutic exercise interventions.
4. Design therapeutic exercise interventions to treat impairments and functional limitations in the wrist and hand that are related to stages of recovery after tissue injury.
5. Discuss the background of, indications for, and outcomes after common surgical procedures for soft tissue and joint pathology of the wrist and hand.
6. Explain the goals and appropriate interventions for postoperative management of wrist and hand dysfunction.
7. Establish postoperative rehabilitation programs that include appropriate progressions of therapeutic exercise interventions for common surgical procedures of the wrist and hand.

The wrist is the final link of joints that positions the hand for functional activities. It has the significant function of controlling the length-tension relationship of the multiarticular muscles of the hand as they adjust to various activities and grips.[46] The hand is a valuable tool through which we control and manipulate our environment and express ideas and talents. It also has an important sensory function of providing feedback to the brain.

The anatomy and kinesiology of the wrist and hand are rather complex but are important to know to effectively treat hand problems. The first section of this chapter reviews highlights of the anatomy and function of those areas that the reader should know and understand. Chapter 8 presents information on principles of management; the reader should be familiar with that material before proceeding with establishing a therapeutic exercise program for the wrist or hand. The remaining sections describe common wrist and hand problems, their conservative or surgical management, and exercise techniques and progressions.

▶ Review of the Structure and Function of the Wrist and Hand

Bony Parts (see Fig. 6–33)

Wrist

The bones of the wrist consist of the distal radius, scaphoid (S), lunate (L), triquetrum (Tri), pisiform (P), trapezium (Tm), trapezoid (Tz), capitate (C), and hamate (H).

Hand

Five metacarpals and 14 phalanges make up the hand and five digits.

Joints of the Wrist Complex and Their Movements

The Wrist Complex

The distal radioulnar (RU) joint is not part of the wrist joint, although pain and impairments in this forearm articulation are often described by the patient as wrist pain. Its structure and function were described in Chapter 10.

The wrist joint is multiarticular and is made up of two compound joints. It is biaxial, allowing for flexion (volar flexion), extension (dorsiflexion), radial deviation (abduction), and ulnar deviation (adduction).

The Radiocarpal Joint

The radiocarpal joint is enclosed in a loose but strong capsule, reinforced by ligaments also shared with the midcarpal joint.

The biconcave articulating surface is the distal end of the radius and radioulnar disk (discus articularis); it is angled slightly volarly and ulnarly.

The biconvex articulating surface is the combined proximal surface of the scaphoid, lunate, and triquetrum. The triquetrum primarily articulates with the disk. These three carpals are bound together with numerous interosseous ligaments.

With motions of the wrist, the convex proximal row of carpals slides in the direction opposite the physiological motion of the hand (Box 11–1).

Box 11–1 Arthrokinematics of the Wrist and Hand Joints

Physiological motion	Roll	Slide
Radiocarpal joint: motion of proximal row of carpals		
Flexion of wrist	*Volar*	*Dorsal*
Extension of wrist	*Dorsal*	*Volar*
Radial deviation	*Radial*	*Ulnar*
Ulnar deviation	*Ulnar*	*Radial*
Midcarpal articulation: motion of distal row of carpals		
Flexion of wrist	*Volar*	*C and H dorsal* *Tm and Tz volar*
Extension of wrist	*Dorsal*	*C and H volar* *Tm and Tz dorsal*
Radial deviation	*Radial*	*C and H ulnar* *Rm and Tz dorsal*
Ulnar deviation	*Ulnar*	*C and H radial* *Tm and Tz volar*
Carpometacarpal joints of digits 2-5: motion of proximal phalanx		
Flexion (increased arch)	*Volar*	*Volar*
Extension (decreased arch)	*Dorsal*	*Dorsal*
Carpometacarpal joint of thumb: motion of 1st metacarpal		
Flexion	*Ulnar*	*Ulnar*
Extension	*Radial*	*Radial*
Abduction	*Volar*	*Dorsal*
Adduction	*Dorsal*	*Volar*
Metacarpophalangeal joints of digits 2-5: motion of phalanx		
Flexion	*Volar*	*Volar*
Extension	*Dorsal*	*Dorsal*
Abduction	*Away from center of hand*	
Adduction	*Toward center of hand*	
Interphalangeal joints and MCP joint of thumb: motion of phalanx		
Flexion	*Volar*	*Volar*
Extension	*Dorsal*	*Dorsal*

The Midcarpal Joint

This is a compound joint between the two rows of carpals. It has a capsule that is also continuous with the intercarpal articulations.

The combined distal surfaces of the scaphoid, lunate, and triquetrum articulate with the combined proximal surfaces of the trapezium, trapezoid, capitate, and hamate.

The articulating surfaces of the capitate and hamate are, in essence, convex and slide on the concave articulating surfaces of a portion of the scaphoid, lunate, and triquetrum so that with flexion and extension, as well as radial and ulnar deviation, their combined surfaces slide opposite the physiologic motion (Box 11–1).

The articulating surfaces of the trapezium and trapezoid are concave and slide on the convex distal surface of the scaphoid so that with flexion and extension their combined surfaces slide in the same direction as the physiological motion. Because the trapezoid is bound to the capitate, they cannot slide in opposite directions during radial and ulnar deviation. The trapezii (the trapezium and trapezoid), therefore, slide dorsal on the scaphoid during radial deviation and volar during ulnar deviation.[41]

Physiological motions of the wrist result in a complex motion between the proximal and distal row of carpals. Since the concave trapezii slide dorsal on the scaphoid and the convex capitate and hamate slide volar on the lunate and triquetrum when extending or radially deviating, the resulting motion is a supination twist of the distal row on the proximal row. A pronation twist occurs when flexing or ulnarly deviating as the trapezii slide volar and the capitate and hamate slide dorsal[46] (Box 11–1).

The Pisiform

The pisiform is categorized as a carpal and is aligned volar to the triquetrum in the proximal row of carpals. It is not part of the wrist joint but functions as a sesamoid bone in the flexor carpi ulnaris tendon.

The Ligaments

Stability and some passive movement of the wrist complex are provided by numerous ligaments: the ulnar and radial collateral, the dorsal and volar (palmar) radiocarpal, the ulnocarpal, and the intercarpal.

Joints of the Hand Complex and Their Movements

Carpometacarpal (CMC) Joints of Digits 2 through 5

The joints are enclosed in a common joint cavity and include the articulations of each metacarpal with the distal row of carpals and the articulations between the bases of each metacarpal.

The joints of digits 2, 3, and 4 are plane uniaxial joints; the joint of digit 5 is biaxial. They are supported by transverse and longitudinal ligaments. The 5th metacarpal is most mobile, with the 4th being the next most mobile. The flexion of the metacarpals and additional adduction of the 5th contribute to cupping (arching) of the hand, which improves prehension (Box 11–1).

Carpometacarpal Joint of the Thumb (Digit 1)

This joint is a saddle-shaped (sellar) biaxial joint between the trapezium and base of the first metacarpal. It has a lax capsule and wide ROM, which allows the thumb to move away from the palm of the hand for opposition in prehension activities.

For flexion/extension of the thumb (components of opposition/reposition, respectively) occurring in the frontal plane, the trapezium surface is convex and the base of the metacarpal is concave; therefore, its surface slides in the same direction as the angulating bone (Box 11–1). For abduction/adduction, occurring in the sagittal plane, the trapezium surface is concave and the metacarpal is convex; therefore, the surface of the metacarpal slides in the opposite direction of the physiologic motion (Box 11–1).

Metacarpophalangeal (MCP) Joints of Digits 2 through 5

They are biaxial condyloid joints with the distal end of each metacarpal convex and proximal phalanx concave. The proximal surface of the proximal phalanx rolls and slides in the same direction as the physiological motion (Box 11–1).

Each joint is supported by a volar and two collateral ligaments. The collaterals become taut in full flexion and prevent abduction and adduction in this position.

Interphalangeal (IP) Joints and MCP Joint of the Thumb

There is a proximal (PIP) and distal (DIP) interphalangeal joint for each digit, 2 through 5. The thumb has only one interphalangeal joint although the MCP joint of the thumb is uniaxial and, therefore, functions similar to the IP joints. The MCP joint of the thumb differs in that it is reinforced by two sesamoid bones on the volar surface, which improve the leverage of the flexor pollicis brevis muscle.

Each of these joints is a uniaxial hinge joint. The articulating surface at the distal end of each phalanx is convex; the articulating surface at the proximal end of each phalanx is concave; and therefore, the proximal surface of each phalanx rolls and slides in the same direction as the physiologic motion (Box 11–1).

Each capsule is reinforced with collateral ligaments, which are taut in extension. Going radial to ulnar in digits 2 through 5 there is increasing flexion/extension range in the joints. This allows for greater opposition of the ulnar fingers to the thumb and also causes a potentially tighter grip on the ulnar side of the hand.

Hand Function

Length-Tension Relationships

The position of the wrist controls the length of the extrinsic muscles of the digits.

As the fingers or thumb flex, the wrist must be stabilized by the wrist extensor muscles to prevent the flexor digitorum profundus and flexor digitorum superficialis or flexor pollicis longus from simultaneously flexing the wrist. As the grip becomes stronger, synchronous wrist extension lengthens the extrinsic flexor tendons across the wrist and maintains a more favorable overall length of the musculotendinous unit for a stronger contraction.

For strong finger or thumb extension, the wrist flexor muscles stabilize or flex the wrist so the extensor digitorum communis, extensor indicis, extensor digiti minimi, or extensor pollicis longus muscles can function more efficiently. In addition, there is ulnar deviation; the flexor and extensor carpi ulnaris muscles are both active as the hand opens.[51]

Cupping and Flattening

Cupping of the hand occurs with finger flexion, and flattening of the hand occurs with extension. Cupping improves the ability of the hand to grasp around objects of various sizes, and flattening improves the ability to release objects.

Extensor Mechanism

Structurally, the extensor hood is made up of the extensor digitorum communis tendon, its connective tissue expansion, and fibers from the tendons of the dorsal and volar interossei and lumbricales.[46] Each structure has an effect on the extensor mechanism.

- An isolated contraction of the extensor digitorum produces clawing of the fingers (MCP hyperextension with IP flexion from passive pull of the extrinsic flexor tendons, also called hook position).
- PIP and DIP extension occurs concurrently and can be caused by the interossei or lumbrical muscles through their pull on the extensor hood.
- There must be tension in the extensor digitorum communis tendon for there to be interphalangeal extension. This occurs either by active contraction of the muscle, causing MCP extension concurrently as the intrinsic muscles contract, or by stretch of the tendon, which occurs with MCP flexion.

Grips and Prehension Patterns

The nature of the intended activity dictates the type of grip used.[46,50,51,61]

- ***Power grips*** involve clamping an object with partially flexed fingers against the palm of the hand and with counterpressure from the adducted thumb. Power grips are primarily isometric functions. The fingers are flexed, laterally rotated, and ulnarly deviated. The amount of flexion varies with the object held. The thumb reinforces the fingers and helps make small adjustments to control the direction of the force. Varieties include cylindrical grip, spherical grip, hook grip, and lateral prehension.
- ***Precision patterns*** involve manipulating an object that is not in contact with the palm of the hand between the opposing abducted thumb and fingers. The muscles primarily function isotonically. The sensory surfaces of the digits are used for maximum sensory input to influence delicate adjustments. With small objects, precise handling occurs primarily between the thumb and index finger. Varieties include pad-to-pad, tip-to-tip, and pad-to-side prehension.
- ***Combined grips*** involve digits 1 and 2 (and sometimes 3) performing precision activities, whereas digits 3 through 5 supplement with power.

Hand Control

Control of the Unloaded (Free) Hand

Anatomic factors, muscular contraction, and viscoelastic properties of the muscles influence finger motion.[51,46]

- Clawing motions occur with only extrinsic muscle contractions.
- Closing motions can occur only with extrinsic muscle contractions but also require the viscoelastic force of the biarticular interossei.
- Opening motions require the synergistic contraction of the extrinsic extensor and the lumbrical muscles.
- Reciprocal motion of MCP flexion and IP extension is caused by the interossei. The lumbrical removes the viscoelastic tension from the profundus tendon and assists IP extension.

Power Grip

The muscles primarily function with isometric contractions[46,81]

- Extrinsic finger flexors provide the major gripping force.
- The extensor digitorum provides a compressive force to the MCP joints, which increases stability and also provides a balancing force for the flexors.
- Interossei rotate the 1st phalanx for positioning to compress the external object and also flex the MCP joint.
- Lumbricales do not participate in the power grip (except the 4th).
- The thenar muscles and adductor pollicis provide compressive forces against the object being gripped.

Precision Handling

The primary dynamic function of the muscles includes the following[46,81]

- Extrinsic muscles provide the compressive force to hold the objects between the fingers and thumb.
- For manipulation of an object, the interossei abduct and adduct the fingers, the thenar muscles control movement of the thumb, and the lumbricales help move the object away from the palm of the hand. The amount of participation of each muscle varies with the amount and direction of motion.

Pinch

Compression between the thumb and fingers is provided by the thenar eminence muscles, the adductor pollicis, the interossei, and extrinsic flexors. The lumbricales also participate.[46]

Major Nerves Subject to Pressure and Trauma at the Wrist and Hand

Median Nerve

To enter the hand, this nerve passes through the carpal tunnel at the wrist with the flexor tendons. The carpal tunnel is covered by the thick, relatively inelastic transverse carpal ligament. Entrapment in the tunnel causes sensory changes and progressive weakness in the muscles innervated distal to the wrist resulting in ape-hand deformity (thenar atrophy and thumb in plane of hand) (Tables 11–1 and 11–2). The branch innervating the opponens muscle hooks over the carpal ligament two-thirds of the way up the thenar eminence and can be entrapped separately.[45]

Ulnar Nerve

This nerve enters the hand through a trough formed by the pisiform bone and hook of the hamate bone and is covered by the volar carpal ligament and palmaris brevis muscle. Trauma or entrapment causes sensory changes and progressive weakness of muscles innervated distal to the site resulting in partial claw-hand (benediction hand) deformity (Tables 11–1 and 11–2). Injury to the nerve after it bifurcates leads to partial involvement, depending on the site of injury.[45]

Radial Nerve

This nerve enters the hand on the dorsal surface as the superficial radial nerve, which is sensory only. Injury to it in the wrist or hand causes sensory changes only.[45] Influence of the radial nerve on hand musculature is entirely proximal to the wrist. It innervates extrinsic wrist and hand muscles (see Chapter 9). Injury near the elbow results in wrist drop and inability to actively extend the wrist and fingers. This affects the length-tension relationship of the extrinsic finger flexors resulting in an ineffective grip unless the wrist is splinted in partial extension.

Referred Pain and Sensory Patterns

The hand is the terminal point for several major nerves. Injury or entrapment of these nerves may occur anywhere along their course, from the cervical spine to their termination. What the patient perceives as pain or a sensory disturbance in the hand may be from injury of the nerve anywhere along its course (Table 11–2), or the pain may be from irritation of tissue of common segmental origin such as the zygopophyseal facet joints of the spine. For treatment to be effective, it must be directed to the source of the problem, not to the site where the patient perceives the pain or sensory changes. Therefore, a thorough history is taken and examination of the entire upper quarter must be done, including the cervical spine when referred pain patterns or sensory changes are reported by the patient.[24,52]

Table 11–1 Patterns of Muscle Weakness Associated with Peripheral Nerve Injuries in the Hand

Nerve	Nerve Injury at Wrist and Hand Level	Deformity	Primary Functional Loss
Median (C6-T1)	Opponens pollicis Abductor pollicis brevis Flexor pollicis brevis (superficial head) Lumbricales I & II	Ape hand	Thumb abduction and opposition for tip-to-tip, tip-to-pad, and pad-to-pad prehension
Ulnar (C8-T1)	Abductor digiti minimi Opponens digiti minimi Flexor digiti minimi Lumbricales to 4th and 5th digits Interossei Adductor pollicis Flexor pollicis brevis (deep head)	Partial claw	Use of 4th and 5th digits for spherical and cylindrical power grips, thumb for adduction, and finger abduction and adduction
Radial (C6-T1)	No intrinsic muscle innervation	None	None

Table 11–2 Patterns of Sensory Loss in the Hand with Nerve Injuries

Location of Impingement	Area of Sensory Changes or Loss
Nerve roots	
C6	Thumb and index finger
C7	Index, middle, and ring fingers
C8	Little and ring fingers
Brachial plexus	
Upper trunk or lateral cord	Radial side of hand
Lower trunk or medial cord	Ulnar side of hand
Other sites	Mixed distribution, depending on involved nerves
Peripheral nerves	
Median nerve	Radial 2/3 of palm, palmar surfaces, and dorsum of distal phalanges of 1st, 2nd, 3rd, and half of 4th digits
Ulnar nerve	Ulnar 1/3 of hand, entire 5th digit, and ulnar side of 4th digit
Radial nerve	Radial 2/3 of dorsum of hand and thumb, proximal phalanx of 2nd, 3rd, and half of 4th digit

Joint Hypomobility: Nonoperative Management

Related Diagnoses and Etiology of Symptoms

Pathologies such as rheumatoid arthritis (RA) and degenerative joint disease (DJD), as well as acute joint trauma, affect the joints of the wrist and hand. Impaired mobility and adhesions from immobilization develop in the joints, tendon sheaths, muscles, and surrounding tissues any time the joints are splinted or casted. Chapter 8 describes the etiology of these arthritic and joint symptoms.

Common Diagnoses and Impairments

Rheumatoid Arthritis

The following is a summary of signs and symptoms and resulting impairments typically seen in rheumatoid arthritis (RA).[2,53,64]

- *Acute stage.* Pain, swelling, warmth, and limited motion from synovial inflammation (synovitis) and tissue proliferation, most commonly in the MCP, PIP, and wrist joints bilaterally, as well as inflammation (tenosynovitis) and synovial proliferation in the extrinsic tendons and tendon sheaths.
- Progressive muscle weakness and imbalances in length and strength between agonists and antagonists and between intrinsic and extrinsic muscles of the hand.
- Carpal tunnel syndrome may occur in conjunction with tenosynovitis due to compression of the median nerve from the swollen tissue.
- General systemic as well as muscular fatigue.

Advanced stages. Joint capsule weakening, cartilage destruction, bone erosion, and tendon rupture lead to subluxations and deformities, including:

- Volar subluxation of the triquetrum on the articular disk and ulna with the extensor carpi ulnaris tendon displaced volarly, causing a flexor force at the wrist joint
- Ulnar subluxation of the carpals resulting in radial deviation of the wrist
- Ulnar drift of the fingers at the MCP joints and volar subluxation of the proximal phalanx
- Swan-neck deformity (PIP hyperextension with DIP flexion)
- Boutonnière deformity (PIP flexion with DIP extension)

Osteoarthritis (OA) and Joint Trauma

The following is a summary of signs and symptoms and resulting impairments commonly seen in OA.[95]

- Age and repetitive joint trauma lead to degenerative cartilaginous and bony changes in susceptible joints. Osteoarthritis most commonly involves the trapezioscaphoid articulation, CMC joint of the thumb, and DIP joints of the digits although the effects of trauma can occur in any joint.
- *Acute stage.* Swelling, warmth, and restricted and painful motion.
- *Advanced stages.* Limitation of both flexion and extension in the affected joints with a firm capsular end-feel.
- General muscle weakness, weak grip strength, and poor muscular endurance.

Precaution: After trauma, the therapist must be alert to signs of a fracture in the wrist or hand because small bone fractures may not show on X-ray for up to 2 weeks. Signs include swelling, muscle spasm when passive motion is attempted, increased pain when the involved bone is stressed (such as deviation toward the involved bone), and tenderness on palpation over the fracture site.[24,56]

Postimmobilization Hypomobility

- Decreased ROM, decreased joint play with firm end-feel and pain on overpressure, and tendon adhesions
- Muscle weakness, weak grip strength, decreased flexibility, and poor endurance

Common Functional Limitations/Disabilities

When joint pathology is acute, many prehension activities will be painful, interfering with activities of daily living (ADL) such as dressing, eating, grooming, and toileting, or almost any functional activity requiring gripping and fine-finger dexterity, including writing and typing.

Depending on which joints are involved, the amount of restricted movement and residual weakness, fatigue or dexterity loss, and type of grip or amount of precision handling required, functional loss may be minor or significant.

Joint Management: Protection Phase

General guidelines for managing acute joint lesions are described in Chapter 8 and summarized in Box 8–1. Special concerns for patients with RA and OA are summarized in Boxes 8–6, 8–7, and 8–8.

Joint Protection and Patient Education

Splinting. Use a splint to rest and protect the involved joints. Instruct the patient to remove the splint for brief periods of nonstressful motion throughout the day.

Activity modification. Analyze the patient's daily activities and recommend adaptations or assistive devices to minimize repetitive or excessive stresses on the joints. This is particularly important for patients with chronic arthritic disorders to prevent repetitive trauma or minimize joint deformity. Examples are summarized in Box 11–2 at the end of this section.

Decrease Pain

In addition to physician-prescribed medication or nonsteroidal anti-inflammants and modalities, gentle grade I or II distraction and oscillation techniques may inhibit pain and move synovial fluid for nutrition in the involved joints.

Maintain Joint, Tendon, and Soft Tissue Mobility

Passive, assistive, or active ROM. It is important to move the joints as tolerated because immobility of the hand quickly leads to muscle imbalance and contracture formation or further articular deterioration. Aquatic therapy is an effective method of combining nonstressful, nonweight-bearing exercises with therapeutic heat.

Multiple-angle muscle setting exercises. Do gentle isometrics to all wrist and hand musculature.

Tendon-gliding exercises. Have the patient perform full motion in the uninvolved joints, and as much motion as possible in the involved joints to prevent adhesions between the long tendons or between the tendons and their synovial sheaths.[34] Tendon-gliding exercises are described in the exercise section of this chapter.

Joint Management: Controlled Motion and Return to Function Phases

With joint pathology, increase ROM by utilizing joint mobilization techniques to stretch the capsule[67] as well as passive stretching and muscle inhibition techniques to elongate the periarticular connective tissue and musculotendinous units following the principles described in Chapters 5 and 6. It is also critical to determine if scar tissue has formed in the long tendon sheaths in the hand, and, if so, attempt to re-establish smooth tendon gliding.

Precautions: For patients with RA, modify the intensity of joint mobilization and stretching techniques that are used to counter any restrictions because the disease process and use of steroid therapy weaken the tensile quality of the connective tissue, and consequently, they are more easily torn. Special considerations for dealing with the deforming forces in rheumatoid arthritis are summarized in Box 11–2 at the end of this section.

Increase Joint Play and Accessory Motions

Joint mobilization techniques. Determine which of the articulations of the distal RU, wrist, hand, or digits are restricted because of decreased joint play, and apply grade III sustained or grade IV oscillation techniques to stretch the capsules. See Figures 6–32 through 6–39 and their descriptions in Chapter 6 for mobilizing the distal RU and restricted wrist joints. See Figures 6–41 through 6–43 for mobilizing restricted joints of the hand and digits.

Unlock a subluxated ulnomeniscal-triquetral (UMT) joint. The mechanism of dysfunction is not clear, but some patients describe locking in the wrist and an inability to supinate the forearm. The meniscus may be displaced and be the cause of the blocked motion. The following techniques may free up the motion.

- Volar glide the ulna on a stabilized triquetrum (similar to Fig. 6–38).
- Self-mobilization. Have the patient grasp the distal ulna with the fingers of the opposite hand, place the thumb on the palmar surface of the triquetrum just medial to the pisiform, and then press with the thumb, causing a dorsal glide of the triquetrum on the radioulnar disk and ulna (Fig. 11–1).

Improve Joint Tracking and Pain-Free Motion

Mobilization with movement (MWM) techniques may be applied to increase ROM and/or decrease the pain associated with movement.[57] (The principles of MWM are described in Chapter 6.)

MWM of the wrist. Patient position and procedure: Seated. Stabilize the distal forearm with one hand and apply a pain-free lateral glide to the proximal row of carpals utilizing the web space of your other hand. Have the patient then perform active wrist extension or flexion to the end of the available range, and with his or her free hand apply a passive stretch at the end of the range (Fig. 11–2).

An internal or external rotation of the carpals relative to the radius may need to be combined with the glide to achieve pain-free, end-range loading.

The intercarpal joint may require specific anterior-posterior gliding of one proximal row of carpals relative to its distal row neighbor combined with active physiologic motion to the end of the range. The mobilization and movement are pain-free. While holding the mobilization force, ask the patient to do repetitive gripping activities or resisted wrist motions.

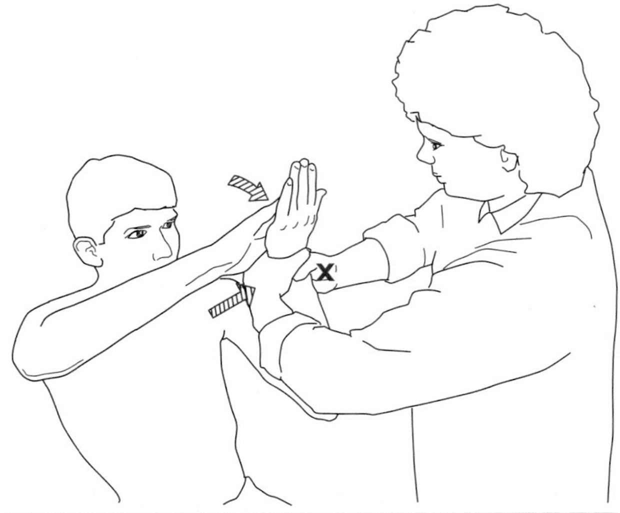

Figure 11–2 Mobilization with movement (MWM) to increase wrist flexion or extension. Apply a lateral glide, while the patient actively flexes or extends the wrist and then applies a passive stretch force with the other hand at the end of the range.

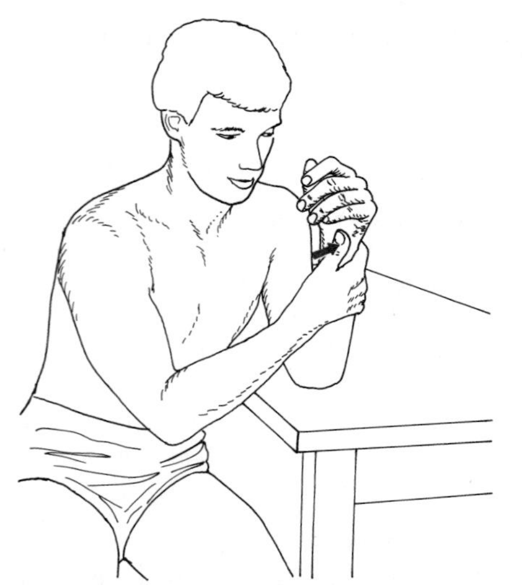

Figure 11–1 Self-mobilization of the ulnomeniscal-triquetral (UMI) joint.

MWM of the MCP and IP joints of the digits. Medially or laterally glide the involved phalanx in a painless direction, then have the patient actively flex or extend the finger and apply a pain-free, end-range stretch.

Internal or external rotation of the more distal phalanx may be required in conjunction with the medial or lateral glide to achieve painless end-range overpressure.[57]

Develop Mobility and Neuromuscular Control in the Musculotendinous Units

Carefully examine the multijoint and intrinsic muscles for restricted motion from contractures or adhesions and poor movement patterns from weakness or imbalances in strength. Stretching, tendon gliding, and strengthening exercises are described in the exercise sections of this chapter. Utilize techniques that specifically address the impairments that the patient has. Once range is gained, it is critical that the patient uses the new range with active ROM and functional activities.

Develop Strength and Function

Neuromuscular control and strength. Progress exercises with controlled and nondestructive forces to increase strength and muscle balance between antagonists, and progress endurance training. With pathologic joints, use caution when applying weights so as not to stress the joints beyond the capability of the stabilizing tissues.

Functional activities. Develop exercises that prepare the patient for functional activities. Consider prehension patterns that will be required for the patient's job, recreational, and daily activities. Include exercises requiring coordination and fine finger dexterity.

Conditioning exercises. Initiate physical conditioning exercises using activities that do not provoke joint symptoms such as aquatic exercises or cycling.

Box 11–2 Joint Protection in the Wrist and Hand

Purpose: performance of daily activities with minimal pain, stress to joints, and energy expenditure. Most of these principles are applicable to any arthritic problem in the hand, but are especially important in the hand affected by rheumatoid arthritis[64,65]

- ***Respect pain.*** Monitor activities; stop when fatigue or discomfort begins to develop. Modify or discontinue any activity or exercise that causes pain that lasts longer than 1 hour after stopping the activity.
- ***Maintain strength and ROM.*** Integrate exercises into daily activities.
  - Look for early signs of muscle tightness in the intrinsic muscles. If tight, initiate stretching. One cause of swan-neck deformity is tight interossei muscles pulling on the extensor tendon, leading to hyperextension of hypermobile PIP joints.
  - Strengthen radial deviation of the MP joints of the fingers to counter the ulnar drifting of the fingers that occur in many functional activities.
- ***Balance activity level and rest.*** More rest than normal will be required during the active phases of the disease of RA. Conserve energy and perform activities in the most economic way or do the most important activities first.
- ***Avoid deforming positions or one position for prolonged periods***
- ***Avoid using strong grasping activities that facilitate the deforming force.*** Typical joint deformities with RA include radial deviation and extension of the wrist and ulnar deviation and volar subluxation of the MP joints. Adaptive suggestions include:
  - Open jars with the left hand or with an assistive device.
  - Cut food with the blade of the knife protruding from the ulnar side of the hand.
  - Stir food with spoon on the ulnar side of the hand.
  - Build up the handles of eating utensils.
  - Use stronger, larger joints whenever feasible. For example carry items in a shoulder bag or over the forearm, or with two hands, rather than with one hand.
  - Avoid twisting or wringing motions with the fingers. Press water out of a rag by opposing the palms of both hands together.

Joint protection. Reinforce use of joint protection techniques as summarized in Box 11–2.

▶ Joint Surgery and Postoperative Management

Long-standing RA or DJD that affects the joints and soft tissues of the wrist and hand can lead to chronic pain, instability and deformity of joints, and restricted ROM, as well as loss of strength in the hand and functional use of the upper extremity. When nonoperative management fails, surgical intervention coupled with individually designed and carefully supervised postoperative rehabilitation is indicated to restore function to the hand and wrist.

Some of the more common surgical options are listed in Box 11–3.

Soft tissue procedures, such as *tenosynovectomy* for chronic tenosynovitis of the extensor and flexor tendons of the wrist, *repair of ruptured tendons, capsulectomy,* or *synovectomy* of the wrist or finger joints, are employed independently when articular surfaces of the involved joints remain intact.[25,34,99,100] If joint deterioration is significant, *arthrodesis, resection arthroplasty,* or *implant arthroplasty,* often performed in conjunction with soft tissue surgery, are the procedures of choice.[3,9,68,79] Some procedures are elected to relieve pain, others to minimize or delay further deformity. For example, if medical management of RA of the wrist fails, tenosynovectomy is performed to

Box 11–3 Surgical Intervention for RA or DJD of the Wrist and Hand

Soft Tissue Procedures

- Synovectomy
- Tenosynovectomy
- Tendon repair, graft, or transfer/realignment
- Nerve decompression
- Capsuloligamentous reconstruction
- Contracture release
  - Capsulectomy/capsulotomy
  - Tendon release
- Soft tissue arthroplasty

Bony Procedures

- Excision/resection arthroplasty
  - Styloidectomy
  - Proximal row carpectomy
- Interpositional, flexible implant arthroplasty
- Total joint arthroplasty
- Arthrodesis

remove proliferated synovium from tendon sheaths and prevent erosion or rupture of tendons before significant deformity and loss of active control of the wrist and fingers occur.[99] If rupture occurs, tendon repairs and transfers can improve function of the hand and delay or prevent the development of fixed deformities or subluxation and dislocation of joints. Limited or complete arthrodesis of the wrist or arthrodesis of an individual joint of a digit, such as the carpometacarpal (CMC) joint of the thumb, are procedures that yield predictable results. Fusion corrects deformity and gives the patient stability and relief of pain with little compromise of function despite the loss of joint motion.[33,34,58] If fusion is inappropriate and pain-free mobility is necessary, several types of arthroplasty, including *proximal row carpectomy, interpositional implant arthroplasty* of individual carpal bones, such as the lunate or scaphoid, the radiocarpal joints or joints of the digits, and *total joint replacement* of the wrist or digits are potential options. In some situations, a combination of surgical procedures is indicated.[3,6,7,8]

The goals of surgery and postoperative management of chronic arthritis and associated deformities include[17,39,68,79,93] (1) restoration of normal or adequate function to the wrist and hand, (2) relief of pain, (3) correction of instability or deformity, (4) restoration of ROM, and (5) improved strength of the wrist and fingers for functional grasp and pinch.

A discussion of postoperative management of several types of arthroplasty follows. Information on surgical management and postoperative rehabilitation of tendon repairs and transfers associated with chronic arthritis is then outlined. Given the complexity of hand rehabilitation, suggested phase-specific guidelines for exercise, founded on principles of tissue healing, must be individualized for each patient and determined by the patient's level of participation in the rehabilitation process and the patient's response to exercise. Successful outcomes are contingent upon close communication among the surgeon, therapist, and patient or patient's family. An effective postoperative rehabilitation program combines early, supervised therapy with patient education and progresses to long-term self-management by the patient.

Radiocarpal Implant Arthroplasty and Total Wrist Replacement

Indications for Surgery

The following are common indications for arthroplasty of the wrist.[6,9,68,79,91,94]

- Severe pain in the wrist region that compromises hand strength and upper extremity function.
- Deterioration of the articular surfaces of the distal radius, carpals, and distal ulna from chronic arthritis (usually RA).
- Marked limitation of motion of the wrist.
- Subluxation or dislocation of the radiocarpal joint.
- Appropriate for *low-demand* upper extremity functional needs.
- Appropriate for patients with bilateral wrist involvement where arthrodesis of both wrists would limit rather than improve overall function.
- Also appropriate for patients with significant stiffness of the ipsilateral shoulder elbow or finger joints in whom unilateral arthrodesis of the wrist would further limit rather than improve functional use of the upper extremity.[6,7,8,9]

Procedures

Background and prosthetic design. Because partial or total arthrodesis of the wrist is often considered the procedure of choice (not just a salvage procedure) for patients with severe pain and instability of the wrist[33,34,58] and because resection arthroplasty of the distal radius or proximal row carpectomy[25] are also suitable options that relieve pain but retain some mobility of the wrist, the use of joint replacement surgery for patients with late-stage arthrosis of the wrist has been limited.[3] Nonetheless, designs of implants and operative techniques for interpositional implant or replacement arthroplasty of the wrist have continued to evolve since Swanson first used an uncemented, double-stemmed, flexible silicone elastomer implant of the radiocarpal joint.[91,94] The early use of silicone implant interposition arthroplasty of the radiocarpal joint was associated with a high, long-term failure rate as the result of poor patient selection, excessive wear of the prosthesis, or cystic changes in bone and, consequently, eventual fracture or loosening of the prosthesis.[11] Although the incidence of these problems is much lower in the wrist than in the MCP and PIP joints,[6] it has also been suggested that as a silicone implant gradually wears (abrades), it may give rise to *particulate synovitis* (silicone synovitis).[40] Subsequent design changes have been made, and flexible implants of the wrist (and digits) are now reinforced with bone-shielding devices (titanium grommets) to improve the long-term durability of the prosthesis.[6,79,91,94] Use of flexible materials other than silicone is also being investigated.[91]

Total joint arthroplasty of the wrist, using rigid materials (metal and high-density polyethylene), is an alternative to flexible implant arthroplasty, particularly for patients with severe deformity and collapse of the wrist joints.[6,7,8,55] The designs can be articulated or nonarticulated. The prosthetic replacements are typically cemented in place, but the use of bioingrowth is also being investigated.[11] Total wrist arthroplasty is preferred over flexible implant arthroplasty in patients with rupture of one or more of the wrist extensor tendons as the result of RA. Design changes have evolved to offset the most serious long-term complication, loosening of the distal component.[7,8,9]

Operative procedures. Both types of wrist arthroplasty, the Swanson interpositional, flexible implant arthroplasty[91] and total wrist replacement,[7,8] require a dorsal incision of the wrist. A concomitant *dorsal clearance* (tenosynovectomy of the extensor tendons) is often necessary.

With a flexible implant arthroplasty after removal of the proximal row of carpals and resection of the distal radius and the base of the capitate, the proximal stem of the double-stemmed prosthesis is placed in the intramedullary canal of the distal radius. The distal stem is placed through the capitate and into the intramedullary canal of the third metacarpal. The prosthesis does not require cement fixation but rather acts as a *dynamic spacer* to maintain joint alignment during healing. Over time it becomes encapsulated as a new fibrous capsule forms.[9,79,91,94]

Total wrist arthroplasty involves resection of the distal portions of the radius and ulna, some of the carpals and a small portion of the proximal aspect of the third metacarpal. The rigid, stemmed prosthetic components are then tightly fit into the reamed intramedullary canals of the third metacarpal and the distal radius. Fixation of the distal component is almost always augmented with cement.[6,7,8,11,34,55,79] In patients with instability and subluxation of the radiocarpal joint, ligament reconstruction is also necessary to improve wrist stability.

In both procedures, flexible implant arthroplasty and total wrist replacement, after closure of the dorsal incision, the hand is placed in a long-arm or short-arm, bulky compression dressing and elevated several days postoperatively to control edema.

Postoperative Management

Immobilization

Flexible implant arthroplasty requires an extended period of immobilization, often 3 to 4 weeks or as long as 6 to 8 weeks, to allow time for encapsulation of the prosthetic spacer to occur.[32,91] After removal of the bulky compression dressing a few days postoperatively, the arm is placed in a long-arm splint and then a short-arm splint with the wrist in a neutral position to 15 degrees of extension and sometimes in slight radial deviation to ensure satisfactory healing of the capsuloligamentous structures that provide wrist stability.

Total wrist replacement with rigid components that are cemented in place involves a similar sequence but with a shorter period of continuous immobilization.[8] Sometimes only 2 weeks of immobilization is necessary if the wrist is stable, but as long as 6 to 8 weeks is required if instability persists even after ligament reconstruction.

If a concomitant repair of the extensor tendons was performed, the immobilizer is fitted with outriggers that have elastic slings to hold the fingers in extension. Even after wrist exercises are initiated the immobilizer is worn for protection between exercise sessions and at night for 6 to 8 weeks postoperatively.

Exercise

As with arthroplasty of other large or small joints, the goals and progression of exercise during each successive phase of rehabilitation after wrist arthroplasty are based on the stages of healing of soft tissues. Stability of the wrist always takes precedence over restoration of wrist mobility. If concomitant tendon repairs were also done, the guidelines and timeframe for exercise are adjusted and special precautions are taken as discussed in a later section of this chapter on extensor tendon rupture in RA.

Exercise: Maximum and Moderate Protection Phases

The emphasis of exercise during the maximum protection phase is to maintain mobility in the fingers and shoulder and in the elbow when the long-arm immobilizer is cut down to a short-arm splint. When the immobilizer can be removed for wrist exercises (between 2 and 6 weeks postoperatively), protection of the wrist is still indicated. The emphasis during the moderate protection (controlled motion) phase of rehabilitation is the restoration of wrist motion without jeopardizing wrist stability.[8,17,32,39,79,91]

- ***Minimize edema in the hand and maintain mobility of adjacent joints.***
  - Active ROM of the shoulder.
  - Active flexion and extension of the fingers with the hand elevated.

- Active ROM of the thumb and elbow when possible.

■ ***Maintain gliding of tendons that cross the wrist.***

- Tendon gliding exercises (see Fig. 11–8*A–E)* with the wrist in neutral.

■ ***Restore mobility of the wrist and forearm.***

- Active pronation and supination of the forearm.
- Active or assisted wrist flexion and extension with the fingers relaxed; emphasize wrist extension more than wrist flexion.

Precautions: Postpone radial and ulnar deviation if wrist stability is questionable.[39] When performing radial and ulnar deviation, avoid wrist flexion with ulnar deviation (the position of wrist deformity).[17]

■ ***Increase mobility of finger joints (if limited preoperatively).***

- Selective use of a low-load, dynamic finger splint(s) during the day or gentle passive stretching to increase finger mobility to at least a functional level at about 6 weeks postoperatively.
- If the joints of the digits are not inflamed, grade II and possibly grade III joint mobilizations and gentle manual stretching of the MCP and IP joints *with the wrist maintained in a neutral position.*

■ ***Prevent atrophy of wrist and finger musculature.***

- Low-intensity, isometric resistance exercises of the wrist and finger musculature.

Precaution: Postpone resisted contractions for at least 6 to 8 weeks if tendons were repaired or transferred.

Exercise: Minimum Protection/Return to Function Phase

During the minimum protection phase, which usually does not begin until 8 to 12 weeks postoperatively, regaining sufficient strength of the entire upper extremity for appropriate functional activities is the priority. In the wrist, emphasize strengthening the wrist extensors more so than the wrist flexors. Patient education focuses on incorporation of joint protection during functional activities (refer to Box 11–2). Use of a cock-up resting splint is advisable at night, particularly if a wrist flexion contracture persists. Although 15 degrees of wrist extension is preferable for a strong functional grasp, the use of manual stretching procedures to increase wrist extension is not consistently advocated so as not to compromise wrist stability.[91]

■ ***Regain functional strength of the hand and wrist.***

- Transition to progressively graded dynamic resistance exercises of the hand and wrist. Emphasize simulated functional movement patterns, such as various types of grasping activities during strengthening exercises.
- Use of the hand for light functional activities usually by 12 weeks postoperatively.

Precautions: Reinforce principles of joint protection through patient education.[17,65] Recommendations include: (1) avoid weight bearing on the operated hand during transfers, ambulation with assistive devices, or other daily living activities, (2) avoid functional activities that place more than 5-lb loads on the wrist; and (3) refrain from high-impact vocational or recreational activities, associated with heavy labor or racquet sports.

■ ***Increase ROM of the wrist to a functional level.***

Note: In patients who exhibit significant postoperative stiffness of the wrist early in a rehabilitation program, stretching activities may be initiated earlier than during the minimum protection phase, possibly at 6 weeks postoperatively.[32]

- Active radial and ulnar deviation if not previously initiated.
- Low-load dynamic splinting of the wrist, emphasizing an increase in wrist extension to at least 15 degrees.
- Possible use of gentle manual passive stretching if the stability of the wrist is sufficient.

Precaution: Motion in excess of 15 to 30 degrees each of wrist flexion and extension may create excessive shear forces on the implants and tends to be associated with higher rates of wrist instability, prosthetic loosening, and premature wear or fracture of the prosthetic components.[91]

Outcomes

A successful outcome after wrist arthroplasty gives the patient a stable, pain-free wrist with functional ROM. Relief of pain after wrist arthroplasty is consistently high.[6] Expected ROM of the wrist is approximately 15 to 30 degrees each of wrist flexion and extension and 5 to 10 degrees each of radial and ulnar deviation.[7,8,91] Patients can expect to use the involved hand for low-demand functional activities, but not heavy manual labor or high-impact recreational activities.

ROM and expected functional use of the hand and wrist as well as long-term failure rates are similar for flexible and rigid wrist arthroplasties. Failure rates continue to be higher for total wrist replacement than replacement arthroplasty of larger joints, such as the shoulder, hip, and knee.[7,8,9,11] For example, prosthetic fracture rates 5 to 10 years postoperatively have been reported at 20%[34] and 22%.[83] If a silicone implant arthroplasty fails, a total wrist replacement is still possible;[6] if a total wrist arthroplasty fails because of mechanical loosening or component fracture, wrist arthrodesis is still a viable alternative.[6,9,33,58]

Metacarpophalangeal (MCP) Implant Arthroplasty

Indications for Surgery

The following are common indications for arthroplasty of the metacarpophalangeal (MCP) joint(s).[9,10,47,68,93]

- Pain at the MCP joint(s) of the hand and deterioration of the joint, usually because of RA
- Instability, possible volar subluxation, and deformity (ulnar drift) of the fingers that cannot be corrected with soft tissue releases alone
- Stiffness and decreased ROM at the MCP joints causing inability to open the hand to grasp large objects

Procedure

Background and prosthetic design. Resection arthroplasty with uncemented implantation or a one-piece flexible (silicone) stemmed prosthesis, which serves as a dynamic spacer and an internal mold, provides a balance of stability and mobility to the MCP joints for patients with late-stage arthritis. The implant, originally developed by Swanson,[10,59,93] becomes encapsulated during the healing process. It maintains internal alignment of the joint and allows early postoperative joint motion. Reconstruction of the collateral ligaments and musculotendinous structures is necessary for stability and active control of joint motion. For implant arthroplasty to be successful, a patient must have intact extensor digitorum communis tendons or repair of these tendons must be performed. The two procedures may be staged, one prior to the other, or performed simultaneously as determined by the surgeon.

As with current-day radiocarpal flexible implants, the MCP silicone implant is reinforced with circumferential titanium grommets to minimize long-term component wear or fracture and the possibility of silicone synovitis.[93] Although the Swanson flexible silicone implant with grommets remains the standard prosthesis for replacement of MCP joints, another silicone implant, designed by Sutter is also in use,[9,47] but with mixed results. A follow-up study noted a high rate (up to 45%) of prosthetic fracture after 3 or more years.[4]

An alternative to flexible implant arthroplasty, total joint replacement with rigid (metal and plastic) components and cemented fixation, has yielded poor results to date because of a high incidence of prosthetic loosening.[9] The use of cementless (bioingrowth) fixation with rigid implants continues to be explored.

Operative procedure. A transverse incision is made over the dorsal aspect of each of the involved MCP joints, and the extensor hood structures and joint capsule are incised. The thick, proliferated synovium is removed. Release of soft tissue contractures (at the volar capsule or collateral ligaments) and repair of the extensor tendons are performed if necessary.

The heads (distal aspect) of the involved metacarpals are excised, and the intramedullary canals of the metacarpal and proximal phalanx are reamed and widened. The flexible, double-stemmed prosthesis is implanted in the intramedullary canal of each involved metacarpal and proximal phalanx. Each joint capsule and collateral ligament are then repaired. The wound is then closed, and a bulky compression dressing is placed around the hand. The MCP joints are held in neutral and slight radial deviation (opposite the position of deformity) and the distal joints (PIP and DIP) in slight flexion. While the compression dressing is in place, the hand is elevated in a sling to control edema.

Note: If the wrist is involved, MCP flexible implant arthroplasty is often combined with *dorsal clearance* (tenosynovectomy) of the diseased synovium of the extensor tendon sheaths of the wrist or arthrodesis of the wrist.[93] A swan-neck deformity of the finger is managed with PIP fusion in 30 to 40 degrees of flexion,[47] but should be done *after,* not before, MCP arthroplasty.[32]

Postoperative Management

As with arthroplasty of the wrist or other joints of the digits, the postoperative rehabilitation program includes phase-specific goals and interventions, including the use of dynamic and static splinting and a supervised exercise program.[17,32,68,93,96] General postoperative guidelines and a progression of exercises are summarized in this section. These guidelines must be individualized for each patient. Ongoing patient education and close communication with the surgeon are essential for effective outcomes.

Immobilization

For the first 2 to 4 days postoperatively, the hand is elevated to control edema and remains in the bulky compression dressing. Continuous immobilization after either flexible implant arthroplasty or cemented or cementless plastic and metal implant arthroplasty is not lengthy. If only an MCP implant has been performed, the hand remains immobilized for a few days. If in addition to the MCP arthroplasty, reconstruction of ruptured extensor tendons has also been performed, the hand remains immobilized longer to protect the repaired or transferred tendons.[34]

When the compression dressing may be removed, the hand is placed in a dynamic MCP extension splint, which consists of a basic dorsal splint with an outrigger (Fig. 11–3). The splint is worn to protect healing structures, prevent recurrent flexion and ulnar drift deformities at the MCP joints, and to control and guide the plane and ROM as soft tissues heal.[54,93,96] The dynamic splint holds the MCP joints in full extension but does not control motion in the IP joints. Slings with rubber bands attached to the outrigger of the splint pull the MCP joints into extension and slight radial deviation but still allow the patient to actively flex the MCP joints within a limited range. The patient wears the dynamic splint throughout the day, including exercise sessions. Protected motion in the dynamic splint is initiated between 3 and 7 days postoperatively when the compression dressing is removed.[9,47,54,93]

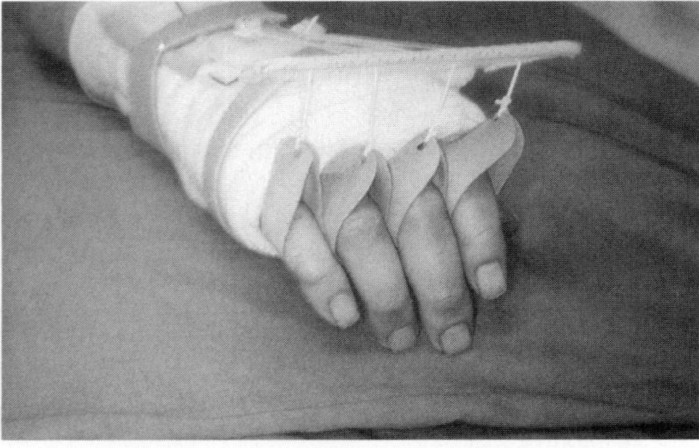

Figure 11–3 A dynamic extension splint with outrigger used after MCP arthroplasty. Courtesy of Janet Bailey, OTR/L, CHT.

At night the patient wears a volar static (resting splint) which holds the wrist in 15 degrees of extension and the fingers in full extension. A block along the ulnar border of the splint prevents ulnar deviation of the fingers. If a flexion contracture or active extensor lag of the MCP joints is present, night splinting is often continued for 3 to 4 months or as long as 1 year.[9,17]

At 2 to 3 weeks a dynamic MCP flexion splint may be indicated and worn intermittently or alternately during the day with the dynamic extension splint if MCP flexion is still limited, particularly in digits 3, 4, and 5.[9,32,98] By 6 weeks postoperatively, dynamic splinting is gradually discontinued unless an active extensor lag or a flexion or extension contracture of the MCP joints persists.[47,98]

Exercise: Maximum Protection Phase

From a few days to 2 to 3 weeks postoperatively, the focus of management is to protect healing structures while applying safe levels of stress to soft tissues to influence organized scar tissue formation and prevent adhesions through protected motion within limited ranges. Early motion assists in reducing postoperative edema and leads to a better long-term outcome in ROM.

Precaution: During this phase of rehabilitation, have the patient perform all hand exercises while wearing the dynamic extension splint until it is permissible to remove the splint for carefully protected movements of the wrist and fingers.

The following goals and exercises are emphasized during the maximum protection phase[17,32,54,98]

- ***Maintain mobility of the shoulder, elbow, and forearm.***
  - Active shoulder, elbow, and forearm ROM
- ***Regain functional ROM of the fingers and maintain gliding of tendons within their sheaths.***
  - Active, pain-free PIP and DIP flexion and extension with the MCP joints held in extension by the dynamic splint.
  - Active, pain-free MCP flexion initially with the IP joints in extension followed by passive extension of the MCP joints by the dynamic splint. Manu-

ally stabilize the IP joints in extension or temporarily splint them in extension with tape and tongue depressors.
- Active opposition of the thumb to each digit.

Precaution: During exercise, avoid lateral pressure of the thumb against the digits, which could contribute to recurrence of an ulnar deviation deformity of the fingers.

- ***Prevent adhesions along the healed incision.***
  - Gentle mobilization of the scar when sutures have been removed.

Exercise: Moderate and Minimum Protection Phases

The goal of the moderate protection phase, which begins at 2 to 3 weeks and extends to 6 weeks postoperatively, is to achieve full *active* extension of the MCP joints (no extensor lag) and sufficient MCP flexion (approximately 45–60 degrees in the index and middle fingers and 70 degrees in digits 4 and 5) as early as possible in this phase of rehabilitation for functional use of the hand.[9,93,98]

Note: Every effort should be made to obtain the desired degrees of flexion by the end of the third week postoperatively, the time at which the reconstructed joint capsules become very tight. Otherwise, it becomes very difficult to gain additional joint ROM.[17,32,93]

During the minimum protection phase, which occurs from 6 to 12 weeks postoperatively, progressive strengthening of the wrist and hand musculature and gradual use of the hand for functional activities are emphasized. In most instances, a patient is allowed full use of the hand for light to moderate functional activities by 12 weeks postoperatively.

- ***Continue to increase ROM and active control of the MCP joints.***
  - Continued active and passive flexion/extension exercises in the dynamic splint.
  - When the dynamic splint can be removed during exercise, begin *active MCP extension* with the wrist in neutral and the IP joints flexed (the intrinsic minus/hook fist position of the hand) to emphasize action of the extensor digitorum communis (EDC) muscle and minimize influence of the intrinsic finger extensors. This movement also promotes gliding of the extrinsic extensors in the tendon sheaths. Emphasize end-range MCP extension by maintaining the extended position briefly with each repetition.
  - Gentle manual passive stretching initially in the dynamic splint and when permissible out of the splint.
- ***Restore ROM of the wrist.***
  - When the dynamic splint can be removed during exercise, initiate active ROM of the wrist, emphasizing wrist extension. Be sure that the fingers are relaxed during wrist motions.
- ***Improve functional strength in the hand and wrist.***
  - Isometric flexion and extension against submaximal manual resistance or a solid object at 6 to 8 weeks postoperatively.
  - Resisted dynamic finger flexion and extension using a variety of exercise devices, such as a small, spring-loaded hand exerciser or exercise putty.
  - Active radial deviation of the digits. Have the patient place the hand on a table, palm down and stabilize the dorsum of the involved hand with the sound hand. Practice sliding or walking the fingers *radially.*[64,65]
- ***Regain use of the hand for functional activities while protecting the operated joints and preventing deformity.***
  - Reinforce principles of joint protection and energy conservation through patient education (see Box 11–2). Emphasize avoidance of stresses on the fingers in an ulnarward direction.
  - Perform simulated functional grasping activities, beginning with light prehension activities.
  - Use the hand for light to moderate functional activities by 12 weeks postoperatively.
  - Modify activities of daily living that could contribute to deforming stresses on the MCP or other involved joints.

Outcomes

A good result provides the patient with pain-free, stable, and properly aligned MCP joints that have adequate mobility for functional use of the hand. Approximately 70 degrees of active flexion of the MCP joints of the ring and little fingers and 45 to 60 degrees of flexion of the index and middle fingers, full active extension, and correction of ulnar drift deformity are considered a good result. This allows the patient to touch the fingertips of the ulnar digits to the palm, which is necessary for grasping small objects. Slightly less MCP flexion in the index and middle fingers is acceptable because limited motion of the MCP joints enhances stability and allows for dexterity and pinch without compromising functional grasp.[9,93]

Pain relief is excellent for most patients after silicone implant arthroplasty. Correction of deformity is also consistent.[47] Although satisfactory improvement of MCP mobility is a predictable outcome after joint reconstruction, grip and pinch strength do not seem to significantly or consistently increase[17] or improve only modestly.[47] The average postoperative extensor lag is 15 degrees, and MCP flexion averages approximately 45 degrees.[47]

The most common long-term complications are mechanical loosening or fracture of prosthetic implants.[9,17,93,98] These complications can be minimized with the practice of principles of joint protection by consistently avoiding heavy loads and deforming forces on the reconstructed joints.

Proximal Interphalangeal (PIP) Implant Arthroplasty

Indications for Surgery

- PIP joint pain and destruction of the joint surfaces (with or without joint subluxation) secondary to OA or post-traumatic arthritis, but less frequently indicated for RA.[1,9,79,92,93] In general, PIP implant arthroplasty is indicated for patients with *isolated* PIP involvement, who are free of MCP joint disease. Implant arthroplasty of contiguous joints (both the MCP and PIP joints) is not recommended.[9,92,93]
- Joint stiffness and decreased ROM that cannot be corrected with soft tissue reconstruction.
- Occasionally for isolated boutonnière deformity or swan-neck deformity[9,34,93] if fusion is not a viable option.
- Lateral stability of the PIP joint is a necessary prerequisite for a successful outcome.

Procedure

Background and prosthetic design. The type of arthroplasty of the PIP joint selected by the surgeon depends on the underlying pathology, the extent of associated impairments and deformities, and the philosophy and experience of the surgeon. Choices include *flexible implant arthroplasty* using a silicone joint spacer; cemented, nonarticulated *surface or total joint replacement arthroplasty,*[1,48] *resection arthroplasty,* or soft tissue reconstruction of the joint. Of these forms of joint surgery, flexible implant arthroplasty is the most common.

Arthroplasty may or may not be preferable to arthrodesis of a PIP joint to improve functional use of the hand. In the ulnar digits, where mobility of the PIP joints is particularly important for functional grasp, arthroplasty is often the procedure of choice.[34] However, in the index finger where stability of the PIP joint is a necessity for many functional activities, arthrodesis is usually preferable.[9,93] If the MCP and PIP joints are involved, as is often the case in patients with RA, the MCP joint is usually replaced but the PIP joint deformity (usually a swan-neck deformity) is corrected by soft tissue reconstruction[93] or fusion.[1]

Operative procedure: flexible implant arthroplasty. A curved incision is made along the dorsal aspect of the PIP joint. Occasionally, a volar (palmar) approach is used. Either a *central slip-sparing approach* (which leaves the central tendon intact) or, when there is significant joint deformity, a *central slip-splinting approach* (where the central tendon is incised longitudinally) is used. The collateral ligaments are either left intact or released and later reattached.

The head of the proximal phalanx and a very small portion of the base of the middle phalanx are resected. The intramedullary canals of the proximal and middle phalanges are reamed and prepared for the prosthetic implant, which is then inserted. Grommets are *not* used with PIP implants.[1]

If necessary, the volar plate is released for a flexion contracture, and the extensor tendon mechanism is repaired. Then the joint capsule is repaired, the wound is closed, and a bulky compression dressing is placed on the hand. The hand is elevated in a sling above the level of the shoulder to minimize edema.

Postoperative Management

Immobilization

The period of time required for immobilization varies, depending on whether or not extensor tendon reconstruction of the fingers was part of the procedure. If no tendon repair was done, only 2 to 3 days of immobilization of the PIP joint is required before exercises are begun. If extensor tendons have been reconstructed or transferred, a longer period of continuous immobilization is necessary to protect the extensor mechanism.

The position of postoperative immobilization of the PIP joint(s) varies with the type of preoperative deformity that existed. Recommended positions of the immobilization are summarized in Table 11–3.[9,93]

Initially, a static, protective splint made of foam-covered plastic or aluminium is worn on the operated PIP joint(s).[97] The splint is removed only for early active exercise. A dynamic splint that permits ROM may also be used in the early phase of rehabilitation. Dynamic splinting to increase PIP ROM may be introduced as early as 3 weeks postoperatively.[1]

Protective splinting with frequent sessions of assisted or active exercises continues during the day for at least 6 to 8 weeks postoperatively and is gradually eliminated by 12 weeks. Night splinting may continue for 3 to 6 months or up to a year to protect the repaired joint(s).

Exercise

The sequence of exercises after PIP arthroplasty emphasizes early protected motion of the operated joints. The time frame for initiation and progression of exercises is based on the type and extent of impairments of the fingers present preoperatively and the type of surgical approach and reconstructive procedures used.

The goals of exercise during each phase of rehabilitation after PIP arthroplasty are similar to the goals already detailed in this chapter for rehabilitation after MCP arthroplasty. Only guidelines and precautions unique to PIP arthroplasty or procedures for associated correction of specific soft tissue deformities of the PIP joints are addressed in this section.

Exercise: Maximum And Moderate Protection Phases

As with MCP arthroplasty, ROM of the unoperated joints is initiated when the hand may be removed from the surgical dressing, and the PIP joint can be placed in a static or dynamic splint. The primary goal of the maximum protection phase of rehabilitation after PIP arthroplasty is to restore mobility of the operated joint(s), initially through early but protected ROM exercises and later in the moderate protection phase (as early as 2–3 weeks) through dynamic splinting or gentle passive stretching. In most instances, the goal is 70 degrees of PIP flexion and full or almost full PIP extension by the end of the moderate protection phase (by 6–8 weeks postoperatively). The following guidelines for exercise are recommended.[9,34,54,92,93]

- ***Restore ROM of the operated joints.***
  - Active or assisted flexion and extension of each PIP joint with the MCP and DIP joints stabilized in neutral to direct motion to the PIP joint (promotes joint mobility and tendon gliding).
  - After a *central slip-sparing approach* (extensor mechanism remains intact), initiate ROM exercises as soon as the bulky dressing has been removed. This may be as early as 1 to 3 days postoperatively.
  - After a *central slip-splitting approach* in a joint with no associated swan-neck or boutonnière deformity, begin ROM exercises 3 to 5 days postoperatively.
  - If a *boutonnière deformity* was corrected (which requires reconstruction of the extensor mechanism), follow the guidelines and precautions described in Box 11–4.
- If a swan-neck deformity was corrected, follow the guidelines and precautions noted in Box 11–5.

Table 11–3 Position of Immobilization After PIP Arthroplasty

Preoperative Deformity	Postoperative Positioning in Splint
PIP flexion contracture	PIP extension
Boutonnière deformity	PIP extension and slight DIP flexion
Swan-neck deformity	10–30 degrees PIP flexion and full DIP extension

Box 11–4 Postoperative Guidelines and Precautions after Correction of a Boutonnière Deformity

Exercise

- Maintain as much extension as possible of the PIP joint through splinting and exercise for 3 to 6 weeks postoperatively.[97] Remove the splint only for exercise and wound care.
- Initiate early DIP flexion exercises with the PIP joint stabilized in extension to maintain the length of the oblique retinacular ligament.[97]
- Begin active or assisted PIP flexion/extension exercises by 10 to 14 days or sooner postoperatively. Stabilize the MCP joint in neutral (on a book or at the edge of a table) during PIP movements.
- Emphasize PIP extension and DIP flexion during exercise.

Precautions

- Avoid hyperextension of the DIP joint.
- Since correction of a boutonnière deformity requires a central slip splitting approach and repair of the extensor mechanism, avoid resisted exercises and stretching of the extensor mechanism of the PIP joint for 6 to 8 weeks or as long as 12 weeks postoperatively.

Box 11–5 Postoperative Guidelines and Precautions after Correction of a Swan-Neck Deformity

Exercise

- Maintain the PIP joint(s) in 10 to 20 degrees[97] or 20 to 30 degrees[34] flexion and the DIP joint(s) in full extension with static digital splinting.
- Initiate active ROM exercises at the PIP and DIP joints several days[34] to 10 to 14 days[97] postoperatively.
- Perform DIP extension exercises with the PIP joint stabilized in slight flexion.
- Stabilize the DIP joint in neutral during PIP ROM exercises.
- Emphasize PIP flexion and DIP extension.

Precautions

- Limit PIP extension to 10 degrees of flexion during exercise to avoid excessive stretch to the volar aspect of the capsule.
- Avoid extreme flexion of the DIP joint.

A central slip-splitting approach is necessary for correction of a swan-neck deformity to allow the tension on the extensor mechanism to be adjusted and to allow greater excursion of the PIP joint into flexion.

Precaution: During ROM exercises avoid lateral stresses to the operated joints that could compromise joint stability.

Exercise: Minimum Protection/ Return to Function Phase

The primary goal of the minimum protection phase shifts from restoration of functional ROM to improving strength in the hand and wrist and gradually incorporating safe but progressive use of the hand into functional activities of daily living. This transition occurs around 6 to 8 or as late as 12 weeks postoperatively. The status of the extensor tendons determines how early resisted exercises are initiated. For optimal results, rehabilitation may need to continue (through adherence to a home program) for 6 months to a year postoperatively.

As with MCP arthroplasty, strengthening exercises can be performed with equipment specifically designed for hand rehabilitation or through graded functional activities that involve resisted movements. Principles of joint protection (see Box 11–2) are integrated into daily living through patient education.

Outcomes

After PIP joint arthroplasty an optimal result provides the patient with a pain-free and mobile but stable and well-aligned joint for functional use of the hand.[9,17,93] Pain relief is the most consistent outcome after PIP arthroplasty.[1] Optimum functional mobility after arthroplasty of the PIP joint is 70 degrees of active flexion and full active extension (no extensor lag) of the reconstructed joint. One surgeon[93] reported that the expected motion after PIP implant arthroplasty ranges from 10 degrees of flexion to 0 degrees extension and 30 to 70 degrees flexion but did not differentiate expected results for each finger. As with MCP arthroplasty, less than 70 degrees of PIP flexion of the index and middle fingers is acceptable and still allows the patient to grasp most objects. In these joints 45 and 60 degrees, respectively, permit functional grasp.

If the extensor tendon mechanism is intact and a central slip-sparing approach is used, which allows early initiation of mobility exercises, approximately 10 degrees greater PIP flexion can be expected than if a central slip-splitting approach is used or repair of extensor tendons is required.[93] If a swan-neck deformity was corrected it is appropriate to allow a slight (up to 10 degrees) flexion contracture to develop at the PIP joint to protect the volar aspect of the joint capsule and avoid recurrence of the deformity.

Patients must continue to avoid forceful grasping and high-impact activities and must practice principles of joint protection for a lifetime to prevent common long-term complications, such as aseptic loosening or fracture of the implant.[1,17,97]

Carpometacarpal (CMC) Arthroplasty of the Thumb

Indications for Surgery

The following are common indications for CMC arthroplasty of the thumb.[9,14,21,34,42,60,72,79]

- Pain at the carpometacarpal (trapeziometacarpal) joint of the thumb because of osteoarthritis or traumatic or rheumatoid arthritis. The majority of CMC arthroplasties are performed for pain and instability associated with degenerative joint disease.
- Dorsoradial subluxation or dislocation of the first metacarpal on the trapezium, leading to a hyperextension deformity at the MCP joint of the thumb.
- Limited ROM, often an adduction contracture of the thumb.
- Decreased pinch and grip strength because of pain in or subluxation of the CMC joint.
- When arthrodesis of the CMC joint is inappropriate.
- Arthroplasty is usually reserved for the patient who requires only low-demand use of the hand.

Procedures

Background and surgical options. Although arthrodesis remains a common surgical option for management of late-stage CMC arthritis of the thumb in patients who use the hand for high-demand activities, a number of soft tissue and bony procedures have been developed to resurface or replace the CMC joint. They may be classified into three broad categories: *tendon interposition arthroplasty with ligament reconstruction;* resurfacing of the metacarpal with a silicone trapezial *interpositional implant arthroplasty* or a titanium condylar implant; and *total replacement arthroplasty* of the CMC joint with a concave proximal component of high-density polyethylene and a convex distal component made of metal, both of which are cemented in place.[9,14,17,21,34,72,79] Of these procedures, total joint replacement is the least frequently elected. If bone stock is poor, as often occurs in RA, cement fixation of rigid prosthetic components usually is not successful.[21] In most instances, soft tissue tendon interposition, resurfacing arthroplasty or, although not as common as in the past, a silicone implant arthroplasty is performed.[9,14,21,34,42,44,60]

There is lack of agreement in the literature whether silicone implant of the first metacarpal or a convex titanium condylar implant of the trapezium are preferable to tendon interposition arthroplasty for isolated CMC joint destruction as the result of OA or post-traumatic arthritis.[9,17,34] Instability (hyperextension) and arthritis of the MCP joint are frequently associated with CMC arthritis. In this situation, the CMC joint is reconstructed by some form of arthroplasty, and concomitant stabilization with a temporary K-wire or arthrodesis of the MCP joint is performed.

Operative overview. In a soft tissue interposition arthroplasty, a dorsal-to-volar incision is made at the base of the thumb. The abductor pollicis longus and extensor pollicis brevis may be reflected, and then the volar capsule is incised longitudinally. A portion of the trapezium and the base of the first metacarpal are resected. Part of the flexor carpi radialis tendon or the palmaris longus is inserted into the trapezial space to act as a soft tissue spacer and stabilize the joint[9,14,34,44,72] The abductor pollicis longus may also be imbricted or advanced to enhance joint stability and function of the abductor postoperatively.[34] The capsule and adjacent soft tissues are then repaired and the wound closed.[9,72]

In a silicone implant arthroplasty, an incision is made from the middle of the first metacarpal to a point just proximal to the styloid process of the radius. The incision runs parallel to the extensor pollicis longus. The capsule is split longitudinally, and the trapezium is excised in pieces. The base of the first metacarpal is squared off, and the intramedullary canal is prepared. The silicone implant is then inserted. The capsule is repaired and the wound closed.[9]

Postoperative Management

Immobilization

In all procedures, the thumb and hand are immobilized postoperatively in a bulky compression dressing and elevated for several days to control edema.

After the compression dressing is removed, the hand is placed in a short-arm thumb spica cast with the thumb immobilized in abduction (40–60 degrees) and slight MCP flexion.[9,34,76,79] The length of time the CMC joint is continuously immobilized is dependent on the surgery. The time frame varies from just 7 to 10 days after total joint arthroplasty, 3 to 4 weeks after tendon interposition arthroplasty[9,17,32,34,76] or as long as 6 weeks after silicone implant arthroplasty.[9,17]

After the cast is removed, a thumb spica splint is worn for a time, usually 2 weeks,[17,32] but removed for exercise. If a K-wire was inserted during surgery to temporarily immobilize the MCP joint to improve stability, it is usually removed at 6 weeks postoperatively.[9] Use of a night splint to stabilize the thumb continues for 8 to 12 weeks or until the joint is stable and essentially pain-free.[17,76]

Exercise

Progression of exercises varies with the type of arthroplasty. Guidelines presented in this section are for *tendon interposition arthroplasty* (still the most common form of CMC arthroplasty) unless otherwise noted.

Exercise: Maximum Protection Phase

During this phase of rehabilitation, after tendon interposition arthroplasty, the CMC joint is continually immobilized. After total joint arthroplasty, ROM maybe initiated during the maximum protection phase, usually at 1 week postoperatively, because of the inherent stability of the cemented prosthesis.[21]

- ***Maintain mobility of the fingers and IP joint of the thumb.***
  - Active ROM of the fingers and IP joint of the thumb while in the thumb spica cast or splint. A thumb spica immobilizer does not allow CMC or MCP motion of the thumb or wrist motion.

Exercise: Moderate and Minimum Protection Phases

- ***Regain mobility of the thumb and wrist.***
  - When it is permissible to remove the spica splint for exercise (usually at 4–6 weeks postoperatively),[17,76] begin active, controlled ROM exercises of wrist and CMC joints.
  - Emphasize CMC extension, abduction, and opposition to the fingers.
  - During active MCP flexion and extension, firmly stabilize the CMC joint.
  - Between 6 and 8 weeks, begin gentle, passive self-stretching exercises or dynamic splinting if limitations in functional ROM persist.

Precaution: Initially refrain from full MCP flexion with thumb adduction (sliding the thumb across the palm to the base of the 5th finger) as this motion places excessive stresses on the ligament reconstruction.[76]

Precaution: When stretching to increase CMC abduction or extension, apply the stretch force to the metacarpal, not the 1st phalanx, to avoid hyperextension or compromise stability of the MCP joint.

- ***Restore grip and pinch strength.***
  - If the CMC joint is stable and reasonably pain-free, gradually introduce strengthening exercises against light resistance in functional patterns at approximately 8 to 10 weeks postoperatively[17,32,76]
  - Use the hand for light to moderate ADL by 8 to 12 weeks postoperatively.[17,32,76]

Outcomes

After undergoing arthroplasty of the CMC joint, the time required to achieve maximum benefit from the surgery is typically 6 to 12 months.[9,32,76] Regardless of the type of CMC arthroplasty, the most consistent benefit of the procedure is relief of pain and, consequently, improved use of the hand for functional activities.[9,14,21,22,34,42] ROM of the thumb may also improve after interposition arthroplasty as the result of pain relief, although preoperative and postoperative ROM has been reported to remain relatively the same.[21,42] Of the current procedures available, total joint arthroplasty produces the best improvement in ROM.[21]

The most successful long-term outcomes have been reported for patients who use the hand primarily for low-demand activities. For example, after silicone implant arthroplasty, satisfactory results have been reported for 80% of patients who typically use the hand for activities that only place light to moderate loads on the thumb.[22]

It is not uncommon for patients to experience discomfort in the region of the CMC joint for up to 1 year after surgery.[32,76] Consequently, improvements in hand function such as pinch and grasp occur very gradually. The most common long-term complications are recurrence of CMC or MCP joint instability and mechanical loosening of implants, which leads to pain and loss of function. This most often occurs in patients who engage in high-demand activities.[9,21,76]

Tendon Rupture Associated with RA: Surgical and Postoperative Management

Background and Indications for Surgery

Ruptures of tendons of the hand are common in patients with chronic tenosynovitis of the tendons of the wrist and hand associated with RA. The actual site of the rupture may be either in the wrist or the hand. When a tendon ruptures, there is a sudden loss of active control of one or more of the digits. Rupture of a single or multiple tendons is usually painless and occurs during unremarkable use of the hand.[34,79,99]

The extensor tendons are affected far more frequently than the flexor tendons. Extensor tendons that most often rupture in order of frequency are the extensor tendons to the small and ring fingers and the extensor pollicis longus (EPL). The most common flexor tendon to rupture is the flexor pollicis longus (FPL).[34,68,79,99]

The causes of rupture include infiltration of proliferative synovium within the tendon sheaths into tendons which subsequently weakens the affected tendon; abrasion and fraying of a tendon as it moves over a bony prominence roughened or eroded by synovitis; or ischemic necrosis caused by direct pressure from hypertrophic synovium particularly at the dorsal retinaculum that compromises blood supply to a tendon. Common sites of abrasion that affect the extensors are the distal ulna and Lister's tubercle and the volar aspect of the scaphoid where it contacts the flexor tendons.[34,68,99]

The indication for surgery is loss of function of the hand. Rupture of a single tendon, such as the extensor digiti minimi, may not impair a patient's function, whereas rupture of multiple tendons simultaneously or over a period of time may cause significant disability.

Procedures

The surgical procedures available for treatment of tendon ruptures in RA vary depending on which tendon(s) has ruptured, the number of ruptured tendons, the location of the rupture, the condition of the tendon at the site of rupture, and the quality of the remaining intact tendons of the hand. Options include:[34,68,99]

- ***Tendon anastomosis (side-to-side tenorrhaphy).*** The ruptured tendon is sutured to an adjacent intact tendon. This is a common option at the wrist for the finger extensor tendons.[99]
- ***Tendon graft reconstruction.*** A portion of another tendon that acts as a "bridge" is inserted between and sutured to the two ends of the ruptured tendon. The palmaris longus tendon is often selected as the donor tendon. A wrist extensor tendon may be selected if a wrist arthrodesis is performed at the time of the tendon reconstruction.
- ***Tendon transfer.*** A tendon is removed from its normal distal insertion and attached at another site. For example, the extensor indicis proprius can be transferred if the extensor pollicis longus has ruptured. A flexor tendon can also be transferred to the dorsal surface of the hand to act as an extensor if multiple extensor tendons have ruptured.
- ***Direct end-to-end repair.*** The two ends of the ruptured tendon are reopposed and sutured together. This option is used only occasionally because the ends of the ruptured tendons in patients with RA have usually frayed and are difficult to suture end-to-end.

Concomitant procedures in the rheumatoid hand include tenosynovectomy, removal of osteophytes from bony prominences, and ligament reconstruction or arthrodesis for instability. If late-stage MCP joint disease is also present and passive extension of the MCP joints is significantly limited, arthroplasty of the involved joints may also be indicated, either simultaneously with the tendon repair or over two separate surgeries as determined by the surgeon. Without adequate joint mobility the repaired extensor tendons will become adherent, resulting in a poor outcome.

Postoperative Management

The guidelines described in this section only apply to management of tendon transfer, reconstruction, or repair of *extensor* tendons in the rheumatoid hand. As mentioned previously, rupture of extensor tendons occurs far more frequently than flexor tendon rupture. As with postoperative management for other surgeries described in this chapter, pain and edema control and exercises for the nonoperated extremities are always essential components of rehabilitation. Tendon transfers and reconstruction are delicate procedures requiring ongoing involvement of the patient in the postoperative program. Therefore, patient education is woven into every phase of rehabilitation.

Immobilization

A bulky compression dressing is applied to the hand and wrist at the time of surgery to control edema. A short-arm, static splint holds the wrist in slight extension and the fingers in neutral to slight flexion at the MCP joints and extension at the IP joints. The surgical compression dressing is removed after several days, and the wrist and hand are then immobilized in a volar splint. Continuous immobilization of the wrist and fingers is maintained for approximately 4 weeks to protect the healing tendons.[54,79,99]

Note: Use of dynamic splinting and early mobilization (a few days after surgery) is not often recommended for tendon reconstruction or transfers in the rheumatoid hand. Tissue healing is typically slower and the risk of rerupture higher postoperatively in patients with long-standing, systemic disease (who likely have been periodically treated with corticosteroids) than in otherwise healthy patients who have sustained an acute laceration or rupture of a tendon in the hand.[28]

Exercise: Maximum Protection Phase

- ***Maintain mobility of the elbow and forearm and unsplinted digits.***
  - While the wrist and fingers or thumb are immobilized, perform active ROM of the elbow and forearm.

- After repair of the extensor pollicis longus (EPL), the thumb is immobilized but the fingers are free to move.
- After repair of one or more finger extensors, all fingers are immobilized in a volar splint, but the thumb is free to move.

▪ ***Re-establish active mobility of tendons and joints of the wrist and digits.***

- When it is permissible to remove the volar splint for exercise, begin active or assisted MCP extension of each of the involved fingers with the wrist and IP joints stabilized in neutral. Briefly hold the extended position to emphasize end-range extension and prevent an extensor lag.

Precaution: Initially have the patient perform MCP extension from slight flexion or neutral not from full, available MCP flexion.

- Begin MCP flexion by having the patient relax the EDC after active extension rather than actively flexing the MCP joints. Progress to active MCP flexion within a protected range with the wrist and PIP joints stabilized.
- Perform active wrist motions with the fingers relaxed.
- With the wrist and MCP joints extended, actively flex (hook fist/intrinsic minus position) and extend (straight hand position) the PIP joints. PIP flexion while in wrist and MCP extension prevents stiffness of the IP joints without placing a stretch on the repaired EDC.[30]

Exercise: Moderate and Minimum Protection Phases

▪ ***Continue to increase active mobility of the operated digits.***

- Continue active extension exercises to prevent an extensor lag at the MCP joints.
- Progress active flexion of the digits if there is no extensor lag.
- Institute dynamic splinting at 8 to 12 weeks intermittently during the day to gently increase MCP flexion if grasp is significantly limited.
- Incorporate active movements of the digits into manual dexterity and coordination activities.

Precaution: Avoid vigorous grasping activities that could potentially place excessive stresses on the reconstructed or transferred tendon.

▪ ***Restore control and strength to the hand for functional activities.***

- Begin *low-intensity* resisted isometric exercises to the MCP extensors at 6 to 8 weeks.
- Use the operated hand for light functional activities to regain functional strength and endurance in the hand.
- At 10 to 12 weeks, add dynamic strengthening exercises against *submaximal* resistance during functional movements of the hand.

▪ ***Practice principles of joint protection during functional use of the hand.***

- Through ongoing patient education, teach or reinforce methods to protect the joint and soft-tissue structures of the hand.
- Discontinue use of splint for protection during the day at 12 weeks, but possibly at a later time at night.

Precaution: Avoid activities or hand postures that combine finger flexion with wrist flexion as this places extreme stress on the reconstructed extensor tendons. If a patient must use the hands for transfer activities, avoid weight bearing on the dorsum of the hand.

Outcomes

The results of surgical intervention and postoperative rehabilitation of ruptured tendons in the rheumatoid hand are highly dependent upon the extent of involvement in the joints and soft tissues of the hand and wrist preoperatively. It is often difficult to sort out postoperative outcomes strictly for repair of ruptured tendons from procedures performed concurrently, such as joint arthroplasty.

A few generalizations can be made. Patients with a recent rupture of a single tendon and who have full passive ROM of the affected joint realize an optimum postoperative outcome, which is full functional grasp and no extensor lag in the involved digit.[34,79,99] The greater the number of tendon ruptures or associated impairments, such as joint contractures, fixed deformities, or joint instabilities, the poorer the results.[34,99]

▶ Repetitive Trauma Syndromes/ Overuse Syndromes

Disorders from cumulative or repetitive trauma in the wrist and hand lead to significant loss of hand function and lost work time.[5] The causes are related to repeated movements over an extended period of time. The resulting inflammation can affect muscle, tendon, synovial sheaths, and nerves. Diagnoses include carpal tunnel syndrome, trigger finger, de Quervain's disease, and tendinitis.

Carpal Tunnel Syndrome

The carpal tunnel is a confined space between the carpal bones dorsally and the flexor retinaculum volarly. The extrinsic finger flexor tendons and median nerve course through the tunnel. Carpal tunnel syndrome is described by the sensory loss and motor weakness that occur when the median nerve is compromised in the carpal tunnel. Anything that decreases the space within the carpal tunnel or causes the contents of the tunnel to enlarge could compress or restrict the mobility of the median nerve causing a compression or traction injury and neurological symptoms distal to the wrist.[37,15]

Etiology of Symptoms

Etiological factors include synovial thickness and scarring in the tendon sheathes (tendinosis), or irritation, inflammation, and swelling (tendinitis) as a result of repetitive wrist flexion, extension, or gripping activities. Swelling of the wrist joint from trauma to the carpals (such as a fall or blow to the wrist), a fracture of the carpals, pregnancy (hormonal changes and water retention), rheumatoid arthritis, or osteoarthritis could decrease the carpal tunnel space. Awkward wrist postures (flexion or extension), compressive forces from sustained equipment usage, and vibration against the carpal tunnel could also lead to median nerve compression.[5]

Because there can be other causes of median nerve symptoms, such as traction, compression, or restricted mobility of the nerve roots in the cervical intervertebral foramen, the brachial plexus in the thoracic outlet, or the median nerve as it courses through the pronator teres muscle, each of these sites must be examined to either rule them out or determine which one of them is contributing to symptom production.[37]

Common Impairments

- Increasing pain in the hand with repetitive use
- Weakness or atrophy in the thenar muscles and first two lumbricales (ape hand deformity)
- Tightness in the adductor pollicis and extrinsic extensors of the thumb and digits 2 and 3
- Sensory loss in the median nerve distribution
- Possible decreased joint mobility in the wrist and MCP joints of the thumb and digits 2 and 3

Common Functional Limitations/Disabilities

- Decreased prehension in tip-to-tip, tip-to-pad, and pad-to-pad activities requiring fine neuromuscular control of thumb opposition
- Inability to perform provoking sustained or repetitive wrist motion, such as cashier checkout scanning, assembly line work, fine tool manipulation, or typing

Nonoperative Management

The intervention is directed to the causative factor. Considerations include:

Splinting. Splint the wrist in the neutral position so that there is minimal pressure in the tunnel and to provide rest from the provoking activity.

Biomechanical analysis. Identify faulty wrist or upper extremity motions. Adapt the environment if possible to reduce the need for faulty motion. Strengthen and increase endurance in stabilizing muscles.

Joint mobilization. If there is restricted joint mobility, mobilize the carpals for increased carpal tunnel space. See Figure 6–39 and its description in Chapter 6.

Tendon-gliding exercises. Teach the patient tendon-gliding exercises to develop mobility in the extrinsic tendons; they should be performed gently to prevent increased swelling. See Figure 11–8 and description in the exercise section of this chapter.

Median nerve mobilization.[16,70] The six positions for median nerve mobilization in the wrist and hand are illustrated in Figure 11–4. Begin with position A and progress to each succeeding position until the median nerve symptoms just begin to be provoked (tingling). That is the maximum position to use. Sustain that position for 5 to 30 seconds without making the symptoms worse. Then alternate between that position and the preceding position. When the patient can be moved into that position without symptoms, progress to the next stretch position, and repeat the mobilizing routine. The mobility exercise should be done 3 to 4 times per day as long as symptoms are not exacerbated. Additional median nerve mobilization techniques, including the entire upper extremity and neck, can be added if symptoms warrant[15] (see Fig. 15–15 and description of principles in Chapter 15 under upper limb tension).

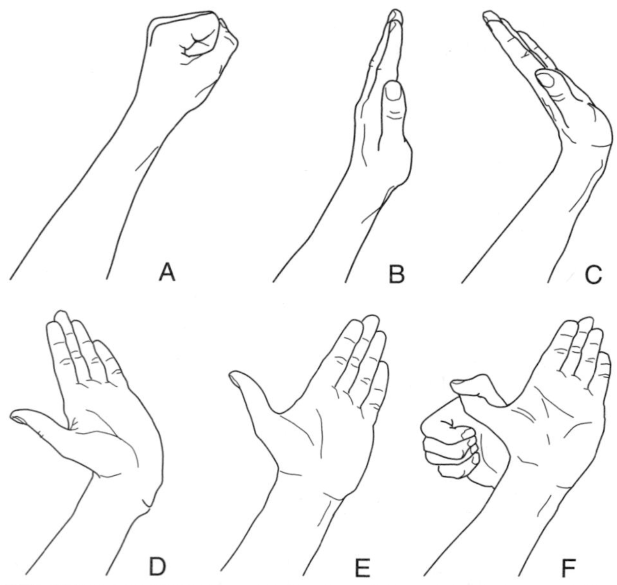

Figure 11–4 Positions for median nerve glides and mobilization: *(A)* wrist neutral with fingers and thumb flexed, *(B)* wrist neutral with fingers and thumb extended, *(C)* wrist and fingers extended, thumb neutral, *(D)* wrist, fingers, and thumb extended, *(E)* wrist, fingers, thumb extended and forearm supinated, *(F)* wrist, fingers, thumb extended, forearm supinated and thumb stretched into extension.

Note: A recent study documented a significant improvement in symptoms in patients treated conservatively with tendon- and median nerve-gliding exercises. Only 43% of patients in experimental group who had the nerve mobilization exercises underwent subsequent surgical release of the carpal tunnel compared to 71% in control group.[70]

Patient education. Teach the patient how to monitor his or her hand for recurrence of symptoms and the provoking factors, and how to modify activities to decrease nerve injury. Usually sustained wrist flexion, ulnar deviation, and repetitive wrist flexion and extension combined with gripping and pinching are the most aggravating motions.

Gentle multiple-angle muscle-setting exercises. Initially, gentle muscle-setting exercises are the only resistance exercises done. It is important that they do not provoke symptoms.

Strengthening and endurance exercises. Add dynamic strengthening and endurance exercises when symptoms are not increased with isometric exercises and there is full tendon- and nerve-gliding without symptoms or edema. Utilize exercises that prepare the patient for return to functional activities. Speed, coordination, endurance, and fine finger dexterity are emphasized when the symptoms are no longer provoked.

Postoperative Management

If conservative measures do not relieve the nerve symptoms, frequently surgical release of the transverse carpal ligament is performed to relieve the compressive forces on the median nerve. Also, any scar tissue is excised. Therapy may be initiated postsurgery if there are restrictions or muscle weakness. Exercises and mobilization techniques are used based on the functional loss.

Pain in the thenar and hypothenar eminences may occur from the release and flattening of the palmar arch. Immediately after surgery there is loss of the wrist pulley in the long finger flexor system due to release of the flexor retinaculum. Therefore, time must be allowed for healing to prevent bowstringing of the flexor tendons at the wrist. The wrist is immobilized 7 to 10 days postoperatively in slight extension with the fingers free to move.

Maximum Protection Phase

Precaution: Avoid active wrist flexion past neutral as well as active finger flexion with the wrist flexed during the first 10 days after surgery. Use extreme caution for up to 3 weeks postoperatively to prevent bowstringing of the flexor tendons through the flexor retinaculum.

- ***Rest and edema control.***
- ***Active tendon- and nerve-gliding exercises.*** Tendon- and nerve-gliding exercises are important to prevent adhesion formation from restricting motion in the carpal tunnel. See Figures 11–4 and 11–8. Include forearm supination and elbow extension as nerve symptoms allow.[5]
- ***Other active exercises.***
  - Active finger and thumb motions with the wrist stabilized in moderate wrist extension
  - Active wrist extension; this may be combined with passive wrist flexion with the splint removed.
  - Active radial and ulnar deviation of the wrist (with the splint removed and wrist supported in slight extension), pronation and supination of the forearm, and all shoulder and elbow motions.

Moderate and Minimum Protection Phases

The stitches are usually removed around the 10th to 12th postoperative day, and more active treatment is allowed.[66] The patient should be able to return to full activity by 6 to 12 weeks. Impairments may include residual weakness and sensory deficits, persistent edema, limited motion, hypersensitivity, and pain.

Suggested interventions include:

- ***Scar tissue mobilization.*** Use soft tissue mobilization to the palmar fascia and scar.
- ***Progressive stretching and joint mobilization of restricted tissue.*** Lengthen the abductor pollicis brevis and opponens pollicis if restricted. Mobilize restricted tendons or nerve tissue (same techniques as described previously except with a stretch force).
- ***Strengthening exercises.*** Begin strengthening exercises 4 weeks after surgery with isometric exercises. Progress to grip and pinch exercises by 6 weeks. Emphasize strength, coordination, and endurance toward functional goals.
- ***Dexterity exercises.*** Begin as soon as signs of motor recovery occur. Suggestions include picking up small objects using pad-to-pad, tip-to-tip, and tip-to pad prehension patterns, turning over cards, stacking checkers, writing, and holding the perimeter of a jar lid and having the thumb move around the edge in a circumduction motion.
- ***Sensory stimulation and discriminative sensory re-education.*** Desensitization of hypersensitive skin is a priority. As the nerve recovers, help desensitize and reprogram awareness.[80]
  - Use multiple types of textures for sensory stimulation (cotton, rough material, sand paper of various grades, Velcro). Have the patient begin manipulating the least irritating texture for 10 minutes. As tolerance improves, progress to the next texture of slightly more irritating but tolerable stimulus. Maximum progress is when the most irritating texture is tolerated.
  - Pattern of recovery after nerve injury is pain (hypersensitivity), perception of slow vibration (30 cps), moving touch, constant touch, rapid vibration (256 cps), and awareness from proximal to distal. Once the hypersensitivity diminishes, begin discriminative re-education by using a moving touch stimulus, such the eraser end of a pencil, and stroke over the area. The patient first watches, then closes his or her eyes and tries to identify where touch occurred. Progress from stroking to using constant touch.
  - When the patient is able to localize constant touch at the fingertips, progress to identification of familiar household objects of various sizes, shapes, and textures.

Patient Education

Instruct the patient to gradually resume use of the hand while monitoring pain, swelling, or any discoloration, and if necessary, modify or temporarily avoid any aggravating activities. While the nerve is recovering or if nerve recovery is incomplete, teach the patient preventive care to avoid injury to the hand (Box 11–6).

Compression in Tunnel of Guyon

Etiology of Symptoms

Injury or irritation of the *ulnar nerve* in the tunnel between the hook of the hamate and pisiform occurs from sustained pressure such as prolonged handwriting or leaning forward onto extended wrists while biking, from repetitive use of the gripping action of the 4th and 5th fingers, as with knitting or tying knots, using pliers and staplers, or from trauma such as falling on the ulnar border of the wrist.

Common Impairments

- Pain and paresthesia along the ulnar side of the palm of the hand and digits in the distribution of the ulnar nerve
- Weakness or atrophy in the hypothenar, interossei, ulnar two lumbricales, adductor pollicis, and deep head of the flexor pollicis brevis muscles (bishop's or benediction hand deformity)
- Tightness in the extrinsic finger flexor and extensor muscles
- Possible restricted mobility of the pisiform

Box 11–6 Patient Instructions for Preventive Care After Nerve Injury

While the nerve is regenerating, or if nerve recovery is incomplete:

- Avoid handling hot, cold, sharp, or abrasive objects.
- Avoid sustained grasps; change use of tools frequently.
- Redistribute hand pressure by building up the size of the handles.
- Wear protective gloves.
- Inspect skin regularly; provide prompt treatment of wounds or blisters.
- Compensate for dryness with massage creams or oils.

Common Functional Limitations/Disabilities

- Decreased grip strength
- Decreased ability to perform provoking activity

Nonoperative Management

Follow the same guidelines as with carpal tunnel syndrome. Modify the provoking activity, avoid pressure to the base of the palm of the hand, and provide rest with a cock-up splint.

Mobilize the ulnar nerve. Move the wrist into extension and radial deviation, and apply overpressure stretch into extension against the ring and little finger. Include forearm pronation and elbow flexion to move the nerve in a proximal direction.

Postoperative Management

After release of the ulnar tunnel, the wrist is immobilized 3 to 5 days; then treatment begins with gentle ROM. Follow the same guidelines as with carpal tunnel surgery but with ulnar nerve mobilization techniques.

Tenosynovitis, Tendinitis

Etiology of Symptoms

Inflammation occurs from continued or repetitive use of the involved muscle, from the effects of RA, from a stress overload to the contracting muscle (such as strongly gripping the steering wheel during a motor vehicle accident), or from roughening of the surface of the tendon or its sheath.

Common Impairments

- Pain whenever the related muscle contracts or whenever there is movement of another joint that causes gliding of the tendon through the sheath.
- Warmth and tenderness with palpation in the region of inflammation.
- In RA, synovial proliferation and swelling in affected tendon sheaths such as over the dorsum of the wrist or in the flexor tendons in the carpal tunnel.[29]
- Frequently there is an imbalance in muscle length and strength or poor endurance in the stabilizing muscles. The fault may be more proximal in the elbow or shoulder girdle, thus causing excessive load and substitute motions at the distal end of the chain.

Common Functional Limitations/Disabilities

Pain that worsens with the provoking activity of the fingers, thumb, or wrist, which may affect grip or repetitive hand motions.

Management: Protection Phase

Follow the guidelines for acute muscle lesions described in Chapter 8, with special emphasis on relieving the stress in the involved musculotendinous unit and maintaining a healthy environment for healing with nondestructive forces.

- Splint the related joints to rest the involved tendon.
- If the tendon is in a sheath, apply cross-fiber massage while the tendon is in an elongated position so mobility develops between the tendon and sheath.
- Perform multiangle muscle-setting techniques in pain-free positions followed by pain-free ROM.
- Instruct the patient in tendon-gliding exercises to prevent adhesions. (These are described in the exercise section of this chapter).

Management: Controlled Motion and Return to Function Phases

- Progress the intensity of massage, exercises, and stretching techniques.
- Assess the biomechanics of the functional activity provoking the symptoms, and design a program to regain a balance in length and strength and endurance of the muscles. Frequently, problems may occur from poor stabilization or endurance in the shoulder or elbow.

▶ Traumatic Lesions in the Hand

Simple Sprain: Nonoperative Management

Etiology of Symptoms

After trauma from a blow or a fall, an excessive stretch force may strain the supporting ligamentous tissue. There may be a related fracture, subluxation, or dislocation.

Common Impairments

- Pain at the involved site whenever a stretch force is placed on the ligament.
- Possible hypermobility or instability in the related joint.

Common Functional Limitations/Disabilities

- With a simple sprain, pain may interfere with functional use of the hand for a couple of weeks if the joint is stressed. There will be no limitation of function if a splint or taping can be worn to protect the ligament and the splint does not interfere with the task.
- With significant tears there will be instability, and the joint may subluxate or dislocate with provoking activities requiring surgery.

Nonoperative Management

- Follow the guidelines in Chapter 8 for treating acute lesions with emphasis on maintaining mobility while minimizing stress to the healing tissue. If immobilization is necessary to protect the part, only the involved joint should be immobilized. Joints above and below should be free to move. This will maintain mobility of the long tendons in their sheaths that cross the involved joint.[11]
- Cross-fiber massage to the site of the lesion may help to prevent the developing scar from adhering and restricting motion.
- Avoid positions of stress and activities that provoke the symptoms while healing.

Lacerated Flexor Tendons of the Hand: Surgical and Postoperative Management

Background and Indications for Surgery

Lacerations of the flexor tendons of the hand are common and can occur in various areas (zones) along the volar surface of the fingers, palm, wrist, and distal forearm. The musculotendinous structures damaged depend on the location and depth of the wound. Damage to one or more tendons may also be accompanied by vascular, nerve, and skeletal injuries that can complicate management. An acute rupture of a flexor tendon may also occur as the result of a closed traumatic injury to the hand.[23,89]

The volar surfaces of the wrist, palm and fingers are divided into five zones; the thumb is divided into three zones (Fig. 11–5). Box 11–7 describes each of the zones of the fingers and thumb.[23,36,76,89,90]

Knowledge of the complex anatomy and kinesiology of the hand is essential to understand the impairments and functional implications caused by damage to the flexor tendons in each of these zones.

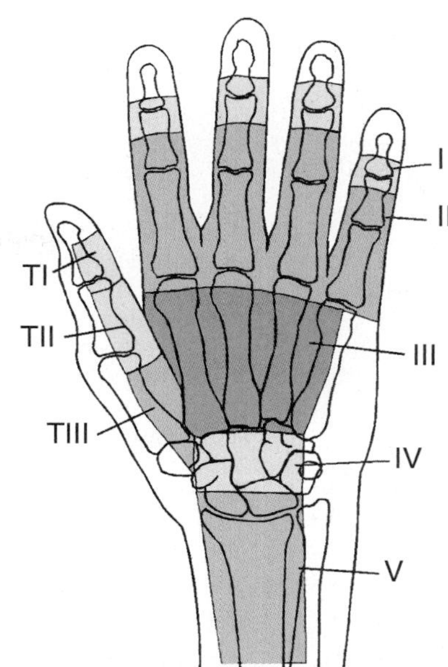

Figure 11–5 Flexor tendon zones; volar aspect of the hand and wrist.

Box 11–8 identifies common impairments associated with damage in each of the zones.

Flexor tendons when severed or ruptured readily retract, thus requiring surgical intervention in most instances to restore function to the hand and prevent

Box 11–7 Flexor Tendon Zones: Anatomic Landmarks

Zones of the Fingers, Palm, Wrist, and Forearm

- I—From the insertion of the FDP on the distal phalanx to just distal of the FDS insertion on the middle phalanx.
- II—From the distal insertion of the FDS tendon to the level of the distal palmar crease (just proximal to the neck of the metacarpals).
- III—From the neck of the metacarpals, proximally along the metacarpals to the distal border of the carpal tunnel.
- IV—The carpal tunnel (area under the transverse carpal ligament).
- V—Area just proximal to the wrist (proximal edge of the carpal ligament) to the musculotendinous junction of the extrinsic flexors in the distal forearm.

Zones of the Thumb

- T-I—From the distal insertion of the FPL on the distal phalanx of the thumb to the neck of the proximal phalanx.
- T-II—From the proximal phalanx, across the MCP joint to the neck of the 1st metacarpal.
- T-III—From the 1st metacarpal to the proximal margin of the carpal ligament.

Box 11–8 Consequences of Injury to the Volar Surface of the Hand, Wrist, and Forearm

- *Zone I.* Only one tendon, the FDP, can be severed as can the A-4 and A-5 retinacular pulleys, which are important for maintaining the mechanical advantage of the FDP for complete finger flexion (full fist).
- *Zone II.* FDS and FDP tendons, a double-layered synovial sheath and multiple pulleys (including A-1) of the flexor retinaculum (the tendinous sheath that approximates the tendons to the underlying bones for full tendon excursion) can all be damaged. Inability to flex the PIP and DIP joints occurs if both tendons are severed. Potential damage to the vincula, the vascular structures that provide blood, and supplement nutrition derived from synovial diffusion, can compromise tendon healing.
- *Zone III.* In addition to loss of the FDP and FDS, damage to lumbricales can disrupt MCP flexion.
- *Zone IV.* Damage in this zone can affect all three extrinsic flexors of the digits, the FDP, FDS, and FPL, which disrupts finger and thumb flexion. Synovial sheath also sustains damage. Nerve injury frequently accompanies laceration in this zone.
- *Zone V.* Laceration in this area can cause major damage to flexor tendons of the digits and wrist, resulting in loss of wrist and digital flexion. Arteries also lie superficial in this zone.
- *Zones T-I and T-II.* Damage to retinacular pulley system of the thumb, synovial sheath in addition to the FPL, and possibly the distal insertion of the FPB can occur; IP and MCP flexion are disrupted.
- *Zone T-III.* Potential damage to the thenar muscles.

deformity. Repair and rehabilitation of lacerations in zone II, traditionally referred to as "no-man's land," pose a particular challenge. Because of the confined space in which the extrinsic flexors of the fingers lie and the limited vascular supply to the tendons in zone II, healing tissues in this area are very prone to excursion-restricting adhesions. Scar tissue formation during the healing process can interrupt tendon-gliding within the synovial sheath and subsequently restrict ROM of the involved fingers. In zone IV (the carpal tunnel), the extrinsic flexor tendons of the digits (FDS, FDP, and FPL) lie in close proximity to each other. An injury in this zone may lead to adherence of adjacent tendons to each other within the carpal tunnel and impairment of differential gliding between the tendons.

Procedures

The mechanism of injury, the type and location (zone) of the laceration, the extent of associated skin, vascular, nerve, and skeletal damage, and the timing of the repair as well as other factors such as a patient's age, health, and lifestyle, all influence the type of surgical repair selected by a hand surgeon.[23,36,89,90] The same factors have a significant impact on rehabilitation and outcomes of a tendon repair.[23,32,76,88,89,90]

Surgical options for repair of lacerations or closed ruptures of flexor tendons can be classified by the *type* of procedure.[23,76,89]

- ***Direct repair.*** An end-to-end repair in which the tendon ends are reopposed and sutured together.
- ***Tendon graft.*** An autogeneous donor tendon, such as the palmaris longus, is sutured in place to replace the damaged tendon. This is necessary when the ends of the severed tendon(s) cannot be brought together without undue tension. Tendon grafts are performed in one or more stages depending on the severity, type, and location of injury.

A straight laceration usually lends itself well to a direct (end-to-end) repair whereas a jagged laceration that frays the tendon may require a tendon graft.

Another method of classifying and describing tendon repairs is the *timing* of the repair. Categories include:[17,23,76,88,89,90]

- ***Primary repair.*** An immediate repair that is done in the first 24 hours after injury.
- ***Delayed primary repair.*** A repair performed by day 10 after injury.
- ***Secondary repair.*** A repair done between 10 days to 3 weeks after injury.
- ***Late reconstruction.*** Surgery performed well beyond 3 to 4 weeks, sometimes months after injury.
- ***Staged reconstruction.*** Multiple separate surgeries performed over a period of weeks or months.[38] A staged reconstruction enables a surgeon to prepare an extensively damaged or scarred tendon bed months prior to a tendon graft so that adhesions are less likely to develop.

A simple, clean, acute laceration of a tendon without associated injuries of the hand is most often managed with a *direct primary repair.*[23,89] However, if the wound is not clean, a *delayed primary repair* allows for medical intervention to reduce the risk of infection. Lengthy delays that necessitate a secondary repair or late reconstruction are often associated with multiple injuries, such as extensive skin loss, fractures that cannot be stabilized immediately, and nerve or vascular damage, as well as scarring and contractures.

The timing of a repair after an acute tendon injury is critical because the severed ends of the tendon begin to soften and deteriorate quickly, and the proximal portion of the tendon retracts. These factors make it difficult to reattach the tendon with a strong repair at its normal length. A delay of up to 10 days yields results equal to an immediate repair. Delays beyond 2 weeks are associated with poorer outcomes.[23,89]

Of the multiple-stage reconstructions for extensive and complex flexor tendon injuries of the hand, the *Hunter two-stage reconstruction passive or active implant* is most widely known. In the first stage of this procedure, the scarred and adherent portions of the damaged flexor tendon are resected. A Hunter implant (rod) made of silicone is then secured in place to act as a tendon spacer around which a new sheath develops over a period of 3 months. In addition, a damaged retinacular pulley system is reconstructed, and any contractures are released during the first surgery. In the second phase, the implant is removed, and a donor tendon (graft) is drawn through the new sheath and sutured in place.[38,89]

Some general aspects of operative procedures for flexor tendon injuries are described in this section. However, careful review of a patient's operative report and close communication with the hand surgeon are the best sources of specific details of each patient's surgery. In a repair of lacerated tendons in zone II, for example, a zigzag approach or lateral incision may be elected by the surgeon, the former being the more common. In a primary repair after the tendon ends are located, prepared, and reopposed, there are a number of very delicate techniques for suturing the tendons.[74,78] Core sutures and possibly epitendinous sutures are used to hold the tendon ends together. The suturing technique and the number of suture strands influence the initial strength of the repair and consequently the type and timing of motion allowable postoperatively.[23,76,89] A larger number of suture strands across the repair site (for example, 4 or 6 strands instead of 2) produces a proportionally stronger repair.[89] Running, locked epitendinous sutures used in addition to core sutures appear to further increase the initial strength of the repair.[74,78]

Suturing technique must also address the vascular supply to the repaired tendon. Nonreactive sutures are placed in the nonvascular volar aspect of the tendon so as not to disturb the vincula, which lies in the dorsal aspect of the tendon and provides a blood supply to the tendon.[23,76,89] When present, as in zones II and IV, the synovial sheath is also repaired to re-establish circulation of synovial fluid, an important source of nutrition to the healing tendons.[89]

After all repairs have been completed, the incision(s) are closed and the hand and wrist are immobilized in a bulky compression dressing and elevated to control edema. The compression dressing remains in place for 1 to 3 days. When the bulky surgical dressing is removed, it is replaced with a light compressive dressing and splint.

Postoperative Management

After surgical intervention for a flexor tendon injury, a strong, well-healed tendon that glides freely is the cornerstone for restoring functional mobility and strength in the hand.[74,77,87,88] Every effort is made to prevent excursion-restricting adhesions from forming while simultaneously protecting the healing of the repaired tendon. Box 11–9 summarizes the factors that contribute to adhesion formation after tendon repair.[23,38,76,89]

Many of the same patient-related and injury-related factors, already noted, that a surgeon weighs when determining the most appropriate operative procedure for a patient's hand injury also influence the complex components and progression of postoperative management. In addition, surgery-related factors including type of repair, suturing technique, and the integrity of the repair, all affect rehabilitation and eventual outcomes. Finally, therapy-related factors, in particular, the use of early mobilization procedures, the quality of splinting, the expertise of the therapist, and ultimately the quality and consistency of the patient's involvement in the rehabilitation process also influence outcomes.

Extensive research has been done on tendon healing, tendon excursion during finger motion, adhesion formation, and the tensile strength of tendon

Box 11–9 Factors that Contribute to Adhesion Formation After Tendon Injury and Repair

- Location of the injury and repair: higher risk in zones II and IV; tendons glide in a closely confined area.
- Extent of trauma: higher risk with extensive trauma and damage to associated structures.
- Reduced blood supply, subsequent ischemia, and reduced nutrition to healing tendons.
- Excessive handling of damaged tissues during surgery.
- Ineffective suturing technique.
- Damage or resection of components of the tendon sheath.
- Prolonged immobilization after injury or repair, which prevents tendon-gliding.
- Gapping of the repaired tendon ends associated with *excessive* stress to the healing tendon.

Box 11–10 Rationale for Early Controlled Mobilization of a Repaired Tendon

- Maintains tendon-gliding and decreases the formation of adhesions that can limit tendon excursion. It has been noted that in the FDS and FDP tendons only 3 to 5 mm of tendon excursion is necessary to prevent loss of joint motion.[27]
- Increases synovial diffusion for tissue nutrition, which increases the rate of tendon healing.
- Controlled stresses that occur with early tendon motion increase the tensile strength of the repaired tendon more rapidly than continuous immobilization.
- Decreases gap formation at the repair site, which, in turn, increases the tensile strength of the repair.
- Decreases edema and postoperative pain.

repairs. A number of sources provide an excellent analysis and summary of this research.[19,23,38,76,88,89] The rationale and components of current-day rehabilitation programs for tendon repair that emphasize early controlled (protected) passive or active motion of the operated digit are based on evidence derived from this basic and clinical research. Box 11–10 summarizes the rationale for early motion after tendon repair.[23,38,76,88,89]

The purpose of this section is to examine and summarize current concepts and approaches to immobilization and exercise associated with rehabilitation after flexor tendon injury and repair, rather than to put forth or ascribe to any one particular protocol. Therapists treating patients after tendon repair should be familiar with many different postoperative protocols or guidelines used by referring hand surgeons as well as those described in the literature. A therapist's knowledge of the basic guidelines and underlying concepts in these protocols is important for effective communication with the surgeon and for patient education. This knowledge enables a therapist to make sound clinical judgments to determine when progression of activities in a protocol preferred by a referring physician is safe or when activities may need to be altered after communication with the surgeon. Remember, a regimented protocol is only safe and effective when there are no postoperative variables, a situation that certainly does not occur in the clinical setting. Detailed descriptions of specific protocols can be found in several publications.*

There are three basic approaches to postoperative management after flexor tendon repair. They are:

- Early passive motion
- Early active motion
- Delayed motion

Key elements of each of these approaches in relationship to immobilization and exercise are presented in this section. Postoperative goals and interventions for pain reduction, edema control, and maintenance of function in uninvolved regions, such as the elbow and shoulder, are consistent with management of other operative procedures previously discussed in this chapter. Patient education is paramount for effective outcomes after hand surgery.

Note: Unless otherwise noted, guidelines described in this section for immobilization and exercise are for injury and primary repair or one-stage tendon grafts of the FDS and/or FDP in zones I, II, and III. Guidelines are similar but not addressed for zones T-I and T-II of the thumb. Postoperative guidelines for multistage or late reconstructions may be progressed in a similar manner or more cautiously. Refer to other resources for this information.[38,76,88]

Immobilization

The *time period,* the *type,* and/or *position* of immobilization must be considered. With only a few exceptions the repaired tendon is continuously immobilized after surgery for *only 1 to 3 days,* the time period the bulky compression dressing is kept in place. The criteria for use of an extended period of continuous immobilization, usually for 3 to 4 weeks in a short-arm cast, are identified in Box 11–11.

The type or method of immobilization usually depends on the preference of the surgeon and the hand therapist, the type of postoperative exercise protocol

Box 11–11 Indications for Use of Prolonged Immobilization and Delayed Motion After Flexor Tendon Repair

- Patients who are unable to comprehend and actively participate in an early controlled motion exercise program. This includes:
  - Children under 7 to 10 years of age[76,88,89]
  - Patients with diminished cognitive capacity associated with head injury, developmental disability, or psychologic impairment
- Patients who have the cognitive ability to understand and follow an early controlled motion program but who are unlikely to adhere to the program
  - The unmotivated patient
  - The overzealous, impatient individual with a history of a previously failed repair
- Patients in whom repair of other hand injuries or surgeries necessitates extended immobilization of the hand

*See references 18, 19, 20, 27, 31, 43, 49, 77, 85, 86, 87, 98.

used, and the stage of rehabilitation based on tissue healing. In the case of prolonged immobilization (3–4 weeks), a plaster cast is typically used. Early controlled motion approaches to rehabilitation that allow motion of the operated digit(s) within a few days after surgery require the fabrication of customized splints. Descriptions of static and dynamic splinting for immobilization and/or exercise are noted in Box 11–12.[18,19,20,27,43,49] Figure 11–6 shows an example of a dorsal blocking splint with dynamic traction. The splint allows active extension of the involved finger; the rubberband passively returns the finger to a flexed position.

Finally, the typical *position of immobilization* is wrist and MCP flexion coupled with PIP and DIP extension. This position prevents full lengthening and undue stress on the repaired FDS and/or FDP tendons while minimizing the risk of IP flexion contractures. The recommended degrees of wrist and MCP flexion differ somewhat from one source to another. Recommended positions range from 10 to 45 degrees of wrist flexion and from 40 to 70 degrees of MCP flexion with the IP joints in extension.[17,18,19,20,23,27,85,88] The wrist is typically positioned in less flexion than the MCP joints. The trend over the years has been to fabricate splints in less wrist flexion than early protocols recommended to increase patient comfort.[88] Positioning after a zone IV repair is typically 70 degrees MCP flexion and a neutral position of the wrist.[88]

Box 11–12 Static and Dynamic Dorsal Blocking Splints: Position and Use

- Static dorsal blocking splint[18,27,85,89]
  - The splint covers the dorsal surface of the entire hand and the distal forearm. (The thumb is free.)
  - Positioned in wrist and MCP flexion and IP extension. Straps hold wrist and fingers in this position.
  - Restricts wrist and MCP extension.
  - Is worn in early phases of rehabilitation.
  - Splint is loosened or removed for early exercises.
- Dorsal blocking splint with dynamic traction[20,43,49,88]
  - Allows early motion of the operated joint while the hand is in the splint.
  - Elastic band (or nylon line with a rubberband) is attached to the nail of the operated finger (or all 4 fingers), passes under a palmar bar that acts as a pulley, and then attaches proximally at the wrist.
  - At rest, the elastic band provides dynamic traction that holds the operated finger in flexion.
  - Allows *active extension* of the IP joints to the surface of the dorsal splint.
  - When PIP and DIP extensors relax, the tension from the elastic band pulls on the finger, causing *passive flexion.*

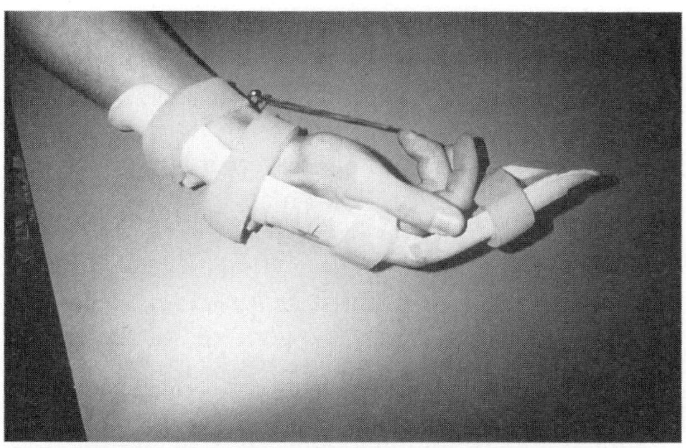

Figure 11–6 A dorsal blocking splint with dynamic traction for early controlled motion after flexor tendon repair.

Exercise: Early Passive Motion Approaches

There are two basic approaches to the use of early passive motion after flexor tendon repair, one based on the work of Duran and Houser,[27] and the other on the work of Kleinert.[43,49] Both approaches emphasize early passive flexion of the IP joints within a protected range to maintain flexor tendon-gliding and prevent tendon adhesions postoperatively. Their original protocols have since been modified. Today most surgeons and therapists use elements of both approaches.[19,20,88,98]

Exercise: Maximum Protection Phase

This phase begins 1 to 3 days postoperatively and continues for the first 3 to 5 weeks.

- If a static dorsal blocking splint is being used, remove it or loosen the stabilization straps to allow joint motion. Begin PROM exercises of the *individual* IP joints of the operated finger(s): passive MCP flexion/extension; DIP flexion/extension with the wrist, MCP, and PIP joints stabilized in flexion; passive PIP flexion/extension with the wrist, MCP, and DIP joints stabilized in flexion. In addition, perform composite MCP, PIP, DIP flexion/extension within the confines of the splint. Composite flexion can include full fist and straight fist positions.

Precaution: It is essential to maintain the wrist and MCP joints in flexion during PROM of the IP joints to avoid excessive stretch to the repair site during IP extension that could cause gapping of the reopposed tendon ends.

- To achieve *differential gliding* of the FDP and FDS tendons, the DIP joint must be flexed and extended separately while the PIP joint is stabilized in flexion.[86,87,88] In this way, as the DIP joint is passively extended, the FDP repair site glides distally, away from the FDS repair.[86,87,88,98]
- If a dynamic traction (rubberband) splint is being used (see Fig 11–6), every hour during the day have the patient perform *active extension* of the operated finger within the confines of the splint. The rubberband returns the finger to a flexed position with each repetition after the finger extensors relax. A manual push into maximum DIP flexion may be added to increase passive flexion.

Note: When a dynamic traction splint is used during the day, a static night splint is worn that holds the IP joints in neutral and the wrist and MCP joints in flexion to prevent IP flexion contractures.

Exercise: Moderate Protection Phase

This phase begins at 3 to 5 weeks and continues until 8 weeks postoperatively with an emphasis on *active flexion of the IP joints.*

- Add active wrist flexion and extension in a dynamic wrist band (cuff) splint, which passively flexes the operated finger(s) with active wrist extension and passively extends the fingers with active wrist flexion. Some dynamic cuff splints limit wrist extension to neutral. These splints use *tenodesis* to passively flex (and extend) the operated digit(s) while permitting some degree of wrist extension (to prevent a wrist flexion contracture) and while keeping the FDP and FDS tendons on a slack for protection.
- Initiate muscle setting of the finger flexors with *"place and hold" exercises.* Passively *place* the patient's fingers in a variety of flexed positions (for example, around different size cones); then have the patient hold the position.
- At 5 to 6 weeks, progress to active composite finger flexion for tendon-gliding in the table top, hook fist, straight fist, and full fist positions and eventually in the straight hand position[18,19,70,88] (see Fig. 11–8 *A–E*).

Note: The recommended positions of the wrist during active finger flexion exercises just described varies, with different sources advocating wrist flexion, extension, or neutral.[18,19,85,88,89]

- Discontinue dynamic traction splinting at 6 to 8 weeks for primary repairs but later for tendon grafts.[76] Use of a static night splint for protection or to decrease a flexion contracture should be continued.

Exercise: Minimum Protection/ Return to Function Phase

This phase begins at approximately 8 weeks postoperatively and is characterized by gradual but progressive strengthening of the hand.

- Full active ROM exercises of the wrist and hand are permissible. Incorporate dexterity exercises of the hand, wrist, and forearm to use active range.
- Low-load resistance exercises to increase strength emphasizing functional patterns of grasp and pinch.
- Sustained grasp exercises to improve muscular endurance.
- Progressive use of the hand for light functional activities (under 5–10 lb resistance).
- Dynamic splinting if flexion contractures persist.
- Full functional use of the hand is typically allowed after 12 weeks (may include lifting over 10 lb with physician approval).

Exercise—Early Active Motion Approach

The primary feature that distinguishes an early active motion from an early passive motion approach is the use of minimum tension, *active contractions of the repaired muscle-tendon units* (FDP and FDS, as well as FPL) within the first 24 to 48 hours postoperatively. In addition, exercises routinely performed in early passive motion approaches are also incorporated into active regimens.[19,31,74,77,78,89] The Indiana regimen[18,19,89,90] and the MAMTT (minimum active muscle tendon tension) approach[31,74,78] are most widely known. Both approaches use "place and hold" exercises as the mechanism of producing early active tension on the repaired tendon. It is hypothesized that gentle tension placed on a repaired tendon by means of a low-intensity muscle contraction, which "pulls" a tendon through its sheath, is a more effective method of creating excursion of the tendon than "pushing" the tendon with passive motion.[31,76,78,89] This approach is becoming more widely accepted because stronger suturing techniques produce a repair that can withstand early stresses.

Precaution: Even proponents of early active mobilization caution that this approach is only recommended for primary tendon repairs in carefully selected patients with access to rehabilitation with an experienced hand therapist.[18,19,89]

Key features of early active mobilization of tendon repairs include the following activities.[18,19,31,77,78,89]

Exercise: Maximum Protection Phase

This phase begins 24 to 48 hours postoperatively and continues to 4 weeks.

- Two different splints are fabricated: a standard static dorsal blocking splint set in wrist and MCP flexion and a dorsal tenodesis splint with a hinged wrist joint that allows full wrist flexion and 30 degrees of extension. The MCP joints are stabilized in 60 degrees of flexion. The tenodesis splint is used *exclusively* for active exercise, and the static dorsal blocking splint is worn at all other times.
- PROM of the fingers with the hand and forearm resting in the static dorsal blocking splint and the straps loosened to allow finger motion. These exercises are the same as those used in the early passive motion approach already described.
- *"Place and hold" exercises* in the tenodesis splint with the palm facing the floor (forearm pronation).[31,78,85] With the *wrist in extension* and MCP joints in flexion, passively place the IP joints in a partially flexed position, and have the patient hold the position independently for 5 seconds. Have the patient relax and allow the wrist to passively flex and the digits to passively extend. Have the patient initially practice this with the uninjured hand or use biofeedback to learn how to hold the position with a minimum of force production in the FDP and FDS. Full PIP and DIP flexion should *not* be emphasized during this early phase.

Note: The wrist is extended and the MCPs are placed in flexion during place and hold exercises because research has indicated that wrist extension is the position in which the IP joints can be moved by contraction of the FDS and FDP with the *least* amount of contraction force and, therefore, a very low level of stress on the repaired tendon.[73]

Precaution: At 3 to 5 weeks, patients who are at greatest risk for tendon rupture are, paradoxically, those who are most flexible and who exhibit no evidence of passive or active restriction (associated with edema or adhesions).[76,89] These patients should be progressed more cautiously than those exhibiting tissue restrictions.

Exercise: Moderate Protection Phase

This phase begins at 4 weeks and continues to 8 weeks.

- Discontinue the tenodesis splint, but retain the static dorsal blocking splint except for exercise until at least 6 weeks.
- Perform the same "place and hold" exercises without the tenodesis splint.
- Initiate tendon blocking and gliding exercises at 5 to 6 weeks.
- Exercises are similar to moderate protection phase of the early passive motion approach.

Precaution: Avoid finger extension combined with wrist extension, as this position places extreme tension on the repaired tendon.

Exercise: Minimum Protection/ Return to Function Phase

This phase begins at 7 to 8 weeks postoperatively.

- Exercise progression is consistent with the early passive motion approaches already described.

Exercise: Delayed Motion Approach

In instances where continuous immobilization of a repaired flexor tendon extends for 3 to 4 weeks (indications already noted in Box 11–11), some degree of tendon healing and adhesion formation will have already occurred by the time exercises can be initiated.

Precaution: Despite the extended period of immobilization, at 3 to 4 weeks the tendon repair must still be protected in a dorsal blocking splint, and exercises must be performed in protected positions and progressed gradually.

Exercises such as PROM, tendon-blocking and tendon-gliding, and AROM can be initiated when the cast is removed. Exercises used in early passive and active motion approaches are appropriate. The reader is also referred to additional resources that provide detailed exercise programs when delayed mobilization is necessary.[17,85,88]

Outcomes

Longitudinal studies of patients who have undergone flexor tendon repairs are numerous in the literature.[23,38,76,89] Findings in these studies indicate that immediate primary and delayed (up to 10 days) primary repairs yield equally positive outcomes.[76] However, late reconstruction and multistage reconstructions, not surprisingly, result in poorer outcomes (less active and passive ROM, greater functional limitations) than primary repairs.[76] This is consistent with the findings that the greater the severity and number of associated injuries, the less favorable the outcomes.[89]

The two most common causes of failure of a flexor tendon repair are, in order of frequency: (1) the development of adhesions, which limit tendon excursion and restrict ROM; and (2) postoperative tendon rupture.[17]

Studies dating back to the 1980s have documented that the use of 4 weeks of uninterrupted immobilization leads to a slower return of tensile strength in the repaired tendon and greater adhesion formation than the use of early mobilization.[23] Although the use of extended immobilization continues to be the treatment of choice for children under 7 to 10 years of age, a recent study indicates that the incidence of chronic contractures or diminished hand function is minimal.[63]

Studies of the use of various approaches to early mobilization after flexor tendon repair demonstrate superior outcomes when compared to the use of extended immobilization.[20,75] Although there continues to be some reluctance to incorporate active mobilization exercises immediately into postoperative rehabilitation because of concerns of tendon rupture, the rate of rupture appears to be equal with early passive and early active mobilization regimens.[89]

Lacerated Extensor Tendons of the Hand: Surgical and Postoperative Management

Background and Indications for Surgery

Laceration and traumatic rupture of the extensor tendons of the fingers, thumb, or wrist are more common than in the flexor tendons.[26] Their superficial location makes the extensor tendons very vulnerable to damage when trauma occurs to the dorsum of the hand. Furthermore, extensor tendons in the hand are substantially thinner than flexor tendons, making them more prone to traumatic rupture.[26,69]

As with the flexor surface, the extensor surface of the hand, wrist, and forearm is divided into zones (Fig. 11–7). The dorsal surface of the fingers and wrist are divided into seven zones, and the thumb is divided into four zones. Each of these zones is identified by specific anatomic landmarks noted in Box 11–13.[26,28,36,69] The odd-number zones correspond to the location of the DIP, PIP, MCP, and wrist joint regions. Although not depicted in Figure 11–7, the dorsal surface of the distal and middle forearm are

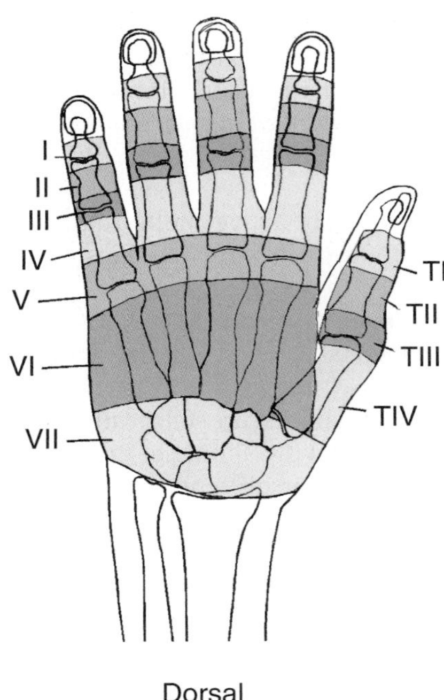

Figure 11–7 Extensor tendon zones; dorsal aspect of the hand and wrist.

Box 11–13 Extensor Tendon Zones: Anatomic Landmarks

Zones of the Dorsal Surfaces of the Fingers, Hand, Wrist and Forearm

- I– DIP joint region
- II–Middle phalanx
- III–PIP joint region
- IV–Proximal phalanx
- V–Apex of the MCP joint region
- VI–Dorsum of the hand
- VII–Wrist region/dorsal retinaculum
- VIII and IX–Distal and middle forearm

Zones of the Thumb

- T-I–IP joint region
- T-II–Proximal phalanx
- T-III–MCP joint region
- T-IV–Metacarpal
- T-V–Carpometacarpal joint region

often identified as zones VIII and IX, respectively. The area at the CMC joint of the thumb is often identified as zone T-V.

The extensor mechanism of the hand and wrist is complex. The structural characteristics of these mechanisms vary in each zone. Damage in one zone produces compensatory imbalances in adjacent zones. Knowledge of the anatomy and kinesiology of the extensor mechanism is basic to an understanding of how a patient's physical impairments and functional limitations occur according to the structures damaged in each zone. Box 11–14 identifies key structures and characteristic impairments associated with tendon rupture or laceration by zone.[26,28,69,86,87] Of all the extensor zone injuries in zones III and VII pose the greatest surgical and rehabilitation problems and challenges.

Depending on the type and location of injury to the extensor mechanisms and the extent of associated skeletal, joint vascular, or nerve damage, surgery may or may not be indicated. The extensor mechanisms has many soft tissue attachments along its various structures, making it far less likely to retract when lacerated or ruptured than flexor tendons.[26,69] Consequently, with a rupture (closed injury) or a simple laceration at a peripheral zone the tendon is typically reopposed and managed by uninterrupted immobilization in a splint or cast for 6 weeks as it heals.[26,69] For example, this is a common course of treatment for a closed rupture of the terminal extensor tendon in zone I, resulting in a *mallet finger* (or thumb) deformity.

Nevertheless, surgical intervention, even for a simple distal tendon injury, may be needed to restore active ROM, muscular balance, strength, and function to the hand and prevent contractures and deformity. Although the extensor muscles of the digits are substantially weaker than the flexors, an intact extensor mechanisms is essential for functional grasp.

Box 11–14 Consequences of Injury to the Dorsal Structures of the Hand and Wrist

Zones I and II: Damage to the terminal extensor leads to inability to actively extend the DIP joint (extensor lag) and eventual DIP flexion contracture and deformity (mallet finger). A swan-neck deformity secondary to an unopposed central slip and migration of the extensor mechanisms proximally may also develop. Damage in those zones is usually the result of a closed rupture rather than a laceration.

Zones III and IV: Damage to the central slip tendon and possibly the lateral bands results in an inability to actively extend the PIP joint from a 90-degree flexed position. Flexion contracture of the PIP joint and eventually a boutonnière deformity develop as the lateral bands slip volarward and cause hyperextension of the DIP joint.

Zone V: Damage to the common extensor tendons (EDC), extensor indicis proprius (EIP), and extensor digiti minimi (EDM), and sagittal bands that surround the MCP joints causes inability to actively extend the MCP joints, eventually resulting in MCP flexion contractures.

Zones VI and VII: The juncturae tendium along the dorsum of the hand (VI) and the dorsal retinaculum (VII) under which multiple extensor tendons of the wrist and digits pass in close proximity can be damaged. A bowstring effect occurs in the extensor tendons if the retinaculum, which acts as a pulley, is lacerated. The synovial sheath through which the tendons glide in zone VII can also be damaged, subsequently compromising synovial diffusion and nutrition to the tendons. Injuries in zones VI and VII can result in loss of extension of the digits and wrist.

T-I and T-II: Damage to the EPL and possibly the EPB (if laceration is in the proximal region of the proximal phalanx) leads to loss of hyperextension of the IP joint (mallet thumb deformity) and weakened MCP extension.

T-III and T-IV: Damage to EPB leads to weakened MCP extension and transfers extension forces to IP joint leading to a flexion deformity of the MCP joint and a hyperextension deformity of the IP joint if the EPL is intact.

Procedures

Surgical options for extensor tendon repair or reconstruction include either a direct (end-to-end) repair or a reconstruction. Tendon transfer is also a common option. As with flexor tendon repair, surgeries are classified as *primary* (immediate or delayed up to 10 days), *secondary,* or *staged.* These terms have already been defined in the previous section of this chapter that dealt with flexor tendon repair and rehabilitation. Operative procedures for ruptured extensor tendons associated with RA have also been described previously in this chapter.

Although similarities of definition exist between extensor and flexor tendon procedures, there are substantial differences in operative techniques used to repair extensor versus flexor tendons. These difference are largely based on the fact that extensor tendons are morphologically thinner than flexor tendons. Extensor tendon repairs, therefore, are more prone to gaping, have less tensile strength, and are more likely to rupture than flexor tendon repairs. Stronger suturing techniques, specifically designed for extensor tendon repair and reconstruction, are being used more frequently, thus allowing early postoperative mobilization of the repaired tendon while lessening concerns of gapping and rupture.[26,28,84]

Operative procedures for repair of lacerated or ruptured extensor tendons vary significantly in the distal versus the proximal zones. In this section only a description of a repair of a zone III/IV laceration (the most common cause of injury in these zones) is presented simply as an example. A closed rupture of the extensor mechanism in zone IV is usually managed nonoperatively. Detailed descriptions of primary repairs and late reconstruction of extensor tendon injuries for all zones of the hand, wrist, and forearm can be found in several resources.[13,26,36,69]

With an acute laceration of the PIP joint and middle phalanx, the wound often enters the joint space. Therefore, the area must be debrided and cleansed and treated with antibiotics. The central slip is then managed with a direct repair.[26,36] The severed tendon is repaired and then sutured into the fibrocartilaginous dorsal plate of the middle phalanx, which is thicker and holds sutures better than the central slip and, therefore, produces a stronger repair.[26] If damaged, the lateral bands are also repaired. If a boutonnière deformity is evident or likely to develop, a K-wire is inserted to immobilize the PIP joint in extension (usually for 3 weeks) and is then removed. After closure of the area, a bulky compression dressing immobilizes the repaired tissues and controls edema.

Postoperative Management

Rehabilitation after extensor tendon repairs progresses more conservatively than after flexor tendon repair. Two general approaches to rehabilitation are described in the literature: prolonged, uninterrupted immobilization or, in very selective situations, early controlled passive or active motion beginning in the first few postoperative days. Although the former is still used more often, there is a growing use of early mobilization after primary extensor tendon repairs. In *acute primary repairs* in zones III-VII, the use of dynamic splinting[12,29,38,71] or minimum active muscle contractions[31] for a limited amount of tendon-gliding in the early phase of tissue healing is dependent on the type of suturing technique used by the surgeon, careful patent selection, and a patient's postoperative access to supervised rehabilitation and education with an experienced hand therapist.[26,28,98] Late reconstruction, which is more complex and usually involves tendon grafts, is managed with continuous extended immobilization,[13] not early mobilization.

Immobilization

Immobilization is typically maintained with a volar splint after the bulky surgical dressing is removed a few days postoperatively. The joints immobilized and the positions of immobilization are based on the location (zone) of the injury and repair and the structures involved. With some exceptions, the joints are immobilized in an extended position to protect the repair from excessive stretch and potential gapping. For example, in a zone III/IV injury, the PIP is held in extension, but the DIP is immobilized in slight flexion. Several resources provide detailed information on immobilization and splinting after extensor tendon repairs.[28,88]

Exercise: Delayed Mobilization Approach

If a traditional approach to postoperative management of extensor tendon repairs is used, exercises are delayed for at least several weeks after surgery. Special considerations and precautions for exercise using a delayed mobilization approach are summarized by zones in Box 11–15.[17,28,32,84,87,88]

Guidelines for resistance exercises to strengthen the hand and continuation of splinting for protection or use of dynamic splinting are not addressed in Box 11–15. In general, resistance to the repaired muscle-tendon unit is not initiated until 8 to 12 weeks postoperatively regardless of the site of the repair. Emphasis is first placed on gradually strengthening the extensors. After 10 to 12 weeks *low-intensity* resisted grasp and pinch is initiated to gradually strengthen the flexors if no extensor lag is present.

Exercise: Early Mobilization Approach

Despite the known problems associated with extended immobilization (tendon adhesions, decreased tensile strength of the repair, and joint contractures), the reported benefits attributed to early mobilization, and studies that indicate that early controlled motion can be used safely, the use of early, controlled passive or active motion after extensor tendon repair has been more limited than after flexor tendon repair.[26] Because the flexors of the hand are so much stronger than the extensors, there is continued concern that if the immobilization is removed in the early phase of rehabilitation, inadvertent, uncontrolled grasping could easily cause gapping or rupture of a recently repaired extensor tendon. Nonetheless, the literature reflects that as stronger suturing techniques continue to be developed, there is a growing trend to incorporate ele-

Box 11–15 Special Considerations for Exercise After Extensor Tendon Repair and Extended Immobilization

Zones I and II

- PIP and MCP AROM while the DIP is immobilized for 4 weeks postoperatively.
- When splint can be removed for exercise, perform active DIP extension and flexion with the MCP and PIP joints stabilized in neutral. Briefly hold the extended position with each repetition.
- Emphasize active extension more than flexion to avoid an extensor lag.

Precaution: Increase flexion of the DIP joint *very gradually,* initially limiting flexion to 20 to 25 degrees during the first week of exercise. The strong FDP can easily place excessive stress on terminal extensor tendon and cause gapping or rupture of the repair.

Zones III and IV

- If the lateral bands were intact, begin DIP AROM 1 week postoperatively while the PIP joint is immobilized in extension in a volar splint or cylinder cast. Early DIP motion prevents loss of extensibility of the lateral bands and oblique retinacular ligaments and loss of mobility of the DIP joint.
- If the lateral bands were damaged and repaired, postpone DIP ROM until 4 to 6 weeks postoperatively.
- At a minimum of 4 weeks but more often at 6 weeks, the volar splint is removed for active ROM of the PIP joints with the MCP joints stabilized. Emphasize active extension more than flexion.

Precautions: Progress PIP flexion in *very gradual* increments; limit PIP flexion to 30 degrees the first week of PIP ROM exercises.[28]

- If the wrist and MCP joints have been immobilized postoperatively, include active ROM of the wrist with the MCP and PIP joins stabilized and active MCP ROM with the wrist and PIP joints stabilized in extension.

Zones V and VI

- When the volar splint can be removed for exercise (between 3 and 4 weeks or as late as 6 weeks postoperatively), begin active or assisted MCP extension and passive flexion with the wrist and IP joints stabilized in neutral and the forearm pronated. Briefly hold the extended position with each repetition. Let the extensors relax to flex the MCP joints.
- Add carefully controlled active MCP flexion within a protected range with the wrist stabilized in extension.
- Emphasize active MCP extension more than flexion to prevent an extensor lag.

Precaution: Initially limit active MCP flexion to 30 degrees in the index and middle fingers and 35 to 40 degrees in the ring and small fingers.

- During IP flexion and extension exercises, stabilize the MCP joints in neutral and the wrist in slight extension.
- Combine active MCP extension with active PIP flexion (hook fist position) and PIP extension (straight hand position).
- Incrementally progress to full fist position over several weeks if no extensor lag develops.

Zone VII

- If the wrist extensors are intact and only extrinsic finger extensors have been repaired, follow guidelines for zone V/VI repairs.
- If the wrist extensors were repaired, begin active wrist extension from neutral to full extension in a gravity-eliminated position (forearm in midposition) at 3 to 4 weeks.
- Incrementally increase wrist flexion beyond neutral between 5 and 8 weeks postoperatively.
- Perform radial and ulnar deviation with the wrist in neutral.

ments of early passive or active tendon mobilization into rehabilitation programs for carefully selected patients who have undergone extensor tendon repairs.[12,28,71,84]

The literature indicates that zone III/IV extensor tendon repairs when managed with continuous immobilization for 3 to 6 weeks postoperatively are particularly prone to adhesion formation and only marginal postoperative results (high incidence of extensor lag and limited PIP flexion).[62] Zone IV with its broad tendon-bone interface over which the extensor tendon must glide is a site of significant tendon adherence.[28] For these reasons, a number of approaches to early controlled mobilization of *primary* zone III/IV repairs has been set forth.[28,29,36] Guidelines for early mobilization of zones V, VI, and VII have also been proposed and detailed in the literature.[28,30,84,88]

The following are key elements of an early mobilization approach using immediate active short-arc motion after a repair of the central slip.[28,29]

- Use of a customized static volar splint applied as soon as the surgical dressing is removed and used between exercise sessions; holds only the PIP and DIP joints in 0 degrees extension; wrist and MCP joints are free. Use of a resting splint for at least 6 weeks postoperatively for protection is also indicated.
- Fabrication of two volar template splints worn only during exercise; the PIP splint limits PIP flexion to 30 degrees and DIP flexion to the same protected range during exercise.

- Patient taught concepts of minimum active muscle tendon tension (MAMTT) to protect healing tissues during tendon excursion.
- AROM of PIP and DIP joints initiated within the limits allowed by the exercise splints during the first few days after surgery; MCP positioned in neutral and wrist in 30 degrees flexion during active PIP flexion/extension; PIP stabilized in neutral during active DIP flexion/extension.
- PIP exercise splint revised during the second week of exercise to allow 40 degrees of flexion if no extensor lag is present. PIP flexion allowed by splint incrementally increased by 10 degrees each week thereafter. Patient ideally reaches 70 degrees by end of 4th week.
- By 6 weeks, low-intensity resisted exercises initiated and gradual use of the hand for functional activities.

Outcomes

Primary repairs of acute injuries of an extensor tendon (rupture or laceration) whether repaired immediately or delayed for approximately 10 days yield equally good results.[26] As with flexor tendon injuries, the greater the extent of associated skeletal, joint, vascular, or nerve injuries, the poorer the results of repair. For example, 64% of patients with simple zone I injuries had good results whereas only 47% of patients with associated skeletal or joint injuries had good result.[62] Overall, repairs of distal injuries (zones I-IV) have less favorable results than repairs of more proximal injuries (zones V-VIII).[62]

Although a traditional approach using extended immobilization (between 3 and 6 weeks depending on the zone of injury) continues to be used, particularly for distal injuries, every effort is made to minimize the period of immobilization. Growing use of early controlled mobilization with dynamic splinting or minimum tension active muscle contractions has been shown to be safe and to result in better outcomes after primary repair than results after delayed mobilization. For example, in studies of zones III-VII repairs[12,29,71] there was no incidence of rupture of the repair. Use of early controlled mobilization as compared to prolonged immobilization leads to a lower incidence of extension contractures (inability to fully grasp) and extensor lag.[29] An early motion approach also enables a patient to safely use the hand for functional activities more quickly.[71]

▶ Techniques for Tendon and Muscular Mobility

Active motion of the digits and wrist is used to maintain or to develop mobility between the multijoint musculotendinous units and other connective structures in the wrist and hand. Because adhesions between the various structures can become restrictive or incapacitating, tendon-gliding exercises are used whenever possible after surgical interventions and during or after periods of immobilization after injury to the hand to develop or maintain mobility. They are not stretching techniques although, if there are restrictions, stretching may also be utilized (stretching techniques are described in the next section). The exercises described here may also be used to develop neuromuscular control and coordinated movement.

Flexor Tendon-Gliding Exercises

These exercises are designed to maintain or develop free gliding between the flexor digitorum profundus and superficialis tendons and between the tendons and bones in the wrist, hand, and fingers.[72a,82] This is particularly important when there has been immobilization after trauma, surgery, or a fracture, and scar tissue or adhesions develop. There are five positions in which the fingers move during tendon-gliding exercises: straight hand (all the joints are extended), hook (claw) fist (MCP joints are extended, IP joints are flexed), full fist (all the joints are flexed), table top, also known as the intrinsic plus hand (MCP joints are flexed, IP joints are extended), and straight fist (MCP and PIP joints are flexed, IP joints are extended) (Fig. 11–8). The following progression is suggested.

1. Initiate the exercises with the wrist in neutral position.
2. Once full range of the finger motions is achieved, progress to doing the gliding exercises with the wrist in flexion and in extension to establish combined finger and wrist mobility.
3. Full excursion and tendon-gliding of all the extrinsic muscles are accomplished by starting with the wrist and fingers in full extension and moving to full wrist and finger flexion then reversing the motion.

Hook (Claw) Fist Position

Have the patient move from the straight hand to the hook fist position by flexing the DIP and PIP joints

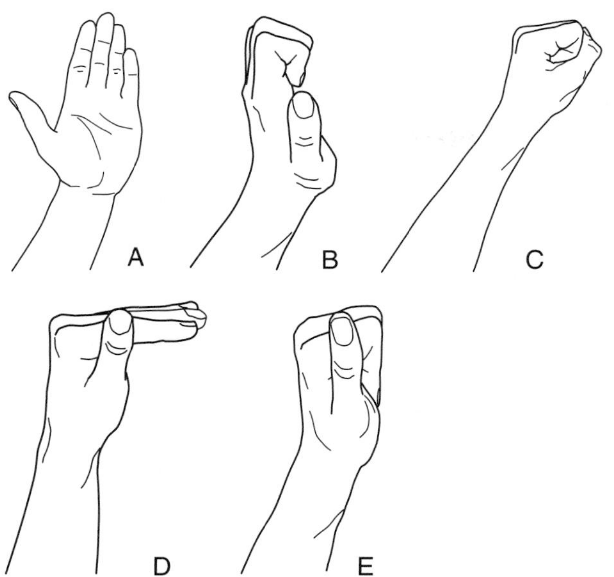

Figure 11–8 The five finger positions used for flexor tendon gliding exercises; *(A)* straight hand, *(B)* claw fist (hook), *(C)* full fist, *(D)* table top (intrinsic plus), and *(E)* straight fist.

while maintaining MCP extension (Fig. 11–8*A* and *B*). Maximum gliding occurs between the profundus and superficialis tendons and between the profundus tendon and the bone. (There is also gliding of the extensor digitorum communis tendons; this motion will be used with the extensor gliding exercises.)

Full Fist

Have the patient move to the full fist position by flexing all the MCP and IP joints simultaneously (Fig. 11–8*C*). Maximum gliding of the profundus tendon with respect to the sheath and bone as well as over the superficialis tendon occurs.

Straight Fist (Sublimis Fist)

Have the patient move to the table top position by flexing the MCP joints then flexing the PIP joints while maintaining the DIP joints in extension (Fig. 11–8*D* and *E*). Maximum gliding of the superficialis tendon occurs with respect to the flexor sheath and bone.

Thumb Flexion

Have the patient flex the MCP and IP joints of the thumb full range. This promotes maximum gliding of the flexor pollicis longus.

Flexor Tendon-Blocking Exercises

Blocking exercises not only develop gliding of the flexor tendons with respect to the sheaths and related bones, but they also require neuromuscular control of individual joint motions. Therefore, they use the mobility gained by the flexor tendon-gliding exercises and are a progression of the flexor tendon-gliding exercises.

Patient position and stabilization: Sitting with the forearm supinated and back of the hand resting on a table. The opposite hand provides stabilization and "blocking" against unwanted movement. Each finger performs the exercise separately.

Precaution: These exercises should not be used in the early stages after tendon repair because of the stress placed on the tendons. Progress to manual resistance as the tissues heal and can tolerate resistance.

Isolated MCP Flexion (Lumbricales and Palmar Interossei)

- Have the patient flex only the MCP joint of one digit (Fig. 11–9*A*).
- If necessary, the rest of the fingers are stabilized in extension against the table with the other hand.
- With improved control, the hand does not have to be stabilized against the table.

PIP Flexion (Flexor Digitorum Superficialis)

- Have the patient stabilize the proximal phalanx of one digit with the other hand, and if possible, flex just the PIP joint of the one digit while keeping the DIP joint extended and all the rest of fingers on the table (Fig. 11–9*B*).
- If the patient has difficulty doing this, the other digits are stabilized in extension with the other hand.

DIP Flexion (Flexor Digitorum Profundus)

- The middle phalanx of one digit is stabilized with the other hand.
- Have the patient attempt to flex just the distal phalanx (Fig. 11–9*C*).
- Vary this exercise by increasing the range of MCP and PIP flexion to where the patient just begins to lose DIP motion; stabilize in this position and have the patient attempt the DIP flexion.

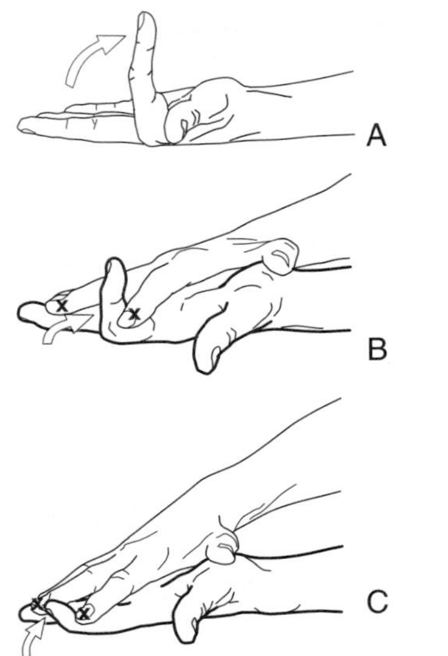

Figure 11–9 Flexor tendon blocking exercises; *(A)* isolated MCP flexion of one digit, *(B)* isolated PIP flexion (flexor digitorum superficialis) of one digit, and *(C)* isolated DIP flexion (flexor digitorum profundus) of one digit.

Full Fist

When full independent tendon-gliding is available, the patient should be able to make a full fist. Progress the exercises described by adding resistance.

Extensor Exercises to Reduce Extensor Lag

The extrinsic finger extensors (extendor digitorum communis, extensor digitorum indicis, and extensor digiti minimi) are more superficial than the flexor tendons and, therefore, more easily damaged. Their prime function is to extend the MCP joints. Extension of the IP joints requires active interaction with the intrinsic muscles of the hand via the extensor mechanism. Adhesions within their sheaths at the wrist or between tendon and bone restrict tendon-gliding both proximally (restricting active finger extension) and distally (restricting active and passive finger flexion). When full passive range of extension is available, but the person cannot actively move the joint through the full range of extension, it is called an *extensor lag*. This can result from weakness, but is frequently caused by adhesions that prevent gliding of the tendons when the muscles contract. One of the purposes of the following exercises is to maintain mobility and thus prevent adhesions. The exercises are also used to regain control of finger extension. Stretching and mobilization of the adhesions are described the next section.

Isolated MCP Extension

- Have the patient move from the full fist position (Fig. 11–8*C*) to the hook fist position (Fig. 11–8*B*).
- If the patient has difficulty maintaining the IP joints in flexion, have him or her hook the fingers around a pencil while extending the MCP joints.
- Begin with the wrist in neutral, and progress to positioning the wrist in flexion and extension while doing the MCP extension.

Isolated PIP and DIP Extension

Extension of the interphalangeal joints requires intrinsic as well as extensor digitorum control.

- For strongest participation of the lumbricales, stabilize the MCP joint in flexion while the patient attempts IP extension, moving from the full fist position (Fig. 11–8*C*) to the table top position (11–8*D*).
- Progress to stabilizing the palm of the hand on the edge of a table (or block) with either the PIP or DIP joint partially flexed over the edge.
- Have the patient extend the involved phalanx through the ROM.

Terminal Range Extension of IP Joints

- Progress to the terminal range by stabilizing the entire hand, palm side down on a flat surface, and have the patient extend the involved phalanx into hyperextension.
- If there is not enough range available, place a pencil or block under the proximal phalanx or middle phalanx so the PIP or DIP can go through greater range (Fig. 11–10).

Extensor Tendon-Gliding Exercises

Differential gliding:

- Teach the patient to passively flex the MCP and IP joints of one digit with the opposite hand while actively maintaining the other digits in extension.

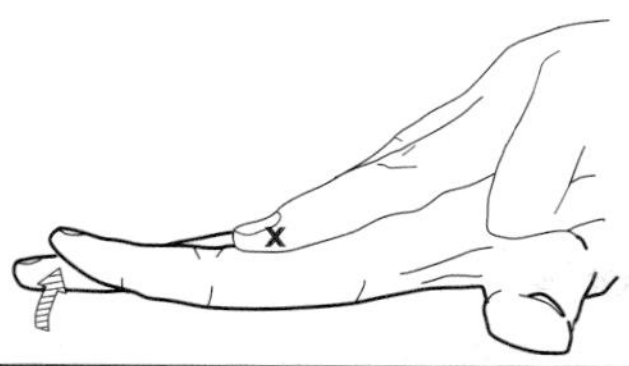

Figure 11–10 Terminal extension of the PIP joint. The MCP joint is stabilized in extension, and the patient lifts the middle and distal phalanges off the table.

- If the patient has difficulty doing this, begin with the involved hand resting on a table with the palm up. Stabilize three of the four digits against the table while passively flexing one of the digits (Fig. 11–11). Then instruct the patient to attempt to actively keep the fingers against the table while one of the digits is passively flexed.

Tendon-Gliding Progression

Instruct the patient to actively maintain the fingers in extension with the fingers spread out, and then actively flex each finger in turn while the other fingers remain extended.

Long Horn Sign

Have the patient flex the middle and ring fingers while maintaining extension of the index and little fingers. This promotes isolated control of the extensor indicis and extensor digiti minimi tendons and promotes their gliding on the extensor digitorum communis tendons.

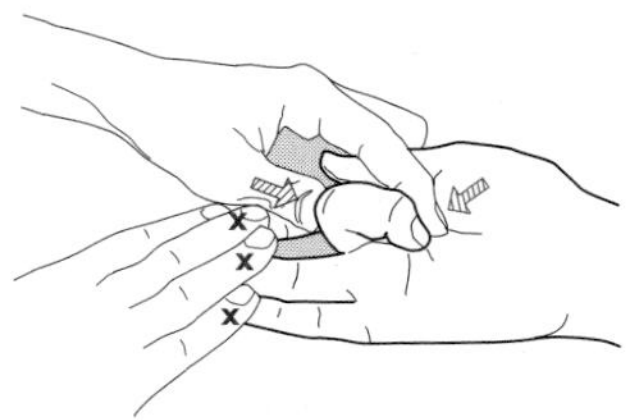

Figure 11–11 Differential gliding of the extensor digitorum tendons. Move each digit into flexion while stabilizing the other digits in extension.

Exercise Techniques to Increase Flexibility and Range of Motion

Stretching the muscles and connective tissue structures in the wrist and hand requires knowledge of the unique anatomic relationships of the multijoint musculotendinous units and the extensor mechanism of the digits. These are described in the first section of this chapter. The principles and techniques of stretching are presented in Chapter 5, and special note is made of the importance of stabilization when stretching the multijoint muscles of the hand and fingers. This is re-emphasized here. In addition, because scarring and adhesions can restrict tendon-gliding and therefore, motion of the digits, stretching techniques that address these restrictions are also presented in this section. Before stretching muscle or connective tissue there should be normal gliding of the joint surfaces to avoid joint damage. Use joint mobilization techniques to stretch the joint capsule and restore gliding (see Chapter 6).

Note: Patient position for most wrist and hand exercises is sitting with the forearm supported on a treatment table unless otherwise noted.

General Stretching Techniques

It is important that when stretching to increase wrist flexion or extension, the fingers must be free to move so that the extrinsic finger flexor and extensor musculotendinous units do not restrict motion at the wrist. Similarly, when stretching ligaments and other periarticular connective tissues across individual finger joints, it is important that there is no tension on the multijoint tendons. The following techniques are initially applied by the therapist and then are taught to the patient to perform in a home exercise program when he or she understands how to safely apply the stretch force and stabilization.

To Increase Wrist Extension

- Have the patient place the palm of the hand on a table with the fingers flexed over the edge. The other hand stabilizes the back of the hand against the table. Have the patient then move the forearm up over the stabilized hand (similar to Fig. 11–13 except the fingers are over the edge of the table so that they are free to flex and the stretch occurs only at the wrist).

- Have the patient place the palms of the hands together at right angles to each other and allow the fingers to intertwine and flex. Instruct the patient to press the restricted hand in a dorsal direction with the palm of the other hand and sustain the stretch.

To Increase Wrist Flexion

- Have the patient place the back of the hand on a table. The other hand provides stabilization against the palm of the hand. Have the patient move the forearm up over the stabilized hand.
- Have the patient sit with the forearm pronated and resting on a table and wrist at the edge of the table. The patient then presses the hand toward flexion with the opposite hand.
- Have the patient place the dorsum of both hands together. With the fingers relaxed, have the patient move the forearms so that the wrists flex toward 90 degrees.

To Increase Flexion or Extension of Individual Joints in the Fingers or Thumb

To increase extension at any one joint the patient's forearm is supinated; to increase flexion, the forearm is pronated and the phalanx to be stretched at the edge of the table. Show the patient how to apply the force against the distal bone while the proximal bone is stabilized against the table.

Stretching Techniques of the Intrinsic and Multijoint Muscles

Self-Stretching the Lumbricales and Interossei Muscles

Have the patient actively extend the MCP joints and flex the IP joints and apply a passive stretch force at the end of the range with the opposite hand (Fig. 11–12*A*).

Self-Stretching the Interossei Muscles

Have the patient place the hand flat on a table with the palm down and the MCP joints extended. Instruct the patient to abduct or adduct the appropriate digit and apply the stretch force to the distal end of the proximal phalanx. Stabilization is provided by fixating against the adjacent digit.

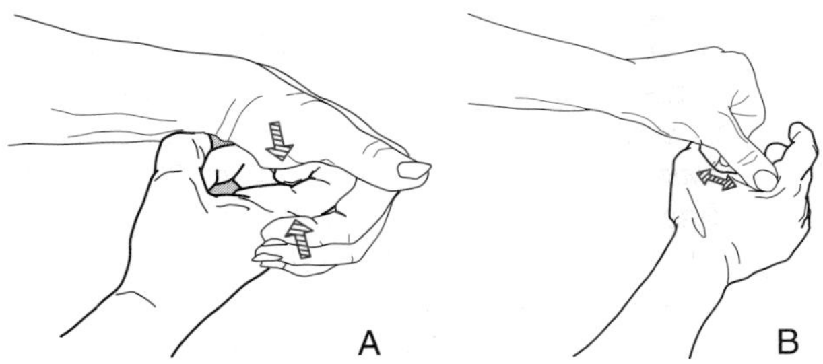

Figure 11–12 Self-stretching *(A)* the lumbricales with MCP extension and IP flexion; and *(B)* the adductor pollicis with CMC abduction of the thumb. To increase thumb abduction it is critical to that the stretch force is applied against the metacarpal head not the proximal or distal phalanges.

Self-Stretching the Adductor Pollicis

Have the patient rest the ulnar border of the hand on the table and abduct the thumb perpendicular to the palm of the hand. Instruct the patient to apply the stretch force with the crossed thumb and index or long finger of the other hand against the metacarpal head of the thumb and index finger and attempt to increase the web space (Fig. 11–12*B*).

Precaution: It is critical that the patient does not apply the stretch force against the proximal or distal phalanx. This would stress the ulnar collateral ligament of the MCP joint of the thumb and lead to instability at that joint with poor functional usage of the thumb. Abduction occurs at the CMC joint at the articulation between the metacarpal and the trapezium.

Manual Stretching of the Extrinsic Muscles

Because they are multijoint muscles, the final step is to elongate each tendon of the extrinsic muscles over all the joints simultaneously, but *do not* initiate stretching procedures in this manner because joint compression and damage can occur to the smaller or less stable joints. Begin by allowing the wrist and more proximal finger joints to relax; stretch the tendon unit over the most distal joint first. Stabilize the distal joint at the end of the range, then stretch the tendon unit over the next joint. Then stabilize the two joints, and stretch the tendon over the next joint. Progress in this manner until the desired length is reached.

Precaution: Do not let the PIP and MCP joints hyperextend as the tendons are stretched over the wrist.

Self-Stretching the Flexor Digitorum Profundus and Superficialis

Have the patient begin by resting the palm of the involved hand on a table and first extend the DIP joint, using the other hand to straighten the joint; keeping it extended, have the patient then straighten the PIP and MCP joints in succession. If the patient can actively extend the finger joints to this point, the motion should be performed unassisted. With the hand stabilized on the table, have the patient then begin to extend the wrist by bringing the arm up over the hand. The patient goes just to the point of feeling discomfort, holds the position, then progresses as the length improves (Fig. 11–13).

Self-Stretching the Extensor Communis

The fingers are flexed to the maximum range, beginning with the distalmost joint first and progressing until the wrist is simultaneously flexed. The opposite hand applies the stretch force.

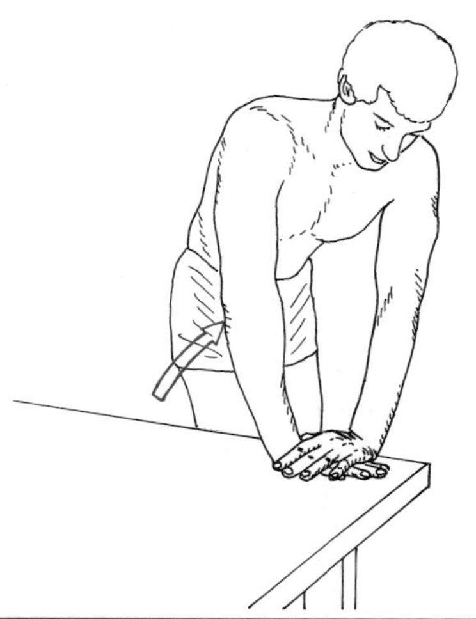

Figure 11–13 Self-stretching of the extrinsic finger flexor muscles, showing stabilization of the small distal joints. To isolate stretch to the wrist flexors, allow the fingers to flex over the edge of the table.

Techniques to Mobilize Scar Tissue (Adhesions) that Restrict Gliding of Long Finger Flexor Tendons

Adhesions between the tendons and their sheaths or between tendons and underlying bones will restrict tendon-gliding in both a proximal and distal directions so that the joints distal to the scar do not move when the muscle contracts. Proximal gliding of the tendons is best achieved through active contraction of the extrinsic muscles. Distal gliding is achieved through passive stretch by extending the finger joints distal to the site of the adhesions.[82]

- Begin the stretching routine by stretching the tendon in a distal direction, followed by active tendon-gliding exercises. Tendon-gliding exercises were described in the previous section (see Fig. 11–8).
- Apply cross-fiber friction massage at the site of the adhesion while the tendon is in its stretched position.[24]

Techniques to Mobilize Scar Tissue (Adhesions) that Restrict Gliding of Extensor Tendons and the Extensor Mechanism

As with the flexor tendons, if the extensor tendons or extensor mechanism has restricted mobility because of adhesions, muscle action will not be transmitted through the mechanism to extend the joint or joints distal to the restriction. Without free gliding, an extensor lag may result. As defined earlier, an extensor lag is the loss of active extension when there is full passive extension.

- Stretch the adhesion in a distal direction by flexing the joint distal to the site. Follow this by having the patient attempt to actively extend the joint and put tension on the scar in a proximal direction.

Precaution: If the extensor lag increases (i.e., flexion increases, but there is no active extension through that increased range), the tendon distal to the adhesion may be stretching and not the adhesion. Do not continue with the passive stretching into flexion, but emphasize friction massage applied to the scar tissue.

- Apply cross-fiber friction massage at the site of the adhesion with the tendon kept taut by holding the joint at the end of its flexion range.[24] Apply the friction massage in a distal and proximal direction.

Exercises to Develop and Improve Muscle Performance, Neuromuscular Control, and Coordinated Movement

Exercises described in this section are for use during the controlled motion and return to function phases of rehabilitation when the tissues are in the subacute and chronic stages of healing and require only moderate or minimum protection. In addition to the conditions already described in this chapter, imbalances in length and strength of the wrist and hand muscles can occur as the result of a variety of causes, such as nerve injury, trauma, disuse, or immobilization. Selection of appropriate exercises to develop fine finger dexterity or to develop strength and muscular endurance for strong or repetitive gripping can be made from the following exercises or their adaptations. Exercises for shoulder, elbow, and forearm strength should also be included to restore proper function in the upper extremity.

Techniques to Strengthen Muscles of the Wrist and Hand

If musculature is weak, use progressive strengthening exercises, beginning at the level of the patient's ability. Use active-assistive, active, or manual resistive ROM as described in Chapters 2 and 3 of this text. Progress to mechanical resistance.

To Strengthen Wrist Musculature

Allow the fingers to relax. Exercise the wrist muscles in groups if their strength is similar. If one muscle is weaker, the wrist should be guided through the range desired to minimize the action of the stronger muscles. For example, with wrist flexion, if the flexor carpi radialis is stronger than the flexor carpi ulnaris, instruct the patient to attempt to flex the wrist toward the ulnar side as you guide the wrist into flexion and ulnar deviation. If the muscle is strong enough to tolerate resistance, apply manual resistance over the fourth and fifth metacarpals.

Wrist Flexion (Flexor Carpi Ulnaris and Radialis) and Extension (Extensor Carpi Radialis Longus and Brevis and Extensor Carpi Ulnaris)

Patient position: Sitting with the forearm supported on a table and grasping a weight or elastic resistance that is secured on the floor. The forearm is pronated to resist extension (see Fig. 10–12) or supinated to resist flexion.

Wrist Radial Deviation (Flexor and Extensor Carpi Radialis Muscles and Abductor Pollicis Longus), and Ulnar Deviation (Flexor and Extensor Carpi Ulnaris Muscles)

Patient position: Standing, holding a bar with a weight on one end. To resist radial deviation the weight is on the radial side of the wrist (Fig. 11–14*A*); to resist or ulnar deviation the weight is on ulnar side of the wrist (Fig. 11–14*B*).

Functional Progressions

Progress to controlled patterns of motion requiring stabilization of the wrist for functional hand activities such as repetitive gripping, picking up and releasing objects of various sizes and weights, and opening and closing the screw lid on a jar. Develop endurance and progress to the desired functional pattern by loading the upper extremity to the tolerance of the wrist stabilizers. When the stabilization begins to fatigue, stop the activity.

To Strengthen Weak Intrinsic Musculature

Note: Imbalance from weak intrinsic muscles leads to a claw hand.

MCP Joint Flexion with IP Joint Extension (Lumbricales)

- Begin with the MCP joints stabilized in flexion. Have the patient actively extend the PIP joint

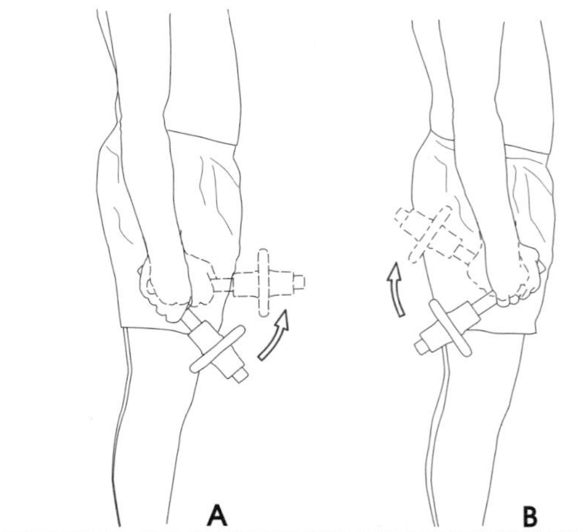

Figure 11–14 Mechanical resistance to strengthen *(A)* radial deviation and *(B)* ulnar deviation of the wrist using a weighted bar.

against a resistive force on the middle phalanx. Progress the resistive force to the distal phalanx. The resistance may be applied manually or with rubberbands.

- Have the patient start with the MCP joints extended and the PIP joints flexed; then actively push the fingertips outward, performing the desired combined motion (Fig. 11–15*A* and *B*). For resistance have the patient push the fingers into the palm of the other hand (Fig 11–15*C*), or push the fingers into exercise putty with the desired motion.
- Begin with all the finger joints extended. Have the patient maintain the IP joints in extension and flex the MCP joints to the tabletop position. Apply resistance against the proximal phalanx.

Isolated or Combined Abduction/Adduction of Each Finger (Dorsal and Volar Interossei)

- Have the patient rest the palm of the hand on a table. Give resistance at the distal end of the proximal phalanx, one finger at a time, for either abduction or adduction.
- To resist adduction, have the patient interlace the fingers of both hands (or with your hand) and squeeze the fingers together or squeeze exercise putty between two adjacent fingers.
- To resist abduction, place a rubberband around two digits, and have the patient spread them apart.

Abduction of the Thumb (Abductor Pollicis Brevis and Longus)

- The patient rests the dorsum of the hand on a table. Apply resistance at the base of the first phalanx of the thumb as the patient lifts the thumb away from the palm of the hand.
- Place a rubberband or band of exercise putty around the thumb and base of the index finger, and have the patient abduct the thumb against the resistance.

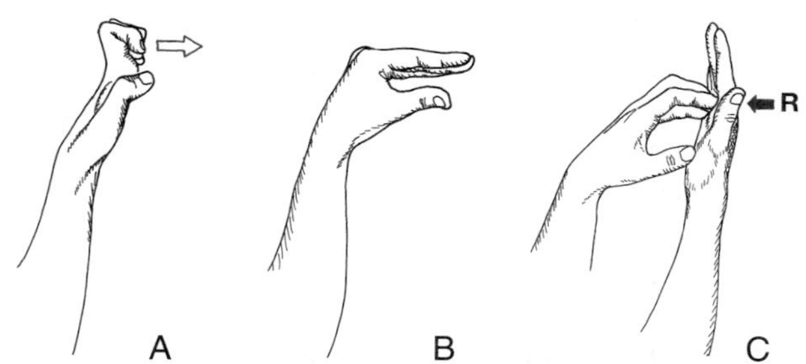

Figure 11–15 To strengthen intrinsic muscle function for combined MCP flexion and IP extension, the patient begins with *(A)* MCP extension and IP flexion and *(B)* pushes his fingertips outward. The same motion is resisted by *(C)* pushing the fingertips against the palm of the other hand.

Opposition of the Thumb (Opponens Pollicis)

- Have the patient use various prehension patterns such as tip-to-tip and tip-to-pad with the thumb opposing each digit in succession, and pad-to-side with the thumb approximating the lateral side of the index finger.
- Use elastic resistance, or have the patient pinch exercise putty, a pliable ball, or a spring-loaded clothespin.

To Strengthen Weak Extrinsic Musculature of the Fingers

Note: The wrist must be stabilized for the action of the extrinsic hand musculature to be effective. With inadequate wrist strength for stabilization, manually stabilize it during exercises and splint it for functional usage.

Metacarpophalangeal Extension (Extensor Digitorum Communis, Indicis, and Digiti Minimi)

Have the hand resting on a table with the palm down and digits over the edge. Place a small strap over the distal end of the proximal phalanx with a small weight hanging down from it or secure an elastic resistance band around the proximal phalanx, and have the patient extend the MCP joint.

Interphalangeal Flexion (Flexor Digitorum Profundus and Superficialis)

Teach the patient to apply self-resistance by starting with the hands pointing in opposite directions and placing the pads of each finger of one hand against the pads of each finger of the other hand (or against your hand). He or she then curls the fingers against the resistance provided by the other hand (Fig. 11–16). The same technique is used to resist thumb flexion.

Mechanical Resistance Techniques for Combined Intrinsic and Extrinsic Muscle Function

Note: Proper stabilization is important; either the patient's stabilizing muscles must be strong enough or the weakened areas must be supported manually. If a weight causes

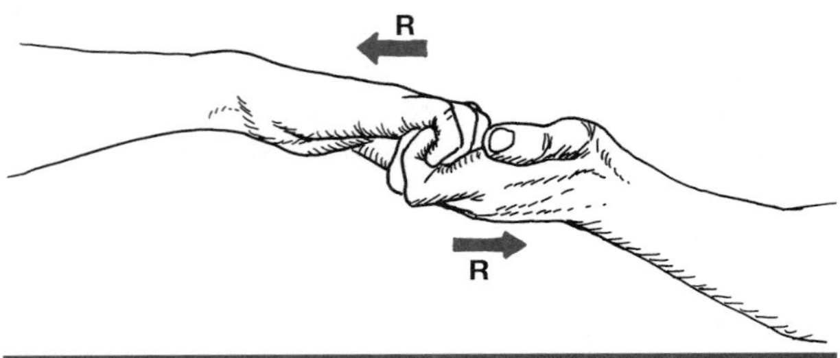

Figure 11–16 Self-resistance to strengthen extrinsic finger flexor muscles.

stress because the patient cannot control it, the exercise will be detrimental rather than beneficial.

Towel or Newspaper Crumple

Spread a towel out on a table. Have the patient place the palm of the hand down at one end of the towel. While maintaining contact with the heel of the hand, he or she crumples the towel into the hand. The same exercise can be carried out by placing a stack of newspapers under the hand. The patient crumples the top sheet into a ball (and tosses it into a basket for coordination and skill practice), then repeats it with each sheet in succession.

Disk Weight

Have the patient grasp the disk in the manner described in each of the following exercises.

- With the forearm pronated (palm down), pick up a disk with the tips of all five digits spread around the outer edge. Have the patient hold the position for isometric resistance. To increase the effect of the resistance to the flexors, have the patient extend one digit at a time.
- Pick up the side of the disk weight with either tip-to-tip or pad-to-pad prehension of thumb and fingers.
- The hand is placed palm down on the table; place a weight on the dorsum of the fingers; the patient hyperextends the fingers by lifting the weight.

Other Resistance Aids

Resistive devices such as putty, spring-loaded hand resistance, and various grades and sizes of soft balls can be used for specific muscles or general strengthening. Observe the pattern used by the patient and be sure he or she does not substitute or develop damaging forces.

Fine-Finger Dexterity

Functional use of the hand for manipulating small objects or skillfully controlling delicate devices requires use of the thumb in opposition to the index and middle fingers. Have the patient perform activities such as picking up small objects of various sizes, twisting nuts on and off bolts, drawing, writing, tying, opening, and closing small bottles or boxes, and typing on a keyboard.

Functional Activities

Progress to specific patterns of activity needed for ADL, job activities, hobbies, or recreational function. For the patient to return to independent function using the hand, he or she must not only have neuromuscular control and strength but must have muscular endurance, coordination, and fine finger dexterity for the desired activity. This requires careful questioning and analysis of the patient's desired outcomes. Each of the power grips and prehension patterns should be considered. Exercises should be adapted to meet the goals.

Independent Learning Activities

CRITICAL THINKING AND DISCUSSION

1. Falling on an outstretched hand can cause several injuries including posterior shoulder dislocation, radial head subluxation (pushed elbow), Colles' fracture, and scaphoid fracture. Complications can develop including reflex sympathetic dystrophy and carpal tunnel syndrome. Describe the mechanism and typical clinical signs and symptoms for each of these injuries, and identify how to recognize the development of complications.
2. Review all the power grips and prehension patterns, and identify the primary muscles that function when performing each action.
3. Summarize the sensory and motor impairments, deformities, and functional limitations that occur in the wrist and hand as the result of a lesion of: (a) the median nerve, (b) the radial nerve, and (c) the ulnar nerve.
4. Differentiate between a boutonnière deformity and a swan-neck deformity of the fingers. What are the underlying factors that contribute to these deformities? After surgical repair of each of these

deformities, how should an exercise program be designed to increase hand function but prevent recurrence of these deformities?

5. Identify key structures by zone in the hand and wrist that could be damaged as the result of a laceration at each zone of the dorsal and volar aspects of the hand and wrist. What functional impairments will occur as the result of damage in each zone?
6. Make a case for the use of early controlled motion after surgical repair of a flexor or extensor tendon injury. Also identify circumstances in which the use of early controlled motion would be inadvisable or not possible.
7. Analyze and summarize the similarities and differences in the components and progression of exercise programs after flexor or extensor tendon repairs using early controlled mobilization versus delayed mobilization approaches.

LABORATORY PRACTICE

1. Mobilize each forearm, wrist, and finger joint with joint mobilization and passive stretching techniques.
2. Practice each tendon-gliding exercise, and identify the purpose for each one.
3. Teach your partner strengthening exercises for each muscle or muscle group in the hand using resistance putty.
4. Identify three alternative resistance devices that can be used to strengthen each muscle and patterns of motion in the hand.
5. Observe someone tying laces on a shoe, identify the muscles functioning, and design an exercise program that could be used to develop neuromuscular control or strengthen each the muscles.

CASE STUDIES

1. A patient is referred to you early in the development of symptoms that stem from RA. He currently is in remission after his first serious flare of the disease and desires a home exercise program to safely improve the use of his hands. He is a salesman who travels frequently. He keeps his records on computer. His grip strength is reduced 50%; he has 25% loss of joint ROM, and decreased joint play in the wrist, MCP, and IP joints. Detectable synovial hypertrophy is minimal, and there are no joint subluxations. Consider what precautions should be followed with this disease to prevent the deforming forces of improperly applied exercises and daily forces. Establish a program of intervention for this patient.
2. A new patient is referred to you 2 months after Colles' fracture. Her hand is swollen and sensitive to touch, and she currently is developing contractures and weakness in the hand related to reflex sympathetic dystrophy (see Chapter 9). Joint contractures exist in the forearm, wrist, and hand. You determine that the patient is in the second stage of the disease. Establish a plan for intervention.
3. A patient with RA who has just undergone MCP implant arthroplasties of the ring and small fingers has been referred to you for an exercise program. The patient has been wearing a dynamic extension splint for the past 3 weeks that allows active MCP flexion and assists MCP extension. The patient is now allowed to remove the splint for active ROM of the wrist and hand. Your evaluation reveals that the patient has an extensor lag and also has restricted flexion of the fingers. Design and progress an exercise program for this patient. What precautions should be incorporated into each phase of the program?
4. A patient has been referred to you who underwent a ligament reconstruction tendon interposition arthroplasty for post-traumatic arthritis of the CMC joint of the thumb 4 weeks ago. The thumb spica cast was removed at 3 1/2 weeks postoperatively, and the patient is now wearing a thumb spica splint that may be removed for exercise. Develop and progress an exercise program for the patient. The patient has already returned to his/her position in an office. The patient would like to be able to resume golf on a recreational basis.
5. An 8-year-old child who sustained a zone II laceration of the index and middle fingers of the nondominant hand while carving a pumpkin has been referred to you after surgical repair of the FDP and FDS tendons. The child's hand has been immobilized in a cast for 3 weeks after the repair in a position of wrist and finger flexion. The child is now wearing a dorsal blocking splint that may be removed for exercise. The child's active and passive extension is now significantly limited. Design and progress an exercise program for this child. Identify activities that the child must do under direct supervision and those that he/she may do independently.

REFERENCES

1. Amadio, PC, and Murray, PM: Arthroplasty of the proximal interphalangeal joint. In Morrey, BF (ed): Reconstructive Surgery of the Joints, Vol 1, ed 2. Churchill Livingstone, New York, 1996, p 267.
2. Anderson, RJ: Rheumatoid arthritis: clinical and laboratory features. In Klippel, JF (ed): Primer on Rheumatic Diseases, ed 11. Arthritis Foundation, Atlanta, 1997, p 161.
3. Ballard, WT, and Buckwalter, JA: Operative treatment of rheumatic disease. In Klippel, JH (ed): Primer on Rheumatic Diseases, ed 11. Arthritis Foundation, Atlanta, 1997, p 447.
4. Bass, RL, Stern, PJ, and Nairus, JG: High implant fracture incidence with Sutler silicone metacarpalphalangeal joint arthroplasty. J Hand Surg 21A:813, 1996.
5. Baxter-Petralia, P, and Penney, V: Cumulative trauma. In Stanley, BG and Tribuzi (eds): Concepts in Hand Rehabilitation. FA Davis Co, Philadelphia, 1992, p 419.
6. Beckenbaugh, RD: Arthroplasty of the wrist. In Morrey, BF (ed): Reconstructive Surgery of the Joints, ed 2. Churchill Livingstone, New York, 1996, p 387.
7. Beckenbaugh, RD: Total wrist arthroplasty. In Lichtman, DM, and Alexander, AH (eds): The Wrist and Its Disorders, ed 2. WB Saunders, Philadelphia, 1997, p 643.
8. Beckenbaugh, RD: Total wrist arthroplasty. In Cooney, WP, Linschied, RL, and Dobyns, JH (eds). The Wrist: Diagnosis and Operative Treatment, Vol 2. CV Mosby, St Louis, 1998, p 924.
9. Berger, RA, Beckenbaugh, RD, and Linschied, RL: Arthroplasty of the hand and wrist. In Green, DP, Hotchkiss, RN, and Pederson, WC (eds): Green's Operative Hand Surgery, Vol 1, ed 4. Churchill Livingstone, New York, 1999. p 147.
10. Blair, WF, Schurr, DG, and Buckwalter, JA: Metacarpophalangeal joint implant arthroplasty with Silastic spacer. J Bone Joint Surg Am 66:365, 1984.
11. Bosco, JA, Byrnum, DK, and Bowers, WH: Long-term outcome of Volz total wrist arthroplasties. 9: 25, 1994.
12. Browne, EZ Jr, and Ribick, CA: Early dynamic splinting for extensor tendon injuries. J Hand Surg 14A:72, 1989.
13. Burton, RI, and Melchior, JA: Extensor tendons—late reconstruction. In Green, DP, Hotchkiss, RN, and Pederson, WC (eds): Green's Operative Hand Surgery, Vol 2, ed 4. Churchill Livingstone, New York, 1999, p 1988.
14. Burton, RI, and Pellegrini, VD: Surgical management of basal joint arthritis of the thumb. II. Ligament reconstruction with tendon interpositional arthroplasty. J Hand Surg 11A:324, 1986.
15. Butler, DS: Mobilization of the Nervous System. Churchill Livingstone, New York, 1991.
16. Byron, PM: Upper extremity nerve gliding programs used at the Philadelphia Hand Center. In Hunter, JM, Mackin, EJ, and Callahan, AD (eds): Rehabilitation of the Hand: Surgery and Therapy, Vol II, ed 4. CV Mosby, St. Louis, 1995, p 951.
17. Calandruccio, JH, Jobe, JT, and Akin, K: Rehabilitation of the hand and wrist. In Brotzman, SB (ed): Clinical Orthopedic Rehabilitation. Mosby, St. Louis, 1996, p 1.
18. Cannon, N: Post flexor tendon repair protocol. Indiana Hand Center Newsletter 1: 13, 1993.
19. Cannon, NM: Diagnosis and Treatment Manual for Physicians and Therapists, ed 4. Hand Rehabilitation Center of Indiana, Indianapolis, 2001.
20. Chow, JA, et al: A combined regimen of controlled motion following flexor tendon repair in "no man's land." Plast Reconstr Surg 79(3): 447, 1987.
21. Cooney, WF III: Arthroplasty of the thumb axis. In Morrey, BF (ed): Reconstructive Surgery of the Joints, Vol 1, ed 2. Churchill Livingstone, New York, 1996, p 313.
22. Creighton, JJ, Steichen, JB, and Strickland, JW: Long-term evaluation of silastic trapezial arthroplasty in-patients with osteoarthritis. J Hand Surg 16A:510, 1991.
23. Culp, RW, and Taras, JS: Primary care of flexor tendon injuries. In Hunter, JM, Mackin, EJ, and Callahan, AD (eds): Rehabilitation of the Hand: Surgery and Therapy, Vol 1, ed 4. CV Mosby, St. Louis, 1995, p 417.
24. Cyriax, J: Textbook of Orthopaedic Medicine, Vol 1. Diagnosis of Soft Tissue Lesions, ed 8. Bailliere Tindall, London, 1982.
25. Degnan, GG, and Lichtman, DM: Soft tissue arthroplasty about the wrist. In Lichtman, DM, and Alexander, AH (eds): The Wrist and Its Disorders, ed 2. WB Saunders, Philadelphia, 1997, p 609.
26. Doyle, JR: Extensor tendons—acute injuries. In Green, DP, Hotchkiss, RN, and Pederson, WC (eds): Green's Operative Hand Surgery, Vol 2, ed 4. Churchill Livingstone, New York, 1999, p 1950.
27. Duran, RJ, and Houser, RC: Controlled passive motion following flexor tendon repair in zones II and III. In AAOS Symposium on Tendon Surgery in the Hand. CV Mosby, St. Louis, 1975.
28. Evans, RB: An update on extensor tendon management. In Hunter, JM, Mackin, EJ, and Callahan, AD (eds): Rehabilitation of the Hand: Surgery and Therapy, Vol 1, ed 4. CV Mosby, St. Louis, 1995, p 565.
29. Evans, RB: Early active short arc motion for the repaired central slip. J Hand Surg 19A: 991, 1994
30. Evans, RB, and Burkhalter, WE: A study of the dynamic anatomy of extensor tendons and implications for treatment. J Hand Surg 11A: 774, 1986.
31. Evans, RB, and Thompson, DE: The application of stress to the healing tendon. J Hand Ther 6: 262, 1993.
32. Falkenstein, N, and Weiss-Lessard, S: Hand Rehabilitation: A Quick Reference Guide and Review. CV Mosby, St. Louis, 1999.
33. Feldon, PG, Nalebuff, EA, and Terrono, AL: Partial wrist fusions: intercarpal and radiocarpal. In Lichtman, DM, and Alexander, AH (eds): The Wrist and Its Disorders, ed 2. WB Saunders, Philadelphia, 1997, p 652.
34. Feldon, PG, Terrono, AL, et al: Rheumatoid arthritis and other connective tissue diseases. In Green, DP, Hotchkiss, RN, and Pederson, WC (eds): Green's Operative Hand Surgery, Vol 2, ed 4. Churchill Livingstone, New York, 1999, p 1651.
35. Foreman, S, and Gieck, J: Rehabilitative management of injuries to the hand. Clin Sports Med 11:239, 1992.
36. Germann, G, Sherman, R, and Levin, LS: Decision Making in Reconstructive Surgery: Upper Extremity. Springer-Verlag, Berlin, 2000.
37. Hunter, JM, Davlin, LB, and Defus, LM: Major neuropathies of the upper extremity: The median nerve. In Hunter, JM, Mackin, EJ, and Callahan, AD (eds): Rehabilitation of the

Hand: Surgery and Therapy, Vol II, ed 4. CV Mosby, St. Louis, 1995, p 905.
38. Hunter, JM, et al: Staged flexor tendon reconstruction using passive and active tendon implants. In Hunter, JM, Mackin, EJ, and Callahan, AD (eds): Rehabilitation of the Hand: Surgery and Therapy, Vol 1, ed 4. CV Mosby, St. Louis, 1995, p 477.
39. Jeter, E, Degnan, GG, and Lichtman, DM: Postoperative wrist rehabilitation. In Lichtman, DM, and Alexander, AH (eds): The Wrist and Its Disorders. CV Mosby, St. Louis, 1997, p 709.
40. Jolly, SL, et al: Swanson silicone arthroplasty of the wrist in rheumatoid arthritis: a long-term follow-up. J Hand Surg 17A: 142, 1992.
41. Kapandji, IA: The Physiology of the Joints, Vol I. Churchill-Livingstone, Edinburgh, 1970.
42. Katarinicic, JA, and Cooney, III, WP: Alternative reconstruction procedures for arthritis of the thumb. In Moorey, BF (ed): Reconstructive Surgery of the Joints, Vol 1, ed 2. Churchill Livingstone, New York, 1996, p 339.
43. Kleinert, HE, Kutz, JE, and Cohen, MJ: Primary repair of zone 2 flexor tendon lacerations. In AAOS Symposium on Tendon Surgery in the Hand. CV Mosby, St. Louis, 1975.
44. Kleinman, WB, and Eckenrode, JF: Tendon suspension sling arthroplasty for thumb trapeziometacarpal arthritis. J Hand Surg 16A: 983, 1991.
45. Kopell, H, and Thompson, W: Peripheral Entrapment Neuropathies, ed 2. Robert E Krieger, Huntington, NY, 1976.
46. Levangie, P, and Norkin, C: Joint Structure and Function: A Comprehensive Analysis, ed 3. FA Davis, Philadelphia, 2001.
47. Linscheid, RL, and Beckenbaugh, RD: Arthroplasty of the metacarpophalangeal joint. In Morrey, BF (ed): Reconstructive Surgery of the Joints, Vol 1, ed 2. Churchill Livingstone, New York, 1996, p 287.
48. Linschied, RL, et al: Development of a surface replacement arthroplasty for proximal interphalangeal joints. J Hand Surg 22A: 286, 1997.
49. Lister, GD, Kleinert, HE, et al: Primary flexor tendon repair followed by immediate controlled mobilization. J Hand Surg 2: 441, 1977.
50. Long, R, et al: Intrinsic-extrinsic muscle control of the hand in power grip and precision handling. J Bone Joint Surg Am 52:853, 1970.
51. Long, C: Normal and Abnormal Motor Control in the Upper Extremities. Final Report. Case Western Reserve University, Cleveland, OH, 1970.
52. Magee, DJ: Orthopedic Physical Assessment, ed 3. WB Saunders, Philadelphia, 1997.
53. Marx, H: Rheumatoid arthritis. In Stanley, BG, and Tribuzi, SM (eds): Concepts in Hand Rehabilitation. FA Davis Co, Philadelphia, 1992, p 395.
54. Melvin, J: Rheumatic Disease in the Adult and Child: Occupational Therapy and Rehabilitation, ed 3. FA Davis, Philadelphia, 1989.
55. Meuli, HC, and Fernandez, DL: Uncemented total arthroplasties. J Hand Surg 20A: 115, 1995.
56. Morgan, RL, and Lindner, MM: Common wrist injuries. Am Family Physician 55(3): 857, 1997.
57. Mulligan, BR: Manual Therapy "NAGS", "SNAGS", MWM'S: etc., ed 4. Plane View Press, Wellington, 1999.
58. Nalebuff, EA, Terrono, AL, and Feldon, PG: Arthrodesis of the wrist: Indications and surgical technique. In Lichtman, DM, and Alexander, AH (eds): The Wrist and Its Disorders, ed 2. WB Saunders, Philadelphia, 1997, p 671.
59. Nalebuff, EA: Silicone arthroplasty of the metacarpophalangeal joint. In Blair, WF and Steyers, CM (eds): Techniques in Hand Surgery. Williams & Wilkins, Baltimore, 1996, p 936.
60. Nalebuff, EA: The rheumatoid thumb. In Strickland, JW (ed): The Hand and Upper Limb, Vol 2. The Thumb. Churchill Livingstone, New York, 1994, p 171.
61. Napier, JR: The prehensile movements of the human hand. J Bone Joint Surg Br 38:902, 1956.
62. Newport, ML, Blair, WF, and Steyers, CM Jr.: Long term results of extensor tendon repair J Hand Surg 15A:961, 1990.
63. O'Connell, SJ, et al: Results of zone I and zone II flexor tendon repairs in children. J Hand Surg 19A:48, 1994.
64. Phillips, CA: Rehabilitation of the patient with rheumatoid hand involvement. Phys Ther 69:1091, 1989.
65. Phillips, CA: Therapist's management of patients with rheumatoid arthritis. In Hunter, JM, Mackin, EJ, and Callahan, AD (eds): Rehabilitation of the Hand: Surgery and Therapy, Vol II, ed 4. CV Mosby, St. Louis, 1995, p 1345.
66. Provinciali, L, Giattini, A, et al: Usefulness of hand rehabilitation after carpal tunnel surgery. Muscle and Nerve 23:211, 2000.
67. Randall, T, Portney, L, and Harris, BA: Effects of joint mobilization on joint stiffness and active motion of the metacarpal-phalangeal joint. J Orthop Sports Phys Ther 16:30, 1992.
68. Richterman, I, and Keenan, MA: Surgical interventions. In Walker, JM, and Helewa, A: Physical Therapy in Arthritis. WB Saunders, Philadelphia, 1996, p 95.
69. Rosenthal, EA: The extensor tendons: anatomy and management. In Hunter, JM, Mackin, EJ, and Callahan, AD (eds): Rehabilitation of the Hand: Surgery and Therapy, Vol 1, ed 4. CV Mosby, St. Louis, 1995, p 519.
70. Rozmaryn, LM, Dovelle, S, et al: Nerve and tendon gliding exercises and the conservative management of carpal tunnel syndrome. J Hand Ther 11:171, 1998.
71. Saldama, MJ, et al: Results of acute Zone III extensor tendon injuries treated with dynamic extension splinting. J Hand Surg 16A: 1145, 1991.
72. Saunders, RJ: Thumb carpometacarpal joint arthroplasty. In Clark, GL, et al (eds): Hand Rehabilitation: A Practical Guide. Churchill Livingstone, New York, 1998, p 363.
72a. Saunders, SR: Physical therapy management of hand fractures. Phys Ther 69:1065, 1989
73. Savage, R: The influence of wrist position on the minimum force required for active movement of the interphalangeal joints. J Hand Surg 13B:262, 1988.
74. Savage, R, and Risitano, G: Flexor tendon repair using a "six strand" method of repair and early active motion. J Hand Surg 14B:396, 1989.
75. Schenk, RR, and Lenhart, DE: Results of zone II flexor tendon lacerations in civilians treated by the Washington regimen. J Hand Surg 21A:984, 1996.
76. Schneider, LH: Flexor tendons—Late reconstruction. In Green, DP, Hotchkiss, RN, and Pederson, WC (eds): Green's Operative Hand Surgery, Vol 2, ed 4. Churchill Livingstone, New York, 1999, p 1898.
77. Silfverskiöld, KL, May, EJ, and Thornvall, AH: Flexor digito-

rum profundis excursions during controlled motion after flexor tendon repair in zone II. A prospective clinical study. J Hand Surg 17A:122, 1992.

78. Silfverskiöld, KL, and May, EJ: Flexor tendon repair in zone II with a new suture technique and an early mobilization program combining passive and active flexion. J Hand Surg 19A:53, 1994.
79. Simmons, BP, Millender, LH, and Nalebuff, EA: Surgery of the hand. In Sledge, CB, et al (eds): Arthritis Surgery. WB Saunders, Philadelphia, 1994.
80. Skirven, T: Nerve Injuries. In Stanley, BG, and Tribuzi, SM (eds): Concepts in Hand Rehabilitation. FA Davis, Philadelphia, 1992, p 322.
81. Smith, LK, Weiss, EL, and Lehmkuhl, LD: Brunnstrom's Clinical Kinesiology, ed 5. FA Davis, Philadelphia, 1996.
82. Stanley, B: Therapeutic exercise: maintaining and restoring mobility in the hand. In Stanley, BG, and Tribuzi, SM (eds): Concepts in Hand Rehabilitation. FA Davis, Philadelphia, 1992, p 178.
83. Stanley, JK, and Tolat, AR: Long-term results of Swanson Silastic arthroplasty in the rheumatoid wrist. J Hand Surg 18B:381, 1993.
84. Steinberg, B: Extensor tendon repair. In Clark, GL, et al (eds): Hand Rehabilitation: A Practical Guide, ed 2. Churchill Livingstone, New York, 1998, p 93.
85. Steinberg, B: Flexor tendon repair. In Clark, GL, et al (eds): Hand Rehabilitation: A Practical Guide, ed 2. Churchill Livingstone, New York, 1998, p 103.
86. Stewart, KM: Review and comparisons in the postoperative management of tendon repair. Hand Clin 7(3): 447–460, 1991.
87. Stewart, KM: Tendon injuries. In Stanley, BG, and Tribuzi, SM (eds): Concepts in Hand Rehabilitation. FA Davis, Philadelphia, 1992.
88. Stewart, KM, and van Strien, G: Postoperative management of flexor tendon injuries. In Hunter, JM, Mackin, EJ, and Callahan, AD (eds): Rehabilitation of the Hand: Surgery and Therapy, Vol 1, ed 4. CV Mosby, St. Louis, 1995, p 433.
89. Strickland, JW: Flexor tendons—Acute injuries. In Green, DP, Hotchkiss, RN, and Pederson, WC (eds): Green's Operative Hand Surgery, Vol 2, ed 4. Churchill Livingstone, New York, 1999, p 1851.
90. Strickland, JW: Flexor tendon injuries: I. Foundations of treatment. J Am Acad Orthop Surg 3: 44, 1995.
91. Swanson, AB, and Swanson, G deGroot: Implant arthroplasty in the carpal and radiocarpal joints. In Lichtman, DM, and Alexander, AH (eds): The Wrist and Its Disorders, ed 2. WB Saunders, Philadelphia, 1997, p 616.
92. Swanson, AB, and Swanson, G deGroot: Flexible implant resection arthroplasty of the proximal interphalangeal joint. Hand Clin 10: 261, 1994.
93. Swanson, AB, Swanson, G deGroot, and Leonard JB: Postoperative rehabilitation programs in flexible implant arthroplasty of the digits. In Hunter, JM, Mackin, EJ, and Callahan, AD (eds): Rehabilitation of the Hand: Surgery and Therapy, Vol 2, ed 4. CV Mosby, St. Louis, 1995, p 1351.
94. Swanson, AB, Swanson, GD, and Maupin, BK: Flexible implant arthroplasty of the radiocarpal joint. Surgical techniques and long-term study. Clin Orthop 187:94, 1984.
95. Swanson, AB: Pathogensis of arthritic lesions. In Hunter, JM, Mackin, EJ, and Callahan, AD (eds): Rehabilitation of the Hand: Surgery and Therapy Vol 2, ed 4. CV Mosby, St. Louis, 1995, p 1307.
96. Theisen, L: Metacarpophalangeal joint arthroplasty. In Clark, GL, et al (eds): Hand Rehabilitation: A Practical Guide, ed 2. Churchill Livingstone, New York, 1998, p 349.
97. Theisen, L: Proximal interphalangeal and distal interphalangeal joint arthroplasty. In Clark, GL, et al (eds): Hand Rehabilitation: A Practical Guide, ed 2. Churchill Livingstone, New York, 1998, p 355.
98. Waite, J: Physical therapy management of patients with wrist and hand disorders. Orthop Phys Ther Clin North Am 8:135, 1999.
99. Wood, MB: Soft tissue reconstruction. In Cooney, WP, Linscheid, RL, and Dobyns, JH (eds): The Wrist: Diagnosis and Operative Treatment, Vol 2. CV Mosby, St. Louis, 1998, p 887.
100. Wynn Parry, CB, and Stanley, JK: Synovectomy of the hand. Br J Rheumotol 32:1089, 1993.
101. Zohn, D, and Mennell, J: Musculoskeletal Pain: Principles of Physical Diagnosis and Physical Treatment. Little, Brown, Boston, 1976.

Chapter 12

The Hip

OBJECTIVES

After studying this chapter, the reader will be able to:

1 Identify important aspects of the hip structure and function for review.

2 Establish a therapeutic exercise program to manage soft tissue and joint lesions in the hip that are related to stages of recovery after an inflammatory insult to the tissues, recognizing unique circumstances in the hip and pelvis for their management.

3 Discuss the background of, indications for, and outcomes of common surgical procedures for joint pathology and fractures of the hip.

4 Develop a postoperative program that includes appropriate goals and therapeutic exercise interventions for management of common surgical procedures of the hip.

The hip is often compared with the shoulder in that it is a triaxial joint, able to function in all three planes, and that it is also the proximal link to its extremity. In contrast to the shoulder, which is designed for mobility, the hip is a stable joint, constructed for weight bearing. However, to carry out activities of daily living (ADL) in what is considered a "normal" manner, at least 120 degrees of hip flexion and at least 20 degrees each of abduction and external rotation are necessary.[65] Forces from the lower extremities are transmitted upward through the hips to the pelvis and trunk during gait and other lower extremity activities. The hips also support the weight of the head, trunk, and upper extremities.

The initial section of this chapter reviews highlights of the anatomy and function of the hip and its relation to the pelvis and lumbar spine. Chapter 8 presents information on principles of management; the reader should be familiar with that material as well as the components of an effective examination of the hip and pelvis before determining a diagnosis and proceeding to establish a therapeutic exercise program.

Review of the Structure and Function of the Hip

Bony Parts: Proximal Femur and the Pelvis (see Fig. 6–45)

The Femur

The shape of the femur is designed to bear body weight and to transmit the ground reaction forces. In the frontal plane there is an angle of inclination (normally 125 degrees) between the axis of the femoral neck and shaft of the femur. The angle of torsion formed by the transverse axis of the femoral condyles and the axis of the neck of the femur ranges from 8 to 25 degrees, with an average angle of 12 degrees. There is also a slight bowing of the shaft in the sagittal plane.[44]

The Pelvis

Each innominate bone of the pelvis is formed by the union of the ilium, ischium and pubis bones and, therefore, is a structural unit. The right and left innominate bones articulate anteriorly with each other at the pubic symphysis and posteriorly with the sacrum at the sacroiliac joints.[44] Slight motion occurs at these three joints to attenuate forces as they are transmitted through the pelvic region, but the pelvis basically functions as a unit in a closed-chain.

Hip Joint

Characteristics

- The hip is a ball-and-socket (spheroidal) triaxial joint, supported by a strong articular capsule that is reinforced by the iliofemoral, pubofemoral, and ischiofemoral ligaments. The two hip joints are linked to each other through the bony pelvis and to the vertebral column through the sacroiliac and lumbosacral joints.[44,80]

- The concave bony partner, the acetabulum, is located in the lateral aspect of the pelvis and faces laterally, anteriorly, and inferiorly. The acetabulum is deepened by a ring of fibrocartilage, the acetabular labrum. The articular cartilage is horseshoe-shaped, being thicker in the lateral region where the major weight-bearing forces are transmitted. The central portion of the acetabular surface is nonarticular.
- The convex bony partner is the spherical head of the femur, which is attached to the femoral neck. It projects anteriorly, medially, and superiorly.

Arthrokinematics

Motions of the femur. The convex femoral head slides in the direction opposite the physiologic motion of the femur, so that with hip flexion and internal rotation the articulating surface slides posterior, with extension and external rotation it slides anterior, with abduction it slides inferior, and with adduction, superior (Box 12–1).

Motions of the pelvis. When the lower extremity is fixated distally, as in standing or during the stance phase of gait, the concave acetabulum moves on the convex femoral head, so the acetabulum slides in the same direction as the pelvis. The pelvis is a link in a closed-chain; therefore, when the pelvis moves, there will be motion at both hip joints as well as the lumbar spine.

Functional Relationships of the Hips and Pelvis in the Kinematic Chain

Changes in the Angle of the Hip and Lumbar Spine with Pelvic Motion

Anterior pelvic tilt (PT). The anterior superior iliac spines of the pelvis move anteriorly and inferiorly and, thus, closer to the anterior aspect of the femur as the pelvis rotates forward around the transverse axis of the hip joints. This results in hip flexion and increased lumbar spine extension (hyperextension).[44]

- Muscles causing this motion are the hip flexors and back extensors.
- When standing, the line of gravity of the trunk falls anterior to the axis of the hip joints; the effect is an anterior PT moment. Stability is provided by the abdominals and hip extensor muscles.

Posterior PT. The posterior superior iliac spines of the pelvis move posteriorly and inferiorly, thus closer to the posterior aspect of the femur as the pelvis rotates backward around the axis of the hip joints. This results in hip extension and lumbar spine flexion.[44]

- Muscles causing this motion are the hip extensors and trunk flexors.
- When standing and the line of gravity of the trunk falls posterior to the axis of the hip joints, the effect is a posterior PT moment. Dynamic stability is provided by the hip flexors and back extensors and passive stability by the iliofemoral ligament.

Pelvic shifting. When standing, a forward translatory shifting of the pelvis results in extension of the hip and extension of the lower lumbar spinal segments. There is a compensatory posterior shifting of the thorax on the upper lumbar spine with increased flexion of these spinal segments. This is often seen with slouched or relaxed postures (see Chapter 16). Little muscle action is required; the posture is maintained by the iliofemoral ligaments at the hip, anterior longitudinal ligament of the lower lumbar spine, and posterior ligaments of the upper lumbar and thoracic spine.

Lumbopelvic rhythm. A coordinated movement between the lumbar spine and pelvis occurs during maximum forward bending of the trunk[11] as when reaching toward the floor or the toes. As the head and upper trunk initiate flexion, the pelvis shifts posteriorly to maintain the center of gravity balanced over the base of support. The trunk continues to forward bend, being controlled by the extensor muscles of the spine, until approximately 45 degrees. At this point for an individual with relatively normal flexibility, the posterior ligaments become taut, and the facets of the zygapophyseal joints ap-

Box 12–1 Summary of Arthrokinematics of the Femoral Head in the Hip Joint

Physiologic Motions of the Femur	Roll	Slide
Flexion	*Anterior*	*Posterior*
Extension	*Posterior*	*Anterior*
Abduction	*Lateral*	*Inferior*
Adduction	*Medial*	*Superior*
Internal rotation	*Medial*	*Posterior*
External rotation	*Lateral*	*Anterior*

proximate. Both of these factors provide stability for the intervertebral joints, and the muscles relax.[82] Once all of the vertebral segments are at the end of the range and stabilized by the posterior ligaments and facets, the pelvis begins to rotate forward (anterior PT), being controlled by the gluteus maximus and hamstring muscles. The pelvis continues to rotate forward until the full length of the muscles is reached. Final range of motion (ROM) in forward bending is dictated by the flexibility in the various back extensor muscles and fasciae as well as hip extensor muscles. The return to the upright position begins with the hip extensor muscles rotating the pelvis posteriorly through reverse muscle action (posterior PT), then back extensor muscles extending the spine from the lumbar region upward. Variations in the normal synchronization of this activity occur because of training (as with dancers and gymnasts), faulty habits, restricted muscle or fascia length, or injury and faulty proprioception.

Lateral PT. Frontal plane pelvic motion results in opposite motions at each hip joint. On the side that is elevated (hip hiking), there is hip adduction; on the side that is lowered (hip drop), there is hip abduction. When standing, the lumbar spine laterally flexes toward the side of the elevated pelvis (convexity of the lateral curve is toward the lowered side).[44]

- Muscles causing lateral pelvic tilting include the quadratus lumborum on the side of the elevated pelvis and reverse muscle pull of the gluteus medius on the side of the lowered pelvis.
- With an asymmetric slouched posture, the person shifts the trunk weight onto one lower extremity and allows the pelvis to drop on the other side. Passive support comes from the iliofemoral ligament and iliotibial band on the elevated side (stance leg).
- When standing on one leg, there is an adduction moment at the hip, tending to cause the pelvis to drop on the unsupported side (hip or pelvic drop). This is prevented by the gluteus medius stabilizing the pelvis on the stance side.

Pelvic rotation. Rotation occurs around one lower extremity that is fixed on the ground. The unsupported lower extremity swings forward or backward along with the pelvis. When the unsupported side of the pelvis moves forward, it is called forward rotation of the pelvis.[44] The trunk concurrently rotates opposite, and the femur on the stabilized side concurrently rotates internally. When the unsupported side of the pelvis moves backward, it is called posterior rotation; the femur on the stabilized side concurrently rotates externally, and the trunk rotates opposite.

Motions, Impairments, and Deformities of the Lower Extremity that Affect the Pelvis and Spine

Reverse muscle action. Hip musculature causes pelvic motion through reverse action. Hip flexors cause an anterior PT; hip extensors, a posterior PT; abductors and adductors, a lateral PT; and rotators cause pelvic rotation. To prevent excessive pelvic motion when moving the femur at the hip joint, the pelvis must be stabilized by the abdominals, erector spinae, multifidus, and quadratus lumborum muscles.

Decreased flexibility in the hip muscles or joints. This will cause weight-bearing forces and movement to be transmitted to the spine rather than absorbed in the pelvis. Tight hip extensors will cause increased lumbar flexion when the thigh flexes. Tight hip flexors will cause increased lumbar extension as the thigh extends. Hip flexion contractures with incomplete hip extension during weight bearing will also place added stresses on the knee because the knee cannot lock while the hip is in flexion unless the trunk is bent forward. Tight adductors cause lateral pelvic tilt opposite and side bending of the trunk toward the side of tightness during weight bearing. The opposite occurs with tight abductors.

Asymmetric Leg Length

- A *unilateral short leg* causes lateral pelvic tilting (drop on the short side) and side-bending of the trunk away from the short side (convexity of lateral lumbar curve toward side of short leg). This may lead to a functional or eventually a structural scoliosis. Causes of a short leg could be unilateral lower extremity asymmetries such as flat foot, genu valgum, coxa vara, tight hip muscles, anteriorly rotated innominate bone, poor standing posture, or asymmetry in bone growth.
- A pathologically large angle of inclination between the femoral neck and shaft of the femur is called coxa valga, and a pathologically smaller angle is called coxa vara. Unilateral coxa valga results in a relatively longer leg on that side and associated genu varum. Unilateral coxa vara leads to a relatively shorter leg with associated genu valgum.
- An increase in the torsion of the femoral neck is called anteversion and causes the shaft of the femur to be rotated medially; a decrease in the torsion is called retroversion and causes the shaft of

the femur to be rotated laterally. Anteversion often results in genu valgum and pes planus. Unilateral anteversion results in a relatively shorter leg on that side; retroversion causes the opposite effects.

The Hip and Gait

Range of hip motion. During the normal gait cycle, the hip goes through a ROM of 40 degrees of flexion and extension (10 degrees extension at terminal stance to 30 degrees flexion at midswing and initial contact). There is also some lateral PT and hip abduction/adduction of 15 degrees (10 degrees adduction at initial contact; 5 degrees abduction at initial swing); and hip internal/external rotation along with pelvic rotation totaling 15 degrees transverse plane motion (peak internal rotation at the end of loading; peak external rotation at the end of preswing). Loss of any of these motions will affect the smoothness of the gait pattern.[67]

Muscle Control During Gait

- *Hip flexors* control hip extension at the end of stance, then contract concentrically to initiate swing.[67] With loss of flexor function, a posterior lurch of the trunk to initiate swing is seen. Contractures in the hip flexors prevent complete extension during the second half of stance; the stride is shortened. The person increases the lumbar lordosis or walks with the trunk bent forward.
- *Hip extensors* control the flexor moment at initial foot contact, and the gluteus maximus initiates hip extension.[67] With loss of extensor function, a posterior lurch of the trunk occurs at foot contact to shift the center of gravity of the trunk posterior to the hip. With contractures in the gluteus maximus, some decreased range occurs in the terminal swing as the femur comes forward, or the person may compensate by rotating the pelvis more forward. The lower extremity may rotate outward because of the external rotation component of the muscle or, the gluteus maximus may place greater tension on the iliotibial band through its attachment, leading to irritation along the lateral aspect of the knee with excessive activity.
- *Hip abductors* control the lateral PT during swinging of the opposite leg.[67] With loss of function of the gluteus medius, lateral shifting of the trunk occurs over the weak side during stance when the opposite leg swings. This lateral shifting also occurs with a painful hip, because it minimizes the torque at the hip joint during weight bearing. The tensor fasciae latae also functions as an abductor and may become tight and affect gait with faulty use.

Musculoskeletal deformities or disorders. Bony and joint deformities change alignment of the lower extremity and, therefore, the mechanics of gait. Painful conditions cause antalgic gait patterns, which are characterized by minimum stance on the painful side to avoid the stress of weight bearing.

Hip Muscle Imbalances and Their Effects

Muscles function through habit. Faulty mechanics from inadequate or excessive length and an imbalance in strength cause hip, knee, or back pain.[75] Overuse syndromes, soft tissue stress, and joint pain develop in response to continued abnormal stresses.

Shortened iliotibial (IT) band with shortened tensor fasciae latae (TFL) or gluteus maximus. Often there are associated postural dysfunctions of an anterior PT posture, slouched posture, or flat back posture (see Chapter 15).

- *Anterior PT posture:* hip musculature imbalances
  - Short TFL and IT band
  - General limitation of hip external rotation
  - Weak, stretched posterior portion of the gluteus medius and piriformis
  - Excessive medial rotation of the femur during the first half of stance with increased stresses on the medial structures of the knee
  - Associated lower extremity compensations including medial rotation of the femur, genu valgum, lateral tibial torsion, pes planus, and hallux valgus
- *Slouched posture:* hip musculature imbalances
  - Shortened rectus femoris and hamstrings
  - General limitation of hip rotators
  - Weak, stretched iliopsoas
  - Weak and tight posterior portion of the gluteus medius
  - Weak, poorly developed gluteus maximus
  - Associated lower extremity compensations including hip extension, sometimes medial rotation of the femur, genu recurvatum, genu varum, and pes valgus
- *Flat back posture:* hip musculature imbalances
  - A shortened rectus femoris, IT band, and gluteus maximus
  - Variations of the above two postures

Dominance of the two-joint hip flexor muscles (TFL, rectus femoris, and sartorius) over the iliopsoas. This may cause faulty hip mechanics or knee pain from overuse of these muscles as they cross the knee.

Dominance of the TFL over the gluteus medius. This leads to lateral knee pain from IT band tension or medial rotation of the femur with medial knee stresses from an increased bowstring effect.

Dominance of hamstring muscles over the gluteus maximus. The gluteus maximus becomes short and range of hip flexion decreases; compensation occurs with excessive lumbar spine flexion whenever the thigh is flexed. Limited mobility in the gluteus maximus also causes increased tension on the IT band with associated trochanteric or lateral knee pain. Overuse of the hamstring muscles causes decreased flexibility as well as muscle imbalances with the quadriceps femoris muscle at the knee. The hamstrings dominate the stabilizing function by pulling posteriorly on the tibia to extend the knee in closed-chain activities. This alters the mechanics at the knee and may lead to overuse syndromes in the hamstring tendons or anterior knee pain from imbalances in quadriceps pull.

Use of lateral trunk muscles for hip abductors. This results in excessive trunk motion and increased stress in the lumbar spine.

Balance and Posture Control

The joint capsule is richly supplied with mechanoreceptors that respond to variations in position, stress, and movement for control of posture, balance, and movement. Reflex muscle contractions of the entire kinematic chain, known as balance strategies, occur in a predictable sequence when standing balance is disturbed and regained. Joint pathologies, restricted motion, or muscle weakness can impair balance and postural control.[17,27]

Nerves in the Hip and Buttock Region

Major Nerves Subject to Entrapment

Sciatic nerve. This nerve forms in the posterior region of the pelvis from the sacral plexus (L-4, L-5, S-1, S-2, and S-3 nerve roots) and leaves the pelvis across the lower edge of the greater sciatic notch. It then passes deep to the piriformis muscle. (Occasionally, it passes over or through the piriformis.) Entrapment results in sensory changes along the lateral and posterior portion of the leg and dorsal and plantar surface of the foot. Progressive weakness also develops in the hamstring muscles, a portion of the adductor magnus muscle, and all the muscles of the leg and foot.[37]

Obturator nerve. This nerve forms within the psoas muscle from nerve roots of L-2, L-3, and L-4 and enters the pelvis anterior to the sacroiliac joint. It then courses through the obturator canal along with the obturator vessels; there, it divides into the anterior and posterior branches. Injury or entrapment results in sensory changes along the medial aspect of the thigh and weakness primarily in the adductor muscles.[37]

Referred Pain from the Hip

The hip is innervated primarily from the L-3 spinal level; hip joint irritation is usually felt along the L-3 dermatome reference from the groin, down the front of the thigh to the knee.[19,47]

Referred Pain Into the Hip and Buttock Region

If painful symptoms are referred to this region from other sources, primary treatment must be directed to the source of the irritation. Common sources of referred pain into the hip and buttock region include:

- Irritation of nerve roots or tissues derived from spinal segments L-1, L-2, L-3, S-1, and S-2
- Lumbar intervertebral and sacroiliac joints

▶ Joint Hypomobility: Nonoperative Management

Related Diagnoses and Etiology of Symptoms

Osteoarthritis (Degenerative Joint Disease)

This is the most common arthritic disease of the hip joint. The etiology may be from aging, joint trauma, repetitive abnormal stresses, obesity, or disease. The degenerative changes include articular cartilage breakdown and loss, capsular fibrosis, and osteophyte formation at the joint margins.[22] These effects usually occur in regions undergoing greatest loading forces, such as along the superior weight-bearing surface of the acetabulum.

Other Joint Pathologies

Rheumatoid arthritis, aseptic necrosis, slipped epiphyses, dislocations, or congenital deformities can also lead to degenerative changes in the hip joint.

Postimmobilization Hypomobility

A restriction in the capsular tissues leading to joint hypomobilities as well as tightness in the surrounding periarticular tissues may occur anytime the joint is immobilized after a fracture or surgery.

Common Impairments

- Pain experienced in the groin and referred along the anterior thigh and knee in the L-3 dermatome.
- Stiffness after rest.
- Limited motion with a firm capsular end-feel. Initially limitation is only in internal rotation; in advanced stages the hip is fixed in adduction, has no internal rotation or extension past neutral, and is limited to 90 degrees of flexion.[19]
- Antalgic gait usually with a compensated gluteus medius (abductor) limp.
- Limited hip extension leading to increased extension forces on the lumbar spine and possible back pain.
- Limited hip extension preventing full knee extension when standing or during gait leading to increased knee stresses.
- Impaired balance and postural control.[27]

Common Functional Limitations/Disabilities

Hip joint impairments interfere with many weight-bearing and ADL activities.[14,28]

Early stages. Progressive pain with continued weight bearing and gait or at the end of the day after repetitive lower extremity activities. The pain may interfere with work (job-specific) or routine household activities that involve weight bearing, such as meal preparation, cleaning, and shopping.

Progressive degeneration. Increased difficulty rising up from a chair, climbing stairs, squatting, and other weight-bearing activities. Restricted routine ADL, such as bathing, toileting, and dressing (putting on pants, hose, socks).

Management: Protection Phase

Chapter 8 describes general principles and plan of care in the treatment of osteoarthritis and rheumatoid arthritis as well as general management of joints during acute, subacute, and chronic stages of tissue injury and repair. In conjunction with the medical management of the disease and inflammation, correction of faulty mechanics is an integral part of decreasing pain in the hip. Faulty hip mechanics may be caused by conditions such as obesity, leg-length differences, muscle length and strength imbalances, sacroiliac dysfunction,[14] poor posture, or injury to other joints in the chain.[9] The following goals and interventions are emphasized during the acute stage of tissue healing and the protection phase of nonoperative management.

Decrease Pain at Rest

- Apply grade I or II oscillation techniques with the joint in the resting position.
- Have the patient rock in a rocking chair to provide gentle oscillations to the lower extremity joints as well as a stimulus to the mechanoreceptors in the joints.[90]

Decrease Pain during Weight-Bearing Activities

- Provide assistive devices for ambulation to help reduce stress on the hip joint. If the pain is unilateral, teach the patient to walk with a single cane or crutch on the side opposite the painful joint.
- If a leg-length asymmetry is causing hip joint stress, gradually elevate the short leg with lifts in the shoe.
- Modify chairs to provide an elevated and firm surface, and adapt commodes with an elevated seat to make sitting and stand-to-sit activities easier.

Decrease Effects of Stiffness and Maintain Available Motion

- Instruct the patient in the importance of frequently moving the hips through their ROM throughout the day. When the acute symptoms are medically controlled, have the patient perform active ROM if he or she can control the motion or with assistance if necessary.
- If a pool is available, have the patient perform ROM in the buoyant environment.
- Initiate nonimpact activities such as swimming, gentle water aerobics, or stationary cycling.

Management: Controlled Motion and Return to Function Phases

As healing progresses and symptoms subside, the emphasis of management includes the following goals and interventions.

Progressively Increase Joint Play and Soft Tissue Mobility

Joint mobilization techniques. Progress joint mobilization to stretch grades (grade III sustained or grade III and IV oscillation) using the glides that stretch restricting capsular tissue at the end of the available ROM (see Box 12–1 and Figs. 6–46 through 6–48 in Chapter 6). Vigorous stretching should not be undertaken until the chronic stage of healing.

Passive stretching, neuromuscular inhibition, and self-stretching techniques. Stretch any range-limiting tissues. Suggested techniques are described in Chapter 5 and in the exercise section later in this chapter.

Improve Joint Tracking and Pain-Free Motion

Mobilization with movement (MWM) techniques[57] may be applied through the use of a mobilization belt to produce a pain-free inferolateral glide and then superimposing motion to the end of the available range. As with all MWM techniques, no pain should be experienced during the application of the technique.

Increase Internal Rotation

- Patient position and procedure: Supine with the involved hip flexed and a mobilization belt secured around the proximal thigh and your pelvis.
- Stabilize the patient's pelvis with the palm of the hand closest to the patient's head.
- Use the mobilization belt to produce a pain-free inferolateral glide while the caudal hand grips around the flexed thigh and shin to create pain-free end-range internal rotation (Fig. 12–1*A*).

Increase Flexion

- Patient position and procedure: Supine with the involved hip flexed and a mobilization belt secured around the proximal thigh and the pelvis.
- Stabilize the patient's pelvis with the palm of the hand closest to the patient's head.
- Use the mobilization belt to produce a pain-free inferolateral glide while the caudal hand grips around the flexed thigh and shin to create pain-free end-range flexion (Fig. 12–1*B*).

Increase Extension

- Patient position and procedure: Supine with the pelvis near the end of the treatment table in the Thomas test position (opposite thigh held against the chest) and a mobilization belt secured around the proximal thigh and your pelvis.
- Stabilize the patient's pelvis with the palm of the hand closest to the patient's head.
- Use the mobilization belt to produce a pain-free inferolateral glide while the caudal hand presses against the extended thigh to create pain-free end-range extension (Figure 12–1*C*).

Increase Extension in Weight Bearing

- Patient position and procedure: Standing with the unaffected foot up on a stool and a mobilization belt secured around the proximal thigh and your pelvis.
- Stabilize the pelvis with both hands, and apply a pain-free lateral glide with the mobilization belt while the patient lunges forward to produce a painless extension of the affected hip (Fig. 12–1*D*).

Progress Strength and Functional Use of Supporting Muscles

- Initiate exercises that develop control of the hip musculature, especially the gluteus maximus,

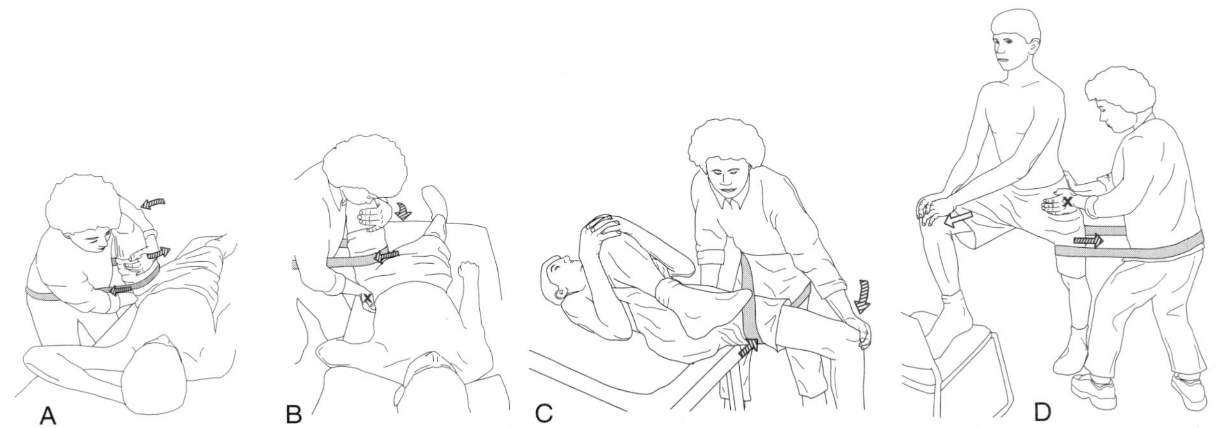

Figure 12–1 Mobilization with movement using an inferolateral glide *(A)* increasing pain-free internal rotation; *(B)* increasing pain-free flexion; *(C)* increasing pain-free extension; *(D)* increasing extension in weight bearing.

gluteus medius, and rotators, and that improve stability and balance when performing weight-bearing activities. Begin with submaximal isometric resistance; progress to dynamic resistance as the patient tolerates movement. If any exercises exacerbate the joint symptoms, reduce the intensity. Also reassess the patient's functional activities and adapt them to reduce the stress.

- Progress to functional exercises as tolerated using closed-chain and weight-bearing activities. The patient may require assistive devices while weight bearing. Use a pool or tank to reduce the effects of gravity to allow partial weight-bearing exercises without stress.
- Develop postural awareness and balance.
- Progress the low-impact aerobic exercise program (swimming or cycling or walking within tolerance).

Patient Education

Help the patient establish a balance between activity and rest and learn the importance of minimizing stressful deforming forces by maintaining muscle strength and flexibility in the hip region.

▶ Joint Surgery and Postoperative Management

Many types of joint surgeries are available to treat chronic joint disease of the hip and some fractures of the hip that compromise the vascular supply to the head of the femur. The procedures include *osteotomy* (which is actually an extra-articular procedure), *arthroscopy,* and arthroplasty of the hip, specifically *hemireplacement* and *total joint replacement* procedures.[38,49,88] *Arthrodesis* and *resection arthroplasty* of the hip are considered salvage procedures after failure of arthroplasty and when revision arthroplasty is contraindicated or not feasible.[49,88] The goals of joint surgery and postoperative management are to provide a patient with (1) a pain-free hip, (2) a stable joint for lower extremity weight bearing and functional ambulation, and (3) adequate ROM and strength of the lower extremity for functional activities.

It is important for the therapist to have a basic understanding of the more common surgical procedures for management of joint disease and deformity and a thorough knowledge of appropriate therapeutic exercise interventions and their progression for an effective and safe postoperative rehabilitation program.

Total Hip Arthroplasty

Indications for Surgery

The following are common indications for total hip arthroplasty (THA), also referred to as total hip replacement (THR):[15,21,25,49,51,88]

- Severe hip pain with motion and weight bearing leading to impaired function and health-related quality of life. This is the result of joint deterioration and loss of articular cartilage associated with rheumatoid or traumatic arthritis, osteoarthritis, ankylosing spondylitis, or osteonecrosis (avascular necrosis).
- Marked limitation of hip motion.
- Instability or deformity of the hip.
- Failure of conservative management or previous hip surgery (femoral stem hemiarthroplasty, total hip replacement, or resurfacing arthroplasty).

Note: THA is usually reserved for patients older than 60 to 65 years of age because the projected life span of current THA procedures is less than 20 years. Patients younger than 60 to 65 years of age who are expected to have low-demand usage may also be candidates for THA after evaluation on a case-by-case basis. These individuals are counseled by the surgeon to anticipate the need for revision arthroplasty later in life.[12,15,25]

Preoperative Management

Preoperative patient education has been advocated as an important aspect of the overall rehabilitation plan for many years.[2,5] Patient-related instruction in past years took place the day before surgery when patients were often admitted to the hospital for preoperative tests. In the current healthcare environment, hospital stays have been shortened dramatically. Preoperative contact with a patient prior to elective surgery now occurs on an outpatient basis individually or in a group several days before surgery. Preoperative management typically includes assessment and documentation of a patient's status as well as patient education about the procedure and what to expect in the early postoperative period.[12,32,49,59,74] Patient information sessions are often coordinated and conducted by a team of professionals from multiple disciplines who are likely to be involved with a patient's postoperative care. Box

Box 12–2 Components of Therapy-Related Preoperative Management: Preparation for Total Hip Arthroplasty

- Examination and evaluation of pain, ROM, muscle strength, balance, ambulatory status, leg lengths, gait characteristics, use of assistive devices, general level of function, perceived level of disability
- Information for patients and their families about joint disease and the operative procedure in nonmedical terms
- Postoperative precautions and their rationale including positioning and weight bearing
- Functional training for early postoperative days including bed mobility, transfers, gait training with assistive devices
- Early postoperative exercises
- Criteria for discharge from the hospital

12–2 summarizes possible components of preoperative management.[12,32,49,59,74]

Procedures

General background. Total hip arthroplasty has been successfully performed since the early 1960s.[13,15,23,25,56] Sir John Charnley,[13] a surgeon from England, is credited with the initial research and clinical application of THA, which subsequently has evolved into contemporary hip arthroplasty. A variety of implant designs, materials, and surgical approaches have been developed and modified over the years since the early replacements.[15,23,25] Total hip implants today are typically an inert metal (cobalt-chrome and titanium) femoral component and a high-density polyethylene acetabular component.

The revolutionary aspect of the early THA procedures was the use of acrylic cement, methyl methacrylate, for prosthetic fixation. Cement fixation allowed very early postoperative weight bearing and shortened the period of rehabilitation, whereas prior to the use of cement fixation patients were subjected to months of restricted weight bearing and limited mobility. Cement fixation continues to be used today but has been noted to have its drawbacks.

A significant postoperative complication, identified a number of years after the first THA procedures were performed, was aseptic (biomechanical) loosening of the prosthetic components at the bone-cement interface. It was shown that loosening subsequently led to a gradual recurrence of hip pain and the need for surgical revision.[15,25,49,54] Patients who most often developed loosening were identified as the younger, physically active patients. In contrast, loosening was not shown to be a particularly prevalent problem in elderly patients or in young patients with multiple joint involvement who typically tended to limit their level of physical activity.[25,71]

The long-term problem of loosening of some cemented implants, most often the acetabular component, gave rise to the development and use of cementless (biological) fixation.[15,25,49,54] Cementless fixation is achieved either by use of porous-coated prostheses that allow osseous ingrowth into the beaded or mesh-like surfaces of an implant or by a cementless press-fit technique.[7,45,68,87] Ingrowth of tissues occurs over a 3- to 6-month period of time with continued bone remodeling beyond that time period.[7,45,68,87]

Improvements in cemented fixation[6,48,53,71,72] as well as uncemented fixation[7,45,68,87] have continued as has debate over the benefits, indications, and disadvantages of both forms of fixation. Cement fixation is routinely used for patients with osteoporosis and poor bone stock and typically with elderly patients.[71,88] In contrast, cementless fixation is more often the choice for the patient under 60 years of age and who is quite physically active.[45,88] In responses to a very low rate of loosening of cemented femoral implants but continued problems of loosening of cemented acetabular components, the use of a hybrid procedure with an uncemented acetabular component and a cemented femoral prosthesis is now being advocated.[60]

The selection of the method of fixation is an important determinant of the progression of postoperative rehabilitation. Box 12–3 summarizes the factors that influence postoperative weight-bearing restrictions after cemented and uncemented THA.

Overview of procedures. A posterolateral, lateral, or anterolateral incision is made along the affected hip.

Box 12–3 Early Postoperative Weight-Bearing Restrictions After Total Hip Arthroplasty (THA)

Cemented THA. *Immediate postoperative weight bearing as tolerated*
Uncemented and hybrid THA. *Restricted weight bearing for at least 6 to 8 weeks*
Trochanteric osteotomy. *Restricted weight bearing at least 6 to 8 weeks or possibly 12 to 16 weeks*
Other considerations. *Stability of the prosthetic implants based on the surgeon's intraoperative evaluation of the quality of the patient's bone, alignment of the implants, degree of deformity, and need for repair of soft tissues or additional skeletal procedures*

The surgical approach affects the degree of exposure available to the surgeon during the operative procedure but also influences postoperative stability of the prosthetic hip and movement restrictions placed on the patient in the early phases of rehabilitation.[1,30,49,88] There is lack of agreement among surgeons as to which is the optimal approach because each has its advantages and disadvantages.[1,30]

- ***Posterolateral approach.*** This is the most frequently used approach for primary THA; the joint is accessed through the interval between the gluteus maximus and medius muscles. Consequently, this approach preserves the integrity of the gluteus maximus, gluteus medius, and vastus lateralis muscles. Trochanteric osteotomy is not necessary. The capsule is incised posteriorly and the short external rotators are released in preparation for hip dislocation. The primary disadvantage of this approach is that it is associated with the highest incidence of postoperative joint instability and resulting subluxation or dislocation of the hip.[41,52,55]
- ***Lateral approach.*** This approach requires a release of up to one-half of the proximal insertion or longitudinal splitting of the gluteus medius muscle as well as longitudinal splitting of the vastus lateralis muscle. It may involve a trochanteric osteotomy. Disruption of the abductor mechanism is associated with postoperative weakness and gait abnormalities (positive Trendelenburg sign).
- ***Anterolateral approach.*** This approach as well as an anterior approach was frequently used for primary THA in the early years of this procedure,[13] but today it is most often reserved for revision arthroplasty or arthroplasty that involves complex reconstruction. It is also indicated for patients with muscle imbalances associated with stroke or cerebral palsy whose standing posture is characterized by hip flexion and internal rotation.[1,30] Patients exhibiting this posturing are at high risk of dislocation with a posterolateral approach. The anterolateral approach provides excellent stability of the hip postoperatively but involves detachment and subsequent repair of the gluteus medius muscle or may necessitate an osteotomy of the greater trochanter for adequate exposure of the hip joint. In addition to the gluteus medius, soft tissues disturbed in an anterolateral approach include the gluteus minimus, tensor fasciae latae, iliopsoas, rectus femoris, and vastus lateralis muscles as well as the anterior capsule.

If a trochanteric osteotomy is performed, the trochanter must then be reattached and wired in place to stabilize the osteotomy site until bone healing occurs. The trochanter is often reattached in a position slightly distal to its normal anatomic position to apply tension on and to improve the mechanical efficiency of the gluteus medius muscle.[1,30] Complications associated with trochanteric osteotomy include nonunion, abductor muscle weakness and greater than usual soft tissue irritation and pain from a considerable amount of internal fixation.

After the hip joint is exposed, the capsule is released and the hip is dislocated. The head of the femur is removed and replaced with a metal intramedullary stemmed prosthesis. The acetabulum is remodeled, and a high-density polyethylene cup is inserted into the prepared acetabulum. To increase the stability of the hip and decrease the risk of postoperative dislocation, the cup replacement may be built up posteriorly or superiorly. The hip is reduced and soft tissues are repaired.

Postoperative Management

Immobilization

After surgery when the patient is lying in bed in the supine position, the operated limb must remain in a position of slight abduction and neutral rotation. An abduction pillow or wedge is usually sufficient, but the operated limb may sometimes be placed in a balanced sling suspension with the thigh and calf supported.[49,88]

Exercise and Functional Training

The use of therapeutic exercise interventions for patients after THA has been reported in the literature for several decades.[5,10,18,31,73] Although the timeframe for and extent of patient-therapist contact have substantially decreased since these early descriptive reports, the ultimate goal of rehabilitation remains the same: to optimize a patient's postoperative level of function. However, specific components, frequency, and progression of the rehabilitation programs have not been consistent or standardized.[20] More often than not rehabilitation programming has centered on protocols developed by and based on the opinions or assumptions of individual surgeons or therapy departments rather than on evidence-based research on the effects of specific exercises or gait-related activities on the hip joint itself or on functional outcomes. In addition, exercise protocols must often be adjusted to meet the needs and abilities of individual patients. Consequently the effectiveness of postoperative exercise has not been clearly supported, in part because of the significant variability of exercise protocols reported in the literature and used in the clinical setting.

A report from the National Institutes of Health (NIH) has identified the need for consistently applied and evaluated long- and short-term intervention strategies for rehabilitation after THA.[64] A recent consensus survey on physical therapy-related intervention for early inpatient total hip (and knee) rehabilitation is a step forward in the development of consistent guidelines for postoperative management.[20] The exercises and functional activities identified in the consensus document were elements common to most postoperative programs and only those agreed upon by the participating physical therapists.

The goals, guidelines, and precautions for exercise for THA discussed in this chapter represent not only those activities identified in the aforementioned consensus survey but also additional exercises selected from other resources in the current literature.[12,49,59] The suggested exercises, functional activities, and precautions are also based on the results of the available, albeit limited, research on the impact of specific exercises and functional activities on the hip joint. For example, several related single-subject studies have measured in vivo forces acting on the hip and acetabular contact pressures during exercise and gait.[26,40a,40b,81] Although these studies involved only two patients after insertion of a femoral endoprosthesis, not a total joint replacement, the results raise questions about assumptions made by clinicians with regard to the selection and progression of common exercises and functional activities during rehabilitation after hip arthroplasty. The results of these studies suggest that active or resistive exercises, performed either statically or dynamically, should be initiated and progressed cautiously. During the acute or postacute phases of rehabilitation some typical exercises, used in preparation for gait and other weight-bearing activities such as maximal effort gluteal setting, unassisted heel slides during the acute phase and manually resisted isometric abduction during the postacute stage of rehabilitation, may actually generate greater acetabular contact pressures than the weight-bearing activities themselves.[26,81]

Exercise: Maximum Protection Phase

In the early postoperative days and weeks after THA, the emphasis of rehabilitation is on prevention and patient education. Selected exercises or activities begin the day of or after surgery. The frequency of treatment by a therapist is often twice a day until the patient is discharged from the hospital.[20] Ideally, the prescribed exercises are performed hourly by the patient. The following goals and interventions apply to the initial postoperative days while the patient is hospitalized through the first few weeks after surgery when the patient is at home or in another healthcare facility.

- ***Prevent vascular and pulmonary complications.***
  - Ankle pumping exercise to prevent venous stasis, thrombus formation, and the potential for pulmonary embolism.
  - Deep breathing exercise and bronchial hygiene to prevent postoperative atelectasis or pneumonia.
  - Continue these two activities until the patient is up and about on a regular basis.
- ***Prevent postoperative dislocation or subluxation of the operated hip.***
  - Patient and caregiver education about motion restrictions, safe bed mobility, transfers, and precautions during other ADL.
  - Monitor the patient for signs and symptoms of dislocation, such as a shortening of the operated lower extremity not previously present.

Precautions: Postoperative precautions to minimize the risk of dislocation of the operated hip after THA are determined by the approach used during the surgery. Box 12–4 summarizes these precautions. (Also refer to Box 12–3 for weight-bearing restrictions.)

Note: The risk of instability is highest in the first month to 6 weeks postoperatively when soft tissues around the hip joint are not yet healed. Dislocation or subluxation occurs most frequently with the posterolateral surgical approach[1,30,41,49,52,55,76] but can also occur with lateral or anterolateral approaches.

- ***Achieve independent functional mobility prior to discharge.***
  - Bed mobility and transfer training integrating weight-bearing and motion restrictions (see Boxes 12–3 and 12–4).
  - Ambulation with an assistive device (usually a walker) immediately after surgery adhering to

Box 12–4 Early Postoperative Motion Precautions After Total Hip Arthroplasty

Posterolateral Approach

ROM

- Avoid hip flexion of more than 80–90 degrees and adduction and internal rotation beyond neutral.

ADL

- Transfer to the sound side from bed to chair or chair to bed.
- Do not cross legs.
- Keep the knees slightly lower than the hips when sitting.
- Avoid sitting in low, soft chairs.
- If the bed at home is low, raise it on blocks.
- Use a raised toilet seat.
- Avoid bending the trunk over the legs when rising from or sitting down in a chair or dressing or undressing.
- For bathing, take showers or use a shower chair in the bathtub.
- When ascending stairs lead with the sound leg. When descending, lead with the operated leg.
- Pivot on the sound lower extremity.
- Avoid activities in standing that involve rotating the body toward the operated extremity.
- Sleep in supine with an abduction pillow; avoid sleeping or resting in side-lying position.

Anterolateral and Lateral Approaches with or without Trochanteric Osteotomy

ROM

- Avoid hip extension, adduction, and external rotation past neutral.
- Avoid the combined motion of flexion, abduction, and external rotation.
- If the gluteus medius was reflected and reattached or if a trochanteric osteotomy was done, do not perform active antigravity hip abduction for at least 6–8 weeks or until approved by the surgeon.

ADL

- Follow precautions noted for a posterolateral approach to avoid excessive flexion and adduction.
- During early ambulation, step to rather than past the operated hip to avoid hyperextension.
- Avoid activities that involve standing on the operated extremity and rotating away from the involved side.

weight-bearing restrictions and gait-related ADL precautions noted in Box 12–4.

Note: Rising from a low chair imposes particularly high loads across the hip joint producing loads approximately 8 times body weight.[65] This places the involved hip at a very high risk of posterior dislocation until soft tissues around the hip joint have healed sufficiently (at least 6 weeks) or until the surgeon indicates unrestricted functional activities are permissable.

- ***Maintain a functional level of strength and muscular endurance in the upper extremities and unoperated lower extremity.***
  - Active-resistive exercises in functional movement patterns.
  - Target muscle groups used during transfers and ambulation with assistive devices.
- ***Prevent reflex inhibition and atrophy of musculature in the operated limb.***
  - *Submaximal* muscle-setting exercises of the quadriceps, hip extensor, and hip abductor muscles, just enough to elicit a muscle contraction.

Precaution: If a trochanteric osteotomy was performed, avoid even low-intensity isometric contractions of the hip abductors in the early postoperative phase unless initially approved by the surgeon and performed strictly at a minimum intensity. (See Box 12–4 for additional precautions after trochanteric osteotomy.)

- ***Regain active mobility and control of the operated extremity.***
  - While in bed, active-assistive (A-AROM) exercises of the hip within protected ranges.
  - Active knee flexion and extension exercises while seated in a chair, emphasizing terminal extension.
  - Progress from assisted to active hip and knee flexion (heel slides), gravity-eliminated hip abduction (if permissible) by sliding the leg on a low-friction surface, and active rotation between external rotation or internal rotation to neutral depending on the surgical approach. Do these exercises while lying supine in bed.
  - Progress to active hip exercises in the standing position with the knee flexed and extended with hands on a stable surface to maintain balance.
  - Perform bilateral closed-chain hip flexion and extension, placing only the allowable amount of weight on the operated extremity.
- ***Prevent a flexion contracture of the operated hip.***
  - Avoid use of a pillow under the knee of the operated extremity.
  - Apply a supine stretch to neutral in the Thomas test position. Pull the uninvolved knee to the chest while relaxing the operated hip or while performing a contraction of the hip extensors on the involved side.

- When rolling to prone-lying is permissible and is also tolerable, rest in prone for a prolonged passive stretch of the hip flexor muscles.

Precaution: Check with the surgeon before initiating a stretch of the hip flexors to neutral if the patient has undergone an anterolateral approach.

Exercise: Moderate and Minimum Protection Phases

Since the patient is typically hospitalized in an acute care facility for only 4 to 5 days postoperatively, the exercises described for the intermediate and late phases of rehabilitation that involve only moderate to minimum protection are a part of a home program that may be taught during home-based therapy, on an outpatient basis, or in an extended care facility. Some degree of moderate protection is indicated for 6 to 12 weeks postoperatively. Full healing of soft tissue and bone continues for a year after surgery.

Restoration of strength, muscular and cardiopulmonary endurance and ROM to functional levels is emphasized in the intermediate and final phases of rehabilitation. Postoperative precautions during ADL are continued for at least 12 weeks and often considerably longer.[49,59] Patient education continues throughout these phases in preparation for a return to anticipated activities in the home, workplace, or recreational setting.

- ***Regain strength and muscular endurance of the operated leg or any other involved areas.***
  - Continue active open- and closed-chain ROM exercises within the permissible ranges.
  - When unsupported standing is permitted, progress bilateral closed-chain exercises such as mini-squats by adding light-grade elastic resistance or while holding light weights in both hands.
  - When full weight bearing is permitted on the involved lower extremity, perform unilateral closed-chain exercises such as forward and lateral step-ups (to a low step) and partial lunges with the involved foot forward.
  - Emphasize increasing the number of repetitions rather than the resistance to improve muscular endurance.

Precaution: Using heavy exercise loads, such as high-intensity weight training, is not appropriate for patients after THA as this may contribute to long-term prosthetic loosening.

- ***Improve cardiorespiratory endurance.***
  - Initiate a nonimpact aerobic conditioning program with progressive cycling, swimming or water aerobics.
- ***Restore functional ROM of the operated hip.***
  - Reduce contractures if they have developed while adhering to motion precautions.
  - Continue or initiate positional stretching to reduce a hip flexion contracture by lying prone or by lying supine in the Thomas position as previously described.
  - Integrate ROM into functional activities.
- ***Progress weight bearing during ambulation, improve balance, and correct gait deviations.***
  - Continue or progress to using a cane in the hand *contralateral* to the operated hip. This may have been initiated as early as 3 weeks postoperatively after a cemented procedure or delayed for 6 to 12 weeks with uncemented fixation or after trochanteric osteotomy.
  - While using a cane, walk over uneven and soft surfaces to challenge the balance system.

Note: Use of a cane in the contralateral hand by patients after a hip replacement has been shown to decrease EMG activity in the hip abductor muscles to a significant degree regardless of whether moderate or near-maximum force is applied into the cane.[63] In the same study, ipsilateral cane use produced no significant decrease in EMG activity in the hip abductor muscles. The degree to which the decreases in EMG activity reflected a reduction in forces imposed on the prosthetic hip joint was not determined in this study. However, in single-subject studies of two different patients with femoral endoprotheses acetabular contact pressures were reduced by use of a cane in the contralateral hand.[26,40a,40b]

- Emphasize correct posture during ambulation (erect trunk, vertical alignment, equal step lengths, and a neutral symmetrical position of the legs).
- Continue cane use until weight-bearing restrictions are discontinued or if the patient exhibits gait deviations, such as a positive Trendelenburg sign on the operated lower extremity, indicating gluteus medius weakness. Cane use is also recommended during extended periods of ambulation to decrease muscle fatigue.

- ***Prepare the patient to return to a full level of functional activities.***
  - Integrate strength and endurance exercises into functional activities, but continue to avoid the application of high loads during exercise. When weight-bearing restrictions have been discontinued, strengthen hip and knee musculature with functional activities such as ascending and descending stairs step over step.
  - Extend the length of time and distances of a low-intensity walking program 2 to 4 days a week.
  - Through patient education reinforce the importance of selecting activities that reduce or minimize the forces and demands placed on the prosthetic hip.

Precaution: During ambulation in the course of daily work- or home-related activities, if the patient must carry a heavy load in one hand, suggest that it be carried in the upper extremity *ipsilateral* to the operated hip to theoretically reduce the stresses imposed over time on the prosthetic hip. The results of research suggest that the forces imposed on the abductor muscles of the prosthetic hip, as measured by EMG, are significantly lower when a load is carried in the arm ipsilateral to the prosthetic hip as compared to when the load is carried in the contralateral arm. This holds true with and without cane usage.[61,62] As the patient's activity level increases, have the patient avoid high-impact activities or activities that impose heavy rotational forces on the operated limb. Both factors can contribute to long-term loosening and wear of the prosthetic implants and eventual failure of the hip replacement.

Outcomes

The asssessment of outcomes of total hip arthroplasty has focused on numerous variables, ranging from patient satisfaction and the impact of THA on function and quality of life to the assessment of prosthetic designs, materials, methods of fixation, and rates of complications. The number of follow-up studies on any one of these areas is extensive. A 1990s NIH report points out that THA and subsequent rehabilitation have resulted in a high degree of success in the categories of pain reduction, improvements in physical function, and health-related quality of life.[43,64] The report goes on to say that THA results in good to excellent long-term results for 90 to 95% of patients.[64] Studies to date indicate that both cemented and cementless THA have yielded equally positive postoperative outcomes in all areas of assessment with the most consistent being a reduction of pain.[45,71]

Patient satisfaction after THA as well as the assessment of pain and perceived level of function as judged by the patient and/or the surgeon generally reflect a marked decrease in pain and improvement in function.[69] Traditionally, patient-related outcomes have been assessed by the surgeon rather than the patient. In the past decade or two, assessing outcomes from a patient's perspective has become increasingly evident in the literature. In a recent study, patients' and physicians' assessments of pain and level of satisfaction were reported to be very similar when patients reported little or no pain. However, as a patient's report of continuing pain increased, the disparity increased between the patient's and the physician's assessment of the level of patient satisfaction.[46] This study points out the need for evaluations by both the patient and the surgeon to fully assess the long-term outcomes of THA and postoperative rehabilitation.

Improvements in level of function occur gradually after THA. Patients typically achieve 90% of their expected level of functional improvement by the end of the first year after surgery. During the next 1 to 2 years patients report additional gains in strength with improvement in function reaching a plateau at approximately 2 to 3 years.[69] In one study, muscle weakness in the operated extremity was noted in all patients at 2 years after surgery with strength in the hip flexors showing the slowest rate of recovery.[78] The investigator suggested that persistent muscle weakness and muscle fatigue during activities that require endurance may increase the stresses placed on the prosthetic implants and contribute to biomechanical loosening of the implant.[78] As such, some patients may benefit from a long-term exercise program even after returning to a full level of functional activity. To prolong the life of the prosthesis, particularly in patients under 50 to 60 years of age, patients are routinely advised to refrain from high-impact sports and recreational activities.[50] If a patient's employment involves heavy labor, vocational retraining or an adjustment in work-related activities is advised.

Despite the success of both cemented and uncemented THA, debate continues as to the benefits and limitations of both types of fixation. What can be said is that as surgical technique, prosthetic designs, and materials continue to improve, the rate of failure because of wear and loosening continues to decrease. The highest rate of loosening continues to occur in the acetabular component.[71,72] In-depth analysis and current information on outcomes of specific prosthetic designs[23] as well as outcome assessments of cemented,[6,48,53,71] uncemented,[7,45,68,87] and hybrid[60] procedures can be found in the references noted.

Finally, in spite of the number of sources in the literature that emphasize the importance of rehabilitation programs or more specifically a postoperative exercise and ambulation program after THA, the impact of these postoperative interventions has not been clearly determined. The NIH reports that there is currently insufficient evidence to determine what constitutes an appropriate level of physical therapy utilization after THA. The report goes on to say that there does appear to be a role for these interventions but that the efficacy of these postoperative programs has not yet been determined.[64] Studies have demonstrated that access to inpatient physical therapy services does[24,58] and does not[42] decrease a patient's length of stay in an acute care facility after THA. The use of physical therapy services after THA has also been shown to increase the probability of discharge to the home setting rather than to another health-care facility.[24]

Studies with control groups that have evaluated the impact of exercise on functional outcomes in patients who have undergone THA are few in number. The few control group studies that do exist have looked at the effect of exercise several months or even a year or two after surgery, not during the first 6 to 12 weeks. One such example is noted here. In a nonrandomized study of the effectiveness of a 6-week home exercise program with patients who were 6 to 48 months post-THA, the two exercise groups (one performing ROM and isometric exercises of the hip, and the other group performing ROM, isometric, and eccentric exercises) increased their walking speed, whereas a control group (no exercise program) did not. Interestingly, strength improvements were noted in all three groups.[77] A great deal more research needs to be done on the effects of exercise on function after THA.

Hemiarthroplasty of the Hip

Indications of Surgery

The following are possible indications for prosthetic replacement of the proximal femur. [1,10,40,48]

- Acute, displaced intracapsular (subcapital, transcervical) fractures of the proximal femur in an elderly patient with poor bone stock and an anticipated low-demand level of activity after surgery[38,51,66,83]
- Failed internal fixation of intracapsular fractures associated with osteonecrosis of the head of the femur[38,51]
- Severe degeneration of the head of the femur (but an intact acetabulum) associated with long-standing hip disease or deformity resulting in disabling pain and loss of function that cannot be managed with nonoperative procedures[38,51,66]

Note: Patients with pre-existing degenerative hip disease who sustain a femoral fracture are candidates for primary THA rather than hemiarthroplasty.[21,51] Acute, severely comminuted intertrochanteric fractures are *infrequently* managed by primary hemiarthroplasty.[51,84]

Procedures

Background. Historically, acute displaced fractures of the proximal femur in the elderly were treated with unipolar (fixed head), uncemented metal-stemmed endoprostheses with marginal results. With the introduction of cement fixation in the 1960s, these results improved.[51] The primary complication associated with the single component unipolar implants, regardless of design or fixation, was progressive erosion of the acetabular cartilage and subsequent pain.

To decrease the problem of acetabular wear, the bipolar hemiarthroplasty was developed. The bipolar design is composed of multiple components: a metal ball and stem femoral prosthesis (which may be modular) that moves within a free-riding polyethylene shell which, in turn, inserts into a metal cup which moves within the acetabulum. The purpose of the multiple-surface, load-bearing design is to displace forces incurred by the acetabulum through the interposed components rather than directly to the acetabulum to lessen the erosion of the acetabular cartilage.[38,51] Both current-day modular unipolar and bipolar prostheses continue to be used today. Considerable differences of opinion exist among surgeons regarding the advantages and disadvantages of one design versus the other.[38,51]

Operative procedure. As with THA, a posterolateral approach is most commonly used. After removal of the head of the femur, the metal-stemmed prosthesis is inserted into the shaft of the proximal femur.

The femoral stem is usually cemented in place, but bioingrowth fixation has also been used. Procedures for closure are consistent with THA.

Postoperative Management

In the literature there are no studies that have examined the effects of comprehensive postoperative exercise programs exclusively for patients who have undergone current-day hemiarthroplasty. This is because, for the most part, considerations and precautions for positioning and ADL as well as the components and progression of the exercise and ambulation program are similar to postoperative management of THA. These guidelines have been detailed in the previous section of this chapter. As with postoperative management after THA, selection and progression of exercises and functional activities after hemiarthroplasty also tend to be based on the opinions of surgeons and therapists as to the potential of specific exercises to remediate impairments and improve functional performance. Consequently, the effectiveness of exercise after hemiarthroplasty also remains unclear. Only limited information on the impact of specific exercises and gait-related activities on the hip joint per se after hemiarthroplasty is available in the literature. Some findings from several single-subject studies of two patients with femoral endoprostheses have already been discussed in rhe previous section of this chapter on THA.[26,40a,40b,81]

Precaution: Given the significant concerns for long-term erosion of acetabular cartilage after hemiarthroplasty, it may be even more critical to avoid exercises that impose the greatest compressive or shearing forces across the hip joint and, therefore, pose the greatest potential for erosion of the cartilaginous surface of the acetabulum. Exercises should be performed initially at a submaximal level and then progressed gradually. *Unassisted* heel slides and *maximum* effort gluteal setting exercises may need to be avoided in the acute phase of postoperative rehabilitation.[81] During the postacute period of rehabilitation exercises, such as maximum effort manually resisted hip abduction may actually generate greater forces across the hip than protected weight-bearing activities.[26]

Outcomes

Present-day modular unipolar and bipolar hemiarthroplasty procedures appear to yield similar results in pain relief, functional outcomes, and type and rate of complications.[38,51] Although acetabular wear was identified as the primary concern after the unipolar replacement used in the 1960s and 1970s, the mechanical effectiveness of the bipolar prosthesis in preventing acetabular erosion has yet to be firmly established.[38] In a recent study of community-dwelling patients age 65 years or older (mean age 80), who had undergone a hemiarthroplasty with either a bipolar implant or a modular unipolar implant, there were no significant differences between the two groups at 1 year and 4 to 5 years of follow-up with regard to functioning in daily activities or rates of dislocation, infection, and mortality.[89] Another study has suggested that joint ROM may decrease over time after bipolar hemiarthroplasty possibly due to the design of the implants. This decreased range was not associated with diminished functional abilities.[34]

Fractures of the Proximal Femur and Postoperative Management

Background

One of the more common musculoskeletal problems in the elderly is fracture of the hip, or more correctly, fracture of the most proximal portion of the femur in the hip joint area.

More than 70% of hip fractures occur in individuals who are more than 70 years of age, and they occur in women significantly more often than in men.[8,38] In the United States, for example, women sustain 84.6% of all hip fractures.[70] Worldwide, the incidence of hip fracture is increasing, in part because of the aging of the population.[8,38,66] Less than 2 to 3% of fractures are sustained by persons who are less than 50 years of age.[38,66] These fractures or fracture-dislocations are usually associated with high-force, high-impact trauma but may also be associated with repetitive microtrauma.[38,66]

Multiple factors contribute to the increasing incidence of hip fracture with age. Osteoporosis, a condition associated with age-related loss of bone density and strength, typically occurs in the proximal femur as well as distal radius and spine.[38,66] Either a sudden twisting motion of the lower extremity or the impact from a fall can cause a pathologic fracture of a fragile proximal femur. Although 90% of all hip fractures in the elderly are associated with a fall,[38] there is always the question of whether trauma from the fall caused the hip fracture or a pathologic fracture of the hip caused the fall. Despite the increasing incidence of osteoporosis with age, the cause of most hip fractures appears to be from impaired functional mobility rather than osteoporosis.[4] Specifically, balance and protective reactions and muscle power deteriorate with age, thus increasing the likelihood of a fall combined with a decreasing ability to absorb the subsequent impact of a fall.[66] Characteristics of falling change with age, which may also increase the risk of hip fracture in the elderly. As walking speed decreases with age, particularly past 70 to 80 years of age, when a loss of balance and fall occurs, an older person usually drops and falls to the side, rather than falling forward on outstretched hands as occurs with faster walking speeds.[38,66]

Hip fracture in the elderly is associated with a high rate of disability because of a loss of independence in mobility.[16] Many patients require long-term nursing care and often are permanently institutionalized in extended care or assisted living facilities. For example, among women who sustain a hip fracture, approximately 15 to 25% lose the ability to live independently within the first year.[8] Although postoperative mortality rates remain high (approximately 20%),[16] improved surgical techniques over the past few decades have decreased the necessity of prolonged immobilization or restricted weight bearing, thus decreasing postoperative complications such as pneumonia and thromboemboli.

The acute signs and symptoms of hip fracture are pain in the groin or hip region or pain with active or passive motion of the hip or with lower extremity weight bearing. The lower extremity appears to be shorter by several centimeters and assumes a position of external rotation.[38,66]

Common sites and types of hip fracture are noted in Box 12–5.[38,51,66,83,84,85] Intracapsular fractures can potentially compromise the vascular supply to the head of the femur which, in turn, increases the risk of delayed healing, nonunion, or osteonecrosis (avascular necrosis) of the head of the femur. These complications occur far more frequently with displaced versus nondisplaced intracapsular fractures.[38,51] Intracapsular fractures are most often sustained by elderly women.[38,51]

In contrast, fracture-dislocation and acetabular trauma is most common in the young, active individual.[38] Most fracture-dislocations occur in a posterior direction. This type of fracture often causes traumatic disruption of the vascular supply to the head of the femur and damage to joint cartilage, resulting in osteonecrosis and post-traumatic arthritis and eventually necessitating prosthetic replacement of the hip joint. However, this need may not arise for many years.

Box 12–5 Common Sites and Types of Hip Fracture

Intracapsular

- Fracture site proximal to the attachment of the hip joint capsule
- May disturb the blood supply to the head of the femur
- Further subdivided into *subcapital* and *transcervical* (femoral neck) fractures
- May be displaced, nondisplaced, or impacted

Extracapsular

- Fracture site distal to the capsule to a line 5 cm distal to the lesser trochanter
- Does not disturb the blood supply to the head of the femur
- Further subdivided into *intertrochanteric* (between the greater and lesser trochanters) or *subtrochanteric* and *stable* or *unstable* (comminuted)

Open Reduction and Internal Fixation of Hip Fracture

Indications for Surgery

Surgical intervention by means of open (or possibly closed) reduction followed by stabilization with internal fixation is indicated for the following types of fractures of the proximal femur.[38,66,83,84,85]

- Displaced or nondisplaced intracapsular femoral neck fractures
- Fracture-dislocations of the head of the femur
- Stable or unstable intertrochanteric fractures
- Subtrochanteric fractures

In the elderly patient, displaced intracapsular fractures are typically treated with prosthetic replacement of the femoral head to avoid a relatively high incidence of nonunion. Some severely comminuted (unstable) intertrochanteric fractures may also be managed in this manner.[38,51,84]

In a few situations, nonoperative management is the treatment of choice. Traction is an appropriate alternative for nonambulatory individuals or for medically unstable patients who cannot undergo a surgical procedure.[38,66] The patient remains in bed in traction just long enough for early healing to occur. Bed to chair mobilization follows. If weight bearing or ambulation is feasible, it is delayed until bone healing is sufficient, usually 10 to 12 or as long as 16 weeks postoperatively.

Procedures

The goal of surgery is to achieve maximum stability and restore alignment of bony structures of the hip. Surgery is indicated in the first 24 to 48 hours after injury particularly with femoral neck fractures where the risk of disruption of the vascular supply to the head of the femur is high. A variety of internal fixation devices are used after open or closed reduction to stabilize the many different types of fractures of the proximal femur. The type and severity of the fracture and associated injuries as well as the patient's age and physical and cognitive status all influence the surgeon's choice of procedure.[38,66] The type of procedure performed, in turn, affects the progression of postoperative management. The most common current-day internal fixation devices used, based on the type of fracture, include the following:[38,66,83,84,85]

- *In situ* fixation with multiple parallel cancellous lag screws or pins for nondisplaced or impacted femoral neck fractures and possibly for displaced femoral neck fractures in active patients less than 65 years of age.
- Dynamic extramedullary fixation with a sliding (compression) hip screw and lateral side plate for stable intertrochanteric fractures; may be combined with an osteotomy for unstable (comminuted) fractures. The dynamic hip screw allows sliding between the screw and plate and creates compression across the fracture site during early weight bearing.
- Static interlocking intramedullary nail fixation or a sliding hip screw coupled with an intramedullary nail for subtrochanteric fractures.

In these procedures, an open lateral approach is used. Aspects of some procedures may be performed percutaneously. Soft tissue disruption differs with each procedure. The tensor fasciae latae (TFL) vastus lateralis or gluteus medius may be incised (parallel to the fibers); a capsulotomy is generally performed with femoral neck fractures.

Postoperative Management

The primary goal of postoperative care is to first get the patient up and moving as quickly as possible and then return the patient to a preinjury level of function.[31,38,66] During the period of fracture healing, which typically extends for 10 to 16 weeks, internal fixation of the fracture site coupled with immediate postoperative rehabilitation activities enables this to happen. Early mobility also minimizes the adverse effects of prolonged bed rest. Despite the well-accepted benefits of early ambulation and exercise, there is always the risk of failure of the internal fixation. Box 12–6 describes signs of possible displacement or loosening of the fracture stabilization device. These signs should be reported immediately to the surgeon.[31,38,66]

In addition to early ambulation, functional mobility, and exercise, postoperative rehabilitation includes patient or caregiver education for wound care, deep breathing and coughing exercises, edema control (use of compressive stockings, an intermittent compression unit or massage), and proper positioning in bed to avoid contractures.

Weight-Bearing Considerations

The amount of early postoperative weight bearing during ambulation and transfers is always determined by the surgeon on an individual basis for each patient. Factors that influence the decision are the patient's age and bone quality, the fracture location and pattern, type of implant used for fixation of the fracture site and, of course, the degree of intraoperative stability achieved.[31,38,40,66] Recommendations range from nonweight-bearing, toe-touch or touch-down weight bearing (less than 10 lb) to weight bearing as tolerated.

Many fixation procedures used today make early weight bearing feasible. Some examples of fractures and fixation procedures in which weight bearing as tolerated is permissible immediately after surgery are:

- Undisplaced, rigidly fixed, or impacted femoral neck fractures managed with *in situ* fixation[38,40,66,83]
- Stable (noncomminuted) intertrochanteric fractures managed with a dynamic (sliding) hip screw and lateral side plate fixation[38,66,84]
- Stable subtrochanteric fractures managed with interlocking intramedullary nailing and bone-to-bone fixation[38,66,85]

Box 12–6 Signs of Possible Failure of the Internal Fixation Mechanism

- Severe, persistent groin, thigh, or knee pain that increases with limb movement or weight bearing
- Progressive limb length inequality (shortening of the involved lower extremity) that was not present immediately after surgery
- Persistent external rotation of the operated limb
- A positive Trendelenburg sign during weight bearing on the involved limb that does not resolve with strengthening exercises

Even when weight bearing is curtailed during ambulation and transfers, the fracture site is still subjected to significant forces. For example, moving in bed, getting up to the side of the bed, and active and resisted ROM exercises all generate forces across the hip that approach or even exceed those incurred during unsupported (full weight bearing) ambulation.[65] With this in mind, in one study, elderly patients with stable as well as comminuted intertrochanteric fractures treated with dynamic hip screw and plate fixation were all allowed to bear weight as tolerated during ambulation with an assistive device immediately after surgery. One year postoperatively there was no significant difference between the rate of implant failure and revision surgery in the patients with stable and those with comminuted fractures. The investigators concluded that at least in elderly patients with comminuted and noncomminuted intertrochanteric fractures that could be stabilized intraoperatively, there was little biomechanical justification for nonweight-bearing restrictions postoperatively.[40] Excluded from this generalization were patients with complex fractures in whom satisfactory intraoperative stabilization could not be achieved, young patients with displaced femoral neck fractures with *in situ* fixation, and patients with severe bone disease, for example, as the result of malignancy.

Exercise

The progression of exercise is dependent on the location and stability of the fracture site, type of repair, and soft tissue traumatized. Some degree of protection during exercise is necessary over the course of soft tissue healing (approximately 6 weeks) and bone healing (between 10 and 16 weeks).[83,84,85] Special considerations for exercise after hip fracture are noted in Box 12–7.[38,66,83,84,85]

Box 12–7 Special Considerations for Exercise and Gait After Internal Fixation of Fractures of the Proximal Femur

- Multiple hip muscles are traumatized by fracture of the hip leading to postoperative pain, reflex inhibition, and weakness. Fractures that involve the following sites cause damage to the following muscles:
  - Greater trochanter: gluteus medius
  - Lesser trochanter: iliopsoas
  - Subtrochanteric region: gluteus maximus
- The tensor fasciae latae (TFL) and vastus lateralis (VL) are usually incised during surgery, causing postoperative pain, inhibition, and weakness during hip abduction and knee flexion.
- Adhesion formation may develop between the incised TFL and VL and restrict motion. Hip adduction and internal rotation and knee flexion place a stretch on the TFL and VL, respectively, during ROM exercises and, therefore, are often painful.
- If there is shortening of the involved limb after fracture and internal fixation, the distance between the distal insertion of the gluteus medius on the greater trochanter and the center of axis of hip motion is often decreased, thus diminishing the mechanical advantage of the muscle and causing weakness and a positive Tendelenburg sign during ambulation.
- Intracapsular fractures typically traumatize the capsule, and internal fixation requires an incision into the capsule (capsulotomy). Both predispose the capsule to postoperative restriction.

Exercise: Maximum Protection Phase

Exercises begin on the first postoperative day. All exercises are performed within the limits of pain. It is reasonable to expect to achieve 80 to 90 degrees of active hip flexion (with the knee flexed) by 2 to 4 weeks postoperatively.[31,38] During the early phase of rehabilitation efforts are directed toward helping the patient learn to transfer and ambulate independently with an assistive device.

- ***Prevent vascular and pulmonary complications.***
  - Active ankle exercises (pumping exercises) performed regularly throughout the day to maintain circulation and prevent thromboemboli.
  - Deep breathing exercises and airway clearance to prevent pulmonary complicaitons.
- ***Improve strength in the upper and sound lower extremities.***
  - Target key muscle groups used to lift body weight during transfers and ambulation with assistive devices.
  - Emphasize closed-chain training to simulate the necessary movement patterns used.
- ***Prevent postoperative reflex inhibition of hip and knee musculature.***
  - Low-intensity isometric exercise of the hip and knee musculature. Depending on the fracture site and its stability, perform submaximal gluteal, abductor, adductor, and quadriceps and hamstring setting exercises.

Precaution: After comminuted subtrochanteric fractures and medial cortex reconstruction, avoid abductor and adductor setting exercises as these contractions place stresses across the fracture site.[85]

- ***Restore dynamic control and active mobility of the involved hip and adjacent joints.***
  - Active-assistive, progressing to active ROM of the

involved hip and knee while lying supine or sitting.

- As pain subsides, add unassisted straight leg lifts in flexion abduction and extension *while standing* on the sound leg and holding on to a stable surface for balance.
- Pelvic tilts and knee-to-chest movements with the *uninvolved* leg to prevent stiffness in the low back region.

Precautions: Hip and even knee motions are quite painful postoperatively; therefore progress ROM exercises very gradually. For example, initially have the patient perform assisted rather than unassisted heel slides, and perform heel slides prior to straight leg raises while lying supine. The shorter moment arm when the knee is flexed places lower rotational loads on the fracture site than a long moment arm.

After subtrochanteric fractures that required medial cortex reconstruction, initially perform only hip flexion and extension and postpone active abduction and adduction for 4 to 6 weeks.[85]

Exercise: Moderate and Minimum Protection Phases

By 6 weeks, soft tissues are healed, and by 8 to 12 weeks, depending on the age and health of the patient, some degree of bone healing has occurred. In most instances at least partial weight bearing is permissible. The emphasis during the intermediate and final phases of rehabilitation focuses on increasing strength and functional control of the involved lower extremity and gradually increasing the patient's level of functional activities. The following goals and activities may be included.

- ***Increase flexibility of any chronically shortened muscles.***
  - Heel cord stretching with a towel or the assistance of a caregiver.
  - Supine stretch in the Thomas test position to elongate the hip flexors
  - Hamstring stretching by sitting on the edge of a table with one leg supported in hip flexion and knee extension and the other in extension over the side of the support surface.
- ***Improve strength and muscular endurance in the lower extremities for functional activities.***

Note: There is lack of agreement whether or not light resistance exercises of the involved hip should be done before the fracture site has fully healed.[31] (Bone healing typically takes 8 to 16 weeks or up to 6 months in some patients.) Communication with the surgeon is advisable before initiating resistance exercises of the hip.

  - As soon as partial weight bearing is permissible, progress to bilateral closed-chain active exercise, such as minisquats and heel raises using a table or walker for support and balance and body weight as the source of resistance. When weight bearing is allowable to tolerance, add lunges and forward and lateral step-ups.
  - Add open-chain hip and knee exercises against light resistance (up to 5 lb) with elastic resistance or cuff weights. Hip extension and abduction are emphasized for a positive impact on ambulation.
- ***Improve postural stability and standing balance.***
  - Follow a progression of balance activities appropriate for the patient's age and desired activity level.
- ***Increase cardiorespiratory endurance.***
  - Stationary bicycling, upper body ergometry, or treadmill walking
  - Progressive ambulation on various types of surfaces
  - Aerobic activities possibly in age-appropriate exercise classes

Outcomes

The true measure of success of surgical intervention and postoperative rehabilitation is the extent to which a patient can return to his or her prefracture level of function. The level of preinjury functional mobility in patients with femoral neck fractures has been shown to be a critical factor in postoperative survival.[32] In one follow-up study of patients after hip fracture, only 33% had regained their preinjury level of function in basic ADL and IADL 1 year postoperatively.[35] Given the advanced age and health status of the "average" patient who sustains a hip fracture, it is not surprising that mortality rates 1 year postoperatively are high, ranging from 12 to 36% depending on the mean age, general health status, and severity of fracture.[38] After 1 year mortality rates are equal to age-matched subjects who have not sustained a hip fracture.[38] Of the patients who survive 1 year postoperatively the ability to independently ambulate (50 feet on an uncarpeted surface) was 83% in one study.[3] In another study 92% of patients returned to independent ambulation, but only 41% regained their prefracture level of ambulation.[39]

The impact of exercise and functional training on

outcomes has also been investigated. The number of visits to physical therapy has been positively associated with the ability to ambulate independently.[3] In another study,[29] the frequency of physical therapy appeared to increase the odds of regaining functional independence and going directly home from an acute care setting after hip fracture surgery. In a third study[79] subjects, most of whom were living in the community and were an average of 7 months postfracture surgery, who participated in a 1-month home exercise program, increased the strength of the knee extensors and increased their walking velocity. In contrast, the results of a study of subjects who received a long-term, home-based, multifaceted rehabilitation program (including extensive ADL and IADL training) for 6 months postoperatively in comparison to a traditional postoperative exercise and ambulation program for an equal period of time demonstrated no significant differences.[86]

Painful Hip Syndromes/ Overuse Syndromes: Nonoperative Management

Related Diagnoses and Etiology of Symptoms

Trochanteric Bursitis

Pain is experienced over the lateral hip and possibly down the lateral thigh to the knee when the iliotibial band rubs over the trochanter. Discomfort may be experienced after standing asymmetrically for long periods with the affected hip elevated and adducted and pelvis dropped on the opposite side. Ambulation and climbing stairs aggravates the condition. Muscle flexibility and strength imbalances and the resulting faulty posture of the pelvis may be the predisposing factors leading to bursal irritation.

Psoas Bursitis

Pain is experienced in the groin or anterior thigh and possibly into the patellar area. It is aggravated during activities requiring excessive hip flexion.

Ischiogluteal Bursitis (Tailor's or Weaver's Bottom)

Pain is experienced around the ischial tuberosities, especially when sitting. If the adjacent sciatic nerve is irritated from the swelling, symptoms of sciatica may occur.

Tendinitis or Muscle Pull

Overuse or trauma to any of the muscles in the hip region can occur from excessive strain while the muscle is contracting (often in a stretched position) or from repetitive use and not allowing the injured tissue to heal between activities. Common problems include hip flexor, adductor, and hamstring strains. Poor flexibility and fatigue may predispose an individual to strain and injury during an activity or sporting event, or sudden falls such as slipping on ice may result in the strain.

Common Impairments

- ***Pain.*** Symptoms occur when the involved muscle contracts, when it is stretched, or when the provoking activity is repeated.
- ***Gait deviations.*** Slightly shorter stance occurs on the painful side. There may be a slight lurch when the involved muscle contracts to protect the muscle.
- ***Imbalance in muscle flexibility and strength.*** Muscle flexibility or dominance in use may be the precipitating factor in many painful hip syndromes. Common imbalances are described on pages 472 and 473. Overuse syndromes are associated with (1) dominance of the tensor fasciae latae and rectus femoris as hip flexors and abductors, with weak gluteus medius and minimus muscles, (2) dominance of the hamstrings over the gluteus maximus, and (3) shortened lateral rotators. Because of the relationship of these muscles with the pelvis and knee, patients may present with low back or knee symptoms.
- ***Decreased muscular endurance.***

Common Functional Limitations/Disabilities

- Inability to do the provoking activity
- Decreased ambulation

Management: Protection Phase

Control Inflammation and Promote Healing

When there is chronic irritation or inflammation from an acute injury, follow the guidelines as described in Chapter 8 with emphasis on rest of the involved tissue by not stressing or putting pressure on it. Have the patient avoid doing the provoking activity, and if necessary, decrease the amount and time walking or use an assistive device.

Develop Support in Related Areas

Initiate exercises to develop neuromuscular control for alignment of the pelvis and hip. Avoid stressing the inflamed tissue. Patient education and cooperation are necessary to reduce repetitive trauma.

Management: Controlled Motion Phase

Note: When the acute symptoms have decreased, initiate a progressive exercise program within the tolerance of the involved tissues that emphasizes regaining a balance in length, neuromuscular control, strength, and endurance in the muscles of the hip and rest of the lower extremity.

Develop a Strong Mobile Scar and Regain Flexibility

Remodel the scar in muscle or tendon by applying cross-fiber massage to the site of the lesion followed by multiple-angle submaximal isometrics in pain-free positions.

Develop a Balance in Length and Strength of the Hip Muscles

Specific exercises are described in the exercise sections of this chapter.

- Stretch any muscles restricting motion with gentle, progressive neuromuscular inhibition techniques. Instruct the patient to do self-stretching with proper stabilization to ensure that the stretches are performed safely and effectively.
- Begin developing neuromuscular control to train the involved muscles to contract and control alignment of the femur. Initially, the emphasis is on control, not strengthening.
- Once the patient is aware of proper muscle control and is able to maintain alignment, progress to strengthening the weakened muscles through the range.
- Muscles not directly injured should be stretched and strengthened if they are contributing to unbalanced forces. The patient may not have good trunk coordination or strength, which may be contributing to the overuse because of compensations in the hip. See Chapter 16 for suggestions for developing control and stabilizing function in the trunk muscles.

Develop Stability and Closed-Chain Function

- Initiate controlled weight-bearing exercises when tolerated. Because the individual is probably standing and walking, he or she may not tolerate much more closed-chain activities than those previously initiated early in the healing stage, so proceed with caution. Carefully observe the exercises so that proper movement patterns are used.
- Use exercises such as biking or partial weight-bearing and weight-shifting activities in the parallel bars. Observe coordination between trunk, hip, knee, and ankle motions, and exercise only to the point of fatigue, substitute motions, or pain in the weakest segment in the chain.

Develop Muscle and Cardiopulmonary Endurance

- For muscle endurance, instruct the patient to safely perform each exercise from 1 to 3 minutes before progressing to the next level of difficulty.
- Determine aerobic activities that will not exacerbate the patient's symptoms. It may be that the patient just needs to modify the intensity or the techniques used in his or her current program.

Patient Education

As soon as the patient has learned the neuromuscular control techniques and correct stretching, strengthening, and aerobic activities, teach home exercise techniques. Provide follow-up instruction for modification and progression of the program.

Management: Return to Function Phase

Progress Strength and Functional Control

- Progress closed-chain and functional training to include balance and muscular endurance for each activity.
- Use specificity principles; increase eccentric resistance and demand for controlled speed if necessary for return-to-work activity or sporting event.
- Progress to patterns of motion consistent with the desired outcome. Use acceleration/deceleration drills and plyometric training; assess the total body functioning while doing the desired activity. Practice timing and sequencing of events.

Return to Function

Prior to returning to the desired function have the patient practice the activity in a controlled environment and for a limited period. As tolerated, introduce variability in the environment and increase the intensity of the endurance activities.

Exercise Techniques to Increase Flexibility and Range of Motion

No matter what the cause, muscle strength or flexibility imbalance in the hip can lead to abnormal lumbopelvic and hip mechanics, which predisposes the patient to or perpetuates low back, sacroiliac, or hip pain. See Chapters 15 and 16 for discussion and treatment of posture impairments and low-back pain. Poor hip mechanics from muscle flexibility and strength imbalances can also affect the knee and ankle during weight-bearing activities, thus causing overuse syndromes or stress to these regions. The exercise techniques in this section are suggestions for correcting limited flexibility of the musculature and periarticular tissues crossing the hip. Principles and techniques of passive stretching and neuromuscular inhibition were presented in Chapter 5 and those of joint mobilization were presented in Chapter 6. Specific manual and self-stretching techniques are described in this section.

Flexibility (self-stretching) exercises, chosen according to the degree of limitation and ability of the patient to participate, can be valuable to reinforce therapeutic interventions performed by the therapist. Not all of the following exercises are appropriate for every patient; the therapist should select each exercise and intensity appropriate for the level of function, and progress each exercise as indicated. Whenever the patient is able to contract the muscle opposite the range-limiting muscle, there are the added benefits of reciprocal inhibition of the shortened muscles as well as training the agonist (the muscle opposite the tight muscle) to function for effective control in the gained ROM.

Techniques to Stretch Range-Limiting Hip Structures

Note: Two-joint muscles can restrict full ROM at the hip. This section describes stretches to increase just hip motions, so the two-joint muscles are kept on a slack across the knee during these stretches. Techniques to stretch the specific two-joint muscles are then described.

To Increase Hip Extension

Prone Press-Ups

Patient position and procedure: Prone with hands on the table at shoulder level. Have the patient press the thorax upward, and allow the pelvis to sag (see Fig. 16–11*A*).

Precaution: This exercise also moves the lumbar spine into extension; if it causes radiating pain down the patient's leg, rather than just a stretch sensation in the anterior trunk, hip, and thigh, it must not be performed.

"Thomas Test" Stretch

- Patient position: Supine with the hips near the end of the treatment table, with both hips and knees flexed, and with the thigh on the side opposite the tight hip held against the chest.
- Procedures: Have the patient slowly lower the thigh to be stretched toward the table in a controlled manner and allow the knee to extend so the two-joint rectus femoris does not limit the range. Do not allow the thigh to rotate outward or abduct. Direct the patient to let the weight of the leg cause the stretch force and to relax the tight muscles at the end of the range. A passive stretch force may be applied manually, or a hold-relax muscle inhibition technique may be used by applying a force to the distal thigh (see Fig. 5–20).

Modified Fencer Stretch

- Patient position: Standing in a fencer's squatlike posture, with the back leg in the same plane as the front leg and the foot pointing forward.
- Procedure: Have the patient first do a posterior PT and then shift the body weight on to the anterior leg until a stretch sensation is felt in the anterior hip region of the back leg (Fig. 12–2).
- If the heel of the back foot is kept on the floor, this exercise may also stretch the gastrocnemius muscle.

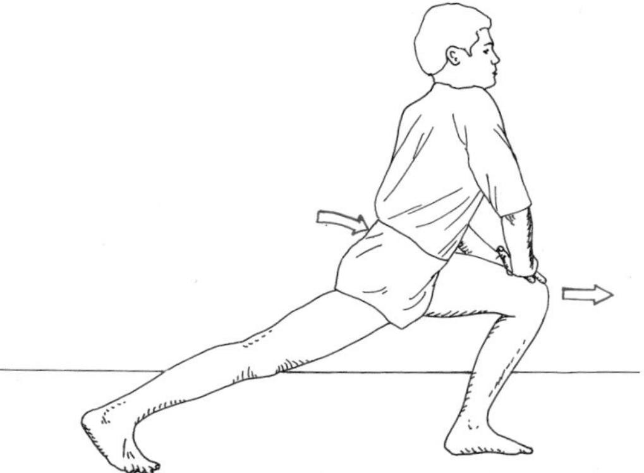

Figure 12–2 Self-stretching of hip flexor muscles and soft tissue anterior to the hip, using a modified fencer's squat posture.

To Increase Hip Flexion

Bilateral Knee to Chest

- Patient position and procedure: Supine; have the patient bring both knees toward the chest and grasp the thighs firmly until a stretch sensation is felt in the posterior hip region.
- Monitor the position carefully because if the pelvis lifts up off the mat, the lumbar spine will flex and the stretch force will be transmitted there instead of the hips.

Unilateral Knee to Chest

- Patient position and procedure: Supine; have the patient bring one knee to the chest and grasp the thigh firmly against the chest while keeping the other lower extremity extended on the mat. This position isolates the stretch force to the hip being flexed and helps stabilize the pelvis.
- To emphasize the gluteus maximus, have the patient pull the knee toward the opposite shoulder.

Quadruped (All Fours) Stretch

- Patient position and procedure: On hands and knees; have the patient rock the pelvis into an anterior tilt, causing lumbar extension, then maintain the lumbar extension and shift the buttocks back in an attempt to sit on the heels. The hands remain forward (Figs. 12–3*A* and *B*).
- It is important not to let the lumbar spine flex while holding the stretch position so that the stretch affects the hip.

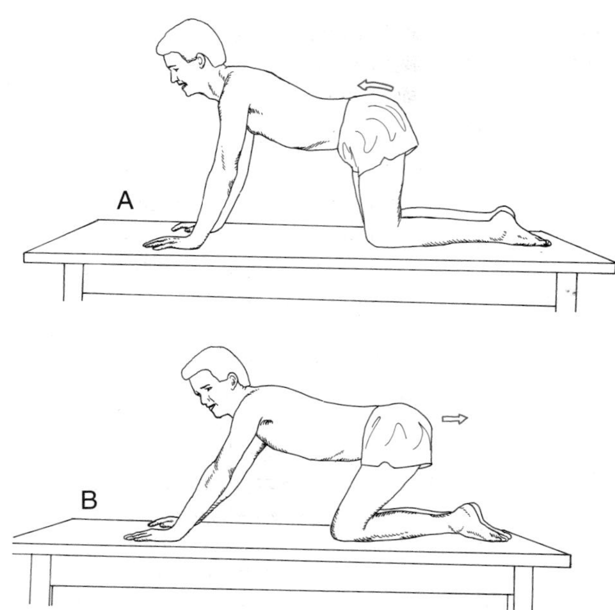

Figure 12–3 Gluteus maximus self-stretch with lumbar spine stabilization. *(A)* The patient on all-4s rocks into an anterior PT, causing lumbar extension. *(B)* While maintaining lumbar extension, the patient shifts the buttocks back, attempting to sit on the heels. When lordosis can no longer be maintained, the end-range of hip flexion is reached and held for the stretch.

Chair Stretch

- Patient position: Sitting in a chair with the pelvis rotated anteriorly and low back extended to stabilize the spine.
- Procedure: Have the patient grasp the front of the chair seat and lean or pull the trunk forward, keeping the back arched so the motion occurs only at the hips.

To Increase Hip Abduction

- Patient position and procedure: Supine with both hips flexed 90 degrees, knees extended and legs and buttocks against the wall. Have the patient abduct both hips as far as possible with gravity causing the stretch force (Fig. 12–4).

To Simultaneously Increase Hip Abduction and External Rotation

- Patient position and procedure: Sitting or supine with soles of feet together and hands on the inner surface of the knees. Have the patient push the knees down toward the floor with a sustained stretch. The amount of stretch can be increased by pulling the feet closer to the trunk.

Precaution: When supine, teach the patient to stabilize the pelvis and lumbar spine by actively contracting the abdominal muscles and maintaining a posterior PT.

- Patient position and procedure: Standing in a fencer's position, but with the hind leg externally rotated. Have the patient shift the weight on to the front leg until a stretch sensation is felt along the medial thigh in the hind leg.

Techniques to Stretch Range-Limiting Two-Joint Muscles

Rectus Femoris Stretches

"Thomas Test" Stretch

- Patient position: Supine with the hips near the end of the treatment table, with both hips and knees flexed and with the thigh on the side opposite the tight hip held against the chest with the arms.

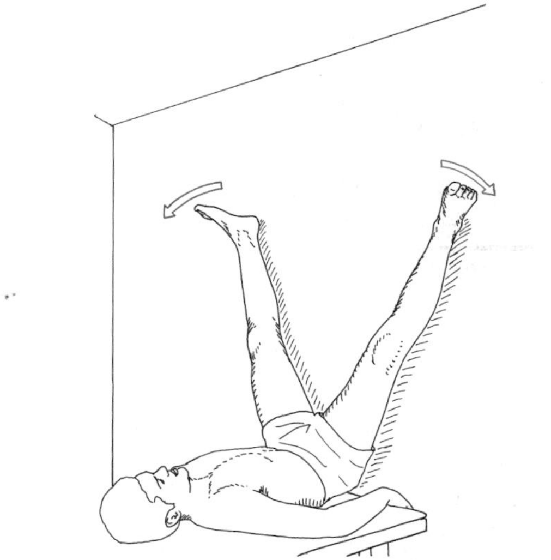

Figure 12–4 Self-stretching of the adductor muscles with the hips at 90 degrees of flexion.

- Procedure: While keeping the knee flexed, have the patient lower the thigh to be stretched toward the table in a controlled manner. Do not allow the thigh to rotate outward or abduct.
- Direct the patient to let the weight of the leg cause the stretch force and to relax the tight muscles at the end of the range. The patient can attempt to further extend the hip by contracting the extensor muscles.

Note: This is the same stretch used to increase hip extension, except to stretch the rectus femoris the knee is kept flexed, so the range for hip extension will be less.

Prone Stretch

- Patient position: Prone with the knee flexed on the side to be stretched.
- Procedure: Have the patient grab the ankle on that side (or place a towel or strap around the ankle to pull on) and flex the knee.
- As the muscle increases in flexibility, place a small folded towel under the distal thigh to further extend the hip.
- Do not let the hip abduct or laterally rotate or let the spine hyperextend.

Standing Stretch

- Patient position: Standing with the hip extended and knee flexed.
- Procedure: Have the patient grasp the ankle.
- Instruct the patient to maintain a posterior PT and not let the back arch or side bend during this stretch (Fig. 12–5).
- If the rectus femoris is too tight to safely stretch in this manner, the patient may place his or her foot on a chair or bench located behind the body rather than grasping the ankle.

Hamstring Stretches

Straight Leg Raising (SLR)

- Patient position: Supine with a towel under the thigh.
- Procedure: Have the patient perform SLR (flex the hip with the knee extended) and apply the stretch force by pulling on the towel to move the hip into more flexion.

Doorway Stretch

- Patient position and procedure: Supine, on the floor, with one leg through a doorway and the other leg (the one to be stretched) propped up against the doorframe. The knee should be kept extended.
- To increase the stretch, have the patient move the buttock closer to the door frame, keeping the knee extended (Fig. 12–6*A*).
- Teach the patient to perform the hold-relax/agonist contraction technique by pressing the

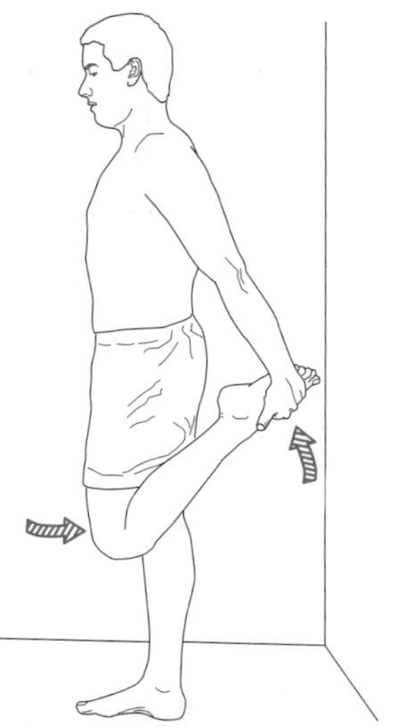

Figure 12–5 Self-stretch of the rectus femoris in standing. The femur is kept in line with the trunk. Care must be taken to maintain a posterior PT and not arch or twist the back.

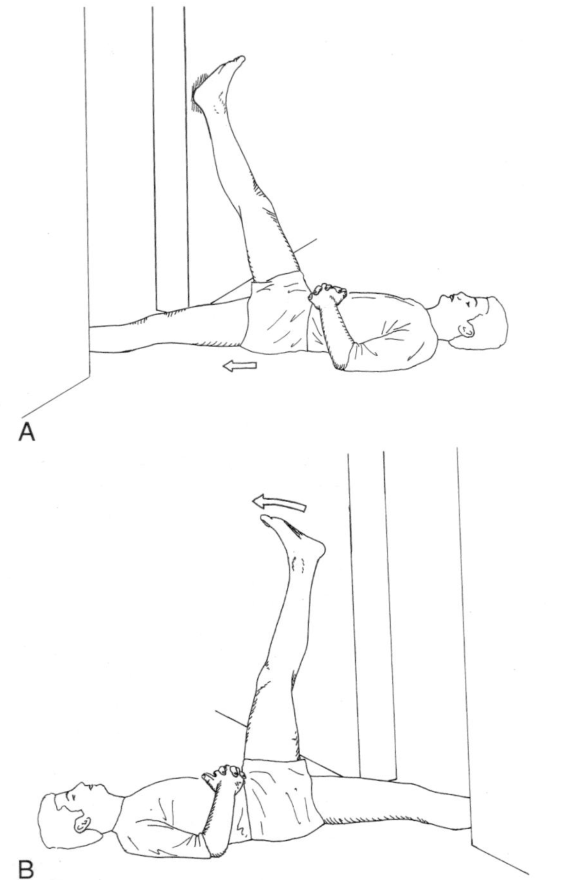

Figure 12–6 Self-stretching of the hamstring muscles. Additional stretch can occur if the person either *(A)* moves the buttock closer to the door frame or *(B)* lifts the leg away from the doorframe.

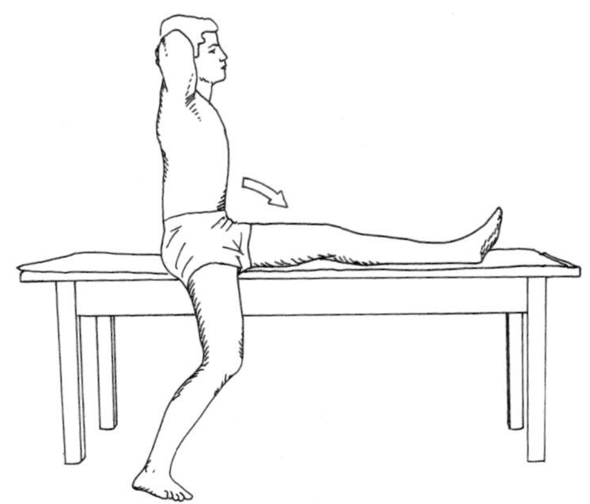

Figure 12–7 Self-stretching of the hamstring muscles by leaning the trunk toward the extended knee, flexing at the hips.

heel of the leg being stretched against the doorframe, causing an isometric contraction, relaxing it, then lifting the leg away from the frame (Fig. 12–6*B*).

- For an effective stretch, the pelvis and opposite leg must remain on the floor with the knee extended.

Chair Stretch

- Patient position: Sitting with the leg to be stretched extended across to another chair, or sitting at the edge of a treatment table, with the leg to be stretched on the table and the opposite foot on the floor.
- Procedure: Have the patient lean the trunk forward toward the thigh, keeping the back extended so that there is motion only at the hip joint (Fig. 12–7).

Bilateral Toe Touching

Precaution: Bilateral toe touching exercises are often used to stretch the hamstring muscles in exercise classes. It is important to recognize that having the patient reach for the toes does not selectively stretch the hamstrings but stretches the low and mid back as well. Toe touching is considered a general flexibility exercise and tends to mask shortening of soft tissues in one region and overstretch areas already flexible. Whether or not a person can touch the toes depends on many factors such as body type, arm, trunk, and leg length, flexibility in the thoracic and lumbar regions, as well as hamstring and gastrocnemius length.[36]

This stretching technique should not be used when the patient has low back impairments since forward bending greatly increases mechanical stress to the tissues of the low back.

- To specifically stretch the hamstrings using the standing forward-bend method, teach the patient to first do an anterior PT to extend the spine, then keep the back stable and bend only at the hips ("hinge at the hips") and go only through the range of forward bending where the spine can be maintained in extension.
- To discourage the "toe touch" idea, instruct the patient to place the hands on the hips when bending forward.
- The stretch sensation should be felt in the hamstring region.

To Stretch the Tensor Fasciae Latae

Standing Stretch

- Patient position: Standing with the side to be stretched toward a wall and the hand on that side placed on the wall.
- Procedure: Have the patient extend, adduct, and externally rotate the extremity to be stretched and cross it behind the other extremity.
- With both feet on the floor, have the patient shift his or her pelvis toward the wall, and allow the normal knee to bend slightly (Fig. 12–8). There will be a slight side-bending of the trunk away from the side being stretched.

Side-Lying Stretch

- Patient position: Side-lying, with the leg to be stretched uppermost. The bottom extremity is flexed for support and the pelvis tilted laterally so the waist is against the mat or floor.
- Procedure: Abduct the top leg and align it in the plane of the body (in extension). While maintaining this position, have the patient externally rotate the hip and then gradually lower (adduct) the thigh to the point of stretch.
- It is critical to keep the trunk aligned and not allow it to roll backward, because the hip will then flex and the iliotibial tract will slip in front of the greater trochanter, and an effective stretch will not take place.
- Flex the knee to obtain additional stretch (Fig. 12–9).

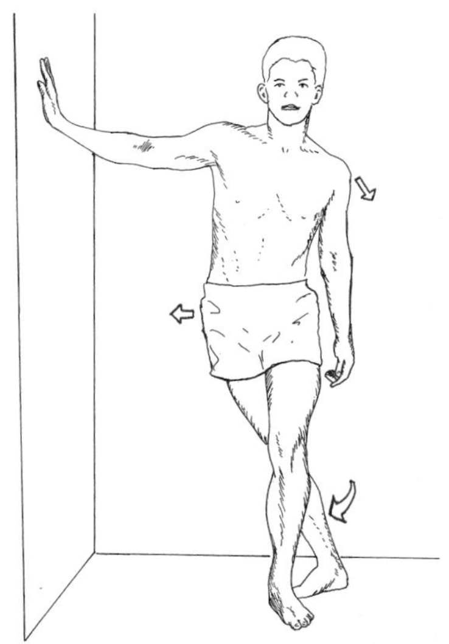

Figure 12–8 Self-stretching of the tensor fasciae latae occurs as the trunk bends away from and the pelvis shifts toward the tight side. Increased stretch occurs when the extremity is positioned in external rotation prior to the stretch.

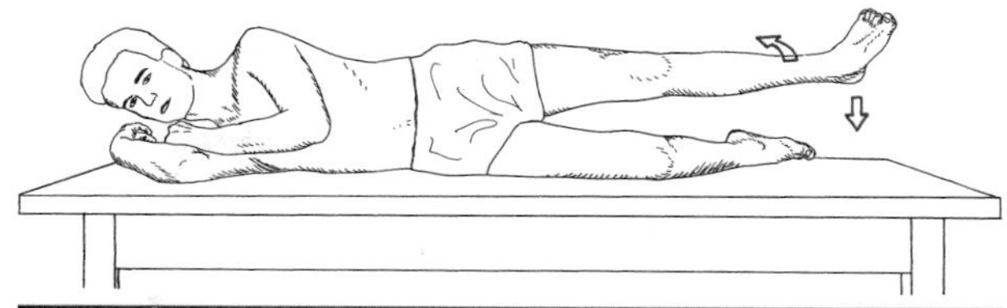

Figure 12–9 Tensor fasciae latae self-stretching: side-lying position. The thigh is abducted in the plane of the body, then it is extended and externally rotated, then slowly lowered. Additional stretch can occur by flexing the knee.

Exercises to Develop and Improve Muscle Performance and Functional Control

During the controlled motion and return to function phases of intervention when only moderate or minimum protection of healing tissues is necessary, it is important that the patient learns to develop control of hip movement while using good trunk stability. For a muscle that has not been properly used or that has been dominated by another muscle, exercises begin with developing patient awareness of muscle contractions and movements through controlled ROM exercises. If muscle shortening has prevented full ROM, development of muscle control in any new range must immediately follow stretching activities. Principles for improving muscle performance as well as techniques for manual resistance exercises and methods of mechanical resistance were described in Chapter 3. Manually applied resistance should be used when muscles are weak or when helping the patient focus on specific muscles. Exercises described in the following sections may be adapted for home exercise programs. Choose exercises that challenge the patient to progress toward the functional goals established during the evaluation.

Nonweight-Bearing Exercises

Even though weight-bearing activities dominate lower extremity function, when a patient is weak or has poor control of specific muscles or patterns of motion, it may be advantageous to begin exercises in the nonweight-bearing position so the individual can learn to isolate muscle activity and learn to control specific motions. In addition, many functional activities have a nonweight-bearing component, such as the swing phase in gait, lifting the leg up to a step when going upstairs, and lifting the lower extremity into a car or onto a bed.

To Develop Control of and Strengthen Hip Abduction (Gluteus Medius and Tensor Fasciae Latae)

Note: Muscle imbalances in the hip that contribute to hip and/or low back pain may be seen if abduction is dominated by the tensor fasciae latae and the stabilizing forces from the gluteus medius are poorly controlled.[75] This will be seen if the patient flexes and internally rotates the thigh when abducting the hip. The posterior fibers of the gluteus medius will need to be trained to contract while the tensor relaxes. Techniques to do this are described below. If the patient has good control of rotation, abduction utilizing the synergy between these muscles is used.

Supine Abduction

This is the easiest position in which to initiate motion since the effects of gravity on the abductors are eliminated.

- Have the patient concentrate on isolated hip abduction while keeping the trunk still. Do not let the femur roll outward into external rotation.
- For very weak patients, provide assistance or place a skate or towel under the leg to minimize the effects of friction.
- If the patient is not strong enough to progress to the side-lying position, place a weight, such as a sandbag, along the outside of the thigh or ankle and have the patient push the weight outward.

Side-Lying Abduction

- Have the patient flex the bottom leg for balance, and then lift the top leg into abduction, keeping the hip neutral to rotation and in slight extension.
- Do not allow the hip to flex or the trunk to roll backward.
- Add ankle weights to provide resistance as the patient's strength improves.

Standing Abduction

- Have the patient bring the lower extremity out to the side while maintaining the trunk in neutral alignment and not letting the hip flex or rotate.
- Add resistance by using pulleys or elastic resistance that is secured on the opposite side.
- While doing this exercise, the abductors on the stationary lower extremity will be experiencing closed-chain resistance.

To Develop Gluteus Medius Control

- Patient position: Side-lying with the leg to be exercised uppermost and the bottom leg flexed for support.
- Procedure: First have the patient practice externally rotating the thigh. This may be done with the hip and knee in slight flexion while the patient lifts the uppermost knee off the mat or with the hip and knee extended while the patient rolls the uppermost extremity outward.
- Once the patient can control external rotation, have him or her extend the hip (without arching the spine) then abduct the top leg (it should be aligned in the plane of the body). The patient then slowly adducts and abducts the thigh against gravity.
- If the tensor fasciae latae is tight, the range into extension or adduction may be limited. Stretching of this muscle should be done prior to this exercise (see Fig. 12–9). It is important that the patient does not let the hip flex or internally rotate during this exercise to minimize action of the tensor fasciae latae.

To Develop Control of and Strengthen Hip Extension (Gluteus Maximus)

Gluteal Muscle Setting

- Patient position and procedure: Prone or supine. Use gluteal setting exercises to increase awareness of the contracting muscle, by instructing the patient to "squeeze" (contract) the buttock.

Leg Lifts While Bending Forward

- Patient position and procedure: Standing at the edge of the treatment table with the trunk flexed and supported on the table. Have the patient alternately extend one hip then the other.
- This is done with the knee flexed to train the gluteus maximus while relaxing the hamstrings. If the hamstrings cramp from active insufficiency, the patient is attempting to use them and should practice relaxing them before progressing with this exercise.
- Progress by adding weights or elastic resistance to the distal thigh.

Quadruped Leg Lifts

- Patient position and procedure: On hands and knees in an all-fours position. Have the patient then alternately extend each hip while keeping the knee flexed (Fig. 12–10).
- Care is taken not to extend the hip beyond the available range of hip extension or the motion will cause stress in the sacroiliac joint or lumbar spine.

To Develop Control of and Strengthen Hip External Rotation

Isometrics

- Patient position and procedure: Prone with knees flexed and about 10 inches apart. Have the patient press the heels together, causing an isometric contraction of the external rotators.

Side-Lying

- Patient position and procedure: Side-lying with both lower extremities partially flexed at the hips and knees and the heel of the top leg resting on the heel of the bottom leg. Have the patient lift the knee of the top leg, keeping the heels together.
- Progress by instructing the patient to extend the top hip and knee, aligning the lower extremity with the trunk, then rolling the leg outward. Progress this to lifting the entire lower extremity into abduction once the hip is externally rotated.
- Do not allow the patient to roll the trunk backward as this exercise is done to minimize substitution with the hip flexor muscles.

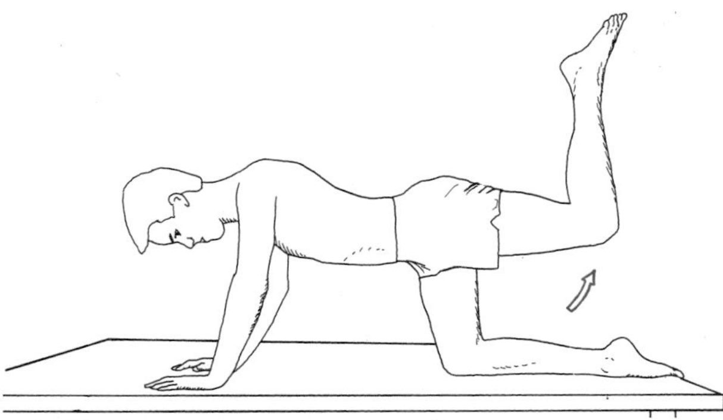

Figure 12–10 Isolated training and strengthening of the gluteus maximus. Starting in the all-fours position, the knee is flexed to rule out substitution by the hamstring muscles. Care is taken not to hyperextend the hip to the point of causing stress to the sacroiliac or lumbar spinal joints.

Standing

- Patient position and procedure: Standing, with feet parallel, about 4 inches apart. Have the patient flex the knees slightly, then externally rotate the thighs (so that the knees are pointing laterally) while keeping the feet stationary on the floor.
- Tell the patient to maintain the external rotation while extending the knees, then relax the rotation slightly until the patellae point forward.

Sitting

- Patient position and procedure: Sitting with knees flexed over the edge of the treatment table. Secure elastic material around the patient's ankle and the table leg on the same side.
- Have the patient move the foot toward the opposite side, pulling against the resistance, causing external rotation of the hip.
- Do not allow substitution with knee flexion or extension or hip abduction.

To Develop Control of and Strengthen Hip Adduction

- Patient position and procedure: Side-lying with the bottom leg aligned in the plane of the trunk and the top leg flexed forward with the foot on the floor or with the thigh resting on a pillow. Have the patient lift the bottom leg upward in adduction. Weights can be added to the ankle to progress strengthening (Fig. 12–11*A*).
- Patient position and procedure: Side-lying with both legs aligned in the plane of the trunk. Have the patient hold the top leg in abduction and adduct the bottom leg up to meet it (Fig. 12–11*B*).

Closed-Chain Weight-Bearing Exercises

Weight-bearing exercises in the lower extremity involve all of the joints in the closed-chain and are therefore not limited to hip muscles. Most activities bring into play antagonistic two-joint muscles in which each muscle is being lengthened across one joint while it is shortening across another, thus maintaining an optimal length-tension relationship. In addition to causing motion, a prime function of the muscles in weight bearing is to control against the forces of gravity and momentum for balance and stability. Therefore, the exercises described in this section include balance and stabilization training as well as strengthening and functional exercises.

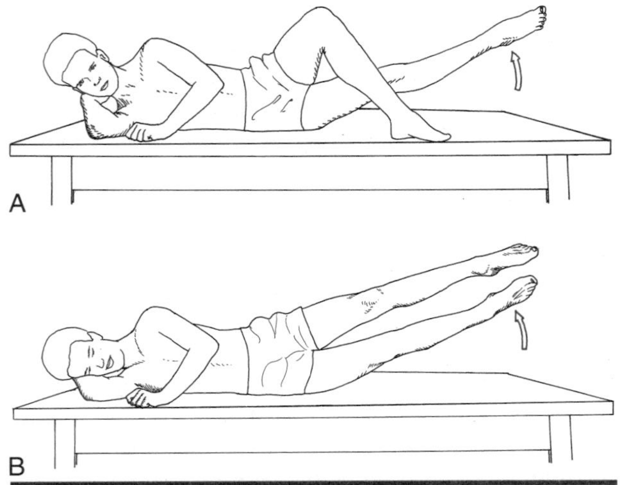

Figure 12–11 Training and strengthening the hip adductors. *(A)* The top leg is stabilized by flexing the hip and resting the foot on the mat while the bottom leg is adducted against gravity. *(B)* The top leg is isometrically held in abduction while the bottom leg is adducted against gravity.

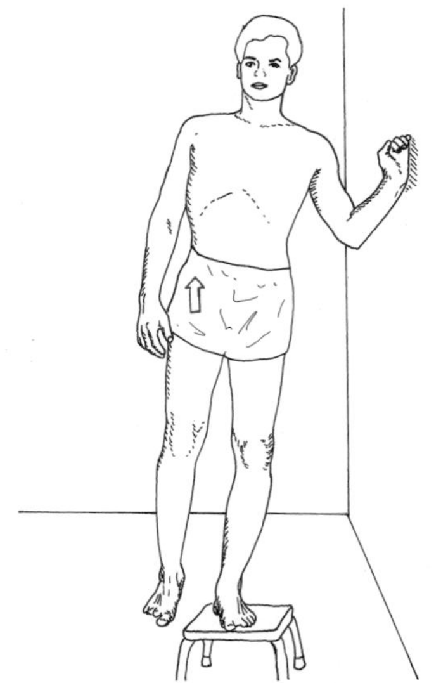

Figure 12–12 Training the hip abductor and hiker muscles for frontal plane strenthening and stability.

Closed-Chain Strengthening and Functional Training

Strengthening and balance activities in weight-bearing postures described in the following section are closely related and are progressed concurrently as the patient is able.

Frontal Plane Resistance

- Patient position and procedure: Standing with one leg on a 2- to 4-inch block. Have the patient alternately lower and elevate the pelvis on the side of the unsupported leg (Fig. 12–12). This develops control in the abductors of the stance leg and hip hikers on the unsupported side.
- Progress by having the patient abduct one leg, then the other, with motion only at the hip but without side bending of the trunk. If the pelvis drops on the unsupported side, the musculature on the supporting limb is too weak for this exercise. If there is good control, place weights around the unsupported ankle for added resistance.

Bridging

- Patient position and procedure: Hook-lying. Have the patient press the upper back and feet into the mat, elevate the pelvis, and extend the hips (Fig. 12–13).
- Apply resistance against the anterior pelvis either manually or by strapping a weighted belt around the pelvis.

Single-Leg Stance Against Resistance

- The patient stands on the involved leg. Place elastic resistance around the thigh of the other extremity, and secure it to a stable upright structure. Progress the exercise by applying the resistance around the ankle if the knee is stable.
- To resist hip flexion, the patient faces away from where the resistance is secured.
- To resist extension, the patient faces toward where the resistance is secured.
- To resist abduction and adduction the patient faces so that the band is directed toward one side, then the other.

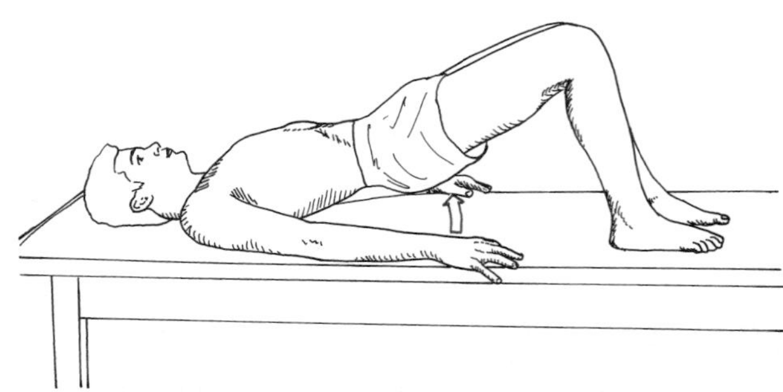

Figure 12–13 Training and strengthening the hip extensor muscles using bridging exercises. Resistance can be added against the pelvis.

- This activity is open-chain on the side of the moving extremity and closed-chain on the weight-bearing side (Fig. 12–14).
- Fatigue is determined when the patient can no longer hold the weight-bearing extremity or pelvis stable.

Step-Ups

- Begin with a low step, 2 to 3 inches in height; progress height as the patient is able.
- Have the patient step up sideways, forward, or backward. Be sure that the entire foot is planted on the step and that the body is lifted, then lowered with smooth motion, not lurching of the trunk or pushing off with the trailing extremity.
- Resistance can be added with a weight belt, with weights in the hands, or around the ankle of the nonweight-bearing leg.

Lunges

- Have the patient stride forward and flex the hip and knee of the forward leg beginning with a small range and progressing to 90 degrees and return upright. Repeat, or alternate legs.
- If the patient has difficulty with balance or control, have him or her use a cane or rod for balance, or begin the activity holding on in the parallel bars or beside a treatment table (Fig. 12–15).
- It is important to instruct the patient to keep the toes pointing forward, bend the knee in the same plane as the feet, and keep the back upright.
- Progressions include using weights in the hands for resistance, taking a longer stride, or lunging forward onto a small step.
- Progress to lunging and picking up objects from the floor.

Note: A patient with an anterior cruciate ligament (ACL) deficiency or a surgically repaired ACL should not flex the knee forward of the toes when performing lunges because this increases the shear force and stress to the ACL. Individuals with patellofemoral compression syndrome will experience increased pain under these circumstances because the compressive force from the body weight is greater when it is kept posterior to the knee. Adapt the position of the knee based on the patient's symptoms and presenting pathology.

Wall Slides

- Have patients rest the back against a wall with feet forward and shoulder-width apart.
- Instruct the patient to slide the back down the wall by flexing the hips and knees and dorsiflexing the ankle, then slide up the wall by extending hips and knees and plantarflexing the ankles (Fig. 12–16*A*).
- If sliding the back directly against the wall causes excessive friction, place a towel behind the patient's back.

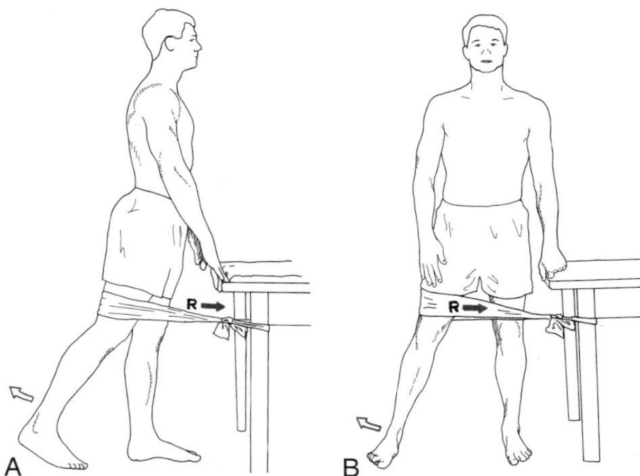

Figure 12–14 Closed-chain exercise with elastic resistance around the opposite leg. *(A)* Resisting extension on the right requires stabilization of anterior muscles of the left side. *(B)* Resisting abduction on the right requires stabilization of the left frontal plane muscles. To increase difficulty, the resistance is moved distally on to the leg.

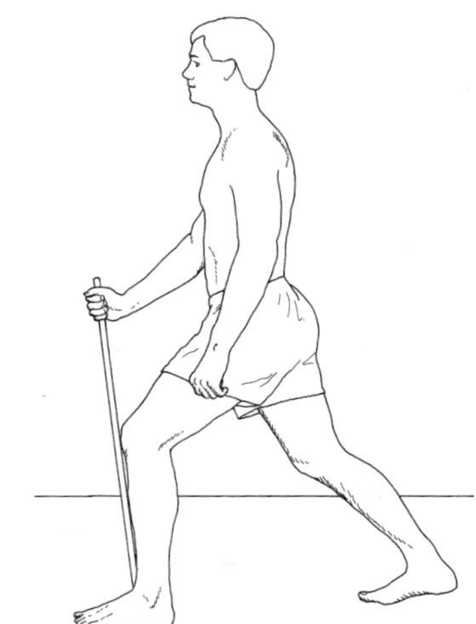

Figure 12–15 Lunge with cane assistance to develop balance and control for lowering body weight.

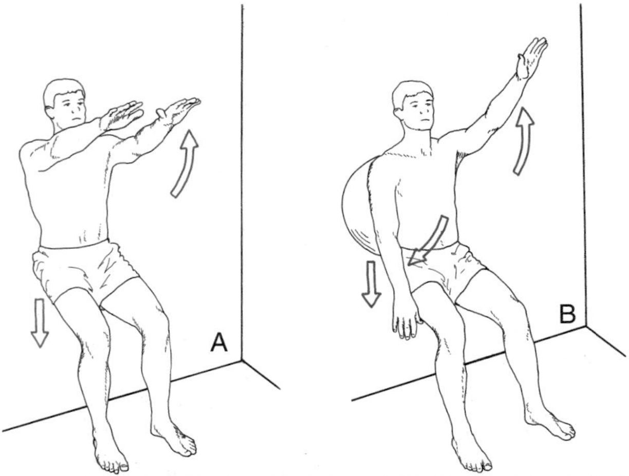

Figure 12–16 Wall slides/partial squats to develop eccentric control of body weight. *(A)* The back sliding down a wall, superimposing bilateral arm motion for added resistance. *(B)* The back rolling a gym ball down the wall, superimposing antagonistic arm motion to develop coordination.

- A large exercise ball (Swiss ball) placed behind the back requires additional control because it is less stable (Fig. 12–16*B*).
- Add arm motions and weights to develop coordination or to add resistance.
- To develop isometric strength have the patient hold the flexed position and superimpose arm motions with weights.

Partial Squats/Mini-Squats

- Have the patient lower the trunk by flexing the hips and knees.
- Add resistance by having the patient hold weights in the hands or use elastic resistance secured under the feet (see Fig. 13–13).
- Progress to safe lifting techniques that involve squatting.

Note: To protect the ACL, knee flexion range is limited from 0 to 60 degrees, and the patient is instructed to lower the hips as if preparing to sit on a chair so that the knees stay behind the toes. To protect a patellofemoral compression problem, instruct the patient to squat only through pain-free ranges and avoid deep knee bends.

Equipment

Mechanical equipment such as a leg press, Total Gym® treadmill, bicycle, slide board, or Profitter™ may be used for strengthening, balance coordination, and endurance.

Postural Control and Balance Activities

As noted earlier, weight-bearing control and balance training begin as soon as the patient tolerates partial weight-bearing. These activities progress with strengthening exercises and are combined whenever possible.

Weight Shifting

- If the patient cannot bear full weight, begin in the parallel bars with part of the weight borne on the hands. An overhead harnessing system can also be used to unweight the lower extremities.
- Have the patient shift anterior to posterior, side to side, and obliquely.
- Add manual resistance to the motion by applying pressure against the patient's pelvis.

Balance Activities with Arm Movements

- Begin with bilateral weight bearing and progress to unilateral weight bearing.
- First have the patient move his or her arms in the sagittal and frontal planes, then progress to the transverse and diagonal planes.
- As the patient demonstrates the ability to balance with simple arm movements, progress to moving the arms and following the movement with the eyes and head. Then progress to moving the entire trunk through planes of motion following the arm motions.

Marching and Resisted Walking

- Once the patient can shift weight and maintain balance with arm movements, have him or her alternately pick up each foot and march in place.
- Progress to moving each leg forward and backward and learning to accept weight onto the moving leg.
- Once the patient can step and walk, progress to resisted walking by applying resistance at the pelvis or have the patient walk against an elastic or pulley resistance secured around the pelvis (Fig. 12–17).

Alternating Isometrics and Rhythmic Stabilization

These exercises develop postural adjustments to applied forces.

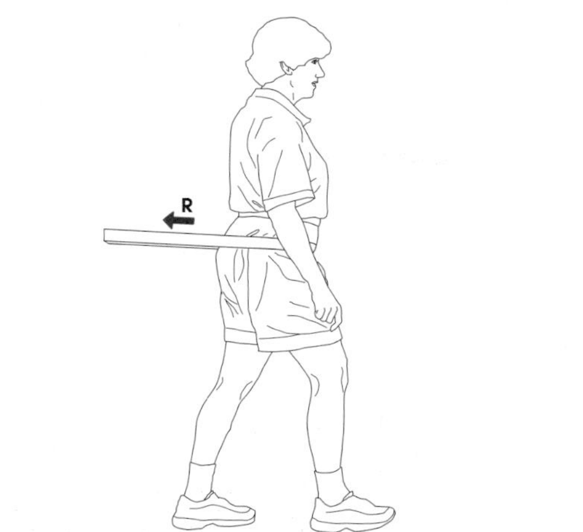

Figure 12–17 Resisted walking using a large elastic resistance band secured around the pelvis.

- Apply manual resistance against the pelvis in alternating directions, and ask the patient to hold (with isometric contractions). There should be little or no movement.
- Vary the force and direction of resistance; also vary where the force is applied by shifting the resistance from the pelvis to the shoulders and eventually against outstretched arms (see Fig. 14–10).
- At first, use verbal cueing; as the patient learns control, apply the varying forces without warning. Progress the patient to unilateral standing.
- Teach the patient a self-applied stabilization technique using elastic resistance secured around the thigh or leg of one extremity and then rapidly moving the extremity forward and backward against the elastic force (see Fig. 12–14 for setup). The rapid motion requires stabilization on the weight-bearing side.

Balance Training on Unstable Surfaces

- The patient stands with bilateral support on foam, a rocker board, wobble board, or BAPS board and begins with single-plane weight shifting forward/backward and side to side.
- Progress by placing the extremities in a diagonal plane and have the patient shift the weight.
- When able, have the patient progress to single-leg activities on an unstable surface.

Advanced Stability and Balance Activities

- Have the patient stand on an unstable surface such as a rocker or wobble board and maintain balance without the edges of the board touching the ground while a partner tosses a weighted ball to the patient from various angles.
- Have the patient hold on to the two ends of an elastic resistance band while someone pulls against it in various directions and with varying speeds.

Simulated Functional Activities

The level of challenge of the exercise program depends on the activities that the patient is required to perform in his or her ADL, IADL, work, or sport-related tasks and, therefore, affects the desired outcomes. An outcome may be simply learning how to safely ambulate forward, backward, and around obstacles or may involve developing a high level of coordination, balance, and skill to climb, perform complicated dance maneuvers, engage in gymnastics, or run and jump. Analyze the patient's exercise techniques, and adapt them whenever necessary to avoid unsafe stresses.

Suggestions for progressive functional training include:

- Increase challenges for ambulation such as having the patient walk on uneven surfaces, turn, maneuver backward, and walk up and down ramps first under supervision, then unassisted. As soon as the patient is able, have him or her practice rising up and sitting down from chairs of various heights and climbing and descending flights of stairs.
- Incorporate exercises that prepare the musculature for safe body mechanics such as repetitive squats and lunges. Progress the exercises by having the patient lift and carry or push and pull various loads as part of the exercise routine. Utilize safe patterns of motion that replicate functional requirements.
- Use agility drills such as maneuvering around and stepping over obstacles. Incorporate running, jumping, hopping, skipping, and side-shuffle drills.
- If the patient is returning to activities that require strength and power, incorporate plyometric drills. For example, have the patient jump from a box or step, flex the hips, knees, and ankles to absorb the impact of landing, and immediately jump back up to the box or step.

- Use maximum eccentric loading. Any of the previously described exercises can be adapted, but it is critical to assist the patient through the concentric phase of the exercise and guard him or her through the eccentric phase since the resis-tance will be great. These are not exercises that the patient can do alone.

Independent Learning Activities

CRITICAL THINKING AND DISCUSSION

1. Describe the function of the primary muscle groups of the hip joint in open- and closed-chain situations. Include their role in stabilizing the pelvis during single leg stance and effects on the spine when the pelvis is moved by the hip musculature.
2. Describe the role of the hip during the gait cycle. Include muscle activity, motion needed, and pathologic gait patterns when there is muscle weakness or restricted motion.
3. Analyze the type of gait deviations a patient might exhibit after internal fixation of a fracture of the proximal femur, total hip arthroplasty, or hemiarthroplasty of the hip.
4. After total hip arthroplasty or internal fixation of a hip fracture, what are the signs that a dislocation of the hip or loss of fracture stabilization has occurred?

LABORATORY PRACTICE

1. Identify and practice the techniques you would use to treat a mobility impairment if the results of your examination included decreased joint play versus restricted flexibility in the hip musculature. Include exercises that could be used in a home exercise program.
2. Demonstrate a progression of exercises to develop control and strength in the gluteus medius muscle after total hip replacement.
3. Develop an exercise routine and progression for an individual with hip muscle weakness who would like to be able to return to work that requires walking, lifting objects weighing up to 45 lb, and climbing ladders with 45-lb weights.

CASE STUDIES

1. Mr. C, 57 years of age, is a mail carrier; he has walked his mail route for 32 years and is proud "that he has no heart problems." Over the past year he has noticed that his hip hurts after sitting for more than 1 hour and that there is a marked increase in pain when first getting up out of a chair and walking. He also has noticed that there is increased discomfort in his hip and knees near the end of each workday. The medical diagnosis is osteoarthritis. Strength testing reveals generally 4/5 on manual muscle tests except the gluteus medius, which is 3+/5. There is mild tightness in the hip flexors, including rectus femoris and tensor fasciae lata. He wants to avoid being a "candidate for total hip replacement surgery."
   - Explain why the patient's job would perpetuate these symptoms.
   - Outline a plan to manage the symptoms; identify measurable goals and interventions you would use to reach the goals.
   - What can the patient do to protect his hip joints?
2. Ms. J, a 31-year-old mother, recreational tennis player, and bowler, is recovering from multiple femoral fractures that she sustained in an automobile accident 3 months ago. There is radiological healing of all the fracture sites, and she is now allowed full weight-bearing and no restrictions in activities. She has significant hip mobility impairments from joint restrictions and muscle weakness.
   - What joint ranges and muscle strength levels will be needed for her to return to her functional activities?
   - Outline a plan to manage the symptoms; identify measurable goals and interventions you would use to reach the goals.
3. Mr. C is a 32-year-old firefighter who strained his hamstrings at the ischial tuberosity while pulling a 250-lb individual out of a burning building. This happened 4 days ago. Currently, he is experiencing considerable pain, is unable to sit on hard surfaces (from pressure as well as flexing the hip), and has pain when rising or lowering self into a chair and climbing or descending stairs. Hip flexion is limited to 90 degrees, straight-leg raising to 45 degrees. He tolerates minimal resis-tance to hip extension or knee flexion. This individual must be able to climb a lad-

der while wearing his gear (weighs 40 lb) and air pack (weighing 40 lb) and carrying a 20-lb hand tool, carry a 175-lb individual across his shoulder, drag a heavy body across the floor, climb five flights of stairs wearing full gear, and run 1/2 mile in 5 minutes to be able to return to work.

- Explain why this patient has impaired function in biomechanical terms.
- Establish goals that reflect treatment of the impairments and desired functional outcomes.
- Design a program of intervention at each stage of tissue healing.
- Design a series of exercises that can be used to prepare Mr. C for return to function once the muscle has healed.

4. A 78-year-old woman who lives at home with her husband has been referred to you for home-based physical therapy. She had a cemented THA with a posterolateral approach 1 week ago and has been home from the hospital for 2 days. She is ambulating with a walker on level surfaces, weight bearing is tolerated.

- Continue progressing her exercise program that was initiated in the hospital.
- Review the precautions she must take for the next 6 to 12 weeks during ADLs.
- Make suggestions on how she or her husband might adapt the home environment to help her adhere to the precautions.

REFERENCES

1. Antoniou, J, Greidanus, NV, and Proprosky, WG: Surgical approaches and anatomic considerations. In Pellicci, PM, Tria, AJ, and Garvin, KL (eds): Orthopedic Knowledge Update, 2. Hip and Knee Reconstruction. American Academy of Orthopedic Surgeons, Rosemont, IL, 2000, p 91.
2. Ball, PB, Wroe, MC, and MacLeod, L: Survey of physical therapy preoperative care in total hip replacement. Phys Ther Health Care 1:83, 1986.
3. Barnes, B, and Dunovan, K: Functional outcomes after hip fracture. Phys Ther 67:1675, 1987.
4. Barrick, EF: Orthopedic trauma. In Kauffman, TL (ed): Geriatric Rehabilitation Manual. Churchill Livingstone, New York, 1999, p 125.
5. Beber, C, and Convery, R: Management of patients with total hip replacement. Phys Ther 52:823, 1972.
6. Berry, DJ, and Chao, EYS: Cemented femoral components. In Morrey, BF (ed): Reconstructive Surgery of the Joints, Vol 2, ed 2. Churchill Livingstone, New York, 1996, p 943.
7. Berry, DJ, and Morrey, BF: Uncemented femoral components. In Morrey, BF (ed): Reconstructive Surgery of the Joints, Vol 2, ed 2. Churchill Livingstone, New York, 1996, p 979.
8. Birage, SJ, Morrow-Howell, N, and Proctor, EK: Hip fracture. Clin Geriatr Med 10:589, 1994.
9. Bullock-Saxton, JE: Local sensation changes and altered hip muscle function following severe ankle sprain. Phys Ther 74:17, 1994.
10. Burton, D, and Imrie, S: Total hip arthroplasty and postoperative rehabilitation. Phys Ther 53:132, 1973.
11. Cailliet, R: Low Back Pain Syndrome, ed 4. FA Davis, Philadelphia, 1988.
12. Cameron, HU, Brotzman, SB, and Boolas, M: Rehabilitation after total joint arthroplasty. In Brotzman, SB: Clinical Orthopedic Rehabilitation. CV Mosby, St Louis, 2000, p 283.
13. Charnley, J: Total hip replacement by low friction arthroplasty. Clin Orthop 72:721, 1974.
14. Cibulka, MT, and Delitto, A: A comparison of two different methods to treat hip pain in runners. J Orthop Sports Phys Ther 17:173, 1993.
15. Coventry, MB: Historical perspective of hip arthroplasty. In Morrey, BF (ed): Reconstructive Surgery of the Joints, ed 2. Churchill Livingstone, New York, 1996, p 875.
16. Craik, RL: Disability following hip fracture. Phys Ther 74:388, 1994.
17. Crutchfield, CA, et al: Balance and coordination training. In Scully, RM, and Barnes, MR (eds): Physical Therapy. JB Lippincott, Philadelphia, 1989.
18. Cullen, S: Physical therapy program for patients with total hip replacement. Phys Ther 53:1293, 1973.
19. Cyriax, J: Textbook of Orthopaedic Medicine, Vol 1. Diagnosis of Soft Tissue Lesions, ed 8. Bailliere Tindall, London, 1982.
20. Enloe, J, et al: Total hip and knee replacement treatment: a report using consensus. J Orthop Sports Phys Ther 23:3, 1996.
21. Fehring, TK, and Rosenberg, AG: Primary total hip arthroplasty: indications and contraindications. In Callaghan, JJ, Rosenberg, AG, and Rubash, HE (eds): The Adult Hip, Vol II. Lippincott-Raven Publishers, Philadelphia, 1998, p 893.
22. Fife, RS: Osteoarthritis, Epidemiology, Pathology, and Pathogensis. In Klippel, JF (ed): Primer on Rheumatic Diseases, ed 11. Arthritis Foundation, Atlanta, 1997, p 216.
23. Finerman, GA, et al: Commentary. In Finerman, GA, et al (eds): Total Hip Arthroplasty Outcomes. Churchill Livingstone, New York, 1998, p 3.
24. Freburger, JK: An analysis of the relationship between utilization of physical therapy services and outcomes of care for patients after total hip arthroplasty. Phys Ther 80: 448, 2000.
25. Galante, JO: An overview of total joint arthroplasty. In Callaghan, JJ, Rosenberg, AG, and Rubash, HE (eds): The Adult Hip, Vol II. Lippincott-Raven Publishers, Philadelphia, 1998, p 829.

26. Givens-Heiss, DL, et al: In vivo acetabular contact pressures during rehabilitation. Part II: post acute phase. Phys Ther 72: 700, 1992.
27. Goldstein, TS: Determining the cause of disability. In Functional Rehabilitation in Orthopedics. Aspen, Gaithersburg, MD, 1995.
28. Gucione, AA: Arthritis and the process of disablement. Phys Ther 74:408, 1994.
29. Gucione, AA, Fogerson, TL, and Anderson, JJ: Regaining functional independence in the acute care setting following hip fracture. Phys Ther 76:818, 1996.
30. Hanssen, AD: Anatomy and surgical approaches. In Morrey, BF (ed): Reconstructive Surgery of the Joints, Vol 2, ed 2. Churchill Livingstone, New York, 1996, p 883.
31. Hielema, F, and Summerfore, R: Physical therapy for patients with hip fracture or joint replacement. Phys Ther Health Care 1:89, 1986.
32. Holt, EM, et al: 1000 femoral neck fractures. The effect of pre-injury mobility and surgical experience on outcome. Injury 25:91, 1994.
33. Howe, JG, and Lambert, B: Critical pathways in total hip arthroplasty. In Callaghan, JJ, Rosenberg, AG, and Rubash, HE (eds): The Adult Hip, Vol II. Lippincott-Raven Publishers, Philadelphia, p 865, 1998.
34. Izumi, H, et al: Joint motion of bipolar femoral prostheses. J Arthroplasty 10:237, 1995.
35. Jette, AM, Harris, BA, and Clearly, PD: Functional recovery after hip fracture. Arch Phys Med Rehabil 68:735, 1987.
36. Kendall, F: Criticism of current tests and exercises for physical fitness. Phys Ther 45:187, 1965.
37. Kopell, H, and Thompson, W: Peripheral Entrapment Neuropathies, ed 2. Robert E Krieger, Huntington, NY, 1976.
38. Koval, KJ, and Zuckerman, JD: Hip Fractures: A Practical Guide to Management. Springer-Verlag, New York, 2000.
39. Koval, KJ, et al: Ambulatory ability after hip fracture. A prospective study in geriatric patients. Clin Orthop 310:150, 1995.
40. Koval, K, et al: Weight bearing after hip fracture: a prospective series of 596 geriatric hip fracture patients. J Orthop Trauma 10:526, 1996.
40a. Krebs, DE, et al: Exercise and gait effects on in vivo hip contact pressures. Phys Ther 71: 301, 1991.
40b. Krebs, DE, et al: Hip biomechanics during gait. J Orthop Sports Phys Ther 28: 51, 1998.
41. Lachiewicz, PF: Dislocation. In Pellicci, PM, Tria, AJ, and Garvin, KL (eds): Orthopedic Knowledge Update, 2. Hip and Knee Reconstruction. American Academy of Orthopedic Surgeons, Rosemont, IL, 2000, p 149.
42. Lang, KE: Comparison of 6- and 7-day physical therapy coverage on length of stay and discharge outcome for individuals with total hip and knee arthroplasty. J Orthop Sports Phys Ther 28:15, 1998.
43. Laupacis, A, et al: The effect of elective total hip replacement on health-related quality of life. J Bone Joint Surg 75A: 1619, 1993.
44. Levangie, P, and Norkin, C: Joint Structure and Function: A Comprehensive Analysis, ed 3. FA Davis, Philadelphia, 2001.
45. Lewallen, DG: Cementless primary total hip arthroplasty. In Pellicci, PM, Tria, AJ, and Garvin, KL (eds): Orthopedic Knowledge Update, 2. Hip and Knee Reconstruction. American Academy of Orthopedic Surgeons, Rosemont, IL, 2000, p 195.
46. Lieberman, JR, et al: Differences between patients' and physicians' evaluation of outcome after total hip arthroplasty. J Bone Joint Surg 78A:835, 1996.
47. Magee, DJ: Orthopedic Physical Assessment, ed 3. WB Saunders, Philadelphia, 1997.
48. Maloney, WJ, and Hartford, JM: The cemented femoral component. In Callaghan, JJ, Rosenberg, AG, and Rubash, HE (eds): The Adult Hip, Vol II. Lippincott-Raven Publishers, Philadelphia, p 959, 1998.
49. Martin, SD, et al: Hip surgery and rehabilitation. In Melvin, JL, and Gall, V (eds): Rheumatologic Rehabilitation Series, Vol 5: Surgical Rehabilitation. American Occupational Therapy Association, Bethesda, MD, p 81, 1999.
50. McGrorey, BJ, Stewart, MJ, and Sim, FH: Participation in sports after total hip and knee arthroplasty: a review of the literature and survey of surgical preferences. Mayo Clin Proc 70B:202, 1995.
51. Meere, PA, DiCesare, PE, and Zuckerman, JD: Hip fractures treated by hip arthroplasty. In Callaghan, JJ, Rosenberg, AG, and Rubash, HE (eds): The Adult Hip, Vol II. Lippincott-Raven Publishers, Philadelphia, 1998, p 1221.
52. Mohler, CG, and Collis, DK: Early complications and their management. In Callaghan, JJ, Rosenberg, AG, and Rubash, HE (eds): The Adult Hip, Vol II. Lippincott-Raven Publishers, Philadelphia, 1998, p 1125.
53. Morrey, BF: Cemented acetabular components. In Morrey, BF (ed): Reconstructive Surgery of the Joints, Vol 2, ed 2. Churchill Livingstone, New York, 1996, p 935.
54. Morrey, RF, and Kavanagh, BF: Cementless joint replacement: Current status and future. Bull Rheum Dis 37:1, 1987.
55. Morrey, BF: Dislocation. In Morrey, BF (ed): Reconstructive Surgery of the Joints, Vol 2, ed 2. Churchill Livingstone, New York, p 1247, 1996.
56. Muller, WE: Total hip prosthesis. Clin Orthop 72:460, 1970.
57. Mulligan, BR: Manual Therapy "NAGS", "SNAGS", MWM'S: etc., ed 4. Plane View Press, Wellington, 1999.
58. Munin, ME, et al: Early inpatient rehabilitation after elective hip and knee arthroplasty. JAMA 279:847, 1998.
59. Munin, MC, et al: Rehabilitation. In Callaghan, JJ, Rosenberg, AG, and Rubash, HE (eds): The Adult Hip, Vol II. Lippincott-Raven Publishers, Philadelphia, 1998, p 1571.
60. Nelson, C, Lombardi, PM, and Pellicci, PM: Hybrid total hip replacement. In Pellicci, PM, Tria, AJ, and Garvin, KL (eds): Orthopedic Knowledge Update, 2. Hip and Knee Reconstruction. American Academy of Orthopedic Surgeons, Rosemont, IL, 2000, p 207.
61. Neumann, DA: An electromyographic study of the hip abductor muscles as subjects with hip prostheses walked with different methods of using a cane and carrying a load. Phys Ther 79:1163, 1999.
62. Neumann, DA: Hip abductor muscle activity in patients with a hip prosthesis while carrying loads in one hand. Phys Ther 76:1320, 1996.
63. Neumann, DA: Hip abductor muscle activity as subjects with hip prostheses walk with different methods of using a cane. Phys Ther 78: 490, 1998.
64. NIH Consensus Development Panel on Total Hip Replacement. JAMA 273:1950, 1995.
65. Nordin, M, and Frankel, VH: Biomechanics of the Hip. In Nordin, M, and Frankel, VH: Basic Biomechanics of the Musculoskeletal System, ed 3. Lippincott Williams & Wilkins, Philadelphia, 2001, p 202.

66. Parker, MJ, Pryor, GA, and Thorngren, K: Handbook of Hip Fracture Surgery. Butterworth-Heinemann, Oxford, 1997.
67. Perry, J: Gait Analysis: Normal and Pathological Function. SLACK Inc., Thorofare, NJ, 1992.
68. Peters, CL, and Dunn, HK: The cementless acetabular component. In Callaghan, JJ, Rosenberg, AG, and Rubash, HE (eds): The Adult Hip, Vol II. Lippincott-Raven Publishers, Philadelphia, 1998, p 993.
69. Poss, R: Total joint replacement: optimizing patient expectations. J Am Acad Orthop Surg 1:18, 1993.
70. Praemer, A, Furner, S, and Rice, DP: Musculoskeletal Conditions in the United States. American Academy of Orthopedic Surgeons, Chicago, 1992.
71. Ranawat, CS, Rasquinna, VJ, and Rodriguez, JA: Results of cemented total hip replacement. In Pellicci, PM, Tria, AJ, and Garvin, KL (eds): Orthopedic Knowledge Update, 2. Hip and Knee Reconstruction. American Academy of Orthopedic Surgeons, Rosemont, IL, 2000, p 181.
72. Ranawat, CS, and Rodriguez, JA: The cemented acetabular component. In Callaghan, JJ, Rosenberg, AG, and Rubash, HE (eds): The Adult Hip, Vol II. Lippincott-Raven Publishers, p 981, 1998.
73. Richardson, R: Physical therapy management of patients undergoing total hip replacement. Phys Ther 55:984, 1975.
74. Roach, JA, Tremblay, LM, and Bowers, DL: A preoperative assessment and education program: implementation and outcomes. Patient Educ Couns 25:83, 1995.
75. Sahrmann, SA: Diagnosis and Treatment of Movement Impairment Syndromes. CV Mosby, St Louis, 2002.
76. Schamerloh, C, and Ritter, M: Prevention of dislocation or subluxation of total hip replacements. Phys Ther 57:1028, 1977.
77. Shashika, H, Matsuba, Y, and Watanabe, Y: Home program of physical therapy: effect on disabilities of patients with total hip arthroplasty. Arch Phys Med Rehabil 77:273, 1996.
78. Sheh, C, et al: Muscle recovery and the hip joint after total hip replacement. Clin Orthop 302:115, 1994.
79. Sherrington, C, and Lord, SR: Home exercise to improve strength and walking velocity after hip fracture: a randomized, controlled trial. Arch Phys Med Rehabil 78:208, 1997.
80. Smith, LK, Weiss, EL, and Lehmkuhl, LD: Brunnstrom's Clinical Kinesiology, ed 5. FA Davis, Philadelphia, 1996.
81. Strickland, EM, et al: In vivo acetabular contact pressures during rehabilitation: Part I. Acute phase. Phys Ther 72:691, 1992.
82. Taylor, JR, and Twomey, LT: Age changes in lumbar zygapophyseal joint. Spine 11(7):739, 1986.
83. Taylor, KW, and Murthy, VL: Femoral neck fractures. In Hoppenfeld, S, and Murthy, VL (eds): Treatment and Rehabilitation of Fractures. Lippincott Williams & Wilkins, Philadelphia, 2000, p 258.
84. Taylor, KW, Hoppenfeld, S: Intertrochanteric fractures. In Hoppenfeld, S, and Murthy, VL (eds): Treatment and Rehabilitation of Fractures. Lippincott Williams & Wilkins, Philadelphia, 2000, p 274.
85. Taylor, KW, and Murthy, VL: Subtrochanteric femur fractures. In Hoppenfeld, S, and Murthy, VL (eds): Treatment and Rehabilitation of Fractures. Lippincott Williams & Wilkins, Philadelphia, 2000, p 288.
86. Tinetti, ME, et al: Home-based multicomponent rehabilitation program for older persons after hip fracture. A randomized trial. Arch Phys Med Rehabil 80:916, 1999.
87. Trousdale, TR, and Cabahela, ME: Uncemented acetabular components. In Morrey, BF (ed): Reconstructive Surgery of the Joints, Vol 2, ed 2. Churchill Livingstone, New York, 1996, p 961.
88. Tsahakis, PJ, Brick, GW, and Poss, R. Surgery of the hip. In Sledge, CB, et al: Arthritis Surgery, WB Saunders, Philadelphia, 1994, p 780.
89. Wathe, RA, Koval, KJ, et al: Modular unipolar versus bipolar prosthesis: a prospective evaluation of functional outcomes after femoral neck fracture. J Orthop Trauma 9:298, 1995.
90. Wyke, B: Neurological aspects of pain for the physical therapy clinician. Physical Therapy Forum, Ohio Chapter APTA Conference, Columbus, OH, 1982.

Chapter 13

The Knee

OBJECTIVES

After studying this chapter, the reader will be able to:

1. Identify important aspects of the knee structure and function for review.
2. Establish a therapeutic exercise program to manage soft tissue and joint lesions in the knee region related to stages of recovery after an inflammatory insult to the tissues, and recognize unique circumstances in the knee and patella for their management.
3. Describe common indications for and expected outcomes of common surgical procedures for pathologies of the knee.
4. Establish a therapeutic exercise program to manage patients following common surgical procedures for the knee.

The knee joint is designed for mobility and stability; it functionally lengthens and shortens the lower extremity to raise and lower the body or to move the foot in space. Along with the hip and ankle, it supports the body when standing, and it is a primary functional unit in walking, climbing, and sitting activities.

Highlights of the anatomy and function of the knee complex are reviewed in the first section of this chapter. To design a therapeutic exercise program for a patient's knee, the reader should be familiar with the principles of management presented in Chapter 8.

Review of the Structure and Function of the Knee

Bony Parts (see Fig. 6–49)

The bones of the knee joint consist of the distal femur with its two condyles, the proximal tibia with its two tibial plateaus, and the large sesamoid bone in the quadriceps tendon, the patella. It is a complex joint both anatomically and biomechanically.[61,70]

Knee Joint Complex

The lax joint capsule encloses two articulations: the tibiofemoral and the patellofemoral joints. Recesses from the capsule form the suprapatellar, subpopliteal, and gastrocnemius bursae. Folds or thickenings in the synovium persist from embryologic tissue in up to 60% of individuals and may become symptomatic with microtraumas or macrotraumas.[9,63]

The Tibiofemoral Joint

Characteristics. The knee joint is a biaxial, modified hinge joint with two interposed menisci supported by ligaments and muscles. Anteroposterior stability is provided by the cruciate ligaments; mediolateral stability is provided by the medial (tibial) and lateral (femoral) collateral ligaments, respectively.[18,61,70,117]

- The convex bony partner is composed of two asymmetric condyles on the distal end of the femur. The medial condyle is longer than the lateral, which contributes to the locking mechanism at the knee.[18,61,70,117]
- The concave bony partner is composed of two tibial plateaus on the proximal tibia with their respective fibrocartilaginous menisci. The medial plateau is larger than the lateral.
- The menisci improve the congruency of the articulating surfaces. They are attached to the joint capsule by the coronary ligaments. The medial meniscus is firmly attached to the joint capsule as well as to the medial collateral ligament, anterior cruciate ligament, and semimembranosus muscle; therefore, it is subject to injury when there is a lateral blow to the knee.

Arthrokinematics. Joint mechanics will be affected by open- and closed-chain positions of the extremity. This is summarized in Box 13–1.

Box 13–1 Summary of Arthrokinematics of the Knee Joint

Physiologic Motion	Roll	Slide
Tibial motion—open-chain		
Flexion	Posterior and medial rotation	Posterior
Extension	Anterior and lateral rotation	Anterior
Femoral motion—closed-chain		
Flexion	Posterior and lateral rotation	Anterior
Extension	Anterior and medial rotation	Posterior

- With motions of the tibia (open kinematic chain), the concave plateaus slide in the same direction as the bone motion.
- With motions of the femur on a fixated tibia (closed kinematic chain), the convex condyles slide in the direction opposite to the bone motion.
- Rotation occurs between the femoral condyles and the tibia during the final degrees of extension. This is called the locking, or screw-home, mechanism.
  - When the tibia moves in an open-chain, terminal extension results in the tibia rotating externally on the femur. To unlock the knee, the tibia rotates internally.
  - When the tibia is fixed with the foot on the ground (closed kinematic chain), terminal extension results in the femur rotating internally (the medial condyle slides further posteriorly than the lateral). Concurrently, the hip goes into extension. Tautness in the iliofemoral ligament, which occurs with hip extension, reinforces the medial rotation of the femur. As the knee is unlocked, the femur rotates laterally. Unlocking of the knee occurs indirectly with hip flexion and directly from action of the popliteus muscle.

The Patellofemoral Joint

Characteristics. The patella is a sesamoid bone in the quadriceps tendon. It articulates with the intercondylar (trochlear) groove on the anterior aspect of the distal portion of the femur. Its articulating surface is covered with smooth hyaline cartilage. The patella is embedded in the anterior portion of the joint capsule and is connected to the tibia by the ligamentum patellae. Many bursae surround the patella.[61,70]

Mechanics. As the knee flexes, the patella enters the intercondylar groove with its inferior margin making first contact, and then it slides caudally along the groove. With extension, the patella slides cranially. If patellar movement is restricted, it interferes with the range of knee flexion and may contribute to an extensor lag with active knee extension.[127]

Knee and Patellar Function

The primary function of the patella is to increase the moment arm of the quadriceps muscle in its function to extend the knee. It also redirects the forces exerted by the quadriceps.

Patellar Alignment

Normal alignment of the patella in the frontal plane is described as having a 15-degree **Q angle.** The Q angle is the angle formed by two intersecting lines: one from the anterior superior iliac spine to the midpatella, the other from the tibial tubercle through the midpatella. The Q angle describes the lateral tracking or bowstring effect that the quadriceps muscles and patellar tendon have on the patella.

Forces Maintaining Alignment

Lateral fixation of the patella is provided by the iliotibial (IT) band and lateral retinaculum; these are opposed by the active medial pull of the vastus medialis obliquis (VMO) muscle. The patellar ligament fixates the patella inferiorly against the active pull of the quadriceps muscle superiorly.[96,99]

Patellar Malalignment and Tracking Problems

Malalignment and tracking problems of the patella may be caused by several factors that may or may not be interrelated.[44a,78]

- ***Increased Q angle.*** This can be from genu valgum, patella alta, pronated feet, wide pelvis, increased femoral anteversion, or external tibial torsion.
- ***Muscle and fascial tightness.*** Tight IT band and lateral retinaculum prevent medial gliding of the patella. Tight ankle plantarflexors result in pronation of the foot when the ankle dorsiflexes, causing medial torsion of the tibia and functional lateral displacement of the tibial tuberosity in relationship to the patella. Tight rectus femoris and hamstring muscles may affect the mechanics of the knee, leading to compensations.[78]
- ***Lax medial capsular retinaculum or an insufficient VMO muscle.*** The VMO may be weak from disuse or inhibited because of joint swelling or pain, leading to poor medial stability.[120] Poor

timing of its contraction, which alters the ratio of firing between the VMO and vastus lateralis muscle, may lead to an imbalance of forces.[108,130] Weakness or poor timing of VMO contractions will increase the lateral drifting of the patella.

Patellar Compression

Patellar contact. The posterior surface of the patella has several facets. It is not completely congruent as it articulates with the trochlear groove on the femur. When the knee is in complete extension (zero degrees), the patella is superior to the trochlear groove. By 15 degrees of flexion the inferior border of the patella begins to articulate with the superior aspect of the groove. As the knee flexes, the patella slides distally in the groove, and more surface area comes in contact. Beyond 60 degrees there is controversy as to whether or not the contact area continues to increase, level off, or decrease.[44,44a] In addition, as the knee flexes past 90 degrees, the quadriceps tendon comes into contact with the trochlear groove as the patella slides inferiorly.

Compression forces. In full extension, because there is no contact of the patella with the trochlear groove, there is no compression of the articular surfaces. In addition, because the femur and tibia are almost parallel, the line of pull of the quadriceps muscle and patellar tendon causes a very small resultant compressive load. The resultant force of the quadriceps and patellar tendon forces rises as the knee flexes, but there is also greater surface area of the patella in contact with the groove to dissipate this force. The joint reaction force on the articular surface rises rapidly between 30 degrees and 60 degrees. There is controversy as to the extent of joint reaction forces in greater degrees of flexion. In closed-chain squatting, the joint reaction force continues to rise until 90 degrees, then levels off or decreases because the quadriceps tendon begins making contact with the trochlear groove and, therefore, dissipates some of the force.[44] In an open-chain with free weights on the distal leg, the greatest joint reaction force is described to occur around 30 degrees of flexion.[44] This is because of the changing moment arm of the resistive force more than the line of pull of the quadriceps and patellar tendons. In an open-chain with variable resistance, the peak stress is at 60 degrees and peak compression at 75 degrees.[32]

Extensor Muscles

- The quadriceps femoris muscle group is the only muscle crossing anterior to the axis of the knee and is the prime mover for knee extension. Other muscles that can act to extend the knee require the foot to be fixated, creating a closed-chain. In this situation, the hamstrings and also the soleus muscles can cause or control knee extension by pulling the tibia posteriorly.
- During standing and the stance phase of gait, the knee is an intermediate joint in a closed-chain. The quadriceps muscle controls the amount of flexion at the knee and also causes knee extension through reverse muscle pull on the femur. In the erect posture, when the knee is locked, the quadriceps need not function when the gravity line falls anterior to the axis of motion. In this case, tension in the hamstring and gastrocnemius tendons supports the posterior capsule.
- The patella improves the moment arm of the extensor force by increasing the distance of the quadriceps tendon from the knee joint axis. Its greatest effect on the leverage of the quadriceps is during extension of the knee from 60 to 30 degrees and rapidly diminishes from 15 to 0 degrees of extension.[46,70]
- The peak torque of the quadriceps muscle occurs between 70 and 50 degrees.[16] The physiological advantage of the quadriceps rapidly decreases during the last 15 degrees of knee extension because of its shortened length. This, combined with its decreased moment arm in the last 15 degrees, requires the muscle to significantly increase its contractile force when large demands are placed on the muscle during terminal extension.[46] During standing, assistance for extension comes from the hamstring and soleus muscles as well as from the mechanical locking mechanism of the knee. In addition, the anterior cruciate ligament and the pull of the hamstring muscle group counter the anterior translation force of the quadriceps muscle.[36,77] During open-chain knee extension exercises in the sitting or supine position, when the resistive force is maximum in terminal extension because of the moment arm of the resistance, a relatively strong contraction of the quadriceps muscle is required to overcome both the physiologic and mechanical disadvantages of the muscle to complete the final 15 degrees of motion.[46] However, it is worth mentioning that the compressive loads on the patella also decrease in terminal extension because of its superior location with respect to the trochlear groove and the resultant force of the line of pull of the quadriceps and patellar tendon.

The therapist needs to be aware of the effect of the resistance and where in the range of motion the muscle is being challenged. During open-chain exercises with fixed resistance when the resistance torque challenges the quadriceps in terminal extension, there will be little challenge midrange where the muscle is capable of generating greater tension.

Flexor Muscles

- The hamstring muscles are the primary knee flexors and also influence rotation of the tibia on the femur. Because they are two-joint muscles, they contract more efficiently when they are simultaneously lengthened over the hip (during hip flexion) as they flex the knee. In closed-chain activities, the hamstring muscles can assist with knee extension by pulling on the tibia.
- The gastrocnemius muscle can also function as a knee flexor, but its prime function at the knee during weight bearing is to support the posterior capsule against hyperextension forces.
- The popliteus muscle supports the posterior capsule and acts to unlock the knee.
- The pes anserinus muscle group (sartorius, gracilis, semitendinosus) provides medial stability to the knee and affects rotation of the tibia in a closed-chain.

The Knee and Gait

Range of motion of the knee during gait. During the normal gait cycle, the knee goes through a range of 60 degrees (0 degrees extension at initial contact or heel strike to 60 degrees at the end of initial swing). There is some medial rotation of the femur as the knee extends at initial contact and just prior to heel-off.[70,101]

Muscle control of the knee during gait. Stability during the gait cycle is normally efficiently controlled.[70,101]

- The quadriceps muscle controls the amount of knee flexion during initial contact (loading response), then extends the knee toward midstance. It again controls the amount of flexion during preswing (heel-off to toe-off) and prevents excessive heel rise during initial swing. With loss of quadriceps function, the patient lurches the trunk anteriorly during initial contact to move the center of gravity anterior to the knee so it is stable or rotates the extremity outward to lock the knee.[122] With fast walking, there may be excessive heel rise during initial swing.
- The hamstring muscles primarily control the forward swing of the leg during terminal swing. Loss of function may result in the knee snapping into extension during this period. The hamstrings also provide posterior support to the knee capsule when the knee is extended during stance. Loss of function results in progressive genu recurvatum.[122]
- The unijoint ankle plantarflexor muscles (primarily the soleus) help control the amount of knee flexion during preswing by controlling the forward movement of the tibia. Loss of function results in hyperextension of the knee during preswing (also loss of heel rise at the ankle and, thus, a lag or slight dropping of the pelvis on that side during the preswing phase).
- The gastrocnemius muscle provides tension posterior to the knee when it is in extension (end of loading response or foot flat, and just prior to preswing or heel-off). Loss of function results in hyperextension of the knee during these periods as well as loss of plantarflexion during preswing or push-off.

Hip and ankle impairments. Because the knee is the intermediate joint between the hip and foot, problems in these two areas will interfere with knee function during gait. Examples:

- Inability to extend the hip will prevent the knee from extending just before terminal stance (heel-off).
- Most of the muscles functioning to control the hip are two-joint muscles that also cross the knee. With asymmetries in length and strength, unbalanced forces may stress various structures in the knee, giving rise to pain when walking or running. For example, a tight tensor fasciae latae or gluteus maximus muscle will increase stress on the IT band, which could lead to lateral knee pain or affect tracking of the patella and lead to anterior knee pain. Overuse of the hamstring muscle group increases posterior translation forces on the tibia requiring compensation in the quadriceps femoris muscle and resulting in anterior knee pain (see Chapter 12).
- The position and function of the foot and ankle affect the stresses transmitted to the knee. For example, with pes planus or pes valgus, there is medial rotation of the tibia and an increased bowstring effect on the patella, increasing the lateral tracking forces.

Referred Pain and Nerve Injuries

Common sources of referred pain. Nerve roots and tissues derived from spinal segments L-3 refer to the anterior aspect, and those from S-1 and S-2 refer to the posterior aspect of the knee.[23] The hip joint, which is primarily innervated by L-3, may refer symptoms to the anterior thigh and knee. Therapeutic exercise for the knee is beneficial only in preventing disuse of the part; primary treatment must be directed to the source of the irritation.

Major nerves subject to injury at the knee. The sciatic nerve divides into the tibial and common peroneal nerves just proximal to the popliteal fossa. These nerves are relatively well protected deep in the fossa.

- Common peroneal nerve (L2-4) becomes superficial where it winds around the fibula just below the fibular head; this is a common site for injury. Symptoms of sensory loss and muscle weakness will be distal to that site.
- Saphenous nerve (L2-4) is a sensory nerve that innervates the skin along the medial side of the knee and leg. It may be injured with trauma or surgery in that region.

Joint Hypomobility: Nonoperative Management

Related Diagnoses and Etiology of Symptoms

Rheumatoid arthritis (RA) and osteoarthritis (OA) as well as acute joint trauma can affect the knee articulations at the tibiofemoral joint. Decreased flexibility and adhesions from immobilization develop in the joints and surrounding tissues any time the joint is splinted or casted. Reflex inhibition and resulting weakness of the quadriceps femoris muscle occurs because of joint distention.[120] Chapter 8 describes the etiology of these arthritic and joint symptoms.

Rheumatoid Arthritis (RA)

Early in the disease, the hands and feet are usually involved first; with progression of RA, the knees may also become involved. The joints become warm and swollen, and limited motion develops. In addition, a genu valgum deformity commonly develops in the advanced stages of this disease.

Osteoarthritis (Degenerative Joint Disease, DJD)

Pain, muscle weakness, and joint limitations progressively worsen. Genu varum commonly develops.

Joint Trauma

Following trauma, immediate swelling indicates bleeding into the joint. Slowly progressive swelling (4 or more hours) indicates serous effusion, which may occur with ligament and meniscal tears. When acute, there will be muscle guarding, weakness, and limited motion from the swelling. When the swelling recedes, examine the knee for ligamentous and meniscal tears.

Joint Restrictions After a Period of Immobilization

When the knee has been immobilized for several weeks or longer, such as after healing of a fracture or postsurgery, the capsule, muscles, and soft tissue develop contractures, and motion becomes restricted. Adhesions may restrict caudal gliding of the patella which will limit knee flexion and may cause pain as the patella is compressed against the femur. An extensor lag may occur with active knee extension if the patella does not glide proximally when the quadriceps muscle contracts.[100] This usually occurs after operative repairs of some knee ligaments, when the knee is immobilized in flexion for a prolonged period.

Common Impairments

With joint involvement, the pattern of restriction at the knee is usually more loss of flexion than extension. When there is effusion (swelling within the joint), the joint assumes a position near 25 degrees of flexion, at which there is greatest capsular distensibility. Little motion is possible because of the swelling. Symptoms of joint involvement, such as distention, stiffness, pain, and reflex quadriceps inhibition may cause extensor (quadriceps) lag in which the active range of knee extension is less than the passive range.[121] Disturbed balance responses have also been reported in patients with arthritis.[133]

Common Functional Limitations/Disabilities

- With acute symptoms and in advanced stages of degeneration there is pain on motion, with weight bearing, and during gait, which may interfere with work or routine household and community activities.
- Limitation or difficulty controlling weight-bearing activities involving knee flexion such as sitting down and rising from a chair or a commode, descending or ascending stairs, stooping, or squatting.[35]

Joint Management: Protection Phase

See Chapter 8 for general guidelines in the management of acute joint lesions as well as specific guidelines for RA and DJD. The following goals and interventions are for treating joint symptoms during the acute stage when protection is necessary.

Control Pain

In addition to using modalities and providing rest with an elastic wrap or splint, use *gentle joint-play oscillation techniques* (grade I) to inhibit the pain. If these techniques increase the pain or swelling, they should not be attempted for several days.

Maintain Soft Tissue and Joint Mobility

Passive, active-assistive or active ROM. Use ROM techniques within the limits of pain and available motion. The patient may be able to perform active ROM in the gravity-eliminated, side-lying position.

Grade I or II tractions or glides. Apply gentle techniques, if tolerated, with the joint in resting position (25 degrees of flexion). Stretching is contraindicated at this stage.

Maintain Muscle Function and Prevent Patellar Adhesions

Multiple-angle, gentle muscle-setting techniques. Include quadriceps femoris and hamstring contractions in pain-free positions. Quad sets may help maintain mobility of the patella when the tibiofemoral joint is immobilized and therefore are routinely taught following surgery or when the joint is immobilized in a cast.

Submaximal closed-chain muscle setting. Begin with the patient sitting and the knee extended as far as possible without provoking pain, and have the patient press the heel on the floor while pressing the thigh into the chair.

Quad sets with leg raising. Vary the angle of knee flexion/extension, including full knee extension, and have the patient perform leg raises; the patient should be able to maintain each knee position without pain.

Note: Leg-raising is a dynamic activity of the hip flexors and is done in conjunction with quad sets to vary the effect of gravity on the quadriceps while it maintains an isometric hold.

Protect the Joint

Partial weight-bearing activities. If necessary during an acute flare of arthritis use crutches, canes, or a walker to distribute forces through the upper extremities while walking.

Patient education. Instruct the patient and family members in good bed positioning to avoid flexion contractures.

Make functional adaptations. To reduce the amount of knee flexion and patellar compression when the person moves from flexion to extension in activities such as standing up from sitting or stair climbing, instruct the patient to minimize stair climbing, to use elevated seats on commodes, and to avoid deep-seated or low chairs.

Joint Management: Controlled Motion and Return to Function Phases

As the inflammation decreases and healing occurs and the joint tissues are able to tolerate increased stresses, the goals of treatment change to deal with the impairments which interfere with functional activities. The patient is progressed through controlled motion exercises and activities with the focus on safely returning to the desired functional outcome.

Decrease the Effects of Stiffness from Inactivity

Instruct the patient to perform active ROM and muscle-setting techniques frequently during the day, especially prior to bearing weight.[35]

Decrease Pain from Mechanical Stress

Continue use of assistive devices for ambulation, if necessary. The patient may progress to using less assistance or may ambulate for periods without assistance. Continue use of elevated seats on commodes and chairs, if needed, to reduce the mechanical stresses imposed when attempting to stand up.[35]

Increase Joint Play and Range of Motion (ROM)

Joint mobilization. When there is loss of joint play and decreased mobility, joint mobilization techniques should be used. Apply grade III sustained or grade IV oscillation techniques to the tibiofemoral and patellofemoral articulations. See Figures 6–50 through 6–55 and their descriptions in Chapter 6. Progress each technique by positioning the joint at the end of its available range before applying the mobilization technique. As range increases, it is important to emphasize the rotational accessory motions that accompany flexion and extension. To increase flexion, position the tibia in medial rotation, and, apply the posterior glide against the anterior aspect of the medial tibial plateau. To increase extension, position the tibia in lateral rotation, and apply the anterior glide against the posterior aspect of the lateral tibial plateau. Medial and lateral gliding of the tibia on the femur may also be done to regain mobility for flexion and extension.[60]

Precaution: Do not increase ROM unless the patient has sufficient strength to control the motion already available. A mobile joint with inadequate muscle control causes poor stability and makes lower extremity weight-bearing function difficult.

Neuromuscular inhibition. When there is decreased flexibility in the muscles affecting knee motion, muscle elongation (inhibition) techniques should be used. Muscles typically involved include hamstrings, quadriceps, and gastrocnemius-soleus complex.

Precaution: Strong muscle contractions may exacerbate joint symptoms; adapt the dosage according to the patient's tolerance level.

Passive stretching. When there is decreased flexibility in the noncontractile soft tissue preventing knee motion, passive stretching techniques should be used.

- Apply a low-intensity, long-duration stretch within the patient's tolerance.

Precaution: Passive stretching using the tibia as a lever tends to exacerbate joint symptoms; use these techniques after joint mobilization so that joint play is available during the stretch.

- Apply soft tissue massage or friction massage to loosen adhesions or contractures. Include deep massage around the border of the patella.

Improve Joint Tracking and Pain-Free Knee ROM Using Mobilization with Movement (MWM)

MWM may be applied to increase ROM and/or decrease the pain associated with movement. Mulligan[85] states that MWMs are more effective with loss of flexion than extension. The principles of MWM are described in Chapter 6.

Lateral or Medial Glides

- Patient position and procedure: Supine for extension or prone for flexion. Apply a pain-free medial or lateral glide to the tibial plateau either by hand or through the use of a mobilization belt. The direction of glide is often in the direction of the pain (i.e., lateral knee pain responds best to a lateral glide of the tibia, and medial knee pain to a medial glide).[85]
- While sustaining the mobilization, ask the patient to move to the end of the available pain-free range of flexion or extension.
- Add pain-free overpressure to achieve the benefit of end-range loading.

Internal Tibial Rotation for Flexion—Manual Technique

- Patient position and procedure: Supine with the knee flexed to the end of its available pain-free range.
- Apply an internal rotation mobilization to the tibia with manual pressure from one hand on the anteromedial tibial plateau simultaneously with pressure from the other hand on the posterolateral tibial plateau, posterior to the fibular head.
- Sustain the internal rotation mobilization, and ask the patient to flex the knee through the use of a mobilization belt looped around the foot. Hold the position at the end of the available pain-free range for several seconds (Fig. 13–1).

Internal Rotation for Flexion—Self-Treatment

- Patient position: Standing with the foot of the involved leg on a chair and knee flexed. Position the foot such that the tibia is internally rotated.
- Have the patient apply the internal rotation pressure against the anteromedial and posterolateral tibial plateaus and shift the weight forward to flex

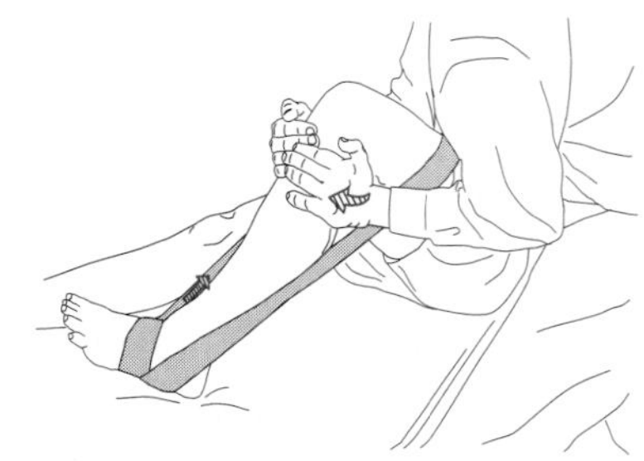

Figure 13–1 MWM with internal tibial rotation to increase knee flexion.

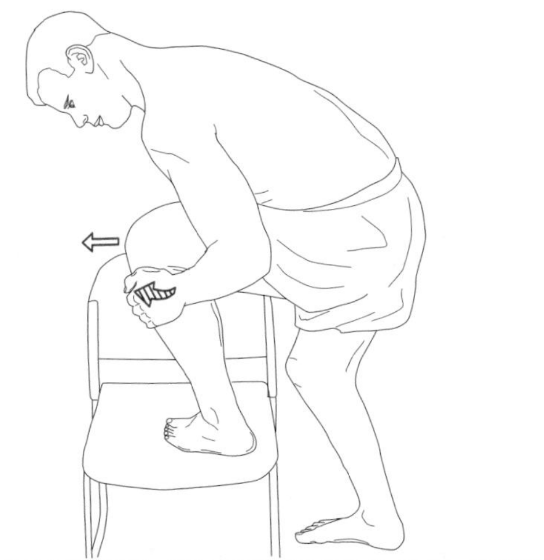

Figure 13–2 Self-treatment using MWM with internal tibial rotation to increase knee flexion.

the knee to the end of the available pain-free range (Fig. 13–2).

Develop Strength and Endurance in Supporting Muscles

Exercises identified in this section are described in detail in the last section of this chapter.

Strengthen the quadriceps femoris and hamstring muscles within the patient's pain-free tolerance. Begin with multiple-angle isometrics, short-arc terminal extension exercises in open- and closed-chain positions, and a moderate progression of repetitions and resistance in wider arcs of motion as long as the motion is pain-free.

- When doing open-chain exercises, patients experience less pain with faster speeds and lighter resistance than when doing the exercises slowly with heavy resistance.
- Resistance through the midrange (45–90 degrees) tends to exacerbate patellofemoral pain because of the compressive forces on the patella. Apply resistance in arcs of motion that are pain-free on either side of the symptomatic range. This could be done using manual or mechanical resistance in the pain-free ranges.

Develop balanced forces through the patella. Because the patellofemoral joint is frequently symptomatic in arthritis of the knee, align patellar forces with patellar mobilization and vastus medialis training.

Strengthen hip- and ankle-stabilizing muscles. Use both open- and closed-chain activities that progress the patient toward functional independence. (See Chapters 12 and 14 for hip and ankle exercises.)

Improve endurance. For muscular endurance, increase repetitions at each resistance level before progressing.

Improve Function

Functional training. Climbing steps, sitting down and rising up from chairs and commodes, and using safe body mechanics to lift objects from the floor are often compromised in individuals with knee arthritis. It is imperative to strengthen the knee musculature using modifications of functional activities and progressing in difficulty as strength improves.

- ***Step-up and step-down exercises (forward, backward, and lateral).*** Begin with blocks or steps 4 to 6 inches in height, and progress to the step height the patient requires for home and community mobility. Progress to functional activities such as climbing stairs or ladders, depending on the desired outcome.
- ***Wall slides and mini-squats to 90 degrees if tolerated.*** Stay within a range that does not exacerbate symptoms or cause crepitation. Practice sitting and sit-to-stand with arm assistance in various chair heights. Determine if chair adaptation is needed for safe function.
- ***Partial lunges.*** This activity is progressed to include lunging to pick up small objects from the floor. Lunges are an effective way to teach body mechanics for an individual with unilateral knee impairment. Concentrate on trunk control during the motion. Have the patient contract the abdominals to stabilize the pelvis during the lunge activity.
- ***Balance activities.*** Balance activities are initiated at the level that the patient can control. Detailed suggestions are outlined in Chapter 12.
- ***Ambulation.*** Decrease use of assistive devices as quadriceps strength improves to a manual muscle test level of 4/5. Practice on a variety of terrains, up and down ramps, and reversing directions, first with assistance, then independently.

Aerobic conditioning. Develop and improve cardiovascular fitness for the individual with joint symptoms by adapting activities to minimize irritating stresses.

- ***Swimming, water aerobics, and aquatic exercises*** provide an environment for improving muscular and cardiovascular pulmonary function with less joint trauma

- ***Bicycling*** is a low-impact form of exercise. Adjust the seat height so that the knee goes into complete extension (but not hyperextension) when the pedal is down. On a stationary bike, use low resistance.
- For some patients, progression to running or jumping rope and other high-impact, faster paced, or more intense activities can be undertaken as long as the joint remains asymptomatic. If joint deformity is present and proper biomechanics cannot be restored, the patient probably cannot progress to these activities.

Patient Education

- Inform the patient about his or her condition, what to expect regarding recovery, and how to protect the joints.
- It is important to emphasize that maintaining strength in the supporting muscles helps protect and stabilize the joint. Balance activities help reduce the incidence of falls. Be sure the patient knows safe exercises to do at home and how to modify them if symptoms are exacerbated by the disease or from overuse.
- Instruct the patient to move the joints and do muscle setting prior to standing to reduce painful symptoms that occur with initial weight bearing.
- With DJD and RA, the patient should be cautioned to alternate activity with rest.

▶ Joint Surgery and Postoperative Management

A range of surgical options for management of arthritis of the knee is available when joint pain and synovitis cannot be controlled with conservative therapy and appropriate medical management or when destruction of articular surfaces, deformity, or restriction of motion have progressed to the point that functional abilities are significantly impaired. The goals of surgery and postoperative management include: (1) reduction of pain, (2) correction of deformity or instability, and (3) restoration of lower extremity function.

The choice of surgical procedure will depend on the patient's signs and symptoms, activity level and age, type of arthritis, severity of joint deterioration or deformity, and involvement of other joints. *Arthroscopic débridement and lavage* are used to remove loose bodies that may be causing swelling and intermittent locking of the knee.[8a,109] *Synovectomy* may be the procedure of choice for a young patient with unremitting joint effusion, synovial proliferation, and pain but with minimal destruction of articular surfaces.[50,87,109] Hypertrophic synovitis most frequently develops in patients with RA or JRA. *Chondroplasty* or *abrasion arthroplasty* procedures are performed to smooth or débride worn articular surfaces. However, in most instances, this procedure appears to be of questionable value as it has not yielded long-term relief of symptoms.[8a,81,109] *Osteochondral autograft transplantation* (OTA), *mosaicplasty*, or *autologous chondrocyte implantation* may be used to repair small, localized lesions of an articular surface of the knee.[10,48,109] The procedures use tissue grafted from a nonweight-bearing, nonarticulating portion of the supracondylar ridge of the lateral femoral articulating sufaces or elsewhere in the knee. Most common sites of transplantation include the medial femoral condyle and the articulating facets of the patella. *Osteotomy* of the proximal tibia, an extra-articular procedure, redistributes weight-bearing forces between the tibia and femur in an attempt to reduce joint pain during weight-bearing activities and delay the need for arthroplasty of the knee.[8a,109] When erosion of articular surfaces becomes severe, *total joint replacement arthroplasty* is the surgical procedure of choice to reduce pain, correct deformity, and improve functional movement.[57,76] Only in very selective situations is *arthrodesis* (fusion) of the knee chosen as a salvage procedure to provide a patient with a stable and pain-free knee.

Regardless of the type of surgery chosen to relieve joint symptoms, a thorough preoperative evaluation followed by exercises and progressive ambulation are necessary components of an effective postoperative treatment plan.

Synovectomy

Indications for Surgery

The following are frequent indications for synovectomy of the knee.[4a,50,89,109]

- Chronic synovitis and joint pain of the knee lasting 6 months or longer secondary to unremitting but early-stage RA or JRA that cannot be controlled by medical management
- Synovial hypertrophy and joint pain secondary to recurrent hemarthrosis associated with hemophilia

- Intact or minimally eroded articular surfaces
- Decreased ROM secondary to chronic synovitis and joint pain
- A means of deferring total joint arthroplasty in the young patient with chronic synovitis

Procedures

An *arthroscopic synovectomy* involves the use of multiple portals for access to and endoscopic removal of as much synovium as possible from all compartments of the knee.[50,109] It is now routinely preferred over an *open synovectomy,* which necessitates an arthrotomy of the knee through a longitudinal medial and/or lateral parapatellar incision(s) of the capsule and, therefore, causes greater postoperative morbidity and a lengthier recovery. It is also more difficult to preserve the menisci with an open approach than an arthroscopic approach.[50] However, an open synovectomy may be performed in conjunction with other open procedures.

Postoperative Management

Postoperative management after arthroscopic synovectomy, summarized in Table 13–1, is progressed based on the patient's signs and symptoms rather than strict adherence to time frames.[92] Exercises and weight-bearing activities are progressed relatively rapidly after arthroscopic synovectomy. A patient often achieves nearly full ROM of the operated knee and is able to ambulate without assistive devices as early as 10 to 14 days postoperatively depending on involvement of unoperated joints. However, a return to a full level of functional activity should be progressed gradually with some degree of protection continuing until joint swelling, limitation of active and passive knee ROM, and muscle weakness are resolved.

Immobilization and Weight Bearing

The knee is immobilized for 24 to 48 hours in a compressive dressing and a posterior splint. During that time the leg is elevated to control postoperative edema. Ambulation with crutches is begun the day after surgery, weight bearing as tolerated. The patient should wear the posterior splint during ambulation until full, active knee extension has been achieved.

Exercise

The goals and exercise interventions commonly included in a postoperative rehabilitation program include the following.[50,87,109] The choices and progression of exercises are based not only on the status of the operated knee but also on the extent of involvement of other joints of the upper or lower extremities.

Exercise: Maximum Protection Phase

- Minimize peripheral edema and decrease the risk of deep vein thrombosis with ankle pumping exercises.
- Regain or maintain neuromuscular control of hip and knee musculature on the operated side, with quadriceps and hamstring setting exercises and straight-leg raises in the supine, prone, and sidelying positions.
- Prevent postoperative contractures and regain full ROM of the knee.
  - Continuous passive motion (CPM), if requested by the surgeon
  - Active-assistive knee flexion and extension exercises within the pain-free ROM
  - Gentle superior and inferior patellar mobilization techniques
  - Gentle inhibition and muscle elongation techniques of the quadriceps and hamstrings
  - Gravity-assisted knee extension with a rolled towel under the ankle and the posterior aspect of the knee unsupported

Exercise: Moderate and Minimum Protection and Return to Function Phases

- Regain or improve control and strength of the knee musculature. Continue setting exercises and straight-leg raising (SLR) exercises, and begin submaximal multiple-angle isometrics against manual resistance. Progress to low-intensity dynamic resistance exercises in an open-chain. Add progressive closed-chain strengthening activities as weight bearing allows. Emphasize control of the quadriceps in full knee extension for safe and efficient ambulation.
- If limitation of motion persists, begin joint mobilization and soft tissue stretching when swelling has subsided.
- Improve cardiorespiratory fitness by encouraging the patient to become involved in or resume low-impact, low-intensity but progressive aerobic conditioning activities such as swimming or bicycling. Incorporate principles of joint protection into work and recreational activities.

Table 13–1 Arthroscopic Synovectomy—Intervention for Each Phase of Rehabilitation

Phase and General Timeframe	Maximum Protection Phase Weeks 1–2	Moderate to Minimum Protection Phases Weeks 3–6	Return-to-Activity Phase Week 6
Patient Presentation	• Patient should enter rehabilitation within 2 days postoperatively • Postoperative compressive dressing • Minimal postoperative pain • ROM minimally limited • Weight bearing as tolerated	• Minimum pain • Full weight bearing • Near full ROM • Joint effusion controlled	• Muscle function 70% of noninvolved side • No symptoms of pain or swelling in the previous phase
Key Examination Procedures	• Pain assessment (0–10 scale) • Monitor for hemarthrosis • ROM • Muscle control • Soft tissue palpation • Patellar mobility	• Pain assessment • Joint effusion—girth • ROM • Muscle strength • Patellar mobility • Gait analysis	• Pain assessment • Muscle strength • Patellar alignment/stability • Functional status
Intervention	• A-AROM and AROM • Patellar mobilization (grades I and II) • Muscle setting: quadriceps, hamstrings, and adductors (may augment with E-stim) • SLRs - four positions (assisted to unassisted) • Flexibility program hamstrings, plantarflexors, IT band • Ankle pumps • Trunk/pelvis strengthening • Pain modulation modalities (cryotherapy) • Compressive wrap to control effusion	• LE flexibility program • Closed-chain strengthening • Limited range PRE • Tibiofemoral joint mobilization if needed • Proprioceptive training • Stabilization exercises • Gait training • Protected aerobic exercise • Swimming or walking program	• Continue previous phase activities and advance as appropriate • Implement exercise specific to functional tasks
Goals	• Control postoperative swelling • Minimize pain • ROM 0–115 degrees • 3/5 to 4/5 muscle strength • Ambulate without assistive device unless weight bearing is delayed • Establish home exercise program	• Swelling control • Full ROM • Full weight bearing • 4/5 to 5/5 strength • Unrestricted ADL • Adherence to home program	• Transition to maintenance program for self-management and prevention • Life-long joint protection

Outcomes

Synovectomy has been shown to be of benefit in alleviating chronic synovitis and joint pain and, in most cases, in improving ROM and postponing joint destruction. After recovery from surgery, joint pain and swelling are reduced in approximately 90 to 95% of patients.[50,87] Long-term results of arthroscopic and open approaches are reported to be comparable. A review of several studies indicates that at 2 to 2.5 years after arthroscopic synovectomy 78 to

90% of patients continued to report a reduction of symptoms and general satisfaction with the procedure.[50,87] However, by 4 to 5 years, positive outcomes for both open and arthroscopic procedures tend to deteriorate to approximately 60 to 70% in the presence of recurrent synovitis.[50,87] Progression of inflammatory joint disease, as reflected by radiographic changes, is also common several years after synovectomy.[50,87] Therefore, there is little evidence to support the claim that synovectomy can reverse the disease process.

Total Knee Arthroplasty

Indications for Surgery

The following are common indications for total knee arthroplasty (total knee replacement).[57,76,109]

- Severe joint pain with weight bearing or motion that compromises functional abilities
- Extensive destruction of articular cartilage of the knee secondary to advanced arthritis
- Gross instability or limitation of motion
- Marked deformity of the knee such as genu varum or valgum
- Failure of nonoperative management or a previous surgical procedure

Procedure

Background and types of total knee arthroplasty. Prosthetic replacement of one or more surfaces of the knee joint began to develop in the late 1950s and early 1960s. Early procedures included replacing only the tibial plateau (hemiarthroplasty).[57,76] The first generation of total knee arthroplasty (TKA) consisted of a noncemented, double-stemmed, fully constrained (hinged) metal prosthesis to replace the articulating surfaces of the distal femur and proximal tibia.[57] This early design had a high failure rate because of progressive biomechanical loosening. Then an unconstrained, multicondylar, metal-to-plastic knee replacement was developed that resurfaced the articulating surfaces of the tibiofemoral joint and was held in place with acrylic cement.[57] From this design, the unicompartmental arthroplasty, which separately resurfaces either the medial or lateral joint surfaces, subsequently evolved.[105] The completely unconstrained TKA was associated with a high incidence of instability.[76] This problem gave rise to the development of a two-component, semiconstrained bicondylar design. This was followed by the development of a three-component, total condylar design that included resurfacing of the patellofemoral joint. These early designs were forerunners of the current-day designs of TKA.[57,76] Numerous modifications of these early designs have since been developed. A therapist's knowledge of the different types of TKA used today enhances communication between the therapist and surgeon and provides a foundation for decisions made during rehabilitation.

Contemporary TKA designs and procedures can be classified in several ways that include: the *number of components or articulations replaced* in the knee (unicomparmental/unicondylar, bicompartmental/bicondylar, and tricompartmental/total condylar); *the degree of constraint* (inherent stability) built into the prothesis (unconstrained, semiconstrained, and fully constrained); the *status of the posterior cruciate ligament* (PCL); and the *method of fixation* (cemented, uncemented or "hybrid"). Most TKA procedures today involve the implantation of a semiconstrained prosthetic system to replace two or three compartments of the knee.[57,76] The designs are commonly composed of a single femoral component with a metal articulating surface and a single all-polyethylene or metal-backed tibial component with a polyethylene articulating surface. The posterior aspect of the patella may or may not be resurfaced with a polyethylene dome-shaped component.[57,76,109] Bicompartmental, unconstrained resurfacing designs (with four separate components) are rarely used today. Unicompartmental replacement is performed today although infrequently; it is an alternative to high tibial osteotomy for the patient with either medial or lateral compartment destruction, who is older than 60 to 70 years of age and leads a relatively sedentary lifestyle and whose weight is close to ideal.[105,110]

Intact medial and lateral collateral ligaments are necessary prerequisites for semiconstrained and unconstrained TKA.[57,76] Fully constrained designs are reserved for the low-demand patient who has marked instability of the knee, extensive bone loss, or severe deformity or who has had multiple revisions of TKA.[57,76] Contemporary fully constrained designs have inherent M-L and A-P stability (no varus/valgus or A-P glide) but some degree of rotation of the tibia on the femur to lessen the problem of progressive loosening of the prosthetic components over time.[57,76]

TKA is also classified as *cruciate-retaining* or *cruciate-excising/substituting* with respect to the

PCL.[49,57,76,109] (During a TKA procedure, the ACL is routinely excised.) If the patient's PCL is intact to provide posterior stability to the knee, one of several cruciate-retaining designs that have little to no congruency and allow some degree of A-P glide are commonly used.[103] If the PCL is deficient, a cruciate-excising/substituting prosthesis, which has inherent posterior stability from the congruency of the components, a posterior prominence in the tibial component, or a cam-post mechanism built into the design, is selected.[49,57,76,110]

Fixation. Total knee arthroplasty is also classified by method of fixation: cemented, uncemented, or "hybrid." Components are either held in place with acrylic cement, bone ingrowth (uncemented), or a combination of approaches to fixation[76,109,134] Initially, almost all total knee replacements relied on cement fixation.[84,109,134] Although cement fixation revolutionized arthroplasty of the knee[57,102] and continues to be the most commonly used method of fixation,[134,141] a long-term complication associated with early designs of cemented prostheses was biomechanical loosening at the bone-cement interface in very active patients.[84,134,141] To counteract this problem, cementless (biological) fixation that relies on rapid growth of bone into the surfaces of a porous-coated or beaded prosthesis was developed.* Recently, the use of a hydroxyapatite coating on the prosthesis has been recommended to enhance biological fixation.[109]

A variety of designs of prostheses have been developed for use with cementless fixation, almost all of which have been cruciate-retaining designs.[57,104] Cementless fixation has been used primarily for the active patient in whom the risk of biomechanical loosening over time is most likely.[84,141] Although it has been demonstrated that the femoral component reliably achieves fixation to bone, the tibial component in cementless procedures as with cemented fixation is prone to loosening.[57,76,104,134] Current-day fixation of the tibial component may be augmented with pegs and screws for additional long-term stability although the value of these designs is debated.[57,141] The "hybrid" TKA, which combines cemented fixation of the tibial component and cementless fixation of the femoral component, is becoming a more frequently used approach to implant fixation.[76]

*See references 57, 76, 84, 103, 104, 109, 134.

Research continues on the biomechanics of TKA, the modifications of designs, the development of better methods of fixation and new materials with better wear qualities, as well as improved surgical techniques and use of sophisticated instrumentation for alignment and placement of prostheses. Ongoing developments in all of these areas will continue to contribute to the success of current-day and improvement of future TKA procedures.[141]

Overview of operative procedure.[20] A longitudinal incision of the skin is made along the anterior aspect of the knee from just proximal to the patella to just distal to the tibial tuberosity. Either a quadriceps-splitting or a quadriceps-sparing approach is used. If a quadriceps-sparing approach is used, the extensor mechanism and patella are shifted, and then an arthrotomy is performed usually along the medial aspect of the patella. The knee is flexed, and osteophytes, menisci, and the ACL are excised. Soft tissue releases and ligament balancing are then done to correct deformity and achieve the best alignment possible.

The tibial and femoral and, if necessary, the patellar surfaces are then prepared for the prosthetic components. After all components are in place, soft tissue tension, collateral ligament balance, ROM, and patellar tracking are checked. The area is thoroughly irrigated, the wound is closed with a suction drain in place, and the area is covered with a sterile dressing.

Postoperative Management

Management of the rehabilitation process for TKA is summarized in Table 13–2. This may include preoperative patient instruction on an individual or group basis.[109] The patient is progressed through the phases of rehabilitation based on examination of signs and symptoms and responses to selected interventions.[92] Accordingly, the timelines reflected in Table 13–2 only are intended to serve as general guidelines.

Immobilization and Early Movement

The knee may be immobilized in a bulky compression dressing for a day postoperatively, or CPM may be initiated immediately or within hours after the procedure because of its effects in controlling hemiarthrosis. Although early CPM use is dependent on the philosophy of the surgeon, it has been recommended after either primary cemented or cementless

Table 13–2 Total Knee Arthroplasty—Interventions for Each Phase of Rehabilitation

Phase and General Time Frame	Preoperative Program	Maximum Protection Phase Weeks 1–2	Moderate/Minimum Protection Phases Weeks 3–6	Return-to-Activity Phase Beyond Week 6
Patient Presentation	• Disabling joint pain • Limited ROM • Limited functional status • Modification of lifestyle • Radiographic evidence of severe arthritic disease • Failed conservative management	• Patient should enter rehabilitation within 2 days postoperatively • Postoperative compressive dressing • Controlled postop pain • ROM 10–60 degrees • Weight bearing as tolerated with cemented—delayed with uncemented prosthesis	• Minimum pain • Full weight bearing except with noncemented • ROM 0–90 degrees • Joint effusion controlled	• Muscle function 70% of noninvolved extremity • No symptoms of pain or swelling in the previous phase
Key Examination Procedures	• Comprehensive knee evaluation including ROM, strength, pain, flexibility, joint crepitation, and functional status • Medical examination including X-ray	• Pain (0–10 scale) • Monitor for hemarthrosis • ROM • Muscle control • Soft tissue palpation • Patellar mobility	• Pain assessment • Joint effusion—girth • ROM • Muscle strength • Patellar mobility • Gait analysis	• Pain assessment • Muscular strength • Patellar allignment/ stability • Functional status
Intervention	• Preoperative strengthening • Preoperative flexibility • Preoperative aerobic conditioning • Postoperative exercise instruction • Postoperative bed mobility and transfers • Gait training with assistive device(s)	• PROM–CPM • A-AROM and AROM • Muscle setting: quadriceps, hamstrings, and adductors (may augment with E-stim) • Patellar mobilization (grades I and II) • Flexibility program hamstrings, calf, IT band • Ankle pumps to minimize risk of DVT • Trunk/pelvis strengthening • Pain modulation modalities • Compressive wrap to control effusion • Gait training	• Patellar mobilization • LE flexibility program • Closed-chain strengthening • Limited range PREs • Tibiofemoral joint mobilization if appropriate and needed • Proprioceptive training • Stabilization exercises • Gait training • Protected aerobic exercise • Swimming program cycling or walking	• Continue as previous phase; advance as appropriate • Implement exercise specific to functional tasks
Goals	• Patient education • Improved strength and aerobic function	• Control postoperative swelling • Minimize pain • ROM 0–90 degrees • 3/5 to 4/5 muscle strength • Ambulate with or without assistive device • Establish home exercise program	• Swelling control • ROM 0–115 degrees or more • Full weight bearing • 4/5 to 5/5 strength • Unrestricted ADL function • Adherence to home exercise program	• Develop maintenance program and educate patient on importance of adherence including methods of joint protection

procedures.[76,104] However, cementless arthroplasty or more complicated revision arthroplasty may require a longer period of immobilization than a cemented procedure to allow ingrowth of bone into the prosthesis. A posterior knee splint may be indicated for use during ambulation until quadriceps control is attained or at night for as long as 12 weeks postoperatively.

Weight Bearing

The extent to which weight bearing is allowable is dependent upon the type of prosthesis implanted and the type of fixation used. If biological fixation has been used, weight bearing is usually restricted to a touch-down level for up to 6 weeks postoperatively and gradually progressed over the duration of rehabilitation. Full weight bearing and ambulation without assistive devices may not be permissible for up to 12 weeks postoperatively.[76]

With cement fixation, weight bearing as tolerated is permissible immediately after surgery and increased to full weight bearing over 6 weeks. The patient should continue to use crutches or a cane through the moderate and minimum protection phases of rehabilitation until adequate strength and stability have been attained in the operated lower extremity. In some instances the patient may be required to wear an immobilizer for a few days during ambulation in the immediate postoperative period.

Exercise

The goals and therapeutic exercise interventions in this section and Table 13–2 are typically included in a rehabilitation program following TKA.[27,31,43,75,109,132] Many of the exercises described for the early phase of rehabilitation are found in a consensus document developed by physical therapists on management of patients during the period of hospitalization after TKA.[31]

Exercise: Maximum Protection Phase

The focus of management during this phase of rehabilitation is to restore ROM (preferably 90 degrees of flexion and full extension by 1 to 2 weeks postoperatively) and prevent postoperative complications. As noted previously, CPM is often initiated by the first day after surgery. It has been suggested that CPM decreases postoperative pain, promotes wound healing, decreases the incidence of deep vein thrombosis, enables patients to regain knee flexion more rapidly during the early postoperative days, and decreases hospital stay, but these benefits have not been consistently supported in the research literature.* Therefore, CPM is recommended as an adjunct to, not a replacement for, a supervised postoperative exercise program.[7] The following goals and exercise interventions are included in the early phase of rehabilitation after TKA.

- Prevent reflex inhibition or loss of strength of knee and hip musculature.
  - Muscle-setting exercises of the quadriceps, hamstrings and hip adductors, possibly coupled with neuromuscular electrical stimulation
  - Assisted progressing to active straight-leg raises in supine, prone, and side-lying positions[58]
- Regain ROM and control of the knee.
  - Active-assistive and active ROM exercises to patient tolerance
  - Heel-slides in supine or sitting to increase flexion
  - Neuromuscular inhibition technique, such as the use of agonist-contraction techniques to decrease muscle guarding, particularly in the quadriceps, and increase knee flexion
  - Gentle inferior and superior patellar gliding techniques
  - Gravity-assisted knee extension in supine by periodically placing a rolled towel under the ankle and leaving the knee unsupported

Precautions: In the early postoperative days, avoid use of a pillow under the knee to avoid development of a knee flexion contracture. Also monitor the impact of knee flexion on the integrity of the incision. Watch for signs of excessive tension on the wound, such as drainage or skin blanching.

- Promote circulation and decrease postoperative edema and pain with ankle pumping exercises immediately after surgery.
- Prevent postoperative pulmonary complications by initiating deep breathing exercises.

Exercise: Moderate Protection Phase

The primary goals of this phase of rehabilitation are to achieve approximately 115 degrees knee flexion and active knee extension to 0 degrees and gradually regain lower extremity strength.

- Increase strength and muscular endurance.

*See references 6, 7, 21, 27, 40, 42, 59, 71, 80.

Note: Depending on the philosophy of the surgeon, exercises against low-intensity resistance may be permissible as early as 2 weeks or as late as 3 months postoperatively.[109]

- Multiple-angle isometrics and low-intensity dynamic resistance exercises of the quadriceps and hamstrings. Adequate strength of the quadriceps is most important for stability of the knee during weight-bearing activities.
- Resisted straight-leg raises in various positions and diagonal patterns should be included to increase the strength of hip musculature with emphasis on the hip extensors and abductors.
- As weight bearing permits, closed-chain exercises including stabilization, wall slides, mini-squats, step-ups (low step), and short-arc lunges to improve stability and functional control of the knee.
- Standing abduction against low-intensity resistance to improve stability of the pelvis.
- Low-intensity PRE against elastic resistance.

- Continue exercises to increase ROM.

- Gentle self-stretching (low-intensity, prolonged stretch) or hold-relax exercises if limited motion persists. Flexibility of the hip flexors, hamstrings, and calf muscles may also need to be increased for standing and ambulation activities.
- When using a stationary bicycle, the patient may first have the seat positioned as high as possible. To increase knee flexion, the seat can be gradually lowered.
- Grade III patellar mobilization techniques to increase knee flexion or extension.

Note: The use of joint mobilization techniques of the tibiofemoral joint to increase ROM may or may not be appropriate, depending on the design of the prosthetic components. It is advisable to discuss the use of these techniques with the surgeon before initiating these techniques.

Exercise: Minimum Protection and Return-to-Activity Phases

From the 6th to 12th week after surgery, the emphasis in rehabilitation is on muscle and cardiorespiratory conditioning so that the patient will have the strength and endurance to return to a full level of functional activities.

- Improve proprioception and balance with activities, such as standing on foam or a rocker or BAPS board, stepping over cups, one-legged balance, walking on an incline/decline, and side-stepping to improve control and ability to maneuver in various directions and on various surfaces.
- Improve cardiorespiratory and muscle endurance with nonimpact activities such as stationary bicycling and aquatic exercises. Gradually progress ambulation and stair-climbing activities using an assistive device as needed.

Outcomes

Almost all patients who undergo total knee arthroplasty report a significant relief of pain with knee motion and weight bearing.[33,53,75,110,116,131] Stiffness may persist for some patients after recovery from surgery.[33] Improvements in ROM are not as predictable. Although patients are encouraged to achieve full functional ROM of the knee (full active extension and at least 90 degrees of flexion) by the time of discharge from the hospital, improvement in ROM may continue up to 12 to 24 months postoperatively.[116] Although use of CPM postoperatively has been shown to increase the rate of return of knee flexion (with no impact on knee extension),[21,109] its use has no significant impact on the long-term improvement of knee ROM.[7,109] Provision of additional physical therapy services (including exercise on a 7-day-per-week versus a 6-day-per-week basis) for patients after TKA surgery has been shown to have no significantly different effect on ROM at the time of discharge.[67] Long-term postoperative follow-up of patients after knee replacement suggests that only minimal improvement occurs in ROM. Patients with restricted ROM preoperatively usually continue to have limited knee flexion or extension postoperatively, despite an aggressive postoperative exercise program.[115,116]

It may take at least 3 months postoperatively for a patient to regain strength in the quadriceps and hamstrings to a preoperative level. Quadriceps weakness tends to persist longer after knee arthroplasty than does knee flexor weakness.[65,116,135] As the patient's level of functional activity continues to increase, further gains in strength and endurance may continue to occur for more than a year postoperatively.[116,135] Lack of full active extension of the knee because of contracture or extensor lag associated with inadequate patellar mobility may be a source of a patient's perception of knee pain or instability during ambulation activities particularly when ascending and descending stairs.[65]

In a study of a group of patients 1 year after TKA surgery, despite a relative absence of pain and some improvement in functional abilities, significant deficits in strength and functional abilities were apparent when compared to age-matched, healthy individuals.[131] The post-TKA patients had less strength of the knee musculature, slower walking and stair-climbing speeds, and a higher perceived level of exertion during activities. The authors pointed out that although the post-TKA patients as a group were heavier than the control group, general physical deconditioning may have strongly contributed to the postoperative group's functional limitations. This study emphasizes the need for inclusion of a low-impact aerobic conditioning program during rehabilitation after TKA.

Extensive research can be found in the orthopedic literature on outcomes assessment of the many variations of prosthetic designs, methods of fixation, types of materials, and surgical techniques. It is often difficult to draw general conclusions because of these many variations.[110] It can be said that the ideal total knee replacement that replicates the normal biomechanics of the knee has yet to be developed.[57,110] Problems such as biomechanical loosening have been significantly reduced with newer prosthetic designs and improvements in surgical techniques.[86,98,110] Polyethylene wear of the patellar and tibial components is a greater long-term complication that may necessitate revision arthroplasty than loosening.[104,109] Instability of the patella, whether or not it has been resurfaced, may complicate postoperative rehabilitation and may require additional surgery to balance soft tissues around the knee.[65]

Both cemented and uncemented approaches to fixation, particularly in the past 5 to 10 years, have yielded comparably favorable outcomes, although cemented fixation continues to be used more prevalently than cementless or hybrid fixation.[104,110] ROM is similar with cemented versus cementless fixation and current-day prosthetic design, averaging 100 degrees of flexion.[104]

▶ Patellofemoral Dysfunction: Nonoperative Management

Related Diagnoses

Historically, the differential diagnosis of patellofemoral pathologies has been plagued with confusion, largely related to the use of broadly inclusive terminology such as chondromalacia patellae and patellofemoral pain syndrome. In an attempt to more clearly identify anatomical structures involved and biomechanical changes leading to dysfunction, several classification systems have been proposed. These classifications include guidelines for intervention based on impairments and functional limitations.[55,139]

Patellofemoral Instability

Instability includes subluxation or dislocation of single or recurrent episodes. There may be an abnormal Q angle, dysplastic trochlea (shallow groove or flat lateral femoral condyle), patella alta, tight lateral retinaculum, and inadequate medial stabilizers (VMO). There may be associated fractures. Usually the instability is in a lateral direction. The dislocation may be from direct trauma to the patella or from a forceful quadriceps contraction while the foot is planted and the femur is externally rotating while the knee is flexed. Recurrent dislocation is usually an indication for surgery to redirect the forces through the patella.

Patellofemoral Pain with Malalignment or Biomechanical Dysfunction

This includes problems that cause an increased functional Q angle such as femoral anteversion, external tibial torsion, genu valgum, and foot hyperpronation. There may be a tight lateral retinaculum, weak VMO, patella alta, patella baja, or dysplastic femoral trochlea. There is usually abnormal patellar tracking, and there may be discordant firing of the quadriceps muscle.[55]

Patellofemoral Pain Without Malalignment

This includes many subcategories that cause anterior knee pain.

Soft tissue lesions. These include plica syndrome, fat pad syndrome, tendinitis, iliotibial band friction syndrome, and bursitis.

- *Plica syndrome* describes a condition related to irritation of remnants of embryological synovial tissue around the patella. With chronic irritation, the tissue becomes an inelastic fibrotic band that is tender on palpation. When acute, the tissue is painful on palpation. The band is usually palpable medial to the patella, although there are variations in its location.[9,63]
- *Fat pad syndrome* involves irritation of the infrapatellar fat pad from trauma or overuse.

- *Tendinitis* of the patellar or quadriceps tendons often occurs from overuse as the result of repetitive jumping. Tenderness occurs along the attachment of the tendon to the patella.
- *Iliotibial (IT) band friction syndrome* is irritation of the IT band as it passes over the lateral femoral condyle. Contributing factors could be tight tensor fasciae latae or tight gluteus maximus (see discussion in Chapter 12). Since the IT band attaches to the patella and lateral retinaculum, it may cause anterior knee pain.
- *Prepatellar bursitis,* also known as housemaid's knee, occurs from prolonged kneeling or recurrent minor trauma to the anterior knee. When inflamed there may be restricted motion from the swelling and pain from direct pressure or pressure from the patellar tendon.

Tight medial and lateral retinacula or patellar pressure syndrome. There is increased contact pressure of the patella in the trochlear groove.

Osteochondritis dissecans of the patella or femoral trochlea. Osteochondral lesions result in pain on the retrosurface of the patella that is worse during squatting, stooping, ambulation, and descending steps. The knee may give way or may lock. There may be loose bodies within the joint.

Traumatic patellar chondromalacia. With chondromalacia there is softening and fissuring of the cartilaginous surface of the patella, which is diagnosed with arthroscopy or arthrogram.[45,58] It may eventually predispose the joint to degenerative arthritis or basal degeneration of the middle and deep zones of the cartilage.[41] Causes of the degeneration may include trauma, surgery, prolonged or repeated stress, or lack of normal stress such as during periods of immobilization.[96]

Patellofemoral osteoarthritis. Osteoarthritis may be idiopathic or posttraumatic and is diagnosed by radiographic changes consistent with degeneration.

Apophysitis. Osgood-Schlatter's disease (traction apophysitis of the tibial tuberosity) and Sinding-Larsen-Johansson syndrome (traction apophysitis on the inferior pole of the patella) occur in adolescence from overuse during rapid growth and are self-limiting conditions.

Symptomatic bipartite patella. Most bipartite patellae are asymptomatic, but trauma may disrupt the chondro-osseous junction leading to symptoms.[55]

Trauma. This category includes *tendon rupture, fracture, contusion,* and *articular cartilage damage* that results in inflammation, swelling, limited motion, and pain with dysfunction whenever contracting the quadriceps such as when stair climbing, squatting, and resisting knee extension.

Etiology of Symptoms

The cause of anterior knee pain may be from direct trauma, overuse, faulty patellar tracking from malalignment due to anatomic variations or soft tissue imbalances, degeneration, or a combination of these factors.* An attempt should be made to determine the causative factors based on the history and comprehensive and sequential examination.

Common Impairments

Impairments that may be associated with patellofemoral dysfunction include:†

- Weakness, inhibition, or poor recruitment or timing of firing of the VMO
- Overstretched medial retinaculum
- Restricted lateral retinaculum, IT band, or fascial structures around the patella
- Decreased medial gliding or medial tipping of the patella
- Pronated foot
- Pain in the retropatellar region
- Tight gastrocnemius soleus, hamstring, or rectus femoris muscles
- Irritated patellar tendon or subpatellar fat pads
- Patellar crepitus, swelling, or locking

Common Functional Limitations/Disabilities

- Pain or poor knee control when descending or ascending stairs
- Pain with walking, jumping, or running interfering during ADL, IADL, work, and community, recreational, or sport activities
- Pain and stiffness with prolonged flexed knee postures such as sitting or squatting

Nonoperative Management of Patellofemoral Symptoms: Protection Phase

When symptoms are acute, treat as any acute joint problem with modalities, rest, gentle motion, and muscle-setting exercises in pain-free positions. Pain

*See references 14, 25, 78, 108, 114, 144, 130, 140.

†See references 14, 25, 68, 78, 108, 114, 130, 140.

and joint effusion inhibit the quadriceps,[124] so it is imperative to reduce irritating forces. Splinting the patella with a brace or tape may unload the joint and relieve the irritating stress.[63]

Nonoperative Management of Patellofemoral Symptoms: Controlled Motion and Return to Function

When signs of inflammation are no longer present, management is directed toward correcting the biomechanical forces that may be contributing to the impairments. Suggestions for correcting faulty patellar alignment or tracking follow.

Increase Flexibility of the Lateral Fascia and Insertion of the IT Band

- ***Patellar mobilization: medial glide*** (Fig. 13–3)[44a,79]
  - Patient position and procedure: Side-lying. Stabilize the femoral condyles with one hand under the femur and glide the patella medially with the base of the other hand.
  - There is usually greater mobility with the knee near extension.
  - To progress stretching, position the knee in greater flexion.
- ***Friction massage around the lateral aspect of the patella***
- ***Medial tipping of the patella*** (Fig. 13–4)

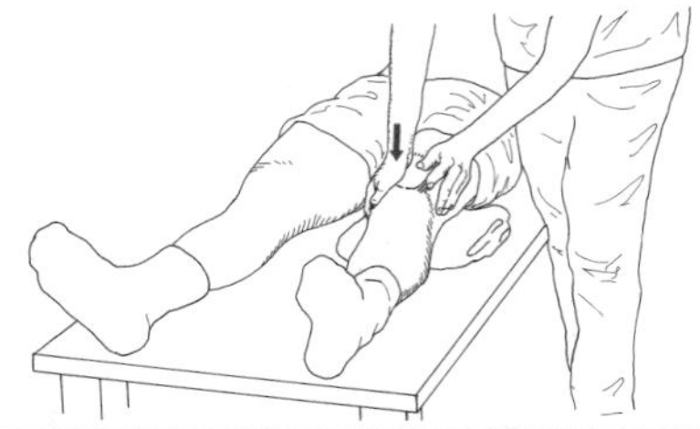

Figure 13–4 Medial tipping of the patella with friction massage along the lateral border.

  - Patient position and procedure: Supine. Place the thenar eminence at the base of the hand over the medial aspect of the patella. A direct posterior force tips the patella medially.
  - While the patella is held in this position, friction massage can be applied with the other hand along the lateral border.
  - Teach the patient to self-stretch in this manner.
- ***Patellar taping***
  - Use tape to realign the patella and apply a prolonged stretch as well as maintain alignment of the patella for nonstressful training.[44a,78,79]
- ***Self-stretching: The insertion of IT band*** (Fig. 13–5)
  - Patient position and procedure: Side-lying with a belt or sheet strapped around the ankle and the other end placed over the shoulder and held in the hand. The hip is positioned in extension, adduction, and slight lateral rotation and the knee in flexion.
  - First flex the knee and abduct the hip; then extend the hip (this ensures that the IT band is over the greater trochanter).

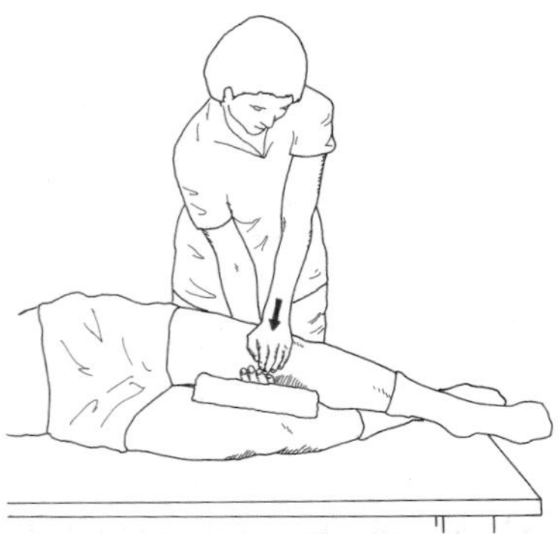

Figure 13–3 Medial glide of the patella.

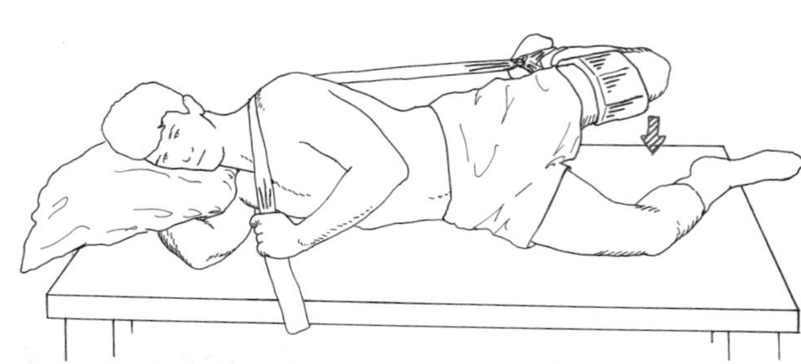

Figure 13–5 Self-stretch to the insertion of IT band.

- The femur is then adducted with slight lateral rotation until tension is felt in the IT band along the lateral knee.
- The patient stabilizes self in this position by holding onto the strap. If tolerated, a 2- to 5-lb weight is placed distally over the lateral thigh for added stretch, and the position is maintained for 20 to 30 minutes.

Stretch Other Tight Structures

Identify any shortened muscles that could be contributing to faulty mechanics, and establish a stretching program. Techniques to increase knee flexion and extension are described in the exercise sections later in this chapter. Techniques to stretch the two-joint muscles that cross the hip and knee are described in Chapter 12, and those that cross the knee and ankle are described in Chapter 14.

Train and Strengthen Functional Control of Knee Extension in Nonweight-Bearing Positions

Note: There is controversy regarding compressive forces and stress in the patellofemoral joint with open-chain exercises.[32,44] The type of resistance (constant, variable or isokinetic) will each require different demands of the quadriceps muscle in terms of maximum effort at various ranges. The resultant force from the quadriceps tendon and patellar tendon and the patellar contact area also vary through the ROM; therefore, stress to articulating surface of the patella varies. There is little or no contact of the patella with the trochlear groove from 0 to 15 degrees of flexion,[32] so pain felt in that range could be from irritation of the patellar fat pads or synovial tissue. Greatest patellar stress is at 60 degrees and compression loads at 75 degrees, so pain may be provoked in these ranges when maximum torque from the resistance force is applied in these ranges.[32] Where the pathology is located affects where in the range the patient feels pain.[44] It is recommended that when examining the patient, the range where pain is felt is noted and that resistance loads which cause pain in that range are avoided.

Vastus medialis obliquis (VMO) emphasis. Although it is not possible to isolate contraction of the VMO, it is accepted that the line of pull of this component of the quadriceps muscle influences the tracking of the patella, and thus, effort is directed toward developing awareness of the VMO contraction during quadriceps muscle activity. Use tactile cues over the muscle belly, electrical stimulation, or biofeedback to reinforce the VMO contraction during open- and closed-chain extension exercises.

Quadriceps setting (quad sets) in pain-free positions. Have the patient set the quads with the knee in various positions while focusing on tension development in the VMO. Because the site of irritation will vary between patients, identify pain-free positions for each patient to ensure nondestructive loading.[32,44]

Quad sets with straight-leg raising (SLR). Because many fibers of the VMO originate on the adductor tendons and medial intramuscular septum, some popular exercise programs suggest that by laterally rotating the femur while performing SLR exercises the adductors will contract and provide a firm base for the VMO,[3,25,78] but EMG studies do not support the claim of increased activity in the VMO.[62]

Progression of resisted isometrics. When the patient tolerates, isometric resistance to knee extension may be utilized in pain-free positions. To determine if there is preferential recruitment of the VMO over the VL, one study looked at five different knee extension exercises in symptomatic and control subjects with various combinations of adduction and medial rotation of the tibia. They found that the VMO:VL ratio was greatest when there was simultaneous resistance to medial tibial rotation and knee extension. The test was conducted with the knee at 70 degrees of flexion and the tibia laterally rotated. The ratio with resisted adduction with extension was less than resisted extension alone.[68] This study did not look at effects on pain or improved function.

Short-arc terminal extension (see Fig. 13–9). Begin with the knee flexed around 20 degrees. If tolerated and the motion is not painful, light resistance is added at the ankle. Strengthening in terminal extension trains the muscle to function where it is least efficient because of its shortened position and where there is minimal patellar compression because it is superior to the femoral groove. This action is needed when lifting the leg into bed and moving the covers, as well as when lifting the leg into a car.

Precaution: If there is irritation of the synovial lining of the suprapatellar pouch or bursa, this exercise may be painful, and should be avoided until the pain subsides.

Train and Strengthen Functional Control of Knee Extension in Weight Bearing Positions

Note: See the last section of this chapter for detailed descriptions of the exercises. The patient should perform the repetitions of the appropriate exercise until symptoms or loss of control just begin in order to develop endurance. It is important to not push beyond that point in order to avoid faulty mechanics or loss of control.

Instruct the patient to focus on the sensation of the VMO contracting while performing the exercises. If weight bearing is painful, begin with partial weight-bearing exercises. Progress to standing exercises as tolerated. A recent study suggests that mini-squats are effective in causing a greater VMO : VL ratio than a maximum voluntary isometric quadriceps contraction.[56] Mini-squats may be useful to improve patellar tracking and are introduced early in the exercise program when weight bearing and partial squatting are tolerated and do not provoke symptoms.

Precaution: Because there are higher patellar compressive loads when the knee is flexed beyond 60 degrees in weight bearing, exercises and activities with the knee flexed greater than this angle may provoke symptoms. Use caution when the patient is ready to progress beyond 60 degrees. Have the patient carefully monitor symptoms and stop the exercise if symptoms develop.

Modify Biomechanical Stresses

If the patient has foot pronation, a foot orthosis may relieve the stresses at the knee.[29] Assess lower extremity mechanics, and modify any faulty patterns.

Educate the Patient

- Until the knee is symptom free, the patient should avoid positions and activities that provoke the symptoms.
- Avoid stair climbing and descending until the muscles are strengthened to a level at which they can function without symptoms.
- The patient should not sit with the knees flexed excessively for prolonged periods.
- Use a home exercise program to reinforce the training, and instruct the patient how to safely progress the exercises.

Functional Activities

Exercises are progressed as described in the exercise section of this chapter as long as the patient is able to maintain control and not exacerbate the symptoms. Use activity-specific drills to prepare the patient to return to the desired activity.

Patellofemoral and Extensor Mechanism Surgery and Postoperative Management

When conservative (nonoperative) management of patellofemoral dysfunction fails, surgery may be indicated. Surgical intervention can be used to alter the alignment of the patellofemoral joint, correct soft tissue imbalances, decrease an abnormal Q angle, improve tracking of the patella, and débride the articular surface of the patella. All of these factors can contribute to chronic patellofemoral pain and crepitation and recurrent dislocation or subluxation of the patella. Before any surgery is chosen, the etiology of symptoms and identification of contributing factors must be determined by a thorough physical examination and arthroscopic and radiographic evaluation. Surgical options include *release of the lateral retinaculum, chondroplasty* or *abrasion arthroplasty* of the patella, *proximal or distal realignment of the extensor mechanism,* and *patellectomy.*[99,101a] A combination of procedures may also be indicated. Only in rare instances is a patellectomy performed, most often as a salvage procedure.[99]

The goals of postoperative rehabilitation are to:[8,37a,73] (1) reduce or control postoperative pain and swelling, (2) prevent or reduce the adverse effects of immobilization, (3) restore postoperative knee ROM quickly and safely, (4) maximize the function of the extensor mechanism, especially the VMO, to restore full active knee extension and prevent a postoperative extensor lag, and (5) educate the patient and possibly alter lifestyle to prevent recurrence of patellofemoral pain and dysfunction.

Lateral Retinacular Release

Indications for Surgery

Although opinion varies, the following are often cited as indications for lateral retinacular release (LRR).[8,37a,39a,99,101a]

- Chronic patellofemoral pain and functional limitations without improvement in symptoms after 6 months of conservative (nonoperative) management including exercise, taping, bracing, anti-inflammatory medication and modification of daily activities.

- Restricting and often tender lateral retinaculum with documented patellar malalignment, specifically a lateral patellar tilt and resulting lateral compression syndrome.[39a,101a]
- Minimal to no evidence of patellofemoral chondrosis or abnormal Q angle.
- Pathology or impairments associated with instability of the patella, which may include lateral subluxation or dislocation, inadequate dynamic medial stabilizers, increased Q angle and inadequate size/shape of the trochlear groove may indicate the need for LRR plus additional surgical procedures.

Procedures

LRR is designed to reduce an identified lateral tilt of the patella, reduce excessive compressive forces on the lateral facet of the patella and, consequently, reduce pain and the risk of lateral subluxation of the patella.[101a] LRR is performed arthroscopically through several parapatellar portals, percutaneously through a 1-cm incision or by an open approach that involves a longitudinal parapatellar incision immediately lateral to the patella.* The procedure "releases" the lateral structures supporting the patellofemoral joint, specifically the superficial and deep portions of the lateral retinaculum and the lateral patellotibial ligament. LRR may be performed alone or in conjunction with synovectomy, chondroplasty, and imbrication of the medial aspect of the capsule or proximal or distal realignment of the extensor mechanism.

Complications associated with LRR include hemarthrosis caused by damage to the lateral superior geniculate artery, medial patellar subluxation as the result of releasing the vastus lateralis too far superiorly, as well as postoperative arthrofibrosis, rupture of the quadriceps tendon, and reflex sympathetic dystrophy.[73,101a] Any of these complications can affect postoperative rehabilitation and compromise outcomes.

Postoperative Management

Postoperative management of LRR is a fairly straightforward intervention process, which progresses quite rapidly, especially after arthroscopic LRR in light of less postoperative tissue morbidity.[8,37a,73,99] The patient is progressed through the phases of rehabilitation based on signs and symptoms and the attainment of phase-specific goals.[92] Management of each phase of rehabilitation is summarized in Table 13–3.

Immobilization

The knee is immobilized in full extension with a compression dressing and patella-stabilizing orthosis or posterior splint for 0 to 3 days.[8,73,99] A Cryo-Cuff®, which combines cold and compression, or another form of cryotherapy is applied to minimize postoperative joint effusion often associated with hemarthrosis. The patient is permitted to ambulate, weight bearing as tolerated with crutches, almost immediately after surgery. When quadriceps control in full knee extension has been achieved, use of assistive devices for ambulation may be discontinued.

Exercise: Maximum Protection Phase

The major emphasis during the acute or maximum protection phase after LRR is prevention of postoperative complications, such as deep vein thrombosis (DVT), control of postoperative joint effusion, restoration of quadriceps function, regaining ROM and adequate patellar mobility to prevent formation of adhesions that could position the patella in the same alignment that was evident preoperatively or even in a more lateral position. Exercises are initiated the day of surgery, even after an open release, including assisted ROM. These exercises, summarized in Table 13–3, are similar to those found in a nonoperative program for management of patellofemoral syndrome, detailed in the previous section of this chapter. For example, after an open release it may be necessary for the patient to wear a removable knee immobilizer or splint that holds the knee in extension during weight-bearing activities. Assisted and active ROM exercises to regain mobility and control of knee flexion and extension are progressed within the patient's comfort level. Exercises to elicit neuromuscular control of the quadriceps can be performed in nonweight-bearing as well as protected weight-bearing positions. As noted in Table 13–3, the use of a felt pad wedge placed under the compression dressing along the lateral border of the patella,[73] which applies a slight medial glide, or the use of McConnell taping[44a,78] to maintain patellar alignment and unload the lateral soft tissue structures may enable the patient to perform knee exercises more comfortably. By the end of the maximum protection phase, by about 2 weeks postoperatively, the goal is to achieve knee motion from 115 degrees of

*See references 15, 37a, 39a, 73, 82, 99, 101a, 106.

Table 13–3 Lateral Retinacular Release—Intervention for Each Phase of Rehabilitation

Phase and General Time Frame	Maximum Protection Phase Weeks 1–2	Moderate Protection Phase Weeks 3–4	Minimum Protection Phase Weeks 5–6	Return-to-Activity Phase Week 6
Patient Presentation	• Patient should enter rehabilitation within 2 days after surgery • Minimum postoperative pain • ROM minimally limited • Weight bearing as tolerated	• Minimum pain, • Full weight bearing • Near full ROM • Joint effusion controlled	• No swelling or tenderness • Good to normal strength • Unrestricted ADL function	• Muscle function 70% of noninvolved extremity • No signs or symptoms of subluxation, pain, or swelling in the previous phase
Key Examination Procedures	• Pain (0–10 scale) • Monitor for hemarthrosis • ROM • Muscle control • Soft tissue palpation • Patellar mobility	• Pain assessment • Joint effusion—girth • ROM • Muscle strength • Patellar mobility • Gait analysis	• Pain assessment • Muscular strength • Patellar alignment/ stability • Functional status	• Pain assessment • Muscular strength • Patellar alignment/ stability • Functional status
Intervention	• A-AROM and AROM • Patellar mobilization (grade I and II) • Muscle setting quadriceps, hamstrings, and adductors (may augment with E-stim) • SLRS—four positions • Flexibility program hamstring, calf, IT band • Ankle pumps • Trunk/pelvis strengthening • Pain modulation modalities • Lateral felt pad to apply medial glide to patella • Compression wrap control effusion	• LE flexibility program • Continued open- and closed-chain strengthening • Limited range PREs • Tibiofemoral joint mobilization if needed • Proprioceptive training • Stabilization exercises • Gait training • Aerobic conditioning program • Swimming or walking program	• Continue LE flexibility • Advance PRE strengthening • Advance closed-chain exercise • Advance proprioceptive training • Advance endurance training • Simulated functional tasks based on signs and symptoms	• Continue stretching and strenghtening; advance as appropriate • Advance agility drills • Advance running drills • Implement drills specific to sport or occupation • Consider bracing for high-demand activity
Goals	• Control postoperative swelling • Minimize pain • ROM 0–115 degrees • 3/5 to 4/5 muscle strength • Ambulate without assistive device • Establish home exercise program	• Swelling control • Full ROM • 4/5 to 5/5 strength • Gradual return to ADL • Adherence to home program	• 70% muscle reconditioning • Educate patient on resuming activity slowly, monitoring signs and symptoms	• Develop maintenance program and educate patient on importance of adherence

Adapted from: Mangine, RE, et al.[73] page 327 with permission.

flexion to full extension as swelling subsides and tissues heal.

Although grade I and II mobilization procedures to maintain patellar mobility should be initiated in the early postoperative period to maintain gliding and to prevent patellofemoral adhesions, these glides should be performed within the patient's pain parameters.[73] With proper instruction the patient can be taught to carry out patellar mobilization procedures at home and should do so regularly throughout the day.

Exercise: Moderate Protection Phase

The moderate protection phase after LRR places emphasis on attaining full active ROM of the knee, developing muscular strength and endurance and reestablishing balance as pain and joint effusion reach a minimal level. Closed- and open-chain exercises are progressed at levels of intensity and positions within the ROM that do not evoke pain. High-speed, submaximal isokinetic training may also be useful.[69] Flexibility exercises for the lower extremity should continue with particular emphasis placed on stretching the IT band. If restricted, the IT band can contribute to excessive compression over the lateral femoral condyle and lateral border of the patella during knee motion. Aerobic conditioning to reestablish cardiorespiratory fitness is also begun during this phase. Available motion and strength are incorporated into progressive functional activities. Any number of exercises, described in the final section of this chapter, as well as individually designed exercises can be incorporated and progressed in a patient's rehabilitation program as long as the selected exercises do not cause a recurrence of patellofemoral symptoms.

Exercise: Minimum Protection and Return-to-Full-Activity Phases

The minimum protection phase is characterized by progression of interventions of the moderate protection phase, and activity-specific training for return to work or sport function is emphasized. The primary focus should be placed on educating the patient to resume activity slowly while monitoring signs and symptoms. The return-to-activity phase concentrates on advanced training for sport or occupational demands. During this phase a maintenance program and compliance plan should be developed. Patients can usually return to a full level of activity by 6 to 8 weeks postoperatively.

Note: Continued use of patellar taping or a patellar tracking orthosis during exercise may be useful during progression of exercise and transition to functional activities.

Outcomes

LRR as an independent procedure can be useful for alleviating or reducing patellofemoral pain if the cause of pain stems from compression of lateral structures of the knee associated with excessive lateral tilt.[37a,39a,99,101a] Comparably favorable outcomes have been reported for arthroscopic and open procedures.[37a] Good to excellent short-term reduction of pain and associated patellofemoral symptoms have been reported for 65 to 75% of patients. Long-term effectiveness of LRR is questionable especially in patients with a history of patellar instability.[99,101a]

Proximal Realignment of the Extensor Mechanism

Indications for Surgery

Proximal realignment of the extensor mechanism is indicated for a combination of the following findings.[53,65,99,106]

- Recurrent lateral dislocation or subluxation of the patella because of extensor mechanism malalignment
- Lateral tracking of the patella and insufficiency of the VMO
- Painful, lateral compressive forces at the patellofemoral joint and persistent lateral tilt of the patella despite an LRR

Procedures

A proximal realignment procedure, which can be performed by an open approach or sometimes arthroscopically, is characterized by an advancement of the vastus medialis to a more central location. The procedure may also include a tightening (imbrication) of the medial capsule.[65,99,101a,106] Sutures are passed through the vastus medialis and medial capsule while visualized. The primary goal is to improve the resting length tension of the VMO. Inadequate transfer of the VMO may result in no change in patellar position, tracking, or a patient's symptoms. Proximal realignment and an LRR may be performed concurrently.

Proximal realignment procedures can result in potential complications. These include significant scarring in the medial capsule and overtightening of the medial capsule and/or VMO leading to excessive medial tracking and potential medial subluxation of the patella. Overtightening may also lead to increased patellar rotation, altering normal patellofemoral biomechanics and resulting in erosion of the articular surface of the patella.[73] The therapist must watch for signs of nerve irritation and/or reflex sympathetic dystrophy during rehabilitation. Entrapment or irritation of the saphenous nerve, as it passes the adductor tubercle and splits at the pes anserine tendon, can occur with procedures involving structures on the medial side of the knee.[22] These complications are more likely to occur with an open rather than an arthroscopic realignment procedure.[73] Surgical advances in proximal realignment procedures by arthroscopic intervention have decreased the morbidity of this surgery.

Postoperative Management

The postsurgical management after proximal realignment follows a similar course as after LRR with the exception of a prolonged maximum protection phase to allow for a more gradual progression of ROM and extended protection of healing soft tissues.[8,73] In the early phases of rehabilitation the therapist must be alert to the presence of inhibition of the VMO. As with postoperative management after LRR and nonoperative management of patellofemoral dysfunction, many of the exercises selected for a patient's rehabilitation focus on recruitment and reconditioning of the quadriceps mechanism as a unit and the VMO in particular.[3,8,19,25,62,73] Of importance is prevention or remediation of an extensor lag (quadriceps lag)[121,127] and development of an appropriate balance of function of the knee musculature.[8,19]

Immobilization and Weight Bearing

The knee is immobilized in a range-limiting orthosis or a posterior splint in full extension up to a week to 10 days. Some surgeons allow protected ROM in the hinged orthosis or removal of the immobilizer for early mobility, while others advocate continuous immobilization for a short period of time after surgery. Only touch-down or toe-touch weight bearing on the operated extremity is permissible for the first 10 to 14 days postoperatively, followed by a gradual progression to 75% weight bearing by 4 weeks. Full weight bearing without assistive devices should be achieved during weeks 8 to 10 but only in the absence of an extensor lag.

Exercise: Maximum Protection Phase

The range-limiting orthosis allows ROM from 0 degrees to only 60 degrees for the first 2 weeks. Range is progressed to 90 degrees by week 3 and 110 degrees by week 4.

Precaution: Too rapid progression of ROM into knee flexion may lead to suture failure in the approximated tissues and result in an inability to control patellar position.[73] Careful monitoring by the therapist is essential.

Early intervention with gentle (grade I and II) mobilization of the patellofemoral and tibiofemoral joints, as well as surrounding soft tissues is recommended to increase ROM, decrease pain and decrease joint effusion.

Exercises similar to those indicated after lateral retinacular release or for nonoperative management of the patellofemoral joint when symptoms are acute may be initiated. Emphasis is placed on repeated pain-free exercises and activation of the VMO, which may be augmented with electrical muscle stimulation and biofeedback. Every effort is made to prevent an extensor lag while simultaneously increasing knee flexion. Patella baja (patella infra), a potential source of an extensor lag,[121,127] must be prevented in the early postoperative period.

Exercise: Moderate Protection Phase

The moderate protection phase after a proximal realignment procedure extends from approximately 4 to 10 weeks postoperatively, as realigned soft tissues continue to heal. The approximate time frame for this phase as with any suggested time frame in a postoperative protocol may be modified based on the patient's signs and symptoms and response to interventions. To begin this phase, which focuses on attaining full knee flexion and improving strength and endurance of the knee musculature, the patient should have minimal pain, full active knee extension, and approximately 110 degrees of knee flexion.

Because knee flexion must be progressed gradually to protect the healing quadriceps mechanism and because substantial emphasis is placed on regaining neuromuscular control of the quadriceps mechanism during the maximum protection phase, low-intensity, prolonged stretching and grade III joint mobilizations may be required in this stage to obtain greater knee flexion. An emphasis on improving strength and endurance throughout the lower extremity through closed- and open-chain exercises must also be emphasized as ROM increases. All exercises to improve muscle performance must be done at a level of intensity and in positions that are pain-free. At the end of the moderate protection phase, the patient should have pain-free functional ROM of the knee (0–135 degrees).[73]

Exercise: Minimum Protection and Return-to-Activity Phases

Individual factors of the patient contribute to the speed of progression to the final phases of the rehabilitation program. These factors include age, general health, severity of symptoms prior to the surgical procedure, presence of other pathology, desired functional outcome, and the patient's adherence to the home exercise program (HEP) and motivation to return to functional activities. Full return to functional activity is expected by 14 to 20 weeks postoperatively. These final phases are characterized by ongoing reinforcement of the HEP, activity-specific training, and participation in gradually more demanding activities. As with previous phases of recovery, exercises and functional activities should not cause recurrence of pain, subluxation, or joint effusion. Patients who continue to report knee pain with provoking activities, such as ascending and descending stairs, should continue to restrict their level of activity until asymptomatic. Efforts should be made to modify the patient's lifestyle to avoid symptom-provoking activities at least on a temporary basis. Refer to the exercise progression previously discussed for advanced nonoperative management and the selected exercises described in the final sections of this chapter.

Distal Realignment of the Extensor Mechanism

Indications for Surgery

The following are indications for distal realignment procedures.[65,99,101a]

- Recurrent dislocation or subluxation of the patella because of extensor mechanism malalignment that cannot be corrected with LRR and proximal realignment procedures.
- Increased Q angle.
- Significant patellofemoral arthrosis.
- Bony procedures are only indicated in the skeletally mature patient.

Procedures

The purpose of the distal realignment procedure is to medially transfer the patellar tendon to reduce the Q angle and improve patellar tracking by decreasing the laterally directed moment, which tends to cause subluxation of the patella with contraction of the quadriceps.[65,99,101a,106] Several techniques of distal realignment have been reported. An osteotomy of the tibial tubercle is preformed; the bony prominence is then transpositioned medially and secured with screw fixation. A concomitant LRR and possibly a medial imbrication are also performed. Occasionally, anteriorization (elevation) of the tibial tubercle is used to reduce shear forces and articular stresses on the patella.[101a] The procedure involves anteriorly displacing the tibial tubercle by means of a bone graft.[101a] In the skeletally immature patient there are distal medialization procedures that involve only soft tissues.

Complications associated with bony distal realignment procedures include nonunion of the transposed bone, osteomyelitis, and inadequate skin closure over the osteotomy site.[101a] In soft tissue and bony procedures patellar adhesions can also occur.

Postoperative Management

Management after a distal realignment procedure is similar to postoperative management after LRR and proximal realignment procedures previously discussed with the major exceptions of the need for delayed weight bearing and a more gradual progression of exercises to allow time for bone healing. Rehabilitation typically begins 2 to 4 days postoperatively. Weight bearing is limited to toe-touch for the first 4 weeks or until radiographic verification of bone callus formation at the osteotomy site has occurred.[8,73] Weight bearing is progressed gradually with full weight bearing permissible at 8 weeks.[73]

A range-limiting orthosis is worn that allows motion from only 0 to 30 degrees of flexion during the first week, to 90 degrees of flexion by the end of the 4th week, and 135 degrees by the end of the 8th week. Return to full activity is based on bone healing. Otherwise exercises are similar to those for nonoperative management and for LRR and proximal realignment procedures. Special attention is given to monitoring wound healing during the early postoperative weeks.

▶ Ligamentous Injuries

Related Diagnoses and Mechanisms of Injury

Ligamentous injuries occur most frequently in individuals between 20 and 40 years of age as the result of sport injuries (e.g., skiing, soccer, and football) but can occur in individuals of all ages. The anterior cruciate ligament (ACL) is the most commonly injured ligament. Often more than one ligament is damaged as the result of a single injury.[57]

Anterior Cruciate Ligament (ACL)

ACL injuries occur from both contact and noncontact mechanisms. The most common contact mechanism is a blow to the lateral side of the knee resulting in a valgus force to the knee. This mechanism can result not only in injury to the ACL, but to the medial collateral ligament (MCL) and the medial meniscus as well. This injury is termed the "unholy triad" injury because of the frequency of these three structures being injured from a common blow. The most common noncontact mechanism is a rotational mechanism in which the tibia is externally rotated on the planted foot. Literature supports that this mechanism can account for up to 78% of all ACL injuries.[90] The second most common noncontact mechanism is forceful hyperextension of the knee.

With prolonged ambulation on a knee that has a deficient ACL, the secondary restraints (lateral collateral ligament and posterolateral joint capsule) are stressed and become lax, and the individual may develop a "quadriceps avoidance gait."[54]

Posterior Cruciate Ligament (PCL)

The PCL is most commonly injured by a forceful blow to the anterior tibia while the knee is flexed, such as a blow to the dashboard or falling onto a flexed knee.

Medial Collateral Ligament (MCL)

Isolated injuries to the MCL can occur from valgus forces being placed across the medial joint line of the knee. While most injuries to the ACL and PCL are complete tears of the ligament, injuries to the MCL can be partial or incomplete and are graded utilizing a I, II, III grading classification of ligament injuries (this is described in Chapter 8).

Lateral Collateral Ligament (LCL)

Injuries to the lateral collateral ligament (LCL) are infrequent, but they usually occur from a traumatic varus force across the knee. It is not uncommon that more than one ligament, joint capsule, and sometimes the menisci are damaged as the result of a single injury.

Ligament Injuries in the Female Athlete

With an increase in the number of female athletes since the passage of Title IX in 1972, a concurrent increase in the number of injuries to female athletes has been seen, most significantly an increase in the number of knee injuries. What is interesting is that when injury to the ACL is sustained in a noncontact manner, a woman is three times as likely to tear the ACL than a man.[4] With the increased number of noncontact ACL injuries in female athletes being reported, the American Academy of Orthopaedic Surgeons published a consensus paper examining the risk factors and prevention strategies of noncontact ACL injuries.[45] The risk factors fall into four major categories: environmental, anatomic, hormonal, and biomechanical.

- *Environmental factors* center on the use of prophylactic knee braces to prevent knee injuries and the shoe-to-surface interface that may improve performance, but may also increase the risk of injury.
- Three *anatomic risk factors* include femoral notch size, ACL size, and lower extremity alignment. Insufficient data relating to each of these factors have resulted in an incomplete understanding of the influence of these factors at this time.
- *Hormonal differences* between males and females have also been postulated to be one possible factor related to increased incidence of female ACL injuries. In 1996, hormone receptor sites for estrogen and progesterone were found in the ACL of humans. Since that time, research has been conducted to study the effects of such hormones on the mechanical properties of the ACL and other musculoskeletal tissues; however, to date, results of multiple studies differ in their conclusions.
- *Biomechanical risk factors* summarized by the consensus panel included: the effect of the total chain (trunk, hip, knee, and ankle) on ACL injuries, awkward or improper dynamic body movements, deceleration and change of direction, and neuromuscular control of the joint.

Common Impairments

- Following trauma, the joint usually does not swell for several hours.
- If tested when the joint is not swollen, the patient feels pain when the injured ligament is stressed.
- If there is a complete tear, instability is detected when the torn ligament is tested.
- If blood vessels are torn, swelling is usually immediate. Once swollen, motion is restricted, the joint assumes a position of minimum stress (usually flexed 25 degrees), and inhibition (shut down) of the quadriceps muscle occurs.[120]

Common Functional Limitations/Disabilities

- When acute, the knee cannot bear weight, and the person cannot ambulate without assistance.
- With complete tear, there is instability, and the knee may give way when weight bearing.

Nonoperative Management: Ligamentous Injuries

Acute sprains and partial ligamentous tears of the knee can be treated conservatively with rest, joint protection, and exercise. After the acute stage of healing, exercises should be geared toward regaining normal ROM, balance control, normalization of gait, and strengthening of muscles that support and stabilize the joint during functional activities. The degree of instability with ligamentous tears will affect the demands the patient can place on the knee when returning to full activity. An intensive rehabilitation program including perturbation training has been shown to be effective in select athletes after ACL injury.[36,37] With extensive damage and in general for those desiring to return to high-level work or sports, surgical repair will probably be necessary for return to a desired level of function.

If the collateral or coronary ligaments are involved, cross-fiber massage to the structure helps align the healing fibers and maintain mobility in them. The MCL is typically managed with a conservative (nonsurgical) approach. Because of the anatomical structure of the MCL (a broad, flat ligament with deep and superficial portions, parallel alignment of collagen fibers, and fan-shaped attachments both proximally and distally), injuries to the MCL heal without surgical intervention if protected.[138] Conservative management of MCL injuries is described in Table 13–4; progression is based on presenting signs and symptoms.[92]

Management: Maximum Protection Phase

- If possible, examine before effusion sets in.
- Treat the injury with cold, compression, and quadriceps-setting exercises.
- When the joint is swollen, treat it like an acute joint lesion. The knee may not fully extend for end-range muscle-setting exercises, so begin the exercises in the range most comfortable for the patient.

Management: Moderate Protection (Controlled Motion) Through Return to Activity

As the swelling decreases, examine the patient for impairments and functional losses. Initiate joint movement, muscle performance, functional activities, and aerobic exercises.

Joint mobility. Use supine wall slides (see Fig. 13–7), patellar mobilizations, and stationary cycling; encourage as much movement as possible. Unless there has been an extended period of immobilization, there should be minimal need to stretch contractures.

Muscle performance. Initiate isometric quadriceps and hamstring exercises and progress to dynamic strengthening and training.

- Straight-leg raising (with high-intensity electrical stimulation if there is an extensor lag)[118]
- Open-chain resistance
- Weight-bearing control and strengthening, balance and stabilization training, partial squats, step-ups, leg press, and heel-rises

Precautions: Open-chain terminal knee extension exercises (from 60 degrees to 0) with resistance applied to the distal leg and squatting between 60 and 90 degrees cause increased anterior translation of the tibia and stress to the ACL. Exercises using either of these activities in the designated ranges should not be attempted with ACL injuries.[45,136,137] Instruct the patient in closed-chain strengthening activities from 60 to 0 degrees and open-chain strengthening from 90 to 60 degrees.[136]

Isolated open-chain knee flexion exercises (hamstring curls) increase posterior translation of the tibia and should not be done with PCL injuries.

Cardiovascular pulmonary conditioning. Utilize a program that is consistent with the patient's goals

Table 13–4 Nonoperative Management of MCL Injuries—Intervention for Each Phase of Rehabilitation

Phase and General Time Frame	Maximum Protection Phase Weeks 1–3	Moderate Protection Phase Weeks 3–6	Minimum Protection Phase Weeks 5–8	Return-to-Activity Phase Weeks 6–10
Patient Presentation	• Joint effusion • Pin-point tenderness • Decreased ROM	• Minimal tenderness • Joint effusion controlled • No increased instability • Full or near full ROM	• No instability • No effusion or tenderness • 4/5 to 5/5 strength (MMT) • Unrestricted ADL function	• No instability • Muscle function 70% of noninvolved extremity • No symptoms of instability, pain, or swelling in the previous phase
Key Examination Procedures	• Pain scale • Joint effusion • Ligament stability • ROM • Muscle control • Functional status • Patellar mobility	• Pain scale • Joint effusion • Ligament stability • ROM • Muscle control/ strength • Functional status	• Ligament stability • Muscle control • Functional status	• Full clinical examination • Ligament stability • Muscle strength • Functional status
Intervention	• PRICE (ice, compression, elevation and protective bracing) • Ambulation training with crutches: weight bearing as tolerated • PROM/A-AROM • Patellar mobilization (grades I and II) • Muscle setting quadriceps, hamstrings, and adductors (may augment with E-stim) • SLRs • Aerobic conditioning	• Continue multiple-angle isometrics • Initiate PRE • Closed-chain strengthening • LE flexibility exercises • Endurance training (bike, pool, ski machine, etc.) • Proprioceptive training • Stabilization exercises • Initiate a walk/jog program at the end of this phase • Initiate skill-specific drills at the end of this phase	• Continue LE flexibility • Advance PRE strengthening • Advance closed-chain exercise • Advance proprioceptive training • Advance endurance training • Isokinetic training (if desired) • Progress running program; full speed jog, sprints, figure-eight running and cutting	• Continue flexibility and strengthening; advance as appropriate • Advance agility drills • Advance running drills • Implement drills specific to sport or occupation • Determine the need for protective bracing prior to return to sport or work
Goals	• Protect healing tissues • Prevent reflex inhibition of muscle • Decrease joint effusion • Decrease pain • Establish home exercise program	• Full pain-free ROM • Restore muscular strength • Normalize gait without assistive device • Normalize ADL function • Adherence to home program	• Increase strength • Increase power • Increase endurance • Improve neuromuscular control • Improve dynamic stability	• Increase strength • Increase power • Increase endurance • Regain ability to function at highest desired level • Transition to maintenance program

(Note: This is based on grade II ligament injury, but may be accelerated for grade I or decelerated for grade III injuries)

Adapted from: Wilk, K and Clancy[138] with permission.

such as biking (begin with a stationary bike), jogging (begin with walking on a treadmill), ski machine, or swimming.

Protective bracing. Bracing may be necessary for weight-bearing activities to decrease stress to the healing ligament or to provide stability where ligament integrity has been compromised. Bracing can be one of two types: range-limiting postoperative type braces that are used to protect healing tissues and discarded in later phases of rehabilitation or functional braces that are used both during rehabilitation and also when returning to functional activities. The patient must be instructed to modify activities until appropriate stability is obtained.

Functional training. Progress to functional training. Suggestions for functional training are described in the exercise section.

Reconstruction of Ligamentous Lesions

Ligamentous structures of the knee provide the key stabilizing forces to accessory motions of the knee. Specifically, these accessory motions are anterior and posterior translation and medial/lateral pivots (valgus/varus). Strong ligamentous support is necessary, in part, because of the shallow design of the concave tibial articulating surface allowing significant translatory motions if unrestrained. Acute traumatic disruption or chronic laxity of the ligaments results in excessive accessory motions of the joint, which can impair functional activities.[13,38,64,83] Although injury to all four of the primary knee ligaments is described in the literature, the ACL is the most frequently injured and surgically repaired.[90] Factors influencing the decision for surgical intervention include the desired level of function to which the patient wishes to return, the presence of additional pathology such as a meniscus tear, the pre-existing condition of joint articular surfaces, and potential exposure to reinjury.[13,34,83,89,126] Acute ligament injuries can lead to chronic instabilities and long-term changes in joint structure and integrity if not adequately managed and monitored.

General indications for ligament surgery. Surgical intervention for ligament injury is indicated if the patient has failed to meet functional goals established in a conservative rehabilitation program, or degenerative changes of the joint are apparent. Many authors[13,39,83,112,125,126] recommend surgical intervention for acute isolated ACL and LCL injuries in recreationally active individuals. This is usually advocated after a brief period of acute injury management. Surgical management of chronic ligament injuries is advocated when the patient's function has become limited, or when secondary pathologies such as meniscus tears, other ligament involvement, or articular surface degeneration have developed.

Types of ligament surgery. Ligamentous surgery, using an arthroscopically assisted or open approach, typically involves an *intra-articular or extra-articular reconstruction* of joint structures or a combination of procedures to restore stability to the knee.[13,64,66,83] In most instances, *direct repair* by means of suturing the torn ligament affords the least acceptable outcome. Direct repair is often unsuccessful because ligaments have a very poor vascular supply, necessitating long periods of immobilization and restricted weight bearing so that the ligament is not disrupted as it heals.

The most successful surgical intervention for ligamentous injury is the intra-articular reconstruction, which has been used most often for anterior or posterior cruciate lesions.[13,64,66,74a,83,89,126] The procedure involves use of an *autograft* (the patient's own tissue), an allograft (donor tissue), or a synthetic graft.[1] The patellar tendon has been shown to have tensile strength initially stronger than the ACL and is the most commonly chosen graft material for intra-articular reconstruction.[38,91] Other substitutes that are not as strong as the patellar tendon are a portion of the IT band or semitendinosus or gracilis tendons. An allograft or synthetic graft is used when an autogenous graft in a previous reconstruction has failed. Drawbacks to the use of allograft tissue include risk of disease transmission, decreased graft strength secondary to graft sterilization procedures, and insufficient availability of graft tissue because of limited resources. Continued advances in graft placement and fixation and improvement and refinement of arthroscopic techniques have all but eliminated the need for long periods of immobilization of the operated knee and protected weight bearing during ambulation.

Extra-articular reconstruction procedures, which involve the transposition of dynamic musculotendinous stabilizers or inert restraints around the knee such as the gracilis or semitendinosus muscle, capsular ligament, or IT band are designed to provide external stability to the knee joint. They were commonly used in the past but are used infrequently today because they do not restore normal arthrokinematics to the knee. Over time, transferred structures often stretch out, resulting in a recurrence of joint instability. Today extra-articular procedures are primarily used as an adjunct to an intra-articular reconstruction in difficult cases or in adolescents who have not reached bony maturity and still have open epiphyses.

General goals of ligament surgery and rehabilitation. The goals of surgery and postoperative rehabilitation after ligament reconstruction are (1) restoration of joint stability and motion, (2) pain-free and stable weight bearing, (3) appropriate postoperative strength and endurance to meet functional demands, and (4) the ability to return to preinjury activities. To meet these goals successful postoperative outcomes start, whenever possible, with a preoperative program including edema control, exercise to minimize atrophy and maintain as much ROM as possible, protected ambulation, and patient education. Exercises are similar to those used for nonoperative management of ligament injuries already discussed. Preoperative exercises should not further irritate the injured tissues or cause additional swelling or pain.[24,100]

The *rate* and *progression* of postoperative rehabilitation programs vary; no one program has been shown to be most effective or most efficient. Emphasis is placed on preventing postoperative complications while always protecting the healing graft. Early controlled motion and weight bearing have been shown to decrease the incidence of postoperative complications, such as contracture, patellofemoral pain, and muscle atrophy,[113,125] and to allow patients to return to activity more quickly without compromising the integrity of the reconstructed ligament.

There is a move away from adherence to strict time-based protocols to management guidelines that are progressed based on the attainment of specific criteria and measurable goals or performance on functional tests.[24,28,51,72,92] For example, an exercise program will be progressed to a higher level only after full active knee extension has been achieved or joint arthrometer testing indicates a particular level of joint stability. It is the responsibility of the therapist to be familiar with testing procedures and to have a thorough understanding of the operative procedure and the impact of exercise on healing structures. Open communication with the surgeon enables the therapist to discuss any precautions or concerns specific to individual patients and procedures.

Intra-Articular Anterior Cruciate Ligament Reconstruction

Indications for Surgery

The following are indications for intra-articular reconstruction of the anterior cruciate ligament (ACL).[1,13,64,83,89,112]

- Complete, acute tear or chronic insufficiency of the ACL leading to abnormal anterior translation of the tibia on the femur and instability or buckling of the knee
- A positive pivot-shift test because an ACL deficit is often associated with a lesion of other structures of the knee, such as the medial collateral ligament (MCL), resulting in rotatory instability of the joint
- Partial tear that results in limitation of functional activities in active individuals
- Failed conservative (nonoperative) management of an ACL tear

Procedures

Over the past 20 years, surgical management of the deficient ACL has evolved and continues to be refined with most procedures now using arthroscopically assisted techniques to reduce tissue morbidity and reduce recovery time. Advances in graft selection, placement, and fixation have also progressed over the years. Today, the most common ACL reconstruction procedure is an arthroscopically assisted or endoscopic procedure using an autograft.[13,34,74a,83] The two most common tissues used for the autograft include a central one-third, bone-tendon-bone patellar tendon graft, or a double hamstring tendon graft.[1,13,39,66,74a,83a,112] A patellar tendon graft, which involves bone-to-bone healing, heals at a faster rate than a hamstring graft, which requires tendon-to-bone healing. In some instances, such as in a revision of a prior ACL repair or when the patient's own tissue is not suitable for graft harvesting, an allograft may be used.[89]

Another technical aspect of surgical intervention for a deficient ACL is graft placement. Precise graft placement is crucial for restoration of joint function. Improper graft placement can lead to loss of ROM postoperatively.[52] A graft placed too far posteriorly may lead to failure to regain full flexion, and a graft placed too far anteriorly may limit extension. Loss of motion into extension may also be caused by an inadequate femoral notch size. A *femoral notchplasty* (an enlarging of the intercondylar notch) is performed to ensure adequate clearance of the graft as the knee extends.

Graft fixation also influences the success of ACL reconstruction. To fixate the graft, bone tunnels are drilled into the femur and tibia at the normal insertion sites of the ACL. The bone plugs of the graft are secured in the prepared tunnels with cortical bone screw fixation.[1,3,39,74a] The bony donor sites are filled with cancellous bone from the drill holes made into the femur and tibia. Proper placement and fit of cortical bone screws allows early tensile forces to be placed across the graft without compromising the security of the graft itself.[66] This, in turn, permits early initiation of weight bearing and ROM of the knee, both typical elements of current-day, accelerated rehabilitation protocols,[51,73a,74a,113] and eliminates the need for prolonged postoperative immobilization and delayed weight bearing historically associated with ACL reconstruction.[12,72,95]

Prior to closure, the knee is moved through the ROM to check the graft's integrity, and the tension on the graft during movement of the knee. The incision is then closed and a small compression dressing is immediately placed on the knee.

Postoperative Management

Just two decades ago, rehabilitation after ACL reconstruction involved long periods of complete immobilization of the knee in a position of flexion and an extended period (often 6–8 weeks) of restricted weight bearing. Return to full activity often took a full year.[12,72] With advances in surgical techniques and a better understanding of tissue healing, early postoperative motion and early weight bearing have become standard after primary intra-articular ACL reconstruction.[12,28,51a,73a,113,129,136] Table 13–5 outlines a contemporary accelerated program for postoperative management after primary ACL reconstruction.

Immobilization and Protective Bracing

With advances in graft fixation, the need for and use of bracing in the early postoperative period has become a point of debate. The surgeon's determination of whether or not postoperative protection with a brace is warranted is based on the type of graft used, intraoperative observations, and an assessment of the patient's expected level of compliance postoperatively.[51,100] If a range-limiting, hinged orthosis is used, the conditions of immobilization and brace use must be addressed.

Position of immobilization. After an intra-articular ACL reconstruction, the knee is placed in a controlled-motion brace that initially is locked in extension or in 5 to 10 degrees of flexion to prevent inadvertent hyperextension.[13,24,28,51,83a,100,113] Even though the greatest stress on the graft occurs between 20 degrees of flexion and full extension of the knee, precise placement of the graft allows the patient to safely extend the knee without disrupting the autograft. If an intra-articular ACL procedure has been combined with an extra-articular procedure, such as a collateral ligament reconstruction, the knee may need to be immobilized in approximately 20 to 30 degrees of knee flexion.

Duration of immobilization and brace use. Continuous postoperative immobilization in a locked brace is typically not necessary after reconstruction with an autogenous graft. In fact, ROM is initiated within a safe range immediately after surgery.[26,28,51,73a,77,94] The protective brace may be locked in extension or 10 degrees of flexion during ambulation the first week after surgery in the event of a fall.[51,100] By week 2 the brace is worn unlocked during ambulation, allowing movement from 0 to 90 degrees. The brace may also be worn during sleep for the first week postoperatively.[100]

Weight Bearing

For the first week after surgery, during ambulation with crutches, weight bearing is limited to between 25 and 50%. Weight bearing is then progressed during the next 2 to 3 weeks based on the patient's symptoms.

Full weight bearing and ambulation without crutches, but while wearing the protective brace, is usually possible by 3 to 4 weeks if weight bearing is pain-free and the patient has achieved full, *active* knee extension and sufficient strength of the quadriceps to control the knee.[51,83a,100] The brace (set to allow motion between 0 and 125 degrees) may need to be worn for ambulation and other weight-bearing activities for 2 to 3 months.

Exercise

The rate and progression of exercise after ACL reconstruction will depend upon the type of surgical procedure and type of graft. Exercise and weight

Table 13–5 ACL Reconstruction—Accelerated Postoperative Intervention for Each Phase of Rehabilitation

Phase and General Time Frame	Maximum Protection Phase Day 1 to Week 4	Moderate Protection Phase Weeks 5–10	Minimum Protection Phase Weeks 11–24	Return-to-Activity Phase 6 months+
Patient Presentation	Postoperative days 1–3 • Postoperative hemarthrosis • Postoperative pain • Decreased ROM • Decreased voluntary quadriceps contraction • Dependent ambulation • Postoperative brace (may or may not have)	• Pain controlled • Joint effusion controlled • No increased joint instability • Full or near full ROM • Fair plus to good muscle strength (3+/5–4/5) • Muscular control of joint • Independent ambulation	• No instability • No swelling • No pain • Good to normal muscle strength (4/5–5/5 on MMT) • Unrestricted ADL function	• No instability • Muscle function 70% of noninvolved extremity • No symptoms of instability, pain, or swelling in the previous phase
Key Examination Procedures	• Pain scale • Hemarthrosis—girth • Ligament stability—joint arthrometer (day 7–14) • ROM • Patellar mobility • Muscle control • Functional status	• Pain scale • Effusion—girth • Ligament stability—joint arthrometer • ROM • Patellar mobility • Muscle strength • Functional status	• Ligament stability—joint arthrometer • Muscle strength • Functional status	• Full clinical examination • Ligament stability • Muscle strength • Functional status
Intervention	**Early: Days 1–14** • PRICE: ice, compression, elevation and protective bracing • Gait training: crutches, weight bearing (25–50%) • PROM/A-AROM (range-limiting braces may or may not be used) • Patellar mobilization (grades I and II) • Muscle setting/ isometrics quadriceps, hamstrings, and adductors at multiple angles (may augment with E-stim) • Assisted SLRs—supine • Ankle pumps **Late: Weeks 2 to 4** • Continue as above • Progress weight bearing: (75% to full); begin closed-chain squats; heel/toe raises • SLRs in four planes • PRE: hamstrings • Initiate open-chain knee extension (range 90°–40°) • Trunk/pelvis stabilization • Aerobic conditioning	**Early: Weeks 5–6** • Multiple-angle isometrics • Advance closed-chain strengthening and PRE • LE stretching program • Endurance training bike, pool, ski machine, etc. • Proprioceptive training: single-leg stance, tilt board, BAPS board • Stabilization exercises, elastic band kicks, band walking **Late: Weeks 7–10** • Continue as above; advance strengthening (include PNF patterns), endurance, and flexibility • Advance proprioceptive training to high speed stepping drills, unstable surface challenge drills, and balance beam • Initiate a walk/jog program at the end of this phase • Initiate plyometric drills: bounding, jumping	• Continue LE stretching program • Advance PRE/ initiate isokinetic training (if desired) • Advance closed-chain exercise and plyometric drills (bouncing, jumping rope, box jumps: double-/single-leg) • Advance proprioceptive training • Progress agility drills (figure-8, skill-specific patterns) • Simulated work or sport-specific endurance training • Progress running program: full speed jogging, sprints, running and cutting	• Continue to progress PRE and flexibility exercises • Advance agility drills • Advance running drills • Implement drills specific to sport or occupation • Determine the need for protective bracing prior to return to sport or work

Table 13–5 ACL Reconstruction—Accelerated Postoperative Intervention for Each Phase of Rehabilitation *(Continued)*

Phase and General Time Frame	Maximum Protection Phase Day 1 to Week 4	Moderate Protection Phase Weeks 5–10	Minimum Protection Phase Weeks 11–24	Return-to-Activity Phase 6 months+
Goals	• Protect healing tissues • Prevent reflex inhibition of muscle • Decrease joint effusion • Decrease pain • ROM 0–125 degrees • Muscular control of ROM • Weight bearing 75% to full • Establish home exercise program	• Full pain-free ROM • Good to normal muscular strength (MMT) • Dynamic control of joint • Normalize gait pattern • Normalize ADL function • Adherence to home program	• Increase strength • Increase power • Increase endurance • Improve neuromuscular control and dynamic stability	• Increase strength • Increase power • Increase endurance • Regain ability to function at highest desired level • Transition to maintenance program

bearing can progress most rapidly after an arthroscopic, autogenous patellar tendon graft reconstruction.[51,100,113,136] Procedures that use less strong grafts, such as a portion of the semitendinosus tendon or IT band[91] or prosthetic graft materials, require a more cautious progression of exercises and weight bearing.

A delicate balance exists in the early postoperative period between adequate protection of healing tissues and prevention of adhesions, contractures, articular degeneration, and muscle atrophy associated with immobilization. Early motion places beneficial stresses that strengthen the graft but must be carefully controlled to avoid stretching the weakened graft, particularly during the early phases of rehabilitation.

Note: In a bone-patellar tendon-bone graft, the tendon graft is actually strongest at the time of implantation. Although at 6 weeks, healing of the bone plugs in the drill holes is relatively complete, the tendon graft first goes through a necrotizing process the first 2 to 3 weeks postoperatively before revascularization commences and maturation gradually occurs.

Most exercises are performed in the range-limiting, protective brace worn in the early and intermediate phases of rehabilitation. Depending on knee stability, either the protective brace or a functional brace may need to be worn during the final phases of rehabilitation particularly during high-speed exercises, such as plyometric training that involves quick changes of direction, or during high-demand functional activities to limit end-range motions.

Exercise: Maximum Protection Phase

Exercises begin the day after surgery, with pain and swelling controlled in a standard manner. The following goals and exercises are emphasized during the first 4 weeks after surgery when considerable protection of knee structures is required.[28,51,73a,100,136] If the patient is wearing a protective brace, it may be removed for muscle-setting and ROM exercises but should be worn during exercises that require weight bearing.

- Prevent reflex inhibition and atrophy of lower extremity musculature.
  - Muscle setting: quadriceps, hamstrings, and hip adductors within the patient's comfort level immediately after surgery.
  - Four-position SLRs, first assisted and then progressing to active hip motion with the knee maintained in extension.
  - Low-intensity, multiple-angle isometrics of the knee musculature.
  - Use of electrical stimulation or biofeedback to augment quadriceps contractions.
  - Stabilization exercises to develop co-contraction while standing with weight bearing distributed to a permissable level on the involved leg. As increased weight bearing is permissible, initiate weight-shifting activities.

Note: A quadriceps contraction with the knee in full extension generates little to no anterior translation of the tibia on the femur, because the knee is in a closed-pack position.

- Regain mobility within a protected range and prevent contractures of the knee. The goal is to achieve 90 degrees of flexion and nearly full extension by the end of the first week.[28,51,83a,100] Full passive extension will not be possible when joint effusion is present. As effusion subsides, the goal is to attain 125 degrees of knee flexion and full extension preferably by 2 to 3 weeks postoperatively. Begin the following activities immediately after surgery or on postoperative day 1.
  - Therapist-controlled PROM or A-AROM within a protected range (0–90 degrees) and within the patient's comfort level.
  - Supine, gravity-assisted, wall slides to increase knee flexion. The involved leg is passively lowered to just the 90-degree position and then *passively* extended to the starting position by the sound leg.
  - Supine, gravity-assisted knee extension. Prop the heel on a rolled towel with the knee unsupported and relaxed.
  - Patellar glides to prevent adhesions.
  - CPM within a limited range (0–90 degrees) if prescribed. Although a valid mechanism for controlling postoperative pain and initiating early motion,[26,77,94] it is used less frequently today than in the recent past.[51] It has been suggested that the CPM unit should be used without a calf band to minimize anterior translation of the tibia and prevent excessive stress to the graft site.[26]
- Begin to restore dynamic control of knee musculature and strengthen adjacent musculature in the later portion of the maximum protection phase.
  - Heel slides in supine.
  - Bilateral, short-arc squats while wearing the protective brace. Weight should be distributed on the involved lower extremity to a permissible level while standing and holding onto a stable surface for support or in a semireclining position on a Total Gym® unit. The value of closed-chain strengthening after ACL reconstruction has been supported by many authors.[5,17,24,51,73a,136]

Precaution: When squatting in an upright position be sure that the knees do not move anterior to the toes as the hips descend because this increases shear forces on the tibia and could potentially place excess stress on the autograft.

  - Assisted, progressing to active knee flexion/extension to 90 degrees while in prone or standing on the sound lower extremity to activate the knee flexors concentrically and eccentrically.
  - While seated on a rolling stool, scoot *forward* to activate the hamstrings concentrically in a closed-chain (see Fig. 13–15).
  - Pool exercises when the incision site is well-healed.
  - Stationary cycling.

Precaution: As noted earlier in this section of the chapter in the discussion of exercises for nonoperative management of the ACL-deficient knee, avoid resisted open-chain, terminal knee extension and closed-chain extension between 60 and 90 degrees of flexion. Contraction of the quadriceps in these positions and ranges causes the greatest anterior tibial translation and can create potentially excessive stress to the graft in the early stage of healing.[32,46,136,138]

Exercise: Moderate Protection Phase

The moderate protection phase begins at about 4 to 5 weeks postoperatively or at a point when pain and joint swelling are well-controlled, and there is no evidence of increased joint instability determined by arthrometer measurements. The patient should already have 110 to 125 degrees of knee flexion and full active knee extension. The emphasis of this intermediate phase is to achieve full ROM and increase strength in the involved lower extremity in preparation for independent functional activities. The hinged, protective brace is worn for gait and most exercises.

Note: By 8 to 10 weeks revascularization of the graft is becoming well-established, and therefore, exercises can be performed more vigorously.

- Regain full ROM of the knee and appropriate flexibility of lower extremity musculature, particularly in the hamstrings and calf muscles with stretching exercises. In the prone-lying position, apply a cuff weight to the ankle with the foot hanging over the edge of a treatment table to apply a sustained stretch and achieve the final degrees of terminal extension. Use grade III joint mobilization techniques to restore full knee flexion.
- Increase strength, control, and endurance in the lower extremities.

- Progressive closed-chain exercises [bilateral squats, standing wall slides against resistance, and unilateral squats or lunges on an inclined sled (such as a Total Gym®)], and step-ups and step-downs, gradually increasing step height.
- PRE on a leg press machine against light resistance and within a protected range.

Precaution: Continue to avoid resisted, closed-chain extension exercises between 60 and 90 degrees of knee flexion and resisted open-chain terminal knee extension exercises with placement of resistance on the distal tibia.

- Improve proprioception, balance, and stability with standing on unstable surfaces and walking activities on uneven surfaces or around objects.
- Regain cardiorespiratory fitness with aerobic conditioning activities. Gradually increase walking distance and speed.

Exercise: Minimum Protection and Return-to-Activity Phases

- From 10 to 24 weeks postoperatively emphasis is placed on incorporating progressively demanding functional activities, such as stair climbing, jogging, and agility drills into the rehabilitation program if the patient has regained approximately 75 to 80% of knee muscle strength. The unlocked knee brace is still worn during most functional activities, particularly the more vigorous activities that involve turning, twisting, or light jumping motions, and simulated work- or sport-specific motions.
- Plyometrics, jumping and hopping, and medium- and high-velocity spectrum isokinetic rehabilitation can also be added to the rehabilitation program.
- By 24 weeks most individuals return to a preinjury activity level. Functional bracing may still be required during high-demand recreational or work-related activities or a high-level maintenance program.

Posterior Cruciate Ligament Reconstruction

Indications for Surgery

Although rupture of the posterior cruciate ligament (PCL) is usually accompanied by damage to other structures in the knee, indications for surgical repair or reconstruction include the following.[2,94a,88,126,129a]

- Complete tear or avulsion of the PCL with posterolateral, posteromedial, or rotary instability of the knee associated with damage to other structures such as the LCL, MCL, ACL, or the menisci.
- "Isolated" PCL rupture and a "3 plus" (>10 or 15 mm) posterior displacement resulting in instability during functional activities.
- Chronic PCL insufficiency associated with posterolateral instability, pain, limitations in functional activities, and deterioration of articular surfaces of the knee.

Note: Many patients with complete PCL tears return to a preinjury level of activity without surgical intervention. There is far less consensus on indications for surgery after PCL injury than after ACL injury.[2,94a,126,129] Reconstructive surgery is a much more common method of treatment of ACL lesions than of PCL lesions.[94a,126]

Procedures

Surgical treatment of a complete, acute tear includes an arthroscopic, arthroscopically assisted, or open primary repair, augmentation, or reconstruction.[129a] Arthroscopically assisted, intra-articular reconstruction procedures for the PCL include a single-bundle or double-bundle bone-central one-third patellar tendon-bone autograft, a hamstring tendon autograft, Achilles tendon allograft, or occasionally, a synthetic graft.[2,88,94a,126,129a] Of these, the patellar tendon graft reconstruction is the most common.

An anterior arthroscopic approach is used to harvest the bone-patellar tendon-bone autograft. The patient is then moved into the prone position, and a small posteromedial curved incision is made at the knee. The posterior joint capsule is incised. Femoral and tibial tunnels are prepared through which the bone plugs of the graft are placed and secured with screw fixation. The graft is secured to the anterior aspect of the medial femoral condyle, advanced through drill holes, and attached to the posterior aspect of the tibial plateau to mimic the function of the PCL. After wound closure, a sterile compression dressing is applied, and the knee is immobilized in full extension.

Postoperative Management

Immobilization, Protective Bracing, and Weight Bearing

The knee is immobilized in a long-leg, hinged brace initially locked in full extension. The immobilizer is worn at all times, even during sleep, for the first 4 weeks to prevent sudden knee flexion. It is removed for gentle exercise during the period of maximum protection. At 4 to 5 weeks the brace is unlocked to allow from 0 to 90 degrees of flexion during functional activities.

Weight bearing is progressed very gradually after PCL surgery.[30,93,94a,129a] Immediately after surgery only toe-touch weight bearing is permissible while wearing the protective brace locked in extension. Weight bearing is gradually progressed to a 25% level at 2 weeks and to a 50% level at 3 to 5 weeks. If quadriceps control is sufficient for full active knee extension and pain and joint effusion are well-controlled, weight bearing is progressed and the brace is unlocked (allowing 0–90 degrees of movement) during ambulation with crutches. Full weight bearing is permitted at approximately 8 weeks, and crutch use is discontinued based on the patient's signs and symptoms.[93,94a]

Exercise

Note: Many of the postoperative exercises in the maximum, moderate, and minimum protection phases after PCL reconstruction are similar to those in a postoperative ACL reconstruction rehabilitation program.[30,93,94]

Precaution: During the first 4 to 6 weeks after surgery all knee flexion exercises should be performed passively. That is, the hamstrings should be essentially inactive during knee flexion activities to avoid the risk of posterior displacement of the tibia on the femur, which could disrupt the healing graft.[93,94a]

Exercise: Maximum Protection Phase

The emphasis in the first phase of rehabilitation is to protect the healing graft and control pain and joint effusion while simultaneously regaining a limited degree of mobility and preventing reflex inhibition of the quadriceps.[30,93,94a,129a] Exercise is initiated immediately after surgery. The maximum protection phase extends for approximately 4 to 5 weeks postoperatively.

- Re-establish control of the quadriceps mechanism to prepare for functional weight-bearing activities and to prevent posterior subluxation of the tibia on the femur when the knee is flexed to more than 50 to 60 degrees.[93,94a]
  - Quadriceps-setting exercises in full knee extension.
  - SLRs only in supine initially while wearing the locked brace.
  - Multiple-angle isometric exercises of the quadriceps from full extension to 25 to 30 degrees of flexion.
  - Active-assistive progressing to active knee extension while seated.
  - Augment quadriceps training with electrical stimulation.
- Regain mobility of the knee.
  - To regain knee flexion, initiate exercises in the sitting position. Hold the patient's leg in a position of knee extension. Have the patient control leg lowering as gravity flexes the knee. This exercise causes knee flexion while the hamstrings are inactive. As pain and joint effusion subside, apply a slight overpressure to the tibia to increase flexion. The patient should be able to achieve 90 degrees of knee flexion by 2 weeks.
  - To regain full passive knee extension, position the patient in a supine position with a rolled towel under the ankle and the knee unsupported to allow gravity to extend the knee.
  - Maintain patellar mobility with grade I and II patellar mobilizations.
  - Maintain flexibility of hip and ankle musculature with gentle stretching

Exercise: Moderate and Minimum Protection Phases

The goals of the moderate protection phase are to progress by approximately 8 weeks postoperatively to full ROM (0–135), full weight bearing and unassisted ambulation while continuing to wear the unlocked protective brace. Strengthening continues to focus on the quadriceps to re-establish full active knee extension and sufficient strength in the quadriceps as well as hip and ankle musculature for functional weight-bearing activities.

At the beginning of this phase if the patient has attained full knee extension and 90 degrees of flexion, 50% weight bearing is permitted. Bilateral closed-chain exercises in the unlocked brace with symmetrical (50%) weight bearing are initiated with mini-squats and heel and toe raises in the parallel bars. Later, these and more advanced closed-chain exercises are performed. Open-chain quadriceps training can also be increased (with continued emphasis in 0 to 25 degree range of knee flexion,[32] unless the patient experiences patellofemoral joint discomfort) during the moderate protection phase. By 9 to 10 weeks postoperatively, the patient can expect to return to light functional activities if full ROM and quadriceps control have been established and there is no evidence of increased posterior displacement.

Precaution: Resisted knee flexion such as hamstring curls are postponed until 9 to 10 weeks postoperatively to avoid excessive posterior shear forces on the knee. When progressing to work- or sport-related activities, the patient should avoid activities that place excessive posterior forces on the knee such as deep squatting or walking down inclines. The need for some degree of protection during exercise and transition to functional activities continues well beyond 6 months after surgery. Return to full activity usually occurs at approximately 9 to 12 months postoperatively.

▶ Meniscal Tears

Related Diagnoses and Mechanisms of Injury

The medial meniscus is more frequently injured than the lateral meniscus. Insult may occur when the foot is fixed on the ground and the femur is rotated internally, as when pivoting, getting out of a car, or receiving a clipping injury. An ACL injury often accompanies a medial meniscus tear. Lateral rotation of the femur on a fixed tibia may tear the lateral meniscus. Simple squatting or trauma may also cause a tear.

Common Impairments

Meniscal tears can cause an acute locking of the knee as well as chronic symptoms with intermittent locking. Pain occurs along the joint line from stress to the coronary ligament, along with joint swelling, and some degree of quadriceps atrophy. When there is joint locking, the knee does not fully extend, and there is a springy end-feel when passive extension is attempted. If the joint is swollen, there is usually slight limitation of flexion or extension. The McMurray or Apley grinding tests may be positive.[42]

Common Functional Limitations/Disabilities

- When the meniscus tear is acute, the patient may be unable to bear weight on the involved side.
- Unexpected locking or giving way during ambulation often occurs, causing safety problems.

Nonoperative Management

- Often the patient can actively move the leg to "unlock" the knee, or the unlocking happens spontaneously.
- Passive manipulative reduction of the medial meniscus (Fig. 13–6). Patient position and procedure: Supine. Passively flex the involved knee and hip and simultaneously internally and externally rotate the tibia. When the knee is fully flexed, laterally rotate the tibia and apply a valgus stress at the knee. Hold the tibia in this position as you extend the knee. The meniscus may click into place. Once reduced, the knee may react as an acute joint lesion. If this occurs, treat as described earlier in this chapter in the section on nonoperative joint management.
- Once acute symptoms decrease, exercises should be performed in open- and closed-chain positions to improve strength and endurance in isolated muscle groups and to prepare the patient for functional activities.

Surgical Management of Meniscal Tears

When a significant tear or rupture of the medial or lateral meniscus occurs or if nonoperative management of a partial tear has been unsuccessful, surgical intervention is often necessary. Every effort is made to retain as much of the meniscus as possible to minimize long-term degeneration of the articular surfaces of the knee. To preserve the load transmission and shock-absorbing functions of the

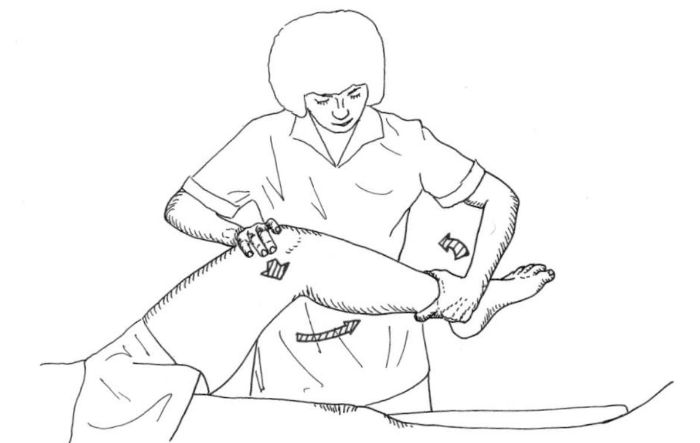

Figure 13–6 Manipulative reduction of a medial meniscus. Internally and externally rotate the tibia as you flex the hip and knee (not shown), then laterally rotate the tibia and apply a valgus stress at the knee as you extend it. The meniscus may click into place.

menisci and reduce stresses on articular surfaces of the knee, surgical *repair of a meniscus* or *partial meniscectomy* is preferable to total meniscectomy.[123,128] A central tear that involves the avascular portion of the meniscus is usually treated with partial meniscectomy,[128] but in some instances a repair using a greater number of sutures is possible.[80a] A peripheral tear that involves the vascular portion of the meniscus is often managed by repair rather than excision of the torn portion. If there is extensive damage to the peripheral and central portions of the meniscus, a total meniscectomy may have to be performed although this is avoided whenever possible.[128] Almost all meniscal tears are evaluated and treated arthroscopically, whether a repair or a partial excision is performed.[128]

Many patients with chronic meniscal lesions have a more successful outcome from surgery and can return to full activity sooner if they participate in a preoperative exercise program. The progression of postoperative rehabilitation and the time required to return to full activity will depend upon the extent and location of the tear and the type of surgical approach and procedure chosen. Rehabilitation proceeds more conservatively after repair of a meniscus or total meniscectomy than after partial meniscectomy. Damage and repair of other soft tissues of the knee also affect the course and progression of rehabilitation after surgery.

Arthroscopic Repair of the Meniscus and Postoperative Management

Indications for Surgery

Repair of a torn meniscus is indicated in the following situations.[80a,123,128] If a lesion occurs in the vascular portion (outer one-third) of the medial or lateral meniscus, surgical repair of the cartilage is indicated. Repair of a central lesion in the relatively avascular portion of the meniscus is a point of debate. Repairs are more successful with acute injuries of a meniscus than with chronic meniscal lesions.[11]

Procedure

Meniscus repair can be performed using an arthroscopic, arthroscopically assisted, or open approach. The decision is generally based on the location and type of tear.[128] Currently, most repairs are performed arthroscopically.[128]

In an arthroscopic approach small incisions are made at the knee for portals, and saline is arthroscopically introduced into the knee joint to distend the knee. The torn portion of the peripheral meniscus is sutured in place. Any loose bodies or debris are endoscopically removed. The knee is irrigated and drained, and then skin incisions at portal sites are closed. A compression dressing is applied. A meniscal repair may be accompanied by repair or reconstruction of other soft tissues of the knee such as the ligaments.

Postoperative Management

The stability of the repair dictates the progression of postoperative management. Exercise and weight bearing can be initiated sooner and progressed more rapidly after a repair of a peripheral tear than a central tear.[80a]

Immobilization, Protective Bracing, and Weight Bearing

The knee is typically immobilized in full extension in a brace immediately after surgery.[128] To protect the sutured cartilage and restrict motion to a safe portion of the range, a controlled-motion orthosis is worn at all times in the early phases of rehabilitation. Depending on the site of the lesion and repair, motion is controlled to allow 0 to no more than 90 degrees of flexion.

Partial weight bearing with crutches is permitted with the brace locked in full extension in the immediate postoperative period. The patient ambulates with crutches using a toe-touch pattern for the first 4 weeks. Weight bearing is progressed gradually. Full weight bearing is possible at 6 to 8 weeks based upon the patient's signs and symptoms.[80a]

Exercise: Maximum Protection Phase

Immediately after surgery, a standard approach (cold, compression, and elevation) to control pain and joint effusion is used. Exercises are begun immediately after surgery with a goal of full active extension by 4 weeks. Knee flexion is restricted by a hinged, controlled-motion brace. Recommendations for maximum flexion during the first 4 weeks vary from 50 to 90 degrees.[11,80a,111,123,128] Goals of management and exercises during the first 4 weeks include:

- Minimize atrophy and re-establish neuromuscular control of knee musculature with comfortable, submaximal quadriceps- and hamstring-setting exercises as soon as possible after surgery. Complement isometric exercises with electrical muscle stimulation or biofeedback. If weight-bearing restrictions allow, initiate bilateral closed-chain exercises such as mini-squats or scooting on a rolling stool.

- Maintain strength in hip musculature on the operated side, with SLR exercises in supine, prone, and side-lying positions.[58]
- Regain mobility with active-assistive and active ROM exercises within a comfortable and protected range, and cautiously progress the exercises while the patient wears the controlled-motion brace. Exercises and manual techniques may include:
  - Heel slides in supine
  - Gravity-assisted knee flexion in sitting
  - Therapist-assisted or self-assisted knee extension in sitting
  - Patellar mobilizations

Exercise: Moderate Protection Phase

A moderate degree of protection is required for an extended period of time (from 5–12 or as long as 16 weeks postoperatively) depending on the stability and location of the tear. By 8 to 9 weeks the patient can discontinue use of crutches if full active knee extension has been achieved.[80a] The patient should achieve full active ROM early in this phase of rehabilitation.

- Progress ROM exercise in flexion and extension in the controlled-motion brace.
- Maintain flexibility of lower extremity musculature with stretching exercises. Consider the use of grade III joint mobilizations to increase knee flexion and extension when joint swelling subsides.
- Increase strength and dynamic control of knee musculature in functional positions with progressive closed-chain exercises such as bilateral mini-squats against elastic resistance or on a Total Gym® unit in a reclining position (see Fig. 3-43) and unilateral terminal knee extension against elastic resistance (see Fig. 13–12).
- Gradually progress open-chain knee flexion and extension exercises to increase strength with PRE such as *submaximal* resisted knee extension in sitting and hamstring curls in standing; add submaximal, medium- to high-speed isokinetic exercises in a safe, protected range during the later weeks of this phase.
- Increase muscular endurance, general lower extremity conditioning, and cardiorespiratory fitness with stationary bicycling or swimming.
- To re-establish balance, initiate proprioceptive training using weight-bearing activities.
- Gradually resume low-demand functional activities.

Exercise: Minimum Protection and Return-to-Activity Phases

Some degree of protection is still warranted during the minimum protection phase, which typically begins around 12 to 16 weeks and may continue until 6 to 9 months.

- Progress strengthening, stabilization, and balance activities in functional positions with marching, lunges, step-up and step-down exercises, and plyometric training or slide board and balance board exercises.
- Progress strengthening with isokinetic exercises for the lower extremity with velocity spectrum rehabilitation.
- Continue to improve cardiorespiratory endurance and conditioning with aerobic activities such as bicycling, swimming, and walking.
- When meniscal integrity tests are normal, restore functional abilities with simulated activities that mimic functional skills. Add light jogging activities, sprinting, or jumping, if appropriate.

Precaution: Full squatting or lunges should be avoided for at least 6 months. Twisting, turning, and pivoting activities should be progressed cautiously between 4 and 9 months postoperatively to prevent excessive shear forces on the repaired meniscus. Return to full activity varies substantially among patients; in general, a minimum of 6 months of rehabilitation is required for a peripheral repair and as long as 9 months for a central repair.[80a]

Arthroscopic Partial Meniscectomy and Postoperative Management

Indications for Surgery

The following are indications for partial meniscectomy.[18,123,128]

- Any tear of the meniscus that is symptomatic and not considered repairable
- Tears or ruptures of the inner two-thirds (the avascular portion) of the medial or lateral menisci of the knee

- Displacement of the meniscus associated with locking of the knee

Procedure

Small incisions are made at the knee for portals (usually 3), and the knee is injected and distended with saline solution through one of the portals. The torn portion of the meniscus is identified, grasped, and divided endoscopically by knife or by scissors and removed by vacuum. Intra-articular debris or loose bodies are also removed. A soft compression dressing is applied after the knee is irrigated and drained, and skin incisions at portal sites are closed. If the meniscus tear occurs in conjunction with tears or ruptures of other soft tissues of the knee, such as the cruciate or collateral ligaments, surgical management for repair of these structures must also be considered.

Postoperative Management

Immobilization and Weight Bearing

A compression dressing is placed on the knee, but it is not necessary to immobilize the knee postoperatively with a splint or motion-controlling orthosis. For the first few postoperative days, cryotherapy, compression, and elevation of the operated leg are used to control edema and pain. Weight bearing is progressed as tolerated.

Exercise: Maximum and Moderate Protection Phase

Note: Although the ideal situation is to begin exercise instruction on the day of or after surgery, most patients undergo a partial meniscectomy on an outpatient basis, and many do not see a therapist for supervised exercise. If a patient is referred for supervised therapy, the emphasis is usually placed on establishing a home exercise program. Under these circumstances it is preferable to teach the patient initial exercises to reduce atrophy and prevent contracture *preoperatively* so that he or she may initiate the exercises at home immediately after surgery.

There is no need for an extended maximum protection phase postoperatively as there is little soft tissue trauma during surgery. Moderate protection are needed for approximately 3 to 4 weeks. All exercises and weight-bearing activities should be pain-free and progressed gradually during the first few postoperative weeks.[11,111]

- Immediately after surgery begin muscle-setting exercises, straight-leg raises, active knee ROM, and weight bearing as tolerated. Full weight bearing is usually achieved by 4 to 7 days, and 90 degrees of knee flexion and full extension are achieved by 10 days.
- Initiate closed-chain exercises and stationary bicycling a few days after surgery to regain dynamic control and endurance of the knee.

Precautions: Patients who have undergone a partial meniscectomy must be cautioned not to push themselves too quickly. Too rapid progression of exercise will cause recurrent joint effusion and possible damage to articular cartilage of the knee.

Exercise: Minimum Protection and Return-to-Activity Phases

By the 3rd to 4th postoperative week, minimum protection of the knee is necessary, but full active knee ROM should be achieved before progressing to high-demand exercises. Resistance training, endurance activities, functional closed-chain exercises in full weight bearing, and balance training can all be progressed rapidly. Advanced activities such as plyometrics, maximum effort isokinetic training, and simulated high-demand functional activities can be initiated as early as 4 to 6 or 6 to 8 weeks postoperatively.

Precaution: High-impact weight-bearing activities such as jogging or jumping, if included in the program, should be added and progressed cautiously to prevent future or additional articular damage to the knee.

▶ Exercise Techniques to Increase Flexibility and Range of Motion

Strength and flexibility imbalances between muscle groups can occur from a variety of causes, some of which are disuse, faulty joint mechanics, joint swelling, immobilization (from fracture, surgery, or trauma), and nerve injury. Besides the hamstrings and rectus femoris, most of the two-joint muscles crossing the knee primarily function either at the hip or at the ankle, yet they also have an effect on knee function. If there is an imbalance in length or strength in the hip or ankle muscles, there are usually altered mechanics throughout the lower extremity. See also the chapters on the hip and the ankle and foot for a complete picture. When attempting to increase ROM, the mechanics of the tibiofemoral and patellofemoral joints and their importance in lower extremity function must be respected. Because the knee is a weight-bearing joint, the need for stability takes precedence over the need for mobility, although mobility coupled with adequate strength is also necessary for normal function.

Principles of inhibition and passive stretching were presented in Chapter 5, joint mobilization in Chapter 6, and techniques directed toward specific joint restrictions at the knee and patella earlier in this chapter. Additional manual and mechanical stretching and self-stretching techniques to increase knee ROM are described in this section.

To Increase Knee Extension

Decreased flexibility in the hamstring musculature as well as periarticular tissue posterior to the knee can restrict full knee extension. Increasing knee extension is a two-step process; first full extension of the knee is obtained without placing tension on the hamstrings at the hip (hip at or near extension). Once full extension is attained, stretch is then placed on the two-joint hamstring muscle group by progressively increasing hip flexion range (straight leg raising—SLR). Techniques to stretch the hamstrings using SLR are described in the stretching section of Chapter 12.

Neuromuscular Inhibition Techniques

- Patient position and procedure: Supine, with the hip and knee extended as much as possible. Resist knee flexion with an isometric hold using your hand proximal to the ankle; have the patient relax and then passively (or have the patient actively) extend the knee into the end of the range (hold-relax and hold-relax/agonist-contraction techniques respectively).
- Patient position and procedure: Prone with the hip and knee extended as much as possible. Place a small pad or folded hand towel under the femur proximal to the patella to protect the patella from compressive forces. Stabilize the pelvis to prevent hip flexion, and then apply the hold-relax technique to increase knee extension.

Passive Stretching Techniques

Use a low-intensity, long-duration stretch to ensure that the patient stays as relaxed as possible.

- Patient position and procedure: Prone, hips extended with the patient's foot off the edge of the treatment table. Place a rolled towel under the patient's femur just proximal to the patella and a cuff weight around the ankle. As the muscle relaxes, the weight will place a sustained passive stretch on the hamstrings, which will increase knee extension.
- Patient position and procedure: Supine with the knee extended as far as possible. Place a rolled towel or padding under the distal leg to elevate it off the table. Secure a cuff weight across the distal femur for a sustained stretch.

Note: This position is not effective for severe knee flexion contractures; use for restrictions that are near the end of the range of knee extension.

Self-Stretching Technique

Patient position and procedure: Long sitting with the distal leg supported on a rolled towel. Have the patient press down with the hands against the femur just above (not on) the patella to cause a sustained force to increase knee extension.

To Increase Knee Flexion

Before stretching to increase knee flexion, be sure the patella is mobile and is able to glide distally in the trochlear groove as the knee flexes; otherwise, it will restrict knee flexion. Patellar mobilization techniques to increase patellar gliding are described in Chapter 6 (see Figs. 6–54 and 6–55). Once full range of knee flexion is reached, the two-joint rectus femoris and tensor fasciae latae muscles should be stretched across the hip joint. These techniques are described in Chapter 12.

Neuromuscular Inhibition Techniques

Patient position and procedure: Sitting, with the knee at the edge of the treatment table and flexed as far as possible. Resist knee extension with an isometric hold with your hand proximal to the ankle. Have the patient relax, and then passively (or have the patient actively) flex the knee to the end of the range.

Passive Stretching Technique

Patient position and procedure: Sitting, with knee flexed to the end of its available range. Instruct the patient to relax the muscles, and let the weight of the leg cause a low-intensity, long-duration stretch. Apply a manual stretch force or strap a light weight around the distal leg to increase the stretch force.

Self-Stretching Techniques

- ***Gravity-assisted supine wall slides (Fig. 13–7).*** Patient position and procedure: Supine, with buttocks close to the wall and lower extremities vertically resting against the wall (hips flexed, knees extended). Slowly flex the involved knee by sliding the foot down the wall until a gentle stretch sensation is felt; hold in a comfortable position, then slide the foot back up the wall.
- ***Rocking forward on a step (Fig. 13–8).*** Patient position and procedure: Standing, with the foot of the involved knee on a step. The patient rocks forward over the stabilized foot, flexing the knee to the limit of its range. He or she can rock back and forth in a slow, rhythmic manner or hold the stretched position. Begin with a low step or stool; increase the height as more range is obtained.
- ***Sitting (Fig. 13–9).*** Patient position and procedure: Sitting in a chair with the involved knee flexed to the end of its available range and the foot firmly planted on the floor. Have the patient move forward in the chair, not allowing the foot to slide. Have the patient hold the position for a comfortable, sustained stretch to the knee extensors.

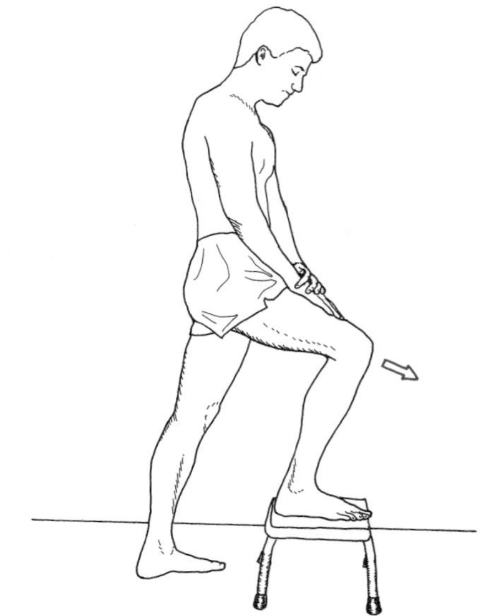

Figure 13–8 Self-stretching rock on step. The patient places the foot of the involved side on a step, then rocks forward over the stabilized foot to the limit of knee flexion to stretch the quadriceps femoris muscle. Use a higher step for greater flexion.

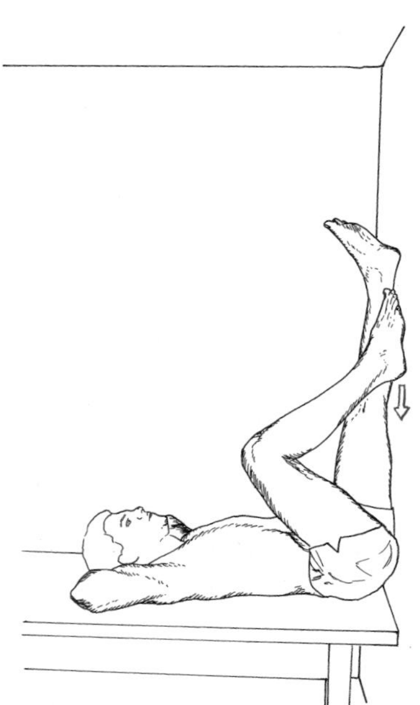

Figure 13–7 Gravity-assisted supine wall slide. The patient flexes the knee to the limit of its range and holds it there for a sustained stretch to the quadriceps femoris muscle.

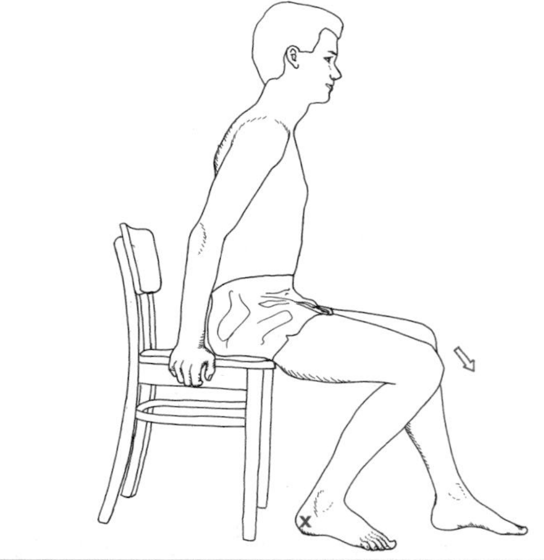

Figure 13–9 Self-stretching in a chair. The patient fixates the foot of the involved leg on the floor, then moves forward in the chair over the stabilized foot to place a sustained stretch on the quadriceps femoris muscle and increase knee flexion.

Exercises to Develop and Improve Muscle Performance and Functional Control

When strengthening exercises for knee musculature are selected, implemented, and progressed in a rehabilitation program, stability of the knee, which involves co-contraction of the quadriceps and hamstrings muscles, and safe patellofemoral and extensor mechanism biomechanics, which allow appropriate patellar tracking, are primary concerns. Once stability and patellar mechanics are well established, coordination and timing of muscle contractions as well as endurance are emphasized. *Closed-chain exercises* with an emphasis on low-intensity (low-resistance) high-repetition activities are more effective than open-chain exercises for improving stability and muscular endurance of the knee for dynamic control during weight-bearing activities.

Although closed-chain control of the knee is essential, remember that the knee functions in both an open- and a closed-chain during most activities of daily living. The quadriceps and hamstrings must contract simultaneously (co-contraction), as well as contract concentrically and eccentrically during functional activities. Therefore, exercises under all of these varying conditions should be incorporated into a comprehensive knee rehabilitation program. It is also important to change the position of the hip during quadriceps- and hamstring-strengthening exercises to affect the length-tension relationship of the rectus femoris and hamstrings.[35] Only after a thorough examination and understanding of a patient's pathology, impairments and functional limitations can a therapist select and design an exercise plan to meet an individual patient's needs.

Considerable research has been done comparing joint reaction forces and muscle function during open- and closed-chain exercises. Comparisons are difficult because of differing research designs and exercise variables.[32] Table 13–6 summarizes results from a recent study comparing two dynamic exercises with recommendations for exercise modification with specific knee impairments. Special adaptations have also been highlighted in the conservative management and surgical management sections of this chapter.

In the exercises that follow, open-chain exercises are described before closed-chain exercises simply because weight bearing after knee injury or surgery is often restricted for a time. Isolated activation of knee musculature is also necessary for ADL that involve open-chain movements such as lifting the leg to get in and out of bed or in and out of a car or flexing and extending the knee for dressing.

Table 13–6 Comparison of Forces and Muscle Action at the Knee During Dynamic Open- and Closed-Chain Exercises[32]

	Open-Chain Exercise Variable resistance: sitting, knee extension machine	Closed-Chain Exercise Variable resistance: squatting, leg-press machine (body moves away from fixed feet)
Rectus femoris development	More effective	Less effective
VMO development	Less effective	More effective for VMO (and VL)
Other muscle development	None	Effective for hamstrings
ACL tensile forces*	ACL under tension <25 degrees	
PCL tensile forces*	PCL under tension between 25–95 degrees (peak at 1.0 × body weight)	PCL under tension throughout range (1.5–2.0 x body weight)
Patellofemoral compression	Peak stress at 60 degrees, peak compression at 75 degrees‡	Compression increases with knee flexion, peaking at 90 degrees†
Tibiofemoral compression	Higher compression (more stability) <30 degrees	Higher compression (more stability) >70 degrees

Recommendations[32,136]

*The 0–25 degree range should be excluded in open-chain exercises following ACL injury, but may be included after PCL injury.

†Squat exercises: exercise only from 0–50 degrees with patellofemoral dysfunctions.

‡Open-chain exercise from 0–30 degrees and 75–90 degrees with patellofemoral dysfunctions. (Note: there is controversy in the literature regarding compressive forces in the patellofemoral joint from 0–30 degrees).

Closed-chain exercises in partial and later in full weight bearing should be initiated as soon as healing allows with progression to balance and proprioceptive training and functional weight-bearing activities.

Nonweight-Bearing Exercises

To Develop Control of Knee Extension and Progress Strength (Quadriceps Femoris)

A wide variety of static and dynamic exercises can be used to improve the function of the quadriceps femoris muscles in an open-chain. Because of variations in muscle fiber orientation and attachments of the knee extensor muscles, individual components of the quadriceps femoris muscle group place different biomechanical stresses on the patella. Emphasis is often placed on isolation and activation of the vastus medialis obliquis (VMO) and vastus medialis (VM) muscles because of their ability to stabilize the patella and to maintain appropriate patellar tracking. Tactile cues, biofeedback, and electrical muscle stimulation over the VMO can reinforce awareness of the muscle contracting for patellar control. In this section, the effectiveness of various quadriceps exercises with regard to training and strengthening the VMO are discussed.

Quadriceps Setting (Quad Sets)

Note: Of the many variations of static and dynamic exercises that have been proposed to selectively train the VMO, quadriceps setting coupled with electrical stimulation or biofeedback has been shown to be most effective.[119]

- Patient position and procedure: Supine, sitting in a chair (with the heel on the floor), or long-sitting with the knee extended (or flexed a few degrees) but not hyperextended. Have the patient contract the quadriceps isometrically, causing the patella to glide proximally; then hold for a count of 10.
- Use verbal cues such as "Try to push your knee back and tighten your thigh muscle" or "Try to tighten your thigh muscle and pull your kneecap up." When the patient sets the muscle properly, offer verbal reinforcement immediately, and then have the patient repeat the activity.
- Have the patient dorsiflex the ankle and then hold an isometric contraction of the quadriceps.[3]

Straight-Leg Raising (SLR)

Note: Straight-leg raising in supine combines dynamic hip flexion with an isometric contraction of the quadriceps. The effective resistance of gravity (or any additional weight added at the ankle) decreases as the lower extremity elevates because of the decreasing moment arm of the resistance force. The rectus femoris is the primary muscle in the quadriceps group that is active during SLR exercise.[119]

- Patient position and procedure: Supine, with the knee extended. To stabilize the pelvis and low back, the opposite hip and knee are flexed and the foot is placed flat on the exercise table.
- Instruct the patient to first set the quadriceps muscle; then lift the leg to about 45 degrees of hip flexion while keeping the knee extended; hold the leg in that position for a count of 10; then lower it.
- As the patient progresses, have the patient lift to only 30 degrees of hip flexion and hold the position. Later, have the patient flex the hip to only 15 degrees. The most significant resistance to the quadriceps is during the first few degrees of SLR.
- To increase resistance, place a cuff weight around the patient's ankle.
- It has been proposed that if SLR in the supine position is coupled with lateral rotation or isometric adduction of the hip, the VMO or VM muscles can be preferentially activated and strengthened.[3,8,16,25,78] The rationale for advocating these exercises is that many fibers of the VMO muscle originate from the adductor magnus tendon.[3,62] Although a number of authors[3,8] have advocated these adaptations to SLR to increase the medially directed forces on the patella, there is lack of research evidence to substantiate the effect. In two quantitative studies comparing quadriceps muscle activity during quad sets and variations of SLR, quad sets were found to be associated with significantly greater VMO or VM activity than several variations of SLR.[62,119]

Straight-Leg Lowering

- Patient position and procedure: Supine. If the patient cannot perform SLR because of a quadriceps lag or weakness, begin by passively placing the leg in 90 degrees of SLR (or as far as the flexibility of the hamstrings allows), and have the patient gradually lower the extremity while keeping the knee fully extended.
- Be prepared to control the descent of the leg with your hand under the heel as the torque created by gravity increases.
- If the knee begins to flex as the extremity is low-

ered, have the patient stop at that point, then raise the extremity upward to 90 degrees.

- Have the patient repeat the motion and attempt to lower the extremity a little further each time while keeping the knee extended.
- Once the patient can keep the knee extended while lowering the leg through the full ROM, SLR exercises can be initiated.

Multiple-Angle Isometric Exercises

- Patient position and procedure: Supine or long-sitting. Have the patient perform bent leg raises with the knee in multiple angles of flexion.
- Patient position and procedure: Seated at the edge of a treatment table. When tolerated, resistance is applied at the ankle either manually or mechanically, to isometrically strengthen the quadriceps in varying degrees of knee flexion. An effective co-contraction with the hamstrings can be activated (except in the last 10–15 degrees of knee extension) by having the patient push the thigh downward into the table while holding the knee in extension against maximum resistance.[47]

Short-Arc Terminal Extension

Note: Although in the past it was thought that the VMO was responsible for the terminal phase of knee extension, it is now well documented that all components of the quadriceps femoris muscle group are active throughout active knee extension and that the VMO primarily affects patellar alignment.[119]

- Patient position and procedure: Supine or long-sitting. Place a rolled towel or bolster under the knee to support it in flexion (Fig. 13–10). The patient can also assume a short-sitting position at the edge of a table with the seat of a chair or a stool placed under the heel to stop knee flexion at the desired angle.

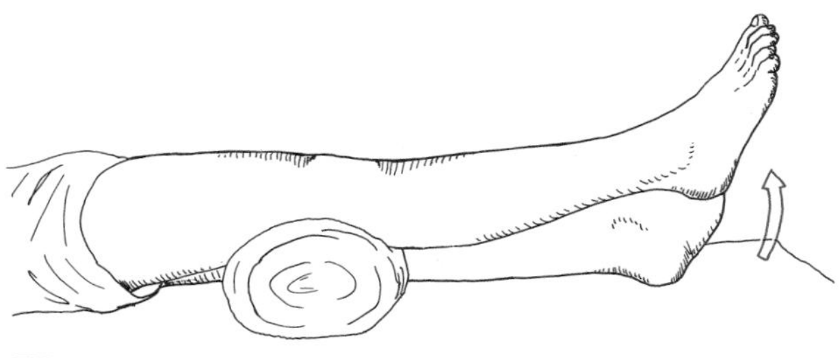

Figure 13–10 Short-arc terminal extension exercise to strengthen the quadriceps femoris muscle. When tolerated, resistance is added proximal to the ankle.

- Begin with the knee in a few degrees of flexion. Progress the degrees of flexion as tolerated by the patient or dictated by the condition.
- Initially have the patient extend the knee only against the resistance of gravity. Later, add cuff weights around the ankle to increase the resistance if the patient does not experience pain or crepitation.

Precaution: When adding resistance to the distal leg, the amount of torque generated by the quadriceps muscle increases significantly in the terminal ranges of knee extension. In this portion of the range the quadriceps has a poor mechanical advantage and poor physiologic length while having to contract against an external resistance force that has a long lever arm. The amount of muscle force generated causes an anterior gliding force on the tibia, which is restrained by the ACL. This exercise is not appropriate for a person with an unstable knee after an ACL injury or during postoperative rehabilitation before the ligament has healed.

- Combine short-arc terminal extension with an isometric hold and/or SLR when the knee is in full extension.
- To prevent lateral shear forces at the knee, have the patient invert the foot as he or she extends the knee.[3,46]

Full-Arc Extension

- Patient position: Sitting or supine.
- Resistance can be applied through the arc of 90 degrees of flexion to full extension.

Note: Resistance from 90 to 60 degrees causes less anterior tibial translation than closed-chain squatting in this range. But resistance applied in open-chain extension from 30 to 0 degrees increases anterior translation more than does performing mini-squats in the same range.[136]

- Apply resistance only in the ranges tolerated by the patient during the controlled-motion, moderate protection phases of treatment. Apply resistance through the full arc of motion only in the later stages of rehabilitation if the knee is pain-free, stable, and asymptomatic. If there is pain, resistance should be applied only through those parts of the range with no symptoms.
- Various forms of mechanical resistance equipment discussed in Chapter 3 can be used to

strengthen the knee extensors in an open-chain. Emphasize high-repetition, low-resistance training with weight-training equipment and medium- to high-speed training with isokinetic equipment to minimize compressive and shear forces to knee joint structures during exercise. The tibial pad against which the patient pushes when extending the knee against resistance can also be placed more proximally than distally on the lower leg to minimize excessive stresses to supporting structures of the knee.

If a cuff weight is applied to the tibia to provide resistance, it will also cause a distraction to the joint and stress on the ligaments when the patient sits or lies supine with the knee flexed to 90 degrees and the tibia over the edge of the treatment table. To avoid this stress to ligaments, place a stool under the foot so it can be supported when the leg is in the dependent position.[18]

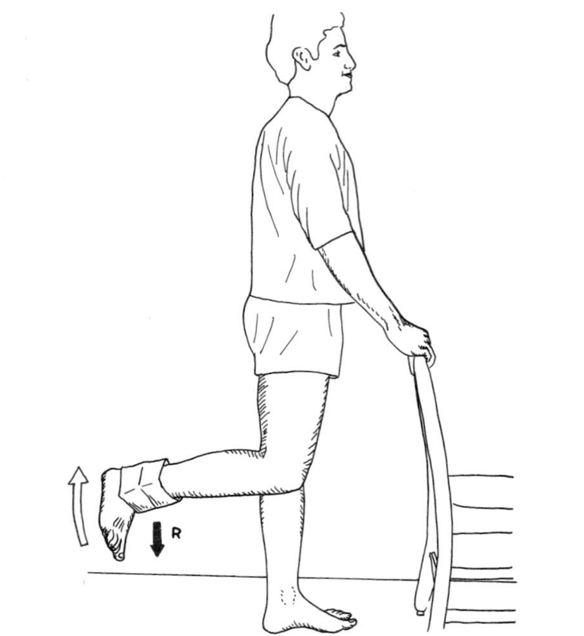

Figure 13–11 Hamstring curls; resistance exercises to the knee flexors with the patient standing. Maximal resistance occurs when the knee is at 90 degrees.

To Strengthen Knee Flexion (Hamstrings)

Hamstring-Setting Exercises (Hamstring Sets)

- Patient position and procedure: Supine or long-sitting, with the knee in extension or slight flexion over a towel roll. Have the patient isometrically contract the knee flexors just enough to feel tension developing in the muscle group by gently pushing the heel into the treatment table and holding the contraction. Have the patient relax and then repeat the setting exercise.

Multiple-Angle Isometric Exercises

- Patient position and procedure: Supine or long-sitting. Apply either manual or mechanical resistance to a static hamstring muscle contraction with the knee flexed to several positions in the ROM.
- Place the tibia in internal or external rotation prior to resisting knee flexion to emphasize the medial or lateral hamstring muscles, respectively.
- Teach the patient to give self-resistance at multiple points in the ROM by placing the opposite foot behind the ankle of the leg to be resisted.

Hamstring Curls (Open-Chain Knee Flexion)

- Patient position and procedure: Standing, holding onto a solid object for balance. Have the patient pick up the foot and flex the knee (Fig. 13–11). Maximum resistance from gravity occurs when the knee is at 90 degrees flexion. Add resistance with ankle weights or a weighted boot. If the patient flexes the hip, stabilize it by having the patient place the anterior thigh against a wall or solid object.
- Patient position and procedure: Prone. Place a small towel roll or foam rubber under the femur just proximal to the patella to avoid compression of the patella between the treatment table and femur. With a cuff weight around the ankle, have the patient flex the knee to only 90 degrees; maximum resistance from gravity occurs when the knee first starts to flex at 0 degrees. If hamstring curls are performed in prone using manual resistance, a weight-pulley system or isokinetic equipment resistance to the knee flexors can be applied throughout the range of knee flexion.

Precaution: Open-chain hamstring curls performed against resistance placed on the distal tibia causes posterior tibial translation. A patient with a PCL injury or reconstruction should avoid this exercise in the early stages of rehabilitation.

Weight-Bearing Exercises

Progressive closed-chain exercises are beneficial for activating and training the musculature of the lower extremity to respond to specific functional demands. As the quadriceps contract eccentrically to control knee flexion or contract concentrically to extend the knee, the hamstrings and soleus function to stabilize the tibia against the forward translating force of the quadriceps at the knee joint. This synergy along with the compressive loading on the joints provides support to the cruciate ligaments.[32,97] In addition, because the hip extends and the ankle plantarflexes as the knee extends (and vice versa) during closed-chain activities, the two-joint hamstrings and gastrocnemius and the one-joint soleus are maintaining favorable length-tension relationships through action at the hip and ankle, respectively.

In a rehabilitation program, closed-chain exercises can be incorporated in an exercise regimen as soon as partial or full weight bearing is safe. Closed-chain strengthening exercises generate fewer shear forces on knee ligaments, particularly anterior tibial translation, than open-chain quadriceps-strengthening activities.[28] Therefore, resistance can be added to closed-chain activities more quickly after injury or surgery than to open-chain exercises while still protecting healing structures such as the ACL. Clinically, closed-chain exercises enable a patient to develop strength, endurance, and stability of the lower extremity in functional patterns sooner after knee injury or surgery than do open-chain exercises. The progression of closed-chain exercises described in Chapter 12 (The Hip) are also appropriately used in knee rehabilitation programs.

If the patient does not tolerate or is not permitted to be full weight bearing, begin exercises in the parallel bars or in a pool to partially unload the body weight. During the healing phase after surgical procedures or with anterior knee pain problems, the knee should be splinted, taped, or braced while exercising. Begin exercises at a level tolerated by the patient and at which there is complete control and no exacerbation of symptoms.

Closed-Chain Isometric Exercises

Setting Exercises

These are done to facilitate co-contraction of the quadriceps and hamstrings.

- Patient position and procedure: Sitting on a chair with the knee extended or slightly flexed and the heel on the floor.
- Have the patient press the heel against the floor and the thigh against the seat of the chair and concentrate on contracting the quadriceps and hamstrings simultaneously to facilitate co-contraction around the knee joint. Hold the muscle contraction, relax, and repeat.
- Co-contraction can be learned more easily or enhanced with biofeedback.

Stabilization Exercises

- Patient position and procedure: Standing, with weight equally distributed. Apply manual resistance to the pelvis in alternating directions as the patient holds the position. This will facilitate isometric contractions of muscles in the ankles, knees, and hips. Increase the speed of application of the resistive forces to train the muscles to respond to sudden shifts in forces.
- Progress the stabilization activity by applying the alternating resistance against the shoulders to develop trunk stabilization and then by having the patient bear weight only on the involved lower extremity while resistance is applied.

Closed-Chain Isometrics Against Elastic Resistance

- Patient position and procedure: Standing on the involved extremity with elastic resistance looped around the thigh of the opposite extremity and secured to a stable object (see Figs. 12–14*A* and *B*).
- Have the patient flex and extend the hip of the nonweight-bearing lower extremity to facilitate co-contraction of muscles and stability of the weight-bearing leg.
- This closed-chain exercise also facilitates proprioceptive input and balance on the weight bearing (involved) lower extremity.

Closed-Chain Dynamic Exercises

Patient position is standing in all of the following exercises.

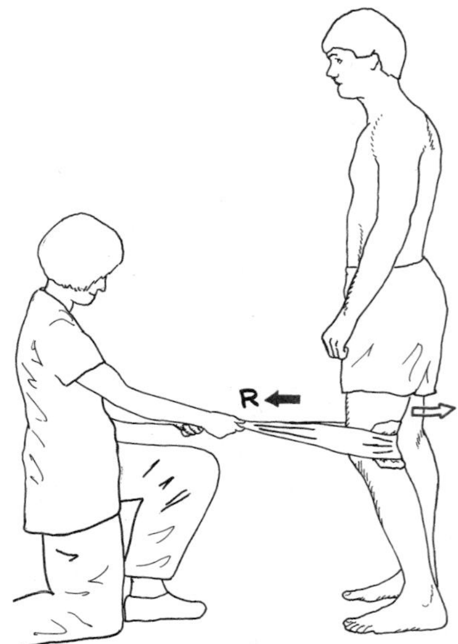

Figure 13–12 Unilateral closed-chain extension.

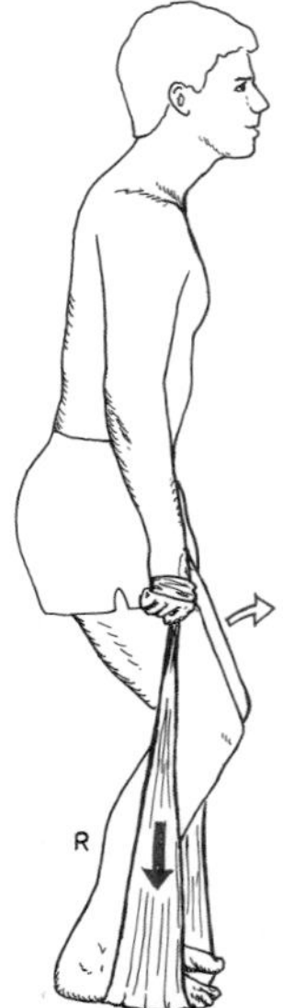

Figure 13–13 Resisted mini-squats; closed-chain short-arc training. Elastic resistance to knee extension is provided for short-arc motion. It is important to use the quadriceps femoris muscles rather than substitute with the hamstring muscles for proper strengthening.

Unilateral Closed-Chain Terminal Knee Extension

Loop elastic resistance around the distal thigh and secure it to a stationary structure (Fig. 13–12). Have the patient actively perform terminal knee extension while bearing partial to full weight on the involved extremity.

Partial Squats, Mini-Squats, and Short-Arc Training

- Begin by having the patient flex both knees up to 30 to 45 degrees, then extend them. Progress by using elastic resistance placed under both feet (Fig. 13–13) or by holding weights in the hands. The patient should maintain the trunk upright and concentrate on the sensation of the quadriceps muscle contracting, not pulling back on the femur with the hip extensors.
- Progress squats to greater ranges of knee flexion in the return-to function phase of treatment if necessary.

Note: Squatting can be accomplished in one of two ways, each with positive and negative effects. Having the knees move anterior to the toes, as the hips descend, increases the shear forces on the tibia and strains the ACL. This can be dangerous if the patient squats while carrying considerable weight or after ACL surgery. Yet this is a more normal method for squatting and maintaining balance over the base of support. Squatting, as if sitting on a chair, in which the tibia remains relatively vertical requires greater trunk flexion to maintain balance and stronger quadriceps contraction to support the load of the pelvis posterior to the knee axis at an angle where patellar compressive loads are great. Yet this method reduces stress on the ACL. Positioning should be based on the patient's symptoms and pathological condition.

- Increase the difficulty of the exercise by performing unilateral resisted mini-squats.

Note: It has been suggested but not documented in research that, if partial squats are performed with the legs slightly externally rotated, the VMO muscle is in an optimal line of pull and may be more readily activated.[8]

Forward, Backward, and Lateral Step-Ups and Step-Downs

- Begin with a low step, 2 to 3 inches in height, and increase the height as the patient is able. Make sure the patient keeps the trunk upright.
- Emphasize control of body weight during concentric (step-up) and eccentric (step-down) quadriceps activity. To emphasize the quadriceps and minimize pushing off with the plantarflexors of the trailing extremity, instruct the patient that the heel is to be the last to leave the floor and first to return or to "keep the toes up."
- Add resistance with a weight belt, with handheld weights or ankle weights around the nonweight-

bearing leg if there is good ligamentous integrity, or place elastic resistance or a belt attached to a pulley system around the patient's hips, and have the patient step up against the resistance force (Fig. 13–14).

Standing Wall Slides

- Patient position and procedure: Standing with back against the wall (see Fig. 12–16*A*); flex the hips and knees and slide the back down and then up the wall, lowering and lifting the body weight.
- As control improves, have the patient move into greater knee flexion, up to a maximum of 60 degrees. Knee flexion beyond 60 degrees is not advocated to avoid excessive shear forces on ligamentous structures of the knee and compressive forces on the patellofemoral joint.
- Isometric training can be added by having the patient stay in the lowered (partial squat) position. If the patient is able, he or she maintains the partial squat and alternately extends one leg and then the other.
- Wall slides performed with a gym ball behind the back decrease stability and require more control (see Fig. 12–16*B*).
- Unpublished data suggest that doing wall slides with a small ball between the knees activates a stronger contraction in the VMO.[74]

Partial and Full Lunges

- Have the patient assume a step-forward stance position and rock his or her body weight forward, allowing the knee to flex slightly, and then rock backward and control knee extension.
- Progress the activity with full lunges (see Fig. 12–15). The patient begins with the feet together, then lunges forward with the involved extremity, beginning with a small stride and small amount of knee flexion, and returns upright by extending the knee and then bringing the foot back beside the other foot. Instruct the patient to keep the flexing knee in alignment with the toes and not to flex beyond a vertical line coming up from the toes. As the patient gains control, the stride length is increased and knee flexion is increased accordingly. Weights can be added to the trunk or in the patient's hands for progressive strengthening. The speed of the activity is also increased as control improves.

Chair Scooting

Patient position and procedure: Sitting on a rolling stool or chair. Have the patient "walk" forward to use the hamstrings or "walk" backwards to utilize the quadriceps. Increase the challenge of the exercise by having the patient steer around an obstacle course, roll the stool across carpeting, or pull against a resistance (such as pulling another person who is also on a rolling stool) (Fig. 13–15).

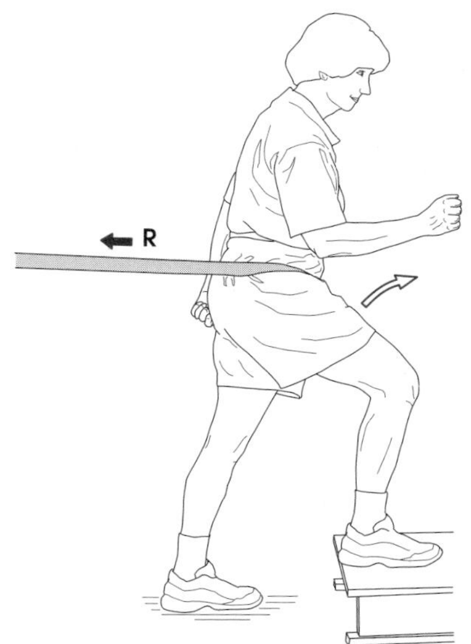

Figure 13–14 Resisted step-ups against elastic resistance or a pulley to strengthen knee extension

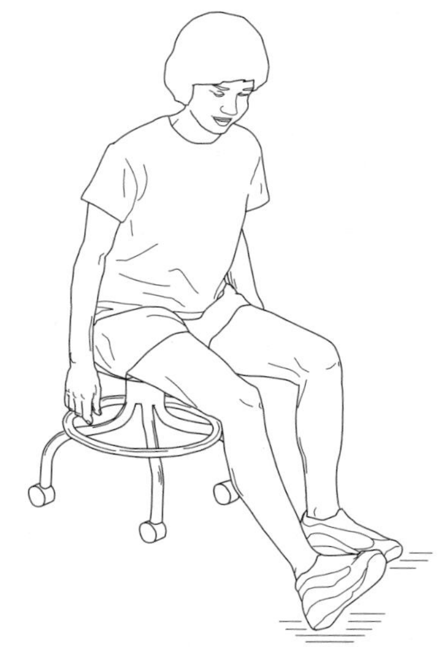

Figure 13–15 Chair scoots to strengthen knee flexion and extension.

Techniques to Simulate Functional Activities, Develop Endurance, Balance, and Progress to Specificity of Training

Activities previously described are progressed for endurance by increasing the number of repetitions or time element at each resistance level. Once control has developed, emphasis is placed on balance, coordination, timing, and skill acquisition specific to the desired activity of the patient. Also refer to the exercises described in the hip chapter for balance stability and training.

Strength and Muscle Endurance Training

Mechanical equipment such as a leg press, Total Gym® unit, isokinetic dynamometer, treadmill, stationary bicycle, and stair-stepping units is useful for strengthening and endurance training and provides motivational feedback to the patient. When implementing isokinetic training for the quadriceps and hamstrings, use velocity-spectrum rehabilitation at medium to fast velocities.[107] Place the tibia pad in a relatively proximal position on the knee to decrease anterior shear forces[137] and program in range-limiting parameters whenever necessary.

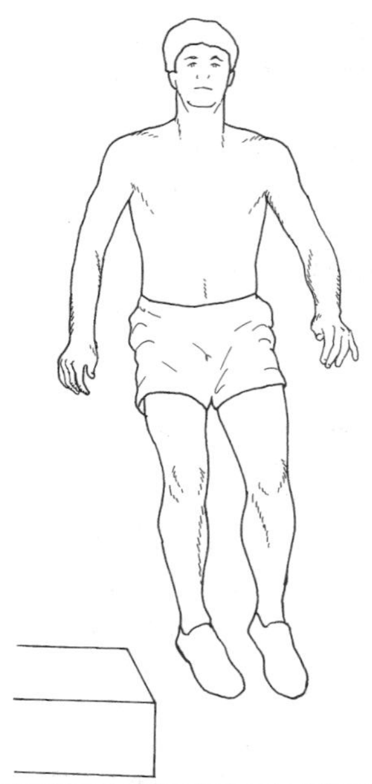

Figure 13–16 Plyometric training using lateral jumps from a step. When the patient lands on the ground, the hips and knees flex, then quickly extend to jump back up on the step. This applies a quick lengthening prior to shortening of the quadriceps muscle.

Conditioning Activities

Activities such as swimming, progressive walking, running, cross-country ski machine training, and biking are designed for general cardiovascular/pulmonary conditioning and are graded to the patient's tolerance.

Balance Activities (Perturbation Training)

Begin as early as weight bearing is allowed with balance activities. Suggestions include:

- Partial weight bearing in parallel bars and shifting weight; progress to full weight bearing.
- Stabilization exercises against alternating resistive forces.
- Stepping and marching in place.
- Balancing with arm movements in sagittal, frontal, and transverse planes, then progressing to diagonal planes.
- Walking; progress to walking in different directions, walking against resistance, and walking on uneven surfaces.
- Bilateral then unilateral stance on a balance (rocker) board, roller board or BAPS board. Increase the challenge by adding destabilizing forces while the patient is balancing such as tossing a weighted ball to the patient or pulling against elastic resistance that the patient is holding.

Plyometric Training

High-speed, stretch-shortening exercises, which are designed to improve power, are appropriate for selected patients intending to return to high-demand functional or recreational activities. Jumping on and off surfaces of varying heights (Fig. 13–16) and incorporating directional changes in the movements are appropriate in the later stages of knee rehabilitation.

Drills

Have the patient begin by stepping over and around objects that are placed on the ground as obstacles. As able, have the patient increase speed moving around the obstacles, or jump or hop over the obstacles. Initiate running, sprinting, jumping, agility drills, and sport-specific simulation drills, and carefully monitor for appropriate progression and correct mechanics.

Work-Related Activities

For a patient returning to a repetitive lifting job, strength in the hip extensors as well as knee extensors is necessary for safe body mechanics. A progression in lifting tasks with squats and lunges should also include use of proper body mechanics. This is described in greater detail in Chapter 16.

Independent Learning Activities

CRITICAL THINKING AND DISCUSSION

1. Observe a functional activity, such as putting on a pair of socks, rising from a chair, or climbing on to a city bus.
   - What ROM is needed in the knee joint? Also include hip and ankle in the analysis.
   - If motion is restricted, what muscles would have decreased mobility; what joint glides would have decreased mobility?
   - What muscles are functioning and what level of strength is needed?
   - Assume there is loss of 50% range and strength, and design an exercise program to progress functional recovery.
2. Describe the function of all the two-joint muscles that cross the knee; include the function of each muscle at its "other joint" and how each muscle can function most efficiently at the knee in terms of its length-tension relationship.
3. Describe the role of the knee musculature during the gait cycle.
   - What ROM is needed, and when during the gait cycle does the maximum degree of flexion and extension occur?
   - During the gait cycle when is each of the muscles active at the knee, and what is their function?
   - What gait deviations occur when there is muscle shortening, muscle weakness, and joint pain? Explain why each deviation occurs.
4. Two patients, both in their 70s, who underwent a TKA procedure 10 days ago because of joint degeneration from OA of the (R) knee have been referred to you in your home health practice. One patient had a cemented TKA and the other had a "hybrid" TKA. How will postoperative management differ or be similar for these two patients?
5. Differentiate among structures that are involved with a lateral retinacular release, a proximal realignment of the extensor mechanism, and a distal realignment procedure. How will these differences have an impact on postoperative rehabilitation?

LABORATORY PRACTICE

1. Design, set up, and then perform a circuit training course for hamstring and quadriceps activation and strengthening and balance exercises. Sequence the activities from basic to advanced. Observe accuracy and safety with each exercise, and note stresses involved.
2. Using mechanical resistance (pulleys, elastic resistance, and free weights), set up exercises to meet each of the following situations.
   - Strengthen the quadriceps with the greatest mechanical torque occurring when the knee is at 90 degrees, at 45 degrees, at 25 degrees.
   - Strengthen the hamstrings with the greatest mechanical torque occurring when the knee is at 90 degrees, at 45 degrees, and at 0 degrees.
3. Review all the joint mobilization techniques for the knee; include basic glides, accessory motions, patellar mobilizations, and mobilization with movement techniques.
   - Identify and practice techniques that increase knee extension, beginning with the knee at 45 degrees and progressing by 15-degree increments until full extension is reached.
   - Do the same for knee flexion, beginning at 25 degrees and progressing at 15-degree increments until full range is achieved. What accessory motions are necessary?
   - What motions will be restricted if the patella does not glide distally?
   - What function will be lost if the patella does not glide proximally?
4. Review and practice soft tissue and patellar mobilization techniques that can be used to increase the mobility of the lateral retinaculum around the patella. How will mobilizing this tissue improve patellar tracking?
5. Identify all the two-joint muscles that cross the knee. Review and practice self-stretching techniques with and without equipment for each of these muscles.

CASE STUDIES

1. Mrs. J is a 49-year-old mother of three children. She is in good health, but recently has experienced considerable right knee pain, especially

after sitting for prolonged periods and then standing up, when descending stairs, and when shopping at the mall for longer than 2 hours. She has a history of a proximal tibial fracture 15 years ago. She reports that it took about a year before relatively normal mobility returned. On examination, you note no obvious deformities or joint swelling. Knee flexion is 125 degrees with firm end-feel and pain on overpressure; extension is 0 degrees with firm end-feel and pain on overpressure. There is a slight decrease in posterior glide accessory motion of the tibia and decreased mobility of the patella on the right compared to the left. Strength of the knee flexors and extensors is 4/5 bilaterally. She complains of pain in the right knee when squatting; pain begins at 45 degrees flexion. She stops when the knees are at 75 degrees, saying it hurts too much. She bends forward from the waist to pick up objects from the floor. She has difficulty lowering herself down to a low chair in a controlled manner.

- List her impairments and functional limitations, and state appropriate goals.
- Develop an exercise program to meet the goals. How will you begin the exercises; how will you progress each exercise and the program?
- Describe a rationale for each manual technique you would use and for each exercise you would teach the patient.

2. Mr. R, 25 years of age, was in a serious automobile accident and sustained multiple femoral and patellar fractures on the left side. His leg was immobilized in a long-leg cast for 3 months, followed by a short leg cast for an additional month. He was allowed to be partial weight bearing when in the short-leg cast. The cast was removed this morning, and now he is to begin his rehabilitation although he will not be allowed to be full weight bearing for an additional month. He describes significant stiffness and discomfort when attempting to flex his knee. Observation reveals significant atrophy in the thigh and leg. There are no open sores and no joint swelling. Range is minimal: flexion to 25 degrees, extension to 20, and no joint play in the tibiofemoral or patellofemoral joints. He demonstrated the ability to do quad and hamstring sets, but strength could not be tested.

- Answer the same questions as in the previous case.
- Even though patients in this and the previous case have restricted motion and demonstrate weakness, what are the differences in your intervention strategies? Are there different precautions that you will follow during treatment? If so, what are they?

REFERENCES

1. Amiel, D, Kleiner, IB, and Akeson, WH: The natural history of the anterior cruciate ligament autograft of patellar tendon origin. Am J Sports Med 14:449, 1986.
2. Anderson, JK, and Noyes, FR: Principles of posterior cruciate ligament reconstruction. Orthopedics 18:493, 1995.
3. Antich, TJ, and Brewster, CE: Modification of quadriceps femoris muscle exercises during knee rehabilitation. Phys Ther 66:1246, 1986.
4. Arendt, E, and Dick, R: Knee injury patterns among men and women in collegiate basketball and soccer. Am J Sports Med 23:694, 1995.
5. Barber-Westin, SD, Noyes, FR, et al: The effect of exercise and rehabilitation on anterior posterior knee displacements after anterior cruciate ligament autograft reconstruction. Am J Sports Med 27:2, 1999.
6. Basso, DM, and Knapp, L: Comparison of two continuous passive motion protocols for patients with total knee implants. Phys Ther 67:360, 1987.
7. Beaupré, LA, et al: Exercise combined with continuous passive motion or slider board therapy compared with exercise only: A randomized controlled trial of patients following total knee arthroplasty. Phys Ther 81:1029, 2001.
8. Bennett, JG: Rehabilitation of patellofemoral joint dysfunction. In Greenfield, BH (ed): Rehabilitation of the Knee: A Problem-Solving Approach. FA Davis, Philadelphia, 1993, p 177.

8a. Bert, JM: Arthoscopic treatment of degenerative arthritis of the knee. In Insall, JN, and Scott, WN (eds): Surgery of the Knee, Vol 1, ed 3. Churchill Livingstone, New York, 2001, p 381

9. Blackburn, TA, Eiland, WG, and Bandy, WG: An introduction to the plica. J Orthop Sports Phys Ther 3:171, 1982.
10. Bobic, V: Autologous osteo-chondral grafts in the management of articular cartilage lesions. Orthopaedics 28:19, 1999
11. Boyce, DA, and Hanley, ST: Functional based rehabilitation of the knee after partial meniscectomy or meniscal repair. Orthop Phys Ther Clin North Am 3:555, 1994.
12. Brewster, CE, Moynes, DR, and Jobe, FW: Rehabilitation for anterior cruciate reconstruction. J Orthop Sports Phys Ther 5:121, 1983.

13. Brodersen, MP: Anterior cruciate ligament reconstruction. In Morrey, BF (ed): Reconstructive Surgery of the Joints, ed 2. Churchill Livingstone, New York, 1996, p 1639.
14. Brody, LT, and Thein, JM: Nonoperative treatment for patellofemoral pain. J Orthop Sports Phys Ther 28:336, 1988.
15. Brossman, J, et al: MR imaging before and after realignment surgery for patellar maltracking comparison with axial radiographs. Skel Radiol 24:191, 1995.
16. Brownstein, BA, Lamb, RL, and Mangine, RE: Quadriceps, torque and integrated electromyography. J Orthop Sports Phys Ther 6:309, 1985.
17. Bynum, EB, Barrick, RL, and Alexander, AH: Open versus closed kinetic chain exercises after anterior cruciate ligament reconstruction: A prospective study. Am J Sports Med 23:401, 1995.
18. Cailliet, R: Knee Pain and Disability, ed 3. FA Davis, Philadelphia, 1992.
19. Campbell, D, and Glenn, W: Rehabilitation of knee flexor and knee extensor muscle strength in patients with meniscectomies, ligamentous repairs and chondromalacia. Phys Ther 62:10, 1982.
20. Carrey, CT, and Tria, AJ: Surgical principles of total knee replacement: Incisions, extensor mechanism, ligament balancing. In Pellicci, PM, Tria, AJ, and Garvin, KL (eds): Orthopedic Knowledge Update, 2. Hip and Knee Reconstruction. American Academy of Orthopedic Surgeons, Rosemont, IL, 2000, p 281.
21. Chiarello, CM, Gunderson, L, and O'Halloran, T: The effect of continuous passive motion duration and increment on range of motion in total knee arthroplasty patients. J Orthop Sports Phys Ther 25:119, 1997.
22. Cooper, DE, DeLee, MD, and Ramamurthy, S: Reflex sympathetic dystrophy of the knee. J Bone Joint Surg 71A:365, 1989.
23. Cyriax, J: Textbook of Orthopaedic Medicine, Vol. 1. Diagnosis of Soft Tissue Lesions, ed 8. Bailliere Tindall, London, 1982.
24. Dietrichson, J, and Souryal, TO: Preoperative and postoperative rehabilitation of anterior cruciate ligament tears. Orthop Phys Ther Clin North Am 3:539, 1994.
25. Doucette, SA, and Goble, EM: The effect of exercise on patellar tracking in lateral patellar compression syndrome. Am J Sports Med 20:434, 1992.
26. Drez, D, et al: In vivo measurement of anterior tibial translation using continuous passive motion devices. Am J Sports Med 19:381, 1991.
27. Ecker, ML, and Lotke, PA: Postoperative care of the total knee patient. Orthop Phys Ther Clin North Am 20:55, 1989.
28. Einhorn, AR, Sawyer, M, and Tovin B: Rehabilitation of intra-articular reconstructions. In Greenfield, BH (ed): Rehabilitation of the Knee: A Problem-Solving Approach. FA Davis, Philadelphia. 1993, p 245.
29. Eng, JJ, and Peirrynowsk, MR: Evaluation of soft foot orthotics in the treatment of patellofemoral pain syndrome. Phys Ther 73:840, 1993.
30. Engle, RP, Meade, TD, and Canner, GC: Rehabilitation of posterior cruciate ligament injuries. In Greenfield, BH (ed): Rehabilitation of the Knee: A Problem-Solving Approach. FA Davis Philadelphia, 1993, p 304.
31. Enloe, J, et al: Total hip and knee replacement programs: a report using consensus. J Orthop Sports Phys Ther 23:3, 1996.
32. Escamilla, RF, et al: Biomechanics of the knee during closed kinetic chain and open kinetic chain exercises. Med Sci Sports Exerc 30:556, 1998.
33. Finch, E, et al: Functional ability perceived by individuals following total knee arthroplasty compared to age-matched individuals without knee disability. J Orthop Sports Phys Ther 27: 255, 1998.
34. Fineberg, MS, Zarins, B, and Sherman, OH: Practical considerations in anterior cruciate ligament replacement surgery. Arthroscopy 16:715, 2000.
35. Fisher, NM, et al: Quantitative effects of physical therapy on muscular and functional performance in subjects with osteoarthritis of the knees. Arch Phys Med Rehabil 74:840, 1993.
36. Fitzgerald, GK, et al: The efficacy of perturbation training in nonoperative anterior cruciate ligament rehabilitation programs for physically active individuals. Phys Ther 80:128, 2000.
37. Fitzgerald, GK, et al: Proposed practice guidelines for nonoperative anterior cruciate ligament rehabilitation of physically active individuals. J Orthop Sports Phys Ther 30:194, 2000.
37a. Ford, DH, and Post, WR: Open or arthroscopic lateral release: Indications, techniques and rehabilitation. Clin Sports Med 16:29, 1997.
38. Fu, FH, et al: Current trends in anterior cruciate ligament reconstruction. Part I: biology and biomechanics of reconstruction. Am J Sports Med 27:821, 1999.
39. Fu, FH, et al: Current trends in anterior cruciate ligament reconstruction. Part II. Operative procedures and clinical correlations. Am J Sports Med 28:124:2000.
39a. Fu, FH, and Maday, M: Arthroscopic lateral release and the patellar compression syndrome. Orthop Clin North Am 23:601, 1992.
40. Goll, SR, Lotke, PA, and Ecker, ML: Failure of CPM as prophylaxis against deep venous thrombosis after total knee arthroplasty. In Rand, JA, and Dorr, LD (eds): Total Arthroplasty of the Knee. Aspen Publishers, Rockville, MD, 1987.
41. Goodfellow, J, Hungerford, D, and Woods, C: Patellofemoral joint mechanics and pathology of chondromalacia patellae. J Bone Joint Surg Br 58:291, 1976.
42. Gose, JC: CPM in the postoperative treatment of patients with total knee replacements. Phys Ther 67:39, 1987.
43. Greene, B: Rehabilitation after total knee replacements. In Greenfield, BH (ed): Rehabilitation of the Knee: A Problem-Solving Approach. FA Davis, Philadelphia, 1993, p 410.
44. Grelsamer, RP, and Klein, JR: The biomechanics of the patellofemoral joint. J Orthop Sports Phys Ther 28:286, 1998.
44a. Grelsamer, RP, and McConnell, J: The Patella: A Team Approach. Aspen Publishers, Gaithersburg, MD, 1998.
45. Griffin, LY, et al: Non-contact anterior cruciate ligament injuries: risk factors and prevention strategies. J Am Acad Orthop Surg 8:141, 2000.
46. Grood, ES, et al: Biomechanics of the knee: Extension exercise. J Bone Joint Surg Am 66:725, 1984.
47. Gryzlo, SM, et al: Electromyographic analysis of knee rehabilitation exercises. J Orthop Sports Phys Ther 20:36, 1994.
48. Hangood, L: Mosaicplasty. In Insall, JN, and Scott, WN (eds): Surgery of the Knee, Vol 1, ed 3. Churchill Livingstone, New York, 2001, p 357.
49. Hanssen, AD, and Stuart, MJ: Posterior cruciate-substituting

and -sacrificing total knee arthroplasty. In Morrey, BF (ed): Reconstructive Surgery of the Joints, ed 2. Churchill Livingstone, New York, 1996, p 1409.

50. Hattrup, SJ: Synovectomy. In Morrey, BF (ed): Reconstructive Surgery of the Joints, ed 2. Churchill Livingstone, New York, 1996, p 1599.
51. Heckman, TP, Noyes, FR, and Barber-Westin, SD: Autogenic and allogenic anterior cruciate ligament rehabilitation. In Ellenbecker, TS: Knee Ligament Rehabilitation. Churchill Livingstone, New York, 2000, p 132.
52. Hefzy, MS, Grood, ES, and Noyes, FR: Factors effecting the region of most isometric femoral attachments. Part II: The anterior cruciate ligament. Am J Sports Med 17:208, 1989.
53. Helfet, AJ: Disorders of the Knee. JB Lippincott, Philadelphia, 1982.
54. Hewett, TE, Blum, KR, and Noyes, FR: Gait characteristics of the anterior cruciate ligament-deficient varus knee. Am J Knee Surg 10:246, 1997.
55. Holmes, SW, and Clancy, WG: Clinical classification of patellofemoral pain and dysfunction. J Orthop Sports Phys Ther 28:299, 1998.
56. Hung, V, and Gross, MST: Effect of foot position on electromyographic activity of the vastus medialis oblique and vastus lateralis during lower-extremity weight-bearing activities. J Orthop Sports Phys Ther 29:91, 1999.
57. Insall, JN, and Clark, HD: Historic development, classification and characteristics of total knee protheses. In Insall, JN, and Scott, WN (eds): Surgery of the Knee, Vol 2, ed 3. Churchill-Livingstone, New York, 2001, p 1516.
57a. Insall, JN, and Easley, ME: Surgical techniques and instrumentation in total knee arthroplasty. In Insall, JN, and Scott, WN (eds): Surgery of the Knee, Vol 2, ed 3. Churchill Livingstone, New York, 2001, p 1553.
58. Jaramillo, J, Worrell, TW, and Ingersoll, CD: Hip isometric strength following knee surgery. J Ortho Sports Phys Ther 20:160, 1993.
59. Johnson, DP: The effect of continuous passive motion on wound healing and joint mobility after knee arthroplasty. J Bone Joint Surg Am 72:421, 1990.
60. Kaltenborn, FM: The Kaltenborn Method of Joint Examination and Treatment, Vol I: The Extremities, ed 5. Olaf Norlis Bokhandle, Oslo, 1999.
61. Kapandji, IA: The Physiology of the Joints, Vol II. Churchill Livingstone, Edinburgh. 1970.
62. Karst, GM, and Jewett, PD: Electromyographic analysis of exercises proposed for differential activation of medial and lateral quadriceps femoris muscle components. Phys Ther 73:286, 1993.
63. Kegerreis, S, Malone, T, and Ohnson, F: The diagonal medical plica: An underestimated clinical entity. J Orthop Sports Phys Ther 9:305, 1988.
64. King, S, and Butterwick, D: The anterior cruciate ligament: A review of recent concepts. J Orthop Sports Phys Ther 8:110, 1986.
65. Kolessar, DJ, and Rand, JA: Extensor mechanism problems following total knee arthroplasty. In Morrey, BF (ed): Reconstructive Surgery of the Joints, ed 2. Churchill Livingstone, New York, 1996, p 1533.
66. Kurosaka, M, Yoshiya, S, and Andrish, JR: A biomechanical comparison of different surgical techniques of fixation in anterior cruciate ligament reconstruction. Am J Sports Med 15:225, 1987.
67. Lang, KE: Comparison of 6- and 7-day physical therapy coverage on length of stay and discharge outcome for individuals with total hip and knee arthroplasty. J Orthop Sports Phys Ther 23:15, 1998.
68. Laprade, J, et al: Comparison of five isometric exercises in the recruitment of the vastus medialis oblique in persons with and without patellofemoral pain syndrome. J Orthop Sports Phys Ther 27:197, 1998.
69. Lennington, KR, and Yanchuleff, TT: The use of isokinetics in the treatment of chondromalacia patellae: A case report. J Orthop Sports Phys Ther 4:176, 1983.
70. Levangie, PK, and Norkin, CC: Joint Structure and Function: A Comprehensive Analysis, ed 3. FA Davis Company, Philadelphia, 2001.
71. Lynch, PA, et al: Deep venous thrombosis and continued passive motion after total knee arthroplasty. J Bone Joint Surg Am 70:11, 1988.
72. Malone, TR, and Garrett, WE: Commentary and historical perspective of anterior cruciate ligament rehabilitation. J Orthop Sports Phys Ther 15:265, 1992.
73. Mangine, RE, Eifert-Mangine, M, et al: Postoperative management of the patellofemoral patient. J Ortho Sports Phys Ther 28:323, 1998.
73a. Mangine, RE, and Kremchek, ET: Evaluation based protocol of the anterior cruciate ligament. J Sport Rehab 6:157, 1997.
74. Mangine, RE, and Quillen, WS: EMG analysis of closed-chain squat with and without hip adduction. Presented at Combined Sections Meeting, American Physical Therapy Association, Seattle, 1999.
74a. Manifold, SG, Cushner, FD, and Scott, WN: Anterior cruciate ligament reconstruction with bone-patellar tendon-bone autograft: Indications, technique, complications, and management. In Insall, JN, and Scott, WN (eds): Surgery of the Knee, Vol 1, ed 3. Churchill Livingstone, New York, 2001, p 665.
75. Manske, PR, and Gleason, P: Rehabilitation program following polycentric total knee arthroplasty. Phys Ther 57:915, 1977.
76. Martin, SD, Scott, RD, and Thornhill, TS: Current concepts of total knee arthroplasty. J Orthop Sports Phys Ther 28:252, 1998.
77. McCarthy, MR, et al: The effects of immediate continuous passive motion on pain during the inflammatory phase of soft tissue healing following anterior cruciate ligament reconstruction. J Orthop Sports Phys Ther 17:96, 1993.
78. McConnell, J: The management of chondromalacia patellae: A long term solution. Austral J Physiother 32:215, 1986.
79. McConnell, J: McConnell Institute Workshop on Management of Patella femoral pain. Columbus, OH, 1994.
80. McInnes, J, and Larson, M: A controlled evaluation of continuous passive motion in patients undergoing total knee arthroplasty. JAMA 268:1423, 1992.
80a. McLaughin, J, et al: Rehabilitation after meniscus repair. Orthopedics 17:463, 1994.
81. Mercier, LR: Practical Orthopedics, ed 4. Mosby-Year Book, Inc, St Louis, 1995.
82. Metcalf, RW: An arthoscopic method for lateral release of the subluxating or dislocating patella. Clin Orthop 167:9, 1982.
83. Mirza, F, et al: Management of injuries to the anterior cru-

ciate ligament: results of a survey of orthopaedic surgeons in Canada. Clin J Sport Med 10:85, 2000.

83a. Mologne, TS, and Friedman, MJ: Arthroscopic anterior cruciate reconstruction with hamstring tendons: Indications, surgical technique, complications and their treatment. In Insall, JN, and Scott, WN (eds): Surgery of the Knee, Vol 1, ed 3. Churchill Livingstone, New York, 2001, p 681.

84. Morrey, BF, and Kavanagh, RD: Cementless joint replacement: Current status and future. Bull Rheum Dis 37:1, 1987.

85. Mulligan, BR: Manual Therapy "NAGS", "SNAGS", "MWM's": etc, ed 4. Plane View Press, Wellington, 1999.

86. Mulvey, TJ, et al: Complications associated with total knee arthroplasty. In Pellicci, PM, Tria, AJ, and Garvin, KL (eds): Orthopedic Knowledge Update 2. Hip and Knee Reconstruction. American Academy of Orthopedic Surgeons, Rosemont, IL, 2000, p 323.

87. Newman, AP: Synovectomy. In Sledge, CB, et al (eds): Arthritis Surgery. WB Saunders, Philadelphia, 1994, p 684.

88. Noyes, FR, and Barber-Westin, SD: Surgical restoration to treat chronic deficiency of the posterolateral complex and cruciate ligaments of the knee. Am J Sports Med 24:415, 1996.

89. Noyes, FR, Barber, SD, and Mangine, RE: Bone-patellar ligament-bone and fascia lata allografts for reconstruction of the anterior cruciate ligament. J Bone Joint Surg (Am) 72:1125, 1990.

90. Noyes, FR, et al: Arthroscopy in acute traumatic hemarthrosis of the knee. Incidence of anterior cruciate tears and other injuries. J Bone Joint Surg (Am) 62:687, 1980.

91. Noyes, FR, Butler, DL, Grood, ES, et al: Biomechanical analysis of human ligament grafts used in knee ligament repairs and reconstructions. J Bone Joint Surg 66A:334, 1984.

92. Noyes, FR, DeMaio, M, and Mangine, RE: Evaluation-based protocol: A new approach to rehabilitation. J Orthop Phys Ther 14:1383, 1991.

93. Noyes, FR, Heckman, TP, and Barber-Westin, SD: Posterior cruciate ligament and posterolateral reconstruction. In Ellenbecker, TS: Knee Ligament Rehabilitation. Churchill Livingstone, New York, 2000, p 167.

94. Noyes, FR, and Mangine, RE: Early knee motion after open and arthroscopic anterior cruciate ligament reconstruction. Am J Sports Med 15:149, 1987.

94a. Noyes, FR, Barber-Westin, SD, and Grood, ES: New concepts in the treatment of posterior cruciate ligament ruptures. In Insall, JN, and Scott, WN (eds): Surgery of the Knee, Vol 1, ed 3. Churchill Livingstone, New York, 2001, p 841.

95. O'Donoghue, DH: Surgical treatment of fresh injuries to the major ligaments of the knee. J Bone Joint Surg 32A:721, 1950.

96. Outerbridge, RE, and Dunlop, J: The problem of chondromalacia patellae. Clin Orthrop Rel Res 110:177, 1975.

97. Palmitier, RA, et al: Kinetic chain exercises in knee rehabilitation. Sports Med 11:402, 1991.

98. Papagelopoulos, PJ, and Rand, JA: Complications and salvage: General survey. In Morrey, BF (ed): Reconstructive Surgery of the Joints, ed 2. Churchill Livingstone, New York, 1996, p 1499.

99. Papagelopoulos, PJ, Sim, FH, and Morrey, BF: Patellectomy and reconstructive surgery for disorders of the patellofemoral joint. In Morrey, BF (ed): Reconstructive Surgery of the Joints, ed 2. Churchill Livingstone, New York, 1996, p 1671.

100. Paulos, LE, Walther, CE, and Walker, JA: Rehabilitation of the surgically reconstructed and nonsurgical anterior cruciate ligament. In Insall, JN, and Scott, WN (eds): Surgery of the Knee, Vol 1, ed 3. Churchill Livingstone, New York, 2001, p 789.

101. Perry, J: Gait Analysis: Normal and Pathological Function. SLACK Inc, Thorofare, NJ, 1992.

101a. Post, WR, and Fulkerson, JP: Surgery of the patellofemoral joint: Indications, effects, results and recommendations. In Insall, JN, and Scott, WN (eds): Surgery of the Knee, Vol 1, ed 3. Churchill Livingstone, New York, 2001, p1045.

102. Rand, JA: Cemented total knee arthroplasty: techniques. In Morrey, BF (ed): Reconstructive Surgery of the Joints, ed 2. Churchill Livingstone, New York, 1996, p 1389.

103. Rand, JA: Posterior cruciate-retaining knee arthroplasty. In Morrey, BF (ed): Reconstructive Surgery of the Joints, ed 2. Churchill Livingstone, New York, 1996, p 1401.

104. Rand, JA: Uncemented total knee arthroplasty: results. In Morrey, BF (ed): Reconstructive Surgery of the Joints, ed 2. Churchill Livingstone, New York, 1996, p 1417.

105. Rand, JA: Unicompartmental total knee arthroplasty. In Morrey, BF (ed): Reconstructive Surgery of the Joints, ed 2. Churchill Livingstone, New York, 1996, p 1487.

106. Riegler, HF: Recurrent dislocations and subluxations of the patella. Clin Orthop 227:201, 1988.

107. Sandor, SM, Hart, JAL, and Oakes, BW: Case study: Rehabilitation of a surgically repaired medial collateral knee ligament using a limited motion cast and isokinetic exercise. J Orthop Sports Phys Ther 7:154, 1986.

108. Scaepanski, TL, et al: Effect of contraction type, angular velocity, and arc of motion on VMO:VL EMG ratio. J Orthop Sports Phys Ther 14:256, 1991.

109. Schulco, T, et al: Knee surgery and rehabilitation. In Melvin, JL, and Gall, V (eds): Rheumatologic Rehabilitation Series, Vol 5: Surgical Rehabilitation. American Occupational Therapy Association, Bethesda, MD, 1999, p 121.

110. Scott, RD, et al: Long-term results of total knee replacement. In Pellicci, JM, Tria, AJ, and Garvin, KL (eds): Orthopedic Knowledge Update, 2. Hip and Knee Reconstruction. American Academy of Orthopedic Surgeons, Rosemont, IL, 2000, p 301.

111. Seto, JL, and Brewster, CE: Rehabilitation of meniscal injuries. In Greenfield, BH: Rehabilitation of the Knee: A Problem-Solving Approach. FA Davis, Philadelphia, 1993.

112. Shelbourne, KD, and Urch, SE: Primary anterior cruciate ligament reconstruction using the contralateral autogenous patellar tendon. Am J Sports Med 18:651, 2000.

113. Shelbourne, KD, and Nitz, P: Accelerated rehabilitation after anterior cruciate ligament reconstruction. J Orthop Sports Phys Ther 15:256, 1992.

114. Shelton, GL, and Thigpen, LK: Rehabilitation of patellofemoral dysfunction: A review of literature. J of Orthop Sports Phys Ther 14:143, 1991.

115. Shoji, H, and Solomonov, M: Factors affecting postoperative flexion in total knee arthroplasty. Clin Orthop 13:643. 1990.

116. Smidt, GL, Albright, JP, and Deusinger, RH: Pre- and postoperative functional changes in total knee patients. J Orthop Sports Phys Ther 6:25, 1984.
117. Smith, LK, Weiss, EL, and Lehmkuhl, LD: Brunnstrom's Clinical Kinesiology, ed 5. FA Davis Company, Philadelphia, 1996.
118. Snyder-Mackler, L, et al: Strength of the quadriceps femoris muscle and functional recovery after reconstruction of the anterior cruciate ligament. J Bone Joint Surg (Am) 77:1166, 1995.
119. Sodeberg, GL, and Cook, TM: An electromyographic analysis of quadriceps femoris muscle setting and straight leg raising. Phys Ther 63:1434-1438, 1983.
120. Spencer, JD, Hayes, KC, and Alexander, IJ: Knee joint effusion and quadriceps reflex inhibition in man. Arch Phys Med Rehabil 65:171, 1984.
121. Sprague, R: Factors related to extension lag at the knee joint. J Orthop Sports Phys Ther 3:178, 1982.
122. Steindler, A: Kinesiology of the Human Body Under Normal and Pathological Conditions. Charles C Thomas, Springfield, IL, 1955.
123. Stone, RC, Frewin, PR, and Gonzales, S: Long term assessment of arthroscopic meniscus repair. A two to six year follow-up study. Arthroscopy 6:73, 1990.
124. Stratford, P: Electromyography of the quadriceps femoris muscles in subjects with normal and acutely effused knees. Phys Ther 62:279, 1982.
125. Strum, GM, et al: Acute anterior cruciate ligament reconstruction. Analysis of complications, Clin Orthop Rel Res 253:184, 1990.
126. Stuart, MJ: Posterior cruciate ligament reconstruction. In Morrey, BF (ed): Reconstructive Surgery of the Joints, ed 2. Churchill Livingstone, New York, 1996, p 1651.
127. Tamburello, T, et al: Patella hypomobility as a cause of extensor lag. Research presentation. Overland Park, KS, May 1985.
128. Torchia, ME: Meniscal tears. In Morrey, BF (ed): Reconstructive Surgery of the Joints, ed 2. Churchill Livingstone, New York, 1996, p 1607.
129. Tovin, BJ, et al: Comparison of the effects of exercise in water and on land on the rehabilitation of patients with intra-articular anterior cruciate ligament reconstructions. Phys Ther 74:710, 1994.
129a. Veltri, DM, and Warren, RF: Isolated and combined posterior cruciate ligament injuries. J Am Acad Orthop Surg 1:57, 1993.
130. Voight, ML, and Wieder, DL: Comparative reflex response times of vastus medialis obliquis and vastus lateralis in normal subjects and subjects with extensor mechanism dysfunction. Am J Sports Med 19:131, 1991.
131. Walsh, M, et al: Physical impairments and functional limitations: a comparison of individuals 1 year after total knee arthroplasty with control subjects. Phys Ther 78:248, 1998.
132. Waters, EA: Physical therapy management of patients with total knee replacement. Phys Ther 54:936, 1974.
133. Wegener, L, Kisner, C, and Nichols, D: Static and dynamic balance responses in persons with bilateral knee osteoarthritis. J Orthop Sports Phys Ther 25:13, 1997.
134. Whiteside, LA: Fixation in total knee replacement: bone ingrowth. In Pellicci, PM, Tria, AJ, and Garvin, KL (eds): Orthopedic Knowledge Update, 2. Hip and Knee Reconstruction. American Academy of Orthopedic Surgeons, Rosemont, IL, 2000, p 275.
135. Wigren, A, et al: Isokinetic muscle strength and endurance after knee arthroplasty with the modular knee in patients with osteoarthritis and rheumatoid arthritis. Scand J Rheumatol 12:145, 1983.
136. Wilk, KE, and Andrews, JR: Current concepts in the treatment of anterior cruciate ligament disruption. J Orthop Sports Phys Ther 15:279, 1992.
137. Wilk, KE, and Andrews, JR: The effects of pad placement and angular velocity on tibial displacement during isokinetic exercise. J Orthop Sports Phys Ther 17:24, 1993.
138. Wilk, KE, and Clancy, WG: Medial collateral ligament injuries: diagnosis, treatment, and rehabilitation in knee ligament injuries. In Engle, RP (ed): Knee Ligament Rehabilitation. Churchill Livingstone, New York, 1991, p 71.
139. Wilk, KE, et al: Patellofemoral disorders: A classification system and clinical guidelines for nonoperative rehabilitation. J Orthop Sports Phys Ther 28:307, 1998.
140. Woodall, W, and Welsh, J: A biomechanical basis for rehabilitation programs involving the patellofemoral joint. J Orthop Sports Phys Ther 11:535, 1990.
141. Wright, TM: Biomechanics of total knee design. In Pellicci, PM, Tria, AJ, and Garvin, KL (eds): Orthopedic Knowledge Update, 2. Hip and Knee Reconstruction. American Academy of Orthopedic Surgeons, Rosemont, IL, 2000, p 265.

Chapter 14

The Ankle and Foot

OBJECTIVES

After studying this chapter, the reader will be able to:

1 Identify important aspects of the structure and function of the ankle and foot for review.

2 Establish a therapeutic exercise program to manage soft tissue and joint lesions in the ankle and foot related to stages of recovery after an inflammatory insult to the tissues, recognizing unique circumstances in the ankle and foot for their management.

3 Describe common indications and an overview of operative procedures for common soft tissue injuries and late-stage joint disease of the ankle and foot.

4 Develop and progress therapeutic exercise interventions after surgical repair or reconstruction of soft tissues and joints of the ankle and foot.

The joints, ligaments, and muscles of the ankle and foot are designed to provide stability as well as mobility in the terminal structures of the lower extremity. The foot must bear the body weight during standing with a minimum of muscle energy expenditure. The foot also must be able to adapt to absorb forces and accommodate to uneven surfaces, and then it must be able to become a rigid structural lever to propel the body forward during walking or running.

The anatomy and kinesiology of the ankle and foot are complex, but it is important to understand and be able to apply this information to effectively treat impairments in this region of the body. The first section of this chapter reviews highlights of these areas that the reader should know and understand. Chapter 8 presents information on principles of management; the reader should be familiar with that material before proceeding with establishing a therapeutic exercise program for the ankle and foot.

Review of the Structure and Function of the Ankle and Foot

Bony Parts (see Figs. 6–49 and 6–58)

Leg

The tibia and fibula make up the leg. These two bones are bound together by an interosseous membrane along the shafts of the bones, by strong anterior and posterior inferior tibiofibular ligaments that hold the distal tibiofibular articulation together, and by a strong capsule that encloses the proximal tibiofibular articulation. These two bones do not rotate around each other as do the radius and ulna in the upper extremity, but there is slight movement between the two bones that allows greater movement of the ankle joints.

Foot

The foot is divided into three segments:

Hindfoot. The talus and calcaneus make up the posterior segment.

Midfoot. The navicular, cuboid, and three cuneiforms make up the middle segment.

Forefoot. Five metatarsals and 14 phalanges make up the anterior segment. Each toe has three phalanges except for the large toe, which has two.

Motions of the Foot and Ankle

Primary Plane Motions

Sagittal plane motion. *Dorsiflexion* is movement in a dorsal direction; *plantarflexion* is movement in a plantar direction around a frontal axis.[11,12,55]

Frontal plane motion. *Inversion* is turning inward and *eversion* is turning outward around a sagittal axis. Normally, an inward and outward motion is described by the terms *abduction* and *adduction*, but because the foot is at a right angle to the leg, abduction and adduction are not used here.[11,12]

Transverse plane motion. *Abduction* is movement away from the midline, and *adduction* is movement toward the midline. In the foot this motion occurs around a vertical axis.[11,12,55]

Triplanar Motions Occurring About Oblique Axes

Triplanar motion occurs at each articulation of the ankle and foot. The definitions are descriptive of the movement of the distal bone on the proximal bone. When the proximal bone moves on the stabilized distal bone as occurs in closed-chain mechanics, the motion of the proximal bone is opposite, although the relative joint motion is the same as defined.

Pronation. This is a combination of dorsiflexion, eversion, and abduction.

Supination. This is a combination of plantarflexion, inversion, and adduction.

Note: The terms *inversion* and *supination,* as well as eversion and pronation, are often interchanged.[46] This text will use the terms as defined above.

Joints and Their Characteristics

The characteristics of each joint in the leg, ankle, and foot dictate how they contribute to their function.[37,45,55,60]

The Tibiofibular Joints

Anatomically, the superior and inferior tibiofibular joints are separate from the ankle but provide accessory motions that allow greater movement at the ankle; fusion or immobility in these joints will impair ankle function.

Superior tibiofibular joint. This is a plane synovial joint made up of the fibular head and a facet on the posterolateral aspect of the rim of the tibial condyle; the facet faces posteriorly, inferiorly, and laterally.

Inferior tibiofibular joint. This is a syndesmosis with fibroadipose tissue between the two bony surfaces; it is supported by the crural tibiofibular interosseous ligament and the anterior and posterior tibiofibular ligaments.

Accessory motions. With dorsiflexion and plantarflexion of the ankle, there are slight accessory movements of the fibula.[25]

- As the ankle plantarflexes, the lateral malleolus (fibula) rotates medially and is pulled inferiorly, and the two malleoli approximate. At the superior joint, the fibula slides inferiorly. The opposite occurs with dorsiflexion.
- As the foot supinates, the head of the fibula slides distally and posteriorly (external rotation); with pronation, the head of the fibula slides proximally and anteriorly (internal rotation).

The Ankle (Talocrural) Joint

This is a synovial hinge joint supported by a structurally strong mortise, which is the distal articulating surfaces of the tibia and tibial and fibular malleoli. The tibia and fibula are held together by an interosseous membrane and by the anterior and posterior talofibular ligaments. The ankle, along with the subtalar joint, is supported medially by the deltoid ligament and laterally by the anterior and posterior talofibular and calcaneofibular ligaments.

- The concave articulating surface is the mortise. The fibular malleolus extends farther distally and posteriorly than the tibial malleolus so that the mortise angles outward and downward. This causes the axis of motion to be rotated laterally 20 to 30 degrees and inclined downward 10 degrees. The surface of the mortise is congruent with the articulating surface of the body of the talus.
- The convex articulating surface is the body of the talus. The surface is wedge-shaped, being wider anteriorly, and is also cone-shaped, with the apex pointing medially.
- As a result of the orientation of the axis and shape of the talus when the foot dorsiflexes, the talus also abducts and slightly everts (pronation); when the foot plantarflexes, the talus also adducts and slightly inverts (supination). With physiologic motions of the foot, the articulating surface of the talus slides in the opposite direction (Box 14–1).

Subtalar (Talocalcaneal) Joint

This is a uniaxial joint with an oblique axis of motion lying approximately 42 degrees from the transverse plane and 16 degrees from the sagittal plane, which allows the calcaneus to pronate and supinate in a triplanar motion on the talus. Frontal plane inversion (turning heel inward) and eversion (turning heel outward) can be isolated only with passive motion. The subtalar joint is supported by the medial

Box 14–1 Arthrokinematics of the Ankle and Foot Joints

Physiologic motion	Roll	Slide
Talocrural joint: motion of talus		
Dorsiflexion	Anterior	Posterior
Plantarflexion	Posterior	Anterior
Subtalar joint: motion of calcaneus (posterior articulating surface)		
Supination with inversion	Medial	Lateral
Pronation with eversion	Lateral	Medial
Talonavicular joint: motion of navicular (open-chain)		
Supination	Plantar and medial	Plantar and medial
Pronation	Dorsal and lateral	Dorsal and lateral
Metatarsophalangeal and interphalangeal joints: motion of the phalanges		
Flexion	Plantar	Plantar
Extension	Dorsal	Dorsal

and lateral collateral ligaments, which also support the talocrural joint, by the interosseous talocalcaneal ligament in the tarsal canal, and by the posterior and lateral talocalcaneal ligaments. In closed-chain activities, the joint attenuates the rotatory forces between the leg and foot so that, normally, excessive inward or outward turning of the foot does not occur.

- There are three articulations between the talus and calcaneus; the posterior is separated from the anterior and middle by the tarsal canal. The canal divides the subtalar joint into two joint cavities.
- The posterior articulation has its own capsule; the facet on the bottom of the talus is concave, whereas the opposing facet on the calcaneus is convex.
- The anterior articulations are enclosed in the same capsule as the talonavicular articulation, forming the *talocalcaneonavicular* joint.[37] Functionally, these articulations work together. The facets of the anterior and middle articulations on the talus are convex, whereas the opposing facets on the calcaneus are concave.
- With physiologic motions of the subtalar joint, the convex posterior portion of the calcaneus slides opposite to the motion; the concave anterior and middle facets on the calcaneus slide in the same direction, similar to turning a doorknob. With eversion, as the calcaneus rolls laterally the posterior articulating surface slides medially, and with inversion, the posterior articulating surface slides laterally (see Box 14–1).

Talonavicular Joint

Anatomically and functionally part of the talocalcaneonavicular joint, this joint is supported by the spring, the deltoid, the bifurcate, and the dorsal talonavicular ligaments. The triplanar motions of the navicular on the talus function with the subtalar joint, resulting in pronation and supination. In the weight-bearing foot this occurs as the head of the talus drops plantarward and medially, resulting in a pliable foot and a decreased medial longitudinal arch. The opposite accessory motions occur with supination, resulting in a rigid foot and an increased medial longitudinal arch.

- The head of the talus is convex; the proximal articulating surface of the navicular is concave. With physiological motions of the foot, the navicular slides in the same direction as the motion of the forefoot. In the open-chain motion of pronation, the navicular slides dorsally and laterally (abduction and eversion), and with supination it slides volarly and medially (adduction and inversion) (see Box 14–1).
- In the weight-bearing foot (closed-chain), this articulation is influenced by what is happening in the subtalar joint.[37]
  - During pronation, as the calcaneus everts, it cannot also dorsiflex and abduct with the foot on the ground, so the talus plantarflexes and inverts on the calcaneus. This downward and inward motion of the talar head results in an upward and outward motion of the navicular and a flattening in the medial longitudinal arch (and pliable foot).
  - During supination, the opposite occurs. The calcaneus inverts, and the talus dorsiflexes and everts, resulting in the navicular plantarflexing, inverting and adducting. The overall effect is an increase in the medial longitudinal arch and a structurally stable foot.

Transverse Tarsal Joint

This functionally compound joint between the hind- and midfoot includes the anatomically separate talonavicular and calcaneocuboid joints.

- *Talonavicular joint* (described in the previous section).
- The *calcaneocuboid joint* is saddle-shaped. The articulating surface of the calcaneus is convex in a dorsal-to-plantar direction and concave in a medial-to-lateral direction; the articulating surface of the cuboid is reciprocally concave and convex.

- The transverse tarsal joint participates in the triplanar pronation/supination activities of the foot and makes compensatory movements to accommodate variations in the ground. Passive accessory motions include abduction/adduction, inversion/eversion, and dorsal/plantar gliding.

The Remaining Intertarsal and Tarsometatarsal Joints

These are plane joints whose functions reinforce those of the hindfoot.

The Metatarsophalangeal (MTP) and Interphalangeal (IP) Joints of the Toes

These joints are the same as the metacarpophalangeal and interphalangeal joints of the hand except that, in the toes, extension range of motion (ROM) is more important than is flexion (the opposite is true in the hand). Extension of the MTP joints is necessary for normal walking. Also, the large toe does not function separately as does the thumb.

Functional Relationships of the Ankle and Foot

Ankle. Normally, an external torsion exists in the tibia so that the ankle mortise faces approximately 15 degrees outward. With dorsiflexion, the foot moves up and slightly laterally; with plantarflexion, the foot moves down and medially.[37] Dorsiflexion is the close-packed, stable position of the talocrural joint. Plantarflexion is the loose-packed position. This joint is more vulnerable to injury when walking in high heels because of the less stable plantarflexed position at the same time that the subtalar and transverse tarsal joints are in their close-packed (rigid) position.

Supination. In the closed-chain, weight-bearing foot, supination of the subtalar and transverse tarsal joints with a pronation twist of the forefoot (plantarflexion of the first and dorsiflexion of the fifth metatarsals) increases the arch of the foot and is the close-packed or stable position of the joints of the foot. This is the position the foot assumes when a rigid lever is needed for propelling the body forward during the push-off phase of ambulation.[37,55]

Pronation. During weight bearing, pronation of the subtalar and transverse tarsal joints causes the arch of the foot to lower, and there is a relative supination of the forefoot with dorsiflexion of the first and plantarflexion of the fifth metatarsals. This is the loose-packed or mobile position of the foot and is assumed when the foot absorbs the impact of weight bearing and rotational forces of the rest of the lower extremity and when the foot conforms to the ground.[12]

Interdependence of leg and foot motions. In the weight-bearing foot, subtalar motion and tibial rotation are interdependent. Supination of the subtalar joint results in or is caused by lateral rotation of the tibia, and conversely, pronation of the subtalar joint results in or is caused by medial rotation of the tibia.[37,55]

Arches. The arches of the foot are visualized as a twisted osteoligamentous plate, with the metatarsal heads being the horizontally placed anterior edge of the plate, and the calcaneus being the vertically placed posterior edge. The twist causes the longitudinal and transverse arches. When bearing weight, the plate tends to untwist and flatten the arches slightly.[37]

- Primary support of the arches comes from the spring ligament with additional support from the long plantar ligament, the plantar aponeurosis, and short plantar ligament. During push-off in gait, as the foot plantarflexes and supinates and the metatarsal phalangeal joints go into extension, increased tension is placed on the plantar aponeurosis, which helps increase the arch. This is called the windlass effect.
- In the normal static foot, muscles do little to support the arches, yet without muscle tension the passive support stretches, and foot pronation increases under weight-bearing loads. Muscles contribute to support during ambulation.

Abnormal foot postures. A person with a varus deformity of the calcaneus (observed nonweight-bearing) may compensate by standing with a pronated (or everted) calcaneus posture.[11,13] *Pes planus, pronated foot,* and *flat foot* are terms often interchanged to mean a pronated posture of the hindfoot and decreased medial longitudinal arch. *Pes cavus* and *supinated foot* describe a high-arched foot.[46]

Muscle Function in the Ankle and Foot

Plantarflexors. Plantarflexion is primarily caused by the two-joint gastrocnemius muscle and the one-joint soleus muscle; they attach to the calcaneus via the Achilles tendon.

Secondary plantarflexors. Other muscles passing posteriorly to the axis of motion of plantarflexion contribute little to that motion, but they do have other functions.

- Tibialis posterior is a strong supinator and invertor that helps to control and reverse pronation during midstance of gait.
- Flexor hallucis longus and flexor digitorum longus flex the toes and help support the medial longitudinal arch. To prevent clawing of the toes (MTP extension with IP flexion), intrinsic muscles must also function at the MTP joints.
- Peroneus longus and brevis primarily evert the foot, and the longus gives support to the transverse and lateral longitudinal arches during weight-bearing activities.

Dorsiflexors. Dorsiflexion of the ankle is caused by the tibialis anterior muscle (which also inverts the ankle), the extensor hallucis longus and extensor digitorum longus (which also extend the toes), and the peroneus tertius muscles.

Intrinsic muscles. Intrinsic muscles of the foot are similar to the hand in their functioning of the toes (except there is no thumb-like function in the foot), and they also provide support to the arches during gait.

Stability in standing. In normal standing, the gravitational line falls anteriorly to the axis of the ankle joint, creating a dorsiflexion moment. The soleus muscle contracts to counter the gravitational moment through its pull on the tibia. Other extrinsic foot muscles help stabilize the foot during postural sway.

The ankle and foot during gait.[37,47] During the normal gait cycle, the ankle goes through a ROM of 35 degrees: 15 degrees of dorsiflexion occurs at the end of midstance, and 20 degrees of plantarflexion occurs at the end of stance.

Joint Function of the Ankle and Foot During Gait

Shock-absorbing, terrain-conforming, and propulsion functions of the ankle and foot.

- During the loading response (heel strike to foot flat), the heel strikes the ground in neutral or slight supination. As the foot lowers to the ground it begins to pronate to its loose-packed position.[21] The entire lower extremity rotates inward, which reinforces the loose-packed position of the foot. With the joints in a lax position, they can conform to variations in the ground contour and absorb some of the impact forces as the foot is lowered.
- Once the foot is fixed on the ground, dorsiflexion begins as the tibia comes up over the foot; the tibia continues to rotate internally, which reinforces pronation of the subtalar joint and loose-packed position of the foot.
- During midstance and continuing through terminal stance, the tibia begins to rotate externally, which initiates supination of the hindfoot and locking of the transverse tarsal joint. This brings the foot into its close-packed position, which is reinforced as the heel rises and the foot rocks up onto the toes causing toe extension and tightening of the plantar aponeurosis (windlass effect). This stable position converts the foot into a rigid lever, ready to propel the body forward as the ankle plantarflexes from the pull of the gastrocnemius-soleus muscle group.

Muscle Control of the Ankle During Gait

- The ankle dorsiflexors function during the initial foot contact and loading response (heel-strike to foot flat) to counter the plantarflexion torque and to control the lowering of the foot to the ground. They also function during the swing phase to keep the foot from plantarflexing and dragging on the ground. With loss of the dorsiflexors, foot slap occurs at initial foot contact, and the hip and knee flex excessively during swing (or else the toe drags on the ground).
- The ankle plantarflexors begin functioning near the end of midstance and during terminal stance and preswing (heel-off to toe-off) to control the rate of forward movement of the tibia and also to plantarflex the ankle for push-off. Loss of function results in a slight lag of the lower extremity during terminal stance with no push-off.

Major Nerves Subject to Pressure and Trauma

The foot is where several major nerves terminate.[32] Injury or entrapment of the nerves may be anywhere along their course, from the lumbosacral spine to near their termination. For treatment to be effective, it must be directed to the source of the problem. Therefore, a thorough history is obtained, and a selective tension examination is performed when referred pain patterns, sensory changes, or muscle weakness are reported by the patient.[8]

Common Peroneal Nerve

After it bifurcates from the sciatic nerve in the knee region, it passes between the biceps femoris tendon and lateral head of the gastrocnemius muscle and then comes laterally around the fibular neck and passes through an opening in the peroneus longus muscle. Pressure or force against the nerve in this region can cause a neuropathy. Sensory changes occur in the distal lateral surface of the leg and dorsum of the foot (except the little toe); muscles affected may include the dorsiflexors of the ankle and evertors of the foot (peroneus longus and brevis, tibialis anterior, extensor digitorum longus and brevis, extensor hallucis longus, and peroneus tertius).

Posterior Tibial Nerve

This nerve occupies a groove behind the medial malleolus along with the tendons of the tibialis posterior, flexor hallucis longus, and flexor digitorum longus muscles; the groove is covered by a ligament, forming a tunnel. Entrapment usually from a space-occupying lesion is known as a *tarsal tunnel syndrome.* Sensory innervation includes the plantar surface of the foot and toes and the dorsum of the distal phalanges. Muscles affected include the intrinsic muscles of the foot (abductor hallucis, flexor hallucis brevis, lumbricales, interossei, and quadratus plantae); weakness and postural changes in the foot (pes cavus and clawing of the toes) may occur.

Plantar and Calcaneal Nerves

These branches of the posterior tibial nerve may become entrapped as they turn under the medial aspect of the foot and pass through openings in the abductor hallucis muscle. Overpronation presses the nerves against these openings. Irritation of the nerves may elicit symptoms similar to acute foot strain (tenderness at the posteromedial plantar aspect of the foot), painful heel (inflamed calcaneal nerve), and pain in a pes cavus foot. The degree of muscle weakness will depend on which of the branches is involved.

Common Sources of Segmental Sensory Reference in the Foot

- Lumbosacral spine
  - Vertebral joints between L-4 and L-5 or between L-5 and S-1 vertebrae
  - Nerve roots L-4, L-5, and S-1
- Dermatomal reference from tissue derived from the same spinal segments as L-4, L-5, and S-1

Joint Hypomobility: Nonoperative Management

Related Diagnoses

Chapter 8 provides a general discussion of arthritic conditions, postimmobilization stiffness, and etiology of symptoms. The following is specific to joint conditions in the ankle and foot:

Rheumatoid arthritis (RA). This pathology commonly affects the forefoot and hindfoot and, less frequently, the ankle.[7] Involvement may occur in the talocrural, subtalar, and MTP joints of the foot leading to instabilities and painful deformities that increase with the stress of weight bearing.

Degenerative joint disease (DJD) and joint trauma. Degenerative symptoms occur in joints that are repetitively traumatized, and acute joint symptoms are often seen in conjunction with ankle sprains.[54]

Postimmobilization stiffness. Contractures and adhesions in the capsular tissues leading to joint hypomobilities as well as in the surrounding periarticular tissues may occur any time the joint is immobilized after a fracture or surgery.

Gout. Symptoms commonly affect the metatarsophalangeal joint of the great toe, causing pain during terminal stance so that there is a shorter stance and lack of smooth push-off.

Common Impairments

In RA, many of the following impairments and deformities occur with progression of the disease.[10,58] With DJD and post-immobilization stiffness, only the affected joint or joints will be limited.[8]

- ***Restricted motion.*** When symptoms are acute, there is swelling and restricted, painful motion; when chronic, there is restricted motion, decreased joint play, and a firm capsular end-feel in the affected joint.
  - ***Talocrural joint.*** Passive plantarflexion is more limited than dorsiflexion (unless the gastrocnemius-soleus muscle group is also shortened, in which case dorsiflexion will be limited accordingly).
  - ***Subtalar and transverse tarsal joints.*** Progressive limitation of supination develops until eventually the joint fixes in pronation with flattening of the medial longitudinal arch. The close-packed position of the tarsals (supination) becomes more and more difficult to assume during the terminal stance (push-off) phase of gait.
  - ***MTP joint of the large toe.*** Gross limitation of extension and some limitation of flexion develop; the rest of the MTP joints are variable. Lack of extension restricts the terminal stance phase of gait with an inability to rock up onto the metatarsal heads. This exacerbates the pronation posture

and inability to supinate the foot during push of in gait.

- ***Hallux valgus.*** This deformity develops as the proximal phalanx shifts laterally toward the second toe. Eventually the flexor and extensor muscles of the great (large) toe shift laterally and further accentuate the deformity. The bursa over the medial aspect of the metatarsal head may become inflamed and the bone hypertophies causing a painful bunion.
- ***Hallux rigidus.*** Narrowing and eventual obliteration of the first MTP joint space occurs with progressive loss of extension. This affects terminal stance, not allowing the foot to roll over the metatarsal heads and great toe for normal push-off. Instead the individual turns the foot outward and rolls over the medial aspect of the large toe. This faulty pattern accentuates hallux valgus and foot pronation, and usually the MTP joint is quite painful.
- ***Dorsal dislocation of the proximal phalanges on the metatarsal heads.*** If this occurs, the fat pad, which is normally under the metatarsal heads, migrates dorsally with the phalanges, and the protective cushion on weight bearing is lost, leading to pain, callus formation, and potential ulceration.
- ***Claw toe (MTP hyperextension and IP flexion) and hammer toe (MTP hyperextension, PIP flexion, and DIP hyperextension).*** These result from muscle imbalances between the intrinsic and extrinsic muscles of the toes. Friction from shoes may cause calluses to form where the toes rub.
- ***Decreased mobility in the proximal and distal tibiofibular joints.*** Restricted accessory motion in these joints usually occurs with periods of immobilization and will limit ankle and subtalar joint motion.[33]
- ***Muscle weakness and decreased muscular endurance.*** Inhibition from pain and decreased use of the extremities lead to impairment of muscle function.
- ***Impaired balance and postural control.*** The sensory receptors in the ankle joints and ligaments, as well as in the muscle spindles provide important information for posture and movement, known as the *ankle strategy.* The ankle strategy is used in balance control during perturbations.[22,51] Faulty feedback and balance deficits occur when there is instability, muscle impairments, or arthritis.
- ***Gait deviations.*** If there is pain on weight bearing, there will be a short stance phase, reduced single limb support, and decreased stride length on the side of involvement. Because of the restricting motion and loss of effective plantarflexion and supination in the arthritic foot, as well as pain in the forefoot area under the metatarsal heads, there is an ineffective push-off during terminal stance. Little or no heel rise occurs; instead the person lifts up the involved foot.

Common Functional Limitations/Disabilities

- ***Painful weight bearing.*** When symptoms are acute, weight-bearing activities will be painful, preventing independent ambulation and causing difficulty rising from a chair and ascending and descending stairs.
- ***Decreased ambulation.*** When symptoms are subacute or chronic with joint restrictions and weakness, ambulation will be decreased. At best there will be limitations on distance and speed, and the person may require use of assistive devices for ambulation; at worst the person will be unable to ambulate and, therefore, be bound to a wheelchair for mobility.
- ***Impaired balance.*** Impaired balance may lead to frequent falling or fear of falling and thus restricted community ambulation.

Management of Joint Hypomobility: Protection Phase

Management will depend on the signs and symptoms present. Follow the general outline as presented in Chapter 8 and summarized in Box 8–1 for acute joint problems. Suggested interventions for the various goals are described in this section.

Joint Protection and Patient Education

- ***Joint protection.*** Instruct the patient in the importance of protecting the feet from deforming weight-bearing forces and trauma imposed by improperly fitting footwear. Use orthotics and well-constructed shoes to help protect the joints by realigning forces and providing support from faulty foot postures.[38,40]
- ***Ambulation.*** Instruct the patient in safe use of assistive devices to decrease the effects of weight bearing and pain.

Decrease Pain

In addition to physician-prescribed medication or nonsteroidal anti-inflammatory medications and modalities, gentle grade I or II distraction and oscillation techniques may inhibit pain and move synovial fluid for nutrition in the involved joints.

Maintain Joint and Soft Tissue Mobility and Muscle Integrity

- ***Passive, active-assistive, or active ROM.*** It is important to move the joints as tolerated. If active exercises are tolerated, they are preferred for the benefits of muscle action.
- ***Aquatic therapy.*** Aquatic therapy is an effective method of combining nonstressful buoyancy-assisted exercises with therapeutic heat.
- ***Muscle setting.*** Apply gentle multiangle muscle-setting techniques in pain-free positions and at an intensity that does not exacerbate symptoms.

Joint Management: Controlled Motion and Return to Function Phases

Examine for signs of decreased muscle flexibility, joint restrictions, muscle weakness, and balance impairments. Initiate exercises and mobilization procedures at a level appropriate for the condition of the patient.

Precautions with RA: Modify the intensity of joint mobilization and stretching techniques that are used to counter any restrictions because the disease process and use of steroid therapy weaken the tensile quality of the connective tissue. Therefore, it is more easily torn. It may be necessary to continue joint protection with orthotics, proper fitting shoes, and assistive devices for ambulation.[58] Encourage the patient to be active, but also respect pain and fatigue.

Increase Joint Play and Accessory Motions

Joint Mobilization Techniques

Determine which of the articulations are restricted owing to decreased joint play, and apply grade III sustained or grade III and IV oscillation techniques to stretch the limitations. See Figures 6–56 through 6–65 and their descriptions in Chapter 6 for techniques to mobilize the leg, ankle, and foot articulations. Mobilizing the toes is the same as the fingers (see Figs. 6–42 through 6–44).

Note: Since weight-bearing forces and joint changes with arthritis accentuate pronation, mobilizing to increase pronation usually should not be undertaken in the arthritic foot. Perform these techniques only in the stiff foot after immobilization when the foot does not effectively pronate during the loading response in gait. In addition, extension of the great toe to at least 50 degrees is important during terminal stance for normal push off and development of the windlass effect in gait.[37,47]

Improve Joint Tracking of the Talocrural Joint

Apply mobilization with movement (MWM) techniques to increase ROM and/or decrease pain associated with movement.[43] (The principles of MWM are described in Chapter 6.)

Plantarflexion MWM

- Patient position: Supine with hip and knee flexed and heel on the table.
- Procedure: Stand at the foot of the table facing the patient and contact the patient's anterior tibia with the palm of your hand (for the right foot use the left hand). Produce a pain-free graded posterior glide of the tibia on the talus. The patient should now be unable to plantarflex.
- While maintaining the posterior tibial glide grip the talus with your other hand (for the right foot, use the right hand) and create a passive end-range plantarflexion movement, causing the talus to roll anteriorly.
- The sustained plantarflexion must be painless. Repeat three to four times in sets of six to 10 and reassess to confirm improved range (Fig. 14–1).

Dorsiflexion MWM

- Patient position and procedure: Standing with the affected foot placed on a chair or stool. Kneel on the floor facing patient with a mobilization belt around your buttocks and the patient's Achilles tendon (padded with towel).
- Place the web space of both hands around the neck of the talus with the palms on the dorsum of the foot. Hold the foot down and back and the subtalar joint in neutral pronation/supination.
- Use the belt to produce a pain-free graded anterior gliding force to the ankle joint
- While maintaining this mobilization, have the patient lunge forward bringing the affected ankle into dorsiflexion and causing painless end-range loading. Repeat in sets of six to 10 and reassessing for effect (Fig. 14–2).

Increase Mobility of the Soft Tissue and Muscles

Perform passive stretching and inhibition techniques as described in Chapter 5. Self-stretching techniques are described later in this chapter.

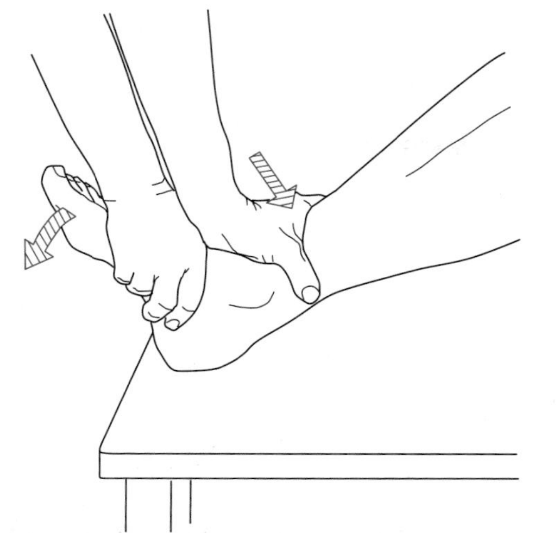

Figure 14–1 Mobilization with movement to increase ankle plantarflexion. Maintain a posterior glide of the tibia while moving the talus into planterflexion. This should not cause pain.

Regain a Balance in Muscle Strength and Prepare for Functional Activities

Begin resistive exercises at a level appropriate for the weakened muscles. Begin with isometric resistance in pain-free positions, and progress to dynamic resistance exercises through pain-free ranges using

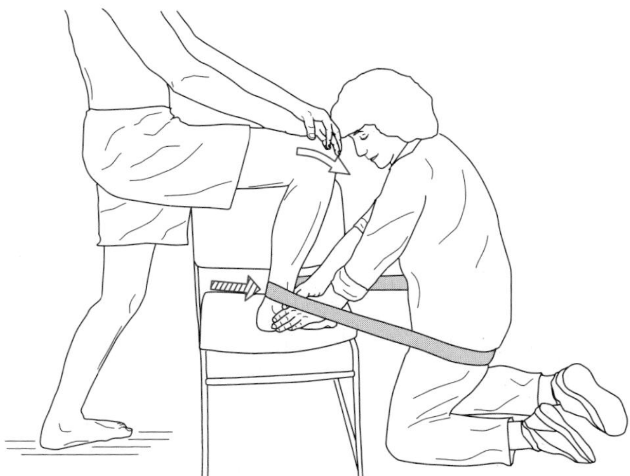

Figure 14–2 Mobilization with movement to increase ankle dorsiflexion. Maintain an anterior glide of the tibia with the mobilization belt while the patient lunges forward to move the ankle into dorsiflexion. This should not cause pain.

open- and closed-chain exercises. Resistive exercises are described later in this chapter. Low-load, weight-bearing exercises may be initiated in a pool or tank and progressed to full weight bearing as tolerated. Develop exercises that prepare the patient to return to functional activities.

Stimulate Balance and Proprioception

Initiate protected balance exercises, and progress the intensity as tolerated. Determine the level of stability and safety during ambulation and continue use of assistive devices if necessary to help prevent falls.

Develop Cardiovascular/Pulmonary Fitness

Low-impact aerobic exercises should be initiated early in the treatment program and progressed as the patient is able. Repetitive exercises in a pool (water aerobics), swimming, treadmill walking, and bicycling may be within the patient's tolerance. A person with degenerative or rheumatoid arthritis should not do high-impact (jumping, hopping, and jogging) aerobic exercises.

Patient Education

Progress the home exercise program to the level of the patient's abilities. Teach the patient to be aware of signs of systemic fatigue (especially in RA), local muscle fatigue, and joint stress, and how to modify exercises and activities to remain active within safe levels. Emphasize the importance of daily ROM and endurance activities and joint protection, including avoidance of faulty foot and ankle postures. For patients with RA, teach them to be aware of signs and symptoms of the disease so that proper measures can be taken to protect the feet and minimize deforming forces.

► Joint Surgery and Postoperative Management

Chronic arthritis of the ankle and foot can lead to severe pain, limitation of motion, gross instability or deformity, and significantly impaired function of the lower extremities. Surgical management includes *arthroscopic débridement or cheilectomy* (removal of osteophytes most often along the dorsum of the MTP joint or the anterior aspect of the tibiotalar joint), *soft tissue reconstruction, synovectomy, arthrodesis, total joint replacement,* or *excision arthroplasty* with or without implant. The choice of surgery depends upon the degree of articular damage, the severity of joint deformity or instability, and the postoperative functional goals of the patient. For example, soft tissue procedures coupled with excision or implant arthroplasty or arthrodesis may be appropriate surgical options for late-stage joint destruction and deformity of the forefoot, most often at the MTP joints.[2,7] Arthrodesis, such as a *triple arthrodesis* or a *subtalar arthrodesis,* provides pain-free weight bearing and stability of the fused joint(s). It is the procedure of choice for most patients, particularly those with high functional demands, but sacrifices mobility of one or more joints of the ankle. Pain-free compensatory movements must be available in adjacent joints to absorb weight-bearing forces during ambulation. Arthroplasty of the ankle, which is used far less frequently than arthrodesis, is an alternative for patients with severe bilateral disease but low functional demands in whom bilateral ankle fusions would be impractical and would dramatically restrict functional mobility such as ascending or descending stairs or rising from a chair.

The goals of joint surgery and a postoperative rehabilitation program include (1) relief of pain with weight bearing and joint motion, (2) stability of the ankle and foot joints for ambulation and functional activities, (3) improvement of joint motion and strength, and (4) correction of deformity.[2,7,53,69] The rehabilitation program includes postoperative exercise, gait training with assistive devices, fabrication of foot orthoses, and patient education including information on shoe fit and selection, as well the appropriate choices of recreational and daily living activities.[7]

Total Ankle Replacement Arthroplasty

Indications for Surgery

The following are frequent indications for total joint replacement of the ankle although at the present time no consensus exists.[7,30,53,54,56,67,69]

- Severe tibiotalar joint deterioration and disabling pain secondary to RA or DJD
- Marked limitation of motion of the ankle joints bilaterally
- An alternative to arthrodesis for the patient with low-intensity functional demands but good ligamentous stability at the ankle

Note: The components of a total ankle arthroplasty do not improve stability of the ankle. Patients with a very unstable ankle, vascular deficiency, inadequate bone density, a neuropathic joint, muscle imbalances at the ankle, or active infection are not appropriate candidates for this procedure.[30,54,69] In contrast, the patient with bilateral ankle or ipsolateral hindfoot arthritis who will require or has had a triple arthrodesis is a good candidate for total ankle arthroplasty.[54]

Procedure

Total ankle arthroplasty, first performed in the 1970s and into the 1980s, involved the use of a two-component metal-to-plastic implant held in place with cement fixation.[30,53,54,67,69] Current-day total ankle arthroplasty involves two- or three-component designs and relies on bioingrowth (cementless) fixation.[30,53,54,56] A hydroxyapatite coating on the implant surfaces increases the rate of bone ingrowth. The tibial implant, made of metal, has a beaded outer surface and a plastic articulating surface. The talar surface, also made of metal, has a beaded outer surface and metal articulating surface. The design of a total ankle prothesis allows dorsiflexion, plantarflexion, and a small degree of rotation of the foot on the tibia.[30,54]

An anterior midline incision or sometimes a posterior incision is made to expose the joint surfaces. Minimal bone is excised prior to insertion of the implants. After insertion of the implants, soft tissues are repaired, and the wound is closed. A bulky compression dressing is placed on the foot and ankle to control joint swelling and peripheral edema.

Postoperative Management

Immobilization and Weight Bearing

Because biological fixation is now routinely used, the ankle is immobilized in a well-padded, short-leg splint in a neutral position for at least 3 weeks if the prosthetic implants have a hydroxyapatite coating or approximately 6 weeks for beaded implants without a coating.[54] Intially the patient must remain non-weight-bearing on the operated foot (3–6 weeks) and then may progress to partial weight bearing and eventually full weight bearing while wearing a short-leg splint. The immobilizer may be discontinued when the patient's ankle is pain-free while full weight bearing during ambulation. The foot is elevated at all times in the early postoperative period when the patient is in bed. Elevation prevents or minimizes edema, which can contribute to poor wound healing.

Exercise: Maximum Protection Phase

- While the ankle is immobilized, begin isometric (muscle-setting) exercises of the ankle musculature, gluteal, and quadriceps muscles. Gentle active-resistive hip and knee exercises can also be performed in preparation for walking.[59]
- Strengthen the nonoperated lower extremity and upper extremities by resisted exercises in preparation for ambulation.
- Regain ROM when it is permissible to remove the immobilization and if wound healing is sufficient. Initiate active, open-chain dorsiflexion and plantarflexion. The patient will need about 10 degrees of dorsiflexion and 25 degrees of plantarflexion for normal walking and about 50 to 60 degrees of ankle motion for ascending and descending stairs.[53] If the design of the prosthetic components allows, active open-chain inversion, eversion, and circumduction can also be initiated.

Note: There is a lack of evidence and consensus as to whether ROM exercises should be intiated a few days postoperatively or delayed for several weeks until there is evidence of bone ingrowth into the implants. It is also unclear whether early protected motion has a positive impact on ROM outcomes (greater long-term ROM) or if it is detrimental to implant fixation or wound healing.[54]

Exercise: Moderate and Minimum Protection Phases

- Continue ROM exercises. The goal is to achieve 100% of the range observed intraoperatively by 6 weeks.[54]
- Increase strength of ankle musculature in an open-chain with dynamic resistance exercises against light-grade elastic tubing.
- Add strengthening exercises in a closed-chain even when weight bearing must be restricted, by performing ankle motions in a *seated* position with the foot on a BAPS (balance or rocker) board. (See Fig 14–5.) Then when partial or full weight bearing is permissible, progress to bilateral and then unilateral closed-chain exercises to improve strength and balance. (A variety of progressive weight-bearing exercises are described in the last section of this chapter.)
- Stretch the plantarflexors, if dorsiflexion is restricted, using towel stretches in a long-sitting position, or have the patient stand on a wedge for an extended period (see Fig. 14–3).
- Initiate and progress a stationary cycling program and progress the speed and distance of ambulation to increase cardiopulmonary fitness and lower extremity muscular endurance. The amount of dorsiflexion required during pedaling can be adjusted by raising or lowering the seat height.
- Gradually return to a desired level of functional activity. Select nonimpact or low-impact activities for joint protection.

Outcomes

The long-term success of total ankle arthroplasty is still in question. Early total ankle arthroplasty afforded pain relief[59] but was associated with a high rate of failure due to poor wound healing, infection and septic as well as biomechanical loosening.[7,30,53,54,56] Although postoperative gains in ROM have been reported to be small (often as little as 5–10 degrees), even small gains can improve functional mobility.[54]

Advances in prosthetic design, improved surgical techniques, use of biological fixation, and more judicious selection of patients are expected to decrease short- and long-term complications and improve outcomes, but long-term follow-up studies are not yet available.[30,53,54]

Arthrodesis at the Ankle and Foot

Indications for Surgery

The following are frequent indications for surgical fusion of selected joints of the ankle and foot.[7,28,53]

- Severe articular damage and pain with weight bearing at any number of joints of the ankle or foot secondary to rheumatoid, degenerative, or post-traumatic arthritis
- Instability of a weight-bearing joint
- Deformity of the toes, foot, or ankle
- Patients with high functional demands and pain-free compensatory movements in adjacent joints
- A salvage procedure after failed total ankle arthroplasty

Procedures

The procedures, all of which provide bony ankylosis by means of bone grafts coupled with internal fixation and external skeletal fixation with compression, vary depending on the joints involved and types of deformity.[2,7,28,53]

Some common procedures include:

Triple arthrodesis of the ankle. This procedure involves stabilization of the hindfoot, usually in 5 degrees of valgus, by fusion of the talocalcaneal, calcaneocuboid, and talonavicular joints. It provides permanent medial-lateral stability and relief of pain in the subtalar joint, but pronation and supination of the ankle are lost.

Arthrodesis of the tibiotalar joint. This procedure involves fusion of the tibia and talus in neutral or approximately 5 degrees of dorsiflexion and 5 to 10 degrees of external rotation of the foot on the tibia. It provides relief of pain and stability at the tibiotalar joint.[28] Dorsiflexion and plantarflexion are lost, significantly affecting the biomechanics and speed of gait. The forefoot must be stable and pain-free to compensate for the loss of motion at the ankle.

Note: Bilateral tibiotalar arthrodesis is usually not appropriate as it makes it difficult to get up from a chair or to ascend or descend stairs.

Arthrodesis of the first toe. Fusion of the first MTP joint for *hallux rigidus* and *hallux valgus* provides relief of pain during ambulation. If the lateral MTP joints are also involved, MTP fusion should be performed after, not before, excision or implant arthroplasty of those joints.[2,7] The position of fusion is 15 to 30 degrees of MTP extension, which allows adequate push-off during ambulation and enables the patient to wear some types of commercially available shoes.[7]

Arthrodesis of the IP joints of the toes. Fusion of the IP joints of the toes in a neutral position for *hammer toes,* usually occurring in the second and third toes, provides relief of pain for ambulation and correction of deformities of the toes.

Postoperative Management

- The fused joints are immobilized for approximately 6 to 12 weeks. The patient must be nonweight-bearing for at least 6 weeks and then may progress to partial weight bearing in an immobilizer.
- Active ROM exercises must be performed to maintain mobility in any other joints affected by arthritis.
- The patient should be advised of proper shoe selection, modification, and fit when the immobilization device is discontinued. The use of custom-made foot orthoses may also be indicated for support, relief of pressure, or shock absorption.[7]

Outcomes

The long-term results of arthrodesis of the ankle or joints of the hindfoot or forefoot depend on the joints that are fused as well as disease and deformity of nonfused joints. Arthrodesis remains the procedure of choice for pain, instability, and arthrosis of the tibiotalar and subtalar joints.[7,53,54] When healing is complete, pain relief and stability are predictable outcomes, resulting in improved functional mobility.

Nevertheless, arthrodesis of involved joints imposes increased stresses on and eventual deterioration of contiguous joints, potentially leading to long-term loss of function.[54] Careful shoe selection, use of foot orthoses, and modification of ADL may improve the long-term outcomes (beyond 7–10 years) after arthodesis.[54]

▶ Overuse Syndromes/ Repetitive Trauma Syndromes

Related Diagnoses and Etiology of Symptoms

An overuse syndrome is a local inflammatory response to stresses from repetitive microtrauma, which may be from faulty alignment in the lower extremity, muscle imbalances or fatigue, changes in exercise or functional routines, training errors, improper footwear for the ground or functional demands placed on the feet, or a combination of several of these factors.[18] The syndrome occurs because continued demand is placed on the tissue before it has adequately healed, so the pain and inflammation continue. A common cause predisposing the foot to overuse syndromes is abnormal pronation of the subtalar joint. The abnormal pronation could be related to a variety of causes including excessive joint mobility, leg-length discrepancy, femoral anteversion, external tibial torsion, genu valgum, or muscle flexibility and strength imbalances.

Tendinitis and Tenosynovitis

Any of the tendons of the extrinsic muscles to the foot may become irritated as they approach and cross over the ankle or where they attach in the foot. Pain occurs during or after repetitive activity. When the foot and ankle are tested, pain is experienced at the site of the lesion as resistance is applied to the muscle action and also when the involved tendon is placed on a stretch or palpated.[3,18,44] A common site for symptoms is proximal to the calcaneus in the Achilles tendon or its sheath (Achilles tendinitis or peritendinitis). Symptoms may develop when the person switches from high-heeled shoes to low-heeled shoes and then does a lot of walking.[18,34] Symptoms in the anterior or posterior tibialis tendons, or peroneus tendons, are also associated with athletic activities such as running, tennis, and basketball.[36,44,50] Usually there is a hypomobile gastrocnemius-soleus complex and abnormal foot pronation.

Plantar Fascitis

Pain is usually experienced along the plantar aspect of the heel where the plantar fascia inserts on the medial tubercle of the calcaneus. The site of the injury is very tender to palpation. Excessive pronation of the subtalar joint, which may be reinforced by hypomobile gastrocnemius-soleus muscles, predisposes the foot to abnormal forces and irritation of the plantar fascia. Conversely, stress forces on the fascia can also occur with an excessively high arch (cavus foot). Pressure transmitted to the irritated site with weight bearing or stretch forces to the fascia, as when extending the toes during push-off, causes pain.

A heel spur may develop at the site of irritation on the calcaneus causing pain whenever the heel is on the ground. The individual usually avoids heel-strike during the loading response of gait.

Shin Splints

This term is used to describe activity-induced leg pain along the posterior medial or anterior lateral aspects of the proximal two-thirds of the tibia. It may include different pathologic conditions such as musculotendinitis, stress fractures of the tibia, periosteitis, increased pressure in a muscular compartment, or irritation of the interosseous membrane.

Anterior shin splints. Most common is overuse of the anterior tibialis muscle. A hypomobile gastrocnemius-soleus complex and a weak anterior tibialis muscle, as well as foot pronation, are associated with anterior shin splints. Pain increases with active dorsiflexion and when the muscle is stretched into plantarflexion.

Posterior shin splints. A tight gastrocnemius-soleus complex and a weak or inflamed posterior tibialis muscle, along with foot pronation, are associated with posterior medial shin splints. Pain is experienced when the foot is passively dorsiflexed with eversion and with active supination. Muscle fatigue with vigorous exercise, such as running or aerobic dancing, may precipitate the problem.

Common Impairments

- Pain with repetitive activity, on palpation of the involved site, when the involved musculotendinous unit is stretched, and with resistance to the involved muscle
- Pain with weight-bearing activities and gait
- Muscle length-strength imbalances, especially tight gastrocnemius-soleus muscle group
- Abnormal foot posture (may be from faulty footwear)

Common Functional Limitations/Disabilities

- Decreased distance or speed of ambulation
- Restriction of sport or recreational activities
- Limited ability to wear nonsupportive footwear

Management of Overuse/Repetitive Trauma Syndromes: Protection Phase

While inflamed, the leg or foot symptoms should be treated as an acute condition with rest and appropriate modalities[9] (see Chapter 8). Immobilization in a cast or splint with the foot slightly plantarflexed or a heel lift inside the shoe may be used to relieve stress.[36,50]

- Apply cross-friction massage to the site of the lesion.
- Initiate gentle muscle-setting contractions or electrical stimulation to the involved muscle in pain-free positions.
- Teach active ROM within the pain-free ranges.
- Instruct the patient to avoid the activity that provokes the pain.
- Use supportive taping of the arch of the foot to provide relief of symptoms.

Management: Controlled Motion and Return to Function Phases

When symptoms become subacute, the entire lower extremity as well as the foot should be examined for abnormal alignment or muscle flexibility and strength imbalances. Eliminating or modifying the cause is important to prevent recurrences. Orthotic devices may be necessary to correct alignment.[11,36,38,50] Therapeutic exercises may be helpful to increase flexibility, and, in general, improve muscle performance. Detailed descriptions of stretching and strengthening exercises for the ankle and foot are in the last sections of this chapter.

Stretch Range-Limiting Structures

- The gastrocnemius-soleus muscle complex is frequently hypomobile with foot problems and should be stretched. Restricted mobility causes the foot to pronate when the ankle dorsiflexes.
- With plantar fasciitis and heel spurs, mobilize the plantar fascia with deep massage across the plantar fascia. Instruct the patient to roll a ball or cylinder under the medial longitudinal arch of the foot for self-stretching.

Improve Muscle Performance

- Begin with resistive isometric and progress to resistive dynamic (including isokinetic) exercises to the foot and ankle in open- and closed-chain activities. Develop a balance in strength between the muscle groups, especially the invertors and evertors for medial and lateral support.
- With plantar fasciitis, the intrinsic muscles need to be strengthened. Include exercises that require toe control such as scrunching tissue paper or a towel and picking up marbles and other small objects with the toes.
- In addition to general strengthening of the extrinsic and intrinsic muscles of the foot, place emphasis on muscular endurance, and train the muscles to respond to eccentric loading.

Patient Education

- Teach prevention. This includes:
  - Gentle repetitive warm-up activities followed by stretching of tight muscles prior to intense exercise.
  - Use of proper foot support for the ground conditions (this cannot be overemphasized).
  - Allow time for recovery from microtrauma after high-intensity workouts.

Note: With plantar fasciitis the patient experiences the greatest pain when first bearing weight, especially in the morning and after prolonged sitting. Teach the patient to do ROM exercises (especially dorsiflexion) or alphabet writing with the foot for several minutes prior to standing.

▶ Traumatic Soft Tissue Injuries

Sprains and Minor Tears of Ligaments

Mechanisms and Sites of Injuries

After trauma, the ligaments of the ankle may be stressed or torn. The most common type of ankle sprain is caused by an inversion stress and can result in a partial or complete tear of the anterior talofibular (ATF) ligament;[23,27,52] the posterior talofibular ligament (PTF) is torn only with massive inversion stresses. If the inferior tibiofibular ligaments are torn after stress to the ankle, the mortise becomes unstable. Rarely do the components of the deltoid ligament become stressed; there is greater likelihood of an avulsion from or fracture of the medial malleolus with an eversion stress. Depending on the severity of injury, the joint capsule may also be involved, and intra-articular pathology, including articular cartilage lesions, may also occur,[31] resulting in symptoms of acute (traumatic) arthritis.

Common Impairments

- Pain when the injured tissue is stressed in mild to moderate injuries
- Excessive motion or instability of the related joint with complete tears
- Proprioceptive deficit manifested as decreased ability to perceive passive motion and development of balance impairments[15]
- Related joint symptoms and reflex muscle inhibition

Common Functional Limitations/Disabilities

- When symptoms are acute, may not be able to bear weight, thus requiring assisted ambulation
- Recurrences of injuries with instabilities; may have increased incidence of falling and safety problems

Nonoperative Management: Protection Phase

See Chapter 8 for principles of treatment during stages of inflammation and repair.

- If possible, examine the ankle before joint effusion occurs. To minimize the swelling, use compression, elevation, and ice. The ankle should be immobilized in neutral or in slight dorsiflexion and eversion.
- Patient instruction
  - Teach the patient the importance of RICE (rest, ice, compression, and elevation) and to apply the ice every 2 hours during the first 24 to 48 hours.
  - Teach partial weight bearing with crutches to decrease the stress of ambulation.[17,49,68]
  - Teach muscle-setting techniques and active toe curls to help maintain muscle integrity and assist with circulation.

Controlled Motion Phase

- As the acute symptoms decrease, continue to provide protection for the involved ligament with a splint during weight bearing. Fabricating a stirrup out of thermoplastic material and holding it in place with an elastic wrap or Velcro straps provide stability to the joint structures while allowing for the stimulus of weight bearing for proprioceptive feedback and proper healing.[49] Commercial splints such as an air splint are also available to provide medial-lateral stability while allowing dorsiflexion and plantarflexion.[29]

- Apply cross-fiber massage to the ligaments as tolerated.
- Use grade II joint mobilization techniques to maintain mobility of the joint.
- Teach the patient exercises to be done within tissue tolerance at least three times per day. Suggestions include:
  - Nonweight-bearing AROM into dorsiflexion and plantarflexion, inversion and eversion, toe curls and writing the alphabet in the air with the foot.
  - Sitting with the heel on floor and scrunching paper or a towel and picking up marbles with the toes.
  - If there are adhesions developing in the healing ligament, have the patient actively move the foot in the direction opposite the line of pull of the ligament. For the anterior talofibular ligament, the motion is plantarflexion and inversion. Also stretch the gastrocnemius-soleus muscle group for adequate dorsiflexion. Progress to weight-bearing stretches when the patient's recovery allows.
  - As swelling decreases and weight-bearing tolerance increases, progress to strengthening, endurance and stabilization exercises; include isometric resistance to the peroneals, bicycle ergometry, and partial to full weight-bearing balance board exercises. Have the patient wear a brace or splint that restricts end-range motion to control the range and prevent excessive stress on the healing ligament.[17]

Return to Function Phase

- Progress strengthening exercises by adding elastic resistance to foot movements in long-sitting (open-chain) and sitting with the heel on the floor for partial weight bearing. Use isokinetic resistance if a unit is available.
- Progress stabilization and balance training for ankle stability, coordination, and reflex response with full weight-bearing activities on a rocker, wobble, or BAPS board.[16,51,70] Depending on the final goals for rehabilitation, train the ankle with weight-bearing activities such as walking, jogging, and running and with agility activities such as controlled twisting, turning, and lateral weight shifting.
- When the patient is involved in sports activities, the ankle should be splinted, taped, or wrapped, and proper shoes should be worn to protect the ligament from reinjury.[17]

Complete Ligament Tears: Surgical Repair and Postoperative Management

A third degree (grade 3) sprain of the lateral ankle, which usually occurs as the result of a severe inversion injury, often causes a complete tear or rupture of the anterior talofibular (ATF) ligament and less frequently disruption of the calcaneofibular (CF) ligament.[14,34,63] A transverse fracture of the lateral malleolus or an avulsion fracture of the base of the fifth metatarsal may also occur with severe inversion injuries.[14,44,52] A complete tear of one or more ligaments causes marked mechanical instability and functional instability (giving way) of the ankle (reported to be as high as 20% after ankle sprain[6]), which significantly impairs an individual's daily activities.[6,14,34,44,48,63] Surgical repair or reconstruction of acutely injured or chronically lax lateral ankle structures may be required to return a patient to a desired level of function. The goal of surgery and postoperative management is to restore joint stability but retain functional ROM of the ankle.[14,19,52,61,63]

Indications for Surgery

The following are frequent indications for surgical repair or reconstruction of the soft tissues of the lateral aspect of the ankle.[14,34,48,57,61,63]

- Acute third degree lateral ankle sprain resulting in a complete tear of the ATF and/or CF ligaments.
- Chronic functional instability of the ankle that is characterized by "giving way" during activity and remains unresolved after conservative management.

Procedures

Types of procedures. There are a number of open and arthroscopic surgical procedures that may be used to repair and reconstruct the lateral ligaments and associated structures of the ankle. They include the modified Brostrom, Chrisman-Snook, Evans, and Watson-Jones procedures.[6,14,19,21,48,57,61,63]

These procedures may involve a direct end-to-end suturing (anatomic repair) combined with imbrication (plication) of lax ligaments for a double layer of reinforcement, or reinsertion of the ligament to bone. Stability is augumented by pulling the fascia of the extensor retinaculum proximally over the repaired structures and suturing it to the fibula. The lateral complex may also be reinforced with a peroneus brevis tendon autograft when the quality of repair of the injured structures is insufficient for satisfactory stabilization.

Operative overview. An arthroscopy is first performed to assess the extent of intra-articular pathology, because a high percentage (93%) of patients with complete tears of one or more lateral ligaments also exhibit associated joint pathology, including articular cartilage lesions.[31] After arthroscopy an obilique or vertical incision is made at the lateral aspect of the ankle. Torn or ruptured structures are identified, repaired, and reinforced. ROM is checked prior to wound closure. The goal is to retain full ROM. The foot and ankle are then placed in a compressive dressing and well-padded, short-leg cast and elevated for control of joint swelling and peripheral edema.

Postoperative Management

In the past decade there has been a trend to allow early postoperative weight bearing while the ankle is immobilized and early but protected ROM after lateral ligament reconstruction. Exercise progression after surgery is similar to that used for nonoperative management of lateral ankle sprains.

Immobilization and Weight Bearing

The ankle is immobilized in 0 degrees of dorsiflexion and slight eversion for 4 to 6 weeks. Initially the patient must remain nonweight-bearing on the operated extremity. During the first 1 to 2 weeks after surgery a walking cast is placed on the foot and ankle, enabling the patient to begin progressive weight bearing as tolerated.[14,44] At 3 to 4 weeks the walking cast is removed and replaced with an air splint or ankle brace, which is worn for an additional 4 to 8 weeks.[14]

Exercise: Maximum Protection Phase

- While the ankle is immobilized, perform active or gentle resisted exercises of the hip and knee on the involved side to maintain strength in the lower extremity.
- Gentle, pain-free muscle setting of the ankle musculature is also appropriate when the ankle is immobilized. Place emphasis on isometric contractions of the peroneal muscle.
- Initiate pain-free, assisted or active dorsiflexion and plantarflexion to begin to regain ROM as soon as the immobilizer may be removed for exercise as determined by the surgeon (possibly by 4 or as late as 6 weeks postoperatively).
- When weight bearing is permissible and if the immobilizer, such as a splint, allows some degree of dorsi- and plantarflexion, begin mini-squats in bilateral stance.

Precaution: Intiation of early motion requires careful patient education to ensure that ROM is progressed very gradually and to avoid excessive stress on the healing tissues of the lateral ankle complex. Have the patient postpone inversion and supination movements until 6 to 8 weeks postoperatively.

Exercise: Moderate and Minimum Protection Phases

By 6 to 8 weeks postoperatively only moderate protection of healing structures is necessary as joint symptoms subside. Emphasis is placed on gradual restoration of ankle ROM as well as improving strength, endurance, neuromuscular control and balance responses in the involved ankle. In the final phase of rehabilitation when only minimal protection is required, the emphasis of management is a gradual return to functional activities by 12 to 18 weeks postoperatively or when the strength of ankle musculature reaches 80 to 90% compared to the noninvolved lower extremity.

- Increase strength of all ankle muscles in open- and closed-chain positions. After surgical repair of the lateral ligaments, improving strength of the evertors is particularly important for increased support of the ankle. Isometric strengthening of the evertors can be achieved by having the patient cross the ankles and press the lateral borders of the feet together. Dynamic strengthening of the evertors against elastic resistance is also appropriate (see Fig. 14–7).
- Retrain neuromuscular control, balance, and stability at the ankle with exercises first on a soft surface, such as foam, and then on a balance board. Begin with bilateral and progress to unilateral standing activities.

Note: Balance training has been shown to be an effective means of improving joint proprioception and single leg standing ability in patients with funtionally unstable ankles[51,70] and therefore is also appropriate after lateral ligament reconstruction.

- Continue active ROM exercises, adding eversion and then inversion.
- Perform grade III joint mobilizations to increase dorsiflexion and plantaflexion but avoid stretch mobilization of the subtalar joint in a lateral direction.
- Add gentle manual or self-stretching activities to restore muscle flexibility. Initially open-chain stretching or closed-chain stretching in a *seated* position is advisable because closed-chain stretching with the patient standing imposes significant ground reaction forces on the repaired ligaments. Emphasize restoration of dorsiflexion and plantarflexion before inversion and eversion.
- Initiate swimming, stationary bicycling or treadmill walking to improve muscular endurance and cardiopulmonary fitness.
- Further progression of exercises is similar to exercises associated with conservative (nonoperative) management of ankle sprains. Include dynamic resistance exercises as well as progressive closed-chain functional activities.
- Taping the ankle or inserting a slight lateral lift in the shoe may be useful to prevent reinjury during high-demand functional activities.[34,40,44]

Outcomes

A successful postoperative outcome after lateral ankle reconstruction is an ankle that has full mobility but remains stable and pain-free during functional activities. At this time, an open approach and reconstruction provides more predictable long-term results than arthroscopic procedures.[6] In some instances, although not an optimal result, a slight loss of inversion (possibly 10 degrees) occurs.[61]

A review of the literature of patients with chronic lateral ankle instability indicated that 87 to 95% of patients report good to excellent results after surgery.[48] Equally good results have been reported in a postoperative follow-up study of ballet dancers.[19] Another study compared two types of lateral ankle reconstruction, one using anatomic repair (Brostrom procedure) and the other involving augmentation with the pero-neus brevis (Chrisman-Snook).[21] Both procedures yielded good to excellent results in 80% of patients, but the latter was associated with a higher rate of complications.

Rupture of the Achilles Tendon: Surgical Repair and Postoperative Management

Rupture of the Achilles tendon usually is the result of a sudden and forceful eccentric contraction of the gastrocnemius and soleus muscles (triceps surae).[24,34,44] It occurs most frequently in older adults (>40 years of age) with compromised blood supply to the tendon. In young, active individuals a rupture can occur during high-intensity weight-bearing activities such as jumping and landing activities or movements that require rapid deceleration. The tendon usually ruptures proximal to the distal insertion of the tendon on the calcaneus.[20] A complete rupture leads to pain, swelling, and significant weakness in plantarflexion and is associated with a positive Thompson test (absence of reflexive plantarflexion when the patient is prone-lying and the calf is squeezed).[66] Although rupture of the Achilles tendon can be managed conservatively, surgery is indicated when the torn fragments cannot be reapposed with positioning and immobilization.[5,34,44,57,65]

Indications for Surgery

- Complete rupture of the Achilles tendon in which end-to-end apposition cannot be achieved by conservative means.[5]
- More frequently indicated for the active individual who wishes to return to high-demand functional activities.[5]

Procedures

There are a considerable number of surgical options for repair of a ruptured Achilles tendon.[4,5,41,42,57] The repair is usually performed 1 week after the injury to allow time for the tendon ends to consolidate, making repair easier. Either an open or percutaneous approach can be used.[64] Acute ruptures are usually managed with a direct repair in which the ends of the torn tendon are reopposed and sutured together. The repair site may or may not be reinforced by some method of tissue augmentation such as a plantaris tendon graft. Late-stage reconstruction of a chronic rupture routinely requires reinforcement by an autograft, allograft, or tendon transfer.

In an open procedure, an incision is made at the distal leg just medial to the gastrocnemius muscle. The tendon ends are identified and then reopposed and sutured together while the ankle is maintained in a neutral position. Prior to closure the ankle is moved through the ROM to assess the stability of the repair. A posterior splint and compressive dressing are applied after closure.

Postoperative Management—Early-Motion Approach

Traditional postoperative management, which is still the most commonlyly used approach, requires 6 to 8 weeks of continuous immobilization with the ankle held in slight plantarflexion for 3 to 4 weeks and then in a neutral position for an additional 3 to 4 weeks. The patient must remain nonweight-bearing on the operated extremity for the first 3 to 4 weeks while the ankle is immobilized in plantarflexion. Remobilization of the ankle typically begins at 6 to 8 weeks.

Extended immobilization, traditionally thought to be necessary to protect the healing tendon, has been shown to lead to significant deficits in strength, particularly in the plantarflexors, and a loss of ROM of the ankle.[3,24,41,64,65] In recent years for carefully selected patients, there has been a trend to minimize the period of continuous postoperative immobilization and initiate early ankle ROM within a protected range and early weight bearing in a functional orthosis.[3,20,24,39,41,42,62] This approach to postoperative management has been advocated only if the surgical repair of the Achilles tendon includes some form of augmentation to reinforce the repair.[4,39,41,42,62]

Note: The postoperative management discussed in this section reflects an *accelerated/early motion,* rather than traditional, approach to exercise after an augmented reconstruction with specialized suturing. The approach emphasizes early, protected but not aggressive ROM, combined with progressive weight bearing. Application of knowledge of the stages of tissue healing is particularly important to safely stress yet protect the healing tissues. Close communication among the surgeon, therapist, and patient is essential for success with this approach to postoperative management.

Regardless of whether a traditional (delayed-motion) or an early motion apprach to postoperative management is employed, careful attention to wound healing and elevation of the operated leg to control joint swelling and peripheral edema are essential in the early postoperative weeks.

Immobilization and Weight Bearing

After surgery, the patient wears a short-leg (bootlike) functional dorsal orthosis that is hinged and can be locked or adjusted and initially holds the ankle in slight plantarflexion.[6,20] The orthosis is worn at all times except when removed for wound care and exercises. It is adjusted to neutral by 2 weeks postoperatively. During the first 2 weeks after surgery, the patient must remain nonweight-bearing on the operated extremity. Then weight bearing is initiated in the protective orthosis and gradually progressed from partial to weight bearing as tolerated. When the patient is able to ambulate on level surfaces without pain while full weight bearing on the operated extremity, the protective boot is discontinued (usually by 8–10 weeks postoperatively.) Patients may wear a 1-cm heel lift to decrease ground reaction forces during functional activities after discontinuing the functional splint.[41]

Exercise: Maximum Protection Phase

The following exercises are implemented to prevent reflex inhibition of muscle and minimize joint swelling or stiffness and loss of mobility of soft tissues. Despite the initiation of early motion, considerable protection of the repaired tendon is required for the first 4 to 6 weeks.

- Within the first day or two after surgery perform submaximal, pain-free muscle setting of the ankle while wearing the immobilizer. First implement low-intensity, isometric inversion and eversion, and by 3 to 4 weeks, add gently resisted isometrics of the dorsiflexors and plantarflexors. When permissible, perform the same sequence of isometric exercises while out of the immobilizer.
- While wearing a hinged, functional orthosis that allows limited dorsiflexion or when the short-leg splint may be removed for exercise (as early as a few days to 2–4 weeks after surgery),[3,39,41,62] begin toe flexion and extension and very gentle assisted or active ROM exercises of the operated ankle *within a protected, pain-free range.*

Precaution: Initially perform protected ROM exercises only for a few repetitions twice a day. Limit dorsiflexion to only minus 5 degrees of neutral with the knee flexed and extended. Progress dorsiflextion very cautiously. At 2 weeks active dorsiflexion to neutral is permissable.

- After 2 to 4 weeks (once partial weight bearing is permissible), perform active ankle ROM while in a seated position and the foot resting on a small rocker board.
- With the ankle in a relaxed position, perform

grade I and II joint mobilization (distraction) techniques.

- At 4 to 5 weeks (at the end of the maximum protection phase) initiate very *gentle* open-chain stretching with a towel to gradually increase dorsiflexion with the knee flexed and extended.
- Improve or maintain cardiopulmonary fitness with upper extremity ergometry if available. As weight bearing is progressed, initate a stationary cycling program while wearing the range-limiting brace. Raise the seat height to accommodate for limited dorsiflexion.

Exercise: Moderate Protection/Controlled Motion Phase

By this phase of rehabilitation (usually by 6 weeks postoperatively) the patient may bear weight as tolerated on the operated extremity. The emphasis is now placed on exercises performed in weight-bearing positions.

- Over the next 6 weeks progress to bilateral, lower extremity strengthing exercises in a closed-chain. (Examples: heel raises while seated, mini-squats, double-leg stance heel raises, and partial lunges.)
- Initiate balance and proprioceptive training and stabilization exercises in double-leg stance
- Continue to progress active ROM of the ankle, and by 6 to 8 weeks postoperatively add open-chain, low-intensity resisted ROM of the ankle against a light grade of elastic resistance.
- Add a standing stretch to increase dorsiflexion with the knee flexed and extended when full weight bearing is permissible.
- Increase muscular and cardiopulmonary endurance with level-surface treadmill walking or continue a stationary cycling program.

Exercise: Minimum Protection/Return to Function Phase

- By 10 to 16 weeks, progress closed-chain strengthening activities such as double-leg and single-leg heel raises with the knee extended and slightly flexed and step-ups.
- Perform treadmill walking at a slight incline; increase velocity and distance. For a further challenge ambulate on uneven surfaces.
- Gradually add controlled eccentric strengthening of the gastrocnemius-soleus complex such as descending stairs, step over step.
- By 18 to 20 weeks perform bilateral, progressing to unilateral, heel raises and drops *over the edge of a step.*
- Eventually progress to jogging, bouncing, jumping, and hopping activities and plyometric training.
- A return to high-demand work- and sport-related activity is permissible by 5 to 6 months if strength and endurance are 90 to 95% of the unoperated lower extremity and all motions are pain-free.

Outcomes

Rehabilitation using early motion and weight bearing as compared to traditional management with prolonged immobilization and delayed weight bearing appears to be equally safe. Early follow-up studies have reported no increased incidence of rerupture with early motion.[3,26,39,41] Although early reports are promising, no determination can yet be made on whether early motion and weight bearing enables a patient to return to a full level of functional activity sooner than if managed with a traditional approach.[24,26,39,41]

Exercise Techniques to Increase Flexibility and Range of Motion

Loss of flexibility in the ankle and foot can be from a variety of causes. Restoration of motion may be necessary to correct alignment or for normal mechanics in walking and running to occur. Joint mobilization techniques are used to increase accessory motion of the joint surfaces; these techniques were referred to earlier in this chapter and are described in detail in Chapter 6. Manual passive stretching and neuromuscular inhibition techniques were described in Chapter 5. This section emphasizes self-stretching techniques.

Increase Dorsiflexion of the Ankle

The muscles that restrict dorsiflexion of the ankle are the one-joint soleus and the two-joint gastrocnemius. To effectively stretch the gastrocnemius, the knee must be extended while dorsiflexing the ankle. To isolate stretch to the soleus the knee must be flexed while dorsiflexing in order to take tension off the gastrocnemius. Most of the following stretching exercises can be adapted with the knee in flexion or extension so that both of the plantarflexor muscles can be stretched.

Precaution: When a patient uses weight-bearing exercises to stretch the plantarflexor muscles, shoes with arch supports should be worn or a folded washcloth can be placed under the medial border of the foot to minimize the stress to the arches of the foot.

- Patient position and procedure: Long-sitting (knees extended) or with the knees partially flexed. Have the patient strongly dorsiflex the feet, attempting to keep the toes relaxed.
- Patient position and procedure: Long-sitting or with the knee partially flexed and with a towel or belt under the forefoot. Have the patient pull the foot into dorsiflexion.
- Patient position and procedure: Sitting with the foot flat on the floor. Have the patient slide the foot backward, keeping the heel on the floor.
- Patient position and procedure: Standing. Have the patient stride forward with one foot, keeping the heel of the back foot flat on the floor (the back foot is the one being stretched). If necessary have the patient brace his or her hands against a wall. To provide stability to the foot, the patient partially rotates the back leg inward so the foot assumes a supinated position and locks the joints. He or she then shifts body weight forward onto the front foot. To stretch the gastrocnemius muscle, the patient keeps the knee of the back leg extended; to stretch the soleus, he or she flexes the knee of the back leg.
- Patient position and procedure: Standing on an inclined board with feet pointing upward and heels downward (Fig. 14–3). Greater stretch will occur if the patient leans forward. Because the body weight is on the heels there is little stretch on the long arches of the feet. Little effort is required to maintain this position for extended periods.
- Patient position and procedure: Standing, with the forefoot on the edge of a step or stool and heel over the edge. Have the patient slowly lower the heel over the edge (heel drop).

Precaution: This stretch may create muscle soreness because it requires that the patient control an eccentric contraction of the plantarflexors.

Increase Inversion

- Patient position and procedure: Sitting, with the foot to be stretched placed across the opposite knee. Have the patient grasp the mid- and hindfoot with the opposite hand; lift the foot into inversion. Emphasize turning the heel inward and not just twisting the forefoot.

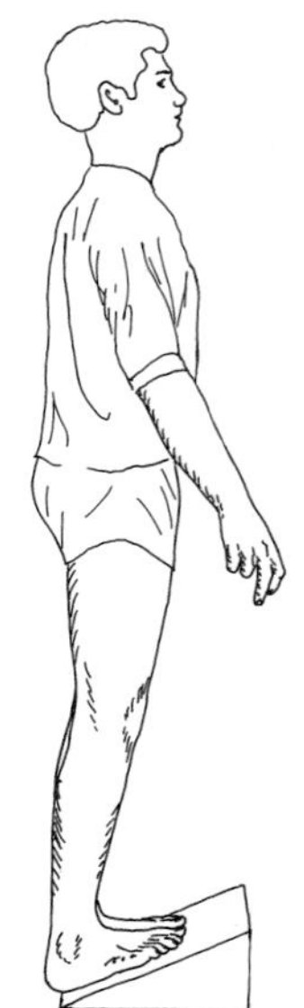

Figure 14–3 Self-stretching the ankle into dorsiflexion (stretching the gastrocnemius muscle).

- Patient position and procedure: Long-sitting with a towel or belt under the foot. Have the patient pull on the medial side of the towel to cause the heel and foot to turn inward (Fig. 14–4). This technique can also be used to turn the foot outward by pulling on the lateral side of the towel. It is important that the motion includes the heel and not just the forefoot.
- Patient position and procedure: Sitting or standing, with feet pointing forward. Have the patient roll to the lateral border of each foot so the soles are turned inward.

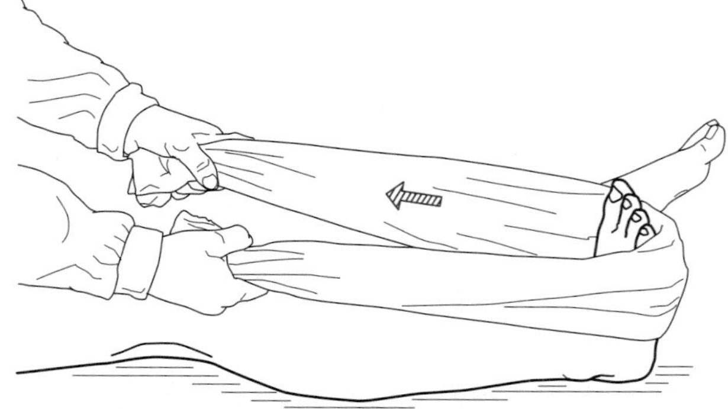

Figure 14–4 Self-stretching the foot into inversion using a towel by pulling on the towel on the medial side of the foot.

- Patient position and procedure: Standing or walking, with the involved foot on a slanted board, placing the lateral aspect of the foot to be stretched on the lower side and the medial side of the foot on the top side of the board. Bilateral stretching can be accomplished if hinged planks are placed in an inverted-V position and the patient stands or walks on them.

Increase Ankle Plantarflexion and Eversion

It is not common for these two motions to be restricted because of the effects of gravity when supine or the body's weight when standing. Eversion, which is a component of pronation, is the loose-packed position of the foot and is perpetuated with weight bearing. The exception for restricted talocrural plantarflexion is when there is a capsular pattern at the joint as a result of arthritis. If the restriction is from joint hypomobility, it is treated with joint mobilization techniques. If there is restriction of eversion, a stretching technique was described previously with use of a towel or belt around the foot.

Increase MTP Flexion and IP Extension

Tight extrinsic muscles of the toes occur with claw toes and hammer toes, causing the MTP joints to extend and IP joints to flex. There is often weakness in the intrinsic muscles.

- Patient position and procedure: Sitting, with the foot crossed onto the opposite knee. Show the patient how to stabilize the foot under the metatarsal heads (MTP joints) with the thumbs, and passively flex the MTP joints by applying pressure against the proximal phalanges. Or have the patient attempt active flexion of the MTP joints, assisting the motion if necessary.
- Patient position and procedure: Sitting with the foot crossed onto the opposite knee. Teach the patient to stabilize the proximal phalanx of the involved toe and passively stretch the long flexors across each joint by moving the middle and or distal phalanx into extension.
- Patient position and procedure: Standing with the toes over the edge of a stool or book and the MTP joints at the edge. Have the patient attempt to flex the MTP joints, keeping the IP joints of the toes extended.

Stretch the Plantar Fascia of the Foot

- Patient position and procedure: Sitting with the foot placed across the opposite knee. Teach the patient to use his or her thumbs to apply deep massage horizontally and longitudinally across the plantar surface of the foot.
- Patient position and procedure: Sitting with a ball or small roller (or bottle) under the foot. Have the patient roll the foot forward and backward across the curved surface, using as much pressure as is comfortable. Pressing down on the knee with one or both hands can exert additional force.

Exercises to Develop and Improve Muscle Performance and Functional Control

Causes of strength and flexibility imbalances in the ankle and foot include disuse, immobilization, nerve injury, and progressive joint degeneration. In addition, imbalances occur from the weight-bearing stresses that are imposed on the feet. Imbalances can be the cause or the effect of faulty lower extremity mechanics. Because the lower extremities bear weight, realignment by strengthening exercises alone is of limited value. Strengthening exercises undertaken in conjunction with conscious correction, appropriate stretching, balance training, and other necessary measures (such as using orthotic inserts or adaptations for shoes, bracing, splinting, or surgery) improve alignment so that structurally safe weight bearing is possible. In addition, observation of the types of shoes and surfaces that the person uses for walking or sports activities may be a lead to the source of faulty mechanics, which can then be adjusted. (Techniques of orthopedic adaptations for shoes, bracing, and splinting are beyond the scope of this text.)

Most functional demands on the ankle and foot occur in weight-bearing postures. Kinesthetic input from skin, joint, and muscle receptors and the resulting joint and muscle responses are different in open- and closed-chain activities; therefore, whenever possible, use of progressive weight-bearing exercises is important to simulate functional activities.[15,35] In addition to the exercises described in this section, refer to Chapter 12 for total lower extremity functional exercises performed in the standing position that influence muscle control at the hip, knee and ankle.

Activities for Active Mobility and to Develop Neuromuscular Control

- Patient position and procedure: Long-sitting or with the knees partially flexed. Have the patient practice contracting each of the major muscles while concentrating on their actions; for example, dorsiflexion with inversion (anterior tibialis), plantarflexion with inversion (posterior tibialis), and eversion (peroneus muscles).

- Patient position and procedure: Long-sitting or with the knee partially flexed. Instruct the patient to "draw" the alphabet in space leading with the toes but moving at the ankle. For variety have the patient "print" using capital letters, then with lower case letters, or "write" words such as his or her name or address.
- Patient position and procedure: Sitting on a chair or low mat table with feet on the floor. Place a number of small objects, such as marbles or dice, to one side of the involved foot. Have the patient pick up one object at a time by curling the toes around it and then placing it in a container on the other side of the foot. This emphasizes the plantar muscles as well as inversion and eversion.
- Patient position and procedure: Sitting or standing, with feet on the floor. Have the patient curl the toes against the resistance of the floor. Place a towel or tissue paper under the feet, and have the patient attempt to wrinkle it up by keeping the heel on the floor and flexing the toes.
- Patient position and procedure: Sitting, with the feet on the floor. Have the patient attempt to raise the medial longitudinal arch while keeping the forefoot and hindfoot on the floor; lateral rotation of the tibia should occur but not abduction of the hips. The activity is repeated until the patient has consistent control, then it is performed while standing as a progression.
- Patient position and procedure: Sitting with a tennis ball placed between the soles of the feet. Instruct the patient to roll the tennis ball back and forth from heel to forefoot.
- Patient position and procedure: Sitting with both feet or just the involved foot on a rocker or balance board. Have patient perform controlled ankle and foot motions (with or without the assistance of the normal foot) into dorsiflexion and plantarflexion and inversion and eversion (Fig. 14–5). If the equipment permits the patient can also perform circumduction in each direction. Progress this activity to the standing position to further develop control and to develop balance.
- Have the patient practice walking while concentrating on placement of the feet and shifting the body weight with each step. The patient begins by accepting body weight on the heel, then shifting the weight along the lateral border of the foot to the fifth metatarsal head and across to the first metatarsal head and great toe for push-off.

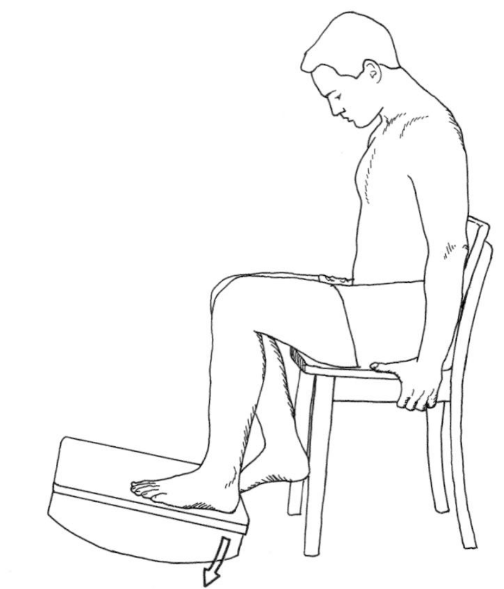

Figure 14–5 Using a rocker board to develop control of ankle motions with the patient sitting. When both feet are on the board, the normal foot can assist the involved side. With only the involved foot on the board, the activity is more difficult.

Open-Chain Strengthening Exercises

All of the following exercises in this section are performed without weight bearing through the foot and ankle.

Plantarflexion

Patient position and procedure: Long-sitting with the leg resting on a rolled towel to slightly elevate the heel off the treatment table. Hold onto the ends of elasticized material that is looped under the forefoot. Have the patient plantarflex the foot against the resistance (Fig. 14–6).

Isometric Eversion and Inversion

Patient position and procedure: Long-sitting or sitting in a chair with knees flexed

- To resist eversion, the ankles are crossed; instruct the patient to press the lateral borders of both feet together against each other.
- To resist inversion, the medial borders of the feet are placed beside each other; instruct the patient to press the medial borders of the feet against each other.

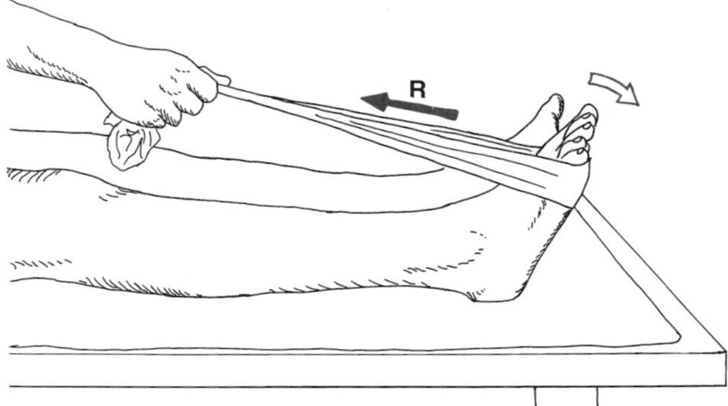

Figure 14–6 Resisting the ankle plantarflexor muscles with an elasticized material.

Eversion and Inversion with Elastic Resistance

Patient position and procedure: Long-sitting, supine, or sitting with the feet resting on the floor.

- To resist eversion, place a loop of elasticized material around both feet and have the patient evert one or both feet against the resistance (Fig. 14–7). Instruct the patient to keep the knees still and just turn the foot outward and not allow the thigh and leg to abduct or externally rotate.
- To resist inversion, tie the elastic material to a structure on the lateral side of the foot. Again, instruct the patient to keep the legs stationary and just turn the foot inward with care to avoid adduction and internal rotation of the thigh.

Adduction with Inversion and Abduction with Eversion Using Weights

Patient position and procedure: Sitting with the foot on the floor. Place a towel under the forefoot and a weight on the end of the towel (Fig. 14–8). Have the patient pull the weighted towel along the floor with the forefoot by keeping the heel fixed on the floor and swinging the foot either inward or outward.

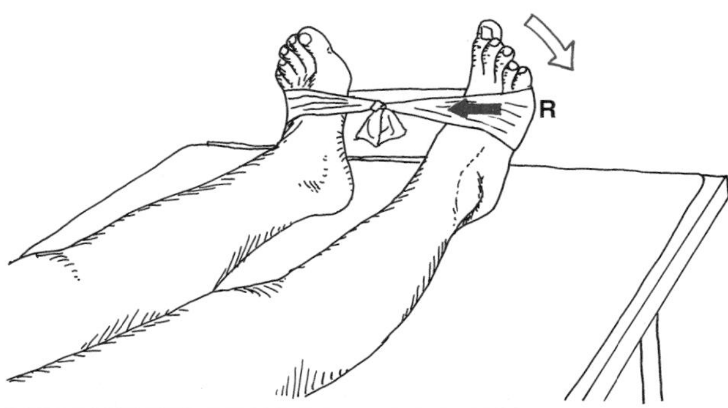

Figure 14–7 Resisting the evertor muscles of the foot with an elasticized material.

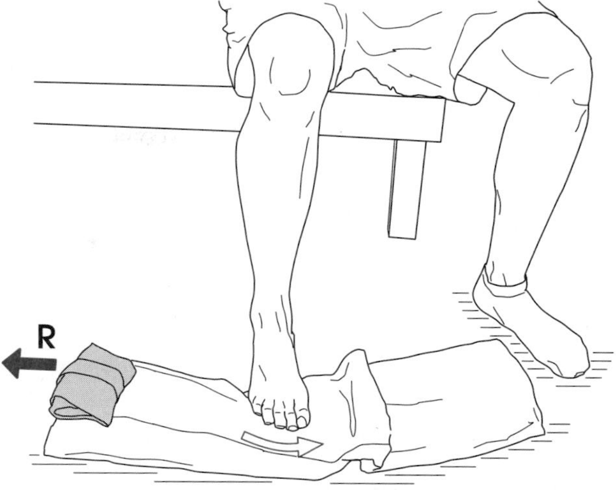

Figure 14–8 Resisting adduction and inversion with a weight on the end of the towel. The heel is kept stationary while a windshield wiper motion of the foot is used to pull the towel along the floor. Abduction with eversion is resisted by placing the weight on the towel on the medial side of the foot.

Dorsiflexion

Patient position and procedure: Long-sitting or supine with a rolled towel under the distal leg to slightly elevate the heel. Tie elasticized material to the foot end of the bed (or other object), and place a loop over the dorsum of the foot. Have the patient dorsiflex against the resistance (Fig. 14–9).

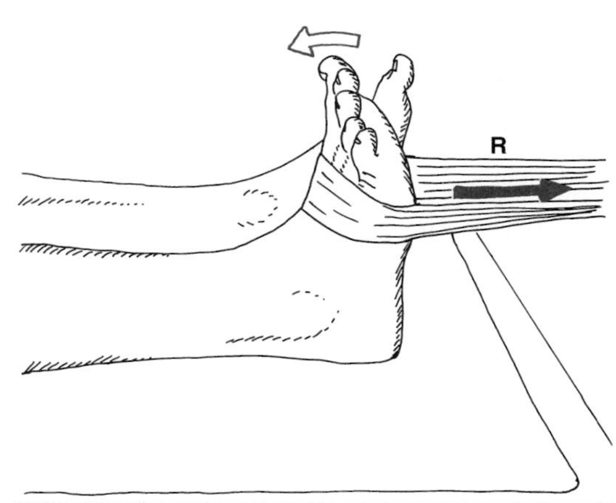

Figure 14–9 Resisting the ankle dorsiflexor muscles with an elasticized material.

All Ankle Motions

Position of patient: Sitting in a chair or standing. Place one or both feet in a box filled with sand, foam, dry peas, dry beans, or other similar type material to offer resistance to various foot motions. Have the patient plantarflex, dorsiflex, invert and evert the foot and ankle, and curl the toes either with the foot on top or with the foot dug into the medium.

Weight-Bearing Exercises for Strength, Balance, and Function

For these exercises, the patient position is standing. If the patient does not initially tolerate full weight bearing without reproduction of symptoms, begin by standing in the parallel bars or in a pool to reduce weight-bearing forces. Refer to Box 3–7 which outlines general guidelines for progresssion of closed-chain exercises.

Stabilization Exercises

- Apply resistance to the patient's pelvis in various directions while he or she attempts to maintain control. At first, use verbal cues, then resist without warning, Also increase the speed and intensity of the perturbation forces.
- A variation is to have the patient hold onto a wooden dowel rod or cane with both hands. Apply the resistance through the rod in various directions and with varying intensities and speeds as the patient attempts to remain stable (Fig. 14–10).
- Progress to standing only on the involved foot.

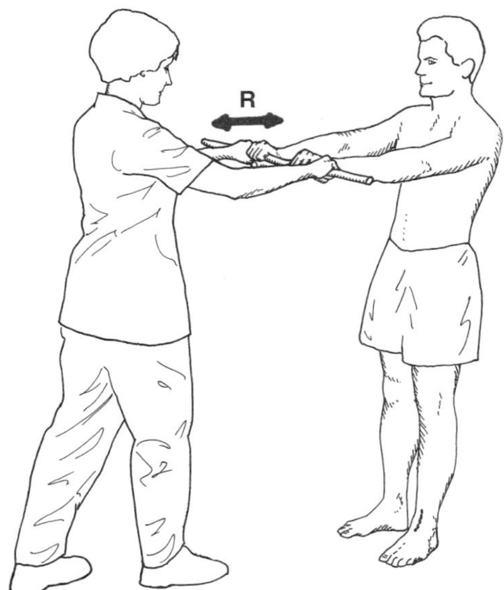

Figure 14–10 Stabilization exercises with the patient standing and maintaining balance against the alternating resistance forces from the therapist. The therapist applies force through the rod in backward/forward, side-to-side, and rotation directions.

Dynamic Strength Training

Have the patient perform bilateral toe raises, heel raises, and rocking outward to the lateral borders of the feet. Progress to unilateral toe raises, heel raises, and lateral border standing. When tolerated, resistance is added with a weight belt or handheld weights.

Resisted Walking

- Have the patient walk on heels and on toes against resistance.
- Apply resistance against the patient's pelvis, or have the patient walk against a pulley weight or elastic resistance fixed around the pelvis (see Fig. 12–17).

Balance Activities

Early balance activities are described in detail in Chapter 14. Begin with partial weight bearing in the parallel bars if necessary; progress to full bilateral weight bearing, then unilateral weight bearing. Have the patient shift body weight, stand and balance while performing various arm motions, march in place, walk, and finally progress to walking on uneven surfaces.

A rocker or balance board can be used several different ways to stimulate balance reactions. If necessary, begin with the patient supporting himself or herself with both hands in the parallel bars or by holding onto a stable object. Initially, both feet are on the board. Increasing the size of the half sphere or rocker under the board will increase the difficulty of the balance activity. Progress to unilateral stance on the board.

- Have the patient rock the feet forward and backward, then side to side while attempting to control the motion and maintain balance.
- Instruct the patient to maintain balance and not let the edges of the board hit the ground (Fig. 14–11). As the patient learns to control the board, impose various challenges while he or she maintains balance on the board. Examples:
  - Have the patient move the arms forward, backward, and overhead.
  - Have the patient do various arm motions against

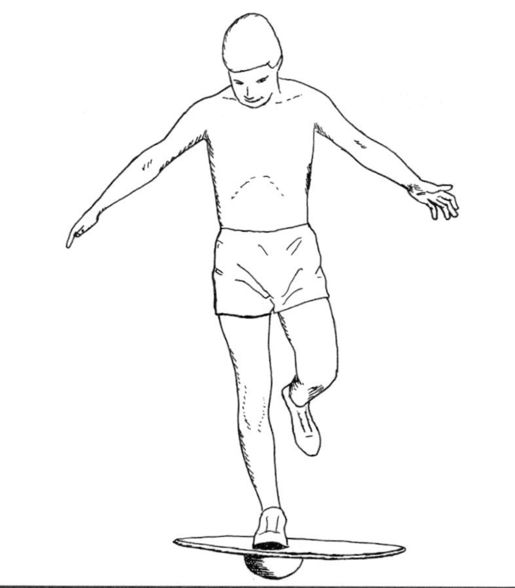

Figure 14–11 Advanced training for balance and coordination on a balance board requires that the patient not hold on while balancing with one leg.

elastic resistance, with free weights, or while controlling a Bodyblade® (see Fig. 3–48).
- Toss a ball (unweighted or weighted) back and forth to the patient.
- Have the patient hold onto elastic resistance while you pull the resistance in various directions.

Simulation and Practice for Return to Functional Activities

Using the principle of specificity of training, replicate whatever functional activity the individual requires, first in controlled patterns, then with increased velocity and decreased control.

Functional strengthening. Lifting, pushing, and pulling heavy objects requires ankle strength as well and hip, knee, and trunk strength. Develop exercises that involve the total body to develop safe body mechanics. Include squatting and lunging to lift objects from the floor, pushing or pulling weighted carts, and climbing and descending steps and ladders while carrying weights. Modify techniques if substitute motions occur.

Endurance. Develop endurance by increasing the amount of time spent performing various drills.

Power. Develop power with plyometric drills such as jumping and hopping. Progress to jumping off and back onto boxes of various heights.

Agility and skill. Develop an obstacle course and have the patient maneuver around or up and over the obstacles, first walking, then running, skipping, or jumping. Include forward, backward, and side-to-side maneuvers.

Independent Learning Activities

CRITICAL THINKING AND DISCUSSION

1. Observe how the foot and ankle function as a unit in several activities such as walking up steps, walking on uneven surfaces, and walking in high-heeled shoes vs. low-heeled shoes.
   - What motions occur in the talocrural, subtalar, transverse tarsal, and metatarsophalangeal joints? Describe the mechanics.
   - What muscles are functioning and what level of strength is needed to move or control each joint?
2. Describe the role of the ankle and foot during the gait cycle.
   - What ROM is needed at the ankle and what muscles are acting to cause or control the motion? What other forces are causing or controlling motion at the ankle?
   - What gait deviations occur if there is muscle-shortening or weakness at the ankle?
   - After a unilateral arthrodesis of the talocrural joint (ankle fused in neutral) what deviations will occur in the gait cycle?
   - Describe the mechanics and function of pronation and supination in the foot during the gait cycle. Explain how the gait cycle would be affected if a patient had flexible flat feet versus rigid supinated feet.
3. Compare and contrast an exercise program for a patient who has had a repair or reconstruction of torn lateral ligaments of the ankle versus a patient who has had a repair of a ruptured Achilles tendon. How will precautions and selection of exercises differ after these two types of surgical repairs?
4. Discuss the benefits and limitations of total ankle arthroplasty versus arthrodesis of the ankle for the patient with RA.

LABORATORY PRACTICE

1. Review all the joint mobilization techniques for the leg, ankle, and foot; include basic glides,

accessory motions, and mobilization with movement techniques.

- Identify and practice techniques that you could use to increase ankle plantarflexion; begin with the ankle at zero, and progress at 15-degree increments until full plantarflexion is reached.
- Do the same for ankle dorsiflexion, subtalar inversion and subtalar eversion, and metatarsophalangeal extension.

2. Set up a circuit-training course for the foot and ankle musculature to increase strength, muscular endurance, stability, and balance. Sequence the activities from basic to advanced, and observe accuracy and safety with each exercise. Identify other muscles in the lower extremity, trunk, or arms that are also being affected by the exercises.

CASE STUDIES

1. Mr. C has a 10-year history of rheumatoid arthritis. Currently, medication is managing his acute symptoms so that he is able to walk with a cane. His complaints are increased pain after walking 15 minutes and considerable stiffness along with generalized weakness. You observe his gait: he walks with a short step and has no push-off. Ankle ROM: dorsiflexion 10 degrees, plantarflexion 15 degrees, inversion 0, eversion, 8 degrees. He stands with a pronated foot, has dorsal migration of the first phalanges and moderate hammer toes. He tolerates moderate resistance in all his musculature within the limited range, although he is unable to demonstrate toe walking or do bilateral toe raises even one time.
   - List his impairments and functional limitations and state goals.
   - Develop a program of intervention to meet the goals. How will you initiate the intervention? What techniques will you use and how will you progress them?
   - Describe rationale for each manual technique you would use, and for each exercise you would teach the patient.
   - Identify any precautions you will use and that you will teach the patient.

2. Sally S., a college student, sustained a bootline fracture of the tibia and fibula as the result of a fall while snow skiing. She was immobilized in a long-leg cast for 6 weeks, followed by a short-leg cast for 4 weeks. She was allowed partial weight bearing while wearing the short-leg cast. The cast was removed this morning. She described significant stiffness and discomfort when attempting to move her foot. Observation reveals atrophy in the calf, no edema or joint swelling. ROM in the ankle and foot is minimal, and there is no gliding of the fibula at the proximal or distal tibiofibular joints. Strength could not be tested, although the patient can activate all muscles.
   - Answer the same questions as in Case #1.
   - Even though both patients have restricted motion and demonstrate weakness, what are the differences in your intervention strategies and in the precautions you will follow?
   - How will you determine the progression of weight-bearing activities?

3. Ron W. is a 35-year-old computer programmer who plays basketball at the local recreation center. He sustained a massive inversion strain of his right ankle when landing on the foot of an opponent after jumping to rebound the basketball. He wrapped the ankle and iced it for two days. On the third day he went for an x-ray. No fractures were detected, but he does have a grade 2 instability of the anterior talofibular ligament. Observation reveals swelling and discoloration in the anterior and lateral ankle region. He experiences a marked increase in pain with inversion and plantarflexion tests, with anterior gliding of the talus, and with palpation over the involved ligament. Because of muscle guarding, strength was not tested.
   - Identify impairments, goals, and an intervention strategy for this patient.
   - Describe how his program will be progressed.
   - Ron wants to know how soon he can return to playing his favorite sport. What criteria will you use to make this judgment, and how will you protect his ankle when he does return?

REFERENCES

1. Cailliet, R: Foot and Ankle Pain, ed 3. FA Davis, Philadelphia, 1997.
2. Campbell, DC II, and Papagelopoulos, PJ: Reconstruction of the great toe: implant and nonimplant options. In Morrey, BF (ed): Reconstructive Surgery of the Joints, Vol 2, ed 2. Churchill Livingstone, New York, 1996, p 1811.
3. Carter, T, Fowler, P, and Blokker, C: Functional postoperative treatment of Achilles tendon repair. Am J Sports Med 20:459, 1992.
4. Cetti, R, Henricksson, LO, and Jacobsen, KS: A new treatment of ruptured Achilles tendons. Clin Orthop 308:155, 1994.
5. Cetti, R, et al: Operative versus nonoperative treatment of Achilles tendon rupture: A prospective randomized study and review of the literature Am J Sports Med 21:791, 1993.
6. Colville, MK, and Grundol, RJ: Anatomic reconstruction of the lateral ankle ligaments using a split peroneus brevis tendon graft. Am J Sports Med 23:210, 1995.
7. Cracchiolo, A, Janisse, D, and Gall, V: Rheumatoid arthritis in the foot and ankle: Surgery and rehabilitation. In Melvin, JL, and Gall, V (eds): Rheumatologic Rehabilitation Series, Vol 5: Surgical Rehabilitation. American Occupational Therapy Assoc., Bethesda MD, 1999, p 165.
8. Cyriax, J: Textbook of Orthopaedic Medicine, Vol 1. Diagnosis of Soft Tissue Lesions, ed 8. Bailliere Tindall, London, 1982.
9. DeLacerda, F: Iontophoresis for treatment of shinsplints. J Orthop Sports Phys Ther 3: 183, 1982.
10. Dimonte, P, and Light, H: Pathomechanics, gait deviations and treatment of the rheumatoid foot. Phys Ther 62:1148, 1982.
11. Donatelli, R, et al: Biomechanical foot orthotics: A retrospective study. J Orthop Sports Phys Ther 10:205, 1988.
12. Donatelli, RA: Normal anatomy and biomechanics. In Donatelli, RA: The Biomechanics of the Foot and Ankle, ed 2. FA Davis, Philadelphia, 1996, p 3.
13. Donatelli, RA: Abnormal biomechanics. In Donatelli, RA: The Biomechanics of the Foot and Ankle, ed 2. FA Davis, Philadelphia, 1996, p 34.
14. Gabrielsen, TA, and Kitaoka, HB: Ankle injuries. In Morrey, BF (ed): Reconstructive Surgery of the Joints, Vol 2, ed 2. Churchill Livingstone, New York, 1996, p 1743.
15. Garn, SN, and Newton, RA: Kinesthetic awareness in subjects with multiple ankle sprains. Phys Ther 68:1669, 1988.
16. Gauffin, H, Trupp, H, and Odenieck, P: Effect of ankle disk training on postural control in patients with functional instability of the ankle joint. Int J Sports Med 9:141, 1988.
17. Glasoe, WM, et al: Weight-bearing immobilization and early exercise treatment following a grade II lateral ankle sprain. J Orthop Sports Phys Ther 29:394, 1999.
18. Greenfield, B, and Johnson, M: Evaluation of overuse syndromes. In Donatelli, R (ed): The Biomechanics of the Foot and Ankle, ed 2. FA Davis, Philadelphia, 1996, p 189.
19. Hamilton, WG, Thompson, FM, and Snow, SW: The modified Brostrom procedure for lateral ankle instability. Foot Ankle 14:1, 1993.
20. Heinrichs, K, and Haney, C: Rehabilitation of the surgically repaired Achilles tendon using a dorsal functional orthosis. A preliminary report. J Sport Rehabil 3:292, 1994.
21. Hennrikus, WL, et al: Outcomes of the Chrisman-Snook and modified Brostrom procedures for chronic lateral ankle instability: A prospective, randomized comparison. Am J Sports Med 24:400, 1996.
22. Horak, F, and Nashner, L: Central programming of postural movements: Adaptations to altered support surface configuration. J Neurophysiol 55:1369, 1986.
23. Howell, DW: Therapeutic exercise and mobilization. In Hunt, GC (ed): Physical Therapy of the Foot and Ankle. Churchill-Livingstone, New York, 1988.
24. Hunter, S, and Prentice, WE: Rehabilitation of ankle and foot injuries. In Prentice, WE (ed): Rehabilitation Techniques in Sports Medicine, ed 3. WCB/McGraw-Hill, Boston, 1999, p 490.
25. Kapandji, IA: The Physiology of the Joints, Vol 11, ed 5. Churchill-Livingstone, Edinburgh, 1980.
26. Kauranen, KJ, and Leppilahti, JI: Motor performance of the foot after Achilles rupture repair. Int J Sports Med 22:154, 2001.
27. Kay, DB: The sprained ankle: Current therapy. Foot Ankle 6:22. 1985.
28. Kile, TA: Ankle arthrodesis. In Morrey, BF (ed): Reconstructive Surgery of the Joints, Vol 2, ed 2. Churchill Livingstone, New York, 1996, p 1771.
29. Kimura, IF, et al: Effect of the air stirrup in controlling ankle inversion stress. J Orthop Sports Phys Ther 190, 1987.
30. Kitaoka, HB, and Johnson, KA: Ankle replacement arthroplasty. In Morrey, BF (ed): Reconstructive Surgery of the Joints, Vol 2, ed 2. Churchill Livingstone New York, 1996, p 1757.
31. Komenda, G, and Ferkel, RD: Arthroscopic findings associated with the unstable ankle. Foot Ankle Intern 20:708, 1999.
32. Kopell, H, and Thompson, W: Peripheral Entrapment Neuropathies, ed 2. Robert E Krieger, Huntington, NY, 1976.
33. Kramer, P: Restoration of dorsiflexion after injuries to the distal leg and ankle. J Orthop Sports Phys Ther 1:159, 1980.
34. Kuland, DN: The Injured Athlete. JB Lippincott, Philadelphia, 1988.
35. Lattanza, L, Gray, GW, and Kantner, R: Closed vs open kinematic chain measurements of subtalar joint eversion: Implications for clinical practice. J Orthop Sports Phys Ther 9:310, 1988.
36. Leach, RE, James, S, and Wasliewski, S: Achilles tendinitis. Am J Sports Med 9:93, 1981.
37. Levangie, PK, and Norkin CC: Joint Structure and Function: A Comprehensive Analysis, ed 3. FA Davis Company, Philadelphia, 2001.
38. Lockard, MA: Foot orthoses. Phys Ther 68:1866, 1988.
39. Mandelbaum, BR, Myerson, MS, and Forster, R: Achilles tendon ruptures: a new method of repair, early range of motion, and functional rehabilitation. Am J Sports Med 23:392, 1995.
40. McPoil, TG: Footwear. Phys Ther 68:1857, 1988.
41. Mortensen, NH, Skov, O, and Jensen, PE: Early motion of the ankle after operative treatment of a rupture of the Achilles tendon. A prospective, randomized clinical and radiographic study. J Bone Joint Surg Am 81:983, 1999.
42. Motta, P, Errichiello, C, and Pontini, I: Achilles tendon rupture.

A new technique for surgical repair and immediate movement of the ankle and foot. Am J Sports Med 25:172, 1997.
43. Mulligan, BR: Manual Therapy "NAGS", "SNAGS", "MWM's": etc, ed 4. Plane View Press, Wellington, 1999.
44. Mulligan, EP: Lower leg, ankle and foot rehabilitation. In Andrews, JR, Harrelson, GL, and Wilk, KE (eds): Physical Rehabilitation of the Injured Athlete, ed 2. WB Saunders, Philadelphia, 1998, p 261.
45. Novick, A: Anatomy and biomechanics. In Hunt, GC, and McPoil TG, (eds): Physical Therapy of the Foot and Ankle, Churchill Livingstone, New York, 1995, p 11.
46. Oatis, CA: Biomechanics of the foot and ankle under static conditions. Phys Ther 68:1815, 1988.
47. Perry, J: Gait Analysis: Normal and Pathological Function. SLACK Inc, Thorofare, NJ, 1992.
48. Peters, WJ, Trevino, SG, and Renstrom, PA: Chronic lateral ankle instability. Foot Ankle 12:82, 1991.
49. Quillen, W: An alternative management protocol for lateral ankle sprains. J Orthop Sports Phys Ther 2:187, 1981.
50. Reynolds, NL, and Worrell, TN: Chronic Achilles peritendinitis: etiology, pathophysiology, and treatment. J Orthop Sports Phys Ther 13:717, 1991.
51. Rozzi, SM, et al: Balance training for patients with functionally unstable ankles. J Orthop Sports Phys Ther 29:478, 1999.
52. Salter, RB: Textbook of Disorders and Injuries of the Musculoskeletal System, ed 3. Williams & Wilkins, Baltimore, 1999.
53. Saltzman, CL, and Johnson, KA: Surgery of the ankle and foot. In Sledge, CB, et al (eds): Arthritis Surgery. WB Saunders, Philadelphia, 1994, p 818.
54. Saltzman, CL, et al: Total ankle replacement revisited. J Orthop Sports Phys Ther 30:56, 2000.
55. Sammarco, GJ, and Hockenbury, RT: Biomechanics of the foot and ankle. In Nordin, M, and Frankel, VH (eds): Basic Biomechanics of the Musculoskeletal System, ed 3. Lippincott Williams & Wilkins, Philadelphia, 2001, p 222.
56. Scholz, KC: Total ankle arthroplasty using biological fixation components compared to ankle arthrodesis. Orthopedics 10:125, 1987.
57. Schon, LC, and Ouzounian, TJ: The ankle. In James, MH (ed): Disorders of the Foot and Ankle. Medical and Surgical Management, ed 2. WB Saunders, Philadelphia, 1991.
58. Shrader, JA: Nonsurgical management of the foot and ankle affected by rheumatoid arthritis. J Orthop Sports Phys Ther 29:703, 1999.
59. Smith, CL: Physical therapy management of patients with total ankle replacement. Phys Ther 60:303, 1980.
60. Smith, LK, Weiss, EL, and Lehmkuhl, LD: Brunnstrom's Clinical Kinesiology, ed 5. FA Davis, Philadelphia, 1996.
61. Snook, GA: Lateral ankle reconstruction for chronic instability. In Torg, JS, Welsh, RP, and Shephard, RJ (eds): Current Therapy in Sports Medicine, ed 2. BC Decker, Toronto, 1990.
62. Solveborn, S, and Moberg, A: Immediate free ankle motion after surgical repair of acute Achilles tendon ruptures. Am J Sports Med 22:607, 1994.
63. Spigel, PV, and Seale, KS: Surgical interventions. In Donatelli, RA: The Biomechanics of the Foot and Ankle, ed 2. FA Davis, Philadelphia, 1996, p 352.
64. Steele, G, Harter, R, and Ting, A: Comparison of functional ability following percutaneous and open surgical repairs of acutely ruptured tendons. J Sport Rehabil 2:115, 1993.
65. Sullivan, JM: Rupture of the Achilles tendon. In Torg, JS, Welsh, RP, and Shephard, RJ (eds): Current Therapy in Sports Medicine, ed 2. BC Decker, Toronto, 1990.
66. Thompson, TC, and Doherty, JH: Spontaneous rupture of tendon of Achilles: A new clinical diagnostic test. J Trauma 2:126, 1962.
67. Unger, AS, Inglis, AE, and Mow, CS: Total ankle arthroplasty in rheumatoid arthritis: A long-term follow-up study. Foot Ankle 8:173, 1988.
68. Wallace, L, Knortz, K, and Esterson, P: Immediate care of ankle injuries. J Orthop Sports Phys Ther 1:46, 1979.
69. Waugh, T: Arthroplasty rehabilitation. In Goodgold, J (ed): Rehabilitation Medicine. CV Mosby, St Louis, 1988, p 457.
70. Wester, JU, et al: Wobble board training after partial sprains of the lateral ligaments of the ankle: A prospective, randomized study. J Orthop Sports Phys Ther 23:332, 1996.

Chapter 15

The Spine and Posture: Structure, Function, and Management Guidelines

OBJECTIVES

After studying this chapter, the reader will be able to:

1. Identify major components of spinal structure and function for review.
2. Define and describe normal and abnormal postures and common pain syndromes related to impaired posture.
3. Describe pathology and pathomechanics of the intervertebral disk and related conditions, and describe signs and symptoms of disk lesions and fluid stasis.
4. Describe the pathomechanical relationship of the intervertebral disk and facet joints and related pathologies including segmental instability, stenosis and spinal nerve root and spinal cord involvement.
5. Identify and describe common pathologies and impairments of the zygapophyseal (facet) joints of the spine.
6. Describe the mechanics of muscle and other soft tissue injuries in the spine.
7. Describe common nerve mobility impairments.
8. Recognize the differences between patients who are sensitive to various postures and or movement patterns.
9. Identify indications and contraindications for therapeutic exercise interventions in the treatment of various spinal and postural pathologies, impairments, and functional limitations.
10. Establish goals and treatment interventions for patients with spinal and postural symptoms and functional limitations based on impairments, stage of healing, and anticipated functional outcome.
11. Establish treatment interventions for managing patients with torticollis, tension headaches, temporomandibular joint dysfunction, and nerve tension impairments.

In theory, treating the tissues of the spinal column and trunk is the same as treating tissues of the extremities. The major complicating factor in the spine is the close proximity of key structures to the spinal cord and nerve roots. The challenge for the therapist is to recognize the complex functional relationships of the facet joints, the intervertebral joints, the muscles, the fascia, and the nervous system and know how to examine and evaluate the individual who presents with pain and functional limitations. Activity, rather than prolonged bed rest, is now accepted as important in the management of patients with spinal and postural pain,[2,73] but defining what is safe activity during the process of healing and rehabilitation is the task of the therapist. With knowledge of the biomechanics, pathomechanics, and precautions of various pathologies of spinal structures the therapist can determine specific therapeutic, nondestructive movements that may be more beneficial for early recovery, functional return to activities, and prevention of recurrences than general exercise. The approach to treatment of spinal and postural problems has changed considerably in the past several years. Therapists have always known the importance of "proximal stability for distal mobility," but emphasis is shifting from traditional dynamic exercises to specific exercises and activities that develop awareness and neuromuscular control in the musculature that provides the proximal stability.

Outcome studies have been inconclusive as to the

most effective programs and techniques of intervention, so the professional community has begun to recognize the need to better categorize patients for treatment. The medical model of diagnosis does not lend itself to direct therapeutic exercise intervention strategies, particularly because patients' complaints of back or neck pain often do not relate to specific pathologies.[99] Efforts are being made to determine the most effective way to categorize patients with symptoms affecting the spine and trunk function in order to be more accurate with outcome research. The reader is referred to the review article by Riddle in which various systems of patient classification are described and critiqued.[85] The approach that is described in this text is a blend of current and traditional thinking.[2,22,23,85]

The content of this chapter has two major emphases. The first focuses on highlights of the anatomy, function, posture, pathology, and pathomechanics of the spine and posture. These are reviewed in the first eight sections. The second emphasis focuses on principles and guidelines for managing patients with spinal and postural problems that interfere with normal functional activities. The sections in the second half include principles of interventions for the broad categories of acute, subacute, and chronic conditions, and then expand on principles of interventions for specific conditions. Techniques geared toward treating unique impairments are described within these sections. General, therapeutic exercise techniques of intervention for all spinal and postural impairments are described in Chapter 16. Both chapters are written with the assumption that the reader has completed or is concurrently taking a course in examination and evaluation of posture and the spine.

▶ Review of the Structure and Function of the Spine

Physiologic Curves

The adult spine is divided into four curves: two *primary* or posterior curves, so named because they are present in the infant and the convexity is posterior, and two *compensatory* or anterior curves, so named because they develop as the infant learns to lift the head and eventually stand, and the convexity is anterior.

- Anterior curves are in the cervical and lumbar regions. **Lordosis** is a term also used to denote an anterior curve, although some sources reserve the term lordosis to denote abnormal conditions such as those that occur with a sway back.[24]
- Posterior curves are in the thoracic and sacral regions. **Kyphosis** is a term used to denote a posterior curve. Kyphotic posture refers to an excessive posterior curvature of the thoracic spine.[24]
- The line of gravity transects the spinal curves, which are balanced anteriorly and posteriorly. Deviation of one portion of the spinal column results in shifting of another portion to compensate and maintain balance.
- The flexibility of the curves gives the vertebral column 10 times the resistance to axial compression forces as that of a straight column.[44,103] Flexibility and balance in the spinal column are necessary to withstand the effects of gravity and other external forces.

Functional Components

Functionally, the spinal column is divided into anterior and posterior pillars.[18,44]

- The anterior pillar, made up of the vertebral bodies and intervertebral disks, is the hydraulic, weight bearing, shock-absorbing portion.
- The posterior pillars, made up of the articular processes and facet joints, are the gliding mechanism for movement. Also part of the posterior unit are the two vertebral arches, two transverse processes, and a central posterior spinous process. Muscles attach to the processes from which they cause and control motion.

Motions of the Spinal Column

Motion of the spinal column is described both globally and at the functional unit or motion segment. The *functional unit* is two vertebra and the joints in between (typically, two zygapophyseal joints and one intervertebral disk). Generally, the axis of motion for each unit is in the nucleus pulposus of the intervertebral disk. Because the spine can move from top down, or bottom up, motion at a functional unit is defined as what is occurring with the anterior portion of the body of the superior vertebra.

- ***Sagittal plane motion.*** Flexion (forward bending) and extension (backward bending). With flexion, the anterior portion of the bodies approximate and the spinous processes separate; with extension the bodies separate and the spinous processes approximate.
- ***Frontal plane motion.*** Lateral flexion (side bend-

ing) left or right. With side bending the lateral edges of the vertebral bodies approximate on the side toward which the spine is bending and separate on the opposite side.

- ***Transverse plane motion.*** Rotation to the right results in relative movement of the body of the superior vertebrae to the right and its spinous process to the left; the opposite occurs with rotation to the left. If movement occurs from the pelvis upward, the motion is still defined by what the top vertebra is doing.
- ***Anterior/posterior shear.*** Shear occurs when the body of the superior vertebra translates forward or backward on the one below.
- ***Lateral shear.*** Lateral shear occurs when the body of the superior vertebra translates sideways on the one below.
- ***Distraction/compression:*** Separation or approximation occurs with a longitudinal force, either away from or toward the vertebral bodies.

Structure and Function of the Intervertebral Disks

The intervertebral disk, consisting of the annulus fibrosus and nucleus pulposus, is one component of a three-joint complex between two adjacent vertebrae. The structure of the disk dictates its function.[18,43,54a,56a,58,59]

The annulus fibrosus. The outer portion of the disk is made up of dense layers of collagen fibers and fibrocartilage. The collagen fibers in any one layer are parallel and angled around 60 to 65 degrees to the axis of the spine, with the tilt alternating in successive layers.[35,48] Because of the orientation of the fibers, tensile strength is provided to the disk by the annulus when the spine is distracted, rotated, or bent. This structure helps restrain the various spinal motions as a complex ligament. The annulus is firmly attached to adjacent vertebrae, and the layers are firmly bound to one another. Fibers of the innermost layers blend with the matrix of the nucleus pulposus. The annulus fibrosus is supported by the anterior and posterior longitudinal ligaments.

The nucleus pulposus. The central portion of the disk is a gelatinous mass that normally is contained within but whose loosely aligned fibers merge with the inner layer of the annulus fibrosus. It is located centrally in the disk except in the lumbar spine where it is situated closer to the posterior border than the anterior border of the annulus. Aggregating proteoglycans, normally in high concentration in a healthy nucleus, have a great affinity for water. The resulting fluid mechanics of the confined nucleus functions to evenly distribute pressure throughout the disk and from one vertebral body to the next under loaded conditions. Because of the affinity for water, the nucleus imbibes water when pressure is reduced on the disk and water is squeezed out under compressive loads. These fluid dynamics provide transport for nutrients and help maintain tissue health in the disk.

With flexion (forward bending) of a vertebral segment, the anterior portion of the disk is compressed, and the posterior is distracted. The nucleus pulposus generally does not move in a healthy disk but may have a slight distortion with flexion, potentially to redistribute the load through the disk.[51] Asymmetric loading in flexion results in distortions of the nucleus toward the contralateral posterolateral corner, where the fibers of the annulus are more stretched.[4]

The cartilaginous end-plates. End-plates cover the nucleus pulposus superiorly and inferiorly and lie between the nucleus and vertebral bodies. Each one is encircled by the apophyseal ring of the respective vertebral body. The collagen fibers of the inner annulus fibrosus insert into the end-plate and angle centrally, thus encapsulating the nucleus pulposus. Nutrition diffuses from the marrow of the vertebral bodies to the disk via the end-plates.[76]

Inert Structures: Influence on Movement and Stability

When a structure limits movement in a specific direction, it provides stability in that direction.[18,44]

The Slant, Direction, and Joint Capsules of the Articulating Facets

Cervical region. In the cervical spine, the facets are generally in the frontal plane, with some oblique angulation toward the transverse plane, allowing relatively free forward bending (flexion) and backward bending (extension). From the second cervical vertebra to the third thoracic vertebra, side bending and rotation of the vertebrae always occur together and are toward the same side whether in the upright position or in the forward-bent position.

Thoracic region. In the upper thoracic spine, the facets are in the frontal plane with slight angulation toward the sagittal plane. In the lower thoracic spine, they lie more in the sagittal plane. Rotation, side bending, and forward bending are allowed to various degrees by the facets but are restricted by the ribs. The facets markedly restrict backward bending along with the spinous processes. The upper three or four thoracic vertebrae function with the cervical spine on side bending and rotation. The remainder of the thoracic vertebrae function similarly to the lumbar vertebrae so that when upright, side bending of the vertebrae results in vertebral rotation in the opposite direction for the vertebrae below the third thoracic level.

Lumbar region. In the lumbar spine, the facets are typically in the sagittal plane with some curvature in the frontal plane, although variations in shape and orientation occur,[11] allowing some forward, backward, and side bending, but limiting rotation except in the lower lumbar segments. At the end of the range of forward bending, the facet surfaces in the frontal plane approximate and provide stability against further movement and shear.[100] When upright, side bending occurs with rotation in opposite directions. When forward bent, side bending and rotation of the vertebrae occur together in the same direction.

The Ligaments

- The ligaments posterior to the axis of motion limit forward bending (flexion) of the spinal segments. Ligaments subjected to highest strains with forward bending are the interspinous and supraspinous ligaments. The capsular ligaments, ligamentum flavum, and posterior longitudinal ligament also become taut and stabilize the spine at the end of the flexion range.[78]
- The anterior longitudinal ligament limits backward bending.
- The contralateral intertransverse ligaments, as well as ligamentum flavum and capsular ligaments, limit side bending.
- The capsular ligaments limit rotation.

The Thoracolumbar (Lumbodorsal) Fascia

The thoracolumbar fascia is an extensive fascial system in the back that consists of several layers.[10,11,30–32,64]

- It surrounds the erector spinae and quadratus lumborum, thus providing support to these muscles when they contract[31] (Fig. 15–1).
- The aponeurosis of the latissimus dorsi and fibers from the serratus posterior inferior, internal obliques, and transverse abdominis muscles blend together at the lateral raphe of the thoracolumbar fascia, so that contraction in these muscles increases tension through the angled fascia, causing stabilizing forces for the lumbar spine[31] (Fig. 15–2). This functional relationship is described in the following section.
- Passive tension in the posterior layer of the fascia occurs with forward bending of the lumbar spine on the pelvis or posterior tilt of the pelvis. The increased tension supports the lower lumbar vertebrae.[11]

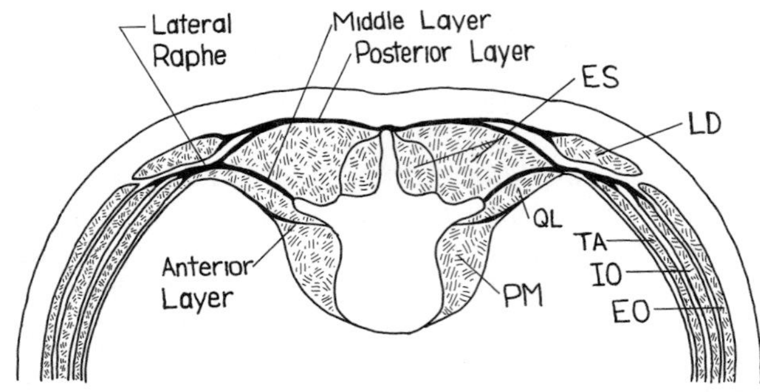

Figure 15–1 Transverse section in the lumbar region showing the relationships of the three layers of the thoracolumbar fascia to the muscles in the region and their attachments to the spine. ES = erector spinae; TA = transversus abdominus; IO = internal obliques; EO = external obliques; LD = latissimus dorsi; PM = psoas major; QL = quadratus lumborum muscles.

The Shape and Slant of the Spinous Processes

With extension, the spinous processes approximate. This is especially evident in the thoracic region with the overlapping spinous processes that limit extension.

The Relative Size of the Intervertebral Disk and Bodies

The greater the ratio of disk thickness to vertebral body height, the greater the mobility. The cervical spine ratio is 2:5 and is most mobile; the thoracic ratio is 1:5 and is least mobile; the lumbar ratio is 1:3.[44]

The Annulus Fibrosus of the Intervertebral Disk

The organized concentric rings of the annulus provide tensile strength to the disk. Movement is allowed, yet some fibers will be taut whichever direction the spinal column bends, twists, or shears, and therefore will behave similarly to ligaments.[11]

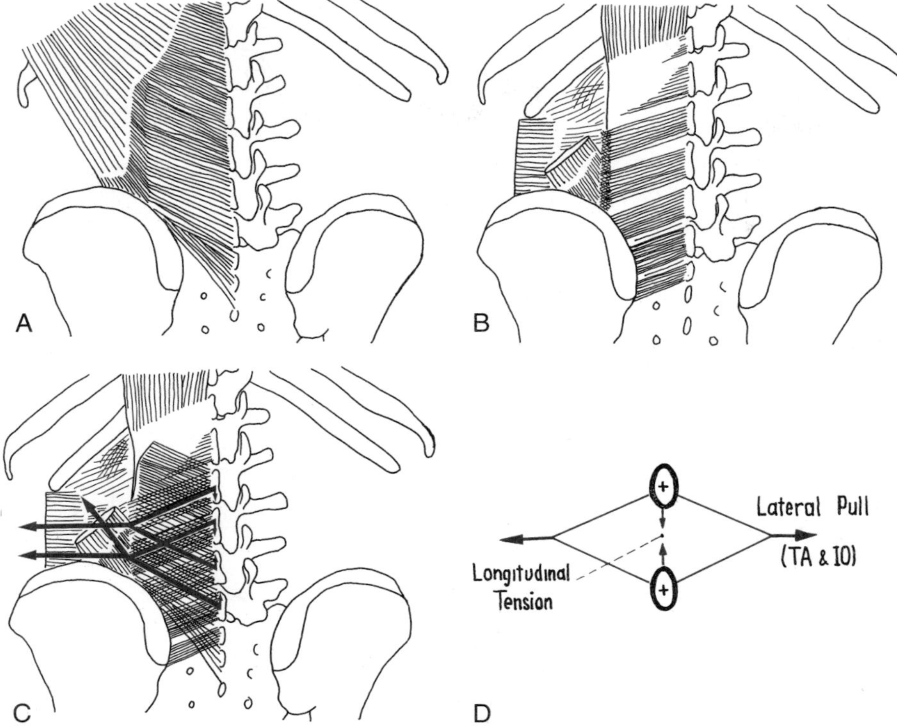

Figure 15–2 Orientation and attachments of the posterior layer of the thoracolumbar fascia. From the lateral raphe, *(A)* the fibers of the superficial lamina are angled inferiorly and medially, and *(B)* the fibers of the deep lamina are angled superiorly and medially. *(C)* Tension in the angled fibers of the posterior layer of the fascia is transmitted to the spinous processes in opposing directions, resisting separation of the spinous processes. *(D)* Diagrammatic representation of a lateral pull at the lateral raphe, resulting in a tension between the lumbar spinous processes that oppose separation, thus providing stability to the spine. (*A, B,* and *C* adapted from Bogduck and MacIntosh,[10] pp 166–167, 169 with permission; *D* adapted from Gracovetsky, Farfan, and Helleur,[30] p 319 with permission).

The Ribs in the Thoracic Region

The ribs limit all motions of the thorax.

- During side bending, the thorax is elevated and enlarged to the contralateral side (side of the convexity) and is compressed on the ipsilateral side.
- During rotation, the ribs protrude posteriorly on the side on which the vertebral body rotates and are flattened on the contralateral side.

Muscles

Muscles with normal elasticity do not cause limitations of spinal movement. When they develop contractures, they restrict movement opposite to their direction of contraction. Muscles provide dynamic stability and control of the spine as described in the following section.

Neuromuscular Function: Dynamic Stabilization

The muscles of the neck and trunk not only act as prime movers or as antagonists to movement caused by gravity during dynamic activity but are the primary stabilizers of the spine.[10,11,30–32,64,100] Without the dynamic stabilization from muscle the spine would collapse in the upright position. The muscles of the neck and trunk are activated and controlled by the nervous system, which is influenced by peripheral and central mechanisms in response to fluctuating forces and activities. Greater percentages of type I fibers than type II fibers are found in all back muscles, which is reflective of their postural and stabilization function.[74] Inactivity has been shown to change muscle fiber composition (decrease size) and may be one reason for decreased function in patients with low back pain.[74]

Muscle Control in the Lumbar Spine

Muscles of the abdominal wall as well as superficial and deep muscles of the spinal region act to stabilize the spine under varying conditions.[63] The more superficial muscles, the erector spinae (ES), rectus abdominis (RA), and external oblique (EO), function as prime movers with secondary function in stabilization. The deeper (core) muscles, the multifidus, rotatores, tranversus abdominis (TrA), internal oblique (IO), and quadratus lumborum (QL), are closer to the axis and primarily function to stabilize.

The transversus abdominis and internal oblique muscles. These two deep abdominal muscles attach to the thoracolumbar fascia posteriorly (see Fig. 15–1) and through their action develop tension that acts like a girdle of support around the abdomen and lumbar vertebra. Only the TrA is active with both isometric trunk flexion and extension, whereas the other abdominal muscles have decreased activity with resisted extension. This may be related to the stabilization function of the TrA.[21] With rotation, the ipsilateral TrA is selectively active and thus contributes to twisting torques.[21] During the Valsalva maneuver, contraction of the TrA and IO along with the EO muscle are activated to increase the intra-abdominal pressure.[21] The increased intra-abdominal pressure pushes out against these muscles, increasing their length-tension relationship and stabilizing force on the thoracolumbar fascia (Fig. 15–3) as well as assisting in unloading the spine.[32] This mechanism is used in the "bracing maneuver" for spinal stabilization. Voluntary activation of the TrA and IO also occurs with a "drawing in" maneuver.[83] (See Chapter 16 for description of these maneuvers.)

Internal and external oblique muscles. The line of pull of the EO on one side and the contralateral IO work together to cause diagonal trunk rotation with flexion. Internal and external obliques on the same side cause side bending of the trunk. These muscles contract to control against the prime mover force of gravity when bending sideways or backward. The obliques along with the rectus abdominis stabilize against anterior rotation of the pelvis and are therefore important postural muscles.

Rectus abdominis. This muscle is the primary trunk flexor. It, along with the iliopsoas muscle, is the muscle primarily active in sit-up and curl-up exercises[63] and in maintaining a posterior pelvic tilt during leg-lifting or leg-lowering exercises.[84]

The quadratus lumborum. This is an important stabilizer of the spine[63] acting in the frontal and sagittal planes to stabilize the vertebrae against shifting forces. It also stabilizes the ribs against the pull of the diaphragm during inspiration.[8]

The multifidus. This deep, multifascicled dynamic spinal extensor and contralateral rotator of the lumbar spine, functions to stabilize the spine against flexion and rotation moment and contralateral side flexion. It increases spinal stiffness. It is activated

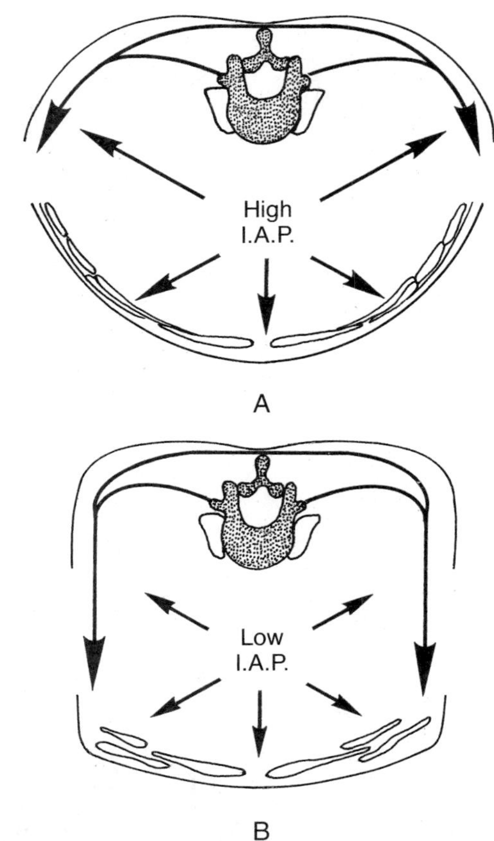

Figure 15–3 *(A)* Increased intra-abdominal pressure (IAP) pushes outward against the transversus abdominus and internal obliques, creating increased tension on the thoracolumbar fascia, resulting in improved spinal stability *(B)* Reduced pressure allows flexion of the spine. (Adapted from Gracovetsky,[32] p 114 with permission)

with the "drawing-in" and "bracing" maneuvers used for spinal stabilization.[83]

The intersegmental muscles (rotators and intertransversarii muscles). These muscles are rich in muscle spindles and may function to sense vertebral position and motion more so than to produce torque for movement. Theoretically they can make small segmental adjustments to stabilize against perturbations.

The superficial erector spinae muscles. The primary trunk extensors do not attach directly to the lumbar vertebrae, but they function as prime movers for spinal extension by pulling the thorax posterior and the prime antagonists to gravity by controlling movement of the trunk during forward-bending activities. When contracting strongly, these muscles generally cause increased compressive and shear forces on the spine.

Iliopsoas (iliacus and psoas major). The iliacus primarily functions as a hip flexor and stabilizer of the pelvis and hip joints.[7] The psoas assists in stabilizing the lumbar spine in the frontal plane, especially when a heavy load is applied to the contralateral side,[7] but in general, this muscle complex does not function as a spinal stabilizer in normal standing.[7,63] Contraction of the psoas increases the compressive load and anterior shear forces on the lumbar vertebrae. It is generally accepted that decreased flexibility in this and the iliopsoas muscle increase lumbar lordosis, anterior pelvic tilt, and a hip flexion posture.

Effect of Poor Postural Support from Trunk Muscles

Little muscle activity is required to maintain upright posture, but with total relaxation of muscles the spinal curves become exaggerated and passive structural support is called on to maintain the posture.

When there is continued end-range loading, strain occurs with creep and fluid redistribution in the supporting tissues, making them vulnerable to injury.[98]

Continual exaggeration of the curves leads to postural impairments and muscle strength and flexibility imbalances as well as other soft tissue restrictions or hypermobility. Muscles that are habitually kept in a stretched position tend to test weaker because of a shift in the length-tension curve; this is known as **stretch weakness.**[46] Muscles kept in a habitually shortened position tend to lose their elasticity. These muscles test strong only in the shortened position but become weak as they are lengthened.[29] This is known as **tight weakness.**[29]

Effect of Limb Muscles on Spinal Stability

Feedforward and spinal stability. The CNS activates the trunk muscles in anticipation of the load imposed by limb movement to maintain stability in the spine.[42] Recent research has demonstrated that there are feedforward postural responses of all trunk muscles preceding activity in muscles that move the extremities[39,40,42] and that anticipatory activation of the transversus abdominis is independent of the other abdominal muscles in various postural tasks.[38] The transversus abdominis and internal and external oblique muscles consistently contract with leg movements, but activation of the rectus abdominis and multifidus action vary with the direction that the lower extremities move.[42] In addition, speed but not direction of arm movements directly affects the activation of the transversus abdominis and internal obliques.[37,41] There are reported differences in patterns of muscle recruitment in patients with low back pain (LBP) with delayed recruitment of the transversus abdominis in all movement directions and delayed recruitment of the rectus abdominis, erector spinae, and oblique abdominal muscles specific to direction of movement compared to healthy subjects.[39]

Without adequate stabilization of the spine, contraction of the limb-girdle musculature will transmit forces proximally and cause motions of the spine that will place excessive stresses on spinal structures and the supporting soft tissue. For example, stabilization of the pelvis and lumbar spine by the abdominal muscles against the pull of the iliopsoas muscle is necessary during active hip flexion to avoid increased lumbar lordosis and anterior shearing of the vertebrae. Stabilization of the ribs by the intercostal and abdominal muscles is necessary for an effective pushing force from the pectoralis major and serratus anterior muscles.

Localized fatigue in the stabilizing spinal musculature may occur with repetitive activity or heavy exertion. There is greater chance of injury in the supporting structures of the spine when the stabilizing muscles fatigue. Marras reports significant changes in motion patterns between the spine and lower extremity joints, as well as significant changes in muscle recruitment patterns with repetitive lifting during an extended period of time, resulting in decreased spinal compression but increased anterior/posterior shear in the lumbar spine.[60]

Imbalances in the flexibility and strength of hip, shoulder, and neck musculature will cause asymmetric forces on the spine and affect posture.

Effects of Breathing on Posture and Stability

Inspiration and thoracic spine extension elevate the rib cage and align the spine. The intercostal muscles function as postural muscles to stabilize and move the ribs as well as function as a dynamic membrane between the ribs to prevent sucking in and blowing out of the soft tissue with the pressure changes during respiration.[8]

Inspiration followed by abdominal muscle contraction unloads the compressive forces on the spine and is a technique frequently used by individuals lifting heavy loads. Using this technique increases the risk of eliciting the Valsalva maneuver, so individuals are taught to slowly exhale while maintaining the abdominal contractions. To reinforce the importance of exhaling during exertion, Hodges et al.[36] found that if a static expulsive effort is maintained (holding breath while contracting the abdominals), activation of the transverse abdominis is delayed. Since activation of the transversus abdominis is important for spinal stability, expiration during exertion is important to reinforce this function.

There is early activation of the transverse abdominis and internal oblique muscles in feedforward stabilization of the spine if there is increased expiratory effort when initiating upper extremity flexion.[36]

Dynamic Support for the Head and Cervical Spine (Fig. 15–4)

The fulcrum of the head on the spine is through the occipital/atlas joints. The center of gravity of the head is anterior to the joint axis and therefore has a flexion moment. The weight of the head is counterbalanced by the cervical extensor muscles.

The mandible is maintained in its resting position with the jaw partially closed through action of the mandibular elevators (masseter, temporalis, and internal pterygoid muscles).

The anterior throat muscles (suprahyoid and infrahyoid muscle groups) assist with swallowing and balancing the jaw against the muscles of mastication. These muscles also function to flex the neck when rising from the supine position. With a forward head posture, they tend to be stretched and weak so that the person lifts the head with the sternocleidomastoid muscles.

The scalene and levator scapulae muscles act as guy wires to counterstabilize against the posterior and anterior translatory forces on the neck.

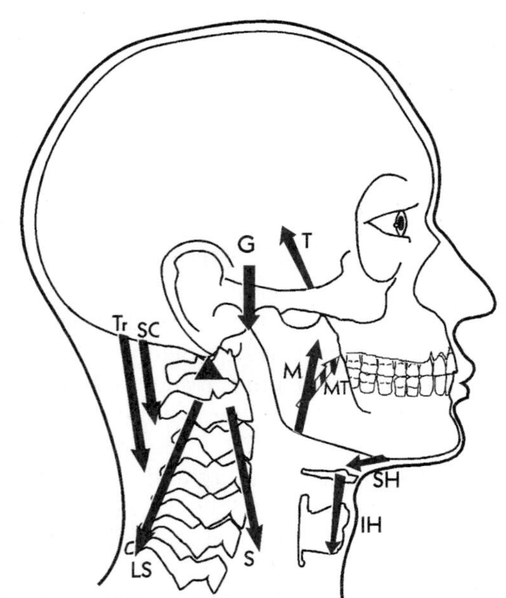

Figure 15–4 Head balance on the cervical spine. The posterior cervical muscles (trapezius and semispinalis capitis) counter the weight of the head. The mandibular elevating muscles (masseter, temporalis, and medial pterygoid) maintain jaw elevation opposing the mandibular depression force of gravity and tension in the anterior throat muscles (suprahyoid and infrahyoid groups). The scalene and levator muscles stabilize against the posterior and anterior translatory forces on the cervical vertebrae. (Tr = trapezius; SC = semispinalis capitis; M = masseter; T = temporalis; MT = medial pterygoid; SH = suprahyoid; IF = infrahyoid; S = scalene; LS = levator scapulae; G = center of gravity; ▲ = axis of motion.)

▶ Posture

Posture Defined

Posture is a "position or attitude of the body, the relative arrangement of body parts for a specific activity, or a characteristic manner of bearing one's body."[94] Ligaments, fasciae, bones, and joints are inert structures that support the body, whereas muscles and their tendinous attachments are the dynamic structures that maintain the body in a posture or move it from one posture to another.

Gravity places stress on the structures responsible for maintaining the body upright in a posture. Normally, the gravitational line goes through the physiological curves of the spinal column and they are balanced. If the weight in one region shifts away from the line of gravity, the remainder of the column compensates to regain equilibrium.

The Equilibrium of Posture

For a weight-bearing joint to be stable, or in equilibrium, the gravity line of the mass must fall exactly through the axis of rotation, or there must be a force to counteract the force of gravity. In the body, the counterforce is provided by either muscle or inert structures.[54a,94] Upright posture usually involves a slight anterior/posterior swaying of the body of about 4 centimeters.

In the standing posture, the following occur:

Ankle. The gravity line is anterior to the joint so it tends to rotate the tibia forward about the ankle. Stability is provided by the plantarflexor muscles, primarily the soleus muscle.

Knee. The normal gravity line is anterior to the joint, which tends to keep the knee in extension. Stability is provided by the anterior cruciate ligament, posterior capsule (locking mechanism of the knee), and tension in the muscles posterior to the knee (the gastrocnemius and hamstring muscles). The soleus provides active stability by pulling posteriorly on the tibia. With the knees fully extended, no muscle support is required at that joint to maintain an upright posture, but if the knees flex slightly, the gravity line shifts posterior to the joint, and the quadriceps femoris muscle must contract to prevent the knee from buckling.

Hip. The gravity line varies with the swaying of the body. When it passes through the hip joint, there is equilibrium, and no external support is necessary. When the gravitational line shifts posterior to the joint, some posterior rotation of the pelvis occurs, which is controlled by tension in the hip flexor muscles (primarily the iliopsoas). In relaxed standing, the iliofemoral ligament provides passive stability to the joint, and no muscle tension is necessary. When the gravitational line shifts anteriorly, stability is provided by active support of the hip extensor muscles.

Trunk. Normally, the gravity line goes through the bodies of the lumbar and cervical vertebrae, and the curves are balanced. Some activity in the muscles of the trunk and pelvis helps maintain the balance. As the trunk shifts, contralateral muscles contract and function as guy wires. Extreme or sustained deviations are supported by inert structures.

Head. The center of gravity of the head falls anterior to the atlanto-occipital joints. The posterior cervical muscles contract to keep the head balanced. In postures in which the head is forward, greater demand is placed on these muscles. At the extreme of flexion, tension in the ligamentum nuchae prevents further motion.

Etiology of Pain in Postural Impairments

The ligaments, facet capsules, periosteum of the vertebrae, muscles, anterior dura mater, dural sleeves, epidural areolar adipose tissue, and walls of blood vessels are innervated and responsive to nociceptive stimuli.[54] Mechanical stress to pain-sensitive structures, such as sustained stretch to ligaments or joint capsules or compression of blood vessels, causes distention or compression of the nerve endings, which leads to the experience of pain. This type of stimulus occurs in the absence of an inflammatory reaction. It is not a pathologic problem but a mechanical one because signs of an acute inflammation with constant pain are not present. Relieving the stress to the pain-sensitive structure relieves the pain stimulus, and the person no longer experiences pain.

Endurance in muscles is necessary to maintain postural control. Sustained postures require continual, small adaptations in the stabilizing muscles to support the trunk against fluctuating forces. Large repetitive motions also require muscles to respond to control the activity. In either case, as the muscles fatigue, the load is shifted to the inert tissues supporting the spine at the end-ranges. With the sustained load, creep and distention occur in the inert tissues, causing mechanical stress.

If the mechanical stresses exceed the supporting capabilities of the tissues, breakdown will occur. If this occurs without adequate healing, overuse syndromes with inflammation and pain will affect function without an apparent injury. In addition, injuries occur more frequently when there is muscle fatigue. Relieving the mechanical stress along with decreasing the inflammation is important.

Pain Syndromes Related to Impaired Posture

Postural Fault and the Postural Pain Syndrome

A **postural fault** is a posture that deviates from normal alignment but has no structural limitations. **Postural pain syndrome** refers to the pain that occurs from mechanical stress when a person maintains a faulty posture for a prolonged period; the pain is usually relieved with activity. There are no abnormalities in muscle strength or flexibility, but if the faulty posture continues, strength and flexibility imbalances will eventually develop.

Postural Dysfunction

Postural dysfunction differs from the postural pain syndrome in that adaptive shortening of soft tissues and muscle weakness are involved. The cause may be prolonged poor postural habits, or it may be a result of contractures and adhesions formed during the healing of tissues after trauma or surgery. Stress to the shortened structures causes pain. In addition, strength and flexibility imbalances may predispose the area to injury or overuse syndromes that a normal musculoskeletal system could sustain.

Postural Habits

Good postural habits in the adult are necessary to avoid postural pain syndromes and postural dysfunctions. Also, careful follow-up in terms of flexibility and posture training exercises is important after trauma or surgery to prevent dysfunctions from contractures and adhesions. In the child, good postural habits are important to avoid abnormal stresses on growing bones and adaptive changes in muscle and soft tissue.

Common Faulty Postures: Characteristics and Impairments

The head, neck, thorax, lumbar spine, and pelvis are all interrelated, and deviations in one region will affect the other areas. In this section, each region and typical impairments are described separately for clarity of presentation. Box 15–1 summarizes common impairments with postural dysfunctions.

Pelvic and Lumbar Region

Lordotic Posture (Fig. 15–5*A*)

This posture is characterized by an increase in the lumbosacral angle (the angle that the superior border of the first sacral vertebral body makes with the horizontal, which optimally is 30 degrees), an increase in the lumbar lordosis, and an increase in the anterior pelvic tilt and hip flexion.[18] This is often seen with an increased thoracic kyphosis and forward head and is called a **kypholordotic posture.**[46]

Potential Sources of Pain

- Stress to the anterior longitudinal ligament.
- Narrowing of the posterior disk space and narrowing of the intervertebral foramen. This may compress the dura and blood vessels of the related nerve root or the nerve root itself, especially if there are degenerative changes in the vertebra or disk.[18]
- Approximation of the articular facets. The facets may become weight bearing, which may cause synovial irritation and joint inflammation.

Potential Muscle Impairments

- Decreased flexibility in the hip flexor muscles (iliopsoas, tensor fasciae latae, rectus femoris) and lumbar extensor muscles (erector spinae)
- Stretched and weak abdominal muscles (rectus abdominis, internal and external obliques, and transversus abdominis)

Common Causes

Sustained faulty posture, pregnancy, obesity, and weak abdominal muscles are common causes.

Box 15–1 Summary of Common Impairments Associated with Postural Dysfunctions

- Pain from mechanical stress to sensitive structures and from muscle tension
- Mobility impairment from restricting muscles, joints, or fascia
- Muscle impairment associated with weakness and poor muscular endurance from sustained faulty postures or disuse
- Insufficient postural control of stabilizing muscles
- Altered kinesthetic sense of posture associated with poor neuromuscular control and prolonged faulty postural habits
- Lack of knowledge of healthy spinal control and mechanics

Relaxed or Slouched Posture (Fig. 15–5*B*)

This posture is also called **swayback.**[46] The amount of pelvic tilting is variable, but usually there is a shifting of the entire pelvic segment anteriorly, resulting in hip extension, and shifting of the thoracic segment posteriorly, resulting in flexion of the thorax on the upper lumbar spine. This results in an increased lordosis in the lower lumbar region, an increased kyphosis in the thoracic region, and usually a forward head. The position of the mid- and upper lumbar spine depends on the amount of displacement of the thorax. When standing for prolonged periods, the person usually assumes an asymmetric stance in which most of the weight is borne on one lower extremity with pelvic drop (lateral tilt) and hip abduction on the unweighted side. This will affect frontal plane symmetry.

Potential Sources of Pain

- Stress to the iliofemoral ligaments, the anterior longitudinal ligament of the lower lumbar spine, and the posterior longitudinal ligament of the upper lumbar and thoracic spine. With asymmetric postures there is also stress to the iliotibial band on the side of the elevated hip. Other frontal plane asymmetries may also be present; (these are described on page 604).
- Narrowing of the intervertebral foramen in the lower lumbar spine that may compress the blood

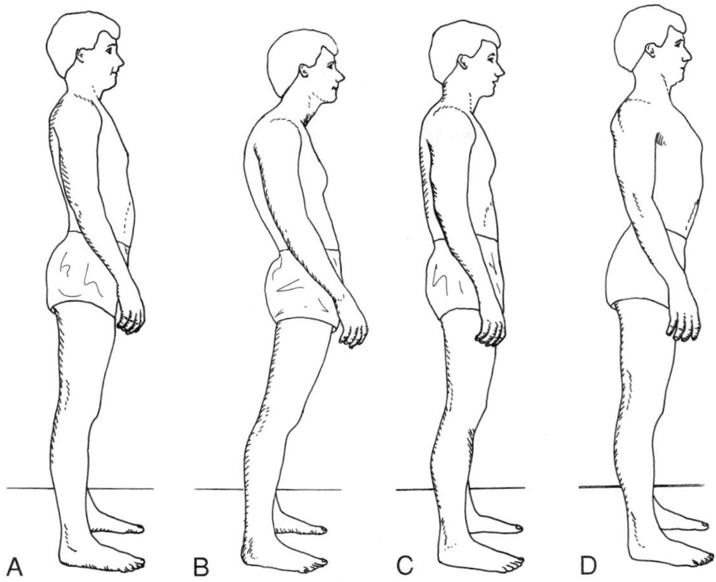

Figure 15–5 *(A)* Lordotic posture characterized by an increase in the lumbosacral angle, an increased lumbar lordosis, an increased anterior tilting of the pelvis, and hip flexion. *(B)* Relaxed or slouched posture characterized by an excessive shifting of the pelvic segment anteriorly, resulting in hip extension, and shifting of the thoracic segment posteriorly, resulting in flexion of the thorax on the upper lumbar spine. A compensatory increased thoracic kyphosis and forward-head placement are also seen. *(C)* Flat low-back posture characterized by a decreased lumbosacral angle, a decreased lumbar lordosis, and a posterior tilting of the pelvis. *(D)* Flat upper back and cervical spine characterized by a decrease in the thoracic curve, depressed scapulae, depressed clavicle, and an exaggeration of axial extension (flexion of the occiput on atlas and flattening of the cervical lordosis).

vessels, dura, and nerve roots, especially with arthritic conditions.
- Approximation of articular facets in the lower lumbar spine.

Potential Muscle Impairments
- Decreased flexibility in the upper abdominal muscles (upper segments of the rectus abdominis and obliques), internal intercostal, hip extensor, and lower lumbar extensor muscles and related fascia
- Stretched and weak lower abdominal muscles (lower segments of the rectus abdominis and obliques), extensor muscles of the lower thoracic region, and hip flexor muscles

Common Causes
As the name implies, this is a relaxed posture in which the muscles are not used to provide support. The person yields fully to the effects of gravity, and only the passive structures at the end of each joint range (such as ligaments, joint capsules, and bony approximation) provide stability. Causes may be attitudinal (the person feels comfortable when slouching), from fatigue (seen when required to stand for extended periods), or from muscle weakness (the weakness may be the cause or the effect of the posture). A poorly designed exercise program, one that emphasizes thoracic flexion without balancing strength with other appropriate exercises and postural training, may perpetuate these impairments.

Flat Low-Back Posture (Fig. 15–5C)

This posture is characterized by a decreased lumbosacral angle, a decreased lumbar lordosis, hip extension, and a posterior tilting of the pelvis.

Potential Sources of Pain
- Lack of the normal physiologic lumbar curve, which reduces the shock-absorbing effect of the lumbar region and predisposes the person to injury
- Stress to the posterior longitudinal ligament
- Increase of the posterior disk space, which allows the nucleus pulposus to imbibe extra fluid and, under certain circumstances, may protrude posteriorly when the person attempts extension.

Potential Muscle Impairments
- Decreased flexibility in the trunk flexor (rectus abdominis and intercostals) and hip extensor muscles
- Stretched and weak lumbar extensor and possibly hip flexor muscles

Common Causes
Continued slouching or flexing in sitting or standing postures; overemphasis on flexion exercises in general exercise programs

Thoracic Region

Round Back or Increased Kyphosis (see Fig. 15–5*B*)

This posture is characterized by an increased thoracic curve, protracted scapulae (round shoulders), and usually an accompanying forward head.

Potential Sources of Pain

- Stress to the posterior longitudinal ligament
- Fatigue of the thoracic erector spinae and scapular retractor muscles
- Thoracic outlet syndrome (see Chapter 9)
- Cervical posture syndromes (see page 603)

Potential Muscle Impairments

- Decreased flexibility in the muscles of the anterior thorax (intercostal muscles), muscles of the upper extremity originating on the thorax (pectoralis major and minor, latissimus dorsi, and serratus anterior), muscles of the cervical spine and head attached to the scapula (levator scapulae and upper trapezius), and muscles of the cervical region
- Stretched and weak thoracic erector spinae and scapular retractor muscles (rhomboids and middle trapezius)

Common Causes

Causes are similar to the relaxed lumbar posture or the flat low-back posture, continued slouching, and overemphasis on flexion exercises in general exercise programs.

Flat Upper Back (Fig. 15–5*D*)

This posture is characterized by a decrease in the thoracic curve, depressed scapulae, depressed clavicles, and a flat-neck posture. It is associated with an exaggerated military posture but is not a common postural deviation.

Potential Sources of Pain

- Fatigue of muscles required to maintain the posture
- Compression of the neurovascular bundle in the thoracic outlet between the clavicle and ribs

Potential Muscle Impairments

- Decreased flexibility in the thoracic erector spinae and scapular retractors and potentially restricted scapular movement, which decreases the freedom of shoulder elevation
- Weak scapular protractor and intercostal muscles of the anterior thorax

Common Cause

Exaggerating the upright posture is a common cause of flat upper back.

Scoliosis

Scoliosis usually involves the thoracic and lumbar regions. Typically, in right-handed individuals, there is a mild right thoracic, left lumbar S-curve, or a mild left thoracolumbar C-curve. There may be asymmetry in the hips, pelvis, and lower extremities.[17]

A **structural scoliosis** involves an irreversible lateral curvature with fixed rotation of the vertebrae (Fig. 15–6*A*). Rotation of the vertebral bodies is toward the convexity of the curve. In the thoracic spine, the ribs rotate with the vertebrae so that there is a prominence of the ribs posteriorly on the side of the spinal convexity and a prominence anteriorly on the side of the concavity. A posterior rib hump is detected on forward bending in a structural scoliosis (Fig. 15–6*B*).[17,56]

A *nonstructural scoliosis* is reversible and can be changed with forward or side bending and with positional changes such as lying supine, realignment of the pelvis by correction of a leg-length discrepancy, or with muscle contractions. It is also called a **functional** or **postural scoliosis.**[17]

Potential Sources of Pain

- Muscle fatigue and ligamentous strain on the side of the convexity.

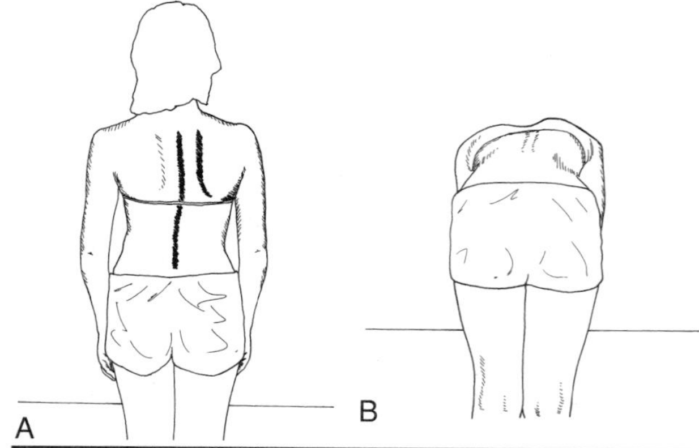

Figure 15–6 *(A)* Mild right thoracic left lumbar structural scoliosis with prominence of the right scapula. *(B)* Forward bending produces a slight posterior rib hump, indicating fixed rotation of the vertebrae and rib cage.

- Nerve root irritation on the side on the concavity.
- Potential muscle imbalances.
- Decreased flexibility in the musculature on the concave side of the curve.
- Stretched and weak musculature on the convex side of the curve.
- If one hip is adducted, the adductor muscles on that side will have decreased flexibility and the abductor muscles will be stretched and weak. The opposite will occur on the contralateral extremity.[46]

Common Causes: Structural Scoliosis

Neuromuscular diseases or disorders (such as cerebral palsy, spinal cord injury, or progressive neurological or muscular diseases), osteopathic disorders (such as hemivertebra, osteomalacia, rickets, or fracture), and idiopathic disorders in which the cause is unknown are common causes of structural scoliosis.

Common Causes: Nonstructural Scoliosis

Leg-length discrepancy, either structural or functional; muscle-guarding or spasm from a painful stimuli in the back or neck; and habitual or asymmetric postures are common causes of nonstructural scoliosis.

Cervical Region

Forward-Head Posture (see Fig. 15–5*B*)

This posture is characterized by increased flexion of the lower cervical and the upper thoracic regions, increased extension of the occiput on the first cervical vertebra, and increased extension of the upper cervical vertebrae. There also may be temporomandibular joint dysfunction with retrusion of the mandible.[22]

Potential Sources of Pain

- Stress to the anterior longitudinal ligament in the upper cervical spine and posterior longitudinal ligament in the lower cervical and upper thoracic spine
- Muscle tension or fatigue
- Irritation of facet joints in the upper cervical spine
- Narrowing of the intervertebral foramina in the upper cervical region, which may impinge on the blood vessels and nerve roots, especially if there are degenerative changes
- Impingement on the neurovascular bundle from anterior scalene muscle tightness (see also thoracic outlet syndrome in Chapter 9)
- Impingement of the cervical plexus from levator scapulae muscle tightness
- Impingement on the greater occipital nerves from a tight or tense upper trapezius muscle, leading to tension headaches
- Temporomandibular joint pain from faulty head, neck, and mandibular alignment and associated facial muscle tension
- Lower cervical disk lesions from the faulty flexed posture

Potential Muscle Impairments

- Decreased flexibility in the levator scapulae, sternocleidomastoid, scalene, and suboccipital muscles. If the scapulae are elevated, there may also be tight upper trapezius muscles. With temporomandibular joint symptoms, the muscles of mastication may have increased tension.
- Stretched and weakened anterior throat muscles (hyoid becomes fixed because of the stretched position) and lower cervical and upper thoracic erector spinae muscles.

Common Causes

Occupational or functional postures requiring leaning forward or tipping the head backward for extended periods, faulty sitting postures such as working at an improperly placed computer screen, relaxed postures, or the end result of a faulty pelvic and lumbar spine posture are common causes of forward-head posture.

Flat-Neck Posture (Fig. 15–5*D*)

This posture is characterized by a decreased cervical lordosis and increased flexion of the occiput on atlas (this is an exaggeration of axial extension). It may be seen with an exaggerated military posture (flat upper back). There may be temporomandibular joint dysfunction with protraction of the mandible.

Potential Sources of Pain

- Temporomandibular joint pain and occlusive changes.
- Decrease in the shock-absorbing function of the lordotic curve, which may predispose the neck to injury.
- Stress to the ligamentum nuchae.

Potential Muscle Impairments

- Decreased flexibility of the anterior neck muscles.
- Theoretically, the levator scapulae, sternocleidomastoid, and scalene muscles become stretched and weakened.

Common Causes

Exaggeration of the posture for extended periods of time is the common cause of flat-neck posture. This posture is uncommon.

Frontal Plane Deviations from Lower Extremity Asymmetries

Any lower extremity inequality will have an effect on the pelvis that, in turn, affects the spinal column and structures supporting it.[26] When dealing with spinal posture, it is imperative to assess lower extremity alignment, symmetry, foot posture, range of motion, muscle flexibility, and strength. See Chapters 12 through 14 for principles, procedures, and techniques for treating the hip, knee, ankle, and foot. Frontal plane deviations may also be seen with faulty postural habits such as perpetually standing with a pelvic drop on one side as frequently seen with slouched postures. This may result in muscle imbalances in the hip and spine and an apparent leg-length discrepancy.

Characteristic Deviations when Standing with Weight Equally Distributed to Both Lower Extremities (Fig. 15–7)

Elevated ilium on the long leg (LL) side and lowered on the short leg (SL) side is the characteristic deviation.

- This puts the LL in hip adduction with greater shear stress, and the SL in hip abduction with greater compression stress.
- The sacroiliac (SI) joint on the LL side is more vertical with greater shear stress; on the SL side it is more horizontal with greater compression stress.
- Side bending of the lumbar spine toward the LL side, coupled with rotation in the opposite direction.
  - This compresses the intervertebral disk on the LL side and distracts the disk on the SL side, as well as causes a torsional stress.
  - There is extension and compression of the lumbar facets on the LL side (concave portion of curve) and flexion and distraction of the lumbar facets on the SL side (convex portion of curve).

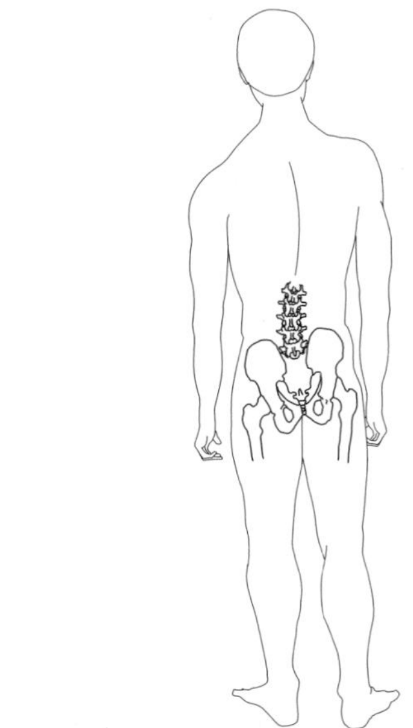

Figure 15–7 Frontal plane asymmetries: pictured is an individual with a long leg and elevated ilium on the right side. Typically on the long-leg side will be seen hip adduction, vertical SI joint, side bending toward and rotation opposite of lumbar spine, and compensations in thoracic and cervical spine.

  - There is narrowing of the intervertebral foramina on the LL side.
- The thoracic and cervical spine have a compensatory scoliosis in the opposite direction.

Potential Sources of Pain

- Greater shear forces occur in the hip and SI joints on the LL side, which increases stress in the supporting ligaments and decreases the load-bearing surface within the joint. Degenerative changes occur more frequently in hips on the LL side.[25]
- Stenosis in the lumbar intervertebral foramina on the LL side may cause vascular congestion or nerve root irritation.
- Lumbar facet compression and irritation on the LL side.
- Disk breakdown from torsional and asymmetric forces.
- Muscle tension, fatigue, or spasm in response to asymmetric loading and response.
- Lower extremity overuse syndromes.

Potential Muscle Impairments

- Decreased flexibility in the hip adductors on the LL side and abductors on the SL side. There may also be asymmetric differences in the iliopsoas, quadratus lumborum, piriformis, erector spinae, and multifidus muscles, with those on the concave side of the curve or LL side having decreased flexibility.

- Stretched and weakened muscles include hip adductors on the SL side, abductors on the LL side, and, in general, muscles on the convex side of the curve.

Common Causes

Asymmetry in the lower extremities may result from structural or functional deviations at the hip, knee, ankle, or foot. Common functional problems include unilateral flat foot and imbalances in the flexibility of muscles. The resulting asymmetric ground reaction forces transmitted to the pelvis and back may lead to tissue breakdown and overuse, particularly as a person ages, becomes overweight, or generally deconditions from inactivity.[81]

▶ Pathology of the Intervertebral Disk

Injury and Degeneration of the Disk

Fatigue Loading and Traumatic Rupture

Breakdown in the annulus fibrosus may occur with fatigue loading over time or with traumatic rupture.[3,4]

Fatigue breakdown. Over time, the annulus will break down as a result of repeated overloading of the spine in flexion with asymmetric forward bending and torsional stresses.[3,4,25,48]

- With torsional stresses, the annulus becomes distorted, most obviously at the posterolateral corner opposite the direction of rotation. The layers of the outer annulus fibrosus lose their cohesion and begin to separate from each other.
- Each layer then acts as a separate barrier to the nuclear material. Eventually, radial tears occur, and there is communication of the nuclear material between the layers.[25]
- With repeated forward bending and lifting stresses, the layers of the annulus are strained; they become tightly packed together in the posterolateral corners, radial fissures develop, and the nuclear material migrates down the fissures.[3,4] Outer layers of annular fibers can contain the nuclear material as long as they remain a continuous layer.[3] After injury, there is a tendency for the nucleus to swell and distort the annulus. Distortion is more severe in the region where the annular fibers are stretched.[4,55] If the outer layers rupture, the nuclear material may extrude through the fissures.
- Healing is attempted, but there is poor circulation in the disk. There may be self-sealing of a defect with the nuclear gel[59] or proliferation of cells of the annulus to seal the defect.[55] Any fibrous repair is weaker than normal and takes a long time because of the relative avascular status of the disk.

Traumatic rupture. Rupture of the annulus can occur as a one-time event or can be superimposed on a disk where there has been gradual breakdown of the annular rings. This is seen most commonly in traumatic hyperflexion injuries.[4]

Axial Overload

Axial overload of the disk usually results in end-plate damage or vertebral body fracture before there is any damage to the annulus fibrosus.[13,58]

Age

Individuals are most susceptible to symptomatic disk injuries between the ages of 30 and 45 years. During this time, the nucleus is still capable of imbibing water, but the annulus weakens from fatigue loading over time and, therefore, is less able to withstand increased pressures when there are disproportionately high stresses. The nuclear material may protrude into the tears of fissures, which most commonly are posterolateral and, with increased pressures, may bulge against the outer annular fibers, causing an annular distortion; or the nuclear material may extrude from the disk through complete fissures in the annulus.[3,14,25,56a]

Degenerative Changes

Any loss of integrity of the disk from infection, disease, herniation, or an end-plate defect becomes a stimulus for degenerative changes in the disk.[37]

- Degeneration is characterized by progressive fibrous changes in the nucleus, loss of the organization of the rings of the annulus fibrosus, and loss of the cartilaginous end-plates.[55]
- As the nucleus becomes more fibrotic, it loses its capacity to imbibe fluid. Water content decreases, and there is an associated decrease in the size of

the nucleus.[57] Acute disk protrusions caused by a bulging nucleus pulposus against the annulus or extrusions of the nucleus through a torn annulus are rare in older people.

- It is possible to have protrusions of the annulus fibrosus without nuclear pressure. Myxomatous degeneration with annular protrusion has been demonstrated in disk lesions in older people.[104]

Effect on Spinal Mechanics

Injury or degeneration of the disk affects spinal mechanics in general.[79] Initially there is increased mobility of the segment with greater than normal flexion/extension and forward and backward translation of the vertebral body.[58] Force distribution through the entire segment is altered, causing abnormal forces in the facets and supporting structures.[15,25,51]

Disk Pathologies and Related Conditions

Disk protrusions (derangements), tissue fluid stasis, diskogenic pain, and swelling from inflammation are conditions that may occur from prolonged flexion postures, repetitive flexion microtrauma, or traumatic flexion injuries. Initially symptoms may be exacerbated when attempting extension but then may be decreased when using carefully controlled extension motions. Several studies have documented that patients with herniated nucleus pulposus who have symptom reduction with an extension approach to treatment respond favorably to conservative nonsurgical treatment.[5,49]

Compression Fracture

Excessive axial compression loads usually cause end-plate or vertebral body fractures.[13,58] Flexion and axial loading usually cause increased pain. Pain occurs without nerve root involvement, although there may be referred pain into the extremities.

Disk Protrusions (Derangements)

A disk protrusion or herniation is any change in the shape of the annulus that causes it to bulge beyond its normal perimeter.

- ***Prolapse*** or contained: a protrusion of the nucleus that is still contained by the outer layers of the annulus and supporting ligamentous structures.
- ***Extrusion:*** a protrusion in which the nuclear material ruptures through the outer annulus and lies under the posterior longitudinal ligament.
- ***Free sequestration:*** the extruded nucleus has moved away from the prolapsed area.

Note: Various authors use these terms differently. The above descriptions are from MacNab.[58] Bogduk[11] defines *prolapse* as a frank rupture of nuclear material into the vertebral canal and *herniation* as the nuclear material being partially expelled into the canal with the majority remaining in a defect in the annulus. Saal[87] describes an *extrusion* as extension of nuclear material beyond the confines of the posterior longitudinal ligament or above and below the disk space as detected on MRI.

Tissue Fluid Stasis

With sustained flexed postures in the spine, the disks, facet joints, and ligaments are placed under sustained loading. The intradiskal pressure increases, and there is compression loading on the cartilage of the facets and a distractive tension on the posterior longitudinal ligament and posterior fibers of the annulus fibrosus. Creep and fluid transfer occur. Sudden movement into extension does not allow for redistribution of the fluids and increases the vulnerability of the distended tissue to injury and inflammation.[98] Symptoms may be similar to those described as disk lesions because they lessen with repeated extension motions and respond to treatment described in the following sections.

Signs and Symptoms of Disk Lesions and Fluid Stasis

Etiology of Symptoms

The disk is largely aneural; not all disk protrusions are symptomatic.

Pain. Symptoms of pain arise from pressure of the protrusion against pain-sensitive structures (ligaments, dura mater, and blood vessels around nerve roots).

Neurologic symptoms and signs. Neurologic signs arise from pressure against the spinal cord or nerve roots. The only true neurologic signs and symptoms are specific motor weaknesses and specific dermatome sensory changes. Radiating pain in a dermatomal pattern, increased myoelectrical activity in the hamstrings, decreased straight-leg raising, and depressed deep tendon reflexes can also be associated with referred pain stimuli from spinal muscles, interspinous ligaments, the disk, and facet joints and, therefore, are not true signs of nerve root pressure.[19,45,67]

Variability of symptoms. Symptoms are variable depending on the degree and direction of the protrusion as well as the spinal level of the lesion.

- Posterior or posterolateral protrusions are most common. With a small posterior or posterolateral lesion, there may be pressure against the posterior longitudinal ligament or against the dura mater or its extensions around the nerve roots. The patient may describe a severe midline backache or pain spreading across the back into the buttock and thigh.
- A large posterior protrusion may cause spinal cord signs such as loss of bladder control and saddle anesthesia.
- A large posterolateral protrusion may cause partial cord or nerve root signs.
- An anterior protrusion may cause pressure against the anterior longitudinal ligament, resulting in back pain. There may be no neurologic signs.
- The most common levels of protrusion are the segments between the fourth and fifth lumbar vertebrae and between the fifth lumbar vertebra and sacrum, although a protrusion may occur at any level.

Shifting symptoms. Symptoms may shift if there is integrity of the annular wall because the hydrostatic mechanism is still intact.[65]

Inflammation. Contents of the nucleus pulposus in the neural canal may cause an inflammatory reaction and irritate the dural sac, its nerve root sleeves, or the nerve roots. The symptoms may persist for extended periods and are not responsive to purely mechanical changes. The back pain may be worse than leg pain on the straight-leg raising test. Poor resolution of this inflammatory stimulus may lead to fibrotic reactions, nerve mobility impairments, and chronic pain.[62,89,91] Early medical intervention with anti-inflammatory agents is usually necessary.[91]

Onset and Behavior of Symptoms

Onset. Onset is usually between 20 and 55 years of age but most frequently from mid 30s to 40s. Except in cases of trauma, symptomatic onset in the lumbar spine is usually associated simply with bending, bending and lifting, or attempting to stand up after having been in a prolonged recumbent, sitting, or forward-bent posture. The person may or may not have the sensation of something tearing.[47,58,65] Although cervical disk lesions are not as prevalent, a prolonged flexed spinal position as in a forward head posture may exacerbate symptoms from a protrusion. Many patients have a predisposing history of a faulty flexion posture.

Pain behavior. Pain may increase gradually when the person is inactive, such as when sitting or after a night's rest. The patient often describes increased pain when attempting to get out of bed in the morning or when first standing up. Symptoms are usually aggravated with activities that increase the intradiskal pressure, such as sitting, forward bending, coughing, or straining or when attempting to stand after being in a flexed position. Usually, symptoms are lessened during walking.[47,58,65]

Acute pain. When there is inflammation during the acute phase, the pain is almost always present but varies in intensity, depending on the person's position or activity.

When there is a lumbar disk lesion, initially discomfort is noticed in the lumbosacral or buttock region. Some patients experience aching that extends into the thigh. In the cervical spine, initially pain is noticed in the midscapular and shoulder area. Numbness or muscle weakness (neurological signs) are not noted unless the protrusion has progressed to a degree in which there is nerve root, spinal cord, or cauda equina compression.

Objective Clinical Findings in the Lumbar Spine

Note: The following information relates to a contained posterior or posterolateral nuclear protrusion in the lumbar spine.[47,65] The impairments are summarized in Box 15–2.

Box 15–2 Summary of Common Impairments Related to Disk Protrusions in the Lumbar Spine

- Pain, muscle-guarding
- Flexed posture and deviation away from (usually) the symptomatic side
- Neurological symptoms in dermatome and possibly myotome of affected nerve roots
- Increased symptoms with sitting, prolonged flexed postures, transition from sit to stand, coughing, straining
- Limited nerve mobility, such as straight-leg raising (usually between 30 and 60 degrees)
- Peripheralization of symptoms with repeated forward-bending (spinal flexion) tests

- The patient usually prefers standing and walking to sitting.
- The patient may have a decrease in or loss of lumbar lordosis and may have some lateral shifting of the spinal column.
- Forward bending is limited. When repeating the forward-bending test, the symptoms increase or peripheralize. *Peripheralization* means the symptoms are experienced farther down the leg.
- Backward bending is limited; when repeating the backward-bending test, the pain lessens or centralizes. *Centralization* means the symptoms recede up the leg or become localized to the back. Important exceptions are:[65]
  - If there is a lateral shift of the spinal column, backward bending increases the pain. If the lateral shift is first corrected, then repeated backward bending lessens or centralizes the pain (see Figs 15–9 and 15–10).
  - If the protrusion cannot be mechanically reduced, backward bending peripheralizes or increases the symptoms.
  - If there is an anterior protrusion, backward bending increases the pain and forward bending relieves the pain.
- Testing passive lumbar flexion in the supine position and passive extension in the prone position usually produces signs similar to those of the standing tests, but results may not be as dramatic because gravity is eliminated.
- Pain between 30 and 60 degrees of straight-leg raising is considered positive for interference of dural mobility but not pathognomonic for a disk protrusion.[47,101]
- A contained nuclear protrusion can be influenced by movement because the hydrostatic mechanism is still intact. An extruded or sequestrated nucleus with a complete annular tear disrupts the hydrostatic mechanism and cannot be influenced by movement.[65] Anti-inflammatory intervention by a physician is important to reduce the inflamed tissue in the acute phase. Patients with disk extrusions may respond to conservative measures due to resolution of the inflammation and resorption of the extruded disk material.[87]

Objective Clinical Findings in the Cervical Spine

- Findings are similar as in the lumbar spine except displayed in the respective dermatomes and myotomes of the cervical nerve roots.
- Initially the patient may present with a faulty forward head posture and may hold the head in a guarded side-bent or rotated position away from the symptomatic side.
- Cervical flexion peripheralizes the symptoms; neck retractions (axial extension) may centralize the symptoms.
- There may be nerve mobility impairments.
- Traction may relieve the symptoms.

Pathomechanical Relationships of the Intervertebral Disk and Facet Joints

The Three-Joint Complex

The disk and facets make up a three-joint complex between two adjoining vertebrae and are biomechanically interrelated. Asymmetric disk injury affects the kinematics of the entire unit plus the joints above and below, resulting in asymmetric movements of the facets, abnormal stresses, and eventual cartilage degeneration.[79] As the disk degenerates, there is a decrease in both water content and disk height. The vertebral bodies approximate, and the intervertebral foramina and spinal canal narrow.[15,18]

Initial Changes

Initially, there is increased slack with increased mobility and translation in the spinal segment.[58] Opposition of the facet surfaces changes and the capsules are strained, resulting in irritation, swelling, and muscle spasm.

Altered Muscle Control

Altered joint receptor function negatively affects muscle recruitment in swollen joints.[95] Pain has also been cited as a factor for altered and diminished recruitment patterns in the stabilizing muscles of the spine.[42] Increasing shear forces from poor stabilization especially in the midrange may contribute to segmental hypermobility or instability.[27]

Progressive Bony Changes

Eventually, with the repeated irritation from the faulty mechanics, there are progressive bony changes in the facet and vertebral body margins. Osteophyte formation along the facets and spondylitic lipping and spurring along the vertebral bodies occur, and hypomobility develops.[51,68] These lead to additional narrowing of the associated foramina and spinal canal. In the cervical spine, the uncovertebral joints thicken, roughen, and distort.[86]

Related Pathologies

Segmental Instability

Segmental instability has been described as poor control in the neutral zones within the physiological range of spinal movement because of a decrease in the capacity of the neuromuscular stabilizing system to control the movement.[27,79] Clinically, patients demonstrate difficulty moving in the midranges of spinal motion and may demonstrate a shifting or fluctuation in movement.

Stenosis

Stenosis is a narrowing of a passage or opening. In the spine, stenosis is any compromise of the space in the spinal canal (central stenosis), nerve root canal, or foramen (lateral stenosis) and may be congenital or acquired. The narrowing may be from soft tissue structures such as a disk protrusion, fibrotic scars, or joint swelling or from bony narrowing as with spondylitic osteophyte formation or spondylolisthesis. With progression, neurologic symptoms develop. Extension exacerbates the symptoms.[75]

Neurologic Symptoms

Spinal nerve roots or spinal cord symptoms occur:

- When a protrusion of the disk compresses against the cord or nerve roots
- When there is decreased disk height from degenerative changes[80] or excessive translation of the vertebra from shear forces[58] resulting in a decreased foraminal space
- When there is an inflammatory response from trauma, degeneration, or disease with accompanying edema and stenosis
- When a facet joint subluxes and the nerve root becomes impinged between the tip of the superior articulating facet and the pedicle
- When spondylosis results in osteophytic growth on the articular facets or along the disk borders of the vertebral bodies that decrease spinal canal or intervertebral foraminal size
- When there is spondylolisthesis, or when there is scarring or adhesion formation after injury or spinal surgery

Dysfunction

The cycle of dysfunction from injury, pain, and muscle splinting leads to further restriction of movement, pain, and muscle splinting unless appropriate therapy is introduced. There is additional description of facet joint pathologies in the following section.

Pathology of the Zygapophyseal (Facet) Joints

Facet Joint Characteristics

Facet joints are synovial articulations that are enclosed in a capsule and supported by ligaments; they respond to trauma and arthritic changes similar to any peripheral joint.

Various types of meniscoid-like structures or invaginations of the facet capsules are present in the zygapophyseal joints of the spine. They are synovial reflections containing fat and blood vessels. In some cases, dense fibrous tissue develops as a result of mechanical stresses.[9,10] Some people describe an entrapment of these structures between the articulating surfaces with sudden or unusual movement as a source of pain and limited motion via tension on the well-innervated capsule.[50,96] Bogduk describes the *locked-back mechanism* as being an extrapment of the meniscoids in the supracapsular or infracapsular folds, which then blocks the return to extension from the flexed position.[9,10] It is called an extrapment because the meniscoid fails to re-enter the joint cavity; consequently, it becomes a space-occupying lesion in the capsular folds, causing pain as it impacts and stretches the capsules.

Common Diagnoses and Impairments from Facet Joint Pathologies

The etiology of facet joint pathologies may be from trauma, degenerative, or systemic pathologies. Box 15–3 summarizes the impairments and functional limitations.

Facet Sprain/Joint Capsule Injury

There is usually a history of trauma, such as falling or a motor vehicle accident. The joints react with effusion (swelling), limited ROM, and accompanying muscle splinting. The swelling may cause foraminal stenosis and neurological signs.

Osteoarthritis, Degenerative Joint Disease, Spondylosis

- Usually there is a history of faulty posture, prolonged immobilization after injury, severe

Box 15–3 Summary of Common Impairments and Functional Limitations Related to the Facet Joints

- Pain: When acute, there is pain and muscle guarding with all motions; pain when subacute and chronic is related to periods of immobility or excessive activity.
- Mobility impairments: Usually hypomobility and decreased joint play in affected joints; there may be hypermobility or instability in early stages
- Postural impairments
- Extension may cause or increase neurological symptoms due to foraminal stenosis; therefore, may be unable to sustain or perform repetitive extension activities without exacerbating symptoms
- Any functional activity that requires flexibility or prolonged repetition of trunk motions such as repetitive lifting and carrying of heavy objects may exacerbate symptoms in the arthritic spine

trauma, repetitive trauma, or degenerative changes in the disk.

- In the early stages of degenerative changes, there is greater play, or hypermobility/instability, in the three-joint complex. Over time, stress from the altered mechanics leads to osteophyte formation with spurring and lipping along the joint margins and vertebral bodies. Progressive hypomobility with bony stenosis results.
- Usually, where there is hypomobility, compensatory hypermobility occurs in neighboring spinal segments.
- Pain may occur from the stresses of excessive mobility or from stretch to hypomobile structures. Pain may also occur from encroachment of developing osteophytes against pain-sensitive tissue or from swelling and irritation because of excessive or abnormal mobility of the segments.
- The encroachment of osteophytes on the spinal canal and intervertebral foramina may cause neurologic signs, especially with spinal extension and side bending.[18]
- The degenerating joint is vulnerable to facet impingement, sprains, and inflammation, as is any arthritic joint.
- In some patients, movement relieves the symptoms; in others, movement irritates the joints and painful symptoms increase.

Rheumatoid Arthritis (RA)

- Symptoms of RA can affect any of the synovial joints of the spine and ribs. There is pain and swelling.
- RA in the cervical spine presents special problems. There are neurologic symptoms wherever degenerative change or swelling impinges against neurologic tissue. There is increased fragility of tissues affected by RA, such as osteoporosis with cyst formation, erosion of bone, and instabilities from ligamentous necrosis. Most common of the serious lesions are atlantoaxial subluxation and C-4/5 and C-5/6 vertebral dislocations.[69]
- Pain or neurologic signs originating in the spine may or may not be related to subluxation. Therefore, these signs should be used as a precaution whenever dealing with this disease because of the potential damage to the spinal cord.[69]
- X-ray examinations are important in ruling out instabilities; signs and symptoms alone are not conclusive.

Precaution: Inappropriate movements of the spine could be life-threatening or extremely debilitating because of the potential of subluxations and dislocations to cause damage to the cervical cord or vertebral artery.[69]

Facet Joint Impingement (Blocking, Fixation, Extrapment)

With a sudden or unusual movement, the meniscoid of a facet capsule may be extrapped, impinged, or stressed, which causes pain and muscle guarding. The onset is sudden and usually involves forward bending and rotation.[9,50,98]

- There is loss of specific motions, and attempted movement induces pain. At rest, the individual has no pain.
- There are no true neurologic signs, but there may be referred pain in the related dermatome.
- Over time, stress is placed on the contralateral joint and on the disk, leading to problems in these structures.

▶ Pathology of Muscle and Soft Tissue Injuries: Strains, Tears, and Contusions

Common impairments and functional limitations are summarized in Box 15–4.

General Symptoms from Trauma

Often more than one tissue is injured as a result of trauma. The extent of the tissue involvement may not be detectable during the acute phase.

- There is pain, localized swelling, tenderness on palpation, and protective muscle guarding regardless of whether the injured tissue is inert or con-

Box 15–4 Summary of Common Impairments and Functional Limitations Associated with Muscle and Soft Tissue Injuries

Acute Stage

- Pain and muscle guarding
- Pain with contraction of the muscle or stretch on the muscle
- Interference with ADLs (rolling over, turning, sitting, sit to stand, standing, walking)

Subacute and Chronic Stages

- Muscle weakness
- Restricted flexibility
- Inadequate spinal control and stabilization during functional activities
- Poor postural awareness
- Limited IADLs, work, and recreational activities (difficulty with repetitive or sustained postures, lifting, pushing, pulling, reaching, and holding loads)

tractile. Muscle guarding serves the immediate purpose of immobilizing the region. If the muscle contraction is prolonged, it results in the buildup of metabolic waste products and sluggish circulation. This altered local environment results in irritation of the free nerve endings so that the muscle continues to contract and becomes the source of additional pain (see Fig. 8–1).

- Ligamentous strains cause pain when the ligament is stressed. If torn, there is hypermobility of the segment.
- As healing of the involved structures occurs, there may be adaptive shortening or scar tissue adhering to surrounding tissue and restricting tissue mobility and postural alignment.

Common Sites of Lumbar Strain

A common site for injury in the lumbar region is along the iliac crest. This is where many forces converge around the attachment of the lateral raphe of the lumbodorsal fascia, quadratus lumborum, erector spinae, and iliolumbar ligament (see Fig. 15–2). Injury to this region frequently occurs with falls and with repeated loading of the region during lifting or twisting motions.

Common Sites of Cervical Strain

Common injuries in the neck and upper thoracic region occur with flexion/extension trauma. Serious cervical trauma may result in vertebral fractures and spinal cord injury. Discussion of these injuries is beyond the scope of this text.

Extension injuries. When the head rapidly accelerates into extension, if nothing stops it (such as a headrest in a car), the occiput is stopped by the thorax. The posterior structures, especially the joints, are compressed. The anterior structures (suprahyoid and infrahyoid muscles) are stretched. The mandible is pulled open, the condylar head of the temporomandibular joint translates forward, stressing the joint structures, and the muscles controlling jaw elevation are stretched (masseter, temporalis, and internal pterygoid).

Flexion injuries. When the head rapidly accelerates into flexion and nothing stops it (such as the steering wheel or air bag in a car), the chin is stopped by the sternum. The mandible is forced posteriorly so the condylar head is forced into the retrodiskal pad within the joint. The posterior cervical muscles, ligaments, fasciae, and joint capsules are stretched.

Postural Strain

Strain to the posterior cervical, scapular, and upper thoracic muscles and fasciae is common with postural stresses such as prolonged sitting at a computer terminal, drawing table, or desk.

Emotional Stress

Emotional stresses are often expressed as increased tension in the posterior cervical or lumbar region.

Functional Limitations/Disabilities

Impaired muscle function underlies most spinal problems that demonstrate pain or poor spinal control and stabilization during functional activities. When acute, muscle guarding interferes with basic activities such as rolling over, sitting, standing, and walking. In subacute and chronic conditions, muscle impairments result in poor stabilization and spinal control in prolonged upright postures and activities. Proximal stability of the spine is imperative for most activities and needs to be addressed for improved function.

Principles of Management for the Spine and Posture

At the time of a low back or cervical injury, impairments, functional limitations and disabilities are not known. Usually 80 to 90% of acute injuries resolve within 1 month.[52] Disabilities will be dependent on the extent of the injury. If it involves the spinal cord, levels of complete paralysis may occur. If it involves the nerve roots (also the cauda equina), varying degrees of muscle weakness in specific myotomes may occur, which may or may not interfere with the individual's daily personal and work-related activities. Upper quarter nerve roots affect function of the arms and hands; lower quarter nerve roots affect function of the lower extremities, especially in weight-bearing activities. Studies on chronic-pain syndromes as a result of back injuries seem to conclude that the degree of disability is related to psychologic, economic, and sociological factors and prior incidence of injury more than the actual tissues involved.[34,52] Nerve root involvement and pain provocation with active movements in several directions are more common in patients who develop chronic pain.[34] Discussion of treatment for spinal cord injuries and chronic-pain syndromes is beyond the scope of this book.

Examination and Evaluation

History, systems review, and testing. A history and systems review of the patient is conducted to rule out any serious conditions, to determine if the patient should be referred to another practitioner, or to determine if the patient's condition is appropriate for physical therapy intervention. Then, if safe, tests and measures are conducted to determine if the source of symptoms can be influenced by mechanical changes in position or movement and to establish a baseline of measurements of impairments and functional limitations from which changes can be documented. Examination techniques and procedures are beyond the scope of this text, but a brief summary of concerns in the spinal area is listed to help focus on critical decisions prior to establishing an intervention strategy.

- *Serious "red flag" conditions* that should be referred to a physician for management include spinal cord symptoms and signs, recent trauma where spinal fracture or instabilities have not been ruled out, and serious pain (especially that wakes the individual) that cannot be explained mechanically.
- *Psychologic distress* may interfere with a patient's recovery; therefore, referral to an appropriate professional may be indicated for a multidisciplinary approach in the patient's care.
- *Neurologic symptoms* should be explored in an attempt to relate them to spinal cord, nerve root, spinal nerve, plexus, or peripheral nerve patterns. Causes of nerve root signs frequently seen by physical therapists include intervertebral disk protrusions, bony, soft tissue, or vascular stenosis in the spinal canal or intervertebral foramina, facet joint swelling, and nerve root tension from restricted mobility.
- *Pain patterns* should be explored to determine if they relate to a known pattern. It should be recognized that pain is interpreted many ways and has various meanings to different people; therefore, interpret the information as only one factor when determining cause of the symptoms.

Stage of recovery. Time frames for each stage vary depending on reference used. In general, the acute stage usually lasts less that 4 weeks, subacute stage is 4 to 12 weeks, and chronic stage is greater than 12 weeks.[2]

- ***Acute inflammatory stage.*** The patient experiences constant pain, and there are signs of inflammation. No position or movement completely relieves the symptoms. Medical intervention with anti-inflammatory medications is usually warranted.
- ***Acute stage without signs of inflammation.*** Symptoms are intermittent and related to mechanical deformation. There may be signs of nerve root irritability when the nerve root or spinal nerve is compressed or placed under tension. The patient may be categorized into an extension bias, a flexion bias, or a nonweight-bearing bias based on the presenting posture, movement impairments, or positions of symptom relief. These categories are described in greater detail in the next section. Delitto and associates[22] classify patients as being at this stage if they cannot stand longer than 15 minutes, sit longer than 30 minutes, or walk more than 1/4 mile without worsening of their status.
- ***Subacute stage.*** Usually at this stage, certain movements and postures with some IADLs still provoke symptoms so that a basic life-style cannot fully be resumed such as lifting, vacuuming, gardening, and other activities requiring repetitive movement of loads. A more thorough examination for identification of impairments that could be interfering with recovery is conducted.
- ***Chronic stage.*** When this stage is reached, emphasis is placed on returning the patient to high-level demand activities that require handling

repetitive loads on a sustained basis over a prolonged period of time (from heavy material handling, to repetitive household activities including lifting of small children, to strenuous athletic activities).

Diagnosis, prognosis and plan of care. As mentioned in the introduction to this chapter, specific pathologies and medical diagnoses often do not guide the therapist in appropriate treatment interventions, and that various systems of patient classification for treating musculoskeletal impairments and functional limitations are present in the literature.[2,22,23,85] Material in the remainder of this chapter is organized to reflect an integration of pathological conditions that are presented by the medical model and mechanical biases that are determined during the examination to help the therapist choose an intervention strategy that best helps the patient's recovery. The categories described in this and the following sections are summarized in the following box.

Categories that Direct Intervention

- **General.** Acute, subacute, and chronic spinal conditions
- **Extension bias** (intervertebral disk lesions, flexion load injuries, flexed postural dysfunctions, fluid stasis)
- **Flexion bias** (spondylosis, stenosis, extension load injuries, swollen facets joints)
- **Muscle and soft tissue lesions** (strains, tears, contusions, overuse)
- **Nonweight-bearing bias** (patient does not tolerate being upright for basic ADLs and IADLs)
- **Other selected conditions** affected by the spine (torticollis, tension headache, temporomandibular joint dysfunction, neural mobility impairment)

General Guidelines for Managing Acute Spinal Problems: The Protection Phase

The approach is determined by the patient's responses to the examination maneuvers and what maneuvers provide greatest relief of symptoms. Use of modalities and massage to decrease pain and swelling from the acute symptoms is appropriate during the acute stage. It is also important that the patient becomes an active participant in his or her program. Kinesthetic training, nondestructive movements in the pain-free range, basic stabilization techniques of core musculature (especially the multifidus and deep abdominals), and basic functional training maneuvers are taught if they do not exacerbate the symptoms. Specific techniques for various tissue pathologies or biases are described in the remaining sections of this chapter, and specific techniques for kinesthetic, stabilization, and functional training are described in Chapter 16. Management guidelines for treatment of the patient with acute symptoms are summarized in Box 15–5. The following points are fundamental to all interventions.

1. **Establish a position of symptom relief or comfort.** If a patient is experiencing acute inflammation from a traumatic injury, there will be constant pain, yet often an optimal position of comfort or symptom reduction can be determined in which there is the least amount of stress on the inflamed, irritated, or swollen region. The terms *functional position, neutral position,* or *functional range* are used to describe this position.[70] The functional range may change for the individual as the tissues heal and the person gains mobility and strength in the region. Some pathologic condi-

Box 15–5 Management Guidelines—Acute Spinal Problems/Protection Phase

Impairments and Functional Limitations:
Pain and/or neurological symptoms
Inflammation
Inability to perform ADLs and IADLs
Guarded posture (prefers flexion, extension, or nonweight-bearing)

Plan of Care	Intervention
1. Learn self-management.	1. Engage patient in all activities.
2. Decrease acute symptoms.	2. Modalities, massage, traction as needed. Rest only for first couple days if needed.
3. Demonstrate awareness of neck and pelvic position and movement.	3. Kinesthetic training: cervical and scapular motions, pelvic tilts, neutral spine.
4. Demonstrate safe postures.	4. Practice positions and movement and experience effect on spine. Provide passive support/bracing if needed.
5. Initiate neuromuscular control of stabilizing muscles.	5. Core Technique: drawing-in maneuver. Basic stabilization: with arm and leg motions (passive support, progress to active control).
6. Safely perform basic ADLs and progress to IADLs.	6. Roll, sit, stand, and walk with safe postures. Progress tolerance to sitting >30 min., standing >15 min., and walking >1 mile.

tions typically tend to cause symptoms in one portion of the range and are relieved in another range.[70] The following terms have been popularized based on the work of Morgan[70] and Saal and Saal.[88,91]

Extension Bias

The patient's symptoms are lessened in positions of extension (lordosis). Sustained flexed postures or repetitive flexion motions load the anterior disk region and facet joints, causing fluid redistribution from the compressed areas and swelling and creep in the distended areas. This is frequently the mechanism of symptom production in posterior or posterolateral intervertebral disk lesions or injury to the posterior longitudinal ligament. Whether the pathology is an injured disk or stressed and swollen tissues, repeated extension motions and positions relieve the symptoms by moving the fluid to reverse the stasis (these techniques are described in the section under disk lesions). Some patients may present with a lateral shift, which usually requires correction before extension relieves the symptoms.[65,66]

Flexion Bias

The patient's symptoms are lessened in positions of spinal flexion and provoked in extension. This is often the case when there is compromise of the intervertebral foramen or spinal canal, as in bony spinal stenosis, spondylosis, and spondylolisthesis.

Nonweight-Bearing Bias

The patient's symptoms are lessened when in nonweight-bearing positions such as when lying down or in traction. Symptoms also lessen when spinal pressure is reduced by leaning on the upper extremities (using arm rests to unweight the trunk), by leaning the trunk against a support, or when in a pool. The condition is considered *gravity sensitive*[12] because the symptoms worsen during standing, walking, running, coughing, or similar activities that increase spinal pressure. Often traction or aquatic therapy are the only interventions that minimize symptoms.

2. **Teach awareness of safe postures and effects of movement.** Teach the patient to identify and assume the spinal position that is most comfortable and reduces the symptoms by using pelvic tilts for lumbar positioning and head nods and chin tucks for cervical spine positioning. Corsets or cervical collars are used to provide support during the acute stage if necessary.

   Teach the patient how to use *passive positioning* to help maintain the functional position during the acute stage.

Examples of Passive Positioning

- In *supine*, hook-lying flexes the lumbar spine; legs extended extends the spine. A pillow under the head flexes the neck; a small roll under the neck stabilizes a mild lordosis with the head neutral.
- In *prone*, use of a pillow under the abdomen flexes the lumbar spine; no pillow extends the spine. To maintain the cervical spine in neutral alignment without rotation, a split table or a small towel roll placed under the forehead provides space for the nose so the patient does not turn the head.
- *Sitting* usually causes spinal flexion, especially if the hips and knees are flexed. To emphasize flexion, the feet are propped up on a small footstool; to emphasize extension, a lumbar pillow or towel roll is placed in the low-back region. To unweight the spine, the arms are placed on an armrest or a reclining chair is used.
- *Standing* usually causes spinal extension; to emphasize flexion, one foot is placed on a small stool.

3. **Teach basic stabilization.** The stabilization exercises are described in detail in the "Stabilization Training" section of Chapter 16.

   As soon as tolerated, teach the patient the *drawing-in* maneuver to activate the transversus abdominis. Instruct the patient to draw the "belly button" up and in towards the spine to hollow out the abdominal region. Exhaling may reinforce the correct muscle contraction. Be sure the patient does not inhale nor lift the rib cage and attempt to "suck in" while doing this activity. This may be practiced in the supine, sitting, or all-fours (quadruped) position.

   Teach upper and lower extremity motions with the spine stabilized. If the patient is unable to actively maintain his or her functional position, *passively preposition* the patient as described in the box above. For both cervical and lumbar problems, instruct the patient to first do the drawing-in maneuver then do gentle arm motions within a range that does not exacerbate symptoms. Leg motions require greater lumbopelvic control and are introduced only if symptoms are not exacerbated.

4. **Teach basic functional movements.** Teach the

patient to perform simple movements for ADL while protecting the spine in the functional position; these include rolling from prone to supine and reverse, lying to sitting and reverse, sitting to standing and reverse, and walking. Descriptions of these maneuvers are in the Functional Training/Transferring of Skills section of Chapter 16.

5. **Review precautions.** Review any special precautions for the condition with the patient. Condition-specific precautions are described in the remaining sections of this chapter.

General Guidelines for Managing Subacute Spinal Problems: The Controlled Motion Phase

When the signs and symptoms of the inflammatory process are under control and pain is no longer constant, progress the patient through a program of nondestructive movement to prepare the tissue for functional activities and rehabilitation training, and then initiate activities that can be performed safely. Pain may still interfere with some daily activities, but it is no longer constant. Poor neuromuscular control and stabilization, poor postural awareness and body mechanics, decreased flexibility and strength, and generalized deconditioning may be the underlying impairments at this stage. Intervention during this stage is critical because either the patient feels good and tends to overdo activities and reinjures the tissues, or the patient is fearful and does not adequately resume safe movements so that impairments develop leading to functional restrictions. Either extreme may slow down the recovery process.

Management guidelines for cervical and lumbar problems that require controlled motion interventions are summarized in Box 15–6. The specific techniques and progressions of intervention outlined here are described in detail in Chapter 16.

1. **Pain modulation.** At this stage, use of modalities to modulate pain is not recommended. Emphasis is placed on increasing patient awareness of posture, strength, mobility, and spinal control and their relationship to modulating pain.

2. **Kinesthetic training.** Progress kinesthetic training to include reinforcement techniques so that assuming correct posture becomes habitual. In addition, observe that the patient is actively controlling the spinal position while doing all activities. Motor learning of feedforward control of the deep abdominal muscles prior to activities is practiced in a variety of ways until it becomes habitual. Kinesthetic training overlaps with stabilization exercises

3. **Stretching/mobilization.** Decreased flexibility in joints, muscles, and fascia may restrict the patient's ability to assume normal spinal alignment. Utilize manual techniques to increase muscle, joint, and connective tissue mobility, and instruct the patient in safe, self-stretching techniques.

4. **Dynamic stabilization exercises.** Progress exercises with increased challenges for control,

Box 15–6 Management Guidelines—Subacute Spinal Problems/Controlled Motion Phase

Impairments and Functional Limitations:

Pain: only when excessive stress is placed on vulnerable tissues
Poor neuromuscular control of stabilizing muscles
Flexibility postural awareness
Generalized deconditioning
Inability to perform IADLs for extended periods of time
Poor body mechanics

Plan of Care	Intervention
1. Learn self-management and decrease episodes of pain.	1. Engage patient in all activities emphasizing safe movement and postures. Ergonomic adaptation of work or home environment.
2. Progress awareness and control of spinal alignment.	2. Practice active spinal control in pain free positions and with all exercises and activities. Practice posture correction.
3. Increase mobility in tight muscles/joint/fascia.	3. Joint mobilization/manipulation, muscle inhibition, self-stretching.
4. Develop neuromuscular control, strength and endurance in stabilizing muscles.	4. Progress stabilization exercises; increase repetitions and challenge.
5. Increase dynamic trunk and extremity strength.	5. Initiate dynamic trunk and extremity resistance exercises.
6. Develop general aerobic endurance.	6. Low to moderate intensity aerobic exercises; emphasize spinal bias.
7. Learn techniques of stress relief/relaxation.	7. Relaxation exercises and postural stress relief.
8. Learn safe body mechanics.	8. Functional exercises to prepare for safe mechanics. Practice stable spine lifts, push/pull activities.
9. Develop functional skills.	9. Functional exercises specific to desired outcome emphasizing spinal control, endurance, and timing.

strength, and endurance in the stabilizing muscles. The exercises emphasize movement and resistance to the extremities while maintaining control of the spinal position. When the patient learns good spinal control with the core stabilizing muscles in a variety of stabilization exercise routines, dynamic trunk and neck strengthening exercises such as curl ups, back extension, and cervical motions are introduced. Care is taken to monitor symptoms and modify any activities that exacerbate the problem.

5. **Extremity strengthening.** Initiate upper and lower extremity strengthening exercises in conjunction with trunk feedforward stabilization to prepare for functional training activities. Wall slides, partial squats, partial lunges, pushing, and pulling against resistance are all methods to prepare for lifting, reaching, pushing, and pulling activities.
6. **Aerobic conditioning.** Aerobic capacity is usually compromised after injury. It is important to guide the patient in initiation of or safe return to an aerobic conditioning program. Help the patient identify activities that do not exacerbate spinal symptoms. Suggestions are included in Chapter 16.
7. **Postural stress management and relaxation exercises.** If the patient's symptoms are exacerbated with sustained postural stresses such as sitting at a computer, talking on the phone (head tilted), or repetitive forward bending (shoe salesman), advise the patient in methods to correct the environmental stresses. In addition, frequent changes of position and movement through the pain-free ROM are encouraged. Teach the patient how to consciously relax tension in muscles to relieve stress.
8. **Function.** Once the patient has learned spinal control and stabilization and has developed adequate flexibility and strength for the task, the task is incorporated into the exercise program, and then into the patient's daily life-style.

General Guidelines for Managing Chronic Spinal Problems: The Return to Function Phase

Patients who have been treated through the acute and subacute phases of healing with appropriately graded exercises should have minimal impairments preventing or restricting daily activities. Those individuals who must do heavy material handling (such as a manual laborer, firefighter, caregiver of small children or of patients), or participate in high-demand sport activities may require additional rehabilitative training to safely return to these high-demand activities and to avoid further injury. Impairments in strength, endurance, neuromuscular control, and skill are related to the functional goals of the individual. At this stage, conditioning and spinal control during high intensity and repetitive activities are emphasized. Any underlying impairments that interfere with the desired outcomes must be remediated. Management guidelines for return to function are summarized in Box 15–7. Suggestions for progressing exercise intervention techniques

Box 15–7 Management Guidelines—Chronic Spinal Problems/Return to Function Phase

Impairments and Functional Limitations:

Pain: only when excessive stress is placed on vulnerable tissues in repetitive or sustained nature for prolonged periods
Poor neuromuscular control and endurance in high intensity or destabilized situations
Flexibility and strength imbalances
Generalized deconditioning
Inability to perform high intensity physical demands for extended periods of time

Plan of Care	Intervention
1. Learn spinal control in high intensity and repetitive activities.	1. Practice active spinal control in various transitional and disturbed balance activities.
2. Increase mobility in tight muscles/joints/fascia.	2. Joint mobilization/manipulation, muscle inhibition, self-stretching.
3. Increase dynamic trunk and extremity strength.	3. Progress dynamic trunk and extremity resistance exercises emphasizing functional goals.
4. Develop general cardiovascular endurance.	4. Progress intensity of aerobic exercises.
5. Habitually use techniques of stress relief/relaxation and posture correction.	5. Reinforce motions and postures to relieve stress and any ergonomic changes needed.
6. Return to high level/high intensity activities for prolonged periods of time without exacerbating symptoms.	6. Progressive practice using activity-specific training consistent with desired functional outcome, emphasizing spinal control, endurance, timing, and speed.
7. Develop healthy exercise habits for self-maintenance.	7. Engage patient in all activities and educate as to benefits of maintaining fitness level and safe body mechanics.

from the subacute through chronic stages are described in Chapter 16.

Guidelines for Management of Impairments with an Extension Bias: Intervertebral Disk Lesions, Flexion Injuries, Flexed Postural Dysfunctions, Fluid Stasis

Patients with an extension bias often assume a flexed posture or flexed posture with lateral deviation of the trunk or neck, but during the examination procedure, sustained or repetitive extension maneuvers reduce or relieve their symptoms. McKenzie[65,66] has developed a method of categorizing these patients based on the extent of their pain and/or neurologic symptoms. He has also described the phenomena of peripheralization and centralization that accompany an expanding and receding lesion, frequently attributed to intervertebral disk lesions. Many of the techniques that are used to manage an acute disk lesion have been found to be beneficial in the treatment of fluid stasis from postural stress and to initiate movement with soft tissue injuries when there is symptom relief in extension.[88]

Principles of Management

Effects of Postural Changes on Intervertebral Disk Pressure

Relative changes in posture and activities affect intradiskal pressure. When compared to the level of pressure when standing, intradiskal pressure is least while lying supine, increases by almost 50% during sitting with hips and knees flexed, and almost doubles if leaning forward while sitting.[43,72] Sitting with a back rest inclination of 120 degrees and lumbar support 5 cm in depth provides the lowest load to the disk while sitting.[6,47] Therefore, sitting with the hips and knees flexed or leaning forward should be avoided when there is an acute disk lesion. If sitting is necessary, there should be support for the lumbar spine by reclining the trunk 120 degrees.

Effects of Bed Rest on the Intervertebral Disk

When a person is lying down, compression forces to the disk are reduced, and with time, the nucleus potentially can absorb more water to equalize pressures (imbibition). If lying down with the spine in flexion, the imbibed fluid will accumulate posteriorly in the disk where there is greater space. Then upon rising, body weight compresses the disk with the increased fluid, and intradiskal pressure greatly increases. The pain or symptoms from a disk protrusion are accentuated. To avoid exacerbating symptoms, absolute bed rest during the acute phase should be avoided. Bed rest during the first 2 days when symptoms are highly irritable may be needed to promote early healing, but it should be interspersed with short intervals of standing, walking, and appropriately controlled movement.[102]

Effects of Traction on the Intervertebral Disk

Traction may relieve symptoms from a disk protrusion. It is proposed that the separation of the vertebral bodies may have the effect of placing tension on the annular fibers and posterior longitudinal ligament, thus have a flattening effect on the bulge, or may decrease the intradiskal pressure.[61] If traction relieves symptoms, the time of application must be short, because with the reduced pressure, fluid imbibition may occur to equalize the pressure. Then when the traction is released, the pressure increases and symptoms will be exacerbated.

Effects of Flexion and Extension on the Intervertebral Disk and Fluid Stasis

Rest in a slightly forward-bent position often lessens pain because of the space potential for the nucleus pulposus of the intervertebral disk. The patient may also deviate laterally to minimize pressure against a nerve root. Movement into extension initially causes increased symptoms. In acute disk lesions in which there is protective lateral shifting and lumbar flexion, techniques that cause lateral shifting of the spine opposite to the deviation followed by passive spinal extension (sustained or repetitive) to mechanically compress the protrusion have been found to relieve the clinical signs and symptoms in many patients.[49,65,66]

Patients experiencing pain from fluid stasis after being in a sustained flexed posture also experience relief with movement into extension.

Effects of Isometric and Dynamic Exercise

Isometric activities (resisted pelvic tilt exercises, straining, Valsalva maneuver) as well as active back flexion or extension exercises increase intradiskal pressures above normal and, therefore, *must be avoided* during the acute stage of a disk lesion. Strong muscle contractions also exacerbate symptoms if a muscle has been injured. Therefore, active and resistive extension exercises are avoided during the acute stage.

Effects of Muscle Guarding

Reflex muscle guarding or splinting often accompanies an acute disk lesion and adds to the compressive forces on the disk. Modalities and gentle oscillatory traction to the spine may help decrease the splinting.

Indications, Precautions, and Contraindications for Interventions Utilizing Extension

Indications

- Pain and/or neurologic symptoms that centralize during extension testing maneuvers and peripheralize (worsen) during flexion.
- Flexed postural dysfunctions with limited range into extension.

Precautions and Contraindications to Treatment Using an Extension Approach

- A patient with acute pain in the spinal region that is not influenced by changing the patient's position or by movement must be screened by a physician for signs of serious pathology.
- Any movement that peripheralizes the symptoms signals a movement that is contraindicated during the acute and early subacute period of treatment. Peripheralization with extension motions may indicate stenosis, large lateral disk protrusion, or pathology in a posterior element.[90]
- Extension of the spine is ***contraindicated***[65]:
  - When no position or movement decreases or centralizes the described pain
  - When saddle anesthesia and/or bladder weakness is present (could indicate spinal cord or cauda equina lesion)
  - When a patient is in such extreme pain that he or she rigidly holds the body immobile with any attempted correction
- Flexion of the spine should be avoided:
  - When extension relieves the symptoms
  - When flexion movements increase the pain or peripheralize the symptoms
- Any form of exercise or activity that increases intradiskal pressure, such as the Valsalva maneuver, active pelvic tilt, or trunk-raising exercises, is ***contraindicated*** during the protection phase of treatment when there is a disk lesion.

Techniques of Intervention Using an Extension Approach in the Lumbar Spine

Note: These techniques are used only if the test movements have shown that the postures and movements used improve the symptoms.[47,65] If no test movements decrease the symptoms, this mechanical approach to treatment should not be used.

Acute Phase: Severe Symptoms

If symptoms are severe, bed rest is indicated with short periods of walking at regular intervals. Walking usually promotes lumbar extension and stimulates fluid mechanics to help reduce swelling in the disk or connective tissues. The patient should use crutches, if he or she cannot stand upright, to help relieve the increased pressure of the forward-bent posture.[47]

Acute Phase: Posterior or Posterolateral Disk Protrusion

If repeated flexion test movements increase the symptoms and if repeated extension test movements decrease or centralize the symptoms, all flexion activities should be avoided during the early phases of intervention. Treatment begins with:

Passive Extension

- Patient position and procedure: Prone. If the flexion posture is severe, place pillows under the abdomen for support. Gradually increase the amount of extension by removing the pillows, and then progress by having the patient prop himself or herself up on the elbows, allowing the pelvis to sag (Fig. 15–8). When propping, pillows placed under the thorax help take strain off the shoulders. Wait 5 to 10 minutes between each increment of extension to allow for reduction of water content and size of the bulge. There should be

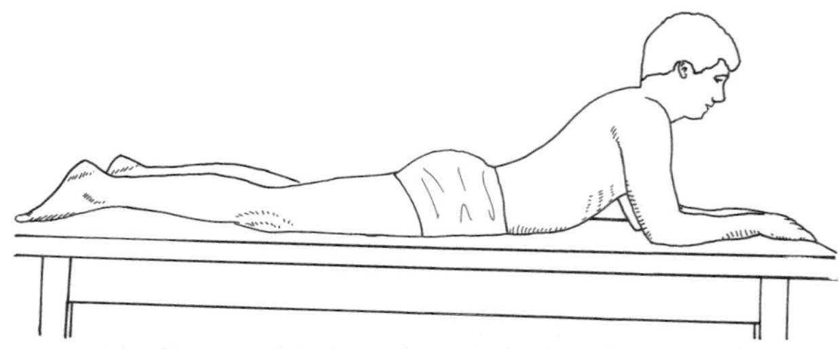

Figure 15–8 Passive lumbar extension accomplished by having the patient prop up on the elbows.

an accompanying centralization of or decrease in symptoms. Progress to having the patient prop himself or herself up on the hands, allowing the pelvis to sag (see Fig. 16–11*A*).

- If the sustained postures are not well tolerated, have the patient perform passive lumbar extension intermittently by repeating the *prone press-ups* (same end position as Fig. 16–11*A*) rather than just propping up.

Precaution: Carefully monitor the patient's symptoms. They should lessen peripherally (i.e., decreased foot and leg symptoms or decreased thigh and buttock symptoms), but may increase in the low back (centralize). If the symptoms progress down the lower extremity (peripheralize), immediately stop the exercises and reassess.[65]

Lateral Shift Correction

If the patient has lateral shifting of the spine (Fig. 15–9), extension alone will not reduce the nuclear protrusion until the shift is corrected. Once the shift is corrected, the patient must extend as described above to maintain the correction. Methods to correct the shift in various positions include the following:

- Patient position and procedure: *Standing* with flexed elbow against the side of the deviated rib cage. Stand on the side to which the thorax is shifted, and place your shoulder against the patient's elbow. Then wrap your arms around the patient's pelvis on the opposite side and simultaneously pull the pelvis toward you while pushing the patient's thorax away (Fig. 15–10). This is a gradual maneuver. Continue with the lateral shifting if centralization of the symptoms occurs.[66] If there is overcorrection, the pain and lateral shift may move to the contralateral side, which is corrected by shifting the thorax back. The purpose is to centralize the pain and correct the lateral shift. Once the shift is corrected, *immediately* have the patient backward-bend (see Fig. 16–11*B*). Again, allow time. Progress to passive extension with prone propping and prone press-ups as previously described.
- Patient position and procedure: *Side-lying* on the side to which the thorax is shifted. Place a small pillow or towel roll under the thorax. The patient remains in this position until the pain centralizes, then rolls prone and begins passive extension with prone propping and prone press-ups.
- Patient position and procedure: *Prone.* Attempt to manually side-glide the thorax and pelvis toward the midline. The forces are in equal and opposite directions. Once the symptoms centralize, instruct the patient to begin passive extension with prone propping and prone press-ups.

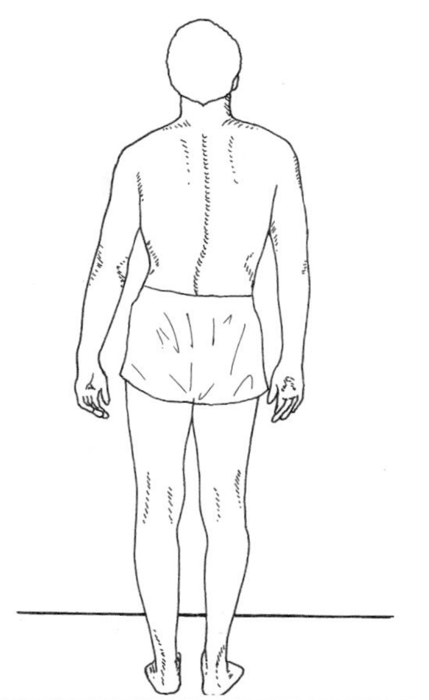

Figure 15–9 Patient with lateral shift of the thoracic cage toward the right. The pelvis is shifted toward the left.

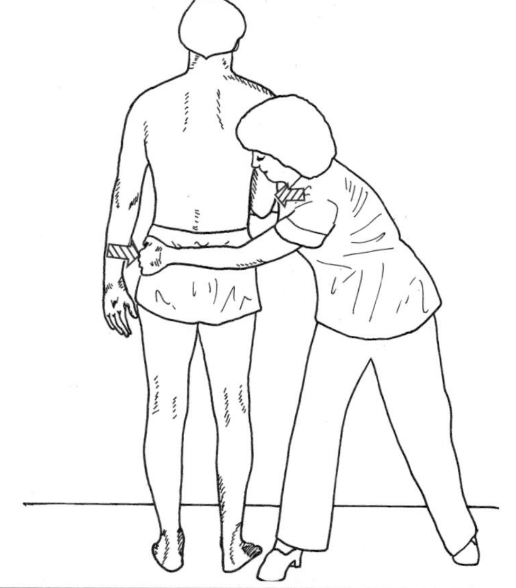

Figure 15–10 A lateral gliding technique used to correct a lateral shift of the thorax is applied against the patient's elbow and thoracic cage as the pelvis is pulled in the opposite direction.

Patient Education

- Help the patient recognize what positions and motions increase or decrease the pain or other symptoms by performing them under supervision.
- Instruct the patient to frequently repeat the extension activities, with lateral shift correction, if necessary, during the first couple of days.
  - Teach *self-correction of the lateral shift.* The patient places the hand on the side of the shifted rib cage on the lateral aspect of the rib cage and places the other hand over the crest of the opposite ilium and then gradually pushes these regions toward the midline and holds (Fig. 15–11).
  - Instruct the patient to correct the shift by side-lying or prone-lying as previously described.
- Caution the patient to immediately stop the activity if pain worsens or peripheralizes during exercises.
- Instruct the patient to maintain an extended posture with passive support while the lesion is healing.
  - While sitting, have the patient use a towel roll or lumbar pillow. This is especially important when riding in a car or sitting in a soft chair.
  - When going to bed, have the patient pin a towel, folded lengthwise four times, around the waist.
- Instruct the patient to avoid flexion activities, lifting, or any other functions that increase intradiskal pressure while symptoms are acute.

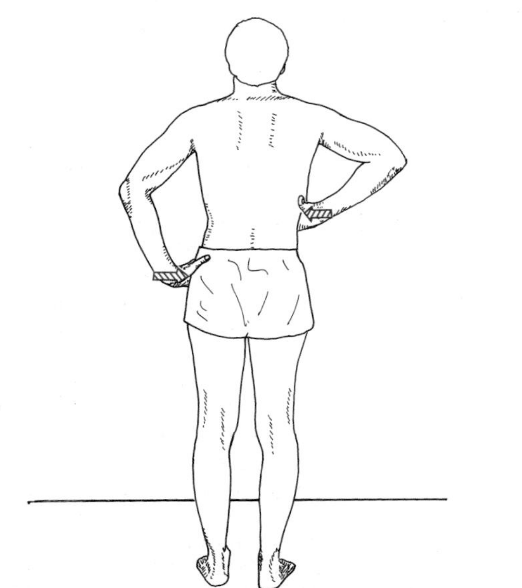

Figure 15–11 Self-correction of a lateral shift.

- Teach safe movement patterns to protect the back as described in the guidelines for treating acute spinal problems (see Box 15–5).

Traction

Traction may be tolerated by the patient during the acute stage and has the benefit of widening the disk space and possibly reducing the nuclear protrusion by decreasing the pressure on the disk or by placing tension on the posterior longitudinal ligament.[92,93]

- Time of the traction should be short; osmotic forces soon equalize. However, upon release of the traction force, there could be an increase in the disk pressure, leading to increased pain.
  - Less than 15 minutes of intermittent traction
  - Less than 10 minutes of sustained traction
- High poundage; greater than half the patient's body weight is necessary for separation of the lumbar vertebrae.
- If there is complete relief initially, often there will be an exacerbation of symptoms later.

Subacute Phase of a Disk Lesion

Usually, the acute symptoms decrease in 4 to 6 days, and the patient learns to control the symptoms. General guidelines for treatment during the subacute phase were previously described (see Box 15–6). The following should be emphasized during this phase of a disk lesion.

- Teach simple spinal movements in pain-free ranges using gentle pelvic tilts. The patient is taught to be aware of how far forward and backward he or she can rock the pelvis and move the spine without increasing symptoms. The pelvic rocking is done in supine, sitting, in the hand-knee all-fours (quadruped), prone-lying, side-lying, and standing. It is important to stay within the patient's ability to control the symptoms. *Instruct the patient to finish all exercise routines with the pelvis tilted anteriorly and the spine in extension.*
- Teach the patient basic stabilization techniques utilizing the core trunk muscles while maintaining control of the extended spinal position and performing simple extremity motions. (These are described in detail at the beginning of chapter 16). It is important to caution against holding the breath and causing the Valsalva maneuver to not excessively increase the intradiskal pressure.
- Encourage activities within the tolerance of the individual, such as walking or swimming.

- Initiate passive straight-leg raising with intermittent dorsi- and plantarflexion to maintain mobility in the nerve roots of the lumbar spine.

Management When Disk Symptoms Have Stabilized

Signs of Improvement

Improvement is noted with loss of spinal deformity, increased motion in the back, and negative dural mobility signs.[47] Loss of back pain with an increase in true neurologic signs is an indication of worsening. The patient is tested to determine the symptoms have stabilized by performing repeated flexion and extension tests with the patient standing, then lying supine and prone as done initially. The tests may be positive for dysfunction (restricted motion, tension) but should not cause peripheralization of the symptoms as when the condition was acute.[65]

Intervention Emphasis

The emphases during this stage are *recovery of function, development of a healthy back care plan,* and *teaching the patient how to prevent recurrences* (see Box 15–7). Suggested exercises to correct the identified impairments are described in Chapter 16. The pain from adaptive shortening will decrease as normal flexibility, strength, and endurance are restored.

In addition, teach the patient these principles:

- Following any flexion exercises, perform extension exercises such as prone press-ups or standing back extension (see Figs. 16–11*A* and *B*).[65]
- If being in a prolonged flexed posture is necessary, interrupt the flexion with backward bending at least once every hour. Also, perform intermittent pelvic tilts.
- If developing symptoms of a protrusion are felt, immediately perform press-ups in the prone position or backward bending while standing to prevent progression of the symptoms.

Techniques to Manage a Disk Lesion in the Cervical Spine

Disk lesions in the cervical spine are less common than in the lumbar spine. Often disk extrusions are an indication for surgery because of potential compromise of the spinal canal and pressure on the spinal cord.[87] Patients may present with peripheral neuropathy and forward-head posture without a diagnosis of disk pathology. Symptoms increase with activities and postures that increase flexion in the lower cervical and upper thoracic spine and decrease with extension in that region (axial extension or neck retraction).[1] Conservative management is similar as in the lumbar spine and follows the same principles described for the lumbar spine in the previous section. Medical management includes pharmacological pain and inflammation control measures.

Acute Phase

Passive Axial Extension (Cervical Retraction).

Patient position and procedure: Begin with the patient supine, with no pillow under the head or neck. Gently nod the patient's head, and allow the neck to flatten against the treatment table. If the neck is deviated or rotated to one side, movement of the head and neck back toward the midline will need to be done first. This may require gentle progressive positioning and take 10 to 20 minutes to accomplish.

Progression: McKenzie advocates progressing the retraction to hyperextension of the cervical spine and then progressing to rotation. Special training in these maneuvers is recommended before using them so that appropriate signs and symptoms can be monitored.[65]

Patient Education

Teach the patient to passively retract his or her head and neck in the sitting position. The patient may gently push against the chin (caution not to push so hard as to cause joint compression of the temporomandibular joint) to direct the motion. This technique has been shown to improve the H-reflex amplitude and may be useful to improve mobility and decrease symptoms of radiculopathy by decompressing nerve roots in the lower cervical spine.[1]

Traction

Cervical traction may relieve the patient's symptoms. As described with lumbar traction, during the acute phase sustained traction should be no longer than 10 minutes, and intermittent traction no longer than 15 minutes in duration. The dosage is at an intensity that causes vertebral separation (at least 15 lb).

Kinesthetic Training for Posture Correction

Instruct the patient in safe mechanics for maintaining the head position. During the acute phase, the patient may need to wear a cervical collar to immobilize the spine. It is important to help the patient identify the posture that centralizes the symptoms and to adjust the collar to maintain that position.

Progression as Symptoms Stabilize

Follow the guidelines described in Box 15–6. The techniques are described in Chapter 16. Faulty cervical and scapulothoracic posture may be present. Emphasize kinesthetic training for postural awareness, dynamic stabilization exercises for postural control with emphasis on the scapular and shoulder muscles, environmental adaptations to reduce postural stresses, and functional activities with safe spinal mechanics.

Guidelines for Management of Impairments with a Flexion Bias: Spondylosis, Stenosis, Extension Load Injuries, Swollen Facet Joints

Patients may present with a flexed posture and be unable to extend because of increased neurologic symptoms and decreased mobility. The flexed position reduces or relieves the symptoms.

Principles of Management

Effect of position. Flexion widens the intervertebral foramina, whereas extension decreases the size of the foramina. Any compromise of the foraminal opening, such as encroachment from bony spurs or lipping or swollen tissue, reduces the space. The patient may describe intermittent nerve root symptoms (intermittent numbness or tingling) whenever the involved segment extends, indicating mechanical compression. Constant nerve root symptoms could be from inflammation and swollen tissue.

Effect of traction. Traction has been demonstrated to widen the intervertebral foramina. Positioning the spine in flexion prior to the application of traction provides the greatest increased space.[18,33,61,82]

Effect of trauma and repetitive irritation. Swelling in the facet joints from macro- or microtrauma leads to compromised foraminal space. With degeneration and increased mobility in a spinal segment, instability could be the cause of repetitive microtrauma leading to swelling and pain.

Effect of meniscoid tissue. The meniscoid tissue of the joint capsule may become impinged with sudden movements. This blocks specific movements such as extension and side bending to the involved side. Manipulation and traction usually relieve the symptoms.

Indications and Contraindications for Intervention Using a Flexion Approach

Indications

Flexion is used if the examination identified that neurologic and/or pain symptoms were eased with flexion and worsened with extension positions or motions.

Contraindications

- Extension and extension with rotation positions, motions, and exercises are ***contraindicated*** if neurologic symptoms or pain worsen with these motions.
- Flexion exercises are ***contraindicated*** if neurologic or pain symptoms peripheralize with flexion or repeated flexion maneuvers.

Techniques of Intervention Utilizing a Flexion Approach

In general, spinal flexion postures and exercises are taught following the guidelines described in Boxes 15–5, 15–6, and 15–7. The following suggestions should also be considered for special conditions.

Management of Acute Symptoms

Rest and Support

- With acute joint symptoms, a cervical collar or lumbar corset may be helpful to provide rest to the inflamed or swollen facet joints.
- Support is also beneficial in management of patients with RA or other disorders associated with hypermobilities or instabilities.
- It is important to discontinue use of such devices as acute symptoms decrease so the muscles can learn dynamic control and to avoid dependency.

Functional Position for Comfort

- For flexion bias in the lumbar spine, the position is usually with the hips and knees flexed so that the lumbar spine flexes.
- In the cervical spine, the position is toward axial extension (upper cervical flexion) with some flexion also in the lower cervical region.
- If there are neurologic signs, the position will provide maximal opening of the intervertebral foramina to minimize impingement of the nerve root.

Traction

- Gentle intermittent joint distraction and gliding techniques may inhibit painful muscle responses and provide synovial fluid movement within the joint for healing.
- Dosages must be very gentle (grade I or II) to avoid stretching the capsules and are best applied with manual techniques during the acute stage.
- With spondylosis or stenosis, if a patient does not have signs of acute joint inflammation but does have signs of nerve root irritation, stronger traction forces may be beneficial to cause opening of the intervertebral foramina, which will help relieve the pressure.

Contraindication. If a patient has RA, traction or joint mobilizations in the spine are potentially dangerous because of ligamentous necrosis and vertebral instability and, therefore, should not be done.[69]

Correction of Lateral Shift If Present

If the patient has a lateral shift of the thoracic region along with symptom relief when in flexion, he or she may be taught self-correction

Patient position and procedure: Standing with the leg opposite the shift on a chair so the hip is in about 90 degrees of flexion. The leg on the side of the lateral shift is kept extended. Have the patient then flex the trunk onto the raised thigh and apply pressure by pulling on the ankle (Fig. 15–12).

Correction of Meniscoid Impingements If Present

If there is entrapped synovial or meniscoid tissue in a facet joint that blocks motion into extension, release of the trapped meniscoid will relieve the pain and accompanying muscle guarding. The joint surfaces need to be separated and the joint capsules made taut.[50] General techniques include:

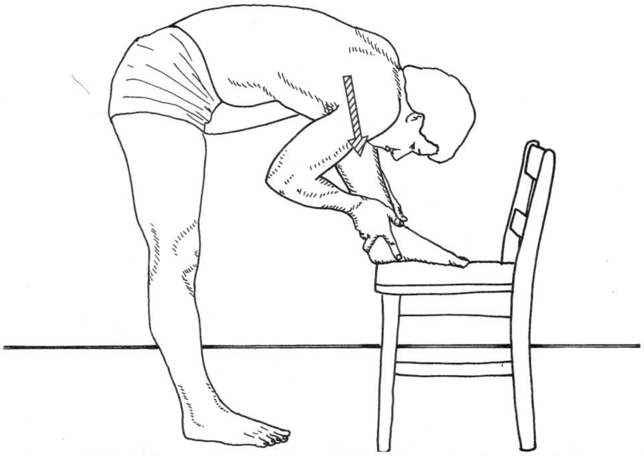

Figure 15–12 Self-correction of a lateral shift when there is deviation of the trunk as it flexes.

Traction

Traction to the spine may be applied manually or mechanically. The patient can also be taught self-traction and positional traction techniques. Techniques of manual traction, self-traction, and positional traction with rotation are described in the stretching section of Chapter 16.

- Traction applied longitudinally along the axis of the spine has the effect of sliding the facets joint surfaces and, thus, places tension on the facet capsules.
- Traction with side bending and rotation of the spine has the effect of distracting the facet joint surfaces as well as placing tension on the capsules.

Spinal Mobilization and Manipulation

These techniques require advanced training and are beyond the scope of this text.

Management When Acute Symptoms Have Stabilized

General guidelines for subacute and chronic spinal problems are summarized in Boxes 15–6 and 15–7. Specific emphasis when treating patients with mobility impairments due to hypo- or hypermobile facet joints include:

- Hypomobile joints require stretching but not if the techniques stress a hypermobile region. Traction techniques may be effective if the hypermobile region is stabilized during stretching. For those trained in joint manipulation techniques, they are effective for selective facet joint stretching and have been found to be an effective part of a total treatment approach when there is instability in specific areas and restricted mobility in neighboring facet joints.[77]
- Emphasis in treatment is on developing dynamic stability through muscle control in the hypermobile regions while gaining mobility in the restricted regions.
- If there are bony changes and osteophytic spurs, the patient should avoid postures and activities of hyperextension such as reaching or looking overhead for prolonged periods of time. Adaptations in the environment might include using a stepstool so that reaching is at shoulder level.

Postures and motions emphasizing flexion of the spine that increase the size of the intervertebral foramina are usually preferred.

- For patients with RA, emphasis is on stabilization and control. Because of the potential instabilities from necrotic tissue and bone erosion, subluxations and dislocations may cause damage to the spinal cord or vascular supply and be extremely debilitating or life threatening.

▶ Guidelines for Management of Muscle and Soft Tissue Lesions: Strains, Tears, Overuse, and Contusions

As previously described, symptoms in soft tissues, including muscles, can occur as a result of direct trauma, strain from sustained or repetitive activities, or as a protective mechanism from injury to joints or other tissues. General guidelines for management follow those presented previously and summarized in Boxes 15–5, 15–6, and 15–7. In addition, specific considerations when treating muscle injury are described in this section.

Management During the Acute Stage: Protection Phase

Modulate Pain and Control Edema and Inflammation

Use appropriate modalities and massage. Passive support may be necessary to relieve the muscles from the job of supporting or controlling the injured part.

Cervical Region

Cervical collars provide passive support. The length of time a collar is worn during the day relates to the severity of the injury and the amount of protection required. Collars often place the neck in a forward-head posture. This causes healing in a faulty position, which leads to future postural problems or painful syndromes. Usually, turning the collar around or cutting down the portion under the mandible allows the neck to assume a correct alignment.

Lumbar Region

Corsets provide passive support. As with the cervical region, the length of time that a corset is worn should be related to the amount of protection required. Some patients tend to become dependent on the corset and continue to wear it even after healing, when it no longer serves its intended purpose. After healing, it is better to strengthen the body's natural corset (deep abdominal muscles) and develop good spinal mechanics (see Chapter 16).

Maintain Muscle Integrity

Identify the functional position in which the patient has reduced symptoms. With a muscle injury, this is often with the muscle in its shortened position. In this position, begin gentle muscle-setting techniques. Dosage is critical; resistance is minimal. Use only enough to generate a setting contraction.

Cervical Region

Patient position and procedure: Supine. Stand at the head of the treatment table, supporting the patient's head with your hands. Start with the guarding muscle in its shortened position. Ask the patient to hold as gentle resistance (light enough to barely move a feather) is applied. Both the contraction and the relaxation should be gradual. There should be no neck movement or jerky resistance.

- If there has been muscle injury, the technique is repeated with the muscle kept in the shortened range for several days before lengthening it.
- If there is no muscle injury, progress the treatment by gradually lengthening the guarding muscle after each contraction and relaxation. Movement is performed only within the patient's pain-free range; no stretching is performed when there is muscle guarding.

Lumbar Region

Patient position and procedure: Prone, with arms resting at the side. Have the patient lift the head. This will initiate a setting (stabilizing) contraction of the lumbar erector spinae muscles. A stronger contraction of the lumbar extensor muscles will occur if the head and thorax are extended. Alternate hip extension will also cause a setting contraction of the lumbar extensor muscles.

- When there is muscle injury, the muscle is kept in this shortened range for several days.
- For progression, if there is no muscle injury or as the muscle heals, gradually allow the muscle to elongate after each contraction by putting a pillow under the abdomen and then extending the thorax on the lumbar spine through a greater range. Elongation is performed only within toler-

ance during the early healing phase. There should be no increase in symptoms.

Alternate position and procedure: Supine. Have the patient press the head and neck into the bed, causing a setting contraction of the spinal extensors.

Maintain Integrity and Promote Relaxation of the Muscles When There Is No Muscle Injury

Reverse muscle action techniques. These techniques are valuable when neck motions cause pain and muscle guarding. The neck is not moved, but the muscles are called on to contract and relax through a functional range. The motions include active scapular elevation, depression, adduction, and rotation and active shoulder flexion, extension, abduction, adduction, and rotation. The shoulder motions may be carried out as circumduction or patterned activities as long as they do not stress the neck.

Traction

Gentle oscillating traction may reflexively inhibit the pain and help maintain synovial fluid and joint-play motion during the acute stage when the muscles do not allow full ROM. Gentle techniques are most effectively applied using manual traction. Position the part with the injured tissue in a shortened position, and use a dosage less than that which causes vertebral separation.

Precaution. Traction techniques may aggravate a muscle or soft tissue injury if the tissue is placed in a lengthened position during the setup or with a high dosage of pull during treatment.[71]

Adapt the Environment

If there are activities or postures that caused the trauma or are continuing to provoke symptoms, identify the mechanism and modify the activity or environment to eliminate the potential of recurrence of the problem.

Management in the Subacute and Chronic Stages of Healing: Controlled Motion and Return to Function Phases

Once acute symptoms are under control, re-examine the patient and determine the impairments and functional limitations. Refer to the general guidelines for management as presented in Boxes 15–6 and 15–7.

▶ Guidelines for Management of Impairments with a Nonweight-Bearing Bias

During examination, some patients do not respond to extension, flexion, or even midrange spinal positions or motions due to the acuity of or mechanical stimuli from their condition. The person is often more comfortable lying down and may have partial or full relief with a traction test maneuver to the painful region of the spine.

For these patients, use of traction procedures or unweighting the body in a pool may be the interventions of choice until the symptoms stabilize.

Management of Acute Symptoms

Traction

Various studies have reported the benefits of traction.[18,33,61,82,93]

- Traction has the mechanical benefit of temporarily separating the vertebrae and causing mechanical sliding of the facet joints in the spine. If done intermittently, this motion may help reduce circulatory congestion and relieve pressure on the dura, blood vessels, and nerve roots in the intervertebral foramina. Improving circulation may also help decrease the concentration of noxious chemical irritants from swelling and inflammation.
- There may be a neurophysiological response via stimulation of the mechanoreceptors that may modulate the transmission of nociceptive stimuli at the spinal cord or brain stem level.

Harness

Various unloading devices may be used such as partially suspending the patient in a harness while he or she performs ambulation on a treadmill or gentle extremity exercises.

Pool

If a person is not fearful of being in a pool, supporting the individual with a buoyant life belt in deep water reduces the effects of gravity on the lumbar spine. If symptoms are reduced, it may be possible to begin and progress gentle stabilization exercises in this buoyant environment to meet some of the goals during the acute and subacute phases. Exercises can also be progressed by using the properties of water for resistance and stretching. (See description of aquatic exercises in Chapter 7.)

Progression

As healing occurs, the patient should begin to tolerate weight bearing. After re-examination and assessment, identify the impairments and functional limitations. If a bias toward flexion or extension is determined, take this into consideration as the program for further intervention is planned.

Management of Selected Conditions

Torticollis (Wryneck, Cervical Scoliosis)

This involves asymmetry in strength or function of the sternocleidomastoid muscle (SCM). There is cervical rotation opposite to and side bending toward the side of the contracting or shortened muscle.

Congenital Torticollis

Causes. Injury may occur in utero or at birth to the SCM, which then becomes fibrotic and shortens. The injury may be from a faulty position of the fetus, nerve injury, or direct trauma to the muscle.

Management. Gentle passive ROM, stretching and positioning are initiated as soon as the diagnosis is made. The head is rotated toward and side-bent away from the side of tightness, using the same technique as for scalene stretches (see Fig. 16–4).

Asymmetric Weakness (Muscle Imbalance)

Causes. A common cause is hemiplegia, in which the stronger muscle turns the head toward the side of weakness. The functional problem may develop into a static limitation if the neck is not periodically taken through full ROM.

Management. If there is innervation and control of the weaker muscle, initiate strengthening exercises. Active or passive ROM is performed several times a day.

Hysterical Torticollis

Causes. There may be many causes; sometimes it is described as the person's turning away from an unpleasant situation.

Management. Intervention consists of resistive exercises to the opposite muscle and ROM to maintain flexibility. Relaxation exercises may be helpful if the person tends to be tense. Close communication is maintained with the psychiatrist or psychologist working with the cause of the disorder.

Tension Headache/Cervical Headache

This usually involves tension in the posterior cervical muscles, pain at the attachment of the cervical extensors, and/or pain radiating across the top and side of the scalp.

Causes

Tension headaches may follow soft tissue injury or may be caused by faulty or sustained postures, nerve irritation or impingement (the greater occipital nerve emerges through the neck extensor muscles where they attach at the base of the skull), or sustained muscle contraction (from faulty posture or emotional tension) leading to ischemia. With cervical headaches, the joints and ligaments of the upper cervical spine are often inflamed or in dysfunction. Headaches may be related to temporomandibular joint dysfunction (see next section) or other kinds of conditions such as allergies or sinusitis, or there may be vascular or autonomic involvement as with migraine or cluster headaches.[74a] Whatever the cause, there usually is a cycle of pain, muscle contraction, decreased circulation, and more pain, which leads to decreased function and potential soft tissue and joint dysfunction.

Management

- Break into the cycle of pain and muscle tension using modalities, massage, and muscle-setting exercises to increase circulation to the part and carry off waste products.
- Evaluate the flexibility and strength of the muscles in the cervical, upper thoracic, and shoulder girdle, and design an exercise program to regain a balance in length and strength in preparation for posture correction and training. Chapter 16 describes these procedures. Be sure there is adequate flexibility in the suboccipital muscles to relieve tension in that region.
- Educate the patient in proper techniques to relieve the source or manage the irritation.
  - If there is impaired posture, teach posture correction and ways to manage posture.
  - If the person is in tension-producing situations, teach relaxation techniques, ROM and muscle-setting techniques, and proper spinal mechanics.

Temporomandibular Joint Dysfunction (Syndrome)

Signs and Symptoms

Pain from a variety of sources is often cited as part of the temporomandibular joint (TMJ) syndrome.[53]

- Pain may occur locally in the TMJ, in the richly vascularized and highly innervated retrodiskal pad located in the posterior region of the joint, or in the ear.
- Pain from muscle spasm or myofascial pain in the masseter, temporalis, or pterygoid internis or externis muscles may be described as a headache or facial pain.
- Tension in the muscles of the cervical spine may itself be painful or cause referenced pain from irritation of the greater occipital nerve that may be described as a tension headache.

Causes

Imbalance occurs between the head, jaw, neck, and shoulder girdle. Causes may be:

- Malocclusion, decreased vertical dimension of the bite, or other dental problems.
- Faulty joint mechanics from inflammation, subluxation of the meniscus (disk), dislocation of the condylar head, joint contractures, or asymmetric forces from jaw and bite imbalances. Restricted motion results from periods of immobilization after reconstructive surgery or fracture of the jaw.
- Muscle spasm in the muscles of mastication, causing abnormal or asymmetric joint forces. Muscle spasm can be the result of emotional tension, faulty joint mechanics, direct or indirect injury, or a postural dysfunction.
- Sinus problems, resulting in the individual's being a mouth breather, which indirectly affects posture and jaw position.
- Postural dysfunctions: With a forward-head posture, there is retraction of the mandible and resulting stretch on the anterior throat muscles. Consequently, there is increased activity in the muscles that close the jaw to counter the changed forces. The muscles and soft tissue in the suboccipital region become tight, and the nerves and joints become compressed or irritated.
- Trauma such as a flexion/extension accident in which the jaw forcefully opens when the head whips back into hyperextension. A direct blow from an auto accident, boxing, a fall or similar trauma, or sustained trauma as occurs in prolonged dental surgery in which the mouth is held open for a lengthy period of time may initiate symptoms in the TMJ or supporting tissue. Excessive stresses such as biting or chewing on large pieces of hard food may also traumatize the joints.

Management

The approach to management depends on the cause. In simple cases in which posture, joint dysfunction, or muscle imbalances are the source of the problem, intervention with therapeutic exercise can directly address the problems. In many cases, a dental referral, otolaryngology referral, or psychological support may be necessary to deal with related pathology. A complete evaluation is necessary prior to the initiation of any treatment.

Modulate Pain and Muscle Guarding

Use modalities, massage, and relaxation techniques. In addition, the person should eat soft foods and avoid items requiring excessive jaw opening or firm biting and chewing motions.

Teach Relaxation of the Facial Muscles, Tongue Proprioception, and Tongue Control

The following are suggested techniques:

- Place the tip of the tongue on the hard palate behind the front teeth and draw little circles or letters on the palate. For additional stimulus, place a Lifesavor® between the tongue and palate then follow the circular edge with the tip of the tongue.
- Place the tip of the tongue on the hard palate and blow air out to vibrate the tongue; making an "r r r r" sound.
- Fill the cheeks with air (mouth closed), then let the air out in a puff.
- Make a "clicking" sound with the tongue on the roof of the mouth. When doing so, the jaw drops open quickly and returns with the teeth slightly apart, and usually the tongue rests on the hard palate behind the front teeth. This is the resting position of the jaw and is also the first step in teaching relaxation exercises. (Relaxation exercises are described in Chapter 16).

Teach Control of the Jaw Muscles

- First, teach recognition of the resting position of the jaw. The lips are closed, teeth slightly apart, and tongue resting lightly on the hard palate behind the front teeth. The patient should breathe in and out slowly through the nose, using diaphragmatic breathing.

- Teach control while opening and closing the jaw through the first half of the ROM. With the tongue on the roof of the mouth, the patient opens the mouth, trying to keep the chin in midline. Use a mirror for visual reinforcement. The patient is also taught to lightly palpate the lateral pole of each condyle of the mandible bilaterally and to attempt to maintain symmetry between movement of the two sides when opening and closing the mouth.
- If the jaw deviates while opening or closing, have the patient practice lateral deviation to the opposite side. The lateral motion should not be excessive or cause pain.
- Progress to applying gentle resistance with the thumb against the chin. Do not overpower the muscles.

Increase ROM If Indicated

- Begin by placing layered tongue depressors between the central incisors. The patient can gradually work to increase the amount of tongue depressors used until he or she can open approximately far enough to insert the knuckles of the index and middle fingers.
- Self-stretching is carried out by placing each thumb under the upper teeth and the index or middle fingers over the lower teeth and pushing the teeth open.

Increase Joint Mobility If Indicated

Patient position and procedures: Supine or sitting, with the head supported and stabilized. Perform joint mobilization techniques with a gloved hand or hands. Determination of dosages and precautions for administration of mobilization techniques are described in Chapter 6.

- ***Unilateral distraction (Fig. 15–13A).*** Use the hand opposite the side on which you are working. Place your thumb in the patient's mouth on the back molars; the fingers are outside and wrapped around the jaw. The force is in a downward (caudal) direction.
- ***Unilateral distraction with glide (Fig. 15–13B).*** After distracting the jaw as described above, pull it in a forward (anterior) direction with a tipping motion. The other hand can be placed over the TMJ to palpate the amount of movement.

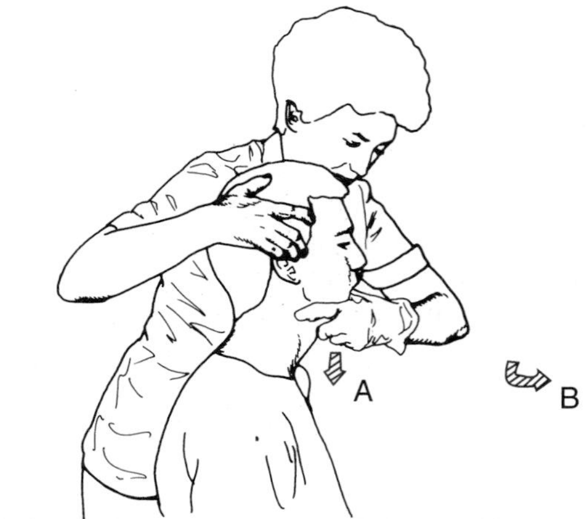

Figure 15–13 Unilateral mobilization of the temporomandibular joint. *(A)* Distraction is in a caudal direction. *(B)* Arrow indicating distraction with glide in a caudal, then anterior direction.

- ***Bilateral distraction (Fig. 15–14).*** If the patient is supine, stand at the head of the treatment table. If the patient is sitting, stand in front of the patient. Use both thumbs, placing them on the molars on each side of the mandible. The fingers are wrapped around the jaw. The force from the thumbs is equal, in a caudal direction.
- ***Self-mobilization:*** Place cotton dental rolls between the back teeth, and have the patient bite down. This distracts the condyles from the fossae in the joints.

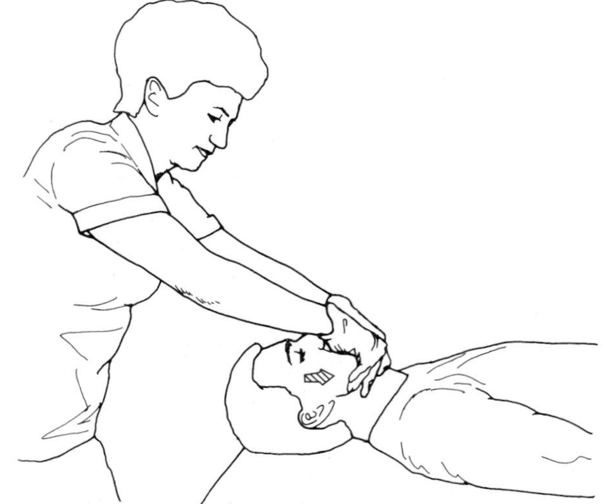

Figure 15–14 Bilateral distraction of the temporomandibular joint with the patient supine.

Correct Muscle Imbalances

Stretch restricting postural muscles, teach relaxation, and then retrain for proper muscle control. Cervical and shoulder postural stretching and retraining exercises are described in Chapters 16 and 8, respectively.

Neural Tension Impairments

If positive nerve tension signs are described by the patient while providing the history and positive signs are detected with testing maneuvers, techniques that are reported to mobilize components of the nervous system may be used to diminish the patient's symptoms.[16] Symptoms described usually include pain and sensory changes when in a stretched position.

Nervous System Mobility Characteristics

Butler[16] describes the peripheral and central nervous systems as a continuous tissue tract; simply stated, it is like an "H" on its side. Structurally and functionally, there is continuity of the connective tissues, of the impulse transmission between the neurons, and with the chemical flow of neurotransmitters. The system is designed to be mobile and deform while at the same time to be able to conduct impulses.

Substantial mobility in the nervous system is needed for an individual to move during functional activities. With movement of an extremity, before there is increased tension within the nerve itself, the whole peripheral nerve moves and there is movement between connective tissues and neural tissues. The mobility is allowed without undue stress on the nerve tissue because:

- The arrangement of the spinal cord, nerve roots, and plexes allows for mobility. If any part of the "H" is placed under tension, the force can be dissipated throughout the system.
- The nerves themselves are wavy and can straighten when tension is applied.
- The connective tissue around the individual nerves and bundles of nerves (epineurium, perineurium, and endoneurium) absorb tensile forces before the nerve itself stretches.

Compressive forces can block nerve impulses, and if sustained can cause nerve damage. The endoneurium helps maintain fluid pressure and may provide cushioning for nerves, especially when close to the surface and subject to greater pressure.

Nerve Injury

Etiology. Biomechanical injuries to the peripheral nervous system occur most commonly from friction, compression, and stretch. Secondary injury could occur from blood or edema. The insult could be acute from trauma or chronic from repetitive trauma or entrapment.

Vulnerable sites. Sites where a peripheral nerve is more vulnerable to compression, friction, or tension include: tunnels (soft tissue, bony, or fibro-osseus), branches of the nervous system (especially if the nerve has an abrupt angle), points where a nerve is relatively fixed, when passing close to rigid structures (across a bony prominence), and at specific tension points.

Types of pathology leading to tension signs. Symptoms can be either pathophysiologic or pathomechanical leading to symptoms of adverse tension on the nervous system.

- ***Intraneural.*** Pathology that affects the conducting tissues (hypoxia, demyelination) or connective tissues of the nerve (scarring of epineurium, irritation of dura mater) may restrict the elasticity of the nervous system itself.
- ***Extraneural.*** Pathology that affects the nerve bed such as blood, adhesions of epineurium to another tissue (such as a ligament), and swelling of tissue adjacent to a nerve (such as foraminal stenosis) may restrict the gross movement of the nervous system in relation to surrounding tissues.

Symptoms and Signs of Nerve Mobility Impairment

History. Vascular and mechanical factors can lead to nerve pathology. Pain is the most common symptom. Sensory responses, reported as stretch pain or paresthesia, occur when in the neural stretch position.[20] Clinical reasoning is used to understand the possible mechanism of injury such as pathologic insult to the nervous tissue or surrounding tissues, or symptoms from movement patterns that place tension on the neural tissues and reproduce symptoms.

Positive signs. Test maneuvers are performed to detect *tension signs*.

- Tension signs are stretch pain or paresthesia that occur when the neurologic system is stretched across multiple joints and is relieved when one of the joints in the chain is moved out of the stretch position.

- Because the test positions place stress across each joint, every joint in the chain must be tested for range, mobility, and symptom provocation prior to nerve tension testing so that any restriction occurring during the test is not from the joint or immediate periarticular tissues.
- The test maneuvers are similar to the treatment maneuvers.

Causes of Symptoms

The symptoms are the result of tension being placed on some component of the nervous system. If compression is preventing normal mobility, tension signs will occur. Restriction in movement can be from inflammation and scarring between the nerve and tissue it runs through or from actual changes within the nerve itself.[16]

Management

Principles of treatment are similar to any mobilization technique.[16]

- The intensity of the maneuver should be related to irritability of the tissue, patient response, and change in symptoms. The greater the irritability, the more gentle the technique.
- If the restriction is primarily tension, the stretch force is applied into the tissue resistance, held for 15 to 20 seconds, released, and then repeated several times.
- Neurologic symptoms of tingling or increased numbness should not last when the stretch is released.
- The application of the techniques requires positioning the individual at the point of tension (symptoms just begin), then either passively or having the patient actively move one joint in the pattern in such a way as to stretch, then release the tension. Moving different joints in the pattern, while maintaining the elongated position on the other joints, changes the forces on the nerves.
- After several treatments and the tissue response is known, the patient is taught self-stretching.

Techniques for the Upper Quadrant

Median Nerve Stretch

Patient position and procedure: Begin with the patient supine; sequentially apply shoulder girdle depression, then slightly abduct the shoulder, extend the elbow, laterally rotate the arm and supinate the forearm. Wrist, finger and thumb extensions are then added; finally the shoulder is taken into greater abduction (Fig. 15–15) The full stretch position includes contralateral cervical side flexion. While maintaining the stretch position, move one joint at a time a few degrees in and out of the stretch position, such as wrist extension and flexion, or elbow flexion and extension.

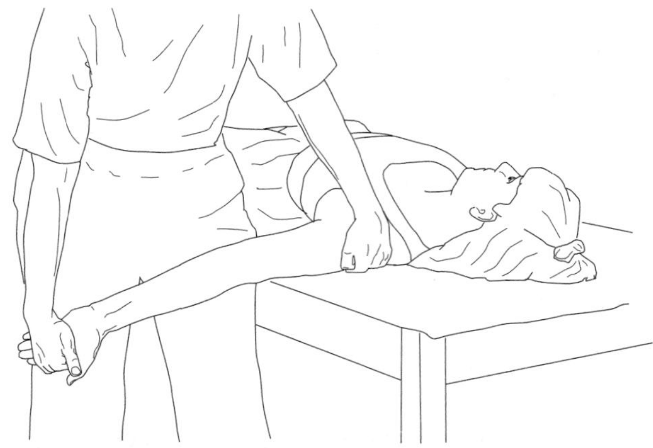

Figure 15–15 Position of maximum stretch on the median nerve includes shoulder girdle depression, shoulder abduction, elbow extension, shoulder external rotation and supination of the forearm, wrist, finger and thumb extension, and finally, contralateral cervical side flexion.

This maneuver is beneficial when examining and treating symptoms related to median nerve distribution, problems with shoulder girdle depression (such as thoracic outlet syndrome), and carpal tunnel syndrome.[16]

Radial Nerve Stretch

Patient position and procedure: Begin with the patient supine; sequentially apply shoulder girdle depression, then slightly abduct the shoulder, extend the elbow, then medially rotate the arm and pronate the forearm. Keep the elbow in extension and add wrist, finger, and thumb flexion, and finally, ulnar deviation of the wrist (Fig. 15–16). The full stretch position includes contralateral side flexion of the cervical spine. While maintaining the stretch position, move one joint at a time a few degrees in and out of the stretch position, such as wrist extension and flexion.

This maneuver is important when examining and treating symptoms that are related to shoulder girdle depression, radial nerve distribution, and disorders such as tennis elbow and deQuervain's syndrome.[16]

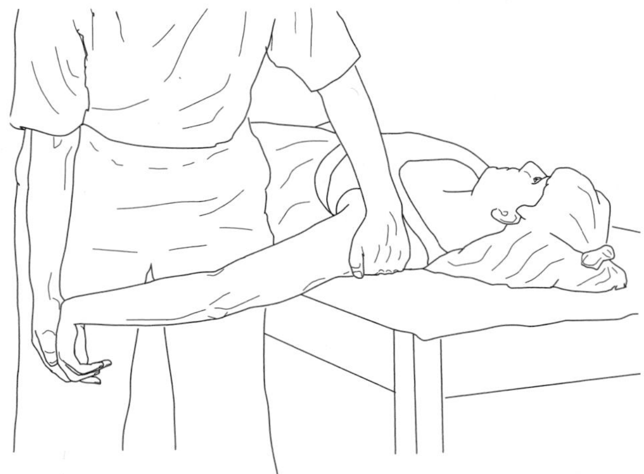

Figure 15–16 Position of maximum stretch on the radial nerve includes shoulder girdle depression, shoulder abduction, elbow extension, shoulder medial rotation and forearm pronation, wrist, finger and thumb flexion, wrist ulnar deviation, and finally, contralateral cervical side flexion.

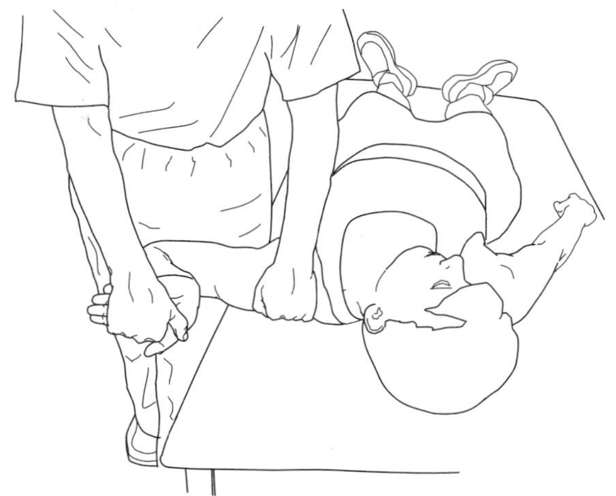

Figure 15–17 Position of maximum stretch on the ulnar nerve includes shoulder girdle depression, shoulder external rotation and abduction, elbow flexion, forearm supination, and wrist extension, and finally, contralateral cervical side flexion.

Ulnar Nerve Stretch

Patient position and procedure: Begin with the patient supine. Sequentially apply wrist extension and forearm supination followed by elbow flexion (full range); then add shoulder girdle depression. Maintain this position and add shoulder lateral rotation and abduction. In the final position the patient's hand is near his or her ear with fingers pointing posteriorly (Fig. 15–17). In the full stretch position, contralateral side flexion of the cervical spine is added. While maintaining the overall stretch position, move one joint at a time a few degrees in and out of the stretch position, such as elbow extension and flexion.

This maneuver is important when symptoms are related to the C-8 and T-1 nerve roots, lower brachial plexus, ulnar nerve, and disorders such as medial epicondylitis.[16]

Techniques for the Lower Quadrant

Straight-Leg Raising (SLR) with Ankle Dorsiflexion

Patient position and procedure: Supine with the lower extremity in the SLR position, add ankle dorsiflexion. Several variations may be done; ankle dorsiflexion, ankle plantar flexion with inversion, hip adduction, hip medial rotation, and passive neck flexion.[16] The maneuver may also be performed long-sitting (slump-sitting position) and side-lying. These various positions of the lower extremity and neck are used to differentiate tight or strained hamstrings from possible sites of restriction or nerve mobility in the lumbosacral plexus and sciatic nerve.[28,97]

Once the position that places tension on the involved neurologic tissue is found, maintain the stretch position, and then move one of the joints a few degrees in and out of the stretch position, such as ankle plantar and dorsiflexion, or knee flexion and extension.

- Ankle dorsiflexion with eversion places more tension on the tibial tract.
- Ankle dorsiflexion with inversion places tension on the sural nerve.
- Ankle plantarflexion with inversion places tension on the common peroneal tract.
- Adduction of the hip while doing SLR places further tension on the nervous system because the sciatic nerve is lateral to the ischial tuberosity; medial rotation of the hip while doing SLR also increases tension on the sciatic nerve (Fig. 15–18).
- Passive neck flexion while doing SLR pulls the spinal cord cranially and places the entire nervous system on a stretch.

Slump-Sitting Stretch

Patient position and procedure: Slump-sitting with neck, thorax, and low back flexed. Extend the knee

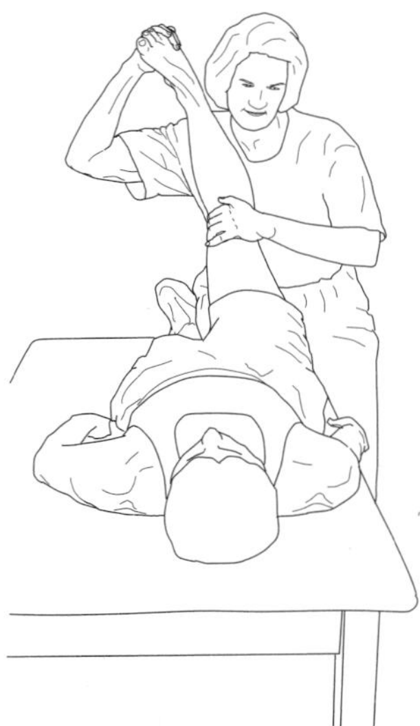

Figure 15–18 Position of stretch on the sciatic nerve includes straight-leg raising with adduction and internal rotation of the hip and dorsiflexion of the ankle.

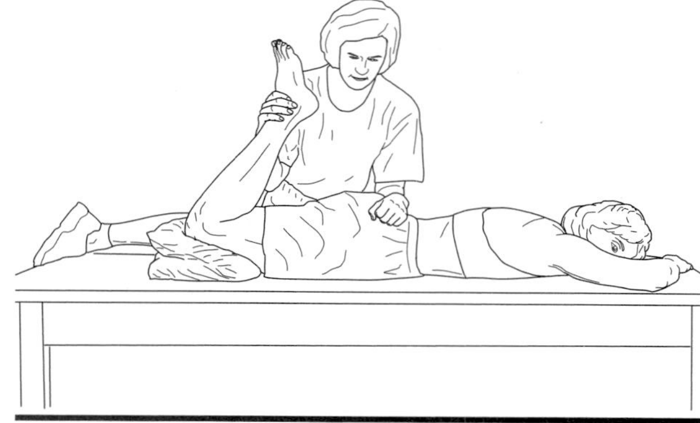

Figure 15–19 Position of stretch on the femoral nerve; prone-lying with the spine neutral, hip extended, and knee flexed.

and dorsiflex the ankle just to the point of tissue resistance and symptom reproduction. Increase and release the stretch force by moving one joint in the chain a few degrees, such as knee flexion and extension, or ankle dorsiflexion and plantarflexion.

Prone Knee Bend Stretch

Patient position and procedure: Prone with the spine neutral (not extended) and the hips extended to 0 degrees. Flex the knee to the point of resistance and symptom reproduction. Pain in the low back or neurological signs are considered positive for upper lumbar nerve roots and femoral nerve tension (Fig. 15–19). Thigh pain could be rectus femoris tightness. It is important not to hyperextend the spine to avoid confusion with facet or compression pain. Flex and extend the knee a few degrees to apply and release tension.

Alternate position and procedure: Side-lying with the involved leg uppermost. Stabilize the pelvis and extend the hip with the knee flexed until symptoms are reproduced. Maintain knee flexion, release, and apply tension across the hip by moving it a few degrees at a time.

Prevention

These maneuvers, especially the SLR with repetitive ankle dorsiflexion and plantarflexion, and the respective upper quadrant maneuvers may be used to prevent restrictive adhesions from developing if done early on in treatment after an acute injury or surgery.

Precautions and Contraindications to Nerve Tension Testing and Treatment

Butler cautions that there is incomplete scientific understanding of the pathology and mechanisms occurring when mobilizing the nervous system.[16] The clinician should always use caution.

Precautions

- Know what other tissues are affected by the positions and maneuvers.
- Recognize the irritability of the tissues involved and do not aggravate the symptoms.
- Identify whether or not the condition is worsening and the rate of worsening. A rapidly worsening condition requires greater care than a slowly progressing condition.
- Use care if there is an active disease or pathology affecting the nervous system.
- Watch for signs of vascular compromise. The vascular system is in close proximity to the nervous system and at no time should show signs of compromise when mobilizing the nervous system.

Contraindications

- Acute or unstable neurologic signs
- Cauda equina symptoms related to the spine including changes in bowel or bladder function and perineal sensation
- Spinal cord injury or symptoms

Independent Learning Activities

CRITICAL THINKING AND DISCUSSION

1. Identify similarities and differences between the anatomy and function of the cervical and lumbar spine. How do these factors affect the way treatment is provided when there is muscle strain, joint irritation, and flexibility imbalances?
2. What are the functional differences between the way the cervical spine and lumbar spine are used in daily activities?
3. Explain how different individuals who sustain back injuries can experience the different symptoms of radiating pain down the leg, numbness and tingling into the foot, deep aching down the leg, or no leg symptoms at all. What do each of these symptoms mean?
4. Explain why some people will experience improved symptoms and function if the emphasis of intervention is spinal extension, whereas others will improve if the emphasis of intervention is spinal flexion.

LABORATORY PRACTICE

1. Practice identifying cervical and lumbar spine positions when in supine, prone, side-lying, sitting, and standing. Determine what is needed to change the position; i.e., if flexion is emphasized, what is needed to cause extension?
2. Identify and feel what happens to the various portions of the spine when moving from one position to another; i.e., rolling supine to prone and return, moving from supine to sit, sit to stand and reverse.
3. Practice methods for developing gentle isometric muscle contractions that could be used during the acute phase of treatment for both the cervical and lumbar spines.

CASE STUDIES

Case 1

A 45-year-old man sustained injuries in a rear-end collision 4 days ago (car hit him going approximately 45 MPH while he was stopped at a stop light). He was in an older car without an air bag or properly positioned headrest, although he was wearing a seatbelt. Initially, he impacted the headrest at the midcervical spine as his neck extended, and then his head flexed forward but did not hit anything. He has been cleared of cervical fractures or instability. Medical history is unremarkable; he is a social drinker and gave up smoking 5 years ago. He is an accountant and usually works long hours at a computer, but has been unable to work since the accident. He presents wearing a cervical collar and has a facial expression of distress. He states he has had difficulty sleeping because the pain wakes him whenever he moves.

Pain: constant posterior cervical pain, headaches, and pain radiating into the shoulder region bilaterally; intermittent tingling in the right thumb, index, and middle finger. Pain rated at 8/10 when at rest, 10/10 when attempting to move.

Positive findings: guarded forward-head posture. Unwilling to move more than 10 degrees into flexion or extension, 25 degrees into side bending bilaterally, and minimal rotation. Gentle traction to the head relieves the neurological symptoms. Palpation tenderness in upper trapezius and posterior cervical and anterior throat muscles bilaterally. Increased tenderness along facet margins of C-4/5, 5/6 and 6/7, right>left.

- From the above impairments and functional limitations, identify goals and interventions for this patient. Describe the techniques you would use, and practice them on a laboratory partner.
- How long do you anticipate the patient will have these symptoms? At what point will you change your goals?

Case 2

Assume you did not see the patient described in Case Study 1 until 4 weeks after the accident. He no longer has constant pain and has returned to work. His complaints are an inability to sit at the computer for more than 1/2 hour before his hand starts to tingle. Numbness occurs after 1 hour of work. Headaches begin within 2 hours of work. Neck and shoulder pain is 6/10 by mid-day at which time he takes NSAIDS so he can continue working. Positive tests include: forward-head posture with forward shoulders, decreased flexibility in the suboccipital muscles, anterior thorax, and internal rotators of the shoulder. Cervical flexion 75%, extension 50%, side bending and rotation 75% bilaterally. Sustained extension of the cervical spine causes tingling into the thumb, index, and middle finger of the right hand. Strength of scapular adductors and lateral rotators of the shoulder is 4/5; myotome testing is normal bilaterally.

- What are your goals and interventions for this patient at this stage?
- After studying the techniques described in Chapter 16, describe the techniques you would use with this patient, and practice them on a laboratory partner.
- For each therapeutic exercise technique, practice progressions, and determine how you would progress this patient so he could work without exacerbation of symptoms.

Case 3

A 55-year-old woman presents with early signs of DJD of the lumbar spine. She has been an active runner since college. Occasionally, she has participated in aerobic dance classes. History is unremarkable. She has three grown children and had no complaints of back pain related to the pregnancies. Current symptoms: Intermittent periods of pain extending from the midlumbar spine, through the right buttock and posterior thigh. The pain begins 15 minutes into her running and progresses to an 8/10 by 25 to 30 minutes. She also complains of increased stiffness after sitting >1 hour, standing >15 minutes, and when waking in the morning and getting out of bed. She is a middle school teacher and track coach for a girl's high school team. Key findings: lordotic posture, with tight low back, hip flexors, and tensor fasciae latae. Strength of lower abdominals is 4/5. Forward bending of the spine increases tension in low back, repeated backward bending and prone press-ups increase buttock pain. Side bending is decreased 25%, with some discomfort with overpressure into right side bending.

- Based on these impairments and limitations, identify the irritability of the condition and determine goals and intervention.
- What are the most important factors to emphasize with this individual to help her manage her symptoms?
- After studying the exercises in Chapter 16, practice the techniques that you would have this patient do. Also, practice how you would progress the techniques and what criteria you would use for progressions.

Case 4

A 42-year-old man presents with a medical diagnosis of herniated nucleus pulposus at the L5/S1 area. Present symptoms began 4 days ago when rising out of bed. He is a sedentary person who plays social golf on the weekends (rides in a cart) and is 50 lb overweight. He has had occasional episodes of low back pain over the past 15 years, but "nothing like this." Medical history: smokes 1 pack of cigarettes/day and is on blood pressure medication. He describes the symptoms as a sharp pain beginning in the left buttock region and radiating down the back of the thigh; there is intermittent paresthesia along the lateral border of his foot, which is noticeable when sitting. He describes considerable increase in symptoms when attempting to rise up from bed, rise up out of a chair, or whenever straining. He has been unable to walk because he cannot stand upright. On observation, you note that the patient is standing with a posterior pelvic tilt and forward-bend of the trunk, and the thorax deviated to the right. Examination maneuvers: all spinal flexion motions increase symptoms; side gliding of the thorax to the left followed by lumbar extension centralizes the symptoms to primarily buttock and low back pain.

- Based on this information, identify the impairments and functional limitations. What type of intervention should be used?
- Develop a sequence of treatment techniques that you would use during the first visit. Include instructions and precautions. Practice the techniques.

REFERENCES

1. Abdulwahab, SS, and Sabbahi, M: Neck retractions, cervical root decompression and radicular pain. J Orthop Sports Phys Ther 30(1):4, 2000.
2. Abenhaim, L, et al: The role of activity in the therapeutic management of back pain: report of the international Paris task force on back pain. Spine 25(4S):1S, 2000
3. Adams, MA, and Hutton, WC: Gradual disc prolapse. Spine 10(6):524, 1985.
4. Adams, MA, and Hutton, WC: The effect of fatigue on the lumbar intervertebral disc. J Bone Joint Surg Br 65(2):199, 1983.
5. Alexander, AH, Jones, AM, and Rosenbaum, DH: Nonoper-

ative management of herniated nucleus pulposus: Patient selection by the extension sign. Orthop Rev 21:181, 1992.
6. Anderson, B, et al: The influence of backrest inclination and lumbar support on lumbar lordosis. Spine 4:52, 1979.
7. Andersson E, et al: The role of the psoas and iliacus muscles for stability and movement of the lumbar spine, pelvis and hip. Scand J Med Sci Sports 5:10, 1995.
8. Basmajian, JV: Muscles Alive, ed 4. The Williams & Wilkins Co, Baltimore, 1979.
9. Bogduk, N, and Engle, R: The menisci of the lumbar zygapophyseal joints: A review of their anatomy and clinical significance. Spine 9(5):454, 1984.
10. Bogduk, N, and MacIntosh, JE: The applied anatomy of the thoracolumbar fascia. Spine 9:164, 1984.
11. Bogduk, N, and Twomey, LT: Clinical Anatomy of the Lumbar Spine. Churchill-Livingstone, New York, 1987.
12. Bondi, BA, and Drinkwater-Kolk, M: Functional stabilization training. Workshop notes, Northeast Seminars, October 1992.
13. Brinckmann, P: Injury of the annulus fibrosus and disc protrusions. Spine 11(2):149, 1986.
14. Burkart, S, and Beresfore, W: The aging intervertebral disk. Phys Ther 59:969, 1979.
15. Butler, D, et al: Discs degenerate before facets. Spine 15:111, 1990.
16. Butler, DS: Mobilisation of the Nervous System. Churchill Livingstone, New York, 1991.
17. Cailliet, R: Scoliosis. FA Davis, Philadelphia, 1975.
18. Cailliet, R: Low Back Pain Syndrome, ed 4. FA Davis, Philadelphia, 1988.
19. Cloward, R: The clinical significance of the sino-vertebral nerve of the cervical spine in relation to the cervical disc syndrome. J Neurol Surg Psychiatry 23:321, 1960.
20. Coppieters, MW, Stappaerts, KH, et al: Addition of test components during neurodynamic testing: effect on range of motion and sensory responses. J Orthop Sports Phys Ther 31(5):226, 2001.
21. Cresswell, AG, Grundstrom, H, and Thorstensson, A; Observations on intra-abdominal pressure and patterns of abdominal intra-muscular activity in man. Acta Physiol Scand 144:409, 1992.
22. Delitto, A, Erhard, RE, and Bowling, RW: A treatment-based classification approach to low back syndrome: identifying and staging patients for conservative treatment. Phys Ther 75(6):470, 1995.
23. DeRosa, CP, and Porterfield, JA. A physical therapy model for the treatment of low back pain. Phys Ther 72:261, 1992.
24. Daniels, L, and Worthingham, C: Therapeutic Exercise for Body Alignment and Function, ed. 2. WB Saunders, Philadelphia, 1977.
25. Farfan, HF, et al: The effects of torsion on the lumbar intervertebral joints: The role of torsion in the production of disc degeneration. J Bone Joint Surg Am 52(3):468, 1970.
26. Friber, O: Clinical symptoms and biomechanics of lumbar spine and hip joint in leg length inequality. Spine 8:643, 1983.
27. Fritz, JM, Erhard, RE, and Hagen, BF: Segmental instability of the lumbar spine. Phys Ther 78(8):889, 1998.
28. George, SZ: Differential diagnosis and treatment for a patient with lower extremity symptoms. J Orthop Sports Phys Ther 30(8):468,2000.
29. Gossman, M, Sahrmann, S, and Rose, S: Review of length-associated changes in muscle. Phys Ther 62:1977, 1982.
30. Gracovetsky, S, Farfan, H, and Helleur, C: The abdominal mechanism. Spine 10:317, 1985.
31. Gracovetsky, S, and Farfan, H: The optimum spine. Spine 11:543, 1986.
32. Gracovetsky, S: The Spinal Engine. Springer-Verlag Wein, New York, 1988.
33. Harris, P: Cervical traction: review of literature and treatment guidelines. Phys Ther 57:910, 1977.
34. Hellsing, AL, Linton, SL, and Kaluemark, M: A prospective study of patients with acute back and neck pain in Sweden. Phys Ther 74:116, 1994.
35. Hickey, DS, and Hukins, DEL: Aging changes in the macromolecular organization of the intervertebral disc: An x-ray diffraction and electron microscopic study. Spine 7(3):234, 1982.
36. Hodges, PW, Gandevia, SC, and Richardson, CA: Contractions of specific abdominal muscles in postural tasks are affected by respiratory maneuvers. J Appl Physiol 83 (3):753, 1997.
37. Hodges, PW, and Richardson, CA: Altered trunk muscle recruitment in people with low back pain with upper limb movement at different speeds. Arch Phys Med Rehabil 80 (9):1005, 1999.
38. Hodges, PW, and Richardson, CA: Transversus abdominis and the superficial abdominal muscles are controlled independently in a postural task. Neurosci Lett 265 (2):91, 1999.
39. Hodges, PW, and Richardson, CA: Delayed postural contraction of transversus abdominis in low back pain associated with movement of the lower limb. J Spinal Disord 11(1):46, 1998.
40. Hodges, PW, and Richardson, CA: Relationship between limb movement speed and associated contraction of the trunk muscles. Ergonomics 40 (11):1220, 1997.
41. Hodges, PW, and Richardson, CA: Feedforward contraction of transversus abdominis is not influenced by direction of arm movement. Exp Brain Res 114(2):362, 1997.
42. Hodges, PW, and Richardson, CA: Contraction of the abdominal muscles associated with movement of the lower limb. Phys Ther 77(2):132, 1997.
43. Jensen, G: Biomechanics of the lumbar intervertebral disc: A review. Phys Ther 60:765, 1980.
44. Kapandji, IA: The Physiology of the Joints, Vol 3. Churchill-Livingstone, New York, 1974.
45. Kellegren J: Observations on referred pain arising from muscle. Clin Sci 3:175, 1983.
46. Kendall, FP, McCreary, EK, and Provance, PG: Muscle Testing and Function, ed 4. Williams & Wilkins, Baltimore, 1993.
47. Kessler, R: Acute symptomatic disk prolapse. Phys Ther 59:978, 1979.
48. Klein, JA, and Hukins, DWL: Collagen fiber orientation in the annulus fibrosus of intervertebral disc during bending and torsion measured by x-ray defraction. Biochem Biophys Acta 719:98, 1982.
49. Kopp, JR, et al: The use of lumbar extension in the evaluation and treatment of patients with acute herniated nucleus pulposus. Clin Orthop 202:211, 1986.
50. Kos, J, and Wolf, J: Intervertebral menisci and their possible role in intervertebral blockage (translated by Burkart, S).

Bull Orthop Sports Med Sect, Amer Phys Ther Assoc 1(3):8, 1976.

51. Krag, MH, et al: Internal displacement distribution from in vitro loading of human thoracic and lumbar spinal motion segments: Experimental results and theoretical predictions. Spine 12:1001, 1987.
52. Krause, N, and Ragland, DR: Occupational disability due to low back pain: A new interdisciplinary classification based on a phase model of disability. Spine 19:1011, 1994.
53. Kraus, SL: TMJ Craniomandibular Cervical Complex: Physical Therapy and Dental Management. Clinical Education Associates, Atlanta, 1986.
54. Lamb, C: The neurology of spinal pain. Phys Ther 59:971, 1979.
54a. Levangie, P, and Norkin, C: Joint Structure and Function: A Comprehensive Analysis, ed 3. FA Davis, Philadelphia, 2001.
55. Lipson, SJ, and Muir, H: Proteoglycans in experimental intervertebral disc degeneration. Spine 6(3):194, 1981.
56. Lovell, WWQ, and Winter, RB (eds): Pediatric Orthopedics, ed 2. JB Lippincott, Philadelphia, 1986.
56a. Lundon, K, and Bolton, K: Structure and function of the lumbar intervertebral disk in the health, aging, and pathologic conditions. J Orthop Sports Phys Ther 31(6):291, 2001.
57. Lyons, G, Eisenstein, SM, and Sweet, MBI: Biochemical changes in intervertebral disc degeneration. Biochem Biophys Acta 673:443, 1981.
58. MacNab, I: Backache. Williams & Wilkins, Baltimore, 1977.
59. Markolf, LK, and Morris, JM: The structural components of the intervertebral disc. J Bone Joint Surg Am 56(4):675, 1974.
60. Marras, WS, and Granata, KP: Changes in trunk dynamics and spine loading during repeated trunk exertions. Spine 22 (21):2564, 1997
61. Matthews J: The effects of spinal traction. Physiotherapy 58:64, 1972.
62. McCarron, RF, et al: The inflammatory effect of nucleus pulposus: A possible element in the pathogenesis of low-back pain. Spine 12:760, 1987.
63. McGill, SM: Low back exercises: evidence for improving exercise regimens. Phys Ther 78(7):754, 1998.
64. McGill, SM, and Norman, RW: Low Back Biomechanics in Industry: The Prevention of Injury Through Safer Lifting, in Grabiner, M (ed): Current Issues in Biomechanics. Human Kinetics Publishers, Champaign, Il, 1993.
65. McKenzie, R: The Lumbar Spine: Mechanical Diagnosis and Therapy. Spinal Publications, New Zealand, 1981.
66. McKenzie, R: Manual correction of sciatic scoliosis. N Z Med J 89:22, 1979.
67. Mooney, V, and Robertson, J: The facet syndrome. Clin Orthop 115:149, 1976.
68. Mooney, V: The syndromes of low back disease. Orthop Clin North Am 14(3):505, 1983.
69. Moneur, C, and Williams, HJ: Cervical spine management in patients with rheumatoid arthritis. Phys Ther 68:509, 1988.
70. Morgan, D: Concepts in functional training and postural stabilization for the low-back injured. Topics in Acute Care and Trauma Rehabilitation 2:8, 1988.
71. Murphy, MJ: Effects of cervical traction on muscle activity. J Orthop Sports Phys Ther 13:220, 1991.
72. Nachemson, A: The lumbar spine: An orthopaedic challenge. Spine 1:59, 1976.
73. Nachemson, A: Recent advances in the treatment of low back pain. Int Orthop 9:1, 1985.
74. Ng, JK-F, et al: Relationship between muscle fiber composition and functional capacity of back muscles in healthy subjects and patients with back pain. J Orthop Sports Phys Ther 27(6):389, 1998.
74a. Nicholson, GG, and Gaston, J: Cervical headache. J Orthop Sports Phys Ther 31(4):184, 2001.
75. Nowakowski, P, Delitto A, and Erhard, RE: Lumbar spinal stenosis. Phys Ther 76:187, 1996.
76. Ogata, K, and Whiteside, LA: Nutritional pathways of the intervertebral disc. Spine 6(3):211, 1981.
77. Olson, KA, and Dustin, J: Diagnosis and treatment of cervical spine clinical instability. J Orthop Sports Phys Ther 31(4):194, 2001.
78. Panjabi, MM, Geol, VK, and Takata, K: Physiologic strains in the lumbar spinal ligaments. Spine 7:192, 1982.
79. Penjabi, MM, Krag, MH, and Chung, TQ: Effects of disc injury on mechanical behavior of the human spine. Spine 9:707, 1984.
80. Porter, RW, Hibbert, C, and Evans, C: The natural history of root entrapment syndrome. Spine 9:418, 1984.
81. Porterfield, JA: Dynamic stabilization of the trunk. J Orthop Sports Phys Ther 6:271, 1985.
82. Pellechia, GL: Lumbar traction: A review of the literature. J Orthop Sports Phys Ther 20:263, 1994.
83. Richardson, CA, et al: Techniques for active lumbar stabilisation for spinal protection: A pilot study. Aust J Physiother 38:105, 1992.
84. Richardson, CA, Toppenberg, R, and Jull, G: An initial evaluation of eight abdominal exercises for their ability to provide stabilisation for the lumbar spine. Aust J Physiother 36:6, 1990.
85. Riddle, DL: Classification and low back pain: A review of the literature and critical analysis of selected systems. Phys Ther 78(7):709, 1998.
86. Russell, EJ: Cervical disk disease. Radiology 177(2):313, 1990.
87. Saal, JS, Saal, JA, and Yurth, EF: Nonoperative management of herniated cervical intervertebral disc with radiculopathy. Spine 21(16):1877, 1996.
88. Saal, JA: Dynamic muscular stabilization in the nonoperative treatment of lumbar pain syndromes. Orthop Rev 19:691, 1990.
89. Saal, JS, et al: High levels of inflammatory phospholipase A2 activity in lumbar disc herniations. Spine 15:674, 1990.
90. Saal, JA, and Saal, JS: Nonoperative treatment of herniated lumbar intervertebral disc with radiculopathy; an outcome study. Spine 14:431, 1989.
91. Saal, JA, Saal, JS, and Herzog, RJ: The natural history of lumbar intervertebral disc extrusions treated nonoperatively. Spine 15:683, 1990.
92. Saunders, JD: Lumbar traction. J Orthop Sports Phys Ther 1:36, 1978.
93. Saunders, HD: Spinal traction. In Saunders, HD: Evaluation, Treatment and Prevention of Musculoskeletal Disorders. Viking, Minneapolis, 1985.
94. Smith, LK, Weiss, EL, and Lehmhuhl, LD: Brunnstrom's Clinical Kinesiology, ed 5. FA Davis, Philadelphia, 1996.
95. Spencer, JD, Hayes, KC, and Alexander, IJ: Knee joint effusion and quadriceps reflex inhibition in man. Arch Phys Med Rehabil 65:171, 1984.

96. Taylor, JR, and Twomey, LT: Age changes in lumbar zygapophyseal joints. Spine 11(7):739, 1986.
97. Turl, SE, and George, KP: Adverse neural tension: a factor in repetitive hamstring strain. J Orthop Sports Phys Ther 27:16, 1998.
98. Twomey, LT: A rationale for the treatment of back pain and joint pain by manual therapy. Phys Ther 72:885, 1992.
99. Twomey, LT: Commentary. Phys Ther 72:270, 1992.
100. Twomey, T, and Taylor, JR: Sagittal movements of the human lumbar vertebral column: A quantitative study of the role of the posterior vertebral elements. Arch Phys Med Rehabil 64:322, 1983.
101. Urban, L: The straight-leg-raising test: A review. J Orthop Sports Phys Ther 2:117, 1981.
102. Waddell, G: A new clinical model for the treatment of low back pain. Spine 12:632, 1987.
103. Wood, P: Applied anatomy and physiology of the vertebral column. Phys Ther 59:248, 1979.
104. Yasuma, T, et al: Histological development of intervertebral disc herniation. J Bone Joint Surg Am 68(7):1066, 1986.

Chapter 16

The Spine: Exercise Interventions for the Neck and Trunk

OBJECTIVES

After studying this chapter, the reader will be able to:

1 Demonstrate safe application of therapeutic exercise techniques to manage patients in the acute, subacute, and chronic stages of healing for rehabilitation of neck and trunk impairments.

2 Explain the purposes for each of the exercises and when they are indicated or contraindicated.

3 Describe the principles of kinesthetic training, flexibility/mobility exercises, core muscle activation, dynamic stabilization training, muscle strengthening, aerobic conditioning, stress relief/relaxation exercises, and functional training for interventions with spinal impairments and explain how they interrelate to each other.

4 Know how to modify basic exercises to safely increase the challenge to the patient.

5 Describe and demonstrate exercise progressions to meet the goals for each phase of rehabilitation.

6 Develop therapeutic exercise programs to meet the goals of intervention for various neck and trunk musculoskeletal impairments of the neck and trunk and related functional limitations.

In Chapter 15, basic anatomy, spinal mechanics, posture, pathomechanics, and common pathologies related to the spine were presented followed by principles of treatment. Interventions were outlined based on stages of healing, and special considerations were presented for conditions that are sensitive to specific postures or movements on spinal testing. Chapter 16 is a continuation of this material in which the techniques of intervention using therapeutic exercise for management of neck and trunk dysfunctions are described.

This chapter is divided into six main sections, each one addressing approaches to meeting one of the primary goals of therapeutic exercise for the neck and trunk as described in Chapter 15. The topics covered include kinesthetic training, flexibility/mobility, muscle performance (including core muscle activation, dynamic stabilization, training, and strengthening), aerobic conditioning, stress relief/relaxation, and functional training.

▶ Basic Principles

It is important to recognize that even though the material in this chapter is presented in separate sections, there is an overlap in use of the techniques described in each section, and there are fundamental techniques basic to all interventions.

Core stabilization. "Proximal stability for distal mobility" is a well-known phrase that is an underlying principle of intervention with therapeutic exercise. The primary functions of the muscles of the trunk are to provide the stabilizing force (core stability) against the effects of gravity so that upright posture can be maintained, and to provide a stable base so that the muscles of the extremities can execute their function efficiently and without undue stress to the spinal structures. Several studies have demonstrated altered or delayed neuromuscular recruitment patterns in the deep stabilizing muscles of the spine during active movement in individuals with low back pain.[9,12,21] and improved ability to recruit these muscles with specific training.[20] Therefore, one of the primary areas of emphasis in rehabilitation of spinal problems is recruiting the postural muscles for stabilization and training them to respond and adapt to various forces and demands imposed on the spine to improve their stabilizing function. Use of the core stabilizing muscles is fundamental when developing awareness of position and movement, and when performing stabilization exercises and basic functional activities (Fig.16–1). The activation of core-stabilizing musculature is then reinforced when developing an aerobic exercise program and when practicing functional activities throughout the rehabilitative process with the anticipation that it will become habitual in all daily activities and functional challenges.

Fundamental techniques. Patients come to treatment with different diagnoses, impairments, and functional limitations and are at different stages of tissue healing, yet all intervention needs to begin with several fundamental techniques because these lay the foundation for developing a stable spine. Interventions then progresses on a continuum at the level of the patient's abilities and willingness to learn. For example, a patient beginning treatment with chronic symptoms will still have to learn safe postures and movements, the effects various postures and movements have on symptoms, how to activate the core-stabilizing musculature. The patient then learns how to use the core stabilizers with fundamental exercises and body mechanics before progressing to exercises that can be tolerated at the chronic stage of healing and returning to desired functional activities. The fundamental techniques for the lumbar spine are summarized in Box 16–1 and are described in the respective sections of this chapter. Many of the same techniques may be used or modified for management of the cervical spine because core stabilization and spinal alignment are also fundamental for cervical rehabilitation.

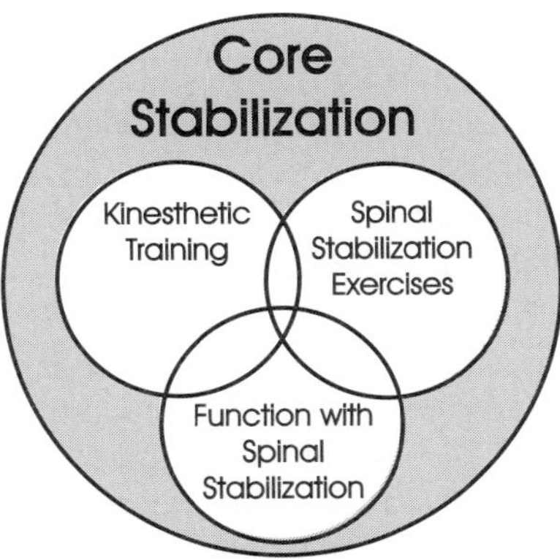

Figure 16–1 Kinesthetic training, stabilization exercises, and functional activities are a part of all spinal rehabilitation programs and are integrated over the background of core stabilization.

Box 16–1 Fundamental Techniques of Intervention for Spinal Rehabilitation

These fundamental techniques are adapted or modified based on patient abilities and responses.

Kinesthetic Training

- Awareness and control of safe spinal motion and neutral spinal position with respect to patient's spinal bias in supine, prone, sitting, and standing positions.
- Awareness of effects of ADLs and extremity motion on the spine (tie in with basic body mechanics).

Muscle Performance

- Core muscle activation: learn *drawing-in* maneuver with spinal control
- Use of active drawing-in maneuver to stabilize spine in neutral spinal position (position of bias) prior to simple extremity motions for basic *dynamic stabilization* exercises
  - Supine, alternating flexion/extension of the upper extremities to 90 degrees
  - Hook-lying, alternating single hip-knee flexion to 90 degrees
  - Hook-lying, alternating leg slides
  - Hook-lying, knee fall out
  - Quadruped or prone, alternating upper extremity flexion
  - Quadruped or prone, alternating leg slide with hip extension
  - Sitting or standing, alternating upper extremity flexion/extension
  - Standing, alternating hip-knee flexion to 90 degrees

Fundamental Body Mechanics, If Needed

Stable spine in position of bias:

- Log roll supine to prone, prone to supine
- Transition from supine to side-lying to sitting and return
- Transition from sit to stand and return
- Walking

In many cases, tissue healing, stages of rehabilitation, and functional expectations parallel each other (Table 16–1) but are not restricted by specific days or weeks.

Patient education. This is a component of every goal and intervention. It encompasses several ideas. First, the patient is a part of identifying the desired outcomes. The patient may need to be educated as to any limitations at each stage of healing so as not to become concerned that the acute symptoms will be forever disabling or so as not to "overdo" exercises and activities during the early subacute phase and cause exacerbation of symptoms. The patient may then need to be challenged to progress beyond perceived limitations in the later stages of recovery. To ensure that each individual develops control over

Table 16–1 Spinal Rehabilitation

The sequence of rehabilitation parallels the stages of healing and functional outcome expectations.

Stage of Tissue Healing:	Acute	Subacute	Chronic
Stage of Rehabilitation:	Early training protection phase	Basic training/controlled motion phase	Intermediate to advanced training/ return to function phase
Functional Expectations:	Control symptoms; ADL if possible	IADL and limited work	Return to work, recreation, sports

and learns how to manage the symptoms, he or she needs to be engaged in all activities at each stage of recovery and is not just a passive recipient of "treatment." The patient will need instruction in how to safely progress self-management beyond the time spent under professional supervision so that he or she can reach the maximum level of functional return. Finally, the patient will need instruction in prevention; this includes safe ways to exercise, safe body mechanics for return to high intensity activities, modification of work and activities to minimize stresses, and recognition of environmental situations that could jeopardize the mechanics of the spine.

Guidelines. In general, the following principles are used in all programs of intervention for spinal problems.

1. Initiate training by developing patient awareness of safe spinal positions and spinal movement in basic positions of supine, prone, side-lying, sitting, and standing as described in the *Kinesthetic Training* section (page 641). Once the patient is aware of spinal positions, have the patient practice basic body mechanics such as rolling, supine to sit, sit to stand, walking and reverse, as described in the *Functional Training* section (page 670), so that safe movement occurs during basic ADLs. Direct the patient's attention to the position of the spine and the feel of the muscles contracting while maintaining the functional position during the activities. Kinesthetic training is a part of all the exercises described in the remaining sections as well.
2. Mobilize and stretch tissues that restrict motion and prevent good alignment so that the muscles can learn stabilization with the spine in proper alignment. Techniques are described in the *Mobility/Flexibility* section (page 644).
3. Activation of the core-stabilizing muscles and stabilization exercises are the foundation for training and are described in detail in the *Muscle Performance* section (page 652). Place emphasis on awareness of muscle contraction and control of spinal position while progressing exercises that use the principles of dynamic stabilization, transitional stabilization, balance, strength, and muscular endurance training. Once the individual learns effective stabilization and management of symptoms, dynamic neck and trunk strengthening exercises are initiated. Most people are familiar with trunk curls, "crunches," and back lifts. The emphasis of therapeutic exercise is safe execution of the exercises combined with respect of the biomechanics of the spine.
4. Initiate aerobic conditioning exercises as soon as the patient tolerates repetitive activity without exacerbating symptoms. Place emphasis on using safe spinal postures while exercising. Aerobic activity increases the patient's feeling of well-being and improves cardiovascular and pulmonary fitness. Principles of aerobic conditioning are detailed in Chapter 4 and briefly summarized in the *Aerobic Conditioning* section of this chapter (page 667).
5. Teach stress relief and relaxation exercises; they serve several purposes. One is to help the individual learn how to relax when feeling stressed, thus preventing unwanted muscle tension and pain. The other is to learn to take frequent breaks from postural stress situations so that muscle tension and tissue fluid stasis do not develop into painful syndromes. These techniques are described in the *Stress Relief and Relaxation* section (page 669).
6. Training skills for good body mechanics, safe work habits, and effective recreational or sport activities. This requires integration of all the preceding sections and advancement of exercises at each level of recovery to meet the goals of the individual. These principles and techniques are described in the last section, *Functional Training* (page 670).

Table 16–2 summarizes these six types of interventions for each stage of rehabilitation. It is important that the reader also has knowledge of various spinal pathologies and special precautions and contraindications (see Chapter 15) so that each patient can safely achieve his or her maximum potential.

▶ Kinesthetic Training Procedures

Goal. The goal of kinesthetic training is to develop proprioceptive awareness of posture, positioning, and safe movement.

Early Training/Protection Phase

Establish a position of symptom relief. This is called the position of bias, the resting position, or neutral spine position. See Chapter 15 for a discussion on spinal bias as it relates to relief of symptoms and common pathologies.

Cervical Spine—Fundamental Techniques

Patient position and procedure: Begin supine, progress to sitting and other functional postures as tolerated.

Table 16–2 Intervention for Each Stage of Rehabilitation

Stages of Rehabilitation	**Early training/protection phase:** *Maximum to moderate protection of injured area, pathologically involved tissues, or painful region*	**Basic training/controlled motion phase:** *Moderate to minimum protection*	**Intermediate to advanced training/return to function phase:** *Minimum to no protection*
KINESTHETIC TRAINING *– proprioceptive awareness* *– posture/positioning*	• Pelvic tilt/cervical retraction: passive → active assist → active in comfortable positions.* • Awareness of what makes symptoms better vs. worse. • Learn neutral spine.	• Active spinal control in supine, prone, quadruped, sitting, standing. • Dynamic maintenance of pain-free position with activities.	• Habitual use of neutral spine in all functional activities.
FLEXIBILITY/MOBILITY *– stretching techniques*	• Movement to relieve fluid stasis. • Trunk stretching: only in pain-relieving positions. • Extremity stretching: stretch UE/LE if no stress to the spine. • Mobilization: grade I and II.	• Gentle spinal movement into painful range. • Stretch U/LE muscles in position of spinal comfort (bias). • Mobilization: progress to grade III.	• Movement into painful ranges to stretch and mobilize as indicated for range of spine and extremities.
MUSCLE PERFORMANCE *– core muscle control* *– dynamic stabilization* *– strengthening* *– muscle endurance*	• Activation of core musculature.* • Stabilization exercises (use of *passive* positioning with pillows, splints, corsets if necessary).*	• Stabilization exercises with *active* control of spine position. • Basic to intermediate. • Low intensity dynamic spinal exercises.	• Stabilization with transitional motions, and functional activities. • Perturbation training. • Progression to dynamic trunk strengthening.
AEROBIC CONDITIONING *– cardiovascular/pulmonary endurance*	• Only if tolerated with maximum protection in position of comfort.	• Low to moderate intensity with moderate to minimal protection. • Use activities that emphasize spinal bias.	• High intensity (target heart rate), multiple times per week.
STRESS RELIEF/RELAXATION EXERCISES	• Only if tolerated.	• Relaxation exercises if needed.	• Reinforcement of motions and postures to relieve stress.
FUNCTIONAL TRAINING *–body mechanics* *– home, community, work* *– recreation, sport* *– skill acquisition/transferring of training*	• Learn safe postures for recumbent, sitting, and standing.* • Learn to stabilize spine while rolling over, moving supine to sit, sit to stand.*	• Exercises to strengthen U/LE while stabilizing spine. • Stable spine body mechanics and environmental adaptations.	• High-intensity functional activities. • Endurance and strengthening activities that replicate return to desired activities. • Practice prevention.

Patient education occurs throughout.
Conscious activation of core trunk stabilizing musculature occurs in all exercises and activities.
*Fundamental techniques for all patients

- Passively move the head and neck with gentle nodding motions of the head into flexion and extension, side bending and/or rotation to find the most comfortable position for the patient. If necessary prop the head and neck with pillows.
- Describe the mechanics of what you are doing to the patient.
- Have the patient identify the change in symptoms as movement occurs in and out of the position of bias.
- Have the patient practice moving into and out of that position to develop control.
- If the patient cannot maintain this position while sitting and standing, wearing a cervical collar may be appropriate during the acute stage.

Lumbar Spine—Fundamental Techniques

Patient position and procedure: Begin supine or hook-lying, then sitting, standing, and quadruped.

- Teach the patient to move his or her pelvis into an anterior and posterior pelvic tilt (PT) through the range that is comfortable.
- Once the patient has moved the pelvis and spine through a safe ROM, instruct him or her to find the position of greatest symptom relief.
- If active movement and control is not possible, teach *passive positioning.* While *supine,* passively position the pelvis in posterior PT by placing the lower extremities in the hook-lying position, or anterior tilt by gently pulling on the extended legs or placing a small roll under the lumbar spine. *Sitting* encourages spinal flexion, if extension is more comfortable instruct the person to use a lumbar pillow for support. *Standing* usually causes spinal extension, if flexion is desired, instruct the person to place one foot up on a stool while standing.

Effects of Movement on the Spine

Once the functional spinal position is determined, it is important for the patient to feel and learn what motions make symptoms better or worse. Generally, movement of the extremities away from the trunk (shoulder flexion and abduction, hip extension and abduction) causes spinal extension; movement of the extremities toward the trunk (shoulder extension and adduction, hip flexion and adduction) cause spinal flexion.

- Have the patient find the neutral or functional spine position then move the arms and then legs to feel the effect on the spine. Control of the spinal position in emphasized; have the patient practice the arm and leg motions and attempt to maintain control of the spinal position.
- If the patient cannot maintain control or the symptoms are made worse, he or she will require passive support or passive positioning (as described under the fundamental techniques) when initiating the stabilization exercises.

Integration with Core Stabilization and Protected Function.

Once awareness of safe positions and movement is learned, teach the patient the fundamental stabilization techniques for developing neuromuscular control of the position (page 654 for cervical spine and page 657 for lumbar spine), and teach the fundamental functional activities of rolling, moving supine to sit, sit to stand, and ambulation (page 670).

Basic Training: Active Control of Posture

Initially, normal alignment may be prevented because of restricted mobility in muscle or connective tissue or malalignment of a vertebral segment, but developing patient awareness of balanced posture and its effects should begin as soon as possible in the treatment program in conjunction with the stretching and muscle-training maneuvers.

Use of Reinforcement Techniques During Treatment

Verbal reinforcement. As you interact with the patient, frequently interpret the sensations of muscle contraction and spinal positions that he or she should be feeling.

Visual reinforcement. Use mirrors so the patient can see how he or she looks, what it takes to assume correct alignment, and then how it feels when properly aligned. Verbally reinforce what the patient sees.

Tactile reinforcement. Help the patient position the head and trunk in correct alignment and touch the muscles that need to contract to move and hold the parts in place.

Teach Proper Control of Movement

Isolate each body segment and train the patient how to move that segment. If one region is out of alignment, it is likely that the entire spine is unbalanced to compensate. Therefore total posture correction should be emphasized. Direct the patient's attention to the feel of proper movement and muscle contraction and relaxation. Use reinforcement techniques as described previously. It may be useful to have the patient assume an extreme corrected posture, then ease away from the extreme toward midposition, and then hold the corrected posture.

Train Axial Extension (Cervical Retraction) to Decrease a Forward-Head Posture

Patient position and procedure: Sitting or standing, with arms relaxed at the side. Lightly touch above the lip under the nose and ask the patient to lift the head up and away (Fig. 16–2*A*). Verbally reinforce the correct movement of tucking the chin in and straightening the spine, and draw attention to the way it feels. Have the patient move to the extreme of the correct posture, then return to midline.

Train Scapular Retraction

Patient position and procedure: Sitting or standing. For tactile and proprioceptive cues, gently resist movement of the inferior angle of the scapulae and ask the patient to pinch them together (retraction). Suggest to the patient to imagine "holding a quarter between the shoulder blades." The patient should not extend the shoulders or elevate the scapulae (Fig. 16–2*B*).

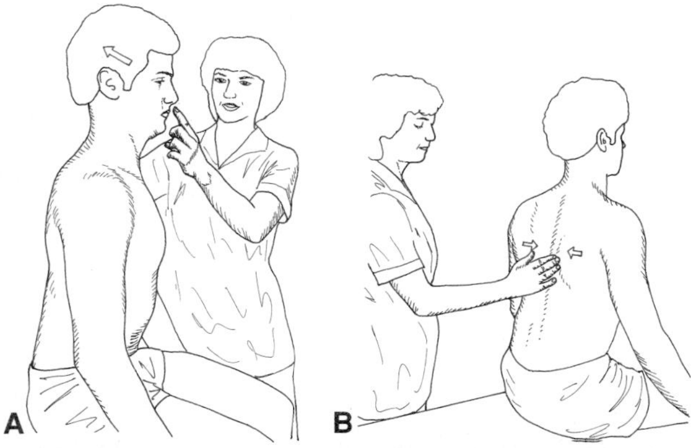

Figure 16–2 Training the patient to correct *(A)* forward-head posture and *(B)* protracted scapulae.

Train Control of the Pelvic Tilt and Balance of the Lumbar Spine

Patient position and procedure: Sitting, then standing with the back against a wall. After the patient has learned pelvic tilt exercises, instruct to practice control of movement of the pelvis and lumbar spine by moving from an extreme lordosis to an extreme flatback and then assuming a mild lordosis. Show that the hand should be able to easily slip between the back and the wall and that he or she can then feel the back with one side of the hand and the wall with the other side. If the patient has difficulty tilting the pelvis, suggest he or she imagines that the pelvis is a bushel basket with a rounded bottom and the waist is the rim of the basket. Have the patient then imagine and practice tipping the basket forward and backward.

Train Control of the Thorax and Lumbar Spine

Patient position and procedure: Standing. The position of the thorax affects the posture of the lumbar spine and pelvis, consequently the feel of thoracic movement is incorporated in posture training for the lumbar spine. As the patient assumes a mild lordotic posture, have him or her breathe in and lift the rib cage (extension). Guide to a balanced posture, not an extremely extended posture. Standing with the back against a wall (as in the pelvic tilt training above) encourages thoracic extension.

Teach Awareness of the Sensation of Assuming a Normal Posture and Developing Spinal Control

Patient position and procedure: Sitting. Instruct the patient to curl the entire spine by first flexing the neck, then the thorax, and then the lumbar spine. Give cues for unrolling by first touching the lumbar spine as the patient extends it, then the thoracic spine as he or she extends it and takes in a breath to elevate the rib cage. Then direct attention to adducting the scapulae while you gently resist the motion, and then lifting the head in axial extension while you give slight pressure against the upper lip. Verbally and visually reinforce the correct posture when it is obtained.

Demonstrate the Relationship of Faulty Posture to the Development of Pain

Have the patient assume the faulty posture and wait. When he or she begins to feel discomfort, point out the posture, and then instruct to correct it and notice the feeling of relief. Many patients will not accept such a simple relationship between stress and pain, so draw their attention to noticing, throughout the day and after a night's rest, what posture they are in when pain comes on and how they can control it with the techniques they have been taught.

Reinforce Learning

It is not possible for a person to always maintain good posture. Therefore, to reinforce proper performance, teach the patient to use cues throughout the day to check posture. For example, instruct the patient to check the posture every time he or she walks past a mirror, waits at a red traffic light while driving a car, sits down for a meal, enters a room, or begins talking with someone. Find out what daily routines the patient has that could be used for reinforcement or reminders; instruct the patient to practice and report the results. Provide positive feedback as the patient becomes actively involved in the relearning process.

Postural Support

If necessary, provide external support with a postural splint or tape to prevent the extreme posture of round shoulders and protracted scapulae. These help train correct muscle functioning by acting as a reminder for the patient to correct posture when he or she slouches. Also, by preventing the position of stretch from occurring, stretch weakness can be corrected. These devices should only be used on a temporary basis for training so that the patient does not become dependent on them.

Intermediate to Advanced Training: Habitual Posture Control

Integrate a progression of postural control into all stabilization exercises, aerobic conditioning, and functional training activities so it is not a separate exercise routine at this stage. Observe the patient as greater challenges to activities are performed, and if necessary, provide reminders to find the neutral spinal position and to initiate contraction of the stabilizing muscles prior to the activity. For example, when reaching overhead, the patient learns to contract the abdominal muscles to maintain a neutral spine position and not allow the spine to extend into a painful or unstable range. This is incorporated into body mechanics such as when going from picking up and lifting to placing an object on a high shelf, or into sport activities when reaching up to block or throw a ball.

▶ Mobility/Flexibility Procedures

Goal. The goal of mobility/flexibility procedures is to increase ROM of specific structures in the neck and trunk.

Stretching is contraindicated in the region of inflamed tissue. If there are postures that relieve symptoms but are difficult to assume because of tissue restriction or fluid stasis, then stretching or repetitive movement into the restricted range may be appropriate. For example, lumbar extension has been shown to relieve symptoms of a disk lesion (see Chapter 15), yet a patient may not be able to get into an extended posture because of a flexed postural dysfunction or swollen tissue. Prone propping and press-ups may stretch the tight tissue as well as compress and massage swollen disk material or fluid stasis to reduce symptoms (see Fig. 15–9 and 16–11).

Another situation in which acute symptoms may be relieved with stretching is with acute nerve root irritation from bony spurs or lipping in an arthritic spine. Reducing pressure on the nerve roots with a stretch traction force, which widens the intervertebral foramina or with procedures that realign the spine in its optimal spinal position may relieve the symptoms.[1]

Decreased mobility in structures in the upper and lower extremities that restrict normal postural alignment may be stretched if the techniques do not stress the area of inflammation.

Stretching is done on a continuum. Critical judgment is used to determine the intensity and duration of stretch based on proximity to the healing tissue and the integrity and tolerance of the tissue. Principles of stretching are described in Chapter 5. Joint mobilization and manipulation techniques may be used to stretch hypomobile facet joint capsules or realign subluxed facets. Specific mobilization/manipulation techniques for the spine are beyond the scope of this text.

The patient is also taught general stress-relieving movements to reduce fluid stasis after being in prolonged postures. These are described in the

Stress Relief/Relaxation section later in this chapter (page 669).

Cervical and Upper Thoracic Region—Stretching Techniques

Increase Thoracic Extension

Self-Stretching

- *Patient position and procedure:* Hook-lying, with the hands behind the head and the elbows resting on the mat. To increase the stretch, place a pad or rolled towel lengthwise under the thoracic spine between the scapulae. Segmental breathing (Chapter 19) can also be used by having the patient start with the elbows together in front of the face, then inhaling as the elbows are brought down to the mat; holding; then exhaling as the elbows are brought together again.
- *Patient position and procedure:* Hook-lying, with both arms elevated overhead. The patient attempts to keep the back flat on the mat while inhaling and expanding the anterior thorax.
- *Patient position and procedure:* Patient supine, with a foam roll placed longitudinally down the length of the spine. If the patient cannot balance on the roll or experiences tenderness along the spinous processes from pressure, tape two foam rolls together. The patient elevates both arms overhead in a "touch down" position and allows gravity to apply the stretch force (Fig. 16–3*A*). The patient then abducts and laterally rotates both shoulders so that the hands are facing the ceiling (Fig. 16–3*B*). This position also stretches the pectoralis major and subscapularis muscles. Breathing exercises can be added to mobilize the ribs.
- *Patient position and procedure:* Sitting on a firm, straight-back chair with the hands behind the head or held abducted and externally rotated 90 degrees. The patient then brings the elbows out to the side as the scapulae are adducted and the thoracic spine is extended (head held neutral, not flexed). To combine with breathing, have the patient inhale as he or she takes the elbows out to the side, and exhale as he or she brings the elbows in front of the face (Fig. 16–4).

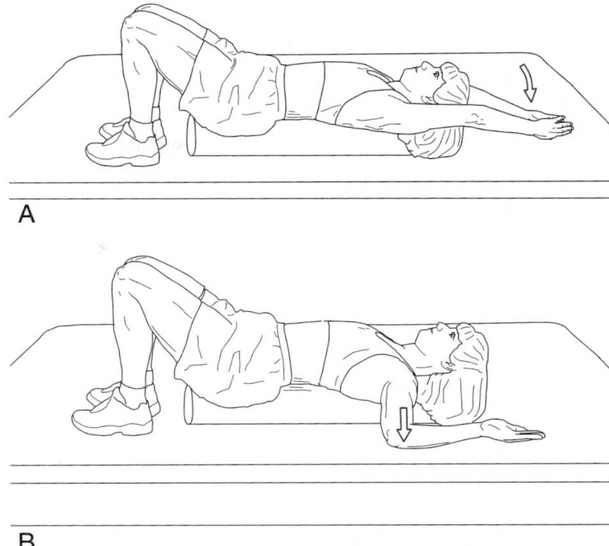

Figure 16–3 Foam roll stretch to increase flexibility of anterior thorax; *(A)* in the "touchdown" position the shoulder extensors are also stretched; *(B)* with the shoulders abducted and laterally rotated the pectoralis major and other internal rotators are also stretched.

Increase Axial Extension (Cervical Retraction)—Scalene Muscle Stretch

Note: Because the scalene muscles are attached to the transverse processes of the upper cervical spine and the upper two ribs, they either flex the cervical spine or elevate the upper ribs when they contract bilaterally. Unilaterally,

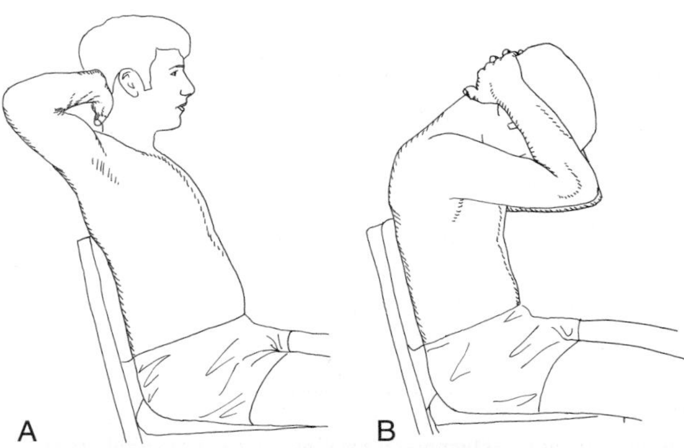

Figure 16–4 *(A)* A stretch is applied to the pectoralis muscles and anterior thorax during inspiration, and *(B)* the patient brings the elbows together to facilitate expiration.

the scalenes side-bend the cervical spine to the same side and rotate it to the opposite side.

Manual Stretch

Patient position and procedure: Sitting. The patient first performs axial extension (tucks the chin and straightens the neck), and then side-bends the neck opposite and rotates it toward the tight muscles. Stand behind the patient and stabilize the upper ribs with one hand over the top of the rib cage on the side of tightness, and stabilize the head with the other hand around the side of the patient's head and face, holding the head against your trunk (Fig. 16–5). The patient inhales and exhales; then hold the ribs down as the patient inhales again. Repeat. This is a gentle, hold-relax stretching maneuver.

Self-Stretching

Patient position and procedure: Standing next to a table and holding onto its underside. The patient positions the head in axial extension, side-bend opposite, and rotation to the same side as the muscle being stretched. Have the patient stabilize the head by placing the opposite hand on the back of the occipital region. To stretch, he or she leans away from the table, inhales, exhales, and holds the stretch position.

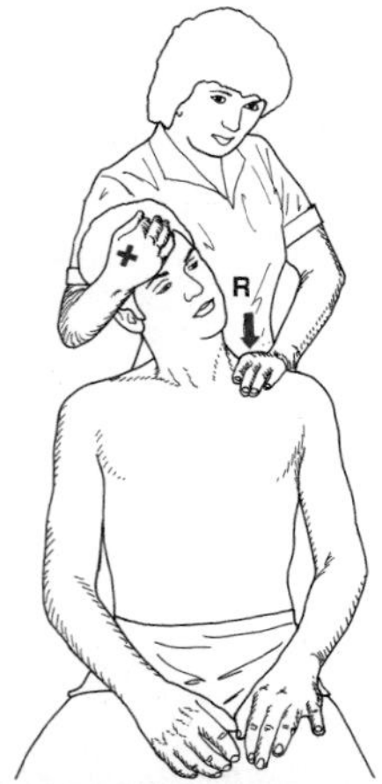

Figure 16–5 Unilateral active stretching of the scalenus muscles. The patient first performs axial extension, then side-bends the neck opposite, and rotates it toward the tight muscles. The therapist stabilizes the head and upper thorax as the patient breathes in, contracting the muscle against the resistance. As the patient relaxes, the rib cage lowers and stretches the muscle.

Increase Axial Extension (Upper Cervical Flexion)—Short Suboccipital Muscle Stretch

Manual Stretch

- *Patient position and procedure:* Sitting. Identify the spinous process of the second cervical vertebra, and stabilize it with your thumb or with the second metacarpophalangeal joint (and the thumb and index finger around the transverse processes). Have the patient slowly nod, doing just a tipping motion of the head on the upper spine (Fig. 16–6). Guide the movement by placing the other hand across the patient's forehead.
- *Patient position and procedure:* Supine. Sit on a stool at the head of the treatment table with your forearms resting on the table. One hand stabilizes the C-2 vertebra by grasping the transverse processes between the proximal portions of the thumb and index finger, and the other hand supports the occiput. Nod the patient's head with the hand under the occiput to take up the slack of the suboccipital muscles, then ask the patient to roll the eyes upward. This causes a gentle isometric contraction of the suboccipital muscles. After holding 6 seconds, ask the patient to roll the eyes downward. As the suboccipital muscles relax, take up the slack by passively nodding the head through any new range. Only motion between the occiput and C-2 should occur. The contraction is gentle in order to not cause overflow into the multisegmental erector spinae and upper trapezius muscles.

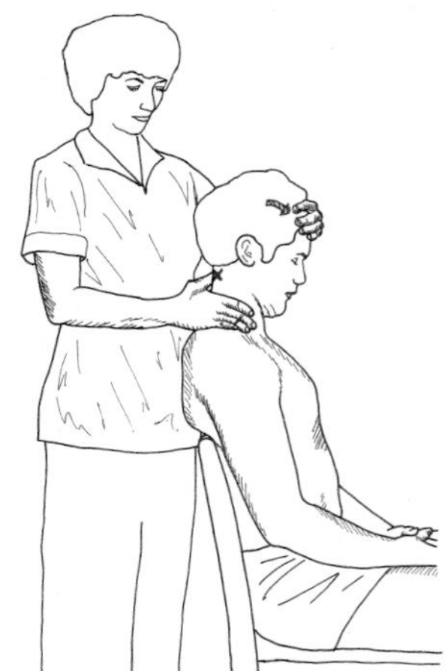

Figure 16–6 Stretching the short suboccipital muscles. The therapist stabilizes the second cervical vertebra as the patient slowly nods the head.

Self-Stretching

Patient position and procedure: Supine or sitting. Instruct the patient to nod the head, bringing the chin toward the larynx until a stretch is felt in the suboccipital area. Putting light pressure under the occipital region with the palm of your hand while tipping the head forward can reinforce the motion.

Increase Scapular and Humeral Muscle Flexibility

Shoulder girdle posture is directly related to cervical and thoracic posture. Techniques to increase flexibility in the shoulder and scapular muscles are described in Chapter 9. Of primary importance are the pectoralis major (see Figs. 9–18 to 9–20), pectoralis minor (see Fig. 9–21), levator scapulae (see Figs. 9–22 and 9–23), and shoulder internal rotator muscles (see Fig. 9–14*A* and *B*).

Manual Traction—Cervical Spine

Traction techniques can be used for the purposes of stretching the posterior ligaments, muscles, and the facet joint capsules and widening the intervertebral foramina.[29] The value of manual traction is that the angle of pull, head position, and placement of the force (via specific hand placements) can be controlled by the therapist, thus the force can be specifically applied with minimum stress to regions that should not be stretched.

Patient position: Supine on a treatment table. The patient should be as relaxed as possible.

Therapist position and hand placement: Standing at the head of the treatment table, supporting the weight of the patient's head in the hands. Hand placement depends on comfort. Suggestions include:

- Place the fingers of both hands under the occiput (Fig. 16–7*A*).
- Place one hand over the forehead and the other hand under the occiput (Fig. 16–7*B*).
- Place the index fingers around the spinous process above the vertebral level to be moved. This hand placement provides a specific traction only to the vertebral segments below the level at which the fingers are placed. A belt around the therapist's hips can be used to reinforce the fingers and increase the ease of applying the traction force (Fig. 16–7*C*).

Procedure: Vary the patient's head position in flexion, extension, side bending, and side bending with rotation until the tissue to be stretched is taut, and then apply a traction force by assuming a stable stance and leaning backward in a controlled manner. If a belt is used, the force is transmitted through the belt. The force is usually applied intermittently with a smooth and gradual building and releasing of the traction force. The intensity and duration are usually limited by the therapist's strength and endurance.

Positional Traction—Cervical Spine

The value of using positional traction is that the primary traction force can be isolated to a specific facet. This may be beneficial when selective stretching is necessary as when the segment above or on the contralateral side is hypermobile and should not be stretched.

Patient position: Supine, lying on the treatment table.

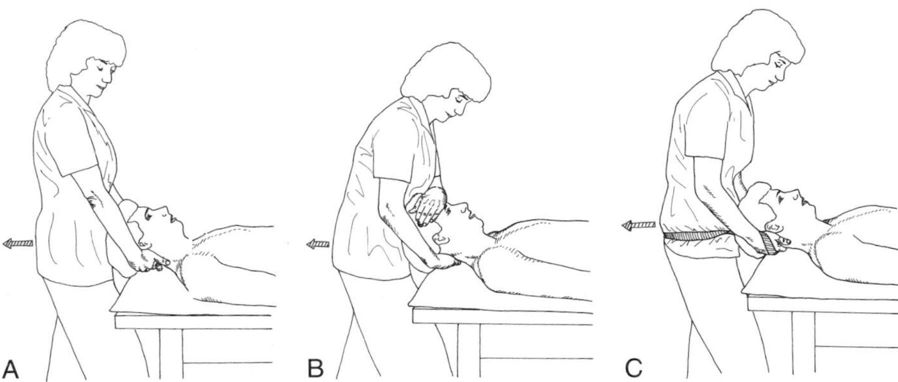

Figure 16–7 Manual cervical traction *(A)* with the fingers of both hands under the occiput, *(B)* with one hand over the frontal region and the other hand under the occiput, and *(C)* using a belt to reinforce the hands for the traction force.

Therapist position: Standing at the head of the treatment table, supporting the patient's head in the hands. Determine the segment to receive the majority of the traction force, and palpate the spinous process at that level.

Procedure: Flex the head until motion of the spinous process just begins at the determined level. Support the head with folded towels at that level of flexion. Then side-bend the head away from the side to be distracted until movement of the spinous process is felt at the desired level. Finally, rotate the head a few degrees toward the side to be distracted. Adjust the towel support to maintain this position for a low-intensity, sustained traction stretch to that facet joint and surrounding soft tissue.[22]

Self-Traction—Cervical Spine

Patient position and procedure: Sitting or lying down. Have the patient place his or her hands behind the neck with the fingers interlocking; the ulnar border of the fingers and hands are under the occiput and mastoid processes. The patient then gives a lifting motion to the head. The head may be placed in flexion, extension, side bending, or rotation for more isolated effects. He or she may apply the traction intermittently or in a sustained manner.

Positional traction can also be used for self-traction. The patient learns to assume the position determined by the therapist as described in the previous procedure.

Other Techniques for Increasing Mobility

Inhibition techniques. Inhibition techniques, as described in Chapter 5, can be used on any muscle group or with any motion. Suggested position for the patient is supine with the therapist standing at the head end of the treatment table supporting the patient's head in the hands. The intensity of resistance should be very gentle and applied smoothly.

Mechanical traction. Various forms of mechanical traction can be used in the clinic and at home. The position, dosage, and duration of traction is determined by the therapist. Instruction for use of the equipment is not described in this text.

Joint mobilization/manipulation. Joint mobilization/manipulation techniques can be used by those trained in the principles and maneuvers. Specific spinal techniques are not described in this text.

Mid- and Lower Thoracic and Lumbar Regions—Stretching Techniques

Increase Lumbar Flexion

Precaution: If flexion of the spine causes a change in sensation or causes pain to radiate down an extremity, reassess the patient's condition to determine if flexion is contraindicated.

Assisted Stretching

Patient position and procedure: Cross-sitting. Have the patient place the hands behind the neck, adduct the scapulae, and extend the thoracic spine. This locks the thoracic vertebrae. Have the patient then lean the thorax forward onto the pelvis, flexing only at the lumbar spine. Stabilize the pelvis by pulling back on the anterior-superior iliac spines (Fig. 16–8).

Self-Stretching

- *Patient position and procedure:* Hook-lying. Have the patient first bring one knee and then the other toward the chest, clasp the hands around the thighs, and pull them to the chest, elevating the sacrum off the mat (Fig. 16–9). The patient should not grasp around the tibia; it places stress on the knee joints as the stretch force is applied.
- *Patient position and procedure:* On hands and knees. Have the patient perform a posterior pelvic tilt without rounding the thorax (concentrate on flexing the lumbar spine, not the thoracic spine),

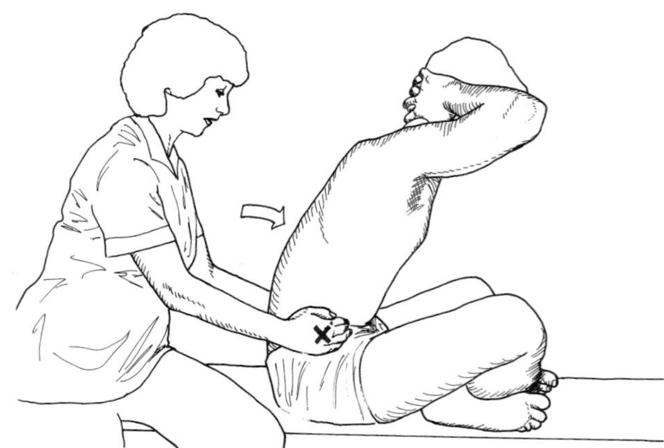

Figure 16–8 Stretching the lumbar spine with the patient stabilizing the thorax in extension and the therapist stabilizing the pelvis.

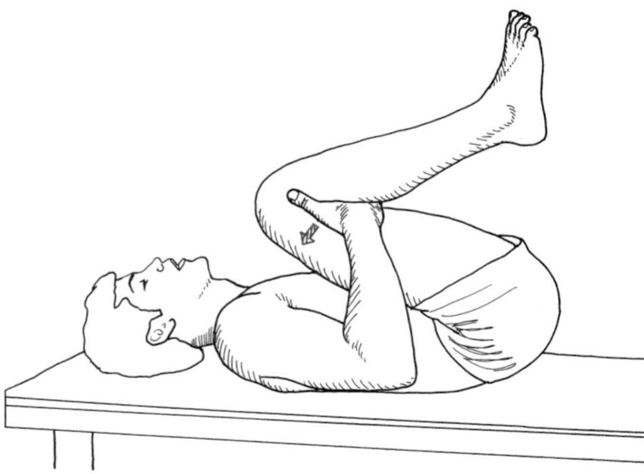

Figure 16–9 Self-stretching the lumbar erector spinae muscles and tissues posterior to the spine. The patient grasps around the thighs to avoid compression of the knee joints.

hold the position, then relax (Fig. 16–10*A*). Repeat; this time bring the hips back to the feet, hold, and then return to the hands and knees position (Fig. 16–10*B*). This also stretches the gluteus maximus, quadriceps femoris, and shoulder extensor muscles.

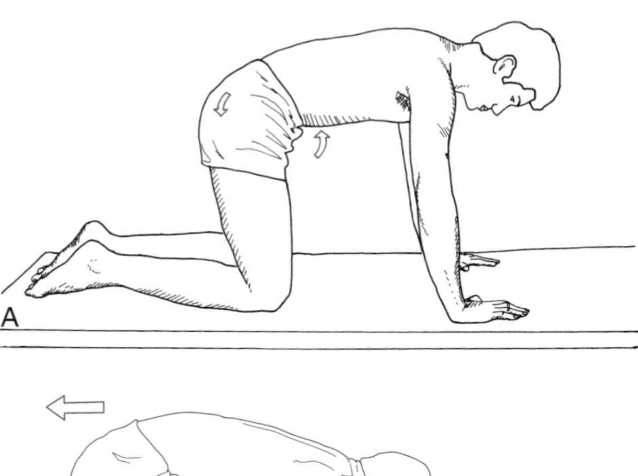

Figure 16–10 Stretching of the lumbar spine. *(A)* The patient performs a posterior pelvic tilt without rounding the thorax. *(B)* The patient moves the buttocks back over the feet for a greater stretch.

- Active trunk flexion exercises (curl-ups) use the principle of reciprocal inhibition and can be used to help stretch lumbar extensor muscles.

Increase Lumbar Extension

Precaution: Do not perform if extension causes a change in sensation or causes pain to radiate down an extremity (see Chapter 15).

Self-Stretching

- *Patient position and procedure:* Prone, with hands placed under the shoulders. Have the patient extend the elbows and lift the thorax up off the mat but keep the pelvis down on the mat. This is a *prone press-up* (Fig. 16–11*A*). To increase the stretch force, the pelvis can be strapped to the treatment table. This exercise also stretches the hip flexor muscles and soft tissue anterior to the hip.
- *Patient position and procedure:* Standing, with the hands placed in the low-back area. Instruct the patient to lean backward (Fig. 16–11*B*).
- *Patient position and procedure:* On hands and knees. Instruct the patient to allow the spine to sag, creating lumbar extension. This, alternated with posterior pelvic tilts, can also be used to teach the patient how to control pelvic motion.
- Any dynamic trunk extension exercises as described in the exercise section may be used as long as the exertion does not increase symptoms.

Increase Lateral Flexibility in the Spine

Stretching techniques to increase lateral flexibility are used for intervention when there is asymmetric flexibility in side bending as well as in the management of scoliosis. It is important to note that stretching has not been shown to correct or halt progression of a structural scoliosis. If these exercises are used for patients with structural scoliosis, they may be beneficial in gaining some flexibility prior to surgical fusion of the spine for correction of a scoliotic deformity. They may also be used to regain flexibility in the frontal plane when muscle or fascial tightness is present with postural dysfunctions. All of the following exercises are designed to stretch hypomobile structures on the concave side of the lateral curvature.

When stretching the trunk, it is necessary to stabilize the spine either above or below the curve. If the patient has a double curve, one curve must be stabilized while the other is stretched.

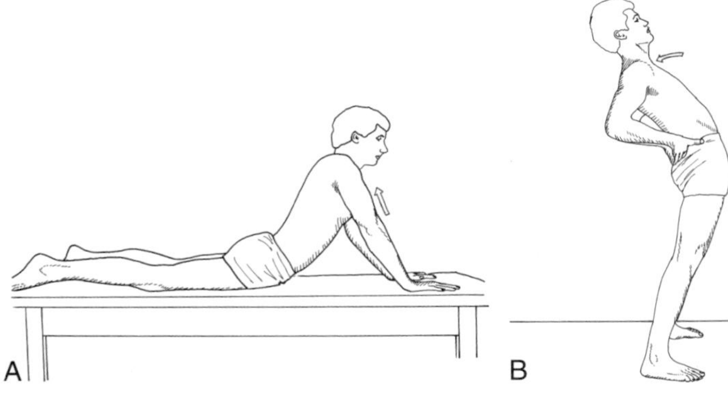

Figure 16–11 Self-stretching of the soft tissues anterior to the lumbar spine and hip joints with the patient *(A)* prone (using a press-up) and *(B)* standing.

- *Patient position and procedures:* Prone. Stabilize the patient at the iliac crest (manually or with a belt) on the side of the concavity. Have the patient reach toward the knee with the arm on the convex side of the curve while stretching the opposite arm up and overhead (Fig. 16–12). Instruct the patient to breathe in and expand the rib cage on the side being stretched.

  To stretch a lumbar curve, have the patient stabilize the upper trunk (thoracic curve) by holding onto the edge of the mat table with the arms. (No shoulder motion should occur.) Lift the hips and legs and laterally bend the trunk away from the concavity (Fig. 16–13).
- *Patient position and procedure:* Heel-sitting. Have the patient lean forward so the abdomen rests on the anterior thighs (Fig. 16–14*A*), the arms are stretched overhead bilaterally, and the hands are flat on the floor. Then have the patient laterally bend the trunk away from the concavity by walking the hands to the convex side of the curve. Hold the position for a sustained stretch (Fig. 16–14*B*).
- *Patient position and procedure:* Side-lying on the convex side of the curve. Place a rolled towel at the apex of the curve, and have the patient reach overhead with the top arm. Stabilize the patient at the iliac crest. Do not allow the patient to roll forward or backward during the stretch. Hold this position for a sustained period of time (Fig. 16–15).
- *Patient position and procedure:* Side-lying over the edge of a mat table with a rolled towel at the apex of the curve and the top arm stretched overhead. Stabilize the iliac crest. Hold this head-down position as long as possible (Fig. 16–16).

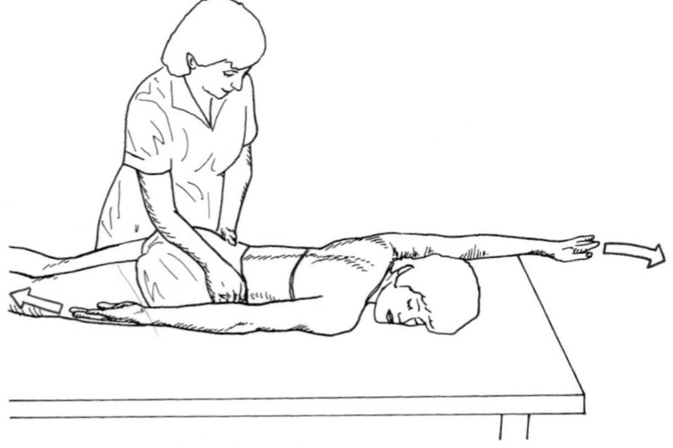

Figure 16–12 Stretching hypomobile structures on the concave side of the thoracic curve. The patient has a right thoracic left lumbar curve. The therapist stabilizes the pelvis and lumbar spine while the patient actively stretches the thoracic curve.

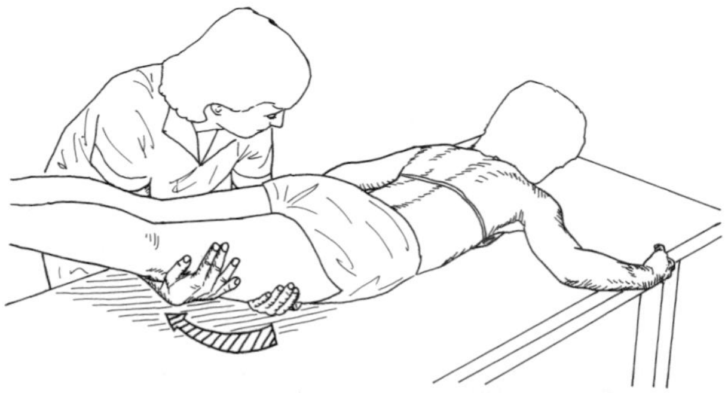

Figure 16–13 Stretching hypomobile structures on the concave side of a left lumbar curve. The patient stabilizes the upper trunk and thoracic curve as the therapist passively stretches the lumbar curve.

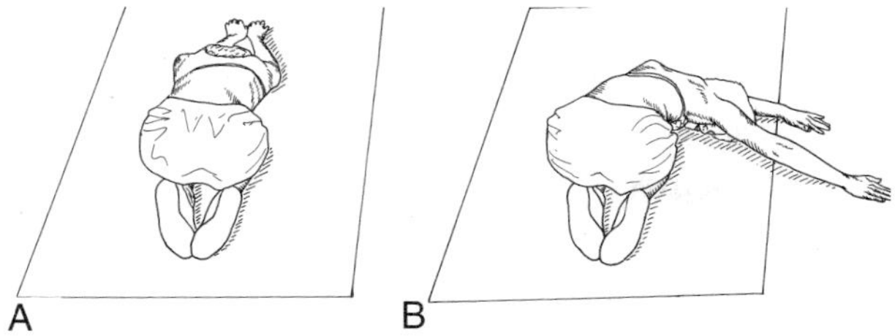

Figure 16–14 *(A)* Heel-sitting to stabilize the lumbar spine. *(B)* Hypomobile structures on the concave side of a right thoracic curve are stretched by having the patient reach the arms overhead and then walk the hands toward the convex side.

Increase Hip Muscle Flexibility

Hip muscles have a direct effect on spinal posture and function because of their attachment on the pelvis. It is important that they have adequate flexibility for proper pelvic and spinal alignment. See Chapter 12 for specific stretching techniques of hip musculature.

Manual Traction—Lumbar Spine

Manual traction in the lumbar region is not as easily applied as in the cervical region. At least one-half of the body weight of the patient must be moved, and the coefficient of friction of the part to be moved also must be overcome to cause vertebral distraction and stretching. It is helpful to place the patient on a split-traction table for ease in moving and stretching the spine.

Patient position: Supine or prone. Stabilize the thorax with a harness that is secured to the head end

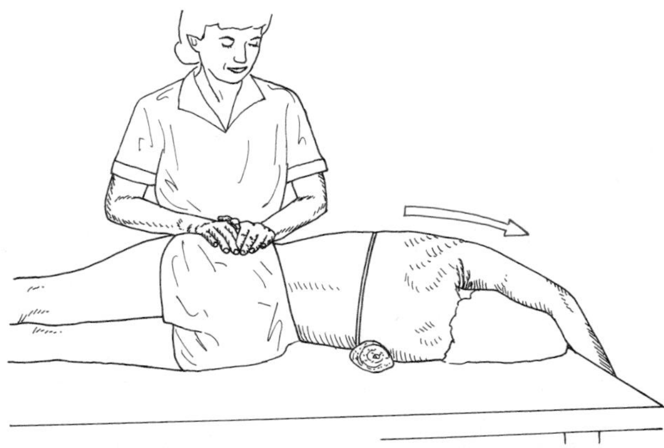

Figure 16–15 Stretching tight structures on the concave side of a right thoracic curve. The patient is positioned side-lying with a rolled towel at the apex of the convexity; the lumbar spine is stabilized by the therapist.

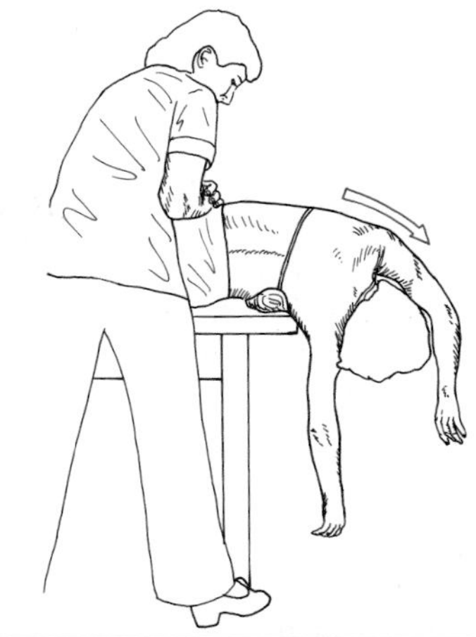

Figure 16–16 Side-lying over the edge of a mat table to stretch hypomobile structures of a right thoracic scoliosis. The therapist stabilizes the pelvis.

of the table, or have an assistant stabilize the patient by standing at the head of the table and holding the patient's arms. Position the patient so that there is maximal stretch on the hypomobile tissue.

- To stretch into extension, extend the hips.
- To stretch into flexion, flex the hips.
- To stretch into side bending, move the lower extremities to one side.

Therapist position and procedures: Position yourself so effective body mechanics and body weight can be used.

- If the lower extremities are extended to emphasize spinal extension, exert the pull at the ankles.
- If the lower extremities are flexed to emphasize spinal flexion, drape the legs over your shoulders, and exert the stretch force with your arms wrapped across the patient's thighs. Alternatively, place a pelvic belt with straps around the patient and manually pull on the straps.

Positional Traction—Lumbar Spine

The value of positional traction is that the primary traction force can be directed to the side on which symptoms occur or can be isolated to a specific facet and is, therefore, beneficial for selective stretching.[22,29]

Patient position: Side-lying, with the side to be stretched uppermost. A rolled blanket is placed under the spine at the level where the traction force is desired; this causes side bending away from the side to be treated and, therefore, an upward gliding of the facets (Fig. 16–17*A*).

Therapist position: Standing, at the side of the treatment table facing the patient. Determine the segment to receive the majority of the traction force, and palpate the spinous processes at that level and the level above.

Procedure:[22] The patient relaxes in the side-bent position. Rotation is added to isolate a distraction force to the desired level. Rotate the upper trunk by gently pulling on the arm on which the patient is lying, while simultaneously palpating the spinous processes with your other hand to determine when rotation has arrived at the level just above the joint to be distracted. Then flex the patient's uppermost thigh, again palpating the spinous processes until flexion of the lower portion of the spine occurs at the desired level. The segment at which these two opposing forces meet now has a maximal positional distraction force (Fig. 16–17*B*).

Other Techniques for Increasing Mobility in the Thoracic and Lumbar Spine

Mechanical traction. Mechanical traction units can provide considerable stretch force to the tissues of the thoracic and lumbar spine. Positioning considerations are as described for manual traction. Instructions for use of the equipment is not part of this text.

Joint mobilization/manipulation. These techniques may be used by those trained in their principles and maneuvers. Techniques for the spine are not described in this text.

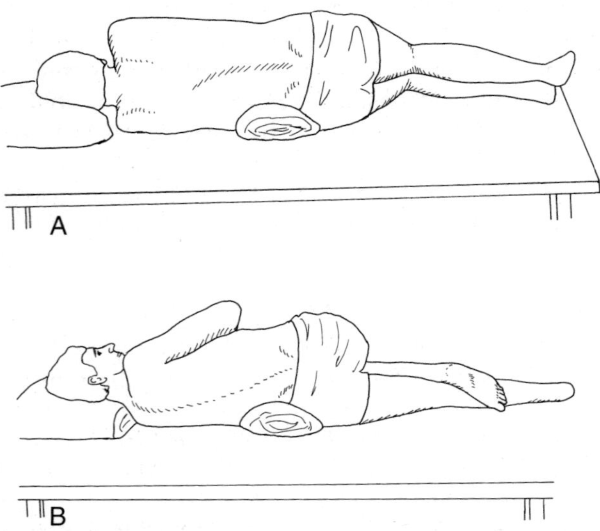

Figure 16–17 Positional traction for the lumbar spine. *(A)* Side bending over a 6- to 8-inch roll causes a longitudinal traction to the segments on the upward side. *(B)* Side bending with rotation adds a distraction force to the facets on the upward side.

▶ Muscle Performance: Stabilization Training, Strengthening, Endurance

Goals. (1) Activate and develop neuromuscular control of spinal stabilization muscles to support the spine during dynamic activities, (2) develop strength and endurance in the postural and stabilizing muscles of the axial skeleton for functional activities, and (3) develop control of balance in stable and unstable situations.

Stabilization training follows the basic principles of motor learning first by developing awareness of muscle contractions and spinal position, then developing control in simple patterns and exercises and progressing to complex, and finally demonstrating automatic maintenance of spinal stability and control in a progression of simple functional activities to complex and unplanned situations.[30] Many of the exercises can be used to accomplish more than one purpose, and there is definite overlap with kinesthetic training and functional training. The choice and progression of exercises described in each of the sections relies on clinical judgment of patient response and attainment of goals not on a strict, time-based protocol or days from injury. The ability of the patient to control the spine in a neutral or nonstressful position is paramount in all the exercises.

There is considerably more research on muscle function and its stabilization action in the lumbar spine. The cervical spine requires more mobility to position the head, yet relies on the thoracic and lumbar spinal regions to provide a base for stability and postural control. Even though there are unique anatomic considerations in the cervical spine, there is overlap between stabilization training for cervical and lumbar problems.

Specific Guidelines

It is important to understand and use the principles and progression of stabilization training for effective instruction.[4,18,26–28,32]

1. Kinesthetic training for awareness of safe motion and positions must precede stabilization training. The functional range and functional position in which symptoms are minimal or absent is used for stabilization exercises.[18] When the condition is not acute, most people find the midrange to be their functional position. It is important to recognize that this position or range is not static, nor is it the same for every person. In addition it may change as the tissues heal and nociceptive stimuli decrease and as flexibility improves.[18]
2. Activation of the deep (core) stabilizing muscles, specifically the transversus abdominis (TrA), internal oblique (IO), and multifidus, is often delayed or absent in patients with back pain.[9,12,21] Learning conscious activation of the stabilizing muscles is the first step in developing habitual activation for spinal control. Three methods are described in the literature for activating the abdominal muscles: the drawing-in maneuver, abdominal bracing, and the posterior pelvic tilt (see Fig. 16–24). According to one study[10] that compared muscle action during these three maneuvers, the drawing-in maneuver is more effective in eliciting a contraction in the TrA and IO than the posterior pelvic tilt or abdominal bracing maneuvers, and it also activates the multifidus muscle. Therefore, the drawing-in maneuver is recommended for teaching the patient how to activate these core stabilizers.

   Once the individual learns correct activation of the core stabilizers with the drawing-in maneuver, this maneuver is used prior to all exercises and activities to develop the early activation and stabilizing function and eventually automatic feedforward stabilization from the muscles.[11] A recent study involving 42 subjects demonstrated that it is possible to consciously and automatically alter abdominal muscle activation with specific exercises.[20]
3. Extremity motions are performed within the tolerance of the trunk or neck muscles to control the neutral or functional position. This is called **dynamic stabilization** because the stabilizing forces in the spinal area must respond to the changing forces coming from the extremities. Exercises that require stabilization against transverse plane rotational forces on the pelvis more consistently activate the oblique abdominal and deep spinal stabilizers than sagittal plane resistive forces.[25]
4. Once control of the position is established and the patient can activate the stabilizing muscles, resistance is applied to the extremities, and repetitions of extremity motions are increased to increase *strength* and *endurance.* The intent is to challenge the trunk muscles to stabilize against these increased forces yet stay within their tolerance and ability to control the spinal position. Repetitions also help develop *habit,* therefore it is important to use careful instructions and provide feedback. Fatigue is determined by the inability of the trunk or neck muscles to stabilize the spine in its functional position. For example:
   - Begin at a resistance force that the patient can repeat for 30 seconds to 1 minute; progress the repetitions to 3 minutes.
   - Progress by adding resistance to or increasing the lever arm of the extremities; initially reduce the time, and again progress to doing the new activity to 3 minutes.
   - Another way to develop endurance in the trunk muscles is to begin exercising at the most difficult level for that patient, then shift to simpler levels of resistance as fatigue begins in order to keep moving. It is important that the patient does not lose control of the functional position.
5. Alternating isometric contractions between antagonists and rhythmic stabilization also enhance stabilizing contractions. When performed while sitting and standing, the alternating contractions and co-contractions also develop control of balance.
6. **Transitional stabilization** develops as the patient moves from one position to another in conjunction with extremity motions. This requires graded contractions and adjustments between the trunk flexors and extensors and requires greater awareness and concentration.[4,18] For example, any motion of the arms or legs away from the trunk tends to cause the spine to extend. The abdominals (trunk flexors) must contract to maintain control of the functional spinal position. This would occur when lifting a load from the floor to overhead. Then as the arms of legs move anteriorly toward the center of gravity, the spine tends to flex; this requires the extensors to contract to maintain the functional position as would occur when lowering a weight to the floor. Greater concentration on maintaining the functional spinal position is necessary when doing more advanced functional activities.

7. Perturbation training, exercising against destabilizing forces or on unstable surfaces, develops neuromuscular responses to improve balance.

Cervical and Upper Thoracic Regions

Fundamental Training of Stabilization Muscles

These are fundamental techniques when initiating stabilization in the cervical spine.

Patient position and procedure: Begin supine with the head and neck in a neutral spine (most comfortable) position, progress to sitting with the back supported on a firm chair. If necessary for the patient with acute symptoms or significant weakness, provide support with a pillow or cervical collar. Use light tactile stimulation to the postural muscles with verbal reinforcement when performed correctly.

- Instruct the patient to flex the shoulders to 90 degrees and return them to the sides. This is repeated for 12 to15 repetitions or for 30 seconds as long as symptoms do not worsen.
- Have the patient abduct the shoulder to 90 degrees, and then externally rotate the shoulder with the arms at the sides, each for 12 to 15 repetitions or 30 seconds.

Stabilization Exercise Progressions for the Cervical Region

Patient positions and procedures: Sitting with back support or standing with the back to a wall and with the cervical spine in its functional position. Progress to standing without support. Begin without weights, and, progress to light weights held in the hands.

- Instruct the patient to reach overhead in flexion and in abduction as far as comfortable.
- Teach diagonal patterns. The second diagonal flexion pattern emphasizes scapular retraction and shoulder lateral rotation, which are important for good posture.
- Progress to reaching forward, outward, and upward using various functional reaching patterns.

Integrate Postural Exercises with Kinesthetic Posture Training

Good postural alignment of the neck begins with the pelvis and lumbar spine and moves on up to scapular and thoracic posture. The thorax must be lifted up from the pelvis and scapula retracted in a comfortable position for the cervical spine to assume an efficient position of axial extension (cervical retraction). Therefore, begin with lumbopelvic control if necessary, and develop thoracic extension, and scapular retraction. When in good spinal alignment, have the patient protract and retract the shoulder girdle by rolling the shoulders forward, then up and back, and pinching the scapulae together. The patient finishes by releasing the extreme position and relaxing the scapulae in a comfortable position but without returning to the slouched position.

Develop control of scapular retraction and shoulder external rotation. These postural muscles are targeted to help maintain good alignment, although it is important to remember that strengthening alone will not correct faulty posture.

Patient position and procedures: Sitting on a chair, mat, or large gym ball, or standing with the spine in its neutral position facing a pulley system or elastic resistance secured at shoulder level and grasping the ends in the hands.

- Initially, have the patient do isolated scapular adduction.
- Progress to shoulder horizontal abduction in a rowing fashion (see Fig. 16–31*B*).
- Progress to more advanced patterns such as shoulder lateral rotation combined with scapular adduction and diagonal patterns (see Figs. 9–33 and 16–31*A*).

Develop cervical retraction (axial extension) and thoracic extension. These exercises also bring in the lumbar extensors as stabilizers.

- *Patient position and procedures:* Prone, with the forehead on the treatment table and the arms at the sides.
- Initially, have the patient lift just the forehead off the mat keeping the chin tucked and maintaining the neutral spinal position (no upper cervical extension). This is a small motion (Fig. 16–18)

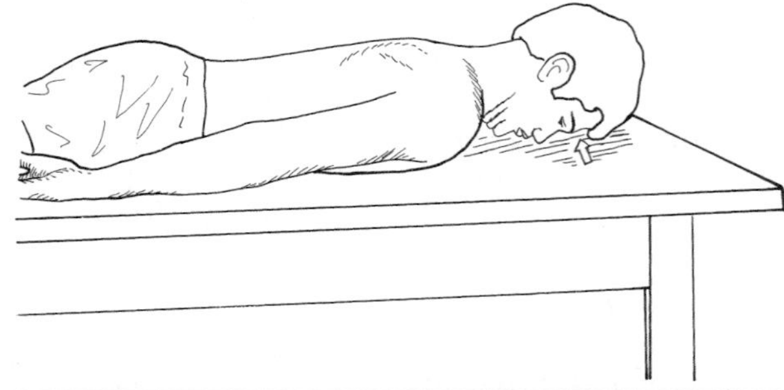

Figure 16–18 Axial extension (cervical retraction) exercises.

- Progress by having the patient lift the upper portion of the chest off the mat.
- Change the arm position from at the side to 90 degrees of abduction and eventually full elevation for increased resistance.

■ *Patient positions and procedures:* Quadruped, over a padded stool or a large gym ball. Have the patient tuck the chin and maintain the eyes focused toward the floor to maintain the functional position.

- Superimpose arm motions while the cervical muscles stabilize the neck and head. Suggestions include reaching out to the side, reaching overhead, and swimming motions.
- Progress by having the patient lift weights in the hands while stabilizing the head and neck position (Fig. 16–19).

■ *Patient position and procedure:* Standing. Place a basketball-sized inflatable ball between the back of the patient's head and a wall.

- Instruct the patient to maintain the position while moving the arms through various ROMs.
- Progress by having the patient maintain the position while lifting free weights in the hands (Fig. 16–20).

Develop cervical flexion. Often with faulty forward-head postures, the patient substitutes using the sternocleidomastoid (SCM) muscles to lift the head rather than the overstretched, weak, suprahyoid and infrahyoid cervical flexors. To correct this muscle imbalance, use gentle motions with a lot of feedback. Emphasize "curling" the head and neck, not lifting the head up.

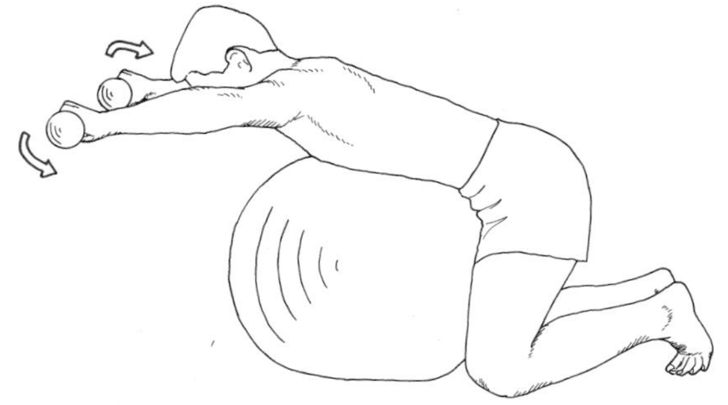

Figure 16–19 Developing spinal extensor stabilization. The patient maintains the head and neck in a neutral position while arm motions provide varying resistive forces. The gym ball provides an unstable surface requiring greater control.

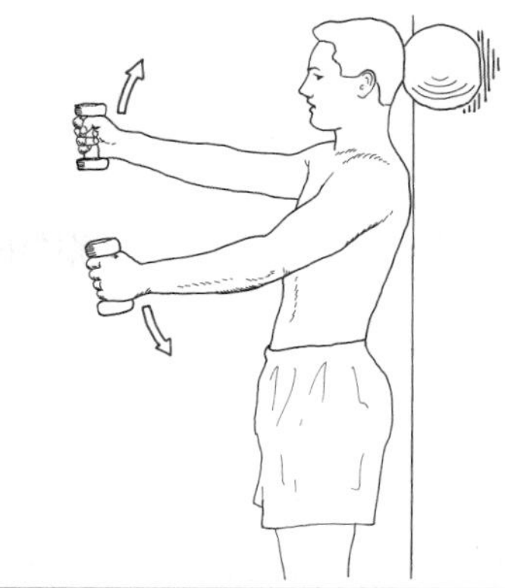

Figure 16–20 Strengthening the cervical and upper thoracic extensor muscles by maintaining control of the soft ball while varying resistance is applied through arm motions.

■ *Patient position and procedure:* Supine. If the patient cannot tuck the chin and curl the neck to lift the head off the mat, begin with the patient on a slant board or large wedge-shaped bolster under the thorax and head to reduce the effects of gravity.

- Have the patient practice tucking the chin and curling the head up. Use assistance until the correct pattern is learned (Fig. 16–21).
- Progress by decreasing the angle of the board or wedge and then adding manual resistance if the patient does not substitute with the SCM.

■ *Patient position and procedure:* Standing with a basketball-sized inflatable ball between the forehead and a wall. Have the patient keep the chin tucked and not go into a forward-head posture. The patient maintains the functional position while superimposing arm motions. Progress by adding weights to the arm motions.

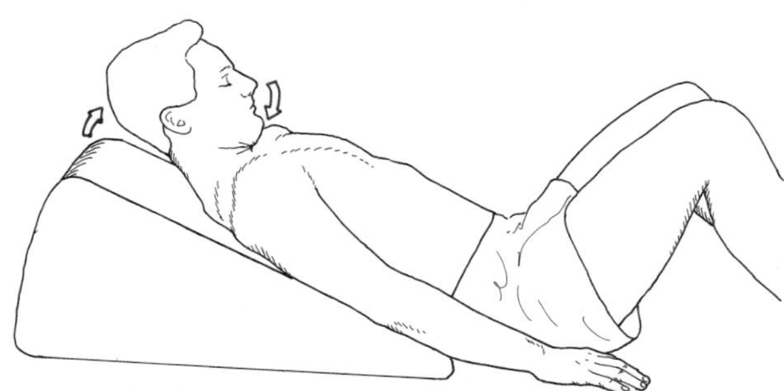

Figure 16–21 Training the short cervical flexors while de-emphasizing the sternocleidomastoid for cervical flexion to regain a balance in strength for anterior cervical stabilization.

- *Patient position and procedure:* Supine with the head over the edge of the mat, the neck maintained in a neutral functional position, and no support to the head. The patient must be able to keep the neck in its safe, functional position to perform this advanced stabilization exercise. He or she holds the position as tolerated. Progress by adding arm motions, then adding weights to the arm motions as tolerated.

Manual Resistance—Cervical Muscles

Patient position and procedures: Supine. Stand at the head end of the treatment table, supporting the patient's head for each exercise.

- Place one hand on the patient's head to resist opposite the motion. Do not resist against the mandible, or the force will be transmitted to the temporomandibular joint. Resistance is given to isolated muscle actions or to general ROMs, whichever best gains muscle balance and function.
- Isometric resistance can be applied with the head in any desired position before applying the resistance. Avoid jerking the neck when applying or releasing the resistance by gradually building up the intensity, telling the patient to match your resistance, holding, and then gradually releasing and, asking the patient to relax.

Self-Resistance—Isometric Exercises/Cervical Region

Patient position: Sitting.

- ***Flexion.*** Have the patient place both hands on the forehead and press the forehead into the palms in a nodding fashion while not moving (Fig. 16–22A).
- ***Side bending.*** Have the patient press one hand against the side of the head and attempt to side-bend, as if trying to bring the ear toward the shoulder but not allowing motion.
- ***Axial extension.*** Have the patient press the back of the head into both hands, which are placed in the back, near the top of the head (Fig. 16–22B).
- ***Rotation.*** Have the patient press one hand against the region just superior and lateral to the eye and attempt to turn the head to look over the shoulder but not allowing motion.

Intermediate and Advanced Training

Basic exercises are progressed by increasing the challenge to the patient with increased resistance, increased repetitions of arm movements, and more challenging patterns of movement. Transitional stabilization and functional activities are emphasized in this stage of rehabilitation.

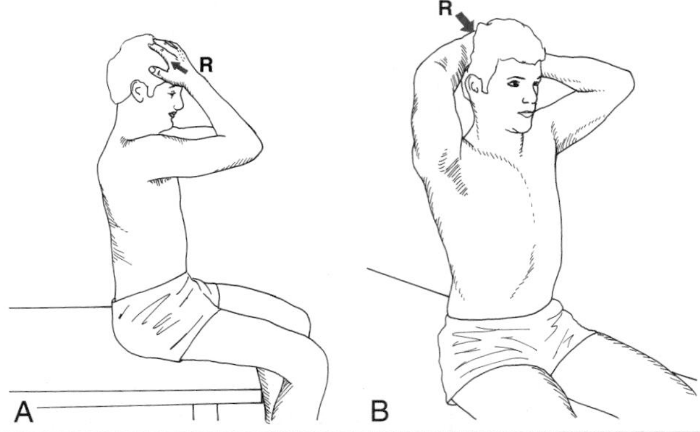

Figure 16–22 Self-resistance for isometric *(A)* cervical flexion and *(B)* axial extension.

Transitional Stabilization for the Cervical and Upper Thoracic Regions

- *Patient position and procedure:* Standing with basketball-sized inflatable ball between the head and the wall. Have the patient roll the ball along the wall, using the head. This requires the patient to turn the body as he or she walks along.
- *Patient position and procedure:* Sitting on a large gym ball. Have the patient walk the feet forward so that the ball rolls up the back and the thorax is resting on the ball (Figs. 16–23*A* and *B*). The head and neck are maintained in a neutral position, and the cervical flexors are emphasized. Have the patient then walk the ball farther so that it is under the head. The extensors are now emphasized (Fig. 16–23*C*). The patient walks the feet forward and backward, alternating stabilization between the flexors and extensors. Progress to advanced training by adding arm motions, and then arm motions with weights in each of the positions.

Note: This activity requires considerable strength in the cervical extensors to support the body weight and should be performed only with advanced training with patients who have been properly progressed to tolerate the resistance.

Functional Exercises

Design exercises that incorporate functional activities. These are patient-specific. Identify what activi-

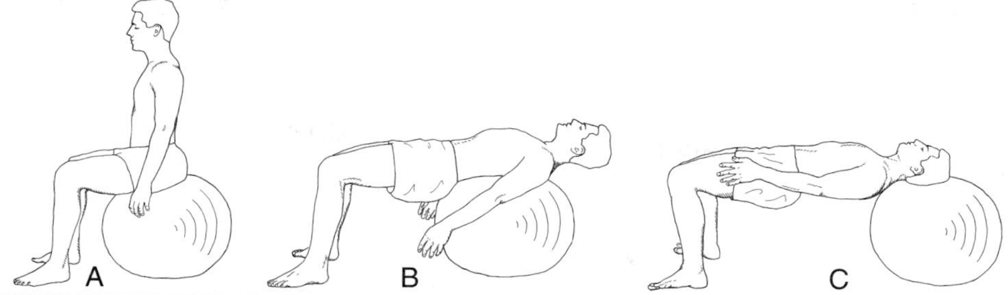

Figure 16–23 Advanced exercises for strengthening the cervical and upper thoracic flexors and extensors as stabilizers. Begin by *(A)* sitting on a large gym ball, then *(B)* walking forward while rolling the ball up the back. With the ball behind the midthoracic area, the cervical flexors must stabilize. Continue walking forward until the ball is *(C)* under the head; the cervical extensors now must stabilize. Walk back and forth between the two positions (*B* and *C*) to alternate control between the flexors and extensors. Progress by adding arm motions or arm motions with weights to increase resistance.

ties stress the neck, and have the patient practice modifications of those activities with the spine kept in a neutral position. Include pushing, pulling, reaching, and lifting. Challenge the patient with increased repetitions and weight and in patterns that replicate functional demands.

Thoracic and Lumbar Regions

Activation of Core Stabilization Musculature

No matter what diagnosis or stage of healing with which a patient presents, prior to the initiation of any trunk exercises, he or she is taught core techniques to activate the deep spinal stabilizers and to train the stabilizers to function under various movement patterns. Once the patient has learned activation of the stabilizers and can demonstrate control of the spine, stabilization exercises are progressed to the level of the patient's abilities. These exercises follow kinesthetic training for safe spinal motion and identification of the functional spinal position as described earlier in this chapter.

Three different techniques of abdominal muscle activation have been described and used in clinical practice: the drawing-in maneuver, abdominal bracing, and posterior pelvic tilt. Studies are showing that each technique differs in the stabilization activity of the abdominal and multifidus muscles.[23] Recent research has demonstrated that the drawing-in maneuver is more selective in coactivating the transversus abdominis and multifidus muscles than the other two techniques.[10,23] The drawing-in maneuver also functions to increase intra-abdominal pressure by inwardly displacing the abdominal wall. Because of this, the drawing-in maneuver is recommended for stabilization training; the other two methods are also described, primarily for information so that the reader can recognize the differences.

Drawing-In Maneuver (Fig. 16–24A)

Patient positions and procedure: Hook-lying, with knees 70 to 90 degrees and feet resting on an exercise mat, or prone-lying. The training can also be done in the quadruped (all fours) or semireclined positions if that is more comfortable for the patient. It is important to progress training to sitting and standing as soon as possible for functional activities. Teach the patient using demonstration, verbal cues, and tactile facilitation.

The patient assumes his or her neutral spinal position and attempts to maintain it while gently drawing in and hollowing the abdominal muscles.[14] There should be a subtle posterior pelvic tilt and flattening of the lumbar spine but no flaring of the lower ribs, bulging out of the abdominal wall, or increased pressure through the feet. Instruct the patient to draw the "belly button" up and in toward the spine to hollow out the abdominal region as exhaling. The individual should not inhale nor lift the rib cage to mimic this activity.

If a patient has difficulty activating the transversus abdominis and internal oblique muscles, the following two techniques of feedback have been shown to assist with learning.[7,13,23,24]

- ***Pressure transducer for clinical testing and visual feedback.*** A small inflatable bladder with pressure sensor (Pressure Bio-Feedback® Chattanooga Pacific) similar to a blood pressure cuff

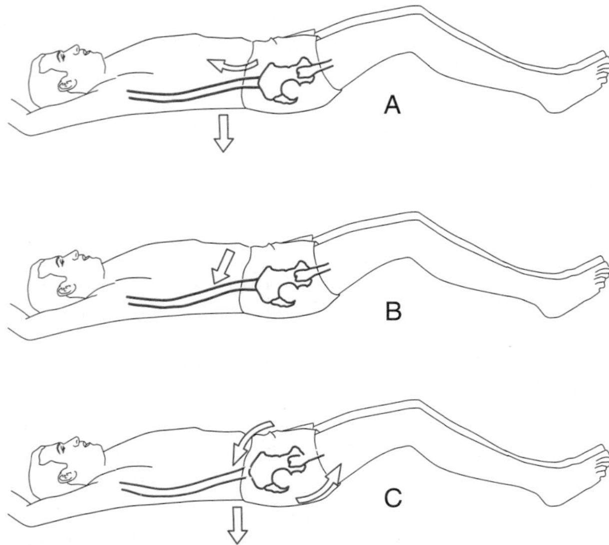

Figure 16–24 Three methods to activate the stabilizing musculature in the lumbar spine; *(A)* drawing-in maneuver where the patient hollows the abdominal region and there is a slight posterior pelvic tilt motion; *(B)* abdominal bracing where setting the abdominal muscles results in flaring laterally around the waist; and *(C)* posterior pelvic tilt where the pelvis is actively tilted posteriorly and the lumbar spine flattens.

is placed under the lumbar spine and inflated to a baseline of 40 mm Hg. Correct activation of the deep abdominals results in a 10-mm Hg increase in pressure. A larger increase occurs with activation of the rectus abdominis and increased lumbar flexion from the posterior pelvic tilt. No change in pressure reflects no activation of the deep muscles.

If used in the prone-lying position, the pressure sensor is placed under the abdomen and is inflated to 70 mm Hg. A decrease of 10 mm Hg during the drawing-in maneuver indicates proper activation of the deep abdominal muscles.

- ***Biofeedback with surface electrodes.*** Surface electrodes is placed over the rectus abdominis and external obliques (near its attachment on the eighth rib) may be used in conjunction with the inflatable cuff. There should be minimal to no activation of these muscles if the drawing-in maneuver is done correctly.

Abdominal Bracing (Fig. 16–24B)

In contrast to the drawing-in maneuver, abdominal bracing occurs by setting the abdominals and actively flaring out laterally around the waist. There is no head or trunk flexion, no elevation of the lower ribs, no protrusion of the abdomen, or pressure through the feet. The patient should be able to hold the braced position while breathing in a relaxed manner. This technique has been taught for a number of years as the method to stabilize the spine, and has been shown to activate the oblique abdominal muscles consistent with their stabilization function.[23]

Posterior Pelvic Tilt (Fig. 16–24C)

Pelvic tilt exercises principally activate the rectus abdominis muscle, which is primarily used for dynamic trunk flexion activity. It is not considered a core spinal stabilization muscle; therefore, it is not emphasized in training for stabilization.[23] It is used primarily to teach awareness of movement of the pelvis and lumbar spine and is activated when the patient explores his or her lumbar ROM with pelvic tilts to find the neutral position or functional spinal range.

Fundamental Training of Stabilization Muscles

Once the patient learns to activate the core stabilizing muscles in the lumbar region, teach him or her to activate the muscles in the neutral spine position and maintain control while superimposing simple arm and leg motions. This is to train the holding capacity of the deep stabilizing muscles.[7,13] If the patient cannot control the position, pre-position him or her using pillows, supports, or corsets. The voluntary contraction, using the drawing-in maneuver, develops the pattern of setting the deep abdominal and multifidus muscles in a feedforward pattern. Continue to use the pressurized cuff for feedback during this early training. To improve the holding capacity of the stabilizing muscles, increase the amount of time the patient does the exercises. It is very important that no exercise is continued if the patient cannot maintain the stabile position. If the deep abdominals cannot stabilize, substitute patterns in the superficial muscles will override the deep muscle activation. Suggested movements:

- ***Alternate shoulder flexion/extension (Fig. 16–25A)***

Patient positions and procedure: Supine hook-lying, sitting, standing, quadruped, or prone-lying. Instruct the patient to preset the deep muscles with the drawing-in maneuver, and then alternately flex and extend each upper extremity, first to 90 degrees,

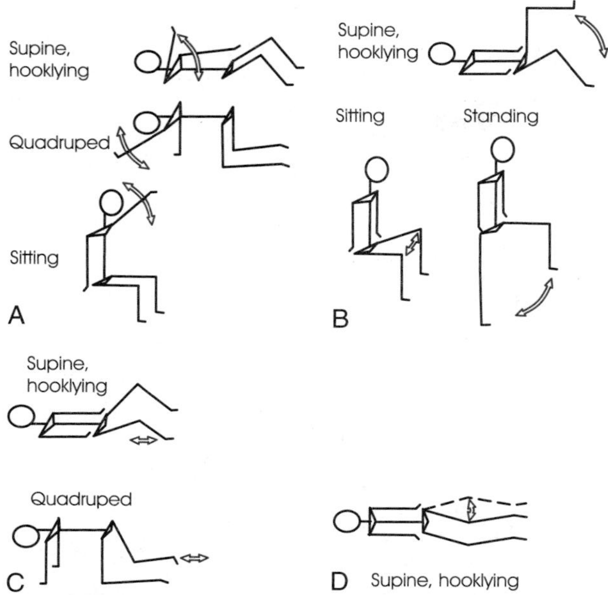

Figure 16–25 Fundamental stabilization exercises; *(A)* alternating arm movements, *(B)* alternating hip-knee flexion with one leg stabilized on the mat, *(C)* alternating leg slides with one leg stabilized on the mat, and *(D)* alternating leg fall-out.

then further if there is good control of the drawing-in maneuver and spinal posture.

Alternate Hip-Knee Flexion to 90 Degrees (Fig. 16–25B)

Patient positions and procedure: Hook-lying, sitting, or standing. Have the patient preset the deep muscles with the drawing-in maneuver, then alternately flex one hip and knee to 90 degrees, and return to the starting position.

Alternate Leg Slides (Fig. 16–25C)

Patient positions and procedure: Hook-lying or quadruped. Remind the patient to preset the deep muscles with the drawing-in maneuver, then alternately slide one leg along the mat toward extension and return. These leg slide exercises require greater control of pelvic rotation and, therefore, greater concentration on the deep stabilizing abdominal muscles.

Leg Fall-Outs (Fig. 16–25D)

Patient position and procedure: Hook-lying. Instruct the patient to use the drawing-in maneuver, then alternately let one knee move away from the midline and return. Keep the feet in the same position; this creates hip rotation and abduction. This motion requires increased control of transverse plane rotation of the pelvis.

Stabilization Exercise Progressions

Once the patient has learned control of his or her neutral spinal position and has developed the ability to do the drawing-in maneuver prior to and during arm and leg movements, increase the intensity and repetitions of the arm and leg movements. This is done to increase strength and muscular endurance in the stabilizing muscles while maintaining the spine in a relatively *static position*. The patient should be able to maintain the neutral spinal position throughout all of the exercises. It is critical to instruct him or her to stop the exercises (or decrease the intensity) as soon as there is a sense that there is loss of control of the stable spinal position. If the patient can maintain good stabilization with decreased intensity then he or she is challenged to do so. Endurance training of the trunk extensor muscles is related to decreased pain and improving function in the early stages of recovery in patients with subacute low back pain.[6]

It is very important not to progress the patient beyond what he or she is able to control in order to develop the proper muscle response. Some of the exercises described in this section provide greater challenge to the abdominal muscles, some to the spinal extensor muscles, and some to both. Isometric resistance to rotation of the trunk brings in the oblique abdominals, transversus abdominis, and deep spinal extensors.[25]

When the patient has developed control, strength, and endurance in the stabilizing muscles, *dynamic trunk strengthening* exercises are initiated at a low intensity. The emphasis is on control and safety.

During this phase of treatment, the patient should be able to return to his or her instrumental activities of daily living (IADL) and limited work activities by incorporating the core stabilization techniques into the activities.

Abdominal Muscles—Emphasis on Stabilization

Patient positions and procedure: Begin supine with arm and leg motions. Adapt the exercises and progress to sitting (at first with, then without back support), kneeling, and eventually standing. These upright postures require increased participation of more extremity muscles for stabilization at the hips, knees, and ankles, respectively and begin training for more functionally related weight-bearing activities. Sitting or lying on an unstable surface such as a large gym ball or wobble board increases the challenge to stabilize the spine. Remind the patient to find and maintain the neutral spinal position and perform the drawing-in maneuver when doing these exercises.

- ***Upper extremity motions (add hand weights as tolerated)***
  - Alternate shoulder flexion; move arms overhead as far as comfortable
  - Bilateral shoulder flexion
  - Bilateral, unilateral, and alternate diagonal patterns; D_1 and D_2 flexion
- ***Lower extremity motions (add ankle weights as tolerated)***
  - Alternate hip-knee extension with one leg stationary on a mat or floor (Fig. 16–26*A*).
  - Alternate hip-knee extension and flexion with both lower extremities moving *(modified bicycle exercise)*. Have the patient start in the 90-90 position (hips and knees each flexed to 90 degrees) and begin with small bicycle motions; progress to larger arcs of motions as he or she demonstrates good stabilization (Fig. 16–26*B*).
- ***Simultaneous Upper and lower extremity motions***
  - One upper extremity flexes overhead while the opposite lower extremity extends; alternate (Fig 16–26*C*).
  - Both upper extremities flex overhead and both lower extremities extend simultaneously then return (upper extremities extend and hips and knees flex). (This is quite advanced and requires strong stabilization.) When able, have the patient pass an object back and forth between the hands and feet.
- ***Elastic resistance or pulley system affixed overhead or behind the patient***
  - Alternate pull-downs; begin with arms overhead and pull down to the sides.
  - Bilateral pull-downs; begin with both arms overhead and pull down simultaneously (Fig 16–27).
  - Bilateral, unilateral, or alternate diagonal pull-downs; D_1 and D_2 extension.
  - When sitting or standing, various patterns of resistance can be obtained by varying the height of the resistance (Fig 16–28).
- ***Unstable surfaces.*** Use a foam roller, large gym ball, or wobble board to increase the challenge of balancing and stabilizing on an unstable surface. A variety of positions can be used such as sitting upright on the ball with the feet on the floor (Fig. 16–29), lying supine with the trunk on the ball and feet on the floor or feet on a low mat, or bridging with just the head on the ball (if the cervical stabilizers are strong) (see Fig. 16–23). If a foam roller is used, the patient is supine with the roller placed longitudinally along the spine. Each of the above exercises may be adapted for use on the unstable surfaces.

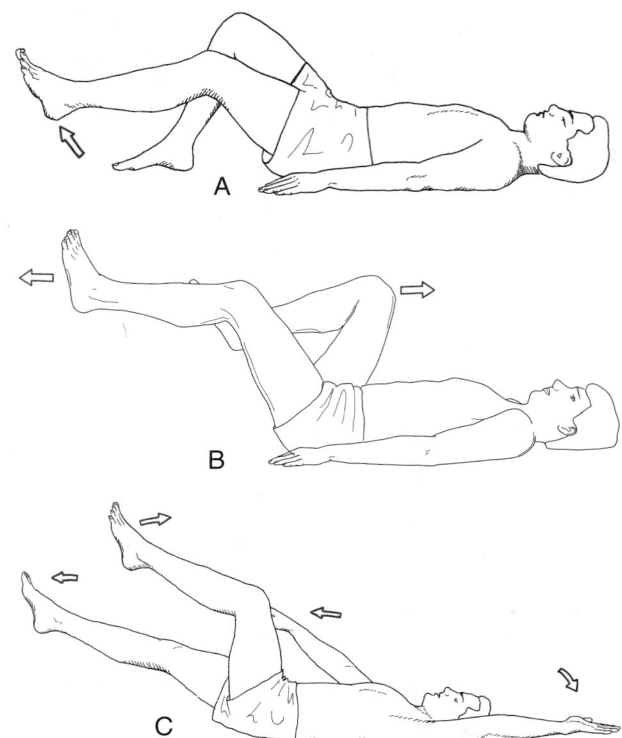

Figure 16–26 Developing abdominal strength as the muscles stabilize the spine in its functional position. *(A)* Light resistance is applied by flexing and extending one lower extremity while the other helps stabilize. *(B)* Increased resistance occurs with the "modified bicycle" (alternating knee flexion and extension). *(C)* A strong controlling action in the abdominals is required when both upper and lower extremities are moving in alternating patterns.

Back Extensor Muscles—Emphasis on Stabilization

Patient positions and procedures: To emphasize the extensors, begin with the patient in the quadruped or prone-lying position. If assistance is needed to

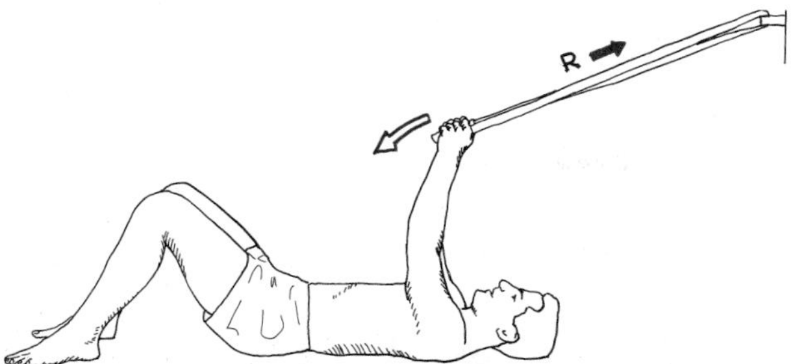

Figure 16–27 Developing the stabilizing action of the abdominal muscles by using pull-down activities against a resistive force from pulleys or elastic bands. This exercise can also be done sitting or standing.

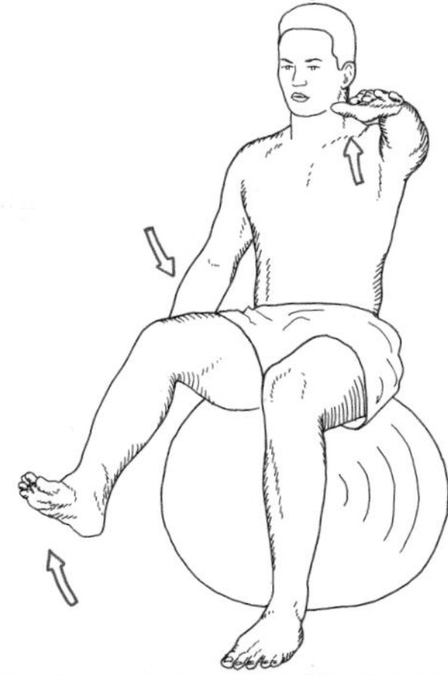

Figure 16–29 Strength, balance, and coordination are required to maintain spinal stabilization while sitting on a gym ball and moving the extremities. This activity is progressed by adding weights to the extremities.

stabilize the spine while in quadruped, position the patient over a padded stool, chair, or large gym ball. It is important to maintain the cervical spine in its neutral position during these exercises. The patient should be able to align the head and focus the eyes on the floor. A small towel roll between the chin and neck may be a helpful reminder to hold the position. If the patient has difficulty controlling the trunk rotation, use a prop, such as a dowel rod placed along the spine, and have the patient attempt to keep it balanced while performing the exercises. It may be helpful to cue the patient to not shift his or her weight as the extremity is moved—this is difficult to do but is effective in bringing in the stabilizing trunk muscles.

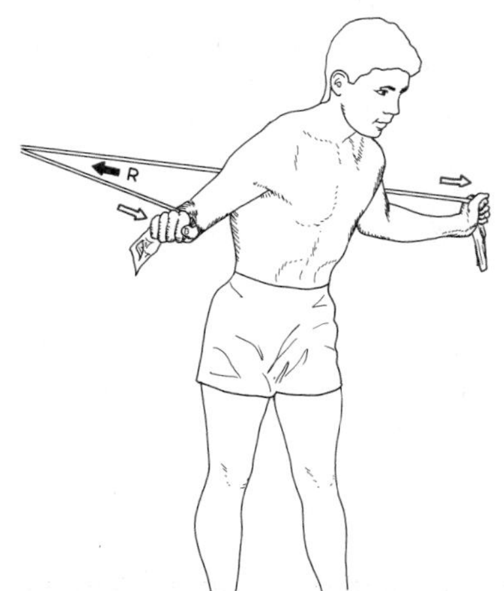

Figure 16–28 Using elastic resistance to train and strengthen the abdominal muscles in the upright position. The drawing-in maneuver to set the stabilizing muscles precedes the movement of the arms forward against the resistance.

The prone position may be difficult in the early stages of healing or if there is significant hip or trunk flexor tightness. If necessary, place a pillow under the abdomen to relieve stress from these restrictions. To maintain the cervical spine in a neutral position, place a small towel under the forehead. Progress to sitting (supported then unsupported), kneeling, and standing.

As with the abdominal musculature, sitting or lying (prone) on an unstable surface such as a large gym ball increases the challenge to the spinal stabilizers. Remind the patient to find and maintain the neutral spinal position and perform the drawing-in maneuver when doing these exercises. As each exercise progresses, light weights are added to the distal end of the extremities.

- ***Upper extremity motions***
  - Alternate shoulder flexion; move arms overhead as far as possible
  - Bilateral shoulder flexion
- ***Lower extremity motions***
  - Alternate leg slides (can only be done when quadruped) (Fig. 16–30*A*).
  - Alternate leg lifts (hip and knee extension). Have the patient begin with very small motions. Caution the patient to not lift the thigh so high as to cause stress to the sacroiliac or spinal joints.
- ***Simultaneous upper and lower extremity motions***
  - One arm reaches overhead while the opposite

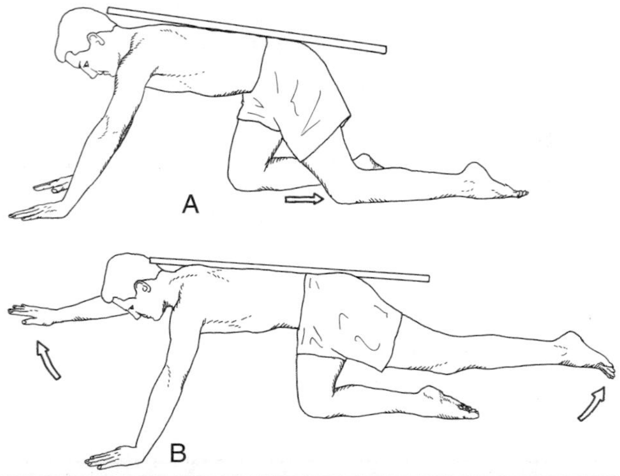

Figure 16–30 Quadruped exercises to develop control and strength in the spinal extensors. *(A)* Light resistance is applied by sliding one lower extremity outward while concentrating on controlling the spine. Balancing a rod on the back provides reinforcement that the trunk is not twisting. *(B)* Greater challenge is provided by lifting the opposite arm and leg simultaneously, then alternating extremities.

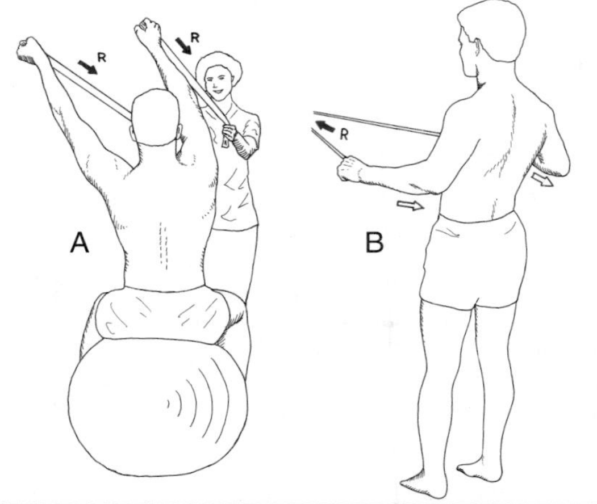

Figure 16–31 Using elastic resistance to train and strengthen the back extensor muscles to stabilize in the upright position *(A)* diagonal patterns while sitting on an unstable surface and *(B)* standing.

lower extremity extends *(bird-dog exercise);* alternate (Fig 16–30*B*)

- If supported by a stool or gym ball, have the patient lift both arms simultaneously and do swimming and reaching motions (see Fig. 16–19)

■ ***Elastic resistance or pulley system secured near the feet of in front of the patient***

- Alternate pull-ups; begin with the arms at the sides and pull up.
- Bilateral pull-ups; pull with both arms to the overhead position simultaneously.
- Bilateral, unilateral, and alternate diagonal pull ups; D_1 and D_2 flexion patterns (Fig. 16–31*A*).
- When sitting or standing, various patterns such as shoulder horizontal abduction can be used by varying the height of the resistance (Fig. 16–31*B*).

■ ***Unstable surfaces.*** Use a large gym ball, foam roller, or wobble board to challenge the patient's balance and develop the stabilizing musculature. Have the patient sit on the ball or roller, or stand on a wobble or balance board. Secure elastic or pulley resistance in front of the patient at various heights, and have him or her do pulling motions (see Fig. 16–31*A*).

Quadratus Lumborum—Emphasis on Stabilization

The quadratus lumborum has been identified as an important stabilizer of the spine in the frontal and transverse planes.[16] Strongest activation of this muscle occurs with the closed-chain side propping position.

Patient position and procedure: Begin side-lying.

- Have the patient prop up on his or her elbow and then lift the pelvis off the mat, supporting the lower body with the lateral side of the knee on the downward side. The position can be maintained for an isometric hold or performed intermittently for a dynamic contraction (Fig. 16–32*A*).
- Progress by having the patient support the upper body with the hand (with the elbow extended) and lateral aspect of the foot of the downward side (Fig. 16–32*B*).

Alternating Isometric Contractions and Rhythmic Stabilization

Patient positions and procedures: Begin with the patient supine in the most stable position. Progress to sitting on a stable surface, sitting on an unstable surface like a large gym ball, kneeling, and then standing. Sitting, kneeling, and standing require stabilizing action in the hip, knee, and ankle musculature, respectively, as well as the spinal muscles. Apply resistance directly against the patient's shoulders or pelvis, against a rod that is held by the patient (see Fig. 9–28), or against the patient's arms or flexed knees.

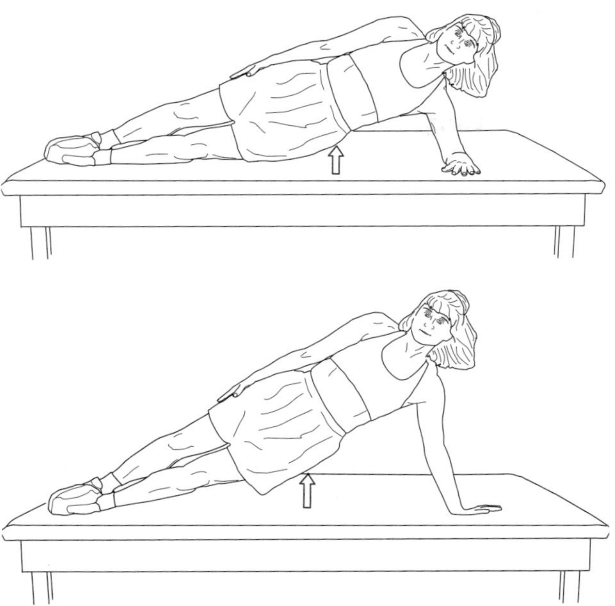

Figure 16–32 Quadratus lumborum stabilization training using closed-chain side-propping; *(A)* on the elbow and knee, and *(B)* on the hand and foot.

- Instruct the patient to find the neutral spine position, and then activate the stabilizing muscles with the drawing-in maneuver prior to the application of the resistive force. Then instruct the patient to "meet my resistance" while applying a force to stimulate isometric contractions. Apply the resistance in alternating directions at a controlled speed while the patient learns to maintain a steady position.
- Initially, provide verbal cues such as "hold against my resistance but do not overpower me; feel your abdominal muscles contracting; now I'm pulling in the opposite direction; match the resistance and feel your back muscles contracting."
- Progress by shifting the directions of resistance without the verbal cues and then by increasing the speed.
- Begin with alternating resistance in the sagittal plane; progress to side-to-side, and then transverse plane resistance. Isometric resistance to trunk rotation (transverse plane resistance) has been shown to be the most effective in stimulating the deep stabilizing muscles.[25]
- Alternating resistance to pelvic rotation can also be done by having the patient assume a modified bridge position. Apply resistance directly to the pelvis while the patient isometrically holds the pelvis and spine in a stable position.

Dynamic Strengthening—Lumbar Muscles

Note: Dynamic exercises of the trunk musculature are not initiated until late in the rehabilitation process and not until after the patient has learned to automatically activate the drawing-in maneuver for stabilization in all functional activities.

Trunk Flexion (Abdominal Muscles)—Supine

Patient position and procedure: Supine or hook-lying with the lumbar spine neutral to flat (posterior pelvic tilt). The spine should not be allowed to extend (arch)—this indicates weakness of the abdominals, and consequently lifting of the trunk occurs from hip flexor action only.[14] When training the abdominals, curl-up exercises should be performed at a slow, controlled rate to activate the stabilizing function of the abdominals.[34]

- ***Curl-ups***
  - First, have the patient perform the drawing-in maneuver to cause a stabilizing contraction of the abdominal muscles and then lift the head. He or she progresses by lifting the shoulders until the scapulae and thorax clear the mat, keeping the arms horizontal (Fig. 16–33). A full sit-up is not necessary because, once the thorax clears the mat, the rest of the motion is performed by the hip flexor muscles.
  - Further progress the difficulty of the curl-up by having the patient change the arm position from horizontal, to folded across the chest, and then to behind the head.

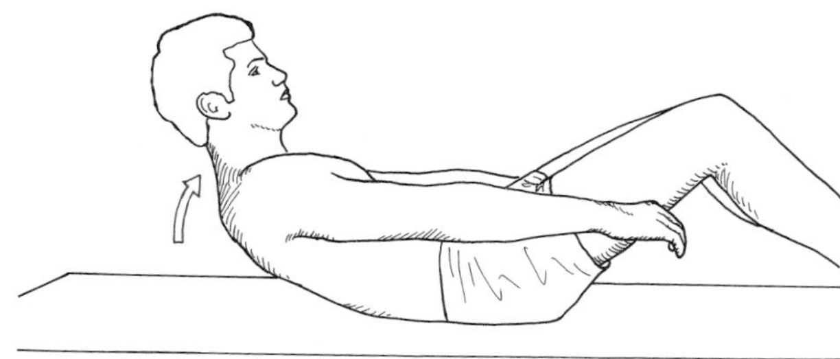

Figure 16–33 The curl-up exercise to strengthen the abdominal muscles. The thorax is flexed on the lumbar spine. The arms are shown in the position for least resistance. Progress by crossing the arms across the chest, then behind the head.

- In all these activities, the low back should not arch; if it does, reduce the progression until the abdominals are strong enough to maintain lumbar flexion.

- ***Curl-downs***
  - If the patient is unable to perform the curl-up, begin with curl-downs by having the patient start in the hook-sitting or long-sitting position and lower the trunk only to the point where he or she can maintain a flat low back, and then return to the sitting position.
  - Once the patient can curl-down full range, reverse and perform a curl-up.
- ***Diagonal curl-ups.*** Have the patient reach one hand toward the outside of the opposite knee while curling up, then alternate. Reverse the muscle action by bringing one knee up toward the opposite shoulder; then repeat with the other knee. Diagonal exercises emphasize the oblique muscles.
- ***Double knee-to-chest.*** To emphasize the lower rectus abdominis and oblique muscles, have the patient set a posterior pelvic tilt, then bring both knees to the chest and return. Progress the difficulty by decreasing the angle of hip and knee flexion (Fig. 16–34).
- ***Pelvic lifts.*** Have the patient begin with the hips at 90 degrees and knees extended then lift the buttocks upward off the mat (small motion). The feet move upward toward the ceiling (Fig. 16–35). The patient should not push against the mat with the hands.

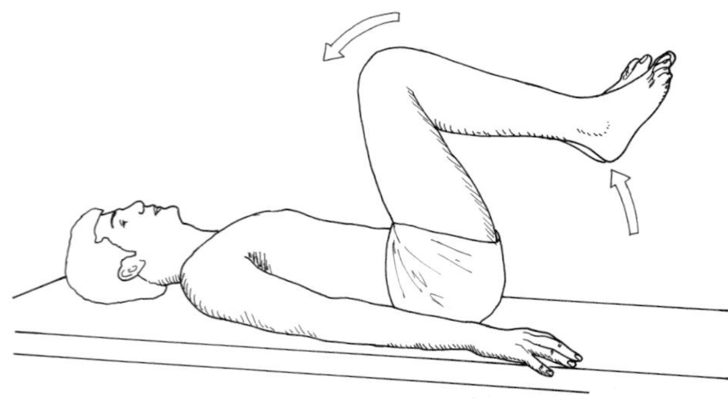

Figure 16–34 Strengthening the abdominal muscles by flexing the hip and pelvis on the lumbar spine. The legs are shown in the position for least resistance. Progress by decreasing the angle of hip flexion until the legs can be lifted with the knees extended.

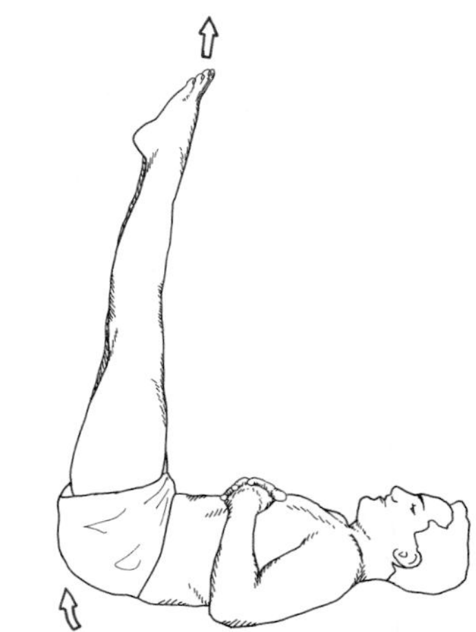

Figure 16–35 Pelvic lifts. Elevating the legs upward toward the ceiling by raising the buttock off the floor emphasizes strengthening the lower abdominal muscles.

- ***Bilateral straight-leg raising (SLR)***
  - This is a progression in difficulty of the double knee-to-chest exercise. It should be undertaken only if the muscles are strong enough to maintain a posterior pelvic tilt.
  - Have the patient begin with legs extended, then perform a posterior pelvic tilt, then flex both hips, keeping the knees extended. If the pelvis and spine cannot be kept stable, the knees should be flexed to a degree that allows control.
  - If the hips are abducted before initiating this exercise, greater stress is placed on the oblique abdominal muscles.

Precaution: The strong pull of the psoas major causes shear forces on the lumbar vertebrae. If there is any low-back pain or discomfort, especially with spinal hypermobility or instability, this exercise should not be performed even if the abdominals are strong enough to maintain a posterior pelvic tilt.

- ***Bilateral straight-leg lowering.*** This can be performed if the bilateral SLR is difficult. Have the patient begin with the hips at 90 degrees and knees extended and then lower the extremities as far as possible while maintaining a flat back, then raise the legs back to 90 degrees. See precaution under the bilateral SLR exercise.

Trunk Flexion (Abdominals)—Sitting or Standing

Patient position and procedures: Sitting or standing. Pulleys or elastic material are secured at shoulder level behind the patient. Progress the resistance as the patient's abdominal strength increases.

- Have the patient hold the handles or ends of the material with each hand and then flex the trunk with emphasis on bringing the rib cage down toward the pubic bone and performing a posterior pelvic tilt, rather than flexing at the hips (Fig. 16–36).
- Have the patient perform diagonal motions by bringing one arm down toward the opposite knee with emphasis on moving the rib cage down toward the opposite side of the pelvis. Repeat the diagonal motion in the opposite direction.

Trunk Flexion (Abdominals)—Unstable Surfaces

Patients with chronic, unilateral low back pain have been shown to have impaired balance.[2] Use of unstable surfaces, such as a gym ball (Fig. 16–37) or balance board, while doing abdominal curl-up exercises has been shown to increase activity in the internal and external obliques as well as rectus abdominis.[33] The presumption is that these muscles generate increased activity to maintain balance on the unstable surfaces. Other suggestions include balancing on a foam roll or BAPS board while performing arm and leg activities or curl-up exercises.

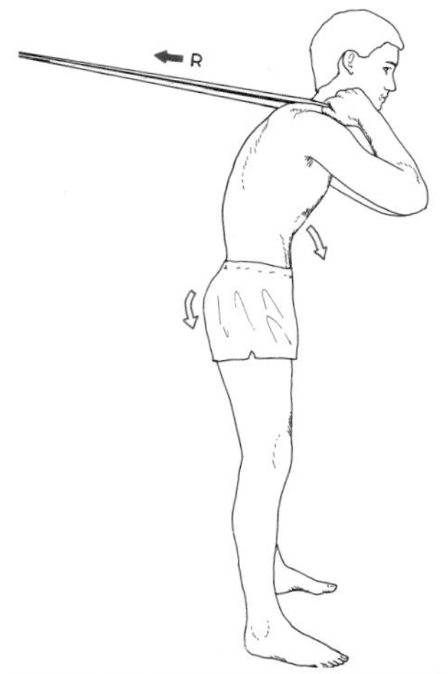

Figure 16–36 Standing trunk flexion against elastic material to strengthen the abdominal muscles. The patient performs a posterior pelvic tilt and approximates the ribs toward the pubis.

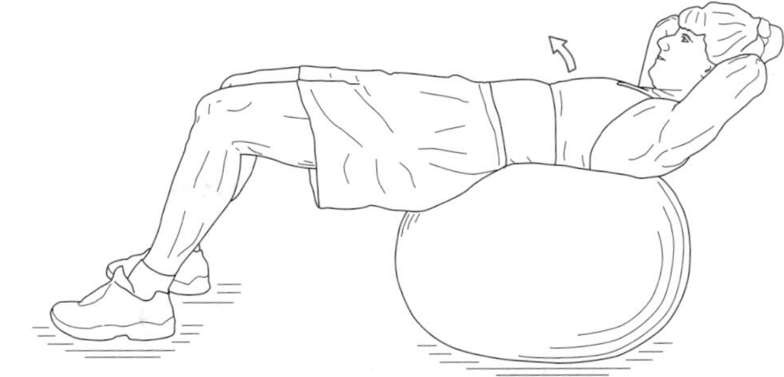

Figure 16–37 Curl-ups on an unstable surface. The unstable surface increases activity in the oblique and rectus abdominis muscles.

Trunk Extension (Thoracolumbar Extensor Muscles)

Resistance can be applied to any of the following recumbent exercises by having the patient hold weights in the hands or by strapping weights around the patient's legs.

Precaution: Because these exercises are performed at the end of the range of spinal extension, patients with spondylosis or other flexion bias conditions may experience increased symptoms and, therefore, should not do them.

- *Patient position and procedure:* Supine, with arms at the sides. Instruct the patient to arch the back by pressing against the mat with the back of the neck and the sacrum (Fig. 16–38).
- *Patient position and procedure:* Prone. Begin with the arms at the side, progress to behind the head or reaching overhead as strength improves. Have the patient tuck in the chin and lift the head and thorax. The lower extremities must be stabilized (Fig. 16–39).

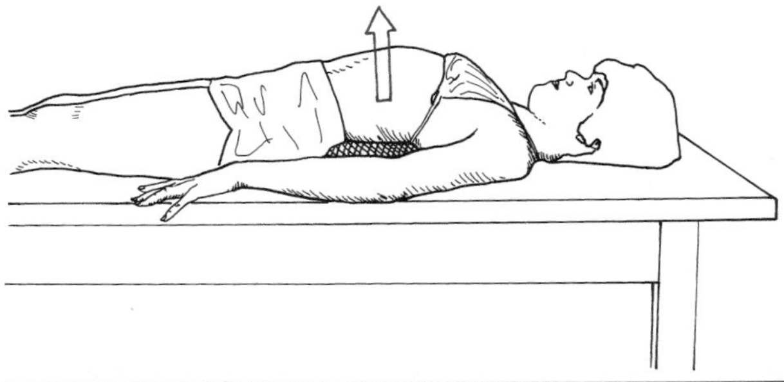

Figure 16–38 Strengthening the back extensors by arching the back against the resistance of the table.

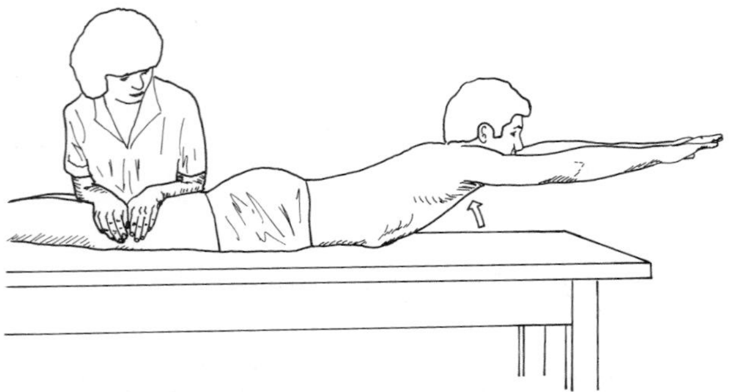

Figure 16–39 Strengthening the back extensors with the arms in position to provide maximal resistance. Additional resistance can be provided by holding weights in the hands.

- ***Leg lifts.*** *Patient position and procedure:* Prone. Initially have the patient lift only one leg, alternate with the other leg, and finally, lift both legs and extend the spine. Stabilize the thorax by having the patient hold onto the side of the treatment table.
- ***"Superman."*** *Patient position and procedure:* Prone. Progress the extension exercises by having the patient lift both upper and lower extremities simultaneously (Fig. 16–40).
- ***Elastic resistance or weighted pulleys.*** *Patient position and procedure:* sitting or standing. Secure pulleys or elastic resistance in front of the patient at shoulder level. Have him or her hold onto the ends of the material or handles and extend the spine (Fig. 16–41).

  For trunk rotation, use a pulley or elastic resistance secured under the foot or to a stable object opposite to the side being exercised. Have the patient pull against the resistance, extending and rotating the back. Change the angle of pull of the resistance to re-create functional patterns specific to the patient's needs (Fig. 16–42).

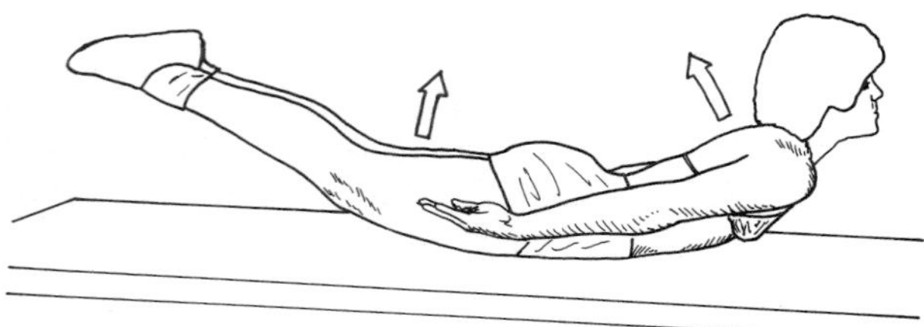

Figure 16–40 Strengthen the trunk and hip extensors by lifting the trunk and legs off the mat simultaneously. Greater resistance can be provided by abducting the shoulders to 90 degrees or by elevating them to 180 degrees ("Superman").

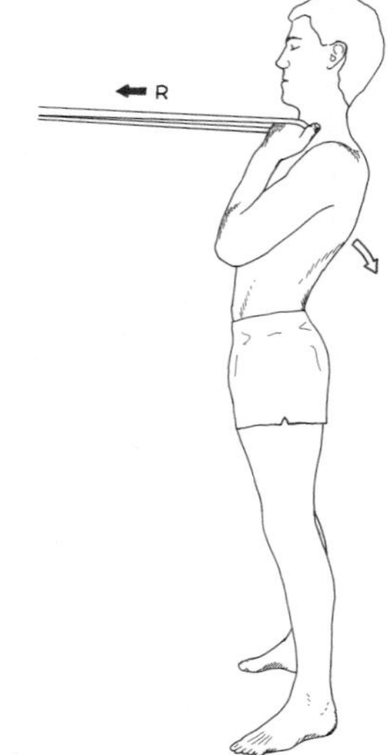

Figure 16–41 Using elastic resistance for concentric eccentric back extension.

Trunk Side Bending (Lateral Trunk Flexor Muscles)

These exercises are used for general strengthening of the muscles that side-bend the trunk. If there is a structural scoliosis, exercise alone has not been shown to halt or change the progression of the curve, but exercise used in conjunction with other

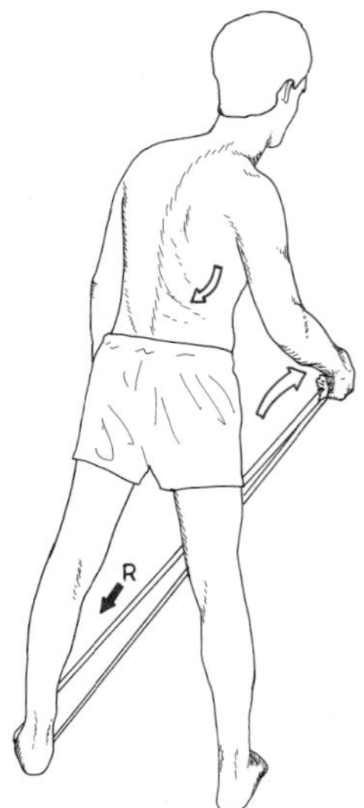

Figure 16–42 Rotation with extension strengthens the back extensors in functional patterns.

methods of correction, such as bracing, is often used.[3,5] When there is a lateral curve, the muscles on the convex side are usually stretched and weakened. The following exercises are described for use as strengthening exercises on the side of the convexity although they may be used bilaterally for symmetrical strengthening.

Stabilization exercises for spinal control as previously described may be beneficial for strengthening and conditioning when there is a scoliosis.

- *Patient position and procedure:* Standing. Place elastic resistance under the foot, or have the patient hold a weight in the hand on the side of the concavity, and then have him or her side-bend the trunk in the opposite direction.
- *Patient position and procedure:* Side-lying on the concave side of the curve with the apex at the edge of the table or mat so that the thorax is lowered. If you have access to a split table with one end that can be lowered, begin with the apex of the curve at the bend of the table. Have the patient place the lower arm folded across the chest and upper arm along the side of the body and side-bend the trunk up against gravity. Progress by having the patient clasp both hands behind the head (Fig. 16–43). Stabilization of the pelvis and lower extremities must be provided.

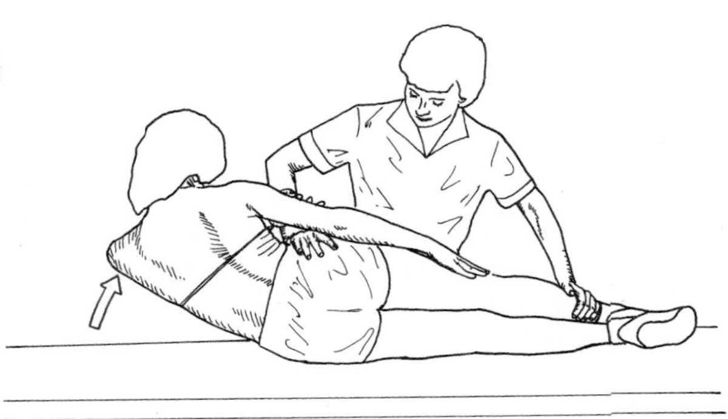

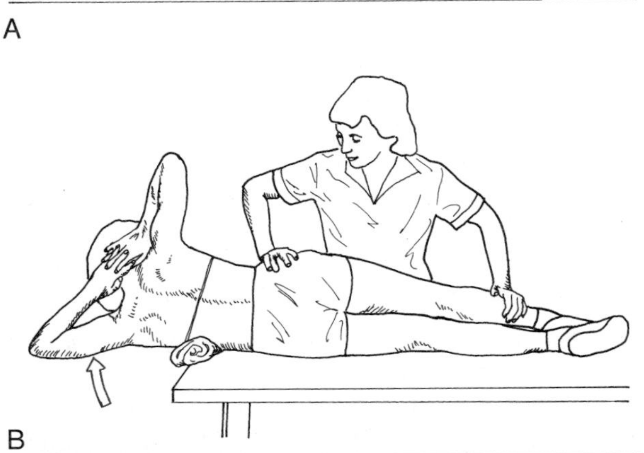

Figure 16–43 Antigravity strengthening of the lateral trunk musculature. There is less resistance if the top arm is at the side and bottom arm is folded across the chest.

Aerobic Conditioning

Goal. The goal of aerobic conditioning is to develop cardiovascular fitness for overall endurance and well-being.

Aerobic conditioning exercises provide many benefits for the patient with spinal symptoms. The activity not only improves cardiovascular endurance but stimulates feelings of well-being and relief of symptoms.[19] Chapter 4 describes aerobic conditioning principles and procedures. Specific precautions and suggestions for medical conditions are also explained. For patients recovering from spinal injuries, surgery, or postural dysfunction, aerobic exercises may be initiated once signs of inflammation no longer exist. Begin with low to moderate intensity, and work with the patient to choose activities that do not place added stress on the recovering spinal structures. If a particular spinal bias has been identified (see Chapter 15), choose exercises that emphasize that spinal bias. A brief summary of the principles is reviewed and guidelines for safe application of common conditioning exercises are described in this section.

Summary of Aerobic Conditioning Principles

1. Establish the target heart rate and maximum heart rate. The maximum heart rate is generally 220 minus the individual's age or may be the symptom-limiting heart rate (that rate where cardiovascular symptoms appear). Target heart rate is between 60% and 80% of the maximum heart rate.
2. Have the patient gradually warm up for 10 to 15 minutes with slow repetitive motions, include full range of available motion of involved joints.
3. Increase the pace of the activity to reach the target heart rate and maintain it for 20 to 30 minutes. Use activities that emphasize the patient's bias (see following sections).
4. Cool down for 5 to 10 minutes with slow, total body repetitive motions and stretching activities.

5. The aerobic activity should be performed three to five times per week.
6. To avoid overuse syndromes to structures of the musculoskeletal system, appropriate equipment, such as correct footwear, should be used for biomechanical support.
7. Always stay within the tolerance of the individual. Overuse commonly occurs when there is an increase in time or effort without adequate rest (recovery) time between sessions. Increase repetitions or time by no more than 10% per week.[15] If pain begins while exercising, heed the warning and reduce the stress.
8. Individualize the program of exercise. All people are not at the same fitness level and, therefore, cannot perform the same exercises. Any one exercise has the potential to be detrimental if attempted by someone not able to execute it properly.

Common Aerobic Exercises and Effects on the Spine

Some aerobic exercises place the spine in end-range positions. These are reviewed so that the reader understands why some activities may be inappropriate for patients with specific conditions. If modifications are possible, they should be considered.

Cycling. Road bikes place the thoracolumbar spine in flexion and upper cervical spine in hyperextension. Use this exercise for patients who have a flexion bias in the lumbar region as long as there are no upper cervical symptoms. Modifications include using a bike that positions the body in a more upright posture such as a mountain bike or hybrid bike. Many stationary bikes also position the individual in upright postures and, therefore, are less likely to precipitate cervical problems.

Walking and running. The upright posture emphasizes normal spinal curves, and lumbar extension is emphasized with walking and running (terminal stance). Emphasize the importance of identifying the neutral spine, activating the drawing-in maneuver, and stabilizing the spine while walking or running. Because conscious control is not possible during the entire exercise time, coach the patient to check his or her posture and muscle control frequently. Walking or running with the cervical spine in retraction (axial extension) and scapulae comfortably adducted, along with a rhythmic arm swing reinforces cervical stabilization. Easy access to treadmills, tracks, or roads and trails make these activities popular.

Stair climbing. Commercial devices that replicate stepping with various grades of resistance are used for strengthening and aerobic conditioning. Regular steps can also be used for aerobic conditioning. This activity requires good pelvic control of the reciprocating lower extremities because lifting the leg on one side emphasizes spinal flexion while the contralateral lower extremity and spine are extending. Coach the patient to maintain the neutral spine with the stabilizing muscles against the rotational forces.

Cross-country skiing and ski machines. This activity, whether out in the cold or on a commercial machine that replicates skiing, is a high-intensity aerobic activity. The kicking motion that accompanies the backward motion of the leg emphasizes spinal extension. It is important to coach the patient to maintain the neutral spine and contract the stabilizing abdominal muscles.

Swimming. The breaststroke emphasizes extension in the cervical and lumbar spinal regions when taking a breath. Coach the patient to not extend the neck full range but keep it neutral and lift the head out of the water as a "solid" unit with the thorax just enough to clear the mouth for the breath.

The freestyle stroke may exacerbate cervical problems because of the repetitive cervical rotation while taking a breath; this stroke also emphasizes lumbar extension with the flutter kick. Teach the patient to breathe using a "log-roll" technique where the whole body rolls toward one side while breathing and then rolls back to the face-down position for the stroke. This requires good spinal stabilization.

The backstroke emphasizes spinal extension via the kicking of the lower extremities and arm motions. The butterfly stroke moves the spine through a full ROM; emphasis is placed on controlling the range with the stabilizing muscles.

Upper body ergometer machines. These machines provide upper extremity resistance and can also be used for aerobic training. Forward motions emphasize spinal flexion and shoulder girdle protraction; backward motions emphasize spinal extension and shoulder girdle retraction. Coach the patient to assume the neutral spinal posture and use the stabilizing muscles prior to and during the use of the ergometer to enhance postural responses. If the machine can be used standing, progression to the standing position will stimulate a total body response.

Step aerobics. Stepping is similar to using stairs or a stair machine except for the jumping and bouncing that is usually added to the more advanced step aerobic programs. The impact may not be tolerated in individuals with intervertebral disk lesions or degenerative joint conditions.

Aerobic dancing. Dancing moves take on many forms, and classes are taught that address various fitness levels and age groups. If possible, review safe movement patterns and help the patient recognize the safe limits of his or her spinal range and abilities.

The "latest popular craze." People like variety and may be attracted to charismatic and energetic figures who demonstrate "new" workout techniques and routines or new exercise machines. Patients may ask for advice as to the value of the activities and techniques. Knowledge and skill in analyzing the biomechanics of the activity and the forces that are imposed through the spine should be used to provide advice about exercise safety. End of range postures and high-velocity stresses (such as vigorous kicking and ballistic motions) may be damaging to vulnerable tissues in the spine and should not be attempted by patients recovering from spinal problems.

▶ Stress Relief and Relaxation

Goals. The goals of stress relief and relaxation are to relax tense muscles and to relieve postural stress.

Note: These techniques are not appropriate to manage acute pain from inflammation, joint swelling, or disk derangements.

Muscle Relaxation Techniques

Active ROM

Whenever discomfort develops from maintaining a constant posture or from sustaining muscle contractions for a period of time, active ROM in the opposite direction aids in taking stress off supporting structures, promoting circulation, and maintaining flexibility. All motions are performed slowly, through the full range, with the patient paying particular attention to the feel of the muscles. Repeat each motion several times.

Cervical and Upper Thoracic Region

Patient position and procedure: Sitting with the arms resting comfortably on the lap, or standing. Instruct the patient to:

- Bend the neck forward and backward. (Backward bending is contraindicated with symptoms of nerve root compression.)
- Side bend the head in each direction; then rotate the head in each direction.
- Roll the shoulders; protract, elevate, retract, and then relax the scapulae (in a position of good posture).
- Circle the arms (shoulder circumduction). This is accomplished with the elbows flexed or extended, using either small or large circular motions with the arms pointing either forward or out to the side. Both clockwise and counterclockwise motions should be performed, but conclude the circumduction by going forward, up, around, and then back, so that the scapulae end up in a retracted position. This has the benefit of helping retrain proper posture.

Lower Thoracic and Lumbar Region

Patient position and procedure: Sitting or standing. If standing, the feet should be shoulder-width apart with the knees slightly bent. Have the patient place the hands at the waist with the fingers pointing backward. Instruct the patient to:

- Extend the lumbar spine by leaning the trunk backward (see Fig. 16–11*B*). This is particularly beneficial when the person must sit or stand in a forward-bent position for prolonged periods.
- Flex the lumbar spine by contracting the abdominal muscles, causing a posterior pelvic tilt: or if there are no signs of a disk problem, the patient can bend the trunk forward while sitting, dangling the arms toward the floor. This motion is beneficial when the person stands in a lordotic or sway-back posture for prolonged periods. "Toe-touching" exercises are not advocated for individuals with low-back impairments due to the stress placed on the low-back structures.
- Side bend in each direction.
- Rotate the trunk by turning in each direction while keeping the pelvis facing forward.

- Stand up and walk around at frequent intervals when sitting for extended periods.

Conscious Relaxation Training for the Cervical Region

Specific techniques for the cervical region develop the patient's kinesthetic awareness of a tensed or relaxed muscle and how to consciously reduce tension in the muscle. In addition, if done with posture training techniques in mind as described earlier in this chapter (page 643), the patient can be helped to recognize decreased muscular tension when the head is properly balanced and the cervical spine is aligned in midposition.

Patient position and procedure: Sitting comfortably with arms relaxed, such as resting on a pillow placed on the lap; the eyes are closed. Position yourself next to the patient to use tactile cues on the muscles and help position the head as necessary. Instruct the patient to:

1. Use diaphragmatic breathing and breathe in slowly and deeply through the nose, allowing the abdomen to relax and expand; then relax and allow the air to be expired through the relaxed open mouth. This breathing is reinforced after each of the following activities.
2. Next, relax the jaw. The tongue rests gently on the hard palate behind the front teeth with the jaw slightly open. If the patient has trouble relaxing the jaw, have him or her click the tongue and allow the jaw to drop. Practice until the patient feels the jaw relax and the tongue rest behind the front teeth. Follow with relaxed breathing as in 1.
3. Slowly flex the neck. As the patient does so, direct the attention to the posterior cervical muscles and the sensation of how the muscles feel. Use verbal cues such as, "Notice the feeling of increased tension in your muscles as your head drops forward."
4. Then slowly raise the head to neutral, inhale slowly, and relax. Help the patient position the head properly, and suggest that he or she note how the muscles contract to lift the head, then relax once the head is balanced.
5. Repeat the motion; again direct the patient's attention to the feeling of contraction and relaxation in the muscles as he or she moves. Imagery can be used with the breathing such as "fill your head with air and feel it lift off your shoulders as you breathe in and relax."
6. Then go through only part of the range, noting how the muscles feel.
7. Next, just think of letting the head drop forward, then tightening the muscles (setting); then think of bringing the head back and then relax. Reinforce to the patient the ability to influence the feeling of contraction and relaxation in the muscles.
8. Finally, just think of tensing the muscles and relaxing, letting the tension go out of the muscles even more. Point out that he or she feels even greater relaxation. Once the patient learns to perceive tension in muscles, he or she can then consciously think of relaxing the muscles. Emphasize the fact that the position of the head also influences muscle tension. Have the patient assume various head postures, then correct them until the feel is reinforced.

External Postural Support

Use of support such as a lumbar pillow while sitting or adaptations of a work station should be used to relieve sustained stressful postures.

Education

Demonstrate the relationship of the patient's faulty posture to the development of pain. Have the patient assume the faulty posture and wait until he or she experiences the stress. Direct the patient's attention to the position or activity when the stress or pain is felt, and relate it to the posture. Then show the patient how to relieve the stress by changing postures or by using the techniques already described. Emphasize practicing posture correction procedures and relaxation techniques.

Modalities and Massage

Minimize or decrease use of modalities and massage once acute symptoms are under control so that the patient learns self-management through exercises, relaxation, and posture retraining and does not become dependent on external applications of interventions for comfort.

▶ Functional Training

Goals. The goals of functional training are to use stabilization techniques in all daily activities and safely progress to functional independence.

Note: Functional training underlies the purpose of therapeutic exercise. The patient learns basic techniques, strengthens muscles, and develops flexibility and endurance to be able to safely function in all daily activities including work, recreation, and athletic pursuits.

Early Training—Fundamental Techniques

Early functional training consists of teaching basic maneuvers needed for ADL such as how to safely roll over, go from lying down to sitting (and reverse), and going from sitting to standing (and reverse). These techniques follow the early kinesthetic training instruction in which the patient learns to find his or her neutral spine and experiences the effect that simple arm and leg motions have on spinal position (see page 642) and the effect that the drawing-in maneuver has for activation of the deep spinal stabilizers (see page 657).

1. **Rolling.** Rolling with a neutral spine requires that the patient first find the neutral spine, perform the drawing-in maneuver, and then roll the trunk as a unit. It may be helpful to suggest that the patient "imagine a steel rod connecting the shoulders and pelvis so as not to twist," or to "roll like a log." Encourage the patient to use his or her arms and top leg to assist the roll.
2. **Supine to sit/sit to lying down.** Have the patient use the log roll maneuver (as described above) to roll from supine to side-lying, while simultaneously flexing the hips and knees and pushing up with the arms. Help the patient focus on stabilizing the trunk with commands like "push up your trunk as if it is a board; do not allow it to twist or bend." The reverse is practiced by coaching the patient to lower oneself down to the side-lying position as a unit first onto the elbow and then shoulder. Once down, the patient can roll to supine or prone-lying using the log-roll technique
3. **Sit to stand/stand to sit.** The patient's level of function dictates how much assistance from the upper extremities is needed. If the hip and knee extensors are not strong enough to elevate the body, the patient will need a chair with armrests so there is some leverage for pushing up, or an elevated seat may be necessary. To use the stable spine technique instruct the patient to find the neutral spine, activate the drawing-in maneuver, and then bend forward at the hips while maintaining the neutral spine position. Help the patient focus on the hip motion while keeping the spine "solid like a board." The reverse is also practiced.
4. **In and out of a car.** This sit-to-stand/stand-to-sit maneuver is often symptom-provoking for patients with low back pain. Once sit to stand can be safely performed, have the patient practice the following. Approach the open car door and seat with the back toward the seat, stabilize the spine in its neutral position with the drawing-in maneuver, bend at the hips and sit down. Once seated, flex both hips and knees and pivot the whole body around as a unit, maintaining a stable spine. Similarly when exiting a car, keep both knees together and pivot the legs and trunk outward as a unit. Once the feet are on the ground, bend at the hips and elevate the trunk as a unit.
5. **Walking.** For some patients walking may provoke symptoms. Coach the patient to use the neutral spine and drawing-in maneuvers to stabilize the spine while walking. It is not possible to maintain conscious control for very long, but remind the patient that whenever he or she begins to feel symptoms, to check the spinal posture and reactivate the drawing-in maneuver.

Basic Techniques—Preparation for Functional Activities

Once the patient has learned to manage his or her symptoms with basic mechanics and symptoms of inflammation are diminished, exercises are initiated that prepare the extremities and trunk for functional activities such as safely lifting, carrying, pushing, pulling, and reaching in various directions. Emphasize strengthening the extremities in functional patterns while maintaining a stable spine. The patient should be able to perform IADLs and limited work activities at this stage. Evaluate the patient's performance, and modify what he or she is doing to include safe spinal postures and correct stabilization. Use the activities in this section to prepare for or advance the patient's function.

Many of the strengthening exercises described in the extremity chapters are appropriate to use in preparation for functional training. With postural problems and recovery from back or neck injuries, it is critical to emphasize the neutral (functional) spinal posture before and during total body exercises. Many of the stabilization and movement patterns described earlier in this chapter can also be progressed in intensity, repetitions, speed, and coordination to prepare for return to functional activities.

Modified Bridging Exercises

These exercises require stabilization of the trunk flexors and extensors in conjunction with strengthening the gluteus maximus and quadriceps muscles. The abdominals function with the gluteus maximus to control the pelvic tilt, and the lumbar extensors stabilize the spine against the pull of the gluteus maximus.

Patient position and procedure: Begin with the patient hook-lying. Have the patient concentrate on maintaining the neutral spinal position while raising and lowering the pelvis, by flexing and extending at the hips (see Fig. 12–13).

- Hold the bridge for isometric control.
- Alternate arm motions; progress by adding weights to the hands.
- Alternate lifting one foot, then the other by marching in place (Fig. 16–44*A*); progress by extending the knee as each leg is lifted. When the patient tolerates greater resistance, add ankle weights and arm motions (Fig. 16–44*B*).

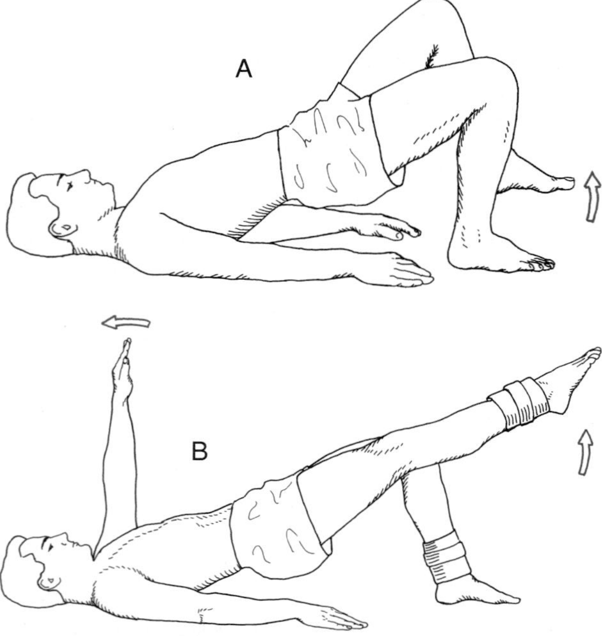

Figure 16–44 Holding a bridge to develop trunk control and gluteus maximus strength while superimposing extremity motions: *(A)* marching in place, *(B)* progressing to extending the extremities. Adding weights to the arms or legs requires greater strength and control.

- Abduct and adduct the thighs without letting the pelvis sag. Progress by placing the feet on a stool, chair, or large gym ball and repeating the bridging activities.

Push-Ups with Trunk Stabilization

Patient position and procedure: Begin prone on a large gym ball. Have the patient walk forward with the hands on the floor until just the thighs are supported by the ball, maintain a stable spinal posture, and perform push-ups with the arms. To progress, walk out farther with the hands until just the legs are supported by the ball (Fig. 16–45).

Wall Slides

These exercises develop strength in the hip and knee extensor muscles to prepare the lower extremities for squatting activities and training in safe body mechanics.

Patient position and procedure: Standing with the back to a wall and the spine held in its neutral position. Place a towel behind the back so it slides easier along the wall. The exercise is more challenging if a large gym ball is placed between the back and the wall (see Fig. 12–16). Have the patient slide his or her back down the wall into a partial squat and hold the position for isometric strengthening of the hip and knee extensors, or move up and down for concentric/eccentric strengthening.

- Superimpose arm motions such as alternating or bilateral shoulder flexion/extension.
- Use handheld weights to add resistance for upper and lower extremity strengthening.

Partial Lunges and Partial Squats

These exercises are described in Chapters 12 (see Fig. 12–16) and 13. They are beneficial for strength-

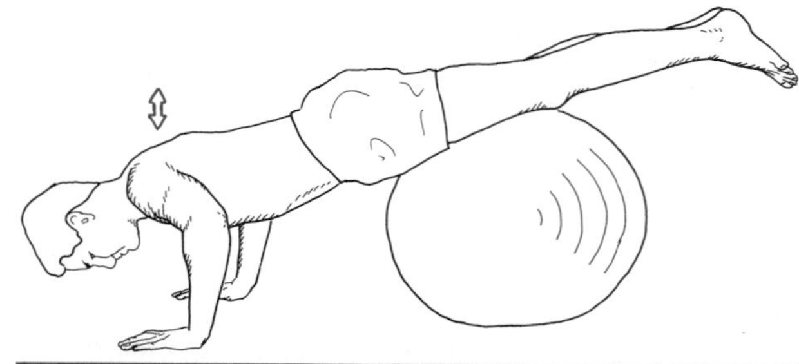

Figure 16–45 Push-up activities with the lower extremities balanced on a gym ball for strengthening the arms and developing trunk control.

ening total body movement in preparation for teaching body mechanics. Add weights to the upper extremities for resistance. Progress by adding arm motions that are synchronized with the leg motions, such as reaching forward and downward to develop coordination and control.

Walking Against Resistance

Secure a weighted pulley or elastic resistance around the patient's pelvis with a belt, or the patient can hold the handles. Have the patient walk forward, backward, or diagonally against the resistive force. Emphasis is placed on spinal control (see Fig. 12–17).

Progress by having the patient push and pull weighted objects, such as a cart or a box on a table; place emphasis on maintaining a stable spinal position while the extremities are loaded (see Figs. 9–43 and 10–16*A*).

Shifting Weight and Turning

Have the patient practice shifting weight forward/backward and side to side while maintaining the neutral spinal position and absorbing the forces with the hips and knees. Practice turning using small steps and rotating at the hips rather than the back. Instruct the patient to imagine two rigid poles connecting each shoulder to each hip that do not allow the spine to twist. Progress by using weights.

Transitional Stabilization Activities

The patient learns to stabilize the spine against alternating trunk motions.

- *Patient position and procedure:* Begin quadruped. Have the patient rock back to rest the buttocks on the heels, then shift the body forward onto the hands in the press-up position. The patient concentrates on controlling the pelvis in its neutral position rather than allowing full spinal flexion when shifting toward the heels or full spinal extension when shifting forward toward the press-up position.
- *Patient position and procedure:* Begin standing. Have the patient reach downward while partially squatting. The tendency is for the spine to flex, so have the patient concentrate on maintaining a neutral spinal position with the spinal extensors. He or she then stands up and reaches overhead. This causes the spine to extend; have the patient concentrate on using the trunk flexors to stabilize in the neutral position. Progress by lifting weights while controlling the neutral posture of the spine.

Body Mechanics

Have the patient practice lifting by squatting down to the object, bringing the object close to the body, positioning the spine in a functional or neutral position, activating the drawing-in maneuver, and then lifting with the hip and knee extensors. Under some circumstances, an individual may be more stable lifting with a lunge technique rather than the squat technique.

The position of the lumbar spine, whether it is flexed, extended, or in midrange, raises several issues. Of the three postures lifting with a neutral spinal posture provides greater stability to the spine[8] and uses both the ligamentous and muscular system to stabilize and control.[31] After a back injury, the preferred lifting posture may have to be adapted, depending on the type of injury and the response of the tissues when stressed.[31]

- When lifting with a flexed lumbar spine (posterior pelvic tilt), support for the spine is primarily from inert structures (ligaments, lumbodorsal fasciae, posterior annulus fibrosus, and facets); there is little muscle activity.
  - This posture may be necessary when stooping to the floor. It may also be the posture of choice for a patient who has injured the back muscles because the muscles are "quiet" when the spine is in flexion.[31]
  - Lifting with the lumbar spine in flexion may pose some problems. When lifting slowly with a flexed spine, the load is maintained on the ligaments, and creep of the inert tissues occurs; this increases the chance of injury if the tissue is already weakened. In addition, with the muscles lengthened and relaxed, they may be at an unfavorable length-tension relationship to quickly respond with appropriate force to resist a sudden change in load. There is greater chance of ligamentous strain when a person lifts with a flexed spine.[10]
- When lifting with an extended (lordotic) lumbar spine, the muscles supporting the spine are more active, which increases the compressive forces on the disk. This posture relieves stress on the ligaments, but for an individual whose back muscles are in poor condition and fatigue quickly, this posture may jeopardize the spine when repeated lifts are performed because the ligaments are not taut and, thus, are not providing support.[31]

Have the patient practice carrying objects close to his or her center of gravity so he or she can feel the balance. When lifting, the closer the object is held to the center of gravity, the less stress is placed on the structures of the back and hip.

Have the patient practice shifting the load from side to side and turning. The action should be directed by the legs while the spine is kept stable with minimal trunk rotation.

Replicate the mechanics of the patient's job setting and practice safe mechanics.

Education for Prevention

- Review the following principles:
  - Avoid any one posture for prolonged periods. If sustained postures are necessary, take frequent breaks and perform appropriate ROM exercises at least every half hour. Finish all exercises by assuming a well-balanced posture.
  - Avoid hyperextending the neck or being in a forward-head posture or forward-bent position for prolonged periods. Find ways to modify a task so it can be accomplished at eye level or with proper lumbar support.
  - If in a tension-producing situation, perform conscious relaxation exercises.
  - Use common sense and follow good safety habits.
- Review flexibility and strengthening exercises appropriate for the patient to maintain adequate ROM and develop adequate strength for good physical conditioning.
- Review the relationship of posture and pain; when experiencing pain, check posture.

Adapt Environment

- Modify the patient's work and home environment.
  - Chairs and car seats should have lumbar support to maintain a slight lordosis. Use a towel roll or lumbar pillow if necessary.
  - Chair height should allow knees to flex to take the pull off the hamstring muscles, support the thighs, and also allow the feet to rest comfortably on the floor.
  - Desk or table height should be adequate to keep the person from having to lean over the work.
  - Work and driving habits should allow frequent changing of posture. If normally sedentary, get up and walk every hour.
- Modify the patient's sleeping environment.
  - Mattress needs to provide firm support to prevent any extreme stresses. If it is too soft, the patient sags and stresses ligaments; if it is too firm, some patients cannot relax.
  - Pillows should be of a comfortable height and density to promote relaxation but should not place joints at an extreme position. Foam rubber pillows tend to cause increased tension in muscles because of the constant resistance they provide.
  - Whether the person should sleep prone, side-lying, or supine is something that must be analyzed for each individual patient. Ideally, a comfortable posture is one that is in the midrange and that does not place stress on any supporting structure. Pain that occurs in the morning is often related to sleeping posture; so, if this is the case, listen carefully to the patient's description of postures when sleeping and see if it relates to the pain. Then attempt to modify the sleep position accordingly.

Intermediate to Advanced Progression

As the patient learns spinal control while doing the exercises, repetitions are increased to develop muscular endurance, and resistance is added to develop strength. If speed and balance are required, these are emphasized. By this stage it is recognized that the individual already knows the basic spinal stabilization techniques and is habitually assuming the neutral spinal position and activating the drawing-in maneuver. Reinforce the importance of this when doing the following activities. It is also recognized that the patient should be able to control greater spinal ROM without experiencing symptoms. Adapt the exercises to replicate return to work or sport-related activities. Examples follow.

Repetitive lifting. The ability to do repetitive lifting throughout the workday is necessary for many jobs and may result in recurrence of symptoms. To prepare for returning to work, progressively increase the repetitions of lifting activities the patient must do to improve muscle endurance. Marras and Granta[17] demonstrated that with repetitive lifting (over a 5-hour period) subjects had a significant change in their lifting pattern and in the muscle recruitment patterns so that there was a decrease in spine stabilization (decreased compression) and an increase in anterior/posterior shear in the lumbar spine. To reduce the risk of recurrence of low back disorders, a patient needs to learn to monitor these changes and be conscious of correcting faulty patterns. Help the patient modify and adapt the stable spine body mechanics that were initiated under basic techniques are adapted to replicate the type of lifting he or she will be doing at home or on the job. Include variations in the lifting tasks to prepare for unexpected situations.

Repetitive reaching. These activities require that the patient learn to assume a comfortable stride and then practice shifting his or her weight forward and backward on the lower extremities rather than bending forward and backward with the spine. Preparatory exercises should include partial lunging forward, sideways, and backward. During practice have the patient use a weight comparable to the real-life situation and go through the action on a repetitive basis, concentrating on spinal control and resting only when control is no longer possible.

Repetitive pushing and pulling. These activities require strong upper extremities and a stable spine. Preparatory activities should include pushing and pulling against elastic resistance or pulley resistance set at heights that replicate the work environment. Progress to pushing and pulling a weighted cart or a weighted box across a table. Reinforce the importance of activating the spinal stabilizers.

Rotation or turning. Turning with a load is a component of most work activity. A person may rotate the spine to reach around to place a load to the side or behind. Rotation may create an unstable situation or may be damaging to the spinal structures. Therefore, it is important to take the rotation out of turning. Have the patient practice a "stable spine turn," which requires motion and control in the hips, or taking steps into the direction of the turn rather than twisting and rotating the back.

Transitioning. Most functional activities require *transitional motions* such as reaching downward to pick up something (spinal flexion), then reaching overhead to place it on a high shelf (spinal extension). Or in sports activities the activity may require moving quickly from a forward-bent position to an extended position with arms overhead (such as dribbling a basketball then shooting). Set up drills that replicate whatever motions are necessary and have the patient practice moving through the patterns while attempting to maintain control of his or her functional spinal position and range.

Transfer of training. Ideally each patient is progressed through rehabilitation to the level of being able to *transfer skills* learned to closely related but new situations. To prepare, provide new learning opportunities for the patient and then assist the patient in analyzing successful adaptations to the new experience.

Independent Learning Activities

CRITICAL THINKING AND DISCUSSION

1. Observe a homemaker or worker doing an activity requiring pushing, pulling, reaching, lifting, or some other repetitive pattern. Analyze what component motions are part of the total pattern and decide if strength, range, endurance, balance, coordination (or a combination) is necessary in the upper extremities, lower extremities, and trunk. Decide what is necessary to make the spine safe while doing this activity, and design an exercise program that encompasses all the components.
2. Go to a health club or exercise class and observe how individuals are performing the exercises. Note which activities cause stress to the spine. How would you modify each exercise? Consider safe use of the equipment, safe biomechanics, and appropriate instruction for the audience. Can you tell the purpose of each exercise (strength, stretch, endurance)? Are the directions appropriately given for the level of participants?
3. Identify and compare the similarities and differences in flexibility and muscle weakness between a person with excessive lumbar lordosis and an anterior pelvic tilt and a person with a slouched posture who stands with the pelvis shifted forward and the thorax flexed. What effect does each pelvic posture have on the hip position, and what muscles would develop restricted mobility? Usually in the slouched posture the thorax and upper lumbar spine are flexed; would the curl-up exercise be beneficial or would it contribute to this problem? Develop an exercise program that addresses the common flexibility and strength impairments without reinforcing the faulty posture.

LABORATORY PRACTICE

1. With a laboratory partner practice the kinesthetic training techniques and core stabilization techniques until you become proficient at performing them and recognizing when they are done

correctly. Then practice teaching them to a family member or friend, and see how well they understand what they are to do.

2. Practice the progression of spinal stabilization exercises described on pages 658 to 663. Start at the easiest level and progress the leg and arm movements until you feel you are at your maximum resistance for stabilization. After resting, time yourself for 1 minute, beginning at the most difficult level of movement. The idea is to keep the spine stable during the entire minute. If you begin to feel you are losing control, decrease the amount of extremity resistance (e.g., going from moving both lower extremities in a reciprocal pattern to moving just one extremity while the other is on the floor). This can also be done for 3 minutes. Were you able to meet the challenge yet keep the spine stable? Did you feel your stabilizing muscles "working?"
3. Practice doing wall slides, partial squats, and partial lunges with a stable spine. When you can do the squat comfortably with a stable spine, practice lifting a box from the floor to table height, then from the floor to shoulder height, and then place it on a shelf at each height. Feel what is happening to your spine. Then repeat the maneuvers with a stable spine, and see if you can control the spinal position with the drawing-in maneuver. When you can do the lunge comfortably, practice lifting small objects from the floor with a lunging technique and stable spine. Finally, practice lifting objects from the floor and turning (using legs and hips to change direction, not spinal rotation) to place the objects on a table or shelf. Feel what is happening to the spine, and repeat doing the activities with a stable spinal posture.

CASE STUDIES

Review the cases described in Chapter 15.

Case 1

Your patient is a 35-year-old computer programmer who is referred to you because of pain symptoms in the right cervical, posterior shoulder, and arm regions as well as discomfort from frequent tension headaches. The symptoms get progressively worse when at work; usually the pain begins within 1 hour and it is 6/10 by lunchtime. The same cycle occurs in the afternoon. There is occasional "tingling" in the thumb and index finger. The symptoms have progressively worsened over the last 3 months, ever since being placed on a priority job. Recreational activities include tennis and reading; the tennis does not cause symptoms, but reading makes the headaches worse.

Examination reveals forward-head and round shoulder posture. Capital flexion 50% range, cervical rotation and side bending are each 80% range, shoulder external rotation is 75 degrees. Restricted flexibility in the pectoralis major, pectoralis minor, levator scapulae, and scalene muscles. Cervical quadrant test reproduces the tingling in the right hand; all other neurologic tests are negative. Strength of the suprahyoid and infrahyoid muscles, scapular retractors, and shoulder lateral rotators is 4/5.

- What is provoking the patient's symptoms and signs? What are the functional limitations? What is the prognosis?
- Identify impairment and functional outcome goals.
- Establish a program of intervention. How will you progress this person to functional independence?

Case 2

A 51-year-old auto mechanic is referred to physical therapy because of pain symptoms in the left buttock and posterior thigh. The symptoms are worse when standing and reaching overhead for more than 15 minutes, which is what he does when working on a car that is up on the racks. Carrying heavy objects (greater than 50 lb), standing and walking for more than 1/2 hour increase the symptoms. There is no precipitating incident, but the symptoms have been recurrent over the past year. Symptoms also increase with the recreational activity of backpacking. Symptoms ease when in the rocker recliner, laying on a couch with knees bent, or when hugging knees to chest.

Examination reveals: sway back posture when standing; decreased flexibility in the low back, gluteus maximus, hamstrings (SLR to 60 degrees), and upper abdominals; increased pain with backward bending. Strength of lower abdominals is 3/5. Able to do repetitive lunges and partial squats for maximum of 20 seconds.

- What is provoking the patient's symptoms and signs? What are the functional limitations? What is the prognosis?
- Identify impairment and functional outcome goals.
- Establish a program of intervention. How will you progress this person to functional independence?

REFERENCES

1. Abdulwahab, SS: Treatment based on H-reflexes testing improves disability status in patients with cervical radiculopathy. Int J Rehabil Res 22(3):207, 1999.
2. Alexander, KM, and Kinney LaPier, TL: Differences in static balance and weight distribution between normal subjects and subjects with chronic unilateral low back pain. J Orthop Sports Phys Ther 28(6):378, 1998.
3. Blount, WP, and Moe, JH. The Milwaukee Brace. Williams & Wilkins, Baltimore, 1980.
4. Bondi, BA, and Drinkwater-Kolk, M: Functional stabilization training. Workshop notes, Northeast Seminars, October 1992.
5. Cassella, MC, and Hall, JE: Current treatment approaches in the nonoperative and operative management of adolescent idiopathic scoliosis. Phys Ther 71:897, 1991.
6. Chok, B, et al: Endurance training of the trunk extensor muscles in people with subacute low back pain. Phys Ther 79(11):1033, 1999.
7. Hagins, M, et al: Effects of practice on the ability to perform lumbar stabilization exercises. J Orthop Sports Phys Ther 29(9):546, 1999.
8. Hart, DL, Stobbe, TJ, and Jaraiedi, M: Effect of lumbar posture on lifting. Spine 12:22, 1987.
9. Hides, JA, Richardson, CA, and Gwendolen, AJ: Multifidus muscle recovery is not automatic after resolution of acute, first-episode low back pain. Spine 21 (23):2763, 1996.
10. Hodges, PW, Richardson, CA, and Jull, G: Evaluation of the relationship between laboratory and clinical tests of transversus abdominis function. Physiother Res Internat 1(1):30, 1996.
11. Hodges, PW, and Richardson, CA: Contraction of the abdominal muscles associated with movement of the lower limb. Phys Ther 77(2):132, 1997.
12. Hodges, PW, and Richardson, CA: Delayed postural contraction of transversus abdominis in low back pain associated with movement of the lower limb. J Spinal Disorders 11(1):46, 1998.
13. Jull, GA, and Richardson, CA: Rehabilitation of Active Stabilization of the Lumbar Spine. In Twomy, LT, and Taylor (eds): Physical Therapy of the Lumbar Spine, ed 2. Churchill Livingstone, New York, 1994.
14. Kendall, F, McCreary, E, and Provance, PG: Muscles: Testing and Function, ed 4. Williams & Wilkins, Baltimore, 1993.
15. Lubell, A: Potentially dangerous exercises: Are they harmful to all? Phys Sports Med 17:187, 1989.
16. McGill, SM: Low back exercises: evidence for improving exercise regimens. Phys Ther 78(7):754, 1998.
17. Marras, WS, and Granata, KP: Changes in trunk dynamics and spine loading during repeated trunk exertions. Spine 22(21):2564, 1997.
18. Morgan, D: Concepts in functional training and postural stabilization for the low-back injured. Topics in Acute Care and Trauma Rehabilitation 2:8, 1988.
19. Nachemson, A: Recent advances in the treatment of low back pain. Int Orthop 9:1, 1985.
20. O'Sullivan, PT, Twomey, L, and Allison, GT: Altered abdominal muscle recruitment in patients with chronic back pain following a specific exercise intervention. J Orthop Sports Phys Ther 27(2):114, 1998.
21. O'Sullivan, P, Twomey, L, Allison, G, et al: Altered patterns of abdominal muscle activation in patients with chronic low back pain. Austral Physiother 43(2):91, 1997.
22. Parris, S: Spinal Dysfunction: Etiology and Treatment of Dysfunction Including Joint Manipulation. Manual of Course Notes, Atlanta, 1979.
23. Richardson, C, Jull, G, et al: Techniques for active lumbar stabilisation for spinal protection: A pilot study. Austral J Physiother 38:105, 1992.
24. Richardson, C, and Jull, G: An historical perspective on the development of clinical techniques to evaluate and treat the active stabilising system of the lumbar spine. Austral J Physiother Monograph 1:5, 1995.
25. Richardson, C, Toppenberg, R, and Jull, G: An initial evaluation of eight abdominal exercises for their ability to provide stabilisation for the lumbar spine. Austral J Physiother 36:6, 1990.
26. Robinson, R: The new back school prescription: Stabilization training part I. Occup Med 7:17, 1992.
27. Saal, JA: The new back school prescription: Stabilization training part II. Occup Med 7:33, 1992.
28. Saal, JA: Dynamic muscular stabilization in the nonoperative treatment of lumbar pain syndromes. Orthop Rev 19:691, 1990.
29. Saunders, HD: Spinal traction. In Saunders, HD: Evaluation, Treatment and Prevention of Musculoskeletal Disorders. Viking, Minneapolis, 1985.
30. Stevans, J, and Hall, KG: Motor skill acquisition strategies for rehabilitation of low back pain. J Orthop Sports Phys Ther 28(3):165, 1998.
31. Sullivan, MS: Back support mechanisms during manual lifting. Phys Ther 69:38, 1989.
32. Sweeney, T: Neck school: Cervicothoracic stabilization training. Occup Med 7:43, 1992.
33. Vera-Garcia, FJ, Grenier, SG, and McGill, SM: Abdominal muscle response during curl-ups on both stable and labile surfaces. Phys Ther 80(6):564, 2000.
34. Wohlfahrt, D, Jull, G, and Richardson, C: The relationship between the dynamic and static function of abdominal muscles. Austral J Physiother 39:9, 1993.

Part III

Special Areas of Therapeutic Exercise

Chapter 17

Principles of Exercise for the Obstetric Patient

Barb Settles Huge, BS, PT · Carolyn Kisner, MS, PT

OBJECTIVES

After studying this chapter, the reader will be able to:

1 Identify and describe the major stages and characteristics of pregnancy, labor, and delivery.

2 Describe the normal physiologic changes of pregnancy in the organ systems and musculoskeletal system.

3 Describe the common postural adjustments to pregnancy.

4 Define diastasis recti and its significance in pregnancy.

5 Describe the examination procedure for diastasis recti and corrective exercise for the condition.

6 Identify other pathologies of the musculoskeletal system related to pregnancy.

7 Describe the structure, function, and significance of the pelvic floor.

8 Explain risk factors for pelvic floor dysfunction.

9 Describe rehabilitation techniques for the pelvic floor.

10 Develop goals and guidelines for an obstetric exercise program in an uncomplicated pregnancy.

11 Explain absolute and possible contraindications to exercise in pregnancy.

12 Establish and/or modify a safe therapeutic exercise program that addresses the changes of pregnancy and aids in preparation for labor.

13 Describe the maternal and fetal responses to exercise.

14 Define cesarean childbirth and high-risk pregnancy.

15 Identify exercise and rehabilitative goals for cesarean and high-risk situations.

16 Describe modifications or additions to exercise programs for the cesarean childbirth or high-risk pregnancy.

During and after pregnancy, female clients present a unique challenge for the physical therapist. Pregnancy is a time of tremendous musculoskeletal, physical, and emotional change and yet, it is a condition of wellness. These women are typically well motivated, willing to learn, and highly responsive to treatment suggestions. For many women, the therapist is able to assess and monitor the physical changes with the primary focus on maintaining wellness. The therapist is also able to examine and treat the client with specific musculoskeletal impairments by incorporating knowledge of injury and tissue healing with knowledge of the changes during pregnancy. In addition, the pregnant woman can be educated, perhaps for the first time, regarding the role of the pelvic floor muscles in musculoskeletal health. This specialized area of treatment in women's health is enjoying great growth within physical therapy. Although all physical therapists can fairly easily incorporate activation of the pelvic floor as a component of trunk strengthening into an exercise program, true expertise can only come with advanced training and mentoring.

This chapter provides the reader with basic information about the physical changes of pregnancy as a foundation for the development of safe and effective exercise programs. The chapter also discusses modification of general exercises to meet the needs of the obstetric client, provides information to assist in the development of an exercise program for an uncomplicated pregnancy, and describes exercises for maintaining pelvic floor health. The ability to educate women about the role of exercise and health promotion provides a significant professional opportunity and responsibility. Cesarean delivery, high-risk pregnancy, and the special needs of clients with these conditions are discussed separately.

Overview of Pregnancy, Labor, and Delivery

Pregnancy

Pregnancy, which spans 40 weeks from conception to delivery, is divided into three trimesters. There are characteristic changes during each trimester.[4,21,41]

Changes During the First Trimester: Weeks 0 Through 12 of Pregnancy

- Implantation of the fertilized ovum in the uterus occurs 7 to 10 days after fertilization.
- The mother may be nauseated or may vomit, is very fatigued, and will urinate more frequently.
- The breast size may increase.
- There is a relatively small weight gain of 0 to 1455 g (0–3 lb is normal).
- Emotional changes may occur.
- By the end of the 12th week, the fetus is 6 to 7 cm long and weighs approximately 20 g (2 oz). The fetus now can kick, turn its head, and swallow and has a beating heart, but these movements are not yet felt by the mother.

Changes During the Second Trimester: Weeks 13 Through 26 of Pregnancy

- The pregnancy now becomes visible to others.
- The mother begins to feel movement at around 20 weeks.
- During this trimester, most women feel very good. Nausea and fatigue have usually disappeared.
- By the end of the second trimester, the fetus is 19 to 23 cm (14 inches) in length and weighs approximately 600 g (1–2 lb).
- The fetus now has eyebrows, eyelashes, and fingernails.

Change During the Third Trimester: Weeks 27 Through 40 of Pregnancy (38–42 Weeks Is Considered Full Term)

- The uterus is now very large and has regular contractions, although these may only occasionally be felt.
- Common complaints during the third trimester are frequent urination, back pain, leg edema and fatigue, round ligament pain, shortness of breath, and constipation.
- By the time of birth, the baby will be 33 to 39 cm long (16–19 inches) and will weigh approximately 3400 g (7 lb, although a range of 5–10 lb is normal).

Labor

Labor is divided into three stages with specific events occurring in each stage.[5,39,42] The exact mechanism for labor induction is not known. Regular and strong involuntary contractions of the smooth muscles of the uterus are the primary symptom of labor. True labor produces palpable changes in the cervix, which are known as effacement and dilation.[42]

- *Effacement* is the shortening or thinning of the cervix from a thickness of 5 cm, or 2 inches, before onset of labor to the thickness of a piece of paper (Fig. 17–1)
- *Dilation* is the opening of the cervix from the diameter of a fingertip to approximately 10 cm, or 4 inches (Fig. 17–1)

Labor: Stage 1

This is the cervical dilation and effacement stage. At the end of this stage, the cervix is fully dilated and the baby is ready to be expelled from the uterus. Stage 1 of labor is divided into three major phases.

1. **Cervical dilation phase.** The cervix dilates from 0 to 3 cm (0–1 inch) and will almost completely efface. Uterine contractions occur from the top down, causing the cervix to open and pushing the fetus downward.

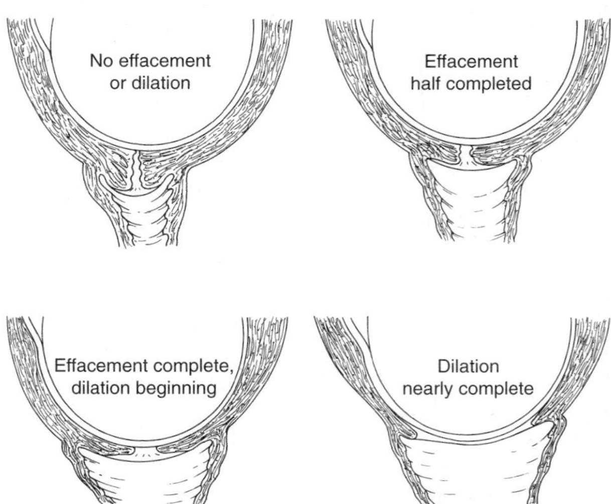

Figure 17–1 Effacement and dilation of the cervix. (From Sandberg,[42] p 192, with permission.)

2. **Middle phase.** The cervix dilates from 4 to 7 cm (1–3 inches). Contractions are stronger and more regular.
3. **Transition phase.** The cervix dilates from 8 to 10 cm (3–4 inches) and dilation is complete. Uterine contractions are very strong and close together.

Labor: Stage 2 (Expulsion of the Fetus—"Pushing")

Intra-abdominal pressure is the primary force expelling the fetus. This pressure is produced by voluntary contraction of the abdominals and diaphragm. Relaxation and stretching of the pelvic floor during stage 2 is also necessary for successful vaginal delivery.

1. **Fetal descent.** Position changes (cardinal movements) by the fetus allow it to pass through the pelvis and be born (Fig. 17–2).

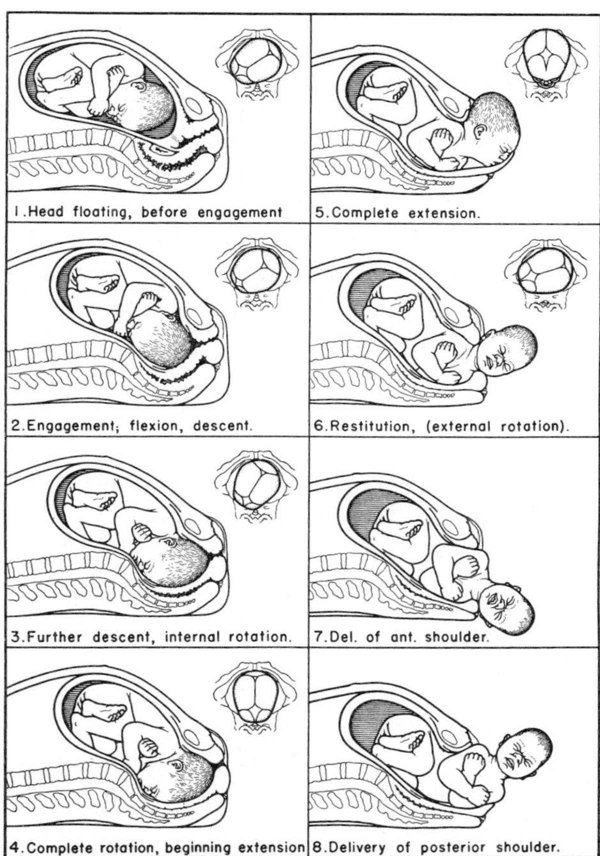

Figure 17–2 Principal movements in the mechanism of labor and delivery, left occiput anterior position. (From Pritchard, J, and MacDonald, P,[40] with permission.)

- ***Engagement.*** The greatest transverse diameter of the fetal head passes through the pelvic inlet (the superior opening of the minor pelvis).
- ***Descent.*** Continued downward progression of the fetus occurs.
- ***Flexion.*** The fetal chin is brought closer to its thorax; this occurs when the descending head meets resistance from the walls and floor of the pelvis and the cervix.
- ***Internal rotation.*** The fetus turns its occiput toward the mother's symphysis pubis when the fetal head reaches the level of the ischial spines.
- ***Extension.*** The flexed fetal head reaches the vulva; the fetus extends its head, bringing the base of the occiput in direct contact with the inferior margin of the maternal symphysis pubis; this phase ends when the fetal head is delivered.
- ***External rotation.*** The fetus rotates its occiput toward the mother's sacrum to allow the fetal shoulders to pass through the pelvis.

2. **Expulsion.** The fetal anterior shoulder passes under the symphysis pubis, and the rest of the body follows.

Labor: Stage 3

1. **Placental stage (expulsion of the placenta)**

- The uterus continues to contract and shrink following delivery; as the uterus decreases in size, the placenta detaches from the uterine wall, blood vessels are constricted, and bleeding slows. This can occur 5 to 30 minutes after fetal expulsion.
- A hematoma forms over the uterine placental site to prevent further significant blood loss; mild bleeding persists for 3 to 6 weeks after delivery.

2. **Uterine involution.** The uterus continues to contract and decrease in size for 3 to 6 weeks after delivery; the uterus always remains a bit enlarged over its prepregnant size.

Anatomical and Physiologic Changes of Pregnancy

Considerable changes occur in the woman's body as the pregnancy progresses.*

Pregnancy Weight Gain

Current recommendations for weight gain during pregnancy are an average of 25 to 27 lb[46] with a distribution as shown in Box 17–1.

*See references 4–6, 26, 34, 37, 39, 41, 46, 48.

Box 17–1 Total Weight Gain (Ranges) for Single Fetus

Fetus	*3.36–3.88 kg*	*(7.5–8.0 lb)*
Placenta	*0.48–0.72 kg*	*(1.0–1.5 lb)*
Amniotic fluid	*0.72–0.97 kg*	*(1.5–2.0 lb)*
Uterus and breasts	*2.42–2.66 kg*	*(5.0–5.5 lb)*
Blood and fluid	*1.94–3.99 kg*	*(4.0–7.0 lb)*
Muscle and fat	*0.48–2.91 kg*	*(1.0–6.0 lb)*
Total:	*9.70–14.55 kg*	*(20.0–30.0 lb)*

Organ Systems

Pelvic Viscera, Fasciae, and Ligaments

- The uterus increases from a prepregnant size of 5 by 10 cm (2 by 4 inches) to 25 by 36 cm (10 by 14 inches). It increases five to six times in size, 3000 to 4000 times in capacity, and 20 times in weight by the end of pregnancy. By the end of pregnancy, each muscle cell in the uterus has increased approximately 10 times its length prior to pregnancy.[48]
- Once the uterus expands upward and leaves the pelvis, it becomes an abdominal organ rather than a pelvic organ.
- Ligaments connected to the pelvic organs are more fibroelastic than ligaments supporting joint structures. The fascial tissues, which surround and enclose the organs in a continuous sheet, also include a significant amount of smooth muscle fibers.[14] The round, broad, and uterosacral ligaments in particular provide suspensory support for the uterus.

Urinary System

- The kidneys increase in length by 1 cm (0.5 inch).
- The ureters enter the bladder at a perpendicular angle because of uterine enlargement. This may result in a reflux of urine out of the bladder and back into the ureter; therefore, there is an increased chance of developing urinary tract infections in pregnancy because of urinary stasis.

Pulmonary System

- Edema and tissue congestion of the upper respiratory tract occur early in pregnancy because of hormonal changes. There is upper respiratory hypersecretion (hormonally stimulated).
- Changes in rib position are hormonally stimulated and occur prior to uterine enlargement. The subcostal angle progressively increases; the ribs flare up and out. The anteroposterior and transverse chest diameters each increase by 2 cm (1 inch). Total chest circumference increases by 5 to 7 cm (2–3 inches) and does not always return to the prepregnant state.
- The diaphragm is elevated by 4 cm (1.5 inch); this is a passive change caused by the change in rib position.
- The respiration rate is unchanged, but the depth of respiration increases.[39]
- Tidal volume and minute ventilation increase, but total lung capacity is unchanged or slightly decreased.[39,48]
- There is a 15 to 20% increase in oxygen consumption; a natural state of hyperventilation exists throughout pregnancy. This occurs to meet the oxygen demands of pregnancy.[39,48]
- The work of breathing increases because of hyperventilation; dyspnea is present with mild exercise as early as 20 weeks into the pregnancy.[39,48]

Cardiovascular System

- Blood volume progressively increases 35 to 50% (1.5–2 liters) throughout pregnancy and returns to normal by 6 to 8 weeks after pregnancy.
- Plasma increase is greater than red blood cell increase, leading to "physiologic anemia" of pregnancy, which is not a true anemia but is representative of the greater increase of plasma volume. The increase in plasma volume occurs as a result of hormonal stimulation to meet the oxygen demands of pregnancy.
- Venous pressure in the lower extremities increases when standing as a result of increased uterine size and increased venous distensibility.
- Pressure in the inferior vena cava rises in late pregnancy, especially in the supine position, because of compression by the uterus just below the diaphragm. In some women, the decline in venous return and resulting decrease in cardiac output may lead to *symptomatic supine hypotensive syndrome.*[16] The aorta is partially occluded in the supine position.
- The heart size increases, and the heart is elevated because of the movement of the diaphragm.
- Heart rhythm disturbances are more common in pregnancy.
- Heart rate usually increases 10 to 20 beats per minute by full term and returns to normal levels within 6 weeks after pregnancy.
- Cardiac output increases 30 to 60% in pregnancy and is most significantly increased when in the left side-lying position. In this position, the uterus places the least pressure on the aorta.

- Blood pressure decreases early in the first trimester. There is a slight decrease of systolic pressure and a greater decrease of diastolic pressure. Blood pressure reaches its lowest level approximately midway through pregnancy, then rises gradually from midpregnancy to reach the prepregnant level approximately 6 weeks after delivery. Although cardiac output increases, blood pressure decreases because of venous distensibility.

Musculoskeletal System

- Abdominal muscles are stretched to the point of their elastic limit by the end of pregnancy. This greatly decreases the muscles' ability to generate a strong contraction and, thus, decreases their efficiency of contraction. The shift in the center of gravity also decreases the mechanical advantage of the abdominal muscles.[48]
- Hormonal influence on the ligaments is profound, producing a systemic decrease in ligamentous tensile strength. This change is primarily a result of change in relaxin and progesterone levels.[46]
- Joint hypermobility occurs as a result of ligamentous laxity and may predispose the patient to joint and ligamentous injury, especially in the weight-bearing joints of the back, pelvis, and lower extremities.
- The pelvic floor muscles must withstand the weight of the uterus; the pelvic floor drops as much as 2.5 cm (1 inch).[37]
- The pelvic floor may be stretched, torn, or incised during the birth process. *Episiotomy* is the term used for an incision made in the perineal body (see Fig. 17–5). It is automatically considered a second-degree laceration by the following classification of perineal lacerations:[40]
  1st degree—only skin
  2nd degree—includes underlying muscle
  3rd degree—extends to anal sphincter
  4th degree—tears into the rectum
- Stretch and compression of the pudendal nerve occurs as the baby's head travels through the birth canal. This compromise to the pudendal nerve is most intense during pushing (the second stage of labor). As a result, the pelvic floor is vulnerable from both a muscular and a neurologic perspective during labor and vaginal delivery.

Thermoregulatory System

- During pregnancy, basal metabolic rate and heat production increase.[16] An increase of 300 kilocalories per day is needed to meet the basic metabolic needs of pregnancy.
- The fasting blood glucose level in pregnant women normally is lower than in nonpregnant women.[16]

Posture and Balance Changes

Center of Gravity

The center of gravity shifts upward and forward because of the enlargement of the uterus and breasts. This requires postural compensations for balance and stability.[30,37,48]

- The shoulder girdle and upper back become rounded with scapular protraction and upper extremity internal rotation because of breast enlargement and postpartum positioning for infant care. Tightness of the pectoralis muscles and weakness of the scapular stabilizers also contributes to this postural change.
- Cervical lordosis increases in the upper cervical spine, and forward-head posture develops to compensate for the shoulder alignment.
- Lumbar lordosis increases to compensate for the shift in the center of gravity, and the knees hyperextend, probably because of the change in the line of gravity.
- Weight shifts toward the heels to bring the center of gravity to a more posterior position.
- Changes in posture do not usually correct spontaneously after childbirth, and the pregnant posture may be maintained as a learned posture. Many child-care activities can also perpetuate faulty posture.

Balance

With the increased weight and redistribution of body mass there are compensations to maintain balance.[37,48]

- The woman usually walks with a wider base of support and increased external rotation at the hips.
- Some activities such as walking, stooping, stair climbing, lifting, and reaching become difficult.
- Some activities requiring fine balance and rapid changes in direction, such as aerobic dancing and bicycle riding, may become inadvisable, especially during the third trimester.

▶ Pregnancy-Induced Pathology

Diastasis Recti

Definition

Diastasis recti is separation of the rectus abdominis muscles in the midline at the linea alba. The etiology of pathology is unknown, but the continuity of the abdominal wall is disrupted (Fig. 17–3). Any separation larger than 2 cm or 2 fingerwidths is considered significant.[3,30]

Incidence

- The condition is not exclusive to childbearing women but is seen frequently in this population. In a study done by Boissonnault and Blaschak,[3] 89 women were tested for separation of the rectus abdominis muscles. The sample included women who were not pregnant, one group for each trimester of pregnancy, and two postpartum groups. The incidence in this study ranged from 0 in the nonpregnant and first trimester women, to 27% in the second trimester, to a high of 66% in the third trimester; also of interest is that 36% of women between 5 weeks and 3 months postpartum continued to display a separation. A second study, done by Bursch,[8] found a significant diastasis in 62.5% of postpartum women tested within 92 hours of delivery.
- Diastasis recti occurs in pregnancy possibly as a result of hormonal effects on the connective tissue and the biomechanical changes of pregnancy. It causes no discomfort.[30]
- It can occur above, below, or at the level of the umbilicus but appears to be less common below the umbilicus.
- It appears to be less common in women with good abdominal tone prior to pregnancy.[3]
- Clinically, a diastasis may be found in women well past their childbearing years and occasionally in men. Routine assessment for this condition is highly recommended and can easily be done in conjunction with abdominal strength testing.

Significance

- The condition of diastasis recti may produce musculoskeletal complaints, such as low back pain, possibly as a result of decreased ability of the abdominal musculature to control the pelvis and lumbar spine.
- Functional limitations can also occur, such as inability to perform independent supine to sitting transitions because of extreme loss of the mechanical alignment and function of the muscle. This finding is not exclusive to childbearing clients.
- In severe separations, the anterior segment of the abdominal wall is composed only of skin, fascia, subcutaneous fat, and peritoneum.[3,8,39] The lack of abdominal support provides less protection for the fetus.
- Severe cases of diastasis recti may progress to herniation of the abdominal viscera through the separation in the abdominal wall.

Diastasis Recti Test

Patient position and procedure: Hook-lying. Have the patient slowly raise her head and shoulders off the floor, reaching her hands toward the knees, until the spines of the scapulae leaves the floor. Place the fingers of one hand horizontally across the midline of the abdomen at the umbilicus (Fig. 17–4). If a

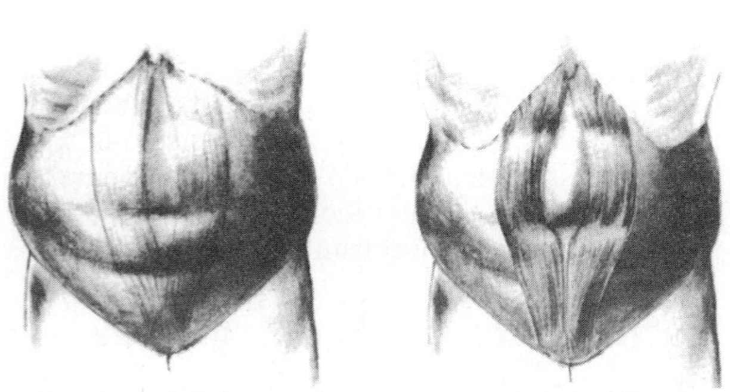

Figure 17–3 Diagramatic representations of diastasis recti. (From Boissonnault, JS, and Kotarinus, RK: Diastasis recti. In Wilder, E [ed]: Obstetric and Gynecologic Physical Therapy. Churchill-Livingstone, New York, 1988, p 397, with permission.)

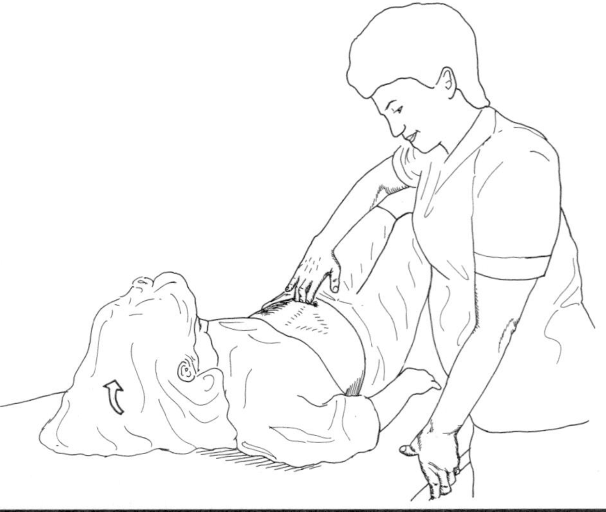

Figure 17–4 Diastasis recti test.

separation exists, the fingers will sink into the gap. The diastasis is measured by the number of fingers that can be placed between the rectus muscle bellies. A diastasis recti can also present as a longitudinal bulge along the linea alba. Since a diastasis recti can occur above, below, or at the level of the umbilicus, test for it at all three areas.

Intervention for Diastasis Recti

- Test all pregnant clients for the presence of diastasis recti prior to performing abdominal exercises.
- Instruct clients to perform a self-diastasis test on or after the third postpartum day for optimal accuracy.[32]
- Teach the client to perform corrective exercise for diastasis recti exclusive of other abdominal exercise until the separation is decreased to 2 cm or less (see page 695).[31] At that time, abdominal exercise can be resumed, but the integrity of the linea alba should be monitored to make sure the separation continues to decrease.

Low Back and Pelvic Pain

Pain commonly occurs because of the postural changes of pregnancy, increased ligamentous laxity, and decreased abdominal function.[1,6,30,35,37,39,48]

Postural Back Pain

- ***Symptoms.*** The symptoms of low back pain usually worsen with muscle fatigue from static postures or as the day progresses; symptoms are usually relieved with rest or change of position.
- ***Intervention.*** Low back pain symptoms can be treated effectively with proper body mechanics, posture instructions, and improvement in work techniques.[16] The use of deep-heating agents, electrical stimulation, and traction is generally *contraindicated* during pregnancy.
- Usually back pain symptoms disappear after pregnancy if proper body mechanics are used during child care and daily activities.
- Women who are physically fit generally have less back pain during pregnancy.[35]

Sacroiliac (Posterior Pelvic) Back Pain

- ***Incidence.*** The incidence of pain in the posterior pelvis is unknown but appears to be fairly common in pregnancy. One study reported a four times greater incidence of posterior pelvic pain than low back pain in pregnant women.[35] Sacroiliac symptoms may be caused by ligamentous laxity coupled with postural adaptations and muscle imbalance.
- ***Symptoms.*** Pain is usually localized to the posterior pelvis and is described as stabbing deep into the buttocks distal and lateral to L-5/S-1. Pain may radiate into the posterior thigh or knee but not into the foot. Symptoms include pain with prolonged sitting, standing, or walking; pain when climbing stairs, turning in bed, unilateral standing, or torsion activities; and pain that is not relieved by rest and frequently worsens with activity. There also may be pubic symphysis discomfort, subluxation, or both.[38]
- ***External stabilization.*** Use of external stabilization such as belts or corsets designed for use during pregnancy helps reduce the posterior pelvic pain, especially when walking.[35]
- ***Exercise and activity modification.*** Exercise must be modified so as not to aggravate the condition. Single-leg weight bearing should be avoided. Activities may need modification to minimize stresses on the symptomatic tissues. For example, getting in and out of a car is done by keeping the legs together, then pivoting the legs and spine as a unit, when side-lying placing a pillow between the knees, and adapting sexual activities to avoid full range of hip abduction. In addition, caution patients to avoid climbing more than one step at a time, swinging one leg out of bed at a time when getting up, or crossing the legs when sitting.

Varicose Veins

Varicosities are aggravated in pregnancy by the increased uterine weight, venous stasis in the legs, and increased venous distensibility.[39]

- ***Symptoms.*** Occasionally, there may be a range of mild discomfort to severe pain in the lower extremities, especially when the legs are in the dependent position.
- ***Intervention.*** If there is discomfort, exercises may need to be modified so that minimal dependent positioning of the legs is required. Elastic support stockings should be worn to provide an external pressure gradient against the distended veins, and the women should be encouraged to elevate the lower extremities as often as possible.

Pelvic Floor Dysfunction

The pelvic floor is a multilayered sheet of muscle stretched between the pubis and coccyx, forming the inferior support to the abdominopelvic cavity. The female pelvic floor is pierced by the urethra, vagina, and rectum.[2,9,22,30,39,44,47–50]

Structure of the Pelvic Floor (Fig. 17–5*A*)

- The pelvic floor musculature is composed of several layers with general attachments to the pubic bone and the coccyx. The structure and action of the muscles of each layer are summarized in Table 17–1.[2,14,49] Laterally, the tissues blend into a fascial layer overlying the obturator internus. Both right and left sides of the muscles contribute fibers to the perineal body (between the vagina and rectum), which is the tissue incised in an episiotomy.
- The pelvic floor complex has a dual nerve supply; the pudendal nerve (from ventral divisions of S-2 to S-4 in the sacral plexus), and direct branches from S-3 and S-4. The pudendal nerve terminates into the perineal branch and the inferior rectal nerve.
- Visual aids are critical in teaching clients about pelvic floor function. Emphasis should be placed on both the sling/hammock and the figure-eight orientation of the musculature (Fig. 17–5).

Note: Advanced study of the anatomy and extensive reading is highly recommended for therapists who wish to specialize in this area. Lack of standard terminology leads to difficulty in communication among healthcare professionals; focus on the function of the pelvic floor as a unit will aid in clarity as learning continues.

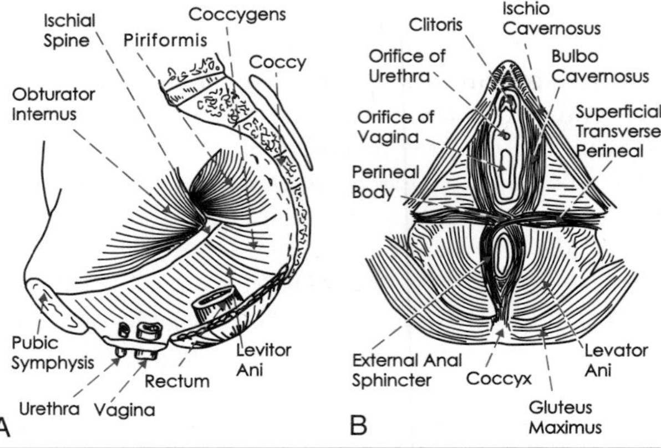

Figure 17–5 Pelvic floor muscles *(A)* sagittal section; note sling/hammock orientation, and *(B)* viewed from below; note figure-eight orientation of the muscles around the vaginal opening and the sphincter.

Functions of the Pelvic Floor

- Provides support for the pelvic organs and their contents
- Withstands increases in intra-abdominal pressure
- Provides sphincter control for the bladder and bowel
- Functions in reproductive and sexual activities

Dysfunction

Contributing Factors

- Childbirth: The process of labor, and particularly vaginal delivery, can produce significant trauma

Table 17–1 Pelvic Floor Anatomy—From Superficial to Deep

Muscle Layer	Structure	Action
Superficial (outlet)	Ischiocavernosus	Clitoral erection
	Bulbocavernosus	Vaginal sphincter
	Superficial transverse perineal	Fixes perineal body
	External anal sphincter	Compression of anal canal
Urogenital diaphragm (perineal membrane)	Deep transverse perineal	
	• Compressor urethrae	Compression of urethra and ventral wall of vagina
	• Urethrovaginal sphincter	Support of the perineal body and introitus
Pelvic diaphragm (primary muscular support)	Levator ani	Prime mover of the pelvic floor; puborectalis aids in closure of the rectum
	• Pubococcygeus	
	• Puborectalis	
	• Iliococcygeus	
	Coccygeus	Flexes coccyx

to the neuromuscular structures of the pelvic floor. The pudendal nerve can be compressed and stretched up to 20% of its length during the second stage of labor.[2] Other risk factors include multiple deliveries, prolonged second stage of labor, use of forceps, third-degree perineal tears, and birth weight over 8 lb.[45]

- Estrogen depletion at menopause, excessive straining because of constipation, and obesity can also contribute to pelvic floor dysfunction.[17]

General Classification

- ***Prolapse.*** A supportive impairment; descent of any of the pelvic viscera out of their normal alignment because of muscular and/or ligamentous deficits and increased abdominal pressure (Fig 17–6); often worsens over time and with subsequent pregnancies.
- ***Urinary or fecal incontinence.*** Involuntary loss of bladder or bowel contents; often a result of both neuromuscular and musculoskeletal impairments; may occur in combination with prolapse.
- ***Pain/hypertonus.*** May be related to delayed healing of perineal lacerations, scar tissue adhesions, or generalized spasm throughout the pelvic floor tissues. Functional limitations include *dyspareunia* (pain with intercourse) and difficulty with elimination.

Intervention for Pelvic Floor Dysfunction

- ***Therapeutic exercise and pelvic floor rehabilitation.*** Teach control and relaxation of the pelvic floor muscles (see exercises beginning on page 697)
  - Neuromuscular re-education is critical as many women have significant proprioceptive impairments in the pelvic floor muscles. Internal techniques of examination and assessment are often indicated for optimal patient outcomes. For example, manual stretch facilitation to the levator ani can be a very effective treatment option. Initially, emphasis on isolated contractions of the pelvic floor is needed, as many clients will exhibit excessive accessory muscle recruitment. Once coordination has improved, the client progresses to integration of pelvic floor activity with ADLs, lumbar stabilization, and other functional exercises.
  - Pelvic floor rehabilitation has not been studied in pregnancy or the immediate postpartum period; however, the use of exercise and biofeedback, including surface EMG for treatment of incontinence in a wider population is well supported.[7,17,36]

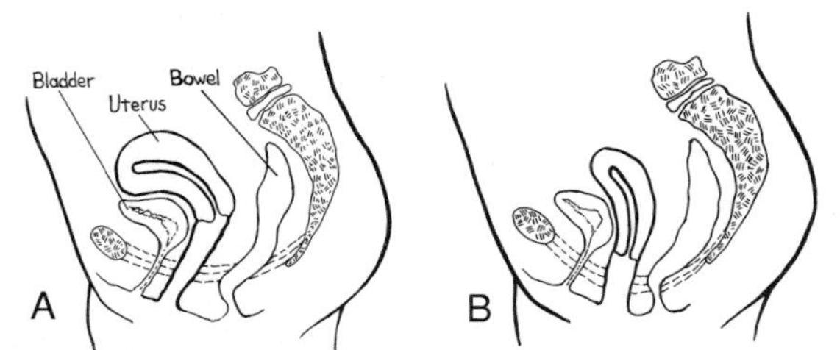

Figure 17–6 *(A)* Good pelvic floor support with a firm base, organs in place. *(B)* Inadequate support and the hammock stage, contents descended.

Modalities and Manual Techniques

Use modalities such as superficial heat, ice, and manual techniques prenatally to relieve discomfort. Transcutaneous electrical stimulation or electrical muscle stimulation may also be used postpartum to modulate pain and to stimulate muscle contractions, respectively.

Joint Laxity

Significance

- All joint structures are at increased risk of injury during pregnancy and during the immediate postpartum period. There is much controversy regarding the impact of postpartum hormone levels, particularly if the woman is nursing. Many women are aware of increased laxity at this time, and also note persistent changes in conjunction with the menstrual cycle.
- The tensile quality of the ligamentous support is decreased and, therefore, injury can occur if women are not educated regarding joint protection.

Interventions for Joint Laxity

- Teach the woman safe exercises to perform during the childbearing year, including modification of exercises to decrease excessive joint stress (see exercise section beginning on page 694).
- Suggest nonweight-bearing or less stressful aerobic activities such as swimming, walking, or biking particularly for women who were exercising minimally before pregnancy.

Compression Syndromes

Causes

Impairments from conditions such as thoracic outlet syndrome (TOS) or carpal tunnel syndrome (CTS) may be caused by one or more of the following in pregnancy: postural changes in the neck and upper quarter, fluid retention, hormonal changes, or circulatory compromise. Overall, women are three times as likely as men to experience carpal tunnel syndrome. Occurrence in pregnancy can be as high as 41%[36] (see Chapter 9 for discussion on TOS, Chapter 11 for discussion on CTS, and Chapter 15 for discussion on posture).

Compression may also occur in the lower extremities because of the weight of the fetus, fluid retention, hormonal changes, or circulatory compromise.

Intervention

- Typical protocols include postural correction exercises, manual techniques, ergonomic assessment, heat, ice, and consideration of splints for carpal tunnel syndrome.
- Carpal tunnel surgery in this population is rare as symptoms generally resolve soon after delivery; a longer course of the problem has been noted in women who breastfeed.[46]

Effects of Aerobic Exercise During Pregnancy

Many women who have been doing aerobic exercises choose to continue exercising during pregnancy to maintain their cardiovascular/pulmonary fitness. Maternal[1,10,15,27,48] and fetal[10–12,16,23,27,48] responses have been reported and influence how the pregnant woman should modify her exercise program.

Maternal Response to Aerobic Exercise

Blood Flow

Aerobic exercise does not reduce blood flow to the brain and heart. It does, however, cause a redistribution of blood flow away from the internal organs and possibly the uterus and toward the working muscles. This raises two concerns: that the reduction in blood flow may decrease the oxygen and nutrient availability to the fetus and that uterine contractions and preterm labor may be stimulated.[10] Stroke volume and cardiac output both increase with steady-state exercise. This coupled with increased blood volume and reduction in systemic vascular resistance during pregnancy may help offset the effects of the vascular shunting.[16]

Respiratory Rate

The maternal respiration rate appears to adapt to mild exercise but does not increase proportionately with moderate and severe exercise when compared with a nonpregnant state. The pregnant woman reaches a maximum exercise capacity at a lower work level than a nonpregnant woman because of the increased oxygen requirements of exercise.

Hematocrit Level

The maternal hematocrit level during pregnancy is lowered; however, it rises up to 10 percentage points within 15 minutes of beginning vigorous exercise. This condition continues for up to 4 weeks postpartum. As a result, cardiac reserve is decreased during exercise.

Interior Vena Cava Compression

Compression of the inferior vena cava by the uterus can occur after the fourth month of pregnancy, altering venous return and cardiac output. It occurs most likely in supine or static standing positions. This has been suggested as a possible cause of *abruptio placentae,* or premature detachment of the placenta from the uterus.[16]

Energy Needs

Hypoglycemia occurs more readily during pregnancy; therefore, adequate carbohydrate intake is important for the pregnant woman who exercises.[12] A caloric intake of an additional 500 calories per day is necessary to support the energy needs of pregnancy and exercise, as opposed to only a 300-calorie-per-day increase for the sedentary pregnant woman.[1]

Core Temperature

Vigorous physical activity and dehydration through perspiration can cause body core temperature to increase. This occurs in anyone who exercises. Concern has been expressed over this occurring in the pregnant woman because of the relationship of elevated core temperature to neural tube defects of the fetus. Studies report that during pregnancy the core temperature of physically fit women decreases during exercise. Apparently they have increased efficiency regulating their core temperature, and thus the thermal stress on the embryo and fetus is reduced.[11,12,16]

Uterine Contractions

Norepinephrine and epinephrine levels increase with exercise. Norepinephrine increases the strength and frequency of uterine contractions. This may pose a problem for the woman at risk of developing premature labor.

Healthy Woman Response

Studies have shown that healthy women who continue to run throughout pregnancy deliver on the average of 5 to 7 days sooner compared with controls.[10,11] Clapp[10–12] recommends that exercise, including weight bearing (even with ballistic motions such as during aerobic dancing), can be performed in mid- and late pregnancy without risk of preterm labor or premature rupture of the membranes. The most recent statement by the American College of Obstetricians and Gynecologists also supports this.[16]

Fetal Response to Maternal Aerobic Exercise

- No human research has conclusively proven a detrimental fetal response to mild-or moderate-intensity maternal exercise. Recent studies[10–12] suggest that even vigorous exercise does not have the detrimental effects on the fetus that once were feared, and therefore, restrictions on exercise because of concerns for the effects on the embryo and fetus have been lessened.[11,16]
- A 50% or greater reduction of uterine blood flow is necessary before fetal well-being is affected (based on animal research). No studies have documented such decreases in pregnant women who exercise, even vigorously. It is suggested that the cardiovascular adaptations in exercising women offset any redistribution of blood to muscles during exercise.[11,16]
- Brief submaximal maternal exercise (up to 70% maternal aerobic power) does not adversely affect fetal heart rate.[16] The fetal heart rate (FHR) usually increases 10 to 30 beats per minute at the onset of maternal exercise. After mild to moderate maternal exercise, the FHR usually returns to normal levels within 15 minutes, but in some cases of strenuous maternal exercise the FHR may remain elevated as long as 30 minutes. Fetal bradycardia (indicating fetal asphyxia) during maternal exercise has been reported in the literature with the return to pre-exercise FHR levels within 3 minutes after maternal exercise, followed by a brief period of fetal tachycardia.[23] The healthy fetus appears to be able to tolerate brief episodes of asphyxia with no detrimental results.
- The fetus has no mechanism such as perspiration or respiration by which to dissipate heat. However, physically fit women are able to dissipate heat and regulate their core temperature more efficiently thus reducing risk.[11,16]
- Newborn children of women who continue endurance exercises into the third trimester of pregnancy are reported to have an average decrease in birth weight of 310 g. There is no change in head circumference or heel-crown length. The decreased weight is proposed to be the result of slightly earlier delivery and less body fat.[11] Further study of these children (up to 5 years of age) has shown slightly better neurodevelopmental status in addition to lean body mass.[12]

Exercise During Pregnancy and Postpartum

Exercise programs during pregnancy and after childbirth are designed to minimize impairments and help the woman maintain or regain function while she is preparing for the arrival of the baby and then caring for the infant.[18,31,34,37,38,48] The potential impairments, functional limitations, and management guidelines related to uncomplicated pregnancies are summarized in Box 17–2. Guidelines and techniques for exercise instruction are included in this section.* Interventions for special situations such as cesarean childbirth and high-risk pregnancy are described in sections following (see pages 700 and 705, respectively).

Guidelines and Precautions for Exercise Instruction

- Suggest to each participant to have a physical examination by a physician prior to engaging in an exercise program.
- Individually examine each woman prior to participation to screen for pre-existing musculoskeletal problems, posture, and fitness level. Exercise levels should not exceed prepregnancy levels.

*See references 1, 16, 18, 28, 30–32, 34, 37, 43, 48.

Box 17–2 Management Guidelines—Pregnancy and Postpartum

Potential Impairments and Functional Limitations:

Stress, pain, and muscle imbalances from faulty postures
Poor body mechanics; related to changing body size and caring for growing child
Changing body image
Lower extremity edema and discomfort from altered circulation, varicose veins
Pelvic floor dysfunction, urinary incontinence from pelvic floor stress, or trauma superimposed on poor proprioceptive awareness
Abdominal muscle stretch, trauma, and diastasis recti
Potential decrease in cardiovascular fitness
Lack of knowledge of body changes and safe exercises to use during pregnancy and after childbirth
Lack of physical preparation (strength, endurance, relaxation) necessary for labor and delivery
Lack of knowledge of appropriate positioning for optimal comfort in labor and delivery
Lack of adequate postpartum rehabilitation

Plan of Care	Interventions
1. Develop awareness and control of posture during and after pregnancy.	1. Stretch, train, and strengthen postural muscle. Posture awareness training.
2. Learn safe body mechanics.	2. Body mechanics in sitting, standing, lifting, and lying as well as transitions from one position to another. Body mechanics with baby equipment and childcare activities. Positioning options for labor and delivery.
3. Develop upper extremity strength for the demands of infant care.	3. Resistive exercises to appropriate muscles.
4. Promote increased body awareness and a positive body image.	4. Body awareness and proprioception activities. Posture reinforcement.
5. Prepare the lower extremities for the demands of increased weight bearing and circulatory compromise.	5. Use of elastic support stockings. Stretching exercises. Resistive exercises to appropriate muscles.
6. Develop awareness and control of the pelvic floor musculature.	6. Awareness of pelvic floor muscle contraction and relaxation. Train and strengthen for muscle control.
7. Maintain abdominal function and prevent or correct diastasis recti pathology.	7. Monitor diastasis recti. Diastasis recti exercises. Safe abdominal-strengthening exercises with diastasis recti protection.
8. Promote or maintain safe cardiovascular fitness.	8. Safe progression of aerobic exercises.[16]
9. Learn about the changes of pregnancy and birth.	9. Client/family instruction. Refer to other disciplines as indicated.
10. Learn relaxation skills.	10. Relaxation techniques.
11. Prevent impairments associated with pregnancy (i.e., low back pain, pelvic floor weakness, decreased circulation).	11. Education about potential problems of pregnancy. Teach prevention techniques and appropriate exercises.
12. Prepare physically for labor, delivery, and postpartum activities.	12. Strengthen muscles needed in labor and delivery, and train responses. Teach comfort measures for labor and delivery.
13. Provide education on safe postpartum exercise progression.	13. Postpartum exercise instruction.
14. Develop awareness of treatment options for pelvic floor dysfunction.	14. Comprehensive approach for prolapse, incontinence, or hypertonus.

- Choose stretching exercises that are specific to a single muscle or muscle group; do not involve several groups at once. Asymmetric stretching or stretching multiple muscle groups can promote joint instability. Avoid ballistic movements.
- Do not allow any joint to be taken beyond its normal physiologic range.
- Use caution with hamstring and adductor stretches. Overstretching of these muscle groups can increase pelvic instability or hypermobility.
- Limit activities in which single-leg weight bearing is required, such as standing leg kicks. Besides possible loss of balance, these activities can promote sacroiliac or pubic symphysis discomfort.
- Do not exceed 5 minutes of supine positioning at any one time after the fourth month of pregnancy to avoid vena cava compression by the uterus. When supine, place a small wedge or rolled towel under the right hip to lessen the effects of uterine compression on abdominal vessels and improve

cardiac output. The wedge turns the patient slightly towards the left (Fig. 17–7).[1,34] This modification is also helpful during examination and treatment when the patient is positioned supine.

- To avoid the effects of postural hypotension, instruct the woman to always rise slowly when moving from lying down to standing positions.
- Discourage breath-holding and avoid activities that increase the tendency to elicit the Valsalva maneuver because this may lead to undesirable downward forces on the uterus and pelvic floor. In addition, breath-holding causes stress to the cardiovascular system in terms of blood pressure and heart rate.
- Break frequently for fluid replenishment. The risk of dehydration during exercise is increased in pregnancy.
- Encourage complete bladder emptying prior to exercise. A full bladder places increased stress on an already weakened pelvic floor.
- Include appropriate warm-up and cool-down activities.
- Adapt or discontinue any exercise that causes pain.
- With postpartum clients in particular, instruct them to avoid the knee-chest position with buttocks elevated above the chest level because of the risk of air embolism.[23,31,32] A pregnant woman is at risk only if bleeding or other symptoms of early placental detachment are present. An air embolism can occur when the buttocks are elevated and the uterus moves superiorly. The pressure change causes air to be introduced into the vagina and uterus, where it can enter the circulatory system through the open placental wound.

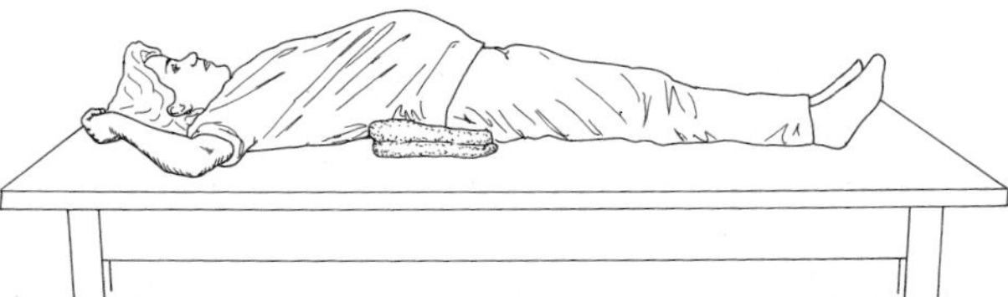

Figure 17–7 To prevent inferior vena cava compression when the patient is lying supine, a folded towel can be placed under the right side of the pelvis so the patient is tipped slightly to the left.

- Observe participants closely for signs of overexertion or complications. The following signs are reasons to discontinue exercise and contact a physician:
  - Pain
  - Bleeding
  - Shortness of breath
  - Irregular heartbeat
  - Dizziness
  - Faintness
  - Tachycardia
  - Back or pubic pain
  - Difficulty in walking
- A suggested sequence for exercise classes is listed in Box 17–3.[1,37,48]

Recommendations for Fitness Exercise

Note: These recommendations are for pregnant women with no maternal or fetal risk factors and are adapted from the American College of Obstetricians and Gynecologists.[16]

- Currently, there are no data in humans suggesting that pregnant women need to decrease their intensity of exercise or lower their target heart rates, but because of decreased oxygen supply, they should modify the intensity according to their symptoms. When fatigued, a woman should stop exercising and never exercise to exhaustion.
- It is preferable to exercise regularly at least 3 times per week rather than intermittently.

Box 17–3 Suggested Sequence for Exercises Classes

1. General rhythmic activities to "warm up"
2. Gentle selective stretching for postural alignment and for perineum and adductor flexibility
3. Aerobic activity for cardiovascular conditioning (15 minutes or less)
4. Postural exercises; upper and lower extremity strengthening and abdominal exercises
5. Cool-down activities
6. Pelvic floor exercises
7. Relaxation techniques
8. Labor and delivery techniques
9. Educational information
10. Postpartum exercise instruction (e.g., when to begin exercises, how to safely progress, precautions) because the client may not be attending a postpartum class

- Use nonweight-bearing aerobic exercises such as stationary cycling or swimming to minimize the risk of injury, but if able, a woman may continue activities such as running and aerobic dancing.
- If the woman cannot safely maintain balance because of the shifting and increasing weight, have her refrain from exercises that could result in falling and injury to herself or the fetus. Have her also refrain from any activity that could result in abdominal trauma.
- Adequate caloric intake for nutrition, adequate fluid intake, and appropriate clothing for heat dissipation are critical.
- Resumption of prepregnancy exercise routines during the postpartum period should be gradual. Physiologic and morphologic changes of pregnancy continue for 4 to 6 weeks postpartum. Encourage continued caution if the woman is nursing.

Precautions and Contraindications to Exercise

There are some circumstances where exercise is contraindicated or requires very specific restrictions and precautions.[1,4,16,32,34,37,48] Guidelines and precautions for intervention when there is a high-risk pregnancy are described later in this chapter.

Absolute Contraindications

- Incompetent cervix: early dilation of the cervix before the pregnancy is full term.
- Vaginal bleeding of any amount.
- Placenta previa: placenta is located on the uterus in a position where it may detach before the baby is delivered.
- Rupture of membranes: loss of amniotic fluid prior to the onset of labor.
- Premature labor: labor beginning prior to the 37th week of pregnancy.
- Maternal heart disease.
- Maternal diabetes or hypertension.
- Intrauterine growth retardation.

Precautions to Exercise

The woman with one or more of the following conditions may participate in an exercise program under close observation by a physician[1,4,32,34] and a therapist as long as no complications arise. Exercises may require modification.

- Multiple gestation (These infants are frequently born prematurely. Because some exercises may precipitate uterine contractions, these patients must be watched closely.[33])
- Anemia: reduction in the number of red blood cells, the amount of hemoglobin, or both (causes a reduction in the oxygen-carrying capacity of the blood)
- Systemic infection
- Extreme fatigue
- Musculoskeletal complaints and/or pain
- Overheating
- Phlebitis
- Diastasis recti
- Uterine contractions (lasting several hours after exercise)

Critical Areas of Emphasis and Selected Exercise Techniques

Posture Exercises

The growing fetus places added stress on postural muscles as the center of gravity shifts forward and upward and the spine shifts to compensate and maintain stability. In addition, after delivery, activities involving holding and caring for the baby stress postural muscles. Muscles that require emphasis for strengthening and stretching are listed. General exercise descriptions are listed in respective chapters. Subsequent sections describe adaptations of exercises specific for the pregnant woman.

Stretching (with caution)

- Upper neck extensors and scalenes (Chapter 16).
- Scapular protractors, shoulder internal rotators, and levator scapulae (Chapter 9).
- Low back extensors (Chapter 16).
- Hip adductors and hamstrings (Chapter 12). Caution: women with pelvic instabilities should not overstretch.
- Ankle plantarflexors (Chapter 14).

Strengthening (Low Intensity)

- Upper neck flexors, lower neck and upper thoracic extensors (Chapter 16)
- Scapular retractors and depressors (Chapter 9)
- Shoulder external rotators (Chapter 9)
- Trunk flexors (abdominals) with modifications noted in this section.
- Hip extensors (Chapter 12)
- Knee extensors (Chapter 13)
- Ankle dorsiflexors (Chapter 14)

Abdominal Muscle Exercises

As pregnancy progresses, the abdominals will undergo extreme overstretching. Therefore, exercise must be adapted to meet the needs of each individual, and periodic re-assessment must be done (approximately every 4 weeks during pregnancy). A check for diastasis recti must always be performed before initiating abdominal exercise.[6,32] Only the head lift or head lift with pelvic tilt exercises should be used until the separation is corrected to 2 cm, or 2 fingerwidths.[32] The following exercises progress from least to most strenuous.

Note: Keep in mind the time limit of 5 minutes with supine positioning when prescribing abdominal exercises during pregnancy.

Corrective Exercises for Diastasis Recti (Fig. 17–8)

- ***Head lift***

  Patient position and procedure: Hook-lying with her hands crossed over midline at the diastasis to support the area. Have her exhale and lift only her head off the floor or until the point just before a bulge appears. Her hands should gently pull the rectus muscles toward midline. Then have the woman lower her head slowly and relax. This exercise emphasizes the rectus abdominis muscle and minimizes the obliques.

- ***Head lift with pelvic tilt***

  Patient position and procedure: Hook-lying. The arms are crossed over the diastasis as above and pulled toward midline. Have her slowly lift her head off the floor while performing a posterior pelvic tilt, then slowly lower her head and relax. All abdominal contractions should be performed with an exhalation so that intra-abdominal pressure is minimized.

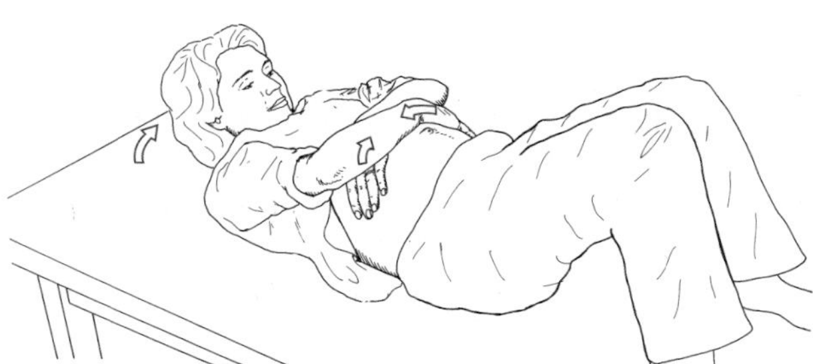

Figure 17–8 Corrective exercise for diastasis recti. The patient pulls with arms toward the midline.

Leg Sliding (Fig. 17–9)[32]

- *Patient position and procedure:* Hook-lying with pelvis in a posterior tilt. Instruct the woman to hold the pelvic tilt as she first slides one foot along the floor until the leg is straight. She stops sliding the foot at the point at which she can no longer hold the pelvic tilt. Have her slowly lift the leg and bring it back to the starting position, then repeat with the other leg. Breathing should be coordinated with the exercise so that abdominal contractions occur with exhalation.[32]
- This exercise can be performed with both legs at the same time only if abdominal muscles can maintain the pelvic tilt through the entire exercise.

Pelvic Tilt Exercise

- *Patient position and procedure:* Quadruped (on hands and knees). Instruct her to perform a posterior pelvic tilt. While keeping her back straight, have her draw in and tighten the abdomen and hold, then release and perform an anterior tilt through partial range.[6,13,15,29]
- For additional exercise, while holding the abdomen in and the back straight, have her laterally flex the trunk to the right (side-bend to the right), looking at the right hip, then reverse to the left.

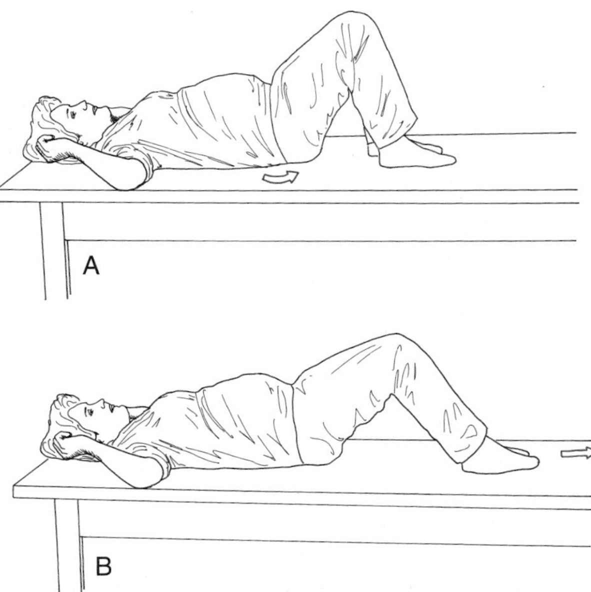

Figure 17–9 Leg-sliding. *(A)* Hook-lying with posterior pelvic tilt. *(B)* Maintain pelvic tilt as the feet slide along the floor away from the body.

- Have the woman practice pelvic tilt exercises in a variety of positions, including side-lying and standing.

Trunk Curls

- Curl-downs and curl-ups are classic abdominal exercises for rectus abdominis strengthening and can be used if tolerated and no diastasis recti is present. Have the woman protect the linea alba with crossed hands (see Fig. 17–8) while performing trunk curls.
- Diagonal curls are carried out to strengthen the oblique muscles. Have the woman lift one shoulder toward the outside of the opposite knee as she curls up and down and protects the linea alba with crossed hands.

Resisted Posterior Pelvic Tilt

- ***Pelvic lifts***

Patient position and procedure: The woman is supine with the lower extremities elevated to 90 degrees. Have her lift the lower extremities upward as the pelvis comes up off the floor (see Fig. 16–35). When this exercise becomes difficult to accomplish during the third trimester as the uterus enlarges and pushes on the diaphragm, it should not be attempted. Once the woman learns pelvic tilt control postpartum, this exercise may be resumed.

- ***Modified bicycle***

Patient position and procedure: The woman is supine with one of the lower extremities flexed and the other partially extended. The lower abdominals stabilize the pelvis against the varying weight of the lower extremities as they are flexed and extended in an alternating pattern as if cycling. The further the lower extremities extend, the greater the resistance. In order to not strain the back, the woman must keep it flat against the floor by controlling the arc of the cycling pattern (see Fig. 16–26*B*).

Precaution: Leg-lowering exercises cause excessive strain on the low back and should not be performed during pregnancy; they may be resumed postpartum with the following precautions and modifications. The legs should be lowered only through the range in which control of the posterior pelvic tilt and flattening of the low back is maintained. If low back strain is felt or if the lumbar spine begins to arch, this exercise should not be performed. The pull of the psoas major may cause a shear force on the lumbar vertebrae, and the supporting ligaments may be strained.

Stabilization Exercises

Exercise progressions for developing dynamic control of the pelvis and lower extremities, as described in Chapter 16, should be initiated and progressed at the intensity that the woman is able to safely control. These may be performed throughout the pregnancy and postpartum period.

Precautions:

- Because the trunk muscles are contracting isometrically while stabilizing, there is a tendency to hold the breath; this is detrimental to the blood pressure and heart rate. Caution the woman to maintain a relaxed breathing pattern and exhale during the exertion phase of each exercise.
- If diastasis recti is present, adapt the stabilization exercises to protect the linea alba as described previously. Any progression of abdominal strengthening exercises should be postponed until the diastasis has been corrected to 2 finger-widths or less.

Pelvic Motion Training

These exercises are helpful in cases of postural back pain; they are beneficial for improving proprioceptive awareness as well as lumbar, pelvic, and hip mobility.[19,29]

"The Pelvic Clock"

Patient position and procedure: Hook-lying, legs may move slightly during exercise. Ask the woman to visualize the face of a clock on her lower abdomen. The umbilicus is 12 o'clock and the pubic symphysis is 6 o'clock.

- Have her begin with gentle movements from 12 to 6 (the basic pelvic tilt exercise)
- Then ask her to move from 3 o'clock (weight shifted to left hip) to 9 o'clock (weight shifted to the right hip)
- Then move in a clockwise manner from 12 o'clock to 3 o'clock to 6 o'clock to 9 o'clock and back to 12 o'clock.

With practice, this will become a very smooth movement and will not require such concentration on each number of the clock. Continue relaxed breathing throughout the exercise and do not force any part of the movement.

Pelvic Clock Progressions

Imagine cutting the face of the clock in half so that there is a right side and a left side, or there is a top half and a bottom half. Have the woman move her pelvis through the arc on the one side and back through the middle of the clock, and then move the pelvis through the opposite side and back through the middle. Initially, the woman may notice asymmetry when comparing the halves; this will improve with time. Adding counterclockwise motions throughout the entire clock and performing the motions in the sitting position are other variations.

Pelvic Floor Awareness Training and Strengthening

Patient position and procedures: Gravity-assisted positioning (hips higher than the heart, such as supported bridge or elbows/knees position) may be indicated initially for some women with extreme weakness and proprioceptive deficits. Positional changes are introduced as strength and awareness improve (supine, side-lying, quadruped, sitting, standing). Significant gains in strength are not likely during pregnancy.

Contract-Relax

The bladder should be empty when performing this exercise. Instruct the woman to tighten the pelvic floor as if attempting to stop urine flow or hold back gas. Hold for 3 to 5 seconds and relax. The pelvic floor muscles are highly susceptible to fatigue, therefore contractions should not be held longer than 5 seconds and with a maximum of 10 repetitions per session.[30,42] When fatigued, substitution with the gluteals, abdominals, or hip adductors may occur. To maximize proprioception and control, it is important to emphasize isolation of the pelvic floor and avoid the substitute muscle actions.

Quick Contractions

Have the woman perform quick, repeated contractions of the pelvic floor muscles while maintaining a normal breathing rate and keeping accessory muscles relaxed. Try for 15 to 20 repetitions per set. This type II fiber response is important to develop in order to withstand pressure from above, especially with coughing or sneezing.

"Elevator" Exercise

Instruct the woman to visually imagine riding in an elevator. As the elevator goes from one floor to the next, contract the pelvic floor muscles a little more. Relax the muscles gradually, as if the elevator were descending one floor at a time. This requires an eccentric contraction and is very challenging.

Hypertonus

When treating women with hypertonus, increase the rest time between pelvic floor contractions and sets. Emphasis on relaxation is equally important for strength training in these clients. Use of surface EMG for feedback is invaluable for enhancing awareness of holding patterns and resting tone.

Modified Upper and Lower Extremity Strengthening

As the abdomen enlarges, it becomes impossible to comfortably assume the prone position. Exercises that are usually performed in the prone position must be modified.

Standing Push-Ups

Patient position and procedure: Standing, facing a wall, feet pointing straight forward, shoulder-width apart, and approximately an arm-length away from the wall. The palms are placed on the wall at shoulder height. Have the woman slowly bend the elbows, bringing her face close to the wall, maintaining a stable pelvic tilt, and keeping the heels on the floor. Her elbows should be shoulder height. She then slowly pushes with her arms, bringing the body back to the original position.

Hip Extension

- Supine bridging (see Fig. 12–13)
- Quadruped leg raising (Fig. 17–10)

Patient position and procedure: On hands and knees (hands may be in fists or palms open and flat). Instruct the woman to first perform a posterior pelvic tilt, then slowly lift one leg, extending the hip to a level no higher than the pelvis while maintaining the posterior pelvic tilt. She then slowly lowers the leg and repeats with the opposite side. The knee may remain flexed or can be straightened throughout the exercise. Monitor this exercise and discontinue if there is stress on the sacroiliac joints or ligaments. If the woman cannot stabilize the pelvis while lifting the leg, have her just slide one leg posteriorly along the floor and return (see Fig. 16–30*A*).

Modified Squatting

These exercises are used to strengthen the hip and knee extensors for good body mechanics and also to help stretch the perineal area for flexibility during

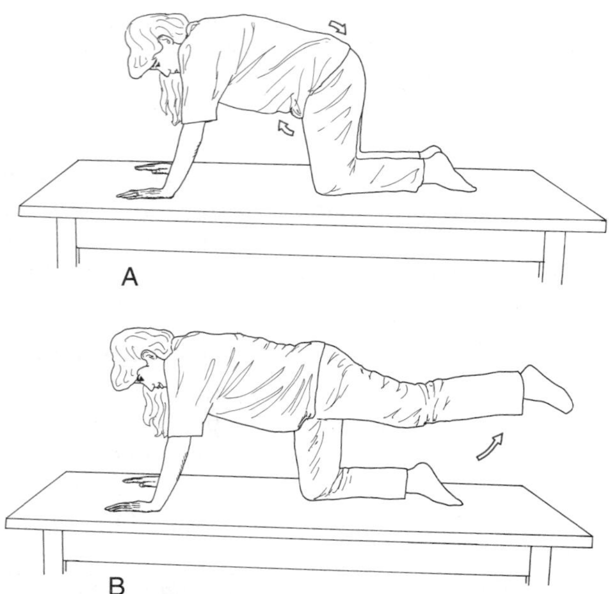

Figure 17–10 All-fours leg-raising. *(A)* Patient assumes quadruped position with posterior pelvic tilt. *(B)* Leg is raised only until it is in line with the trunk.

the delivery process. In addition, if the woman wishes to use squatting for labor and delivery, the muscles *must* be strengthened in advance.

- Instruct the woman to stand with feet shoulder-width apart or wider, facing a counter, chair, or wall on which she can rest her hands for support. She slowly squats as far as is comfortable, keeping knees apart and over the feet and keeping the back straight. To protect her feet, she should wear shoes with good arch support. A woman with knee problems should perform only partial range of the squat.
- Wall slides. The woman stands with her back against a wall and her feet shoulder-width apart. She slides her back down the wall as her hips and knees flex only as far as is comfortable, then slides back up (see Fig. 12–16).

Scapular Retraction

When scapular retraction exercises become difficult in the prone position, the woman should continue strengthening in the sitting position (see Fig. 9–33).

Perineum and Adductor Flexibility

In addition to the modified squatting exercises described above, these flexibility exercises prepare the legs and pelvis for childbirth.[6,13,37]

Self-Stretching

- *Patient position and procedure:* Supine or side-lying. Instruct the patient to abduct the hips and pull the knees toward the sides of her chest and hold the position for as long as is comfortable (at least to the count of 10).
- *Patient position and procedure:* Sitting on a short stool with the hips abducted as far as possible and feet flat on the floor. Have her flex forward slightly at the hips (keeping the back straight), or have her gently press her knees outward with her hands for an additional stretch.

Relaxation and Breathing

Developing the ability to relax requires awareness of stress and muscle tension. Techniques of conscious relaxation allow the individual to control and cope with a variety of imposed stresses by being mentally alert to the task at hand while relaxing tense muscles that are superfluous to the activity. This is particularly important during labor and delivery when there are times that the woman should relax and allow the physiologic processes to occur without excessive tension in unrelated muscles.[32] Relaxation techniques for managing stress are described in Chapters 5 and 16. In addition, the following guidelines are suggested for the pregnant woman in preparation for labor and delivery.

Visual Imagery

Use music and verbal guidance. Instruct the woman to concentrate on a relaxing image such as the beach, mountains, or a favorite vacation spot. Suggest that she focus on the image during the relaxation training so that the image can be called up to the conscious level when recognizing the need to relax.

Muscle Setting

- Have the woman lie in a comfortable position.
- Have her begin with the lower body. Instruct her to gently contract and then relax first the muscles in the feet, then legs, thighs, pelvic floor, and buttocks.
- Next progress to the upper extremities and trunk, then to the head.
- Reinforce the importance of remaining awake and aware of the sensations of the muscles contracting and relaxing. Emphasize "softening" of the muscles as the session continues.
- Add deep, slow, relaxed breathing to the routine.

Selective Tension

Progress the training by emphasizing awareness of muscles contracting in one part of the body while remaining relaxed in other parts. For example, while she is tensing the fist and upper extremity, the feet and legs should be limp. Reinforce the two sensations and the ability to control the tension and relaxation.

Breathing

- General breathing techniques are described in Chapter 19. Slow, deep diaphragmatic breathing is the most efficient method for exchange of air to use with relaxation techniques and for controlled breathing during labor.
- Teach the woman to relax the abdomen during inspiration so that it feels as though the abdominal cavity is "filling up." During exhalation, the abdominal cavity becomes smaller; contraction of the abdominal muscles is not necessary with relaxed breathing.
- To avoid hyperventilation, have her avoid deep, rapid breathing. Caution the woman to decrease the intensity of the breathing if she experiences dizziness or feels tingling in the lips and fingers.

Pelvic Floor Relaxation

- Instruct the woman to contract the pelvic floor as in the strengthening exercise, then allow total voluntary release and relaxation of the pelvic floor.
- This activity is coordinated with breathing. Instruct the woman to concentrate on a slow, deep breath and allow the pelvic floor to completely relax. Relaxation of the pelvic floor is important not only during vaginal delivery, but also for elimination of bowel and bladder contents.[6,22,32]

Relaxation and Breathing During Labor

- ***First stage.*** Once labor begins, the contractions of the uterus progress. Relaxation during the contractions becomes more demanding. Provide the woman with suggested techniques to assist in relaxation.[32]
  - Have moral support from the father, family member, or special friend to provide encouragement and assist with comfort aids.
  - Seek comfortable positions, including walking or lying on pillows; include gentle motions such as pelvic rocking.
  - Breathe slowly with each contraction; use the visual imagery and relax with each contraction. Some women find it helpful to focus their attention on some visual object. Other suggestions include singing, talking, or moaning during each contraction to prevent breath-holding and encourage slow breathing.
  - During the transition (near the end of the first stage) there is often an urge to push. Teach the woman to use quick blowing techniques, using the cheeks, not the abdominal muscles, to overcome the desire to push.
  - Massage or apply pressure to any areas that hurt such as the low back. Using the hands may help distract the focus from the contractions.
  - Apply heat or cold for local symptoms; wipe the face with a wet wash cloth.
- ***Second stage.*** Once dilation of the cervix has occurred, the woman may become active in the birth process by assisting the uterus during a contraction in pushing the baby down the birth canal.[32] Teach her the following techniques:
  - While bearing down, take in a breath, contract the abdominal wall, and slowly breathe out. This will cause increased pressure within the abdomen along with relaxation of the pelvic floor.

Precaution: Tell the woman that if she holds her breath, there will be increased tension and resistance in the pelvic floor. In addition, exertion with a closed glottis, known as the Valsalva maneuver, has adverse effects on the cardiovascular system.

  - For maximum efficiency, maintain relaxation in the extremities, especially the legs and perineum. Keeping the face and jaw relaxed assists with this.
  - Between contractions, perform total body relaxation.
  - As the baby is delivered, just "let go" and breathe with light pants or groans to relax the pelvic floor as it stretches.

Unsafe Exercises During Pregnancy

Bilateral Straight-Leg Raising

This exercise typically places more stress on the abdominal muscles and low back than they can tolerate. It can cause back injury or diastasis recti and, therefore, should not be attempted.

"Fire Hydrant" Exercise

This exercise is performed on hands and knees, and one hip is abducted and externally rotated at a time (the "image" of a dog at a fire hydrant). If the leg is elevated too high, the sacroiliac joint and lumbar vertebrae can be stressed. The exercise can be performed safely if hip abduction remains within the physiologic range (Fig. 17–11). It should be avoided by any woman who has pre-existing sacroiliac joint symptoms or if symptoms develop.

All-fours (Quadruped) Hip Extension

This exercise can be performed safely as explained earlier in this chapter (Fig. 17–10). It becomes unsafe and can cause low back pain when the leg is elevated beyond the physiologic range of hip extension, causing the pelvis to tilt anteriorly and the lumbar spine to hyperextend.

Unilateral Weight-Bearing Activities

Weight bearing on one leg (which includes slouched standing with the majority of weight shifted to one leg and the pelvis tilted down on the opposite side) during pregnancy can cause sacroiliac joint irritation and should be avoided by women with pre-existing sacroiliac joint symptoms. Unilateral weight bearing also can cause balance problems because of the increasing body weight and shifting of the center of gravity. This posture becomes a significant problem postpartum when the woman carries her growing child on one hip. Any asymmetries become accentuated, and painful symptoms develop.

Exercise Critical to the Postpartum Period

After an uncomplicated vaginal delivery, exercise can be started as soon after delivery as the woman feels able to exercise. All prenatal exercises can be performed safely in the postpartum period. Some exercises should be initiated as soon as possible after delivery.[1,30,32,48]

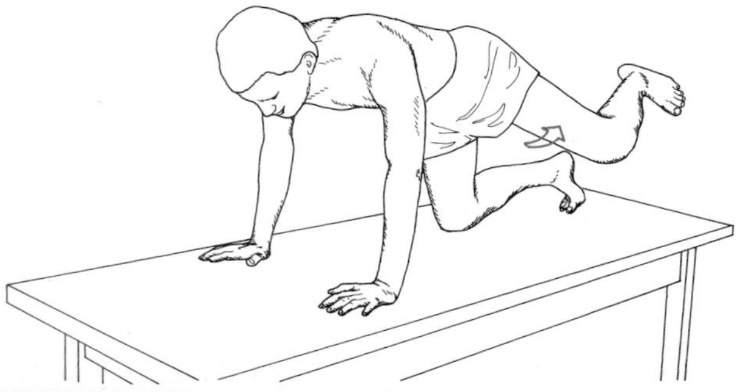

Figure 17–11 The fire hydrant is a potentially damaging exercise. To do this exercise correctly, the individual must stabilize the pelvis midrange, then stop the abduction external rotation motion when the hip has completed its range. The leg should not be "kicked as high as possible," or stress to the hip, sacroiliac joint, and lumbar spine results.

Pelvic floor strengthening. Exercises should be initiated as soon after the birth as possible. These exercises may increase circulation and aid healing.[26]

Diastasis recti correction. Exercises should begin approximately 3 days after delivery and continue until correction to 2 cm is achieved. At that time, more vigorous abdominal exercise can be initiated. Until 3 days postdelivery, the abdominal musculature is too stretched to accurately test for diastasis recti. Therefore, the test should not be done until 3 days postdelivery.[26]

Aerobic and strengthening exercises. As soon as the woman feels able, exercise can be resumed in a progressive program. A physical examination is suggested prior to the onset of vigorous exercise.

Precautions: Since the woman may not be seen for exercise instruction after the delivery, inform her of the following precautions:

- If bleeding increases or turns bright red, exercise should be postponed. Tell her to rest more and allow a longer recovery time.
- Joint laxity may be present for some time after delivery, especially if breast-feeding. Precautions should be taken to protect the joints as described previously.
- Adequate warm-up and cool-down time is important.
- Avoid the prone knee-chest position for at least 6 weeks postpartum because of the risk of air embolism.[31]

▶ Cesarean Childbirth

Definition

A cesarean section is the delivery of a baby through an incision in the abdominal wall and uterus rather than through the pelvis and vagina.[24,34] General, spinal, or epidural anesthesia may be used.

Significance to Physical Therapists

- Cesarean section (C-section) is the single most common operation performed in the United States.[34] The cesarean birth rate in the United

States ranges from 12 to 25% depending on the type of hospital and the population it serves. This has increased greatly over the past 30 years and is the focus of much discussion within obstetrics. The Vaginal Birth After Cesarean (VBAC) movement has been quite visible, as historically more than one-third of all C-sections are repeat procedures. Since the early 1990s, the American College of Obstetricians and Gynecologists (ACOG) has discouraged repeat cesarean delivery as routine practice. Pregnant women need to be informed as to the risks and benefits of each choice in order to make informed decisions.[36] Because of this high incidence, physical therapists must be prepared to address the specific concerns of these clients in all pregnancy-related programming.[6,24,32–34,36,39,41,46]

- Women who have had cesarean deliveries may still require pelvic floor rehabilitation. Many women experience a lengthy labor and trial pushing before a cesarean section is deemed necessary. Therefore, the pelvic floor musculature and tissues are not spared the stress of labor. Also, pregnancy itself creates significant stress on the pelvic floor musculature and tissues.
- Postpartum intervention for the woman who has had cesarean delivery is essentially the same as that of the woman who has had a vaginal delivery. However, a C-section is major abdominal surgery with all the risks and complications of such surgeries, and therefore, the woman will also require general postsurgical rehabilitation.[34,46] Impairments and management guidelines are summarized in Box 17–4.
- Many childbirth preparation classes do not adequately educate and prepare couples for the experience of a cesarean delivery. As a result, the patient with a C-section frequently feels as if her body has failed her, causing her to have more emotional changes than a woman who has experienced a vaginal delivery.

Box 17–4 Management Guidelines—Postcesarean Section

Impairments and Functional Limitations:

Risk of pulmonary complications
Postsurgical pain and discomfort
Risk of vascular complications
Development of adhesions at incisional site
Faulty posture
Pelvic floor dysfunction
Abdominal weakness; diastasis recti
General functional restrictions of postdelivery

Plan of Care	Interventions
1. Improve pulmonary function and decrease the risk of pneumonia.	1. Breathing instruction; coughing and/or huffing.[24,32]
2. Decrease incisional pain associated with coughing, movement, or breast-feeding.	2. Postoperative TENS; support incision with pillow when coughing or breast-feeding. Incisional support with pillow or hands when exercising. Education regarding incisional care and risk of injury.
3. Prevent postsurgical vascular complications.	3. Active leg exercises. Early ambulation.
4. Enhance incisional circulation and healing; prevent adhesion formation.	4. Gentle abdominal exercise with incisional support. Scar mobilization and friction massage.
5. Decrease postsurgical discomfort from flatulence, itching, or catheter.	5. Positioning instruction, massage, and supportive exercises.
6. Correct posture.	6. Posture instruction.
7. Prevent injury and reduce low back pain.	7. Instruction in incisional splinting and positioning for ADL. Body mechanics instruction.
8. Prevent pelvic floor dysfunction.	8. Pelvic floor exercises; education regarding risk factors and types of pelvic floor dysfunction.
9. Develop abdominal strength.	9. Abdominal exercises including corrective exercises for diastasis recti.

Suggested Activities for the Patient with a Cesarean Section

Exercises

- Instruct the woman in all prenatal exercises.
- Instruct the woman to begin preventive exercises as soon as possible during the recovery period.[24,32]
  - Initiate ankle pumping, active lower extremity ROM, and walking to promote circulation and prevent venous stasis.
  - Initiate pelvic floor exercises to regain tone and control of the muscles of the perineum.
  - Deep breathing and coughing or huffing is used to prevent pulmonary complications (see instructions below).
- Progress abdominal exercises slowly. Check for diastasis recti and protect the area of the incision as with diastasis exercises. Initiate nonstressful muscle-setting techniques and progress as tolerated.[24,32]
- Teach posture correction as necessary. Retrain postural awareness and help realign posture in the nonpregnant state. Develop control of the shoulder girdle muscles as they respond to the increased stress of caring for the new baby.
- Reinforce the value of deep diaphragmatic breathing techniques for pulmonary ventilation, especially when exercising, and relaxed breathing techniques to relieve stress and promote relaxation.
- The woman should wait at least 6 to 8 weeks before resuming vigorous exercise. Emphasize the importance of progressing at a safe and controlled pace and not expecting to begin at her prepregnancy level.

Coughing or Huffing

Coughing is difficult because of incisional pain. An alternative is huffing.[32] A huff is an outward breath caused by the upper abdominals contracting up and in against the diaphragm to push air out of the lungs. The abdominals are pulled up and in, rather than pushed out, causing decreased pressure in the abdominal cavity and less strain on the incision. Huffing must be done quickly to generate sufficient force to expel mucus. Instruct the patient to support the incision with a pillow or the hands and say "ha" forcefully and repetitively while contracting the abdominal muscles.

Interventions to Relieve Intestinal Gas Pains

- Abdominal massage or kneading while lying on the left side. This is very effective and typically done with either long or circular strokes. Begin on the right side at the ascending colon, stroking upward, then stroke across the transverse colon from right to left and down the descending colon, then finish with an "S" stroke along the sigmoid colon.
- Pelvic tilting and/or bridging (can be done in conjunction with massage).
- Bridge and twist. Have the patient maintain a position of bridging while twisting hips to the right and left. This position may also facilitate air embolism and should be used with caution in the early postpartum period.
- Partial abdominal curl-up.

Scar Mobilization

Cross-friction massage should be initiated around the incision site as soon as sufficient healing has occurred. This will minimize adhesions that may contribute to postural problems and back pain.

▶ High-Risk Pregnancy

Various factors may lead to high-risk pregnancies that require special care for successful outcomes.[4,25,26,36,37,39,46]

Definition

A high-risk pregnancy is one that is complicated by disease or problems that put the mother or fetus at risk for illness or death. Conditions may be pre-existing, be induced by pregnancy, or be caused by an abnormal physiologic reaction during pregnancy.[25] The goal of medical intervention is to prevent preterm delivery, usually through use of bed rest, restriction of activity, and medications, when appropriate.

High-Risk Conditions

Preterm Rupture of Membranes

The amniotic sac breaks, and amniotic fluid is lost prior to onset of labor. This can be dangerous to the fetus if it occurs before fetal development is complete. Labor may begin spontaneously after the membranes rupture. The chance for fetal infection also increases when the protection of the amniotic sac is lost.

Premature Onset of Labor

Labor that begins prior to 37 weeks of gestation or before completion of fetal development is considered premature. Fetal life is endangered if delivery occurs too early.

Incompetent Cervix

An incompetent cervix is the painless dilation of the cervix that occurs in the second trimester (after 16 weeks gestation) or early in the third trimester of pregnancy. This may lead to premature membrane rupture and delivery of a fetus too small to survive.

Placenta Previa

The placenta attaches too low on the uterus, near the cervix. As the cervix dilates, the placenta begins to separate from the uterus and may present before the fetus, thus endangering fetal life. The primary symptom is intermittent, recurrent, or painless bleeding that increases in intensity.

Pregnancy-Related Hypertension or Pre-Eclampsia

Characterized by hypertension, protein in the urine, and severe fluid retention, pre-eclampsia can progress to maternal convulsions, coma, and death if it becomes severe (eclampsia). It usually occurs in the third trimester and disappears after birth. The cause is not understood.

Multiple Gestation

More than one fetus forms. Complications of multiple gestation include premature onset of labor and birth, increased incidence of perinatal mortality, lower birth weight infants, and increased incidence of maternal complications (e.g., hypertension).

Diabetes

Diabetes can be present before pregnancy or may occur as a result of the physiological stress of pregnancy. *Gestational diabetes,* which presents in pregnancy, affects 4 to 7% of pregnant women and usually disappears after pregnancy, but there remains a greater tendency for development of the disease at some future time.

Unlike many of the previously discussed high-risk conditions, women with gestational diabetes may be appropriate candidates for more traditional physical therapy treatment. Supervised, individualized exercise programs are excellent options for the woman with gestational diabetes. In particular, recumbent bicycling or arm ergometer exercises have been shown to stabilize and lower glucose levels.[36]

Management Guidelines and Precautions for High-Risk Pregnancies

All exercise programs for high-risk populations should be individually established based on diagnosis, limitations, physical therapy examination and evaluation, and consultation with the physician. Activities must address patient needs but should not further complicate the condition.[37,46] Management guidelines for the woman who is confined to bed because of her high-risk status are summarized in Box 17–5.

Develop good rapport with the patient and instill trust. Closely monitor the patient during all activities; re-evaluate her after each treatment and note any changes. It is also important to teach the patient self-monitoring techniques so that she will be alert to adverse reactions and respond appropriately.

- Prolonged static positioning is a primary concern. The position of choice for the high-risk client is left side-lying, which is optimal for reducing pressure on the inferior vena cava and for maximizing cardiac output, thereby enhancing maternal and fetal circulation.
- Some exercises, especially abdominal exercises, may stimulate uterine contractions. If this occurs, modify or discontinue them.
- Monitor and report any uterine contractions, bleeding, or amniotic fluid loss.
- Do not allow the Valsalva maneuver to occur. Avoid any activities that increase intra-abdominal pressure. Body mechanics and postural instruction will stimulate abdominal contractions, so be sure the patient does not strain and closely monitor for adverse symptoms.
- Keep the exercises simple. Have the patient do them slowly, smoothly, and with minimal exertion.
- Many high-risk pregnancies result in cesarean deliveries, so educate the woman about cesarean delivery rehabilitation.
- Incorporate maximum muscle efficiency into each movement.
- Teach the patient self-monitoring techniques.

Suggestions for Exercise Programs with High-Risk Pregnancies

The following are adaptations of exercises that have already been described that should be considered for the bed-bound patient with a high-risk pregnancy.[36,37,46]

Box 17–5 Management Guidelines—High-Risk Pregnancy

Impairments and Functional Limitations[37,46]:

Primary functional limitation is inability to be out of bed and prolonged static positioning with the potential of the following impairments.
Joint stiffness and muscle aches
Muscle weakness and atrophy
Vascular complications including risk of thrombosis and decreased uterine blood flow
Decreased proprioception in distal body parts
Constipation caused by lack of exercise
Postural changes
Boredom
Emotional stress; patient may be at risk of losing the baby
Guilt from the belief that some activity caused the problem or that the patient did not take good enough care of herself
Anxiety about her home situation or the impending birth

Plan of Care	Interventions
1. Decrease stiffness.	1. Positioning instructions; assess for supports. Facilitation of joint motion in available range.
2. Maintain muscle length and bulk.	2. Stretching and strengthening exercises within limits imposed by the physician.
3. Maximize circulation; prevent deep-vein thrombosis.	3. Ankle pumping; ROM.
4. Improve proprioception.	4. Movement activities for as many body parts as possible.
5. Improve posture within available limits.	5. Posture instruction, modified as necessary based on allowed activity level. Bed mobility and transfer techniques if able (avoid Valsalva).
6. Relieve boredom.	6. Vary activities and positioning for exercises.
7. Enhance relaxation.	7. Relaxation techniques/stress management.
8. Prepare for delivery.	8. Childbirth education, breathing training, and exercises to assist and prepare for labor.
9. Enhance postpartum recovery.	9. Exercise instruction and home program for postpartum period. Body mechanics instruction.

Positioning

- Left side-lying to prevent vena cava compression, enhance cardiac output, and decrease lower extremity edema
- Pillows between the knees and under the abdomen
- Supine positioning for short periods, with a wedge placed under the right hip to decrease inferior vena cava compression (Fig. 17–7)
- Modified prone positioning (side-lying, partially rolled toward prone, with pillow under abdomen) to decrease low back discomfort and pressure

Range of Motion (ROM)

- Active ROM of all joints.
- Motions should be slow, nonstressful, and through the full range if possible.
- Teach in a gravity-neutral position if antigravity ROM is too stressful.
- Individualize the number of repetitions and frequency to the woman's condition.
- Include the following exercises with the patient supine with wedge under the right hip or side-lying:
  - Alternate knee to chest
  - Ankle pumping and ankle circles
  - Shoulder, elbow, and finger flexion and extension; reach to ceiling; arm circles
  - Unilateral straight-leg raise in supine or side-lying position
  - Unilateral active ROM in diagonal patterns for the upper and lower extremities
  - Lower extremity abduction and adduction
  - Pelvic tilt, bridging, gluteal setting
  - Abdominal exercises (check for diastasis); these should be very mild and closely monitored
  - Pelvic floor exercises
  - Neck motions: look up/down, turn head left/right
  - Backward shoulder circles

Ambulation/Standing

- Almost always contraindicated; when allowed, usually will be only to use the bathroom

- Good posture in ambulation
- Tip-toe or heel walking
- Gentle, partial-range squatting to stretch quadriceps
- Lower extremity rotation

Relaxation Techniques, Bed Mobility and Transfer Activities

- Moving up, down, side to side in bed
- Log rolling: incorporate neck and upper and lower extremities to aid movement
- Supine to sitting: use log roll technique assisted by arms

Preparation for Labor

- Relaxation techniques
- Modified squatting: supine, sitting, or side-lying with knees to chest
- Pelvic floor relaxation
- Breathing exercises: minimize forced abdominal exhalations

Postpartum Exercise Instruction

Instructions are the same as previously described.

Independent Learning Activities

CRITICAL THINKING AND DISCUSSION

1. Describe three normal changes of pregnancy that will affect exercise tolerance.
2. Explain the clinical significance of diastasis recti, the testing procedure, and the corrective exercise.
3. Differentiate between postural and sacroiliac back pain in the pregnant client.
4. Name five risk factors for pelvic floor dysfunction.
5. What exercise guidelines are most helpful for a woman who has not exercised prior to becoming pregnant?
6. Discuss optimal positioning for an uncomplicated labor and delivery in terms of biomechanics, gravity, and energy conservation.
7. Vaginal delivery places great stretch and compression on which nerve?

LABORATORY PRACTICE

1. Practice giving instructions to a lab partner on how to perform the following exercises. Observe that they are being done correctly. Reverse the experience and provide feedback.
   Diastasis recti exercises
   Pelvic clock exercises
   Breathing and relaxation for the different stages of labor and delivery
2. Practice giving instructions and get verbal feedback as to the success of instructions for the pelvic floor awareness training and strengthening exercises
3. Observe an exercise class for pregnant women. Critique the effectiveness and inclusiveness of the instruction.

CASE STUDIES

Case 1

Ms V. is a 32-year-old pregnant woman referred with a diagnosis of "low back pain," which became severe at 24 weeks' gestation. She reports (L) lumbar/thoracic, (R) anterior rib/pectoral, and cervical symptoms, which are worsening as the pregnancy progresses. Prior to her pregnancy, she wore a custom-made bra (32-MM), which is now much too small and provides inadequate support. Wearing this bra greatly increases her cervical and upper trapezius symptoms. Wearing a sports bra or standing more than 10 to 15 minutes causes increased low back symptoms. Pain is severely limiting her daily activities both at home and in the community. She has difficulty climbing stairs, grocery shopping, doing laundry, and other household chores. She is wakened at night by pain and also reports LE numbness at night. She is a single mother of a 6-year-old son. Pertinent medical history includes: weight gain of 100 lb with her previous pregnancy; C-section delivery; removal of fibrocystic breast tissue three times. No systemic medical conditions or medications other than prenatal vitamins. Current weight: 238 lb, height: 5′4″. Clinical findings:

Marked postural asymmetry: forward-head/shoulders with internal rotation at both shoulder joints, significant lordosis (cervical and lumbar), recurvatum bilaterally, decreased longitudinal arches, increased base of support with excessive ER at both hips.

All dynamic movements are pain inhibited: frequent weight shift and asymmetrical transitions, antalgic gait pattern with increased ER of hips. Lumbar extension and (L) cervical rotation most limited by pain and spasm.

Diastasis recti of 9 cm noted above umbilicus; abdominal strength 3-/5

Pelvic landmarks difficult to assess due to adipose tissue; leg lengths appear equal. Slight tenderness over pubic symphysis with palpation.

- Identify the impairments and functional limitations
- Identify goals that deal with impairments and functional limitations
- Develop a treatment plan to meet the goals; identify specific interventions and parameters, number of times she will be seen, and any follow-up or referrals that you believe will be necessary.

Case 2: Late Effects of Multiple Pregnancies and Disuse Atrophy

Mrs. W is a 71-year-old woman with an 11-year history of urinary incontinence and urgency. She experiences frequent, large-volume accidents, using 8 to 10 large incontinence pads and 8 panty liners/day for garment protection. Voiding frequency is 13 to 16 times every 24 hours. She also reports constipation and straining for evacuation, which improves with increased fiber intake. Caffeine intake is 2 servings per day. Mrs. W is a nonsmoker. She is much less active with social and community activities as a result of this problem. Urodynamic testing revealed diminished bladder capacity at 150 cc and confirmed the diagnosis of detrusor instability.

Pertinent medical history includes nine pregnancies and seven live births (G9, P7) with one breech presentation. LBP and "sciatic nerve problems" of long-standing were reported with lumbar fusion done when she was 44 and 48 years of age. Other surgical history includes rectocele/cystocele repair when she was 36 and partial hysterectomy when she was 37. Hypertension and asthma are both well controlled with medication. Clinical findings:

Pelvic floor muscle assessment reveals poor sensory awareness decreased resting tone, with a MMT of 2/5. Patient able to hold a contraction 4 seconds and repeat 10 "quick flicks" in 10 seconds. Accessory recruitment of the abdominals noted. Pressure perineometry confirms muscle weakness with 6.35 cm of water pressure generated. Levator ani contraction is enhanced with stretch facilitation to the pelvic floor (R>L).

Abdominal strength is 3/5. Diastasis recti noted above the umbilicus of 4.5cm.

Diaphragmatic breathing pattern present, no Valsalva with exertion.

All dynamic movements of the trunk are mildly restricted because of lumbar fusion.

The patient underwent physical therapy treatments approximately 18 months ago and is independent with her LB program. (Because of insurance limitations of 10 visits, the patient requested primary attention to pelvic floor dysfunction and incontinence.)

- Identify the impairments and functional limitations
- Identify goals that deal with the impairments and functional limitations
- Design a treatment plan to meet the goals; identify specific interventions and parameters, number of times she will be seen, and any follow-up or referrals that you believe will be necessary.

REFERENCES

1. Artal, R, and Wiswell, R: Exercise in Pregnancy. Williams & Wilkins, Baltimore, 1986.
2. Benson, JT (ed.): Female Pelvic Floor Disorders, Investigation and Management, W W Norton, NY, 1992.
3. Boissonnault, J, and Blaschak, M: Incidence of diastasis recti abdominis during the childbearing years. Phys Ther 68:1082, 1988.
4. Boston Children's Medical Center and Feinbloom, R: Pregnancy, Birth and the Newborn Baby, ed 1. Dell Publishing, New York, 1979.
5. Boston Women's Health Book Collective: Our Bodies. Our Selves, ed 2. Simon & Schuster, New York, 1979.
6. Brewer, G: The Pregnancy After 30 Workbook, ed 1. Rodale, Emmaus, PA, 1978.
7. Burgio, KL, Locher, JL, et al: Behavioral versus drug treatment for urge urinary incontinence in older women. JAMA 280:1995, 1998.
8. Bursch, S: Interrater reliability of diastasis recti abdominis measurement. Phys Ther 67:1077, 1987.
9. Chiarelli, P, and O'Keefe, D: Physiotherapy for the pelvic floor. Austral J Physiother 27: 4, 1981.
10. Clapp, JF: A clinical approach to exercise during pregnancy. Clin Sports Med 13:443, 1994.
11. Clapp, JF: Exercise and fetal health. J Dev Physiol 15:9, 1991.
12. Clapp, JF: Exercise during pregnancy: a clinical update. Clin Sports Med April, 19 (2):273, 2000.
13. Dale, B, and Roeber, J: The Pregnancy Exercise Book. Pantheon Books, New York, 1982.
14. DeLancey JOL, Richardson, AC: Anatomy of Genital Support.

In Benson, JT (ed.): Female Pelvic Floor Disorders, Investigation and Management. W W Norton, NY, 1992.

15. De Lyser, F: Jane Fonda's Workout Book for Pregnancy, Birth and Recovery. Simon & Schuster, New York, 1982.
16. Exercise During Pregnancy and the Postpartum Period. ACOG: An Educational Aid to Obstetrician-Gynecologists (Technical Bulletin No 189). Washington, DC, ACOG, 1994.
17. Fantl, JA, Newman, DK, et al: Urinary incontinence in adults: acute and chronic management. Clinical Practice Guideline No. 2, 1996 Update, US Dept of HHS, Public Health Service, AHCPR Publication No. 96-0682, Rockville, MD, March, 1996.
18. Feigel, D: Evaluating Prenatal and Postpartum Exercise Classes. Bulletin of Section on Obstetrics and Gynecology, American Physical Therapy Association 7:12, 1983.
19. Feldenkrais, M: Awareness Through Movement: Health Exercises for Personal Growth, ed 1. Harper & Row, New York, 1972.
20. Feldt, CM: Applying the Guide to Physical Therapist Practice to Women's Health Physical Therapy: Part II. J Section Women's Health, APTA 24:1, 2000.
21. Flanagan, G: The First Nine Months of Life, ed 2. Simon & Schuster, New York, 1962.
22. Frahm, J: Strengthening the Pelvic Floor. Clinical Management in Physical Therapy 5:30, 1985.
23. Freyder, SC: Exercising while pregnant. Journal of Orthopedic and Sports Physical Therapy Association 10:358, 1989.
24. Gent, D, and Gottlieb, K: Cesarean Rehabilitation. Clinical Management in Physical Therapy 5:14, 1985.
25. Gilbert, E, and Harman, J: High-Risk Pregnancy and Delivery, ed 1. CV Mosby, St Louis, 1986.
26. Ingalls, A, and Salerno, M: Maternal and Child Health Nursing, ed 5. CV Mosby, St Louis, 1983.
27. Jarski, RW, and Trippett, DL: The risks and benefits of exercise during pregnancy. J Fam Pract 30:185, 1990.
28. Knee-Chest Exercises and Maternal Death: Comments. Med J Aust 1:1127, 1973.
29. Mandelstam, D: The pelvic floor. Physiotherapy 64:8, 1978.
30. Markowiz, E, and Brainen, H: Baby Dance: A Comprehensive Guide to Prenatal and Postpartum Exercise. Prentice-Hall, Englewood Cliffs, NJ, 1980.
31. Nelson, P: Pulmonary Gas Embolism in Pregnancy and the Puerpurium. Obstet Gynecol Surv 15, 1960.
32. Noble, E: Essential Exercises for the Childbearing Years, ed 3. Houghton Mifflin, Boston, 1988.
33. Noble, E: Having Twins, ed 1. Houghton Mifflin, Boston, 1980.
34. Norwood, C: Cesarean Variations: Patients, Facilities or Policies. Internat J Childbirth Educ 1:4, 1986.
35. Ostgaard, HC, et al: Reduction of back and posterior pelvic pain in pregnancy. Spine 19:894, 1994.
36. Pauls, J: Therapeutic Approaches to Women's Health- A Program of Exercise and Education. Aspen Publishers, Gaithersburg, 1995.
37. Perinatal Exercise Guidelines. Section on Obstetrics and Gynecology, American Physical Therapy Association. 1986.
38. Physical Therapy Assessment and Treatment of the Female Patient. Obstetrical and Gynecological Implications, March 15–21, 1986. Sponsored by Programs in Physical Therapy. Northwestern University Medical School and Section on Obstetrics and Gynecology. American Physical Therapy Association.
39. Position Paper. Section on Obstetrics and Gynecology: Bulletin of Section on Obstetrics and Gynecology, American Physical Therapy Association 8:6, 1984.
40. Pritchard, J, and MacDonald, P (eds): Williams' Obstetrics, ed 16. Appleton-Century-Crofts, Norwalk, CT, 1980.
41. Prudden, S, and Sussman, J: Pregnancy and Back-to-Shape Exercise Program. Workman Publishing, New York, 1980.
42. Sandberg, E: Synopsis of Obstetrics, ed 10. CV Mosby, St Louis, 1978.
43. Santiesteban, A: Electromyographic and dynamometric characteristics of female pelvic floor musculature. Phys Ther 68:344, 1988.
44. Shrock, P, Simkin, P, and Shearer, M: Teaching prenatal exercise: Part II—Exercises to think twice about. Birth Fam J 8:3, 1981.
45. Snooks, SJ, Swash, M, et al: Risk Factors in childbirth causing damage to the pelvic floor innervation. Int J Colorect Dis 1:20, 1986.
46. Stephenson, R, and O'Connor, L: Obstetric and Gynecologic Care in Physical Therapy, ed 2. Slack, Inc. Thorofare, 2000.
47. Tchow, D, et al: Pelvic-floor musculature exercises in treatment of anatomical urinary stress incontinence. Phys Ther 68:652, 1988.
48. Wilder, E (ed): Obstetric and Gynecologic Physical Therapy: Clinics in Physical Therapy, Vol 20, ed 1. New York, Churchill-Livingstone, 1988.
49. Wilder, E (ed.): The Gynecological Manual, APTA, Section on Women's Health, 1997.
50. Zacharin, RF: Pelvic Floor Anatomy and the Surgery of Pulsion Enterocele. Springer-Verlag/Wien, New York, 1985.

Chapter 18

Management of Vascular Disorders of the Extremities

OBJECTIVES

After studying this chapter, the reader will be able to:

1 Differentiate between common acute and chronic vascular disorders of the extremities that occur as a result of a variety of medical or surgical conditions and that affect the arterial, venous, and lymphatic circulatory systems.

2 Describe the clinical signs and symptoms as well as the primary and secondary impairments associated with specific disorders of the peripheral vascular system.

3 Explain the role of exercise in the examination and screening of patients with known or suspected vascular disorders affecting the extremities.

4 Explain the principles for the use of therapeutic exercise for the rehabilitation of patients with specific vascular conditions.

5 Develop guidelines for the management of patients with acute or chronic peripheral vascular disorders resulting in arterial, venous, or lymphatic circulatory dysfunction.

6 Identify any precautions or contraindications that should be included in patient education and considered when incorporating exercise into a patient's rehabilitation program.

7 Describe the vascular, musculoskeletal, respiratory, and integumentary impairments and potential functional limitations that can occur after surgery or adjuvant therapy for breast cancer.

8 Develop guidelines for the management of patients who have undergone surgery for breast cancer.

9 Explain the rationale for the use of therapeutic exercise for the management of patients with lymphedema.

10 Identify and prioritize the types of therapeutic exercise that are appropriate for patients with lymphedema.

11 Discuss the guidelines and important precautions for the use of exercise in a comprehensive lymphatic drainage program.

12 Develop an appropriate sequence and variety of exercises for a patient with upper or lower extremity lymphedema.

Vascular disorders, which cause insufficient circulation to the extremities, can result in significant physical impairments and subsequent loss of function of either the upper or lower extremities. Disturbances of structure or function of the circulatory systems are broadly classified as acute or chronic *peripheral vascular disease* (PVD) and can be caused by a number of underlying pathologies of the arterial, venous, or lymphatic systems, including occlusion, inflammation, vasomotor dysfunction, or neoplasms.[34,40,50] In addition, surgical procedures or radiation therapy necessary for the treatment of some forms of cancer can impair lymphatic circulation.[7,41,67,71]

To contribute to the effective management of patients with vascular disorders, a therapist must possess a sound understanding of the underlying pathologies and the clinical manifestations of many types of arterial, venous, and lymphatic disorders. A therapist must also be aware of the use, effectiveness, and limitations of therapeutic exercise in the comprehensive management and rehabilitation of patients with vascular disorders.

Arterial Disorders

Types of Arterial Disorders

Acute Arterial Occlusion

A thrombus (blood clot), embolism, or trauma can cause acute loss of blood flow to peripheral arteries. The most common location of an arterial embolus is at the femoral-popliteal bifurcation, although an embolus can occur at other arterial bifurcations in the extremities.[34,40] Crush injuries to the vessels of the extremities can also disrupt arterial blood flow and must be repaired quickly to restore circulation and prevent tissue necrosis. If a patient develops an acute arterial occlusion, immediate medical or surgical measures must be taken to maintain viability of the limb. This could include complete bed rest, systemic coagulation therapy, or a thromboembolectomy or reconstructive arterial bypass surgery.[29,34,46,49,59]

Precaution: With an acute occlusion therapeutic exercise is contraindicated. Use of support hose or application of direct heat over painful areas is also contraindicated.[59]

Arteriosclerosis Obliterans (ASO)

ASO, also called *chronic occlusive arterial disease, peripheral arterial occlusive disease,* or *atherosclerotic occlusive disease,* accounts for 95% of all the arterial disorders affecting the lower extremities.[34] It is a chronic disorder, most often seen in elderly patients. It is more common in men than women and is associated with risk factors that include elevated serum cholesterol (above 200 mg/dL), smoking, high systolic blood pressure, obesity, and diabetes mellitus.[15,34,36,70]

ASO is characterized by chronic, progressive occlusion of peripheral circulation, most often in the large and medium arteries of the lower extremities, caused by atherosclerotic plaque formation.[34,70]

Thromboangiitis Obliterans (Buerger's Disease)

This chronic disease, which predominantly is seen in young male patients who smoke, involves an inflammatory reaction of the arteries to nicotine. It initially occurs in the small arteries of the feet and hands, progresses proximally, and results in vasoconstriction, decreased arterial circulation to the extremities, ischemia, and eventual necrosis and ulceration of soft tissues.[29,39,40,50] The inflammatory reaction and resulting signs and symptoms can be controlled if the patient stops smoking.

Raynaud's Disease

This chronic, functional arterial disorder, which occurs more often in women than in men, is thought to be caused by an abnormality of the sympathetic nervous system leading to digital vasospasm, most often affecting the small arteries and arterioles of the fingers and, sometimes, the toes. The vasospasm is brought on by exposure to cold, vibration, or stress. The response is characterized by temporary blanching *(pallor)*, then cyanosis and pain, followed by numbness and a cold sensation of the digits. Symptoms are slowly relieved by warmth.[29,34,40,50,59,76]

When the disorder is primary, it is called *idiopathic Raynaud's disease* or *Raynaud's syndrome;* when it is a secondary complication and associated with another disease (such as scleroderma, systemic lupus erythematosis, rheumatoid arthritis, or vasculitis), it is called *Raynaud's phenomenon.*[50,76]

Clinical Manifestations of Arterial Disorders

The following signs and symptoms are associated with peripheral arterial disorders.

Diminished or Absent Peripheral Pulses

The more occluded or restricted the arterial blood flow and the more diminished the peripheral pulses, the more severe or advanced the arterial disease.[29,34,50,55,59] If collateral circulation is extensive, the patient may not experience pain despite diminished pulses.

Integumentary Changes

A variety of integumentary changes are associated with peripheral arterial disease.[29,34,35,40,46,50,58,59]

- Skin discoloration, including *pallor* at rest or with exercise, or *reactive hyperemia* can develop. Pallor is more evident when the extremity is elevated above the level of the heart for several minutes. Reactive hyperemia occurs when the extremity is then moved to a dependent position. The skin takes on a bright red appearance rather than a normal pink flush. (See test for rubor of dependency later in this chapter.) Pallor of the distal extremity may also occur with exercise. After exercise, cutaneous ischemia causes blanching of the skin as arterial blood flow is diverted to the exercising muscles and away from the surface tissues of the distal extremity.

- *Trophic changes* include a shiny, waxy appearance of the skin and dryness and loss of hair distal to the occlusion.
- *Skin temperature* is decreased.
- *Ulcerations* may develop particularly at weight-bearing areas or over bony prominences.

Sensory Disturbances

Intolerance to heat or cold and paresthesia (initially tingling, then numbness) can develop.[29,49,50,59]

Exercise Pain and Rest Pain

Pain during exercise and, later, pain at rest are associated with progressive peripheral arterial disease and lead to significant disability.[15,29,34,35,36,40,50,59]

Exercise pain. Pain that occurs and gradually increases with exercise, most commonly in the lower extremities, is referred to as *intermittent claudication.*[29,30,31,50,59] It occurs more frequently and with greater intensity as the severity of chronic arterial insufficiency progresses over time. Intermittent claudication is characterized by a feeling of fatigue or weakness in the early stages of arterial disease and, later, as cramping or aching in the musculature that is used during exercise. Pain is located distal to the occluded vessels. The symptoms are caused by insufficient blood supply and activity-induced ischemia in the exercising muscles. Leg pain is typically brought on by walking and gradually subsides when the patient stops walking. Intermittent claudication does not occur with extended periods of standing (as occurs in spinal stenosis)[35] or with prolonged sitting (as is often seen with sciatica.)[11,36]

Although exercise pain occurs most commonly in the calf, it can also occur more proximally. Table 18–1 lists the common sites of intermittent claudication.[11,29,34,35,40,50,59]

Table 18–1 Common Sites of Exercise Pain and Associated Arterial Occlusion

Site of Pain	Occluded Artery
Chronic Arterial Insufficiency	
Calf	Femoral
Foot	Popliteal
Thigh	Iliac
Buttocks or low back	Aortic
Thromboangitis Obliterans	
Arch of the foot	Plantar and tibial
Palm of the hand	Palmar and ulnar

If peripheral vessels such as the popliteal, femoral, or iliac arteries are occluded, symptoms usually occur in one extremity; whereas, if the occlusion is in the lower aorta, symptoms often are present in both extremities as well as the buttocks and low back regions. As the disease progresses, exercise tolerance deteriorates as ischemic pain occurs more readily with activity.

Rest pain. If a burning, tingling sensation gradually occurs in the distal extremities at rest or with elevation, it may be indicative of severe ischemia. Pain frequently occurs at night because the heart rate and volume of blood flow to the extremities decreases with rest.

Sometimes partial or complete relief of pain can be achieved if the leg is placed in a dependent position, for example, over the edge of a bed. Elevation of the limb increases the pain.

Muscle Weakness

Loss of strength, atrophy of muscles, and eventual loss of motor function, particularly in the hands and feet, occur with progressive arterial vascular disease. Loss of motor function is compounded by pain, which further compromises functional strength.[29,59]

Examination and Evaluation of Arterial Sufficiency

A comprehensive examination of a patient with known or suspected peripheral arterial disease is necessary to determine or verify the etiology of a patient's impairments and functional limitations. For example, the origin of a patient's buttock and leg pain or lower extremity weakness could be caused by either vascular or neuromuscular pathologies.[36] The initial and subsequent examinations also provide a basis to determine a patient's status before treatment and the effectiveness of the interventions over time.

Of course, a thorough examination includes a complete history and systems review coupled with specific tests and measures. Some of the examination procedures listed in Box 18–1 and described in this section are commonly used by therapists to indirectly assess arterial blood flow.[4a,46,50,55,58] Other tests, such as angiography or arteriography, are administered by practitioners with specialized training and are interpreted by the patient's physician.

In addition, the examination should also include active and passive range of motion (ROM), neural

Box 18–1 Tests and Measurements of Arterial Sufficiency

- Palpation and comparison of pulses in the involved and uninvolved upper or lower extremities
- Skin temperature
- Skin integrity and pigmentation
- Tests for reactive hyperemia (rubor of dependency)
- Claudication time
- Doppler ultrasonography
- Transcutaneous oximetry
- Magnetic resonance angiography
- Arteriography

tissue mobility, deep tendon reflex (DTR) testing, and strength testing.[15] Other tests of arterial blood flow, such as Doppler ultrasonography or transcutaneous oximetry, which are generally ordered or performed and interpreted by the physician for determination of a medical diagnosis, are also briefly noted at the end of this section.[15,50,59] An understanding of test procedures and their interpretation is important so the therapist can determine an effective plan of care with appropriate interventions and evaluate the patient's response to the treatment program.

Palpation of Pulses

- The basis of any evaluation of the integrity of the arterial system is the detection of pulses in the distal portion of the extremities. Pulses are described as *normal, diminished,* or *absent.* The strength of pulses can also be rated quantitatively from 0 to +3. Even if pulses appear normal, blood flow to the extremity can still be substantially decreased.[14] Pulselessness is a sign of severe arterial insufficiency.
- The femoral, popliteal, dorsalis pedis, and posterior tibial pulses should be palpated in the lower extremities. The radial, ulnar, and brachial pulses are often palpated in the upper extremity.

Note: Pulses are difficult to assess quantitatively by palpation. Other, more accurate and reliable noninvasive tests such as Doppler ultrasound supplement information gained from palpation of pulses.

Skin Temperature

- Temperature of the skin can be grossly assessed by palpation. A limb with diminished arterial blood flow will be cool to the touch.
- If a discrepancy exists between an involved and an uninvolved extremity, a quantitative measurement of skin temperature should be made with an electronic thermometer.

Skin Integrity and Pigmentation

- Diminished or absent arterial blood flow to an extremity causes trophic changes in the skin peripherally.
- The patient's skin is dry and color is diminished (pallor). Hair loss and a shiny appearance to the skin also occur. Skin ulcerations may also be present.

Test for Rubor/Reactive Hyperemia

- Changes in skin color that occur with elevation and dependency of the limb as the result of altered blood flow are determined.
- Procedure.
  - The legs are elevated for several minutes above the level of the heart while the patient is lying supine.
  - Pallor (blanching) of the skin will occur in the feet within 1 minute or less if arterial circulation is poor. The time necessary for blanching to develop is noted.
  - The legs are then placed in a dependent position, and the color of the feet is noted.

Note: Normally, a pinkish flush appears in the feet within several seconds after the legs are placed in a dependent position. In occlusive arterial disease, a bright bluish-red or rubor of the distal legs and feet is evident, which is caused by reduced blood flow in the capillaries. The rubor may take as long as 30 seconds to appear.

- Alternate procedure
  - Reactive hyperemia can also be evaluated by temporarily restricting blood flow to the distal portion of the lower extremity with a blood pressure cuff.
  - This restriction causes an accumulation of CO_2 and lactic acid in the distal extremity. These metabolites are vasodilators and affect the vascular bed of the blood flow-deprived area.[14]
  - When the cuff is released and blood flow resumes to the distal extremity, a normal hyperemia (flushing) of the extremity should occur within 10 seconds. In arteriosclerotic vascular disease it may take as long as 1 to 2 minutes for a flush to appear. However, in vasospastic arterial disease (Raynaud's disease), flushing will occur within the normal timeframe.[14]

- This method of assessing reactive hyperemia is quite painful and is not tolerated well in either normal individuals or patients with occlusive arterial disease.

Claudication Time

- An objective assessment of exercise pain (intermittent claudication) is performed to determine the amount of time a patient can exercise before experiencing cramping and pain in the distal musculature.[31,50,70,81]
- A common test is to have the patient walk at a slow, predetermined speed on a level treadmill (1–2 mph). The time that the patient is able to walk before the onset of pain or before pain prohibits further walking is noted.[31,50,59]
- This measurement should be taken to determine a baseline for exercise tolerance before initiating a program to improve exercise tolerance.

Doppler Ultrasonography

- This noninvasive assessment uses the Doppler principle to determine the relative velocity of blood flow in the major arteries and veins.[29,46,50,55,59] A soundhead, covered with coupling gel, is placed on the skin directly over the artery to be evaluated. An ultrasonic beam is directed transcutaneously to the artery. Blood cells moving in the path of the beam cause a shift in the frequency of the reflected sound.
- The frequency of the reflected sound emitted varies with the velocity of blood flow. This information is transmitted visually onto an oscilloscope or printed tape or audibly, via a loudspeaker or stethoscope.
- Systolic pressure can also be measured at various points in arterial vessels.

Note: Although Doppler ultrasonic evaluations are not commonly performed by therapists, a recent study indicates that therapists who have been trained in the use of the technique have demonstrated competence and accuracy.[55]

Transcutaneous Oximetry

- This procedure provides information about the oxygen saturation of blood by means of a photoelectric device (a pulse oximeter).[34]
- A beam of red and infrared light passes through a pulsating capillary bed, for example, in the fingertip. The ratio of red to infrared transmission varies with the oxygen saturation of the blood. Because it responds only to pulsating objects, it does not detect nonpulsating objects, such as venous blood or skin.

Arteriography

- This is an invasive procedure that involves the injection of a radiopaque dye (contrast medium) directly into an artery.[34,40,46,50]
- The arteries are then radiographically visualized to detect any restriction of movement of the dye in arterial vessels indicating a partial or complete occlusion. Collateral circulation can also be visualized.

Note: Although this is an invasive procedure, it gives a very accurate picture of the location and extent of an arterial obstruction. The procedure is most often done prior to reconstructive arterial bypass surgery.

Magnetic Resonance Angiography

This noninvasive procedure also provides radiographic visualization of arteries without the use of a contrast medium.[34]

Management of Acute Arterial Occlusion

The management of acute occlusion is often a medical or surgical emergency. The viability of the limb will depend on the location and extent of the occlusion and the availability of collateral circulation. Medical or surgical measures must be taken to reduce ischemia and to restore circulation. A common surgical intervention for an acute occlusion is a *thromboembolectomy*. If circulation cannot be significantly improved or restored, gangrene will develop in a very short time, and amputation of the extremity will be necessary.[34,46]

Box 18–2 summarizes the guidelines for management of acute arterial occlusion.[29,44,46,50,59]

Management of Chronic Arterial Insufficiency

Chronic arterial insufficiency can often be conservatively managed by medical and physical means.* Chronic ASO does not usually require emergency medical or surgical care, except in the very advanced stages. Conservative measures are also useful in the management of thromboangitis and Raynaud's disease.

*See references 29, 44, 49, 50, 59, 69, 70, 74, 81.

Box 18–2 Management Guidelines—Acute Arterial Occlusion

Impairments:

Severe ischemia
Severe pain
Potential for tissue necrosis and amputation
Risk of local or systemic infection

Plan of Care	Interventions
1. Decrease ischemia by restoration or improvement of blood flow.	1. Medical: bed rest; complete systemic anticoagulation therapy. Physical: reflex heating of the torso or opposite extremity.[29,50] Positioning the patient in bed, with the head slightly raised, increases the blood flow to the distal portion of the extremity. Note: Thromboembolectomy and reconstructive arterial or bypass graft surgery are alternatives to nonoperative treatment.
2. Protect the limb.	2. The limb must be protected from any trauma. Pressure on skin must be minimized by a special mattress, implementation of a turning schedule, and periodic repositioning of the patient.[29,49,59]

Precautions/Contraindications: With an acute arterial occlusion any form of exercise is *contraindicated.* Local, direct heating of the involved extremity is *contraindicated* because it could easily cause a burn to ischemic tissue. Use of support hose is also *contraindicated* as they may increase peripheral resistance to blood flow. In addition, avoid wearing restrictive clothing that could compromise blood flow.

In all cases, patients must be advised to stop smoking and alter their diet, including limitations or avoidance of salt, sucrose, and alcohol to lower their blood pressure and triglyceride and cholesterol levels. These measures may not cure chronic arterial disorders but will minimize the risk factors.

Related medical disorders are also treated. Diabetes is commonly associated with chronic arteriosclerotic vascular disease and must be recognized and appropriately controlled. Hypertension is also managed with medication, diet, and exercise.[70]

In patients with mild disease, a graded exercise program of walking or bicycling should be initiated to improve exercise tolerance and functional capacity in activities of daily living. A regular program of mild- to moderate-level exercise (commonly a walking program) has been shown to decrease the occurrence of exercise pain (intermittent claudication) in patients with chronic ASO.*

Buerger or Buerger-Allen exercises, which were developed many years ago to progressively promote collateral circulation, involved a series of positional changes of the affected limb (from an elevated to a dependent position) coupled with active ankle dorsiflexion and plantarflexion exercises.[6,49,84] Although these exercises are still occasionally included in some exercise programs for patients with chronic arterial disease, there is little evidence that they are effective in improving blood flow to an extremity.[29,59] They are not advocated by the authors of this text.

Reconstructive vascular surgery, such as bypass grafts, may be indicated for patients with pain at rest. A graded exercise program after revascularization surgery may help maintain peripheral circulation. Patients with vasospastic disease may benefit from sympathetic blocks or sympathectomies to increase blood flow.[50] If patients develop ulcerations and gangrene that cannot be treated medically or with conservative surgical procedures, amputation of the limb will be necessary.[50,60]

Box 18–3 summarizes management guidelines for chronic arterial insufficiency.

Special Considerations for a Graded Exercise Program for Patients with Chronic Arterial Insufficiency

Rationale for Graded Exercise

The following factors related to the body's normal response to exercise are the basis for the use of a

*See references 29, 30, 49, 50, 59, 69, 70, 74, 75, 81.

Box 18–3 Management Guidelines—Chronic Arterial Insufficiency

Impairments:

- Decreased endurance and increased frequency of muscular fatigue with functional activities such as walking
- Pain with exercise or at rest
- Skin breakdown and ulcerations
- Limitation of passive and active motion
- Weakness and disuse atrophy

Plan of Care	Interventions
1. Teach the patient how to minimize or prevent potential impairments and correct impairments or functional limitations currently affecting functional capabilities.	1. Self-management of current or potential impairments through patient education.
2. Communicate with health professionals from other disciplines appropriate for consultation with the patient.	2. Medical or surgical management including medications; nutritional counseling for weight control and to decrease salt, sucrose, cholesterol and caffeine intake; smoking cessation.
3. Improve exercise tolerance for ADL and decrease the incidence of intermittent claudication.	3. Regular, graded aerobic conditioning program of walking or bicycling[31,50,59,69,70,81] (see Chapter 4).
4. Relieve pain at rest.	4. Sleep with the legs in a dependent but supported position over the edge of the bed or with the head of the bed slightly elevated.
5. Prevent skin ulcerations.	5. Proper care and protection of the skin, particularly the feet[14] or hands. Proper nail care.[14] Proper shoe selection and fit.[14] Avoid use of support hose and restrictive clothing. Avoid exposure to extremes of temperature, both hot and cold.
6. Improve vasodilation in affected arteries.	6. Vasodilation by iontophoresis.[2] Vasodilation by reflex heating.[2] *Note:* Although these physical measures have been advocated, their effectiveness is questionable.
7. Prevent or minimize joint contractures and muscle atrophy, particularly if the patient is confined to bed.	7. Repetitive, active ROM against low loads and/or gentle stretching exercises; proper positioning in bed to maintain joint and muscle extensibility.
8. Promote healing of any skin ulcerations that develop.	8. Wound management procedures for treating ischemic ulcers, including electrical stimulation and oxygen therapy.[29,60,61]

graded exercise program to improve the functional status of patients with chronic arterial insufficiency.*

- During an active contraction of a muscle, blood flow temporarily decreases, but a rapid increase in blood flow occurs immediately after the muscle contraction.
- After exercise is ended, there is a rapid decrease in blood flow during the first 3 to 4 minutes. This is followed by a slow decline to resting levels within 15 minutes.
- With repeated, moderate-level exercise, blood flow in muscles can be increased 10 to 12 times the resting values for blood flow.

Note: It has been suggested that regular daily exercise, for example, walking or cycling, will increase the time before the onset of exercise pain. Although it is questionable whether a regular graded exercise program improves collateral circulation in the extremities of humans with vascular disease, it has been demonstrated that exercise performed over time quantitatively improves the efficiency of oxygen utilization in exercising muscles and qualitatively improves a patient's sense of well-being and everyday life. This enables a patient to tolerate exercise over a longer period and to walk longer distances before the onset of exercise pain.†

Exercise Guidelines

- The patient should be encouraged to walk or bicycle as far as possible, without causing intermittent claudication.

*See references 15, 29, 30, 31, 50, 59, 69, 70, 74, 75, 81, 84.

†See references 11, 26, 31, 33, 39, 15, 29, 30, 31, 50, 69, 70, 74, 75, 81, 84.

- The graded endurance exercise should be carried out 3 to 5 days per week.
- The patient should perform mild warm-up and stretching activities prior to initiating walking or bicycling. Warm-up activities could include active pumping exercises of the ankle and toes.
- See Chapter 4 for specific guidelines for establishing an aerobic exercise program.

Precautions:

- A maximum target heart rate should be established. A discussion of maximum target heart rate can be found in Chapter 4.
- The patient should avoid exercising outside during very cold weather.
- The patient must wear shoes that fit properly and that will not cause skin irritations, blisters, or sores.
- Patients with a history of cardiac disease must be monitored closely. An outline of these examination procedures can also be found in Chapter 4.

Contraindications:

- Graded ambulation or bicycling is discontinued if leg pain increases rather than decreases over time.
- Patients with resting pain should not participate in an ambulation or a bicycling program.
- Patients with ulcerations of the feet and wound or fungal infections should not participate in a walking program.

▶ Venous Disorders

Just as arterial disorders of the extremities can be acute or chronic, so can venous disorders.[34,39,40,47] Therapeutic exercise is one aspect of the management of patients with either an acute disease, such as thrombophlebitis, or a chronic disorder, such as varicose veins or chronic venous insufficiency.[29,34,50,59]

Types of Venous Disorders

Acute Thrombophlebitis

This disorder usually affects the lower extremities and is characterized by acute inflammation with partial or complete occlusion of a superficial or deep vein.[29,34,39,40,47] Risk factors associated with thrombophlebitis are listed in Box 18–4. If a *thrombus* (clot) lodges in one of the superficial veins (most commonly the saphenous vein), the condition usually resolves without long-term complications.

A *deep vein thrombosis* (DVT), which is a frequent complication in the lower extremities after surgery (as high as 30%) or with prolonged immobility, illness, or bed rest, is attributed to venous stasis, injury to and inflammation of the walls of a vein, or a hypercoaguable state of blood.[34,40,79] Obesity, pregnancy, increasing age, and malignancy also increase the risk for development of a DVT.[34,40,47] If a thrombus in a deep vein breaks loose and circulates through the blood stream, it is called an *embolus,* which can be life-threatening.

Chronic Venous Insufficiency

This disorder is defined as inadequate venous return over a prolonged period of time. It may begin after a severe episode of DVT, may be associated with varicose veins, or may be the result of trauma to the lower extremities or blockage of the venous system from a neoplasm.[34,40,50] In all of these disorders damaged or incompetent valves in the veins prevent or compromise venous return leading to venous hypertension and stasis in the lower extremities. Chronic pooling of blood in the veins causes inadequate oxygenation of cells and removal of waste products. This, in turn, leads to necrosis of tissues and the development of *venous stasis ulcers.*[34,40,47,60]

Clinical Manifestations of Venous Disorders

Acute Deep Vein Thrombosis: Signs and Symptoms

In the early stages of a DVT, only 25 to 50% of cases can be identified by clinical manifestations, that is, pain, swelling, or heat.[34,40] The temperature of the

Box 18–4 Risk Factors Associated with Thrombophlebitis

- Fracture or postoperative immobilization
- Prolonged bed rest
- Trauma to venous vessels
- Advanced age
- Obesity
- Sedentary lifestyle
- Congestive heart failure
- Malignancy
- Use of oral contraceptives
- Pregnancy

skin of the affected extremity may feel warmer than the noninvolved extremity.

Although edema in the vicinity of the clot may be present, it is usually too deep to palpate. If the clot is in the calf, pain or tenderness of the calf may be felt with passive dorsiflexion of the affected foot *(Homan's sign)*. However, the sensitivity of this test is poor and often reflects a false-negative or false-positive finding.[58,59,79] Only measurement by Doppler ultrasonography, venous duplex screening, or venography can confirm an acute DVT.[47,79]

Chronic Venous Insufficiency: Signs and Symptoms

Dependent, peripheral edema, occurring with long periods of standing or sitting is a common manifestation of chronic venous dysfunction. Edema decreases if the limb is elevated. Patients often report dull aching or tiredness in the affected extremity.[29,34,40,47,50,59,66] If the insufficiency is associated with varicosities, venous distention (bulging) is also notable. The skin becomes less supple over time and takes on a brownish pigmentation.

Examination and Evaluation of Venous Sufficiency

As with arterial disorders, a complete history and systems review help determine the causes of venous disorders. Some specific tests to determine venous sufficiency are listed in Box 18–5 and briefly described in this section.[29,35,47,58,59,66] These tests complement a comprehensive integumentary and neuromuscular examination that includes skin integrity, mobility, color, texture, temperature, vital signs including peripheral pulses, sensation, pain, functional mobility, ROM, strength, and endurance.

Girth Measurements

- Circumferential measurements of the involved and uninvolved limbs are used to determine the extent of edema and effectiveness of interventions over time.[29,50,58,59,65]
- Measurements are taken at predetermined and consistent distances apart, such as 8 or 10 cm apart.

Box 18–5 Tests and Measures of Venous Sufficiency

- Girth measurements of the upper or lower extremities
- Percussion test: compliance of the greater saphenous vein
- Homan's sign
- Response to compression of the limb with a blood pressure cuff
- Doppler ultrasonography
- Venous duplex screening/scanning
- Venography

Competency of the Greater Saphenous Vein (Percussion Test)

- This test is used to evaluate the valves of the saphenous vein and is commonly done in patients with varicosities.
- Procedure:[40,58,59]
  Ask the patient to stand until the veins in the legs appear to fill. While palpating a portion of the saphenous vein below the knee, sharply percuss a portion of the vein above the knee. If valves are not functioning adequately, the examiner will feel a back flow of fluid distalward under the palpating fingertips.

Tests for Deep Vein Thrombophlebitis

These tests determine the possible presence of a thrombus in a lower extremity.

- ***Homan's sign.*** Procedure: With the patient supine and the knee extended, passively dorsiflex the ankle and gently squeeze the posterior calf muscles. If the patient experiences pain in the calf, Homan's sign is positive.[34,40,58,59] However, this is not a definitive test for the presence of a DVT. Homan's sign has been found to be positive in more than 50% of subjects who did not have a DVT. In addition, it has been shown to be positive in fewer than one-third of patients with a confirmed DVT in the calf.[79]
- ***Application of a blood pressure cuff around the calf.*** Procedure:[58] Inflate the cuff gradually until the patient experiences calf pain. A patient with acute thrombophlebitis usually cannot tolerate pressures above 40 mm Hg.

Additional Special Tests

These tests are performed and analyzed by the patient's physician or a practitioner with specialized training.[34,47,50,55,58,59]

- ***Doppler ultrasonography.*** A noninvasive screening device.[34,55,58,59]
- ***Venous duplex scanning.*** The preferred noninvasive medical diagnostic tool.
- ***Venography (phlebography).*** An invasive procedure less commonly used than noninvasive pro-

cedures used for the medical diagnosis of venous thrombosis. It involves injection of radiopaque dye and visualization of the venous system by x-ray.[49]

Prevention of Deep Vein Thrombosis

Every effort should be made to prevent the occurrence of acute thrombophlebitis in patients at risk. The following guidelines may reduce the risk of development of a DVT.[49,79]

- Appropriate medical management often includes prophylactic use of anticoagulants for high-risk patients.
- After surgery, begin ambulation as soon as possible.
- Perform active "pumping" exercises (active dorsiflexion, plantarflexion, and circumduction of the ankle) regularly throughout the day while lying supine in bed. Daily passive ROM is necessary if active exercises and ambulation are not possible because of a medical or surgical condition or significant muscle weakness or paralysis.
- Use compression stockings to support the walls of the veins and minimize venous pooling. For patients on bed rest, use of sequential compression units is indicated.
- Keep lower extremities elevated on a footstool or ottoman when sitting for prolonged periods of time.

Management of Acute Thrombophlebitis

Immediate medical management is essential in this life-threatening disorder. During the initial stages of treatment, the patient is placed on complete bed rest and systemic anticoagulant therapy, and the involved extremity is elevated. Movement of the extremity will cause pain and will increase congestion in the venous channels in the early inflammatory period. Therefore, exercise is contraindicated.

Box 18–6 summarizes the guidelines for management of acute thrombophlebitis.[29,47,50,59]

Management of Chronic Venous Insufficiency and Varicose Veins

Patient education is fundamental in the management of these chronic disorders. The patient must be advised on how to prevent dependent edema, skin ulceration, and infections. The therapist may be involved in (1) measuring and fitting a patient for a pressure-gradient support stocking; (2) teaching the patient how to put on the stocking before getting out of bed; (3) setting up a program of regular active exercise; and (4) teaching the patient proper skin care.

Box 18–7 summarizes the guidelines for management of chronic venous insufficiency and varicose veins.[29,47,49,50,59,61,66]

Box 18–6 Management Guidelines—Acute Thrombophlebitis

Impairments:

Dull ache or pain usually in the calf
Tenderness, warmth, and swelling with palpation

Plan of Care	Interventions
1. Relieve pain during the acute inflammatory period.	1. Bed rest, pharmacologic management (systemic anticoagulant therapy); elevation of the affected lower extremity, keeping the knee slightly flexed.
2. In later stages, as the acute symptoms subside, regain functional mobility.	2. Graded ambulation with legs wrapped in elastic bandages or when pressure-gradient support stockings are worn.
3. Prevent recurrence of the acute disorder.	3. Continuation of appropriate medical and pharmacologic management. Use of strategies to prevent DVTs.

Contraindications: Passive or active motion or application of moist heat; use of a sequential pneumatic compression pump.

Box 18–7 Management Guidelines—Chronic Venous Insufficiency and Varicose Veins

Impairments:

- Edema
- Increased risk of skin ulcerations and infections
- Aching of involved limb
- Decreased functional mobility, strength, and endurance

Plan of Care	Interventions
1. Teach the patient how to prevent or minimize impairments.	1. Patient education and self-management skills for skin care, self-massage for lymphedema, and a home exercise program.
2. Prevent lymphedema; minimize venous stasis.	2. Use of individually tailored pressure-gradient support stockings donned before getting out of bed in the morning and worn every day. Support garment worn during exercise and ambulation. Light active exercise, such as walking, on a regular basis. Elevate the lower extremities after graded ambulation until the heart rate returns to normal. Avoid prolonged periods of standing still and sitting with legs dependent. Elevate involved limb(s) above the level of the heart (about 30–45 degrees) when resting or sleeping (see Box 18-9 for additional methods to prevent lymphedema).
3. Increase venous return and reduce lymphedema if already present.	3. Use intermittent mechanical compression pump and sleeve with involved limb elevated for several hours a day. Manual massage to drain edema. Stroke in a distal-to-proximal direction clearing the proximal nodes and areas of lymphedema first, then the middle, and finally the distal areas. Relaxation and active ROM (pumping exercises) of the distal muscles while involved limb is elevated.
4. Prevent skin abrasions, ulcerations, and wound infections.	4. Proper skin care (see Box 18–9).

Lymphatic Disorders

One of the primary functions of the lymphatic system, which consists of lymph vessels and nodes, is to collect and clear excess tissue fluid from interstitial spaces and return it to the venous system.[39] Edema is a natural consequence of trauma to and healing of soft tissues. If the lymphatic system is compromised and does not function efficiently, lymphedema develops and impedes wound healing.[39] **Lymphedema** is an excessive and persistent accumulation of extravascular and extracellular fluid and proteins in tissue spaces.[18,22,28,53] It is caused by a disturbance of the water and protein balance across the capillary membrane. An increased concentration of proteins draws greater amounts of water into interstitial spaces leading to lymphedema.[28,41] In addition, many disorders can cause the load on lymphatic vessels to exceed their transport capacity and to subsequently cause lymphedema.[41,47,53]

Disorders of the Lymphatic System Leading to Lymphatic Insufficiency

Disorders of the lymphatic transport system can cause either primary or secondary lymphedema.[34] Remember, lymphedema is not a disease, but rather a symptom of a malfunctioning lymphatic system. The vast majority of patients seen by healthcare practitioners for management of lymphedema have secondary lymphedema.[71] By far, the most common causes of secondary lymphedema are related to the comprehensive management of cancers of the breast, pelvis, and abdomen.*

Congenital Malformation of the Lymphatic System

Although uncommon, congenital malformations are the cause of primary lymphedema.[34,40]

*See references 7, 16, 18, 34, 40, 41, 71, 72, 77.

Infection and Inflammation

Inflammation of the lymph vessels, *lymphangitis,* or of the lymph nodes, *lymphadenitis,* and enlargement of lymph nodes, *lymphadenopathy,* can occur as the result of a systemic infection or local trauma. Any of these can cause disruption of lymph circulation.[34,40,41]

Obstruction or Fibrosis

Trauma, surgery, and neoplasms can block or impair lymphatic circulation.[34,41,80] Radiation therapy associated with treatment of malignant tumors can also cause fibrosis of vessels.[7,17]

Surgical Dissection of Lymph Nodes

Lymph nodes and vessels are often surgically removed *(lymphadenectomy)* as an aspect of the treatment of a primary malignancy or metastatic disease. For example, axillary lymph node dissection is performed in most types of breast cancer surgeries for the determination of the extent and progression of breast cancer.[17,20,34,45] Likewise, pelvic or inguinal lymph node excision is often associated with the treatment of pelvic or abdominal cancers.[7,71,72]

Chronic Venous Insufficiency

Although they are not lymphatic disorders, chronic venous insufficiency and varicose veins are associated with venous stasis and accumulation of edema in the extremities.[34,40,47,50]

Clinical Manifestations of Lymphatic Disorders

Lymphedema

Location. When lymphedema develops, it is most often apparent in the distal extremities, particularly over the dorsum of the foot or hand.[28,41] The term *dependent edema* describes the accumulation of fluids in the peripheral aspects of the limbs particularly when the distal segments are lower than the heart. In contrast, lymphedema can also manifest itself more centrally, for example, in the axilla, groin, or even the trunk.[28,34,40]

Severity. The severity of lymphedema may be described quantitatively or qualitatively. For example, with unilateral lymphedema, a 1- to 2-cm increase in girth measurements between the involved and noninvolved limbs is classified as mild lymphedema; a 2- to 5-cm increase is moderate lymphedema; and a greater than 5-cm increase is severe lymphedema.[65]

Lymphedema is also described by the severity of changes that occur in skin and subcutaneous tissues. The three categories, *pitting, brawny,* and *weeping* edema, are described in Box 18–8. Although all three types reflect a significant degree of lymphedema, they are listed in order of severity, from least severe to most severe.[20,22,34,40,77]

Increased Girth and Weight of the Limb

As the volume of interstitial fluid in the limb increases, so does the weight and circumferential size of the affected limb.[19,41,50,65] Increased volume, in turn, causes tautness of the skin and susceptibility to skin breakdown.[20,34]

Sensory Disturbances

Paresthesia (tingling, itching, or numbness) or occasionally a mild aching pain may be felt particularly in the fingers or toes. In many instances the condition is painless, and the patient only perceives a sense of heaviness of the limb. Fine finger coordination may also be impaired as the result of the sensory disturbances.[20,41,65,77]

Stiffness and Limited ROM

ROM decreases in the fingers and wrist or toes and ankle or even in the more proximal joints leading to decreased functional mobility of the involved segments.[20,62]

Decreased Resistance to Infection

Wound healing is delayed, and frequent infections, such as cellulitis, may occur.[41,50]

Box 18–8 Types of Lymphedema

Pitting edema	Pressure on the edematous tissues with the fingertips causes an indentation of the skin that persists for several seconds after the pressure is removed. This reflects significant but short-duration edema with little or no fibrotic changes in skin and subcutaneous tissues.
Brawny edema	Pressure on the edematous areas feels hard with palpation. This reflects a more severe form of interstitial swelling with progressive, fibrotic changes in subcutaneous tissues.
Weeping edema	This represents the most severe and long-duration form of lymphedema. Fluids leak from cuts or sores; wound healing is significantly impaired. Lymphedema of this severity occurs almost exclusively in the lower extremities.

Examination and Evaluation of Lymphatic Function

A patient's history, a systems review, and specific tests and measures provide information to determine impairments and functional limitations that can arise from lymphatic disorders and the presence of lymphedema. Key components in the examination process that are particularly relevant when a lymphatic dysfunction is suspected or lymphedema is present are summarized in this section. Other tests and measurements, such as vital signs, ROM, strength, posture, sensory testing, and functional testing, are also appropriate.[4a,5,21,29,50,59,62]

History and Systems Review

- Note any history of infection, trauma, surgery, or radiation therapy.
- Determine onset and duration of lymphedema, delayed wound healing, or previous treatment of lymphedema.
- Identify the occupation or daily activities of the patient. Are long periods of standing or sitting required?

Skin Integrity

- Note the location of the edema, wounds, or scars.
- Note the color and integrity of skin; it may be red or shiny.
- Measure the size of wounds or scars: note stage of healing.
- Note evidence of inflammation or infection.
- Check the mobility of skin and scar tissue. Note any evidence of adherence of underlying tissues.
- Palpate the dependent limb to determine the type and severity of lymphedema and changes in skin and subcutaneous tissues. Note areas of pitting, brawny, or weeping edema.
- When palpating the skin over lymph nodes, note any tenderness of the nodes (cervical, supraclavicular, inguinal). Tenderness may or may not indicate ongoing infection or serious disease.[35] Evidence of warm, enlarged, tender, painless, or adherent nodes should be reported to the physician.

Girth Measurements

- Take circumferential measurements of the involved limb and compare with the noninvolved limb if the problem is unilateral.[19,59,65]
- Identify specific intervals or landmarks at which measurements are taken so that re-examination measurements will be reliable.

Volumetric Measurements

Determine the overall volume of the involved limb by measuring the amount of water displaced as the involved and noninvolved limbs are independently immersed in a tank of water.[5,19,59]

General Considerations for the Prevention and Management of Lymphedema

Prevention of Lymphedema

If a patient is at risk of developing lymphedema secondary to infection, inflammation, obstruction, or surgical removal of lymphatic structures, or chronic venous insufficiency, *prevention* of lymphedema should be the priority of patient management. In some situations, such as after removal of lymph nodes or vessels, preventative measures may need to be taken for a lifetime. Even when a patient takes every measure to prevent edema, it still may develop at some time, particularly after trauma to or surgical removal of lymph vessels. Box 18–9 summarizes precautions and measures to prevent or reduce the risk of lymphedema.[18,20,22,44,62,68,77,80]

Aspects of Management of Lymphedema

Management involves a combination of appropriate medical management and direct therapeutic intervention by a therapist combined with self-management by the patient.

- Comprehensive treatment also includes appropriate pharmacological management for infection control as well as prevention or removal of excessive fluid and proteins.[18,34,40,47]
- To increase lymphatic drainage, the hydrostatic pressures on edematous tissues must be increased.[28] This is accomplished by *external compression of tissues* with manual lymphatic drainage, sequential lymphatic compression machines, or compressive garments.[18,19,20,21,52,62,80]

Note: It appears that compression facilitates the evacuation and reabsorption of fluids but does not increase the reabsorption of proteins in edema.[34]

- Lymphatic and venous return can also be enhanced by *elevation of the involved limb*. Lymphedema, caused by infection or inflammation of the lymphatic system, such as lymphangitis or cellulitis, does not diminish as readily with elevation as does edema secondary to chronic venous insufficiency.[28,34,80]

Box 18–9 Precautions for the Prevention or Self-Management of Lymphedema

Prevention of Lymphedema

- Avoid static, dependent positioning of the lower extremities such as prolonged sitting or standing. Avoid sitting with legs crossed.
- When traveling long distances by car, stop periodically and walk around, or support an involved upper extremity on the car's window ledge or seat back.
- Elevate involved limb(s) and perform repetitive pumping exercises frequently during the day.
- Avoid vigorous, repetitive activities with the involved limb. Avoid carrying heavy loads, such as a suitcase, a heavy backpack or shoulder bag. Avoid use of heavy weights when exercising.
- Wear compressive garments while exercising.
- Avoid wearing clothing that restricts circulation, such as sleeves or socks with tight elastic bands. Do not wear tight jewelry such as rings or watches.
- Monitor diet to maintain an ideal weight and minimize sodium intake.
- Avoid hot environments or use of local heat.
- If possible, avoid having blood pressure taken on an involved upper extremity or injections in either an involved upper or lower extremity.

Skin Care

- Keep the skin clean and supple; use moisturizers, but avoid perfumed lotions.
- Avoid infections; pay immediate attention to a skin abrasion or cut, an insect bite, a blister, or a burn.
- Protect hands and feet; wear socks or hose, properly fitting shoes, rubber gloves, oven mitts, etc.
- Avoid contact with harsh detergents and chemicals.
- Use caution when cutting nails. Women need to use an electric razor when shaving legs or underarm area.
- Avoid hot baths, whirlpools, and saunas that elevate the body's core temperature.

- A comprehensive approach to the management of lymphedema is referred to in the literature by a variety of terms, including *complex lymphedema therapy, complex decongestive physiotherapy,* or *decongestive lymphatic therapy.** Box 18–10 summarizes the components of these programs. These regimens combine manual lymphatic drainage through light, superficial massage and compressive bandaging with active ROM, low-intensity resistance exercises, and good skin hygiene. The overall goal of intervention, when lymphedema has developed, is to improve drainage of obstructed areas and to theoretically channel fluids into unobstructed, collateral vessels.

*See references 12, 13, 23, 24, 27, 56, 57, 73, 86.

Box 18–10 Components of a Decongestive Lymphatic Therapy Program

- Elevation
- Manual lymphatic drainage (massage)
  - Direct intervention by a therapist
  - Self-massage by the patient
- Compression
  - Nonelastic or low-stretch bandages or custom-fitted garments
  - Intermittent, sequential pneumatic compression pump
- Individualized exercise program
  - Active ROM (pumping exercises)
  - Flexibility exercises
  - Low-intensity resistance exercises
  - Cardiovascular conditioning
- Skin care and daily living precautions

Manual lymphatic drainage. This procedure involves slow, very light repetitive stroking and circular massage movements done in a specific sequence with the involved extremity elevated whenever possible.[12,13,23,24,27,51,78,86] Proximal congestion in the trunk, groin, buttock, or axilla is cleared first to make room for fluid from the more distal areas. The direction of the massage is toward specific lymph nodes and usually involves distal to proximal stroking. Fluid in the involved extremity is then cleared, first in the proximal portion, then in the distal portion. Because manual lymphatic drainage is very labor- and time-intensive, methods of self-massage are taught to the patient as soon as possible in a treatment program.

Exercise. *Active ROM, stretching,* and *low-intensity resistance exercises* are interposed with manual drainage techniques.[18,20,23,25,63,64] Exercises should be performed while wearing a compressive garment or bandages. Exercises are performed in a specific sequence, often with the edematous limb(s) elevated. A low-intensity cardiovascular/pulmonary endurance activity, such as bicycling, often follows ROM and strengthening exercises. Specific exercises and a suggested sequence for the upper and lower extremities, compiled from several sources, are described and illustrated in the last section of this chapter.

Elevation. Elevate the involved limb when using a sequential compression pump, when sleeping or resting, or even during sedentary activities. The compressive bandages or garment should be worn during periods of elevation.[13,18,20,62,80]

Compressive bandages, garments, or pumps. No-stretch, nonelastic bandages or low-stretch elastic bandages or garments are recommended because they provide relatively low compressive forces on the edematous extremity at rest. In addition, they provide a higher working pressure with active muscular contractions because of their less yielding nature than high-stretch bandages.[18,20,23,27,80] High-stretch sports bandages, such as Ace wraps, are not recommended for treatment of lymphedema.[13,18,80]

The use of a sequential, pneumatic compression pump on a daily basis may also be recommended in the early stages of treatment of substantial lymphedema.[18,21,27,62]

Skin care and hygiene. Lymphedema predisposes the patient to skin breakdown, infection, and delayed wound healing. Proper skin care and protection of the edematous limb are essential elements of self-management of lymphedema.[18,20,62,80]

Management Guidelines for Lymphatic Disorders

Specific Guidelines

Guidelines for the management of lymphatic disorders are essentially the same as the guidelines already described for the management of chronic venous insufficiency and associated lymphedema (see Box 18–7). As with chronic venous insufficiency, management of lymphatic disorders initially involves direct interventions by a therapist and an emphasis on patient education, followed by life-long prevention and self-management by the patient.

Precautions for the Prevention or Self-Management of Lymphedema

Precautions that patients should take for the prevention of lymphedema and skin breakdown or infection are an important aspect of self-management. Suggestions have already been summarized in Box 18–9.

Use of Community Resources

A valuable resource for patients and healthcare professions is the National Lymphedema Network (www.lymphnet.org). This nonprofit organization provides education and guidance about lymphedema. Another resource is the Lymphedema Internet Network (http://www.lymphedema.org).

▶ Lymphatic Disorders Associated with Treatment of Breast Cancer

According to the American Cancer Society, carcinoma of the breast is the most common form of cancer among women in the United States and is a leading cause of cancer-related death in women, second only to lung cancer.[4] The incidence of breast cancer increases with age;[10,37] in fact, a woman's risk of developing breast cancer during her lifetime is now estimated to be 1 in 8.[1,4,42] Despite important advances in methods of early detection, chemotherapy, radiation therapy, and hormone therapy, as well as the use of less radical surgery, breast cancer continues to be one of the most significant health issues in the United States and throughout the world.[1,4,42]

Tumors that are detected early and that are small and localized can be successfully treated by surgery, radiation therapy, chemotherapy, and hormone therapy. Although the increasing use of radiation therapy in primary treatment has permitted greater use of breast conservation surgeries, such as lumpectomy or quadrectomy, *mastectomy* (removal of the breast) is still the most common surgical procedure for the treatment of breast cancer.[1,4,42]

After a mastectomy and the accompanying excision or radiation of adjacent axillary lymph nodes, a patient is at risk of developing upper extremity lymphedema, loss of shoulder motion, and limited functional use of the arm and hand.* Axillary node dissection interrupts and slows the flow of lymph, which, in turn, can lead to lymphedema of the upper extremity.[17,20,42] Radiation can cause fibrosis in the area of the axilla, which obstructs the lymphatic vessels and contributes to pooling of lymph in the arm and hand.[17,20] Shoulder motion can become impaired as the result of incisional pain, delayed wound healing, and skin ulcerations (associated with radiation therapy), and postoperative weakness of the muscles of the shoulder girdle.[20,62] Fortunately, the impairments and functional limitations experienced by patients following mastectomy are usually temporary and respond well to early therapeutic interventions. To prevent or minimize lymphedema and loss of upper extremity function, a comprehensive approach to postoperative management that emphasizes patient education and includes therapeutic exercise and other direct interventions to prevent or treat lymphedema and other impairments or functional limitations must be implemented.[3,6,7,18,20,32,38,62,68]

As with many cancers, the diagnosis of breast cancer and the ensuing treatments have an enormous emotional impact on patients and their families.[20,77] All therapists should be aware of Reach to

*See references 3, 16, 17, 19, 20, 32, 33, 65, 67.

Recovery, a one-to-one patient education program, sponsored by the American Cancer Society (www.cancer.org). Representatives of this program, most of whom are breast cancer survivors, provide emotional support to the patient and family as well as current information on breast prostheses and reconstructive surgery.

As mentioned previously in this chapter, the National Lymphedema Network (www.lymphnet.org) is another source of information for patients at risk for or who have developed lymphedema postoperatively.

Surgical Procedures

The following types of surgery may be used in the management of breast cancer.[1,3,6,10,32,40,42]

Radical Mastectomy

- A radical mastectomy involves removal of the breast, the pectoralis muscles, chest fascia, and the ipsilateral axillary lymph nodes, followed by chemotherapy and radiation therapy to the involved area. Some of the nerve supply to the chest and shoulder musculature may also be disturbed.
- Radical mastectomy was the most common surgery for breast cancer until the 1970s, but today it is performed only for late-stage, invasive tumors.
- In addition to postoperative lymphedema and limited shoulder mobility, radical mastectomy with the removal of the pectoralis muscles causes significant disfigurement and upper extremity weakness.

Modified Radical Mastectomy

- The entire breast, fascia over the chest muscle, and axillary lymph nodes are removed, but the pectoralis muscles remain intact, which reduces cosmetic deformity and upper extremity weakness and functional limitations.
- Radiation and chemotherapy may be necessary after surgery.
- The modified radical mastectomy is still a common surgical option despite the increasing use of breast conserving surgeries.

Simple Mastectomy

- A simple mastectomy involves surgical removal of the entire breast, but the lymphatic system and pectoralis muscles are preserved.
- Postoperative radiation therapy is used to decrease the regional recurrence of the disease. Even though the lymphatic system remains intact, radiation may cause fibrosis in the lymph vessels and predispose the patient to the development of lymphedema.

Breast-Conserving Surgery

- Options include *lumpectomy* (excision of the mass and some surrounding breast tissue) or *segmental mastectomy* (also known as *quadrectomy;* excision of the affected quadrant of the breast.)
- These procedures, which preserve a portion of the breast, are being increasingly employed in combination with adjuvant therapy as an alternative to mastectomy for patients with stage I or II cancers.[1,42] An aspect of adjuvant therapy, radiation therapy, routinely follows breast-conserving surgery to minimize the risk of recurrence of the disease. At this time, axillary lymph node dissection is also a standard part of breast-conserving surgery, although the extent of removal of nodes is controversial.[1,42] A minimum of a level I axillary node dissection (removal of lymph nodes at the lateral borders of the breast in the axilla) is done for biopsy; more extensive dissection removes the nodes under the pectoralis minor muscle or around the clavicle. In addition, chemotherapy or hormonal therapy may also be employed. There are now multiple, randomized clinical trials that show that the 10- to 20-year survival rate for patients with stage I or II disease who underwent breast-conserving surgery combined with radiation therapy is equivalent to that achieved by patients who underwent mastectomy alone or mastectomy with adjuvant therapy.[1]
- Patients who undergo breast-conserving procedures are still at risk for developing postoperative lymphedema and impaired shoulder mobility because of potential complications from radiation therapy and axillary node dissection.[20,62]

Postoperative Impairments Associated with Breast Cancer Treatment

The following postoperative impairments are associated with breast cancer surgeries. Many of these problems are interrelated and must be considered jointly when a comprehensive postoperative plan of care is developed for the patient.*

*See references 3, 8, 9, 10, 16, 17, 20, 30, 32, 33, 38, 45, 62, 65, 67, 82, 83, 85.

Postoperative Pain

- ***Incisional pain***
  - A transverse incision across the chest wall is made to remove the breast tissue and underlying fascia on the chest musculature. The incision extends into the axilla for lymph node dissection.
  - The sutured skin over the breast area may feel tight along the incision; movement of the arm pulls on the incision and is uncomfortable for the patient.
  - Healing of the incision may be delayed as the result of radiation therapy. Delayed wound healing, in turn, prolongs pain in the area of the incision.
- ***Posterior cervical and shoulder girdle pain***
  - Pain and muscle spasm may occur in the neck and shoulder region as a result of muscle guarding.
  - The levator scapulae, teres major and minor, and infraspinatus are often tender with palpation and can restrict active shoulder motion.
- Decreased use of the involved upper extremity after surgery due to pain sets the stage for the patient to develop a chronic frozen shoulder and increases the likelihood of lymphedema in the hand and arm.

Postoperative Thromboemboli and Pulmonary Complications

- Decreased activity and extended time in bed increase venous stasis and the risk of DVTs, particularly in the lower extremities.
- Risk of pulmonary complications, such as pneumonia, is also higher because of the patient's reduced activity level. Incisional pain may make the patient reluctant to cough or breathe deeply, both of which are necessary postoperatively to keep the airways clear of fluid accumulation in the lungs.

Lymphedema

Patients who undergo any level of lymph node dissection or whose treatment includes radiation therapy remain at risk throughout life for developing ipsilateral upper extremity lymphedema.[20,62] Lymphedema can occur almost immediately after lymph node dissection, during the course of radiation therapy, or many months or even years after treatment has been completed. Estimates of the incidence of lymphedema after lymph node dissection and irradiation range from 7 to 70%.[17,33,65,67] The incidence is higher after radical than after modified radical mastectomy and breast-conserving surgery.[33] One reason for the wide disparity of reported incidence is that some studies only include patients with "measurable" lymphedema of greater than either 2 cm or 2 inches in the involved arm.[67] For those patients who do develop lymphedema, it can cause significant impairment of function in the upper extremity, as well as poor cosmesis and emotional distress.[8,20,33,65,77] Lymphedema is most often evident in the hand and arm or occasionally in the upper chest or back area.[17,20,62,65]

- Removal of the axillary chain of lymph nodes appears to disrupt the normal circulation of lymph and causes swelling of the upper extremity.
- Radiation therapy may lead to the formation of fibrotic scar tissue in the axilla, and sclerosis of vessels may occur as the result of chemotherapy; either can obstruct lymphatic vessels.
- Reduced use of the arm for functional activities and maintaining the arm in a dependent position may also contribute to the development of postoperative lymphedema.

The problems associated with acute and chronic lymphedema have been discussed earlier in this chapter. The more common signs and symptoms and potential impairments associated with lymphedema after breast cancer treatment bear reiteration. They include:

- Increased size of the extremity
- Tautness of the skin and risk of skin breakdown and infection
- Stiffness and decreased ROM, particularly in the fingers wrist and elbow
- Sensory disturbances in the hand
- Decreased use of the involved upper extremity for functional tasks

Chest Wall Adhesions

- Restrictive scarring of underlying tissue on the chest wall can develop as the result of surgery, radiation fibrosis, or wound infection.
- Chest wall adhesions can lead to:
  - Increased risk of postoperative pulmonary complications
  - Restricted mobility of the shoulder on the involved side
  - Postural asymmetry and dysfunction
  - Discomfort in the neck, shoulder girdle, and upper back

Decreased Shoulder Mobility

It is well documented that patients may experience temporary and sometimes permanent loss of shoul-

Box 18–11 Factors That Contribute to Potential Restriction of Shoulder Mobility After Breast Cancer Surgery

- Incisional pain immediately after surgery or associated with delayed wound healing
- Muscle guarding and tenderness of the shoulder and posterior cervical musculature
- Need for protected shoulder ROM until the surgical drain is removed within several days to a week postoperatively
- Fibrosis of soft tissues in axillary region from adjuvant radiation therapy
- Chest wall adhesions
- Temporary or permanent weakness of the muscles of the shoulder girdle
- Rounded shoulders and kyphotic or scoliotic trunk posture associated with age or incisional pain
- Lymphedema and a feeling of heaviness of the upper extremity
- Decreased use of the ipsilateral hand and arm for functional activities

der mobility after surgery or radiation therapy for treatment of breast cancer.* The factors that can potentially limit shoulder motion postoperatively are listed in Box 18–11.

Weakness and Impaired Functional Control of the Involved Upper Extremity

- ***Weakness of the horizontal adductors of the shoulder.***
  - If a radical mastectomy is performed, the pectoralis major muscle is removed.
  - This results in decreased strength and active motion of the upper extremity on the involved side on a permanent basis.
- ***Weakness of the serratus anterior.***
  - The long thoracic nerve can be temporarily traumatized during axillary dissection and removal of the axillary lymph nodes. This results in weakness of the serratus anterior and compromised shoulder stabilization and function. Without the stabilization and upward rotation of the scapula that the serratus anterior normally supplies, active flexion and abduction of the arm will be limited.
  - Faulty shoulder biomechanics and use of substitute motions with the upper trapezius and levator scapulae during overhead reaching activities can then cause subacromial impingement and resulting shoulder pain. This can be a precursor of a frozen shoulder.

*See references 3, 32, 37, 38, 45, 54, 62, 68, 82, 83, 85.

- ***Decreased grip strength.*** Grip strength is often diminished as the result of lymphedema and secondary stiffness of the fingers.

Postural Malalignment

- The patient may sit or stand with rounded shoulders and kyphosis because of pain, skin tightness, or psychological reasons. An increase in thoracic kyphosis associated with aging is commonly seen in the older patient.[37] This contributes to faulty shoulder biomechanics and eventually restricts active use of the involved upper extremity.
- Asymmetry of the trunk and abnormal scapular alignment may occur as the result of a subtle lateral weight shift, particularly in a large-breasted woman.

Fatigue and Decreased Endurance

Patients undergoing radiation therapy or chemotherapy often experience debilitating fatigue.[1,34] Anemia may develop as a result of chemotherapy. Nutritional intake and subsequent energy stores may be diminished, particularly if a patient is experiencing nausea and vomiting for several days after a cycle of chemotherapy. Fatigue may also be associated with depression. As a result, exercise tolerance and endurance during functional activities are markedly reduced.

Psychological Considerations

- A patient undergoing treatment for breast cancer experiences a wide range of emotional and social issues.[8,26,77] The needs and concerns of both the patient and the family must be considered. The patient and family members must cope with the potentially life-threatening nature of the disease as well as a difficult treatment regimen.
- It is common for a patient to feel anxiety, agitation, anger, depression, a sense of loss, and significant mood swings during treatment and recovery from breast cancer.
- Besides the obvious physical disfigurement and altered body image associated with mastectomy, medications such as immunosuppressants and corticosteroids can affect the emotional state of the patient.
- Psychological manifestations affect physical well-being and can contribute to general fatigue, the patient's perception of functional disability, and motivation in treatment.

Management after Surgery for Breast Cancer

General Considerations

Whenever possible, preoperative contact with the patient enables the therapist to screen the patient's posture and mobility, establish rapport with the patient, and teach the patient aspects of self-management, such as deep breathing and coughing, lower extremity pumping exercises, and positioning of the upper extremity.[8,37] This enables the patient to initiate these activities independently as early as the first postoperative day. Because the length of stay for patients after surgery for breast cancer is very short, direct intervention by a therapist should start on the first postoperative day with an emphasis on *prevention* of postoperative complications, impairments, or functional limitations, such as pulmonary complications and thromboemboli, as well as lymphedema and loss of functional mobility of the ipsilateral upper extremity.

As mentioned previously, after lymph node dissection or radiation, the risk of lymphedema is significant. Guidelines and precautions for prevention and self-management of lymphedema have already been summarized (see Box 18–9). Many of these measures can be initiated immediately after surgery and will need to be continued during postoperative radiation therapy and even throughout life.

Early, but protected, assisted or active ROM of the shoulder is the key to preventing chronic, postoperative restriction of shoulder mobility. The postoperative risks that can contribute to restricted shoulder mobility have been summarized previously in Box 18–11 of this chapter.[1,8,20,42,62,64] These risks are highest in the first few postoperative weeks until drains have been removed and the incision has completely healed. Remember, radiation therapy to the axillary and breast areas can delay wound healing beyond the typical 3- to 4-week time period.[1,42] Even after initial healing of the incision, the scar has a tendency to contract and can become adherent to underlying tissues, which, in turn, can restrict shoulder motion.

Although strengthening and endurance exercises are important for both upper extremity function and total body fitness, *moderation* in an exercise program is imperative. Exercises must be progressed gradually, excessive fatigue must be avoided, and energy conservation must be emphasized, especially if the patient is undergoing chemotherapy or radiation therapy.

Precautions: Exercise precautions include:[8,20,64,68]

- The patient should only exercise at a moderate level and should never experience aching in the affected arm after exercise, even if there is no evidence of postoperative lymphedema.
- The *timing* of exercise should be adjusted during cycles of chemotherapy. For example, with some medications, a patient can develop cardiac arrhythmia and, therefore, should not perform aerobic exercises, such as stationary cycling, for 24 to 48 hours after a chemotherapy treatment.
- After completion of chemotherapy or radiation therapy, the patient can gradually return to more physically demanding work and recreational activities.

Although early intervention for the prevention of lymphedema and upper extremity mobility impairments is often advocated by therapists and suggested in descriptive articles in the literature, many patients are not referred for postoperative rehabilitation until after impairments and functional limitations have developed. This may be because only a few studies have rigorously investigated the efficacy of specific interventions or rehabilitation protocols.[62] Subsequently, some physicians may doubt the benefits of therapy or may have concerns that early postoperative ROM may disturb drains or delay wound healing.[75]

Because of the many treatment options and variations in approaches to management of patients after breast cancer surgeries and the relatively limited number of definitive studies, it is difficult for clinicians to make evidence-based decisions of which interventions to include in a patient's treatment plan.[62] Despite these issues, the following recommendations can be drawn from the existing literature.*

- Postoperative lymphedema is best prevented or managed by combining several interventions including exercise, massage, and use of compression bandages, garments and pumps into a patient's comprehensive plan of care.[19,57]
- Inclusion of ROM exercises in a postoperative treatment program has a positive impact on shoulder mobility.[38,54,57,62,82,83]
- Therapeutic intervention within the first few postoperative days does not prolong hospital stays or increase the incidence of postoperative complications, in particular, wound healing.[54,62]

*See references 3, 6, 8, 9, 16, 19, 20, 32, 33, 38, 54, 62, 63, 64, 82, 83.

Guidelines for Postoperative Management After Breast Cancer Surgery

Effective postoperative management, as outlined in Box 18–12, for the patient who has undergone a mastectomy or breast-conserving surgery and who may currently be receiving adjuvant therapy, addresses those impairments and functional limitations that currently exist as well as those problems that could develop in the near future.

Note: The guidelines outlined in Box 18–12 can also be modified to prevent or manage problems that can develop in the trunk and lower extremities after surgery for abdominal or pelvic cancers with accompanying inguinal lymph node dissection.

Box 18–12 Management Guidelines after Surgery for Breast Cancer

Potential Postoperative Impairments:

- Pulmonary and circulatory complications
- Lymphedema
- Restricted mobility of the upper extremity
- Postural malalignment
- Weakness and decreased functional use of the upper extremity
- Fatigue and decreased endurance for functional activities
- Emotional and social adjustments

Plan of Care	Interventions
1. Prepare the patient for postoperative self-management.	1. Interdisciplinary patient education involving all aspects of potential impairments and functional limitations. Self-management activities and preparation for participation in a home program on the first postoperative day.
2. Prevent postoperative pulmonary complications and thromboemboli.	2. Pre- or postoperative instruction in deep breathing, emphasizing maximal inspirations and effective coughing (see Chapter 19). Active ankle exercises (calf pumping exercises).
3. Prevent or minimize postoperative lymphedema.	3. Elevation of the involved upper extremity on pillows (about 30 degrees) while the patient is in bed or sitting in a chair. Wrapping the involved upper extremity with bandages or wearing an elastic pressure gradient sleeve. Pumping exercises of the arm on the side of the surgery. Early ROM exercises. ***Precaution:*** Avoid static, dependent positioning of the arm.
4. Decrease lymphedema if or when it develops.	4. Daily use of a sequential pneumatic compression pump followed by wrapping. Continued elevation of the involved upper extremity while at rest. Compressive bandaging with nonelastic or low-stretch wraps worn continually (during activity and at rest). Manual lymphatic drainage massage. Daily regimen of exercises to reduce lymphedema. Use of custom-fit elastic compression garment when lymphedema is stabilized. Adherence to precautions for skin care (see Box 18–9).
5. Prevent postural deformities.	5. Instruction in proper bed positioning preoperatively or on the first postoperative day, emphasizing midline and symmetric positioning of the shoulders and trunk. Posture awareness training; encourage the patient to assume an erect posture when sitting or standing to minimize a rounded shoulder posture. Posture exercises with an emphasis on scapular retraction exercises.
6. Prevent muscle tension and guarding in cervical musculature.	6. Active ROM of the cervical spine to promote relaxation. Shoulder shrugging and shoulder circle exercises. Gentle massage to cervical musculature.

cont'd on page 728

Box 18–12 Management Guidelines after Surgery for Breast Cancer *(continued)*

7. Prevent restricted mobility of the upper extremity.	7. Active-assistive and active ROM exercises of the shoulder, elbow, and hand initiated as soon as possible but cautiously usually on the first postoperative day. *Note:* Exercise may be initiated even when the drainage tubes and sutures are still in place. After the incision has healed, self-stretching to the shoulder.
8. Regain strength and functional use of the involved upper extremity.	8. Low-intensity isometric exercises of shoulder musculature initiated on the first or second postoperative day. Resistance exercises with a light handheld weight or a light grade of elastic resistance material, emphasizing scapular and glenohumeral musculature. Scapular and glenohumeral stabilization exercises in standing with hands against a table or wall. Upper extremity ergometry initially against minimal and, later, moderate resistance. Use of the involved extremity for light functional activities.
9. Improve exercise tolerance and sense of well-being, and reduce fatigue.	9. Graded, low-intensity aerobic exercise such as walking or cycling.
10. Provide information about resources for patient and family support and ongoing patient education.	10. Resources include: American Cancer Society family support and ongoing patient education (www.cancer.org), National Breast Cancer Coalition; National Lymphedema Network.

Precautions: Shoulder exercise should be performed within a *protected* ROM usually no more than 90 degrees of elevation of the arm until after removal of drains. Observe the incision and sutures carefully during exercises. Avoid any undue tension on the incision or blanching of the scar during shoulder exercises. Avoid exercises with the involved arm in a dependent position. Progress graded exercise program very slowly, particularly if the patient is receiving adjuvant therapy.

▶ Exercises for the Management of Lymphedema

Background and Rationale

As noted previously in this chapter, exercise is just one aspect of a decongestive lymphatic therapy program. The primary reasons for including exercise in the comprehensive treatment of patients with upper or lower extremity lymphedema are to move and drain lymph fluid for the reduction of edema and to improve the functional use of the involved limb or limbs. The exercises employed cover a wide spectrum of therapeutic exercise activities, specifically, deep breathing, relaxation, flexibility, strengthening, and cardiovascular conditioning exercises, as well as lymphatic drainage exercises.*

The rationale for including exercise in a program for the management of lymphedema is based on the following principles: (1) contraction of muscles pumps fluids by direct compression of the collecting lymphatic vessels; (2) exercise reduces soft tissue and joint hypomobility that can contribute to static positioning and lead to lymphostasis; (3) exercise strengthens and prevents atrophy of muscles of the limbs, which improves the efficiency of the lymphatic pump; (4) exercise increases heart rate and arterial pulsations, which, in turn, contribute to lymph flow; (5) exercise should be sequenced to clear the central lymphatic reservoirs before the peripheral areas; and (6) active exercise performed while compression bandages are worn enhances lymph flow and protein reabsorption more efficiently than exercising without bandages.[63]

No one combination or sequence of exercises has been shown to be more effective than another. In fact, there have been virtually no clinical research studies that have looked specifically at the impact of exercise on lymphatic drainage. The rationale for and efficacy of exercise, as well as the components and sequencing of activities are based primarily on assumptions and clinical observations of experienced practitioners who have reported positive

*See references 12, 13, 20, 24, 25, 26, 44, 52, 56, 57, 62, 64, 68, 72, 86.

outcomes as the result of their interventions.[20,23,24,25,26,62,63,68]

Components of Exercise Regimens for Management of Lymphedema

Deep Breathing and Relaxation Exercises

- Deep breathing is interwoven throughout exercise regimens for the management of lymphedema. It has been suggested that the use of abdominal-diaphragmatic breathing assists in the movement of lymphatic fluid as the diaphragm descends during a deep inspiration and the abdominals contract during a controlled, maximum expiration.[20] Changes in intra-abdominal and intrathoracic pressures create a gentle, continual pumping action that moves fluids in the central lymphatic vessels, which run superiorly in the chest cavity and drain into the venous system in the neck.
- Progressive, total body relaxation exercises, originally described by Jacobson[43,48] and summarized in Chapter 5 of this text, are used at the beginning of each exercise session to decrease muscle tension, which may be contributing to restricted mobility and lymph congestion.[20,23] Deep breathing is an integral component of the sequence of relaxation exercises.

Flexibility Exercises

Gentle, self-stretching exercises are used to minimize soft tissue and joint hypomobility, particularly in proximal areas of the body that may contribute to static postures and lymph congestion.

Strengthening and Muscular Endurance Exercises

Both isometric and dynamic exercises using self-resistance, elastic resistance, and weights or weight machines are all appropriate if done against light resistance (initially, 1–2 lb) and by progressing resistance and repetitions gradually. Whether or not lymphedema has developed, it is important to closely monitor the circumferential size and the skin texture of the involved limb to determine whether an appropriate intensity of exercise has been established. Emphasis is placed on improving endurance and strength of central and peripheral muscle groups that enhance an erect posture and minimize fatigue in muscles that contribute to the efficiency of the lymphatic pump mechanism.

Cardiovascular Conditioning Exercises

Activities such as upper extremity ergometry, swimming, cycling, and walking increase circulation and stimulate lymphatic flow.[20] Thirty minutes of aerobic endurance exercises complement lymph drainage exercises. Conditioning exercises are done at a low-intensity (at 40–50% of the target heart rate) when lymphedema is present and at higher intensities (up to an 80% level) when lymphedema has been reduced and exercise is otherwise safe.[20,63]

Lymphatic Drainage Exercises

These exercises, often referred to as *pumping exercises,* move fluids through lymphatic channels. Active, repetitive ROM exercises are performed throughout each session. *The exercises follow a specific sequence to move lymph away from congested areas.*[20,25,26] It is similar to the sequence of massage applied in manual lymph drainage.[51,78] In general, exercises first focus on *proximal* areas of the body to clear central collecting vessels and then involve distal muscle groups to begin to move peripheral edema in a centripedal direction to the central lymph vessels. The affected upper or lower extremity or extremities are held in an elevated position during many of the exercises. Static, dependent postures are avoided. Self-massage is also interspersed throughout the exercise sequence to further enhance drainage. These exercises also maintain mobility of the involved limbs.

Guidelines for Lymphatic Drainage Exercises

The patient should follow these guidelines when performing a sequence of lymphatic drainage exercises. These guidelines apply to management of either upper or lower extremity lymphedema and reflect the combined opinions of several authors and experts in the field.[20,24,25,62,63]

Preparation for Lymphatic Drainage Exercises

- Set aside approximately 20 to 30 minutes for each exercise session.
- Perform exercises BID every day.
- Have needed equipment at hand, such as a foam roll, wedge, or exercise wand.

During Lymphatic Drainage Exercises

- Wear compression bandages or a customized compression garment.
- Precede lymphatic drainage exercises with total body relaxation activities.

- Follow a specified order of exercises.
- Perform active, repetitive movements slowly, about 1 to 2 seconds per repetition.
- Elevate the involved limb above the heart when doing distal pumping exercises.
- Combine deep breathing exercises with active movements of the head, neck, trunk, and limbs.
- Initially, perform a low number of repetitions. Increase repetitions gradually to avoid excessive fatigue.
- Do not exercise to the point where the edematous limb aches.
- Incorporate self-massage into the exercise sequence to further enhance lymph drainage.
- Maintain good posture during exercises.
- When strengthening exercises are added to the lymph drainage sequence, use light resistance and avoid excessive muscle fatigue.

After Lymphatic Drainage Exercises

- If possible, rest with the involved extremity elevated for 30 minutes.
- Set aside time several times per week for low-intensity aerobic exercise activities, such as walking or bicycling for 30 minutes.
- Look carefully for signs of redness or increased swelling in the edematous limb, either of which could indicate that the level of exercise was excessive.

Selected Exercises for Lymphatic Drainage: Upper and Lower Extremity Sequences

The selection and sequences of exercises described in this section and summarized in Box 18–13 are designed to assist in the drainage of upper or lower extremity lymphedema. Many of the individual exercises suggested in lymphedema protocols, such as ROM of the cervical spine and some of the shoulder girdle or upper extremity exercises, are not exclusively used for lymph drainage. They are also used for improving mobility and strength. Several of the exercises highlighted in this section already have been described in previous chapters in this text. Only those exercises or variations of exercises that are somewhat unique or not previously described in this text are explained or illustrated in this section.

Sequence of Exercises

- Total body relaxation exercises are implemented prior to lymphatic drainage exercises.
- Exercises for lymphatic drainage should follow a particular sequence to assist lymph flow. The central and proximal lymphatic vessels, such as the abdominal, inguinal, and cervical nodes, are cleared first with trunk, pelvic, hip, and cervical exercises. Then, for the most part, exercises proceed distally from shoulders to fingers or from hips to toes. If lymph nodes have been surgically removed, for example with a unilateral axillary node dissection for breast cancer or a bilateral inguinal node dissection for cancers of the abdominal or pelvic organs, lymph must be moved to the remaining nodes in the body.

Note: Because no single sequence of exercises has been shown to be more effective than another, the upper and lower extremity sequences of exercises outlined in this section do not reflect the exercises included in any one specific protocol. Rather, the exercise sequences are based on the recommendations of several authors.[20,23,24,25,62,63] Sequences of exercises for upper or lower extremity lymphedema are summarized in the remaining portion of this chapter. Therapists are encouraged to modify or add other exercises to the sequences in this chapter as they see fit to meet the individual needs of their patients.

Exercises Common to Upper and Lower Extremity Sequences

These initial exercises should be included in exercise programs for either unilateral or bilateral upper or lower extremity lymphedema. They are designed to first help the patient relax and then to clear the central channels and nodes.

- ***Total body relaxation***
  - Have the patient assume a comfortable supine position and begin deep breathing. Then, isometrically contract and relax the muscles of the lower trunk (abdominals and erector spinae), then the hips, lower legs, feet, and toes.
  - Then contract and relax the muscles of the upper back, shoulders, upper arms, forearms, wrist, and fingers.
  - Finally, contract and relax the muscles of the neck and face.
  - Relax the whole body for at least a minute.
  - Perform diaphragmatic breathing throughout the entire sequence. Avoid breath-holding and the Valsalva maneuver.
- ***Posterior pelvic tilts and partial curl-ups***
  - Perform with hips and knees flexed, in supine.
- ***Unilateral knee-to-chest movements.*** These exercises are designed to target the inguinal

Box 18–13 Sequence of Selected Exercises for Management of Upper or Lower Extremity Lymphedema

Exercises Common to Upper and Lower Extremity Regimens

Note: Start an upper or lower extremity regimen with these exercises
- Deep breathing and total body relaxation exercises
- Posterior pelvic tilts and partial curl-ups
- Cervical ROM
- Bilateral scapular movements

Upper Extremity Exercises	Lower Extremity Exercises
■ Active circumduction with the involved arm elevated while lying supine	■ Alternate knee to chest exercises
■ Bilateral active movements of the arms while lying supine or on a foam roll	■ Bilateral knees to chest
■ Bilateral hand press while lying supine or sitting	■ Gluteal setting and posterior pelvic tilts
■ Shoulder stretches (with wand, doorway, or towel) while standing	■ Single knee to chest with the involved lower extremity
■ Active elbow, forearm, wrist, and finger exercises of the involved arm	■ External rotation of the hips while lying supine with both legs elevated and resting on a wedge or wall
■ Bilateral horizontal abduction and adduction of the shoulders	■ Active knee flexion of the involved lower extremity while lying supine
■ Overhead wall press while standing	■ Active plantarflexion and dorsiflexion and circumduction of the ankles while lying supine with lower extremities elevated
■ Finger exercises	■ Active hip and knee flexion with legs externally rotated and elevated against a wall
■ Partial curl-ups	■ Active cycling and scissoring movements with legs elevated
■ Rest with involved upper extremity elevated	■ Bilateral knee to chest exercises, followed by partial curl-ups
	■ Rest with lower extremities elevated

nodes. This is important even for upper extremity lymphedema.

- In the supine position flex one hip and knee, and grasp the lower leg. Pull the knee to the chest. Gently press or bounce the thigh against the abdomen and chest about 15 times.
- Repeat the procedure with the opposite lower extremity.

Note: If lymphedema is present in only one lower extremity, initiate the knee-to-chest exercises with the *uninvolved* lower extremity.

- ***Cervical ROM.*** Perform each motion for a count of 5 for five repetitions.
  - Rotation
  - Lateral flexion
- ***Scapular exercises.*** Perform exercise for a count of 5 for five repetitions.
  - Active elevation and depression (shoulder shrugs)
  - Active shoulder rolls
  - Active scapular retraction and protraction. With arms at sides and elbows flexed, bilaterally retract the scapulae, pointing elbows posteriorly and medially. Then protract the scapulae.

Note: Be sure to shrug shoulders as high as possible and then *actively* pull down the shoulders (depress the scapulae) as far as possible

Exercises Specifically for Upper Extremity Lymphedema Clearance

The following sequence of exercises is performed after the general, total body exercises just described. The exercises, which are performed in a proximal to distal sequence, are done specifically for upper extremity lymph clearance.

Note: Periodically during the exercise sequence have the patient perform self-massage to the axillary node area of the *uninvolved* side proceeding from the axilla to the chest.

- ***Active circumduction of the arm (Fig. 18–1).*** While lying supine, flex the involved arm to 90 degrees (reach toward the ceiling), and do active circular movements of the arm about 6 to 12 inches in diameter. Do this clockwise and counterclockwise, five repetitions in each direction.

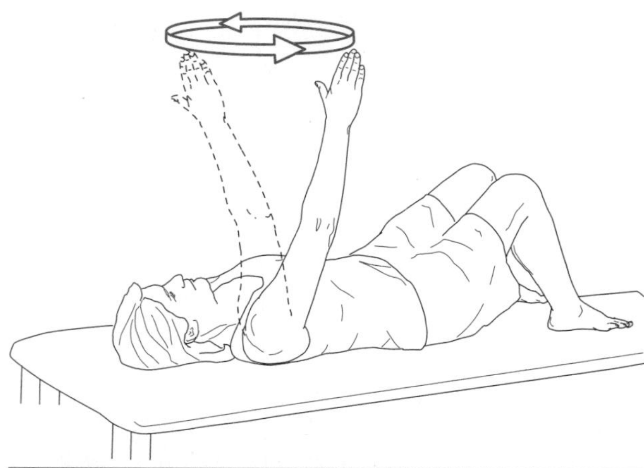

Figure 18–1 Active circumduction of the edematous extremity.

Precaution: Avoid pendular swinging or circumduction of the edematous upper extremity with the arm in a dependent position.

- ***Exercises on a foam roll (Fig. 18–2).*** While lying supine on a firm, foam roll (approximately 6 inches in diameter), perform horizontal abduction and adduction as well as flexion and extension of the shoulder. These movements target congested axillary nodes and are done unilaterally.
- For home exercises if special equipment, such as an Ethyfoam® roller, is not available, have the patient perform these exercises on a foam pool "noodle." Although the diameter is smaller, a towel or folded sheet can be wrapped around the foam "noodle" to increase the diameter of the roll.
- ***Bilateral hand press.*** With arms elevated to shoulder level or higher and elbows flexed, place the palms of the hands together in front of the chest or head. Press the palms together (for an isometric contraction of the pectoralis major muscles) while breathing in for a count of 5. Relax and then repeat up to five times.

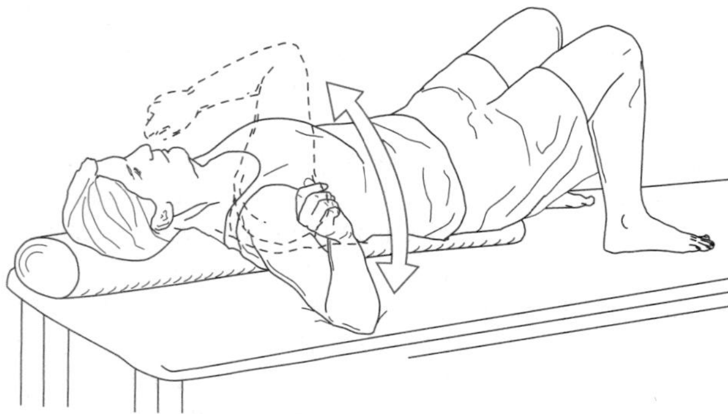

Figure 18–2 Active shoulder exercises on a firm, foam roll.

- ***Wand exercise, doorway or corner stretch, and towel stretch.*** Incorporate several exercises to increase shoulder mobility and to decrease congestion and assist lymph flow in the upper extremity. Hold the position of stretch for several seconds with each repetition. These exercises have been described and are illustrated in Chapter 9.
- ***Unilateral arm exercises with arm elevated***

Note: These exercises are done with the patient seated and the arm supported at shoulder level on a tabletop or countertop or with the patient supine and the arm supported on a wedge or elevated overhead.

  - Shoulder rotation with the elbow extended. Turn the palm up, then down, by rotating the shoulder, not simply pronating and supinating the forearm.
  - Elbow flexion and extension.
  - Circumduction of the wrist.
  - Hand opening and closing.
- ***Bilateral, horizontal abduction and adduction.*** While standing or sitting, place both hands behind the head. Horizontally adduct and abduct the shoulders by bringing the elbows together and then pointing them laterally.
- ***Overhead wall press.*** Face a wall; place one or both palms on the wall with the hands above shoulder level. Gently press the palms into the wall for several seconds without moving the body. Relax and repeat approximately five times.
- ***Wrist and finger exercises.*** If swelling is present in the wrist and hand, repetitive active finger movements are indicated with the arm elevated.
  - After performing the overhead wall press as just described, keep the heel of the hand on the wall and alternatively move all of the fingers away from and back to the wall (Fig. 18–3).
  - In the same position as just described, alternately press individual fingers into the wall, as if playing a piano, while keeping the heel of the hand in contact with the wall.
  - Place the palms of both hands together with the hands overhead or at least above shoulder level. One finger at a time, press matching fingers together and then pull them away from each other.
- ***Partial curl-ups.*** To complete the exercise se-

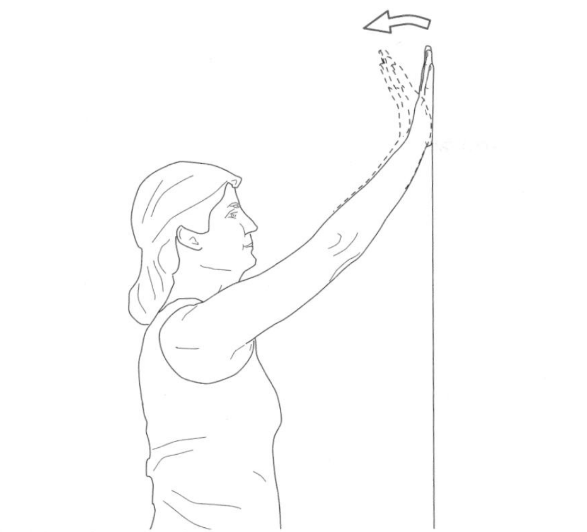

Figure 18–3 Overhead wall press.

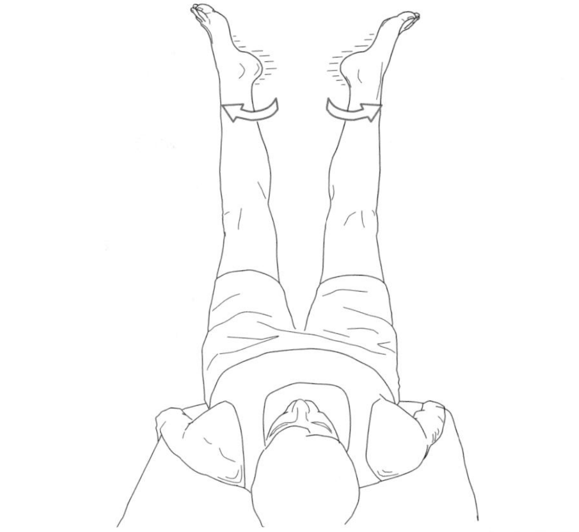

Figure 18–4 Repeated outward rotation of the hips with legs elevated.

quence, perform additional curl-ups (about five repetitions) with hands sliding on the thighs.

- ***Rest.*** Rest in a supine position with the involved arm elevated on pillows for about 30 minutes after completing the exercise sequence.

Exercises Specifically for Lower Extremity Lymphedema Clearance

Note: After completing the general lower body, neck, and shoulder exercises previously described, have the patient perform self-massage first to the axillary lymph nodes on the *involved* side of the body. Then massage the lower abdominal area superiorly to the waist and then laterally and superiorly to the axillary area of the involved side. This sequence is repeated periodically throughout the lower extremity exercise sequence.

- ***Unilateral knee-to-chest movements.*** In the supine position, repeat this exercise for another 15 repetitions. As mentioned previously, if lymphedema is present in only one lower extremity, perform repeated knee to chest movements with the *uninvolved leg first* and then the involved leg.
- ***Bilateral knees to chest.*** In the supine position, flex both hips and knees, grasp both thighs, and gently pull them to the abdomen and chest. Repeat 10 to 15 times.
- ***Gluteal setting and posterior pelvic tilts.*** Repeat five times, holding each contraction for several seconds and then slowly releasing.
- ***External rotation of the hips (Fig. 18–4).*** Lie in the supine position with the legs elevated and resting against a wall or on a wedge. Externally rotate the hips, pressing the buttocks together, and holding the outwardly rotated position. Repeat several times.
- ***Knee flexion to clear the popliteal area.*** While lying in the supine position and keeping the uninvolved lower extremity extended, flex the involved hip and knee enough to clear the foot from the mat table. Actively flex the knee as far as possible by quickly moving the heel to the buttocks. Repeat approximately 15 times.
- ***Active ankle movements.*** With both legs elevated and propped against a wall, or just the involved leg propped against a door frame and the uninvolved leg resting on the floor, actively plantarflex the ankle and curl the toes, and then dorsiflex the ankle and extend the toes as far as possible for multiple repetitions. Then actively circumduct the foot clockwise and counterclockwise for several repetitions.
- ***Wall slides in external rotation (Fig. 18–5).*** With the feet propped up against the wall, legs externally rotated, and heels touching, slide both feet down the wall as far as possible and then back up the wall for several repetitions.
- ***Leg movements in the air (Fig. 18–6).*** With both hips flexed and the back flat on the floor and both

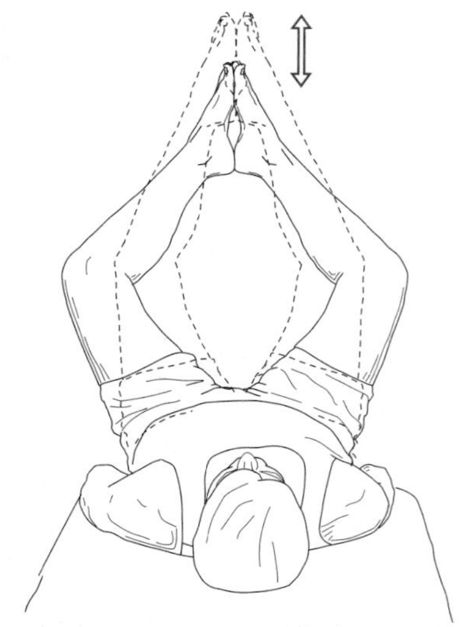

Figure 18–5 Wall slides with hips externally rotated.

feet pointed to the ceiling, alternately move the legs, simulating cycling, walking, and scissoring motions.

- ***Hip adduction across the midline (Fig. 18–7).*** Lie in the supine position with the uninvolved leg extended. Flex the hip and knee of the involved leg. Grasp the lateral aspect of the knee with the contralateral hand; pull the involved knee repeatedly across the midline in a rocking motion.

Note: If lymphedema is bilateral, repeat this exercise with the other lower extremity.

- ***Bilateral knee to chest.*** Repeat bilateral gentle, bouncing movements of the legs previously described.

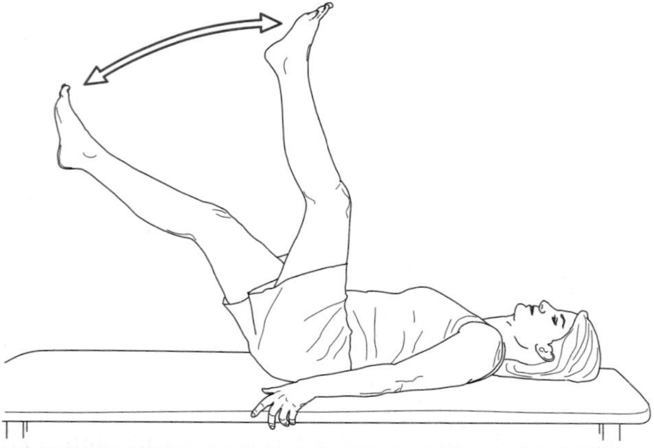

Figure 18–6 Repeated walking movements.

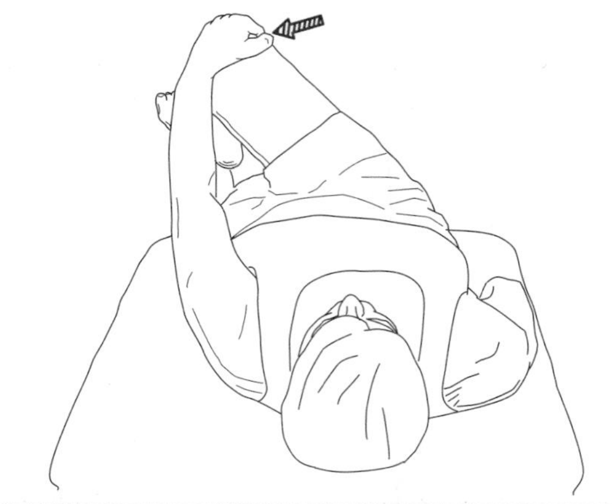

Figure 18–7 Hip adduction across the midline to clear inguinal nodes.

- ***Partial curl-ups.*** To complete the exercise sequence, perform additional partial curl-ups, about five repetitions.
- ***Rest.*** With feet elevated and legs propped up against the wall, rest in this position for several minutes after completing exercises. Then rest the legs partially elevated on a wedge, and remain in this position for another 30 minutes.

Independent Learning Activities

CRITICAL THINKING AND DISCUSSION

1. Differentiate between the signs and symptoms associated with chronic arterial insufficiency and chronic venous insufficiency.
2. You have been asked to participate in a patient education program at your community's cancer society for patients who have undergone surgery for breast cancer. Your responsibility in this program is to help these breast cancer survivors prevent physical impairments and functional limitations associated with their surgery and any related adjuvant therapies. Outline the components of such a program, and explain the rationale for the activities you have chosen to include.
3. What part does a program of exercise and physical activity play in the overall prevention or management of deep vein thrombophlebitis? What are the signs and symptoms of DVT that a patient at risk for this problem must learn to recognize? If you suspect that a patient you are seeing after some type of orthopedic surgery of the lower ex-

tremity has developed a DVT, what questions should you ask the patient, and what should you do before contacting the patient's physician?

4. A patient presents with leg pain that occurs intermittently during the day, but not at night. Describe how you would evaluate the patient's signs and symptoms and determine whether the cause of the pain is vascular or neurological.

LABORATORY PRACTICE

Perform the sequence of exercises and suggested repetitions for the exercise plan you have designed for Case 2 (Ms. L).

CASE STUDIES

Case 1

Mr. A, a 65-year-old man with a 5-year history of Type II diabetes and PVD, has been referred to you in your home health practice to establish a program to help him improve his overall level of physical activity. He enjoys golf, but recently has had difficulty completing a round because of calf pain that occurs when he walks for even short distances along the course. His pain goes away when he stands or sits.

What additional information will you need to secure during the examination and evaluation process? What tests and measurements would be of particular importance? From your evaluation, design a plan of care that includes a program of exercise to help Mr. A improve his level of physical activity and prevent vascular-related complications.

Case 2

Ms. L underwent surgery for metastatic pelvic cancer and lymphadenectomy (lymph node dissection) 3 months ago. She also received a series of radiation therapy treatments as part of her comprehensive oncological management. About 2 weeks ago, she began to notice bilateral swelling in her legs, most notably in her feet and ankles.

She has been referred by her oncologist to the outpatient facility where you work to "Evaluate and Treat" her for her lymphedema. Describe the examination procedures you would use in your evaluation, and then develop a plan of care, including a program of exercise, to help her manage and reduce her lymphedema and prevent potential complications related to the lymphedema.

REFERENCES

1. Abeloff, MD, et al: Breast. In Abeloff, MD, et al (eds): Clinical Oncology, ed 2. Churchill Livingstone, New York, 2000, p 2051.
2. Abramson, DI: Physiologic basis for the use of physical agents in peripheral vascular disorders. Arch Phys Med Rehabil 46:216, 1965.
3. Adcock, JL: Rehabilitation of the breast cancer patient. In McGarvey, CL (ed): Physical Therapy for the Cancer Patient. Churchill-Livingstone, New York, 1990, pp 67–84.
4. American Cancer Society: Cancer Facts and Figures, 1999. American Cancer Society, Atlanta, GA, 1999.

4a. American Physical Therapy Association: Guide to Physical Therapist Practice, ed 2. Phys Ther 81:S1, 2001.

5. Beach, RB: Measurement of extremity volume by water displacement. Phys Ther 57:286, 1977.
6. Beeby, J, and Broeg, PE: Treatment of patients with radical mastectomies. Phys Ther 50:40, 1970.
7. Bergan, JJ: Effect of cancer therapy on lower extremity lymphedema. National Lymphedema Network Newsletter 11(1), January–March 1999.
8. Berkman, S: Fighting back after breast cancer. Advance for Physical Therapists and PT Assistants 11(9):8, May 1, 2000.
9. Bertelli, G, et al: Conservative treatment of postmastectomy lymphedema: A controlled randomized trial. Am Oncology 2(8):575, 1991.
10. Boissonnault, WG: The female genital/reproductive system. In Goodman, CC, and Boissonnault, WG (eds): Pathology: Implications for Physical Therapists. WB Saunders, Philadelphia, 1998, p 559.
11. Boissonnault, WG, and Bass, C: Pathological origins of trunk and neck pain, part two: Disorders of the cardiovascular and pulmonary systems. J Orthop Sports Phys Ther 12:208, 1990.
12. Boris, M, et al: Lymphedema reduction by noninvasive complex lymphedema therapy. Oncology 8:95, 1994.
13. Boris, M, Weindorf, S, and Lasinski, B: Persistence of lymphedema reduction after noninvasive complex lymphedema therapy. Oncology 11:99, 1997.
14. Bottomley, JM: The insensitive foot. In Kauffman, TL (ed): Geriatric Rehabilitation Manual. Churchill Livingstone, New York, 1999, p 266.
15. Brandsma, JW, Robeer, BG, et al: The effect of exercises on walking distance of patients with intermittent claudication: A study of randomized clinical trials. Phys Ther 78:278, 1998.
16. Brennan, MJ: Lymphedema following the surgical treatment of breast cancer: A review of pathophysiology and treatment. J Pain Symptom Managemt 7(2):110–116, 1992.
17. Brennan, MJ, DePompodo, RW, and Garden, FH: Focused review: Postmastectomy lymphedema. Arch Phys Med Rehabil 77(3 supplement):574, 1996.
18. Brennan, MJ, and Miller, L: Overview of treatment options in the management of lymphedema. Cancer Supplement 83:2821, 1998.

19. Bunce, IH, et al: Postmastectomy lymphoedema treatment and measurement. Med J Austral 161:125, 1994.
20. Burt, J, and White, G: Lymphedema: A Breast Cancer Patient's Guide to Prevention and Healing. Hunter House Inc., Publishers, Alameda, CA, 1999.
21. Cameron, MH: Physical Agents in Rehabilitation: From Research to Practice. WB Saunders, Philadelphia, 1999.
22. Casley-Smith, Jr.: Information about Lymphoedema for Patients, ed 6. Lymphoedema Association of Australia, Malvern, Australia, 1997.
23. Casley-Smith, JR: Treatment for lymphedema of the arm—the Casley-Smith method. Cancer Supplement 83:2843, 1998 (December 15).
24. Casley-Smith, JR, and Casley-Smith, JR: Modern treatment of lymphoedema, I: complex physical therapy—the first 200 Australian limbs. Austral J Dermatol 33:61, 1992.
25. Casley-Smith, JR: Exercises for Patients with Lymphedema of the Arm, ed 2. Lymphoedema Association of Australia, Adelade, Australia, 1991.
26. Casley-Smith, JR: Exercises for Patients with Lymphedema of the Leg, ed 2. Lymphoedema Association of Australia, Adelade, Australia, 1991.
27. Connell, M: Complete decongestive therapy. Innovations in Breast Cancer Care 3:93, 1998.
28. Daroczy, J: Pathology of lymphedema. Clin Dermatol 13:433, 1995.
29. Eisenhardt, JR: Evaluation and physical treatment of the patient with peripheral vascular disorders. In Irwin, S, and Tecklin, JS (eds): Cardiopulmonary Physical Therapy, ed 3. Mosby–Year Book, St Louis, 1995, pp 215–233.
30. Ekroth, R, et al: Physical training of patients with intermittent claudication: Indications, methods, and results. Surgery 84:640, 1978.
31. Ernest, E, and Fialka, V: A review of the clinical effectiveness of exercise therapy for intermittent claudication. Arch Intern Med 113:135, 1990.
32. Ganz, PA: Current issues in cancer rehabilitation. Cancer 65(Suppl 3):742–751. 1990.
33. Ganz, PA: The quality of life after breast cancer—solving the problem of lymphedema. N Engl J Med 340:383, 1999.
34. Goodman, CC: The cardiovascular system. In Goodman, CC, and Boissonnault, WG (eds). Pathology: Implications for the Physical Therapist, WB Saunders, Philadelphia, 1998, p 263.
35. Goodman, CC, and Snyder, TEK: Differential Diagnosis in Physical Therapy, ed 3. WB Saunders Co., Philadelphia, 2000.
36. Gray, JC: Diagnosis of intermittent vascular claudication in a patient with a diagnosis of sciatica. Phys Ther 79:582, 1999.
37. Gudas, SA: Neoplasms of the breast. In Kauffman, TL (ed): Geriatric Rehabilitation Manual, Churchill Livingstone, New York, 1999, p 182.
38. Guttman, H, et al: Achievements of physical therapy in patients after modified radical mastectomy compared with quadrantectomy, axillary dissection and radiation for carcinoma of the breast. Arch Surg 125:389–391, 1990.
39. Guyton, AC: Human Physiology and Mechanisms of Disease, ed 6. WB Saunders, Philadelphia, 1997.
40. Hansen, M: Pathophysiology: Foundations of Disease and Clinical Intervention. WB Saunders, Philadelphia, 1998.
41. Harwood, CA, and Mortimer, PS: Causes and clinical manifestations of lymphatic failure. Clin Dermatol 13:459, 1995.
42. Henderson, IC: Breast cancer. In Murphy, GP, Lawrence, W, and Lenhard, RE (eds): Clinical Oncology, ed 2, American Cancer Society, Atlanta, 1995, p 198.
43. Hertling, D, and Jones, D: Relaxation and related techniques. In Hertling, D, and Kessler, RM (eds): Management of Common Musculoskeletal Disorders, ed 3. Lippincott, Philadelphia, 1996, p 140.
44. Hewitson, JW: Management of lower extremity lymphedema. National Lymphedema Network Newsletter 9(3):1, July–September, 1997.
45. Hladiuk, M, et al: Arm function after axillary dissection for breast cancer: A pilot study to provide parameter estimates. J Surg Oncol 50(1):47–52, 1992.
46. Hurst, PAE: Peripheral vascular disease—Assessment and treatment. In Downie, PA (ed): Cash's Textbook of Chest, Heart and Vascular Disorders for Physiotherapists, ed 4. JB Lippincott, Philadelphia, 1987.
47. Hurst, PAE: Venous and lymphatic disease—Assessment and treatment. In Downie, PA (ed): Cash's Textbook of Chest, Heart and Vascular Disorders for Physiotherapists, ed 4. JB Lippincott, Philadelphia, 1987.
48. Jacobson, E: Progressive Relaxation. University of Chicago Press, Chicago, 1929.
49. Kim, DJ, and Ebel, A: Therapeutic exercise in peripheral vascular disease. In Basmajian, JV, and Wolf, SL (eds): Therapeutic Exercise. Williams & Wilkins, Baltimore, 1990, p 371.
50. Knight, CA: Peripheral vascular disease and wound care. In O'Sullivan, SB, and Schmitz, TJ (eds): Physical Rehabilitation: Assessment and Treatment, ed 4. FA Davis, Philadelphia, 2001, p 583.
51. Kurtz, I: Textbook of Dr. Vodder's Manual Lymphatic Drainage, Volume 2: Therapy, ed 2. Karl F. Haug Publishers, Heidelberg, Germany, 1989.
52. Lerner, R: What's new in lymphedema therapy in America? Internat J Angiol 7:191, 1998.
53. Logan, V: Incidence and prevalence of lymphedema: a literature review. J Clin Nurs 4:213, 1995.
54. Lotze, MT, et al: Early versus delayed shoulder motion following axillary dissection. A randomized prospective study. Am Surg 193:288, 1981.
55. MacKinnon, JL: Study of Doppler ultrasonic peripheral vascular assessment performed by physical therapists. Phys Ther 63:30, 1983.
56. Mason, M: The treatment of lymphoedema by complex physical therapy. Austral J Physiother 39:41, 1993.
57. Matthews, K, and Smith J: Effectiveness of modified complex physical therapy for lymphoedema treatment. Austral J Physiother 42:323, 1996.
58. McCulloch, JM: Examination procedure for patients with vascular system problems. Clin Managemt Phys Ther 1:17, 1981.
59. McCulloch, JM: Peripheral vascular disease. In O'Sullivan, SB, and Schmitz, TJ (eds): Physical Rehabilitation: Assessment and Treatment, ed 3. FA Davis, Philadelphia, 1994.
60. McCulloch, JM, Kloth, L, and Feedar, JA (eds): Wound Healing: Alternatives and Management, ed 2. FA Davis, Philadelphia, 1995.
61. McGarvey, CL: Pneumatic compression devices for lymphedema. Rehabil Oncol 10:16–17, 1992.
62. Megens, A, and Harris, S: Physical therapist management of lymphedema following treatment for breast cancer: a critical review of its effectiveness. Phys Ther 78:1302, 1998.
63. Miller, LT: Exercise in the management of breast cancer-

related lymphedema. Innovations in Breast Cancer Care 3(4):101, 1998.
64. Miller, LT: The enigma of exercise: Participation in an exercise program after breast cancer surgery. National Lymphedema Network Newsletter 8(4), October–December 1996.
65. Norman, SA, et al: Development and validation of a telephone questionnaire to characterize lymphedema in women treated for breast cancer. Phys Ther 81:1192, 2001.
66. Peters, K, et al: Lower leg subcutaneous blood flow during walking and passive dependency in chronic venous insufficiency, Br J Dermatol 124(2):177, 1991.
67. Petrek, JA, and Heelan, M: Incidence of breast carcinoma-related lymphedema. Cancer Supplement 83(12):2776, December 15, 1998.
68. Price, J, and Purtell, J: Teaming up to prevent and treat lymphedema. Am J Nursing 7(9):23, 1997.
69. Regensteiner, JG, Steiner, JF, and Hiatt, WR: Exercise training improves functional status in patients with peripheral arterial disease. J Vasc Surg 23:104, 1996.
70. Regensteiner, JG, and Hiatt, WR: Exercise in the management of peripheral arterial disease. In Roitman, JL (ed): ACSM's Resource Manual for Exercise Testing and Prescription, ed 4. Lippincott, Williams & Wilkins, Philadelphia, 2001, p 292.
71. Rockson, SG: Secondary lymphedema of the lower extremities. National Lymphedema Network Newsletter 10(3):1–3, July–September, 1998.
72. Rockson, SG, Miller, LT, and Senie, R: Diagnosis and management of lymphedema. Cancer Supplement 83:2882, 1998.
73. Ross, C: Complex physical therapy: a treatment note. NZ J Physiother 40:19, 1994.
74. Ruell, PA, et al: Intermittent claudication. The effect of physical training on walking tolerance and venous lactate concentration. Eur J Appl Physiol 52:420, 1984.
75. Sidoti, SP: Exercise and peripheral vascular disease. Clin Podiatr Med Surg 9(1):173, 1992.
76. Spencer-Green, G: Raynaud's phenomenon. Bull Rheum Dis 33:1, 1983.
77. Swirsky, J, and Nannery, DS: Coping with Lymphedema. Avery Publishing Group, Garden City Park, NY, 1998.
78. Tappan, FM, and Benjamin, PJ: Tappan's Handbook of Healing Massage. Appleton and Lange, Stamford, CT, 1998.
79. Weinmann, EE, and Salzman, EW: Deep vein thrombosis. N Engl J Med 331:1630, 1994.
80. Weiss, JM: Treatment of leg edema and wounds in patients with severe musculoskeletal injuries. Phys Ther 78:1104, 1998.
81. Williams, LR, et al: Vascular rehabilitation: Benefits of a structured exercise and risk modification program. J Vasc Surg 14:320, 1991.
82. Wingate, L: Efficacy of physical therapy for patients who have undergone mastectomies. Phys Ther 65:896, 1985.
83. Wingate, L, et al: Rehabilitation of the mastectomy patient: A randomized, blind, prospective study. Arch Phys Med Rehabil 70:21–24, 1989.
84. Wisham, LH, Abramson, AS, and Ebel, A: Value of exercise in peripheral arterial disease. JAMA 153:10, 1953.
85. Woods, EN: Reaching out to patients with breast cancer. Clin Managemt Phys Ther 12:58–63, 1992.
86. Zuther, JE: Treatment of lymphedema with complete decongestive physiotherapy. National Lymphedema Network Newsletter, Vol II (2), April 1999.

Chapter 19

Management of Pulmonary Conditions

OBJECTIVES

After studying this chapter, the reader will be able to:

1. Apply knowledge of respiratory structure and function in the management of patients with pulmonary dysfunction.
2. Describe examination procedures pertinent to the evaluation and management of patients with pulmonary dysfunction.
3. Identify the goals, indications, and guidelines for application of breathing exercises and retraining.
4. Describe the procedures and a sequence for teaching a patient specific breathing and chest mobilization exercises.
5. Summarize factors that impair airway clearance and methods of teaching a patient an effective cough.
6. Summarize the goals, indications, precautions, and guidelines for application of postural drainage.
7. Describe the procedure, positions, and techniques of postural drainage.
8. Design comprehensive management strategies for patients with chronic and restrictive pulmonary dysfunction.

Cardiopulmonary physical therapy is a multifaceted area of professional practice that deals with the management of patients of all ages with acute or chronic and primary or secondary cardiopulmonary disorders. Although the cardiovascular and pulmonary systems are inherently linked as they interface with all other body systems, the focus of this chapter is on examination procedures and interventions used for the management of patients with pulmonary dysfunction. In particular, exercise interventions and manual techniques that enhance ventilation and airway clearance are presented.

The goals of cardiopulmonary physical therapy for patients with respiratory dysfunction are to[8,10,16,18]:

- Prevent airway obstruction and accumulation of secretions that interfere with normal respiration.
- Improve airway clearance and ventilation through mobilization and drainage of secretions.
- Improve endurance and general exercise tolerance.
- Reduce energy costs during respiration through breathing retraining.
- Prevent or correct postural deformities associated with respiratory disorders.
- Promote relaxation.
- Maintain or improve chest mobility.
- Improve cough effectiveness.

Treatment settings vary widely. Inpatients may be treated in intensive care, chronic care, and postsurgical units; outpatients may be seen at home or followed in pulmonary clinics or rehabilitation centers.

▶ Review of Respiratory Structure and Function

Respiration is a general term used to describe gas exchange within the body and can be categorized as either external respiration or internal respiration. Basic terms are described here but an in-depth discussion of respiratory physiology, including diffusion and perfusion, goes well beyond the scope or purpose of this text. The reader is referred to several references for further study.[11,20,29,54,57]

External respiration describes the exchange of gas at the alveolar-capillary membrane and the pulmonary capillaries. When a person inhales and air is delivered to the alveoli via the tracheobronchial tree, oxygen diffuses through the alveolar wall and interstitial space and into the bloodstream through the pulmonary capillary walls. The opposite occurs with carbon dioxide transport. *Internal respiration* describes the exchange of gas between the pulmonary capillaries and the cells of the surrounding tissues. Internal respiration occurs when oxygen in arterial blood diffuses from red blood cells into tissues requiring oxygen for function. The reverse occurs with carbon dioxide transport.

Ventilation, as it refers to the respiratory system, is the mass exchange of air to and from the body during inspiration and expiration. This cyclic process requires coordinated ventilatory muscle activity, rib cage movements, and appropriate structure and function of the upper and lower respiratory tracts.[9,20,29,57]

The Thorax and Chest Wall: Structure and Function

The main function of the thoracic cage, also referred to as the chest wall, is to protect the internal organs of respiration, circulation, and digestion and participate in ventilation of the lungs.[46] The thoracic cage provides the site of attachment for the muscles of ventilation to mechanically enlarge the thorax for inspiration or to compress the thorax for expiration.[43] It is also the site of attachment of upper extremity muscles, which function during lifting, pulling, or pushing activities. These activities are usually carried out in conjunction with inspiratory effort.

Along the posterior aspect of the thorax, the dorsal portions of the ribs articulate with the 12 thoracic vertebrae at the costotransverse and costovertebral joints. Along the anterior aspect of the thoracic cage, the first to seventh ribs articulate directly with the sternum via the costal cartilage. The eighth to tenth ribs have cartilaginous attachments to the rib above, whereas the eleventh and twelfth are floating ribs.[43,46]

Muscles of Ventilation

Multiple muscles that attach to the thoracic cage can have an impact on the movement of air in and out of the lungs during either the inspiratory or expiratory phases of breathing.[9,11,43] Box 19–1 lists the muscles of ventilation.[10]

Ventilatory muscles, also referred to as respiratory muscles, can be classified as either primary or accessory.[43,51] The *primary muscles of ventilation* are recruited during quiet (tidal) breathing whereas the *accessory muscles of ventilation* are only recruited during deep, forced, or labored breathing. During quiet inspiration the *diaphragm, scalenes,* and *parasternals* are activated.[43,51] In contrast, no primary ventilatory muscles contract during resting expiration. During deep or forced breathing different accessory muscles of ventilation are recruited, depending on whether inspiration or expiration is occurring as noted in Box 19–1.

Box 19–1 Primary and Accessory Ventilatory Muscles

Inspiration

- Primary muscles: diaphragm, scalenes, parasternals
- Accessory muscles: sternocleidomastoids, upper trapezius, pectoralis major and minor, subclavius, and possibly the external intercostals

Expiration

- Primary muscles: none active during tidal (resting) expiration
- Accessory muscles: the abdominals, including the rectus abdominis, the transversus abdominis and the internal and external obliques, pectoralis major, and possibly the internal intercostals

Inspiration

Diaphragm. The diaphragm, the major muscle of inspiration, is innervated by the phrenic nerve (C-3, C-4, C-5). During relaxed inspiration, it is the primary muscle responsible for movement of air, and under these quiet conditions it performs about 70 to 80% of the work of breathing.[51] As the diaphragm contracts, it moves caudally from its dome-shaped position at rest to increase the capacity of the thoracic cage.

Scalenes. The scalenes, which insert proximally on the transverse processes of the lower five cervical vertebrae and distally on the upper surface of the first two ribs, also are active during quiet inspiration.[43,51] They begin to contract at the onset of inspiration and generate an even greater amount of tension late into the inspiratory cycle as the tension-producing capacity of the diaphragm is decreasing. The scalenes lift the sternum and the first two ribs in a "pump handle" action, which causes an upward and outward action of the upper portion of the rib cage.

Parasternal intercostals. The parasternals, a portion of the internal intercostals, are active during resting inspiration. They function to stabilize the rib cage and prevent an inward movement of the superior aspect of the chest wall.[43,51]

Accessory muscles of inspiration. The sternocleidomastoid (SCM), upper trapezius, pectoralis major and minor, and subclavius muscles are all active during deep or labored inspiration.[10,43,51] These muscles become increasingly active with greater inspiratory effort, which occurs frequently during strenuous physical activity. The accessory muscles of inspiration may become the primary muscles of inspiration and may become active during resting inspiration when the diaphragm is ineffective or weak as the result of pathology. For example, paralysis of the abdominals as the result of a spinal cord injury reduces the support to the viscera (when the patient is in an upright position) which, in turn, allows the diaphragm to assume a flattened rather than a normal dome-shaped position. Thus, diaphragmatic excursion is reduced, and breathing is less efficient, which necessitates recruitment of the accessory muscles of inspiration.

The *SCM muscles* elevate the sternum to increase the anteroposterior (AP) diameter of the thorax. In patients with weakness of the diaphragm, the SCM muscles are required to act as primary muscles of inspiration. The *upper trapezius* muscles elevate the shoulders and, indirectly, the rib cage during labored inspiration. They also fixate the neck so the scalenes have a stable attachment. The *pectoralis major* muscles can act to elevate the rib cage and contribute to inspiration when the arms are overhead.

Expiration

Expiration is a passive process when a person is at rest. When the diaphragm relaxes after a contraction, the diaphragm rises and the ribs drop. The elastic recoil of tissues decreases the intrathoracic area and increases intrathoracic pressure, which causes exhalation. During active expiration, which can be controlled, forced, or prolonged, several accessory muscles groups are active.[10,43,51]

Abdominals. The rectus abdominis, the internal and external obliques, and the transversus abdominis contract to force down the thoracic cage and force the abdominal contents superiorly into the diaphragm. When the abdominals contract, the intrathoracic pressure increases and air is forced out of the lungs. A strong contraction of the abdominals is also necessary for a strong cough. The abdominals are innervated by spinal cord levels T-10 to T-12.

Other accessory muscles of expiration include the pectoralis major muscles (when the distal insertion is inferior to the clavicle and the arm is fixed in position), the *quadratus lumborum,* because of its attachment to the twelfth rib, which enables it to act to stabilize the diaphragm during phonation, and possibly the *internal intercostals,* which may act to depress the rib cage.[43,51]

Mechanics of Ventilation

Movements of the Thorax During Ventilation

Each rib has its own pattern of movement, but generalizations can be made. The ribs attach anteriorly to the sternum (except ribs 11 and 12) and posteriorly to the vertebral bodies, disks, and transverse processes, making a closed kinematic chain. The thorax enlarges in all three planes of movement during inspiration.[9,11,43,51]

Increase in the AP dimension. There is a forward and upward movement of the sternum and upper ribs. This is described as a *pump-handle* motion. The thoracic spine extends (straightens), enabling greater excursion of the sternum.

Increase in the transverse (lateral) dimension. There is an elevation and outward turning of the lateral (midshaft) portions of the ribs. This is described as a *bucket handle* motion. The lower ribs (8–10), which are not attached directly to the sternum, also flare or open outward, increasing the subcostal angle. This is described as *caliper* motion. The angle at the costochondral junction also increases, making the rib segments longer during inspiration.

Increase in vertical dimension. The central tendon of the diaphragm descends as the muscle contracts. This is described as a *piston action.* Elevation of the ribs increases the vertical dimension of the thorax and improves the effectiveness of the diaphragm. At the end of inspiration, the muscles relax; elastic recoil causes the diaphragm to move superiorly. The ribs return to their resting position.

Movement of Air

As noted previously, *ventilation* is the mass exchange of gases to and from the body. During inspiration, as the thorax enlarges, the pressure inside the lungs (alveolar pressure) becomes lower than the atmospheric pressure, and air rushes into the lungs. At the end of inspiration, the muscles relax, and the elastic recoil of the lungs pushes the air out, resulting in expiration.

Note: Breathing exercises, a common intervention for the management of patients with cardiopulmonary conditions as well as neuromuscular and musculoskeletal conditions, are designed to affect the movement of air to and from the lungs.[11,44,48,51]

Compliance

Compliance refers to the distensibility of tissue or how easily the lungs inflate during inspiration. With regard to ventilation, it relates to how easily the lungs inflate or the chest wall expands during inspiration.[20,55,57] Normal lungs are very distensible (compliant), but compliance changes with age and the presence of disease. During the normal aging process lung tissue becomes more compliant. Diseases of the pulmonary system that, for example, cause fibrosis of tissues (alveolar or pleural) make the lungs rigid that is, less compliant, whereas, emphysema, one of the chronic obstructive diseases, makes lung tissue more compliant to pressures.[20,55,57]

Airway Resistance

The amount of resistance to the flow of air through the airways depends on a number of factors.[20,55,57] The bifurcation and branching of airways is a source of airway resistance. The size (diameter) of the lumen of each airway also influences resistance. The diameter of the lumen can be decreased by mucus or edema in the airways, contraction of smooth muscles, and the degree of elasticity or distensibility of the lung parenchyma.

Normally, the airways widen during inspiration and narrow during expiration. As the diameter of the airway decreases, the resistance to airflow increases. In diseases that cause bronchospasm (asthma) or increased mucus production (chronic bronchitis), airway resistance is even greater than normal particularly during expiration.

Flow Rates

Flow rates indicate measurements of the amount of air moved in or out of the airways in a period of time. Flow rates, which are related to airflow resistance, reflect the ease with which ventilation occurs.[20,55,57] *Expiratory flow rate* is determined by the volume of air exhaled divided by the amount of time it takes for the volume of gas to be exhaled.[24]

Flow rates are altered as the result of diseases that affect the respiratory tree and chest wall. For example, in chronic obstructive pulmonary disease, expiratory flow rate is decreased in comparison to normal. That is, it will take a longer than normal period to exhale a specific volume of air.

Anatomy and Function of the Respiratory Tracts

Upper Respiratory Tract

The structures of the upper respiratory tract are the *nasal cavity, pharynx,* and *larynx.*[11,46,63,64] As air is brought into the body, the nasal cavity and pharynx filter and remove particles in the air and begin to humidify and warm it to body temperature. The mucosal lining of these structures has cells that secrete mucus and cells that are ciliated. Cilia and mucus trap particles; a sneeze removes large particles.

With illness and elevated body temperature, the mucous membrane tends to dry out, so the body secretes more mucus. This mucus dries out, and a cycle begins. Action of the cilia is inhibited by drying of mucus. The patient tends to breathe by mouth, which decreases the humidification of mucus and increases its viscosity.

The larynx, which extends from C-3 to C-6, controls airflow, and when it contracts rapidly, the epiglottis prevents food, liquids, or foreign objects from entering the airway.[8,12,16,35,39,42]

Lower Respiratory Tract

The lower respiratory tract is composed of conducting airways of the tracheobronchial tree and the terminal respiratory units. There are approximately 23 generations (branchings) of the structures within the tracheobronchial tree, which extends from the trachea to the terminal respiratory units of the lungs. The structures and branchings of the lower respiratory tract are summarized in Box 19–2.[11,46,63,64]

The initial branchings of the tracheobronchial tree are depicted in Figure 19–1. The first 16 of the airway branchings of the lower respiratory tract primarily conduct air, whereas the last 6 are respiratory airways that end (in the mature lung) in approximately 300 million alveoli.[46,64] The diameter of

Box 19–2 Structures and Branchings of the Lower Respiratory Tract

- Trachea
- Mainstem bronchi: 2
- Lobar bronchi: 5
- Segmental bronchi: 18
- Bronchioles: subsegmental, terminal, and respiratory
- Alveolar ducts and sacs

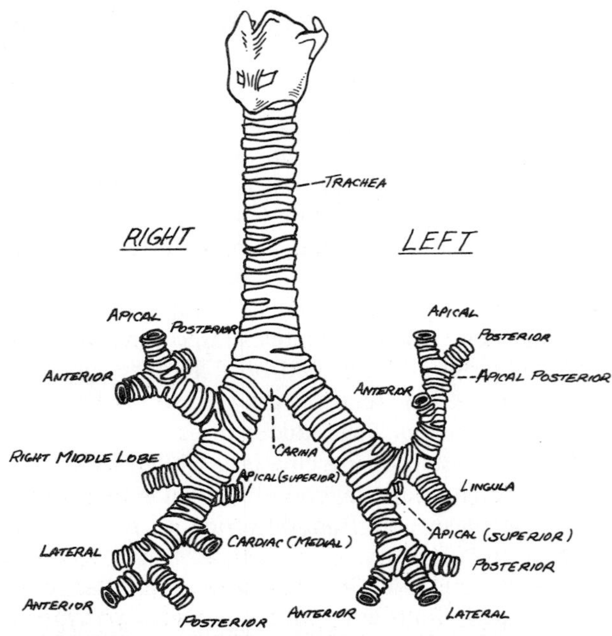

Figure 19–1 Lower respiratory tract—tracheobronchial tree. (From Frownfelter, DL: Chest Physical Therapy and Pulmonary Rehabilitation. Year-Book Medical Publishers, Chicago, 1987, p 26, with permission.)

the airways becomes increasingly smaller with each successive generation of the tracheobronchial tree.

Trachea. The trachea is an oval, flexible tube supported by semicircular rings of cartilage. It extends from C-6 in an oblique, downward direction to the sternal angle level of rib 2 and T-6, at which point it bifurcates. The posterior wall is smooth muscle, and it contains an equal number of ciliated epithelial cells and mucus-containing goblet cells.

Mainstem bronchi. The trachea branches into two mainstream bronchi: the right which is directed almost vertically and the left which is directed more obliquely.

Lobar bronchi. The two mainstem bronchi then divide into five lobar bronchi: three on the right and two on the left. Mainstem and lobar bronchi have a great amount of cartilage, which helps maintain airway patency.

Segmental bronchi. Each of the lobar bronchi divide into two or more segmental bronchi: 10 on the right and 8 on the left. Segmental bronchi have scattered cartilage, smooth muscle, elastic fibers, and a capillary network. The mainstem, lobar, and segmental bronchi have a mucous membrane essentially the same as the trachea.

Bronchioles. Segmental bronchi divide into subsegmental bronchi and bronchioles, which have less and less cartilage and ciliated epithelial cells. These bronchioles divide into the *terminal bronchioles,* which are distal to the last cartilage of the tracheobronchial tree. Terminal bronchioles contain no ciliated cells. Terminal bronchioles divide into *respiratory bronchioles* and provide a transitional zone between the bronchioles and alveoli.

Alveoli. The respiratory bronchioles divide into alveolar ducts and alveolar sacs (Fig. 19–2). One duct may supply several sacs. The ducts contain smooth muscle, which narrows the lumen of the duct with contraction. The alveoli are located in the periphery of the alveolar ducts and sacs and are in contact with capillaries (alveolar-arterial membrane). Gas exchange occurs here.

Summary of Function of the Upper and Lower Respiratory Tracts

- Conducts air to and from the alveolar system for gas exchange
- Helps with humidification and traps small particles to clean the air with the mucosal lining
- Warms the air by the vascular supply
- Moves mucus upward with the cilia
- Elicits the cough reflex to clear the larger airways

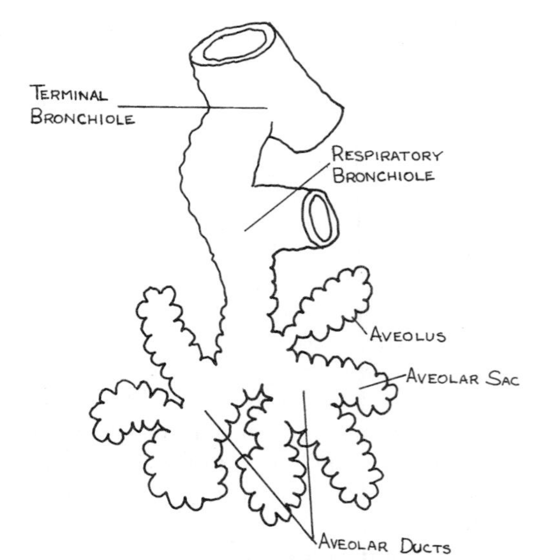

Figure 19–2 Bronchopulmonary segment.

The Lungs and Pleurae

The lungs and pleurae are made up of the following components. The *right lung* has three lobes—the upper, middle, and lower—and 10 bronchopulmonary segments. The *left lung* has two true lobes—the upper and lower—and a slip of lung called the lingula, which is not considered a "true" lobe of the lungs. The left lung has eight bronchopulmonary segments. The lobes of the lungs are depicted in Figure 19–3.

Each lung is covered in *pleura,* a serous membrane known as the *visceral pleura.* This membrane adheres to all surfaces of each lung. The *parietal pleura* lines the inside of the thoracic wall. The parietal pleura is sensitive to pain, but the visceral pleura appears to be insensitive.[25,26] A negative pressure in the minute space between the pleurae serves to keep the lungs inflated. Pleural fluid is found between the pleurae and lubricates the pleurae as they slide on each other during ventilation.

Lung Volumes and Capacities

Pulmonary function tests that measure lung volumes and capacities are performed to evaluate the mechanical function of the lungs (Fig. 19–4). Lung volumes and capacities are related to a person's age, weight, gender, and body position and are altered by disease.[24,55,57] Two or more lung volumes, when combined, are described as a capacity. A basic understanding of these measurements and what the values reflect is useful for the therapist who is treating the patient with pulmonary dysfunction.

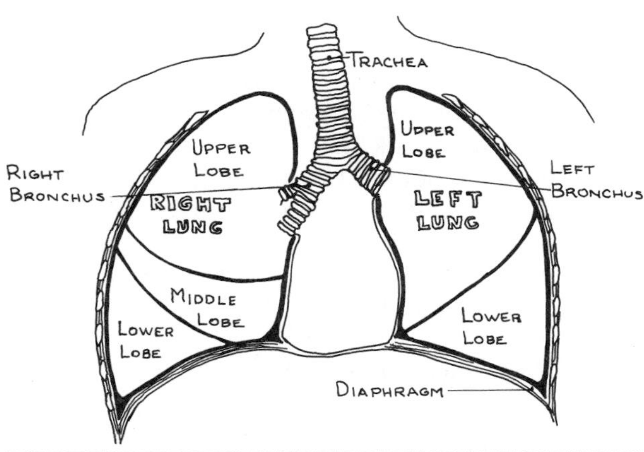

Figure 19–3 Structure of the right and left lungs.

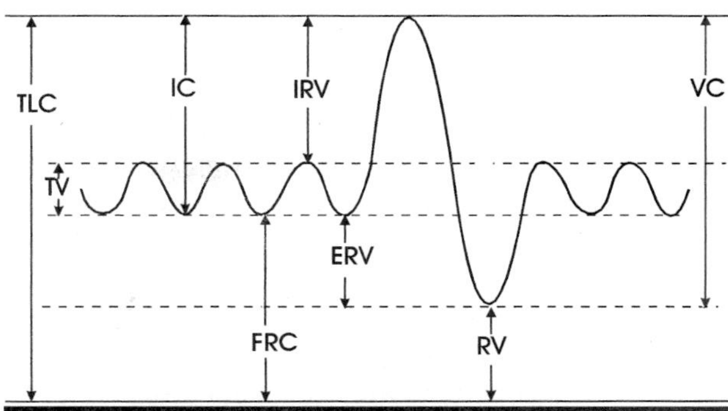

Figure 19–4 Normal lung values and capacities.

Total Lung Capacity (TLC)

- TLC is the total amount of air contained in the lungs after a maximum inspiration.
- The TLC can be subdivided into four volumes: the tidal volume, inspiratory reserve volume, expiratory reserve volume, and residual volume.
- The vital capacity plus the residual volume equal the TLC.
- TLC is approximately 6000 mL in a healthy, young adult.

Tidal Volume (TV)

- The amount of air exchanged during a relaxed inspiration followed by a relaxed expiration.
- In a healthy, young adult, TV is approximately 500 mL per inspiration; approximately 350 mL of the tidal volume reaches the alveoli and participates in gas exchange (respiration).

Inspiratory Reserve Volume (IRV)

- The IRV is the amount of air a person can breathe in after a resting inspiration (approximately 3000 mL).

Expiratory Reserve Volume (ERV)

- The ERV is the amount of air a person can exhale after a normal resting expiration (approximately 1000 mL).

Residual Volume (RV)

- The RV is the amount of air left in the lungs after a maximum expiration (approximately 1500 mL).
- RV increases with age and with restrictive and obstructive pulmonary diseases.

Inspiratory Capacity (IC)

- The IC is the maximum amount of air a person

can breathe in after a resting expiration (approximately 3500 mL).

Functional Residual Capacity (FRC)

- The FRC is the amount of air remaining in the lungs after a resting (tidal) expiration (approximately 2500 mL).
- It is the sum of the ERV and RV.
- This capacity represents the point during ventilation at which the forces that expand the thoracic wall are in balance with the forces that tend to collapse the lungs.[55]

Vital Capacity (VC)

- The VC is the sum of the TV, IRV and ERV. Vital capacity is measured by a maximum inspiration followed by a maximum expiration (approximately 4500 mL).
- Vital capacity decreases with age and is less in the supine position in comparison to an erect posture (sitting or standing).
- VC decreases in the presence of restrictive and obstructive diseases.

▶ Examination

Evaluation of the patient with pulmonary dysfunction and determination of a diagnosis, prognosis, and intervention plan are based on the findings derived from a comprehensive examination, including a history, systems review, and specific tests and measures.[26] The assessment procedures discussed in this section are those commonly performed by a therapist during the examination of a patient with primary or secondary pulmonary dysfunction.[11,12,30,33,71] Other examination procedures not performed by therapists but commonly used in the assessment of a patient with known or suspected pulmonary disease, such as radiographs, evaluation of blood gases, tomography, bronchoscopy, and hematological tests, are not discussed in this section.

Purpose

- Determine a patient's primary and secondary respiratory and ventilatory impairments and how they limit physical function.
- Determine the adequacy of the ventilatory pump and the oxygen uptake/carbon dioxide elimination mechanisms to meet the oxygen demands at rest and during functional activities.
- Ascertain a patient's suitability for participation in a pulmonary rehabilitation program.
- Develop an appropriate level intervention plan for the patient.
- Establish baseline information to measure a patient's progress and the effectiveness of the treatment.
- Determine when to discontinue specific interventions.
- Plan and implement a home program as a basis for self-management.

Components of the Examination

A comprehensive examination of a patient with dysfunction related to pulmonary or chest disorders has many elements. The procedures described in this section are those most often used by a therapist in an initial or ongoing assessment or for modification of therapeutic exercise interventions. More extensive descriptions of examination procedures and the possible implications of those findings for the purposes of a differential diagnosis by a therapist can be found in a number of in-depth resources.[11,12,26,30,33,71]

History and Systems Review

The examination process begins with the patient's history including an interview with the patient as well as family members, if they are available. During the interview the therapist can identify the patient's and/or family members' perception of any functional limitations or disabilities and determine the patient's chief complaints and why the patient is seeking treatment. In preparation for the interview, the medical history and any medical diagnoses are obtained from the patient's medical record, if available, or more generally, from the patient or family. Relevant occupational and social history are obtained; particularly important are on-the-job physical demands, the environment of the workplace, as well as social habits that affect a person's well-being, such as smoking and drinking. Assessment of the home or family environment might include the patient's family responsibilities, the housing situation, and available family support systems. A brief systems review should follow the history.

General Appearance of the Patient

Table 19–1 describes the type of information that can be obtained by visual inspection of the patient and the possible implications of these observations.

Table 19–1 General Appearances of the Patient and Implications

General Appearance	Implications
Level of awareness: (level of consciousness): Alert, responsive, or cooperative versus lethargic, disoriented, or inattentive	Respiratory acidosis, hypercarbia (increased P_{CO_2} level), or hypoxia (decreased P_{O_2} level) can alter level of consciousness
Body Type: Normal, obese, or cachectic	May reflect intolerance to exercise
Color: Cyanosis (bluish appearance) peripherally (nailbeds) or centrally (lips)	Peripheral may indicate low cardiac output; central may indicate inadequate gas exchange in the lungs
Facial signs or expressions: Focused or dilated pupils, nasal flaring, sweating, or distressed appearance	Signs of respiratory distress, fatigue, or pulmonary or musculoskeletal pain
Jugular vein engorgement: Visualization of the jugular venous pulse with the patient supine and the head and neck on pillows at a 45-degree angle	Bilateral distention associated with congestive heart failure/ right-sided heart failure
Hypertrophy of or use at rest of accessory muscles of ventilation: SCM, upper trapezius	Seen in patients with early chronic lung disease or weakness of the diaphragm
Supraclavicular or intercostal retractions occurring with inspiration	Seen in patients with labored breathing
Use of pursed lip breathing (usually with expiraton)	Indicates difficulty with expiration; often seen in patients with chronic obstructive pulmonary disease
Clubbing of digits: Loss of angle between the nail bed and DIP joint	May be linked to increased perfusion
Peripheral edema	Sign of (R) ventricular failure or lymphatic dysfunction

Many of these findings can be noted during the course of the history or during the systems review.

Analysis of Chest Shape and Dimensions

Symmetry of the chest and trunk. Observe anteriorly, posteriorly, and laterally; the thoracic cage should be symmetrical.

Mobility of the trunk. Check active movements in all directions and identify any restricted spinal motions, particularly in the thoracic spine.

Shape and dimensions of the chest. The AP and lateral dimensions are usually 1:2. Common chest deformities include:

- ***Barrel chest.*** The circumference of the upper chest appears larger than that of the lower chest. The sternum appears prominent, and the AP diameter of the chest is greater than normal. Many patients with chronic obstructive pulmonary disorders, who are usually upper chest breathers, develop a barrel chest.
- ***Pectus excavatum (funnel breast).*** The lower part of the sternum is depressed and the lower ribs flare out. Patients with this deformity are diaphragmatic breathers; excessive abdominal protrusion and little upper chest movement occur during breathing.
- ***Pectus carinatum (pigeon breast).*** The sternum is prominent and protrudes anteriorly.

Posture or Preferred Positioning

Patients who have difficulty breathing as the result of chronic lung disease often lean forward on their hands or forearms when sitting or standing and stabilize and elevate the shoulder girdle to assist with inspiration (Fig. 19–5). This increases the effectiveness of the pectoralis and serratus anterior muscles to act as accessory muscles of inspiration by reverse action. Note any postural deformities such as kyphosis and scoliosis and postural asymmetry from thoracic surgery, which could restrict chest movements and ventilation.

Patients with cardiopulmonary dysfunction when resting or sleeping often prefer to be in a head-up rather than a fully recumbent position. Assuming a horizontal position may result in shortness of breath.

Breathing Pattern

Assess the *rate, regularity,* and *location* of ventilation at rest and with activity. A normal respiratory rate is 12 to 20 breaths per minute. This is most accurately determined when the patient is unaware that his or her respiratory rate is being measured, as

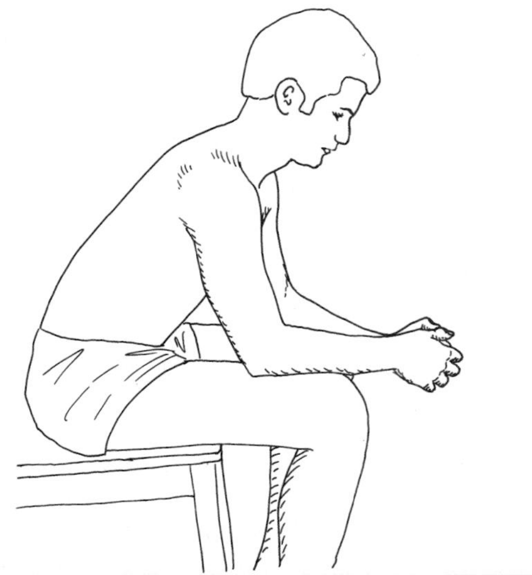

Figure 19–5 A patient who is short of breath at rest or after activity often assumes a forward-bent position with hands or elbows resting on the thighs to reduce or relieve symptoms.

when taking the pulse rate. The normal ratio of inspiration to expiration at rest is 1:2 and with activity, 1:1. Patients with chronic obstructive pulmonary disease (COPD) may have a ratio of 1:4 at rest, which reflects the difficulty these patients have with the expiratory phase of breathing. The normal sequence of inspiration at rest is (1) the diaphragm contracts and descends and the abdomen (epigastric area) rises; (2) this is followed by lateral costal expansion as the ribs move up and out; and, finally, (3) the upper chest rises. The neck muscles that act as accessory muscles of inspiration should be inactive during relaxed inspiration. To assess the sequence have the patient assume a comfortable position (semirecling or supine). Place your hands on the patient's epigastric region and sternum to observe movements in these two areas.

Abnormal Breathing Patterns

The following terms describe variations of abnormal breathing patterns.[11,12,30,33]

- ***Dyspnea.*** Distressed, labored breathing as the result of shortness of breath.
- ***Tachypnea.*** Rapid, shallow breathing; decreased tidal volume but increased rate; associated with restrictive or obstructive lung disease and use of accessory muscles of inspiration.
- ***Bradypnea.*** Slow rate with shallow or normal depth and regular rhythm; may be associated with drug overdose.
- ***Hyperventilation.*** Deep, rapid respiration; increased tidal volume and increased rate of respiration; regular rhythm.
- ***Orthopnea.*** Difficulty breathing in the supine position.
- ***Apnea.*** Cessation of breathing in the expiratory phase.
- ***Apneusis.*** Cessation of breathing in the inspiratory phase.
- ***Cheyne-Stokes.*** Cycles of gradually increasing tidal volumes, followed by a series of gradually decreasing tidal volumes, and then a period of apnea. This is sometimes seen in the patient with a severe head injury.

Chest Mobility

Symmetry of chest movement. Analysis of the symmetry of the moving chest during breathing gives the therapist some information on the mobility of the chest and indirectly indicates what areas of the lungs may or may not be responding. *Procedure:* Place your hands on the patient's chest and assess the excursion of each side of the chest during inspiration and expiration. Each of the three lobar areas can be checked.[11,12,17,30,33,71]

- To check *upper lobe expansion,* face the patient; place the tips of your thumbs at the midsternal line at the sternal notch. Extend your fingers above the clavicles. Have the patient fully exhale and then inhale deeply.
- To check *middle lobe expansion,* continue to face the patient; place the tips of your thumbs at the xiphoid process and extend your fingers laterally around the ribs. Again, ask the patient to breathe in deeply.
- To check *lower lobe expansion,* place the tips of your thumbs along the patient's back at the spinous processes (lower thoracic level), and extend your fingers around the ribs. Ask the patient to breathe in deeply.

Extent of excursion. The extent of chest mobility can be measured by two methods:[17,30,33]

- Measure the girth of the chest with a tape measure at three levels (axilla, xiphoid, lower costal). Document change in girth after a maximum inspiration and maximum expiration.
- Place both hands on the patient's chest or back as

previously described. Note the distance between your thumbs after a maximum inspiration.

Palpation

Palpation of the thorax can provide evidence of dysfunction of the underlying tissues including the lungs, chest wall, and mediastinum.[11,12,30,33,71]

Tactile (vocal) fremitus. This is the vibration felt as the therapist palpates over the chest wall as a patient speaks. *Procedure:* Place the palms of your hands lightly on the chest wall and ask the patient to speak a few words or repeat "99" several times. Normally, fremitus is felt uniformly on the chest wall. Fremitus is increased in the presence of secretions in the airways and decreased or absent when air is trapped as the result of obstructed airways.

Chest wall pain. Specific areas or points of pain over anterior, posterior, or lateral aspects of the chest wall can be identified with palpation. *Procedure:* Firmly press against the chest wall with your hands to identify any specific areas of pain potentially of musculoskeletal origin. Ask the patient to take a deep breath, and identify any painful areas of the chest wall. Chest wall pain of musculoskeletal origin often increases with direct point pressure during palpation and during a deep inspiration.[30,33]

Note: Pain in the anterior, posterior, or lateral region of the chest can be of musculoskeletal, pulmonary, or cardiac origin.[26] Pain of pulmonary origin is usually localized to a region of the chest but may also be felt in the neck or shoulder. Several pulmonary or cardiac conditions can mimic musculoskeletal pain such as pulmonary embolism, pleurisy, pneumonia, pneumothorax, and pulmonary artery hypertension.[26]

Mediastinal shift. The position of the trachea is normally oriented centrally in relationship to the suprasternal notch indicating symmetry of the mediastinum. The position of the trachea shifts as the result of asymmetrical intrathoracic pressures or lung volumes. For example, if the patient has had a lung removed (pneumonectomy), the lung volume on the operated side will decrease, and the trachea will shift toward that side. Conversely, if the patient has a hemothorax (blood in the thorax), intrathoracic pressure on the side of the hemothorax increases, and the mediastinum will shift away from the affected side of the chest.[11,12,30,33]

Procedure: To identify a *mediastinal shift,* have the patient sit facing you with the head in midline and the neck slightly flexed to relax the sternocleidomastoid muscles. With your index finger gently palpate the soft tissue space on either side of the trachea at the suprasternal notch. Determine whether the trachea is palpable at the midline or has shifted to the left or right.

Mediate Percussion

This is an examination technique designed to assess lung density, specifically, air to solid ratio in the lungs.[11,12,30,33]

Procedure: Place the middle finger of the nondominant hand flat against the chest wall along an intercostal space. With the tip of the middle finger of the opposite hand tap firmly on the finger positioned on the chest wall. Repeat the procedure at several points on the right and left and anterior and posterior aspects of the chest wall. This maneuver produces a resonance; the pitch varies with the density of the underlying tissue. The subjective determination of pitch indicates the following:

- The sound will be dull and flat if there is a greater than normal amount of solid matter (tumor, consolidation) in the lungs in comparison with the amount of air.
- The sound will be hyper-resonant (tympanic) if there is a greater than normal amount of air in the area (as in patients with emphysema).
- If asymmetrical or abnormal findings are noted, the patient should be referred to the physician for additional objective tests such as a chest x-ray.

Auscultation of Breath Sounds

Auscultation is a general term that refers to the process of listening to sounds within the body, specifically to breath sounds in an examination of the lungs.[11,12,30,33] Breath sounds occur because of movement of air in the airways during inspiration and expiration. A stethoscope is used to magnify these sounds. Breath sounds should be assessed to:

- Identify the areas of the lungs in which congestion exists and in which airway clearance techniques should be performed.
- Determine the effectiveness of any airway clearance intervention.
- Determine whether or not the lungs are clear and whether or not interventions should be discontinued.

Procedure: When assessing breath sounds, be sure the setting is quiet. Have the patient assume a comfortable, relaxed, sitting position to allow access to the chest wall. Place the diaphragm of the stethoscope directly against the patient's skin along the anterior or posterior chest wall. Be sure that the tubing does not rub together or come in contact with clothing during auscultation, as this contact produces extraneous sounds. Follow a systematic pattern (Fig. 19–6*A* and *B*) and place the stethoscope against specific thoracic landmarks (T-2, T-6, T-10) along the right and left sides of the chest wall. Ask the patient to breathe in deeply and out quickly through the mouth as you move the stethoscope from point to point. Note the quality, intensity, and pitch of the breath sounds.

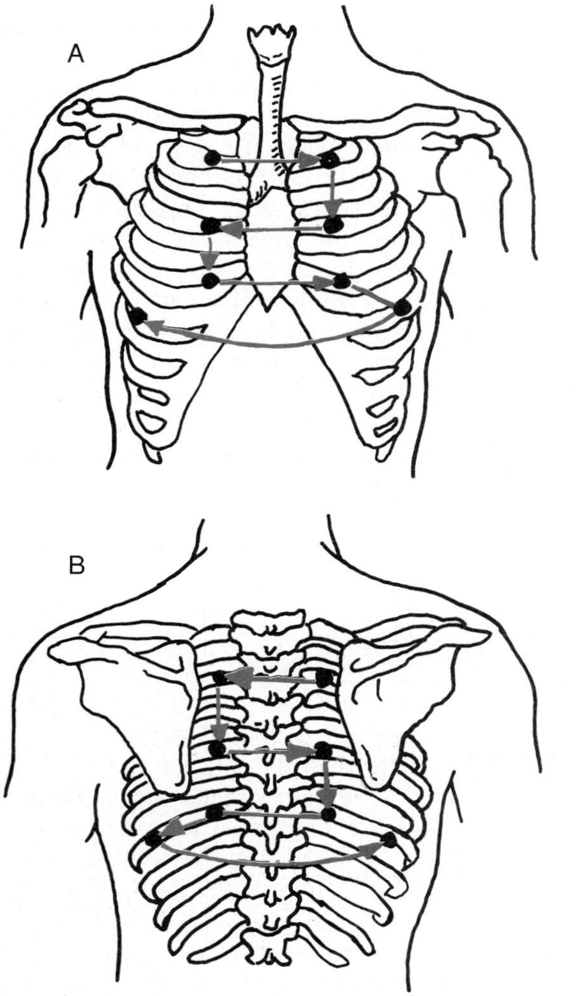

Precaution: Auscultate slowly from one area to another. Allow the patient to breathe in a relaxed manner after several deep breaths to prevent dizziness from hyperventilation. Guard the patient closely to prevent loss of balance if lightheadedness occurs.

Classification of breath sounds. Breath sounds are classified by location, pitch and intensity, and the ratio of sounds heard on inspiration versus expiration. Breath sounds are also identified as normal or adventitious (extra).[12,30,70,71] Normal breath sounds occur in the absence of pathology and are predominantly heard during inspiration. Normal breath sounds are categorized as *vesicular, bronchial,* or *bronchovesicular* based on the location and quality of the sound. They are described in Box 19–3.[5,70] *Adventitious* breath sounds are abnormal sounds in

A

B

Figure 19–6 Pattern of specific thoracic landmarks for auscultation. The diaphragm of the stethoscope is placed along the right and left *(A)* anterior chest wall and the *(B)* posterior chest wall at T-2, T-6, and T-10. (From Frownfelter, DL: Chest Physical Therapy and Pulmonary Rehabilitation. Year-Book Medical Publishers, Chicago, 1987, p 135, with permission.)

Box 19–3 Normal and Adventitious Breath Sounds

Normal Breath Sounds

- ***Vesicular.*** Soft, low-pitched, breezy but faint sounds heard over most of the chest except near the trachea and mainstem bronchi and between the scapulae. Vesicular sounds are audible considerably longer on inspiration than expiration (about a 3:1 ratio).
- ***Bronchial.*** Loud, hollow, or tubular, high-pitched sounds heard over the mainstem bronchi and trachea. Bronchial sounds are heard equally during inspiration and expiration; a slight pause in the sound occurs between inspiration and expiration.
- ***Bronchovesicular.*** Softer than bronchial breath sounds; also heard equally during inspiration and expiration but without a pause in the sound between the cycles. The sounds are heard in the supraclavicular, suprascapular, and parasternal regions anteriorly and between the scapulae posteriorly.

Adventitious Breath Sounds

- ***Crackles.*** Fine, discontinuous sounds (similar to the sound of bubbles popping or the sound of hairs being rubbed between your fingers next to your ear). Crackles, which can be fine or coarse, are heard primarily during inspiration as the result of secretions moving in the airways or in closed airways that are rapidly reopening. The former term for crackles was *rales*.
- ***Wheezes.*** Continuous high- or low-pitched sounds or sometimes musical tones heard during exhalation but occasionally audible during inspiration. Bronchospasm or secretions that narrow the lumen of the airways cause wheezes. The term previously used for wheezes was *rhonchi*.

the lungs that are heard with a stethoscope. Although terminology in the literature is inconsistent, nomenclature most often used was proposed by a joint committee of the American College of Chest Physicians and the American Thoracic Society[5,70] Adventitious breath sounds are categorized as *crackles* or *wheezes.* Box 19–3 describes the location and quality of these breath sounds.

Breath sounds may also be totally absent or substantially diminished over a portion of the lungs. This indicates total or partial obstruction and lack of aeration of lung tissue. The absence of air and collapse of an area of lung tissue is known as *atelectasis.* It may be caused by obstruction of airways, by fluids, mucus, bronchospasm, or compression by tumor. Breath sounds are absent over areas of atelectasis.

Cough and Cough Production

The *strength, depth, length,* and *frequency* of a patient's cough must be assessed. An effective cough is sharp and deep. In the patient with current or potential pulmonary dysfunction a cough can be described as weak, shallow, soft, or throaty. A patient may have a weak, shallow cough as the result of pain or paralysis. A sudden onset of a cough or a sustained cough can be described as paroxysmal or spasmodic. If a cough is substantially weak or ineffective, suctioning may be required to clear the airways.[11,12,30,71]

A cough may be productive or nonproductive in the presence of pathology. The productivity of the cough and secretions produced by the cough must be assessed. Secretions should be checked for:

- Color (clear, yellow, green, blood-stained)
- Consistency (viscous, thin, frothy)
- Amount (minimal to copious)
- Odor (no odor to foul-smelling)

Production of a small amount of clear or white secretions on a daily basis is normal. Copious but clear secretions are common in chronic bronchitis. Yellow, green, and purulent secretions with a strong odor are indicative of some type of infection. Blood-streaked secretions, known as *hemoptysis,* is indicative of some degree of hemorrhage within the lungs. Frothy, white secretions are associated with pulmonary edema and heart failure. When secretions are produced during the course of interventions such as exercise or airway clearance, it is the responsibility of the therapist to document the characteristics of the secretions.

Other Areas of Examination

The examination procedures discussed in this section must be complemented with other examination procedures, which may include:

- Range of motion, particularly of the shoulders and trunk
- Muscle strength
- General endurance and graded exercise testing
- Functional abilities or limitations; the patient's perception of disability
- Use of assistive respiratory equipment

Breathing Exercises and Ventilatory Training

Breathing exercises and ventilatory training are fundamental interventions for the prevention or comprehensive management of acute or chronic pulmonary disorders. For example, these interventions are frequently advocated in the literature for patients with chronic obstructive pulmonary diseases (chronic bronchitis, emphysema, asthma, and cystic fibrosis), for patients with a high spinal cord lesion, for patients who have undergone thoracic or abdominal surgery and are at high risk for acute pulmonary complications, or for patients who must remain in bed for an extended period of time.*

Breathing exercises and ventilatory training can take on many forms including diaphragmatic breathing, segmental breathing, ventilatory muscle training, inspiratory resistance training, incentive spirometry, and breathing techniques for the relief of dyspnea with exertion. The goals of these forms of intervention are listed in Box 19–4.

Research studies indicate that, although breathing exercises or ventilatory muscle training may affect and possibly alter a patient's rate and depth of ventilation, these interventions may not necessarily have any impact on gas exchange at the alveolar level or on oxygenation.[11,32,44,48,56] Therefore, breathing exercises or ventilatory training should be only one aspect of management to improve pulmonary status and to increase a patient's overall endurance and function in daily living activities. Depending on the patient's underlying pathology and impairments, exercises to improve ventilation are often combined with medication, airway clearance,

*See references 3, 7, 11, 13, 14, 31, 35, 38, 39, 44, 48, 52, 53, 56, 61, 63, 69, 72.

Box 19–4 Goals of Breathing Exercises and Ventilatory Muscle Training

- Improve or redistribute ventilation.
- Increase the effectiveness of the cough mechanism and promote airway clearance.
- Prevent postoperative pulmonary complications.
- Improve the strength, endurance, and coordination of the muscles of ventilation.
- Maintain or improve chest and thoracic spine mobility.
- Correct inefficient or abnormal breathing patterns and decrease the work of breathing.
- Promote relaxation and relieve stress.
- Teach the patient how to deal with episodes of dyspnea.
- Improve a patient's overall functional capacity for daily living, occupational, and recreational activities.

the use of respiratory therapy devices, and a graded exercise (conditioning) program.

Guidelines for Teaching Breathing Exercises

1. If possible, choose a quiet area for instruction in which you can interact with the patient with minimal distractions.
2. Explain to the patient the aims and rationale of breathing exercises or ventilatory training specific to his or her particular impairments and functional limitations.
3. Have the patient assume a comfortable, relaxed position and loosen restrictive clothing. Initially, a semi-Fowler's position with the head and trunk elevated approximately 45 degrees, is desirable. By totally supporting the head and trunk and by flexing the hips and knees and supporting the legs with a pillow, the abdominal muscles remain relaxed. Other positions such as supine, sitting, or standing may be used initially or as the patient progresses in treatment.
4. Observe and assess the patient's spontaneous breathing pattern while at rest and later with activity.
5. Determine whether or not ventilatory training is indicated.
6. Establish a baseline for assessment of change, progress, and outcomes of intervention.
7. If necessary, teach the patient relaxation techniques. This will relax the muscles of the upper thorax, neck, and shoulders to minimize the use of the accessory muscles of ventilation. Pay particular attention to relaxation of the sternocleidomastoids, upper trapezius, and levator scapulae muscles.
8. Depending on the patient's underlying pathology and impairments determine whether to emphasize the inspiratory or expiratory phase of ventilation.
9. Demonstrate the desired breathing pattern to the patient.
10. Have the patient practice the correct breathing pattern in a variety of positions at rest and with activity.

Precautions: When teaching breathing exercises, be aware of the following precautions:[11,44,48,56]

- Never allow a patient to force expiration. Expiration should be relaxed and passive or controlled. Forced expiration only increases turbulence in the airways, which can lead to bronchospasm and increased airway restriction.
- Do not allow a patient to take a very *prolonged* expiration. This causes the patient to gasp with the next inspiration. The patient's breathing pattern then becomes irregular and inefficient.
- Do not allow the patient to initiate inspiration with the accessory muscles and the upper chest. Advise the patient that the upper chest should be relatively quiet during breathing.
- Allow the patient to perform deep breathing for only three or four inspirations and expirations at a time to avoid hyperventilation.

Diaphragmatic Breathing

When the diaphragm is functioning effectively in its role as the primary muscle of inspiration, ventilation is efficient and the oxygen consumption of the muscles of ventilation is very low during quiet relaxed breathing.[7,48,54] When a patient substantially relies on the accessory muscles of inspiration, the work of breathing increases. Although the diaphragm controls breathing at an involuntary level, a patient with primary pulmonary disease such as COPD, can be taught breathing control by optimal use of the diaphragm and relaxation of accessory muscles. Controlled breathing techniques, which emphasize diaphragmatic breathing, are designed to improve the efficiency of ventilation, decrease the work of breathing, increase the excursion (descent or ascent) of the diaphragm, and improve gas exchange and oxygenation.[11,38,44,48,56] Diaphragmatic breathing exercises are also used to mobilize lung secretions during postural drainage.[23,47]

Procedure

- Prepare the patient in a relaxed and comfortable position in which gravity *assists* the diaphragm, such as a semi-Fowler's position.
- If you have noted in the examination that the patient initiates the breathing pattern with the accessory muscles of inspiration, start instruction by teaching the patient how to relax those muscles (shoulder rolls or shoulder shrugs coupled with relaxation).
- Place your hand(s) on the rectus abdominis just below the anterior costal margin (Fig. 19–7). Ask the patient to breathe in slowly and deeply through the nose. Have the patient keep the shoulders relaxed and upper chest quiet, allowing the abdomen to rise. Then tell the patient to slowly let all the air out using controlled expiration.
- Have the patient practice this three or four times and then rest. Do not allow the patient to hyperventilate.
- If the patient is having difficulty using the diaphragm during inspiration, have the patient inhale several times in succession through the nose by using a *sniffing* action.[48,56] This action usually facilitates the diaphragm.
- To learn how to self-monitor this sequence, have the patient place his or her own hand below the anterior costal margin and feel the movement (Fig. 19–8). The patient's hand should rise during inspiration and fall during expiration. By placing one hand on the abdomen, the patient can also feel the contraction of the abdominal muscles, which occurs with controlled expiration or coughing.
- After the patient understands and is able to control breathing using a diaphragmatic pattern, keeping the shoulders relaxed, practice diaphragmatic breathing in a variety of positions (supine, sitting, standing) and during activity (walking and climbing stairs).

Note: The effect of diaphragmatic breathing exercises directly on ventilation, oxygenation, and excursion of the diaphragm in normal subjects and in patients with pulmonary disorders remains unclear.[11,38,48,72] Studies have both supported[32,54,58,60] and refuted[54,60] the positive impact of diaphragmatic breathing exercises on each of these areas of function. Despite this, diaphragmatic breathing exercises continue to be an integral part of most cardiopulmonary

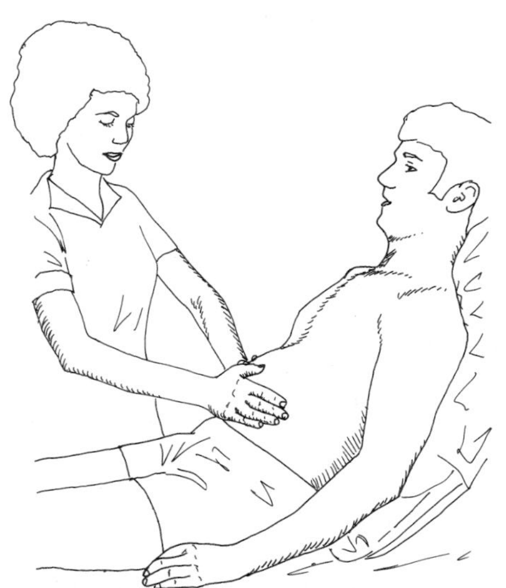

Figure 19–7 The semireclining (as shown) and semi-Fowler's positions are comfortable, relaxed positions in which to teach diaphragmatic breathing.

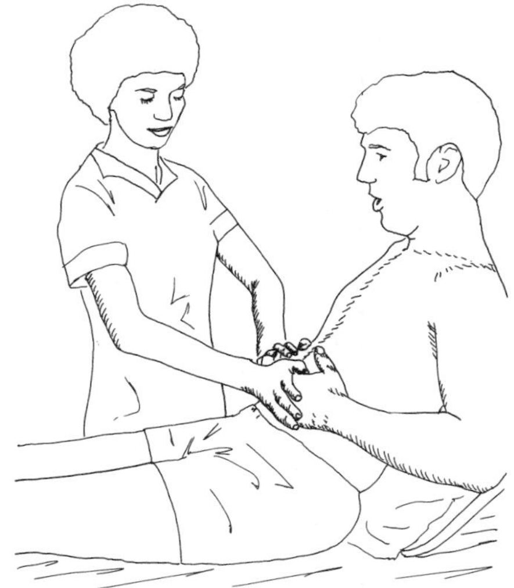

Figure 19–8 The patient places his or her own hands on the abdomen to feel the movement of proper diaphragmatic breathing. By placing the hands on the abdomen, the patient can also feel the contraction of the abdominals, which occurs with controlled expiration or coughing.

physical therapy programs as research on the effects of diaphragmatic breathing continues.

Respiratory Resistance Training

The process of improving the strength or endurance of the muscles of ventilation is known as *respiratory resistance training* (RRT). Other descriptions used to denote this form of breathing exercises are *inspiratory resistance training, diaphragmatic strengthening exercises,* or *flow-controlled endurance training.* This technique usually focuses on training the muscles of inspiration although the use of expiratory muscle training has also been studied and advocated.[27] RRT has been advocated most frequently in the treatment of patients with pulmonary dysfunction associated with weakness, atrophy, or inefficiency of the muscles of inspiration. With support from animal studies, it has been suggested that the principles of overload and specificity of training apply to skeletal muscles throughout the body, including the muscles of ventilation.* In humans, it is not feasible to evaluate morphological or histochemical changes in the diaphragm that may occur as the result of strength or endurance training with invasive procedures. Instead, strength or endurance changes must be assessed indirectly. Increases in respiratory muscle endurance have been measured by maximal voluntary ventilation and decreased reliance on accessory muscles of inspiration. Respiratory muscle strength (either inspiratory or expiratory) has been evaluated indirectly with measurements of inspiratory capacity, forced expiratory volume, inspiratory mouth pressure using a spirometer, vital capacity, and increased cough effectiveness.

Two approaches to respiratory resistance training: diaphragmatic strengthening and inspiratory resistance training, are addressed in this section.

Precaution: Avoid prolonged periods of any form of resistance training for inspiratory muscles. Unlike muscles of the extremities, the diaphragm cannot totally rest to recover from a session of resistance exercises. Use of accessory muscles of inspiration (neck and shoulder muscles) is a sign that the diaphragm is beginning to fatigue.[3,69]

Inspiratory Resistance Training

This form of ventilation muscle training uses specifically designed breathing devices (resistors) to improve the strength and endurance of the muscles of inspiration and decrease the occurrence of inspiratory muscle fatigue. This technique was originally and sometimes still is advocated for patients with primary, acute, or chronic lung disease.[1,2,13,14,41,62] More recently, it has been studied and found to be effective for patients with cervical level spinal cord lesions.[28,45,53,59,68]

Procedure

- The patient inhales through a hand-held resistive training device that he or she places in the mouth. Inspiratory resistive training devices are narrow tubes of varying diameters that provide resistance to airflow during inspiration and, therefore, place resistance on inspiratory muscles to improve strength or endurance. The narrower the diameter of the airway, the greater the resistance.
- The patient inhales through the tube for a specified period of time several times each day. The time is gradually increased to 20 to 30 minutes at each training session to increase inspiratory muscle endurance.
- As the patient's strength and endurance improve, the diameter of the handheld tube is decreased. The commercially available resistive devices have six different diameters to provide levels of resistance appropriate for each patient.

The effectiveness of inspiratory resistance training continues to be investigated. Some studies have indicated that ventilatory muscle strength and endurance have not improved as the result of this type of training, but other studies have shown that respiratory rate decreases and exercise tolerance increases over time.[3,13,14,41,45,53]

Diaphragmatic Training Using Weights

The use of a small weight, such as a sandbag, to strengthen or improve the endurance of the diaphragm is often suggested in the literature by means of the following procedure.[3,22,40,44,59,69]

- Have the patient assume a slightly head-up position or, if possible, a horizontal position.
- Place a small weight (3–5 lb) over the epigastric region of the patient's abdomen.
- Tell the patient to breathe in deeply while trying to keep the upper chest quiet. The resistance should not interfere with full excursion of the diaphragm and normal rise of the epigastric area.
- Gradually increase the time that the patient breathes against the resistance of the weight. The

*See references 1, 2, 27, 28, 38, 41, 53, 59, 60, 65.

weight can be increased when the patient can sustain the diaphragmatic breathing pattern without the use of accessory muscles of inspiration for 15 minutes.

- Trendelenburg positioning can also be used to strengthen the diaphragm. In the head-down position the abdominal contents move superiorly and provide resistance to the diaphragm as it contracts and descends.[69]

Note: Although this method of strengthening the diaphragm is often suggested in the literature for patients with respiratory muscle weakness, the results of a study of normal subjects indicated that the effectiveness of this method of strengthening was questionable.[49] There is also concern that patients who have used this technique have been observed to develop poor breathing patterns.[7] In another study with patients with cervical level spinal cord injuries, abdominal weight training and inspiratory resistance training were both reported to be effective methods of ventilatory muscle training to improve respiratory muscle strength and endurance.[22] In general, there seems to be a trend away from the use of small weights for this type of training in favor of devices, such as resistors, specifically designed for inspiratory muscle training.

Incentive Respiratory Spirometry

Incentive spirometry is a form of ventilatory training that emphasizes sustained maximum inspirations. A synonymous term is *sustained maximum inspiratory maneuver,* which is performed with or without the use of a spirometer.[18,44,48,56] The patient inhales through a spirometer that provides visual or auditory feedback as the patient breathes in as deeply as possible. Incentive spirometry increases the volume of air inspired and has been advocated primarily to prevent alveolar collapse and atelectasis in postoperative patients and to strengthen weak inspiratory muscles in patients with neuromuscular disorders.[8,48] Despite the widespread use of incentive spirometry for the postoperative patient, the effectiveness of its use alone or in addition to general deep breathing and coughing for the prevention of postoperative pulmonary complications is in question.[18,35,65]

Procedure

- Place the patient in a comfortable position (semi-reclining, if possible).
- Have the patient take three to four slow, easy breaths and maximally exhale with the fourth breath.
- Then have the patient place the spirometer in the mouth, maximally inhale through the spirometer, and hold the inspiration for several seconds.
- This sequence is repeated five to ten times several times per day.

Segmental Breathing

It is questionable whether a patient can be taught to expand localized areas of the lung while keeping other areas quiet. It is known, however, the hypoventilation does occur in certain areas of the lungs because of chest wall fibrosis, pain, and muscle guarding after surgery, atelectasis, and pneumonia. Therefore, there are certain instances such as during postural drainage or following thoracic surgery when it is important to emphasize expansion of problem areas of the lung and chest wall.

Lateral Costal Expansion

This is sometimes called *lateral basal expansion* and may be done unilaterally or bilaterally. Emphasizing deep breathing with a focus of movement of this portion of the lower rib cage is thought to facilitate diaphragmatic excursion.[48] It is a particularly useful technique for those patients with a stiff lower rib cage, as is often seen in the patient with chronic bronchitis, emphysema, or asthma.[7]

Procedures. The patient may be sitting or in a hook-lying position. Place your hands along the lateral aspect of the lower ribs to fix the patient's attention to the areas at which movement is to occur (Figs. 19–9 and 19–10).

- Ask the patient to breathe out, and feel the rib cage move downward and inward. As the patient

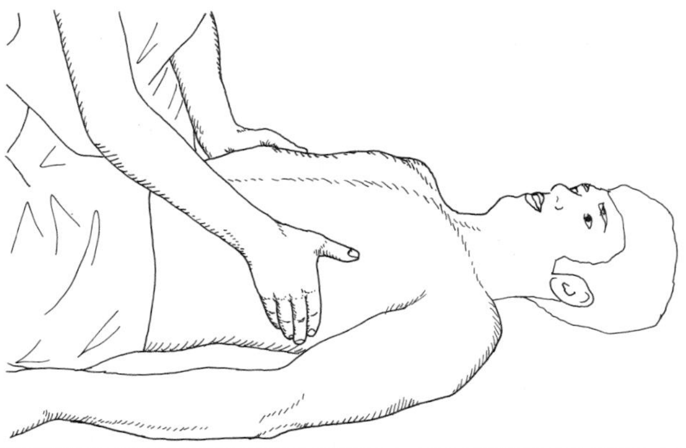

Figure 19–9 Bilateral lateral costal expansion—supine.

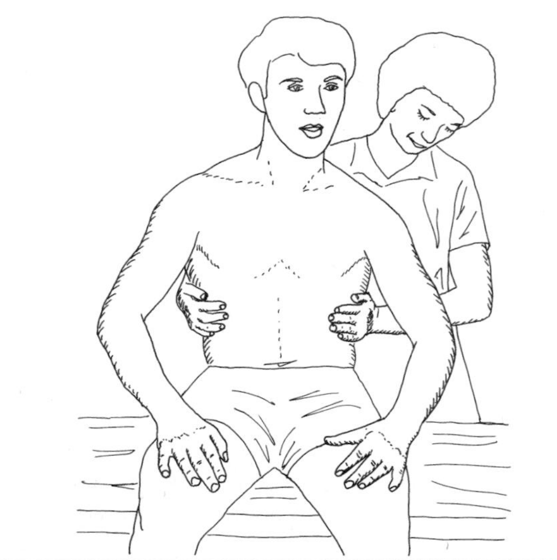

Figure 19–10 Bilateral lateral costal expansion–sitting.

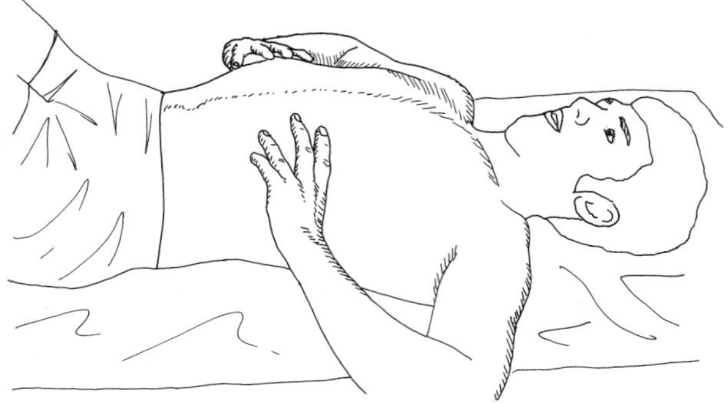

Figure 19–11 The patient applies his or her own manual pressure during lateral costal expansion.

breathes out, place pressure into the ribs with the palms of your hands.

- Just prior to inspiration, apply a quick downward and inward stretch to the chest. This places a quick stretch on the external intercostals to facilitate their contraction.
- Apply *gentle* manual resistance to the lower rib area to increase sensory awareness as the patient breathes in deeply and the chest expands and ribs flare.
- Then, again, as the patient breathes out, assist by gently squeezing the rib cage in a downward and inward direction.
- The patient may then be taught to perform the maneuver independently. He or she may place the hand(s) over the ribs (Fig. 19–11) or apply resistance using a towel or belt (Fig. 19–12*A* and *B*).

Posterior Basal Expansion

This form of segmental breathing is important for the postsurgical patient who is confined to bed in a semi-reclining position for an extended period of time. Secretions often accumulate in the posterior segments of the lower lobes.

Procedure. Have the patient sit and lean forward on a pillow, slightly bending the hips (see Fig. 19–13). Place your hands over the posterior aspect of the lower ribs. Follow the same procedure just described for lateral costal expansion.

Right Middle Lobe or Lingula Expansion

Procedure. While the patient is sitting, place your hands at either the right or the left side of the patient's chest, just below the axilla. Follow the same procedure as described for lateral basal expansion.

Glossopharyngeal Breathing

Glossopharyngeal breathing is a means of increasing a patient's inspiratory capacity when there is severe weakness of the muscles of inspiration.[34,48,50,69] It is taught to patients who have difficulty taking in a deep breath, for example, in preparation for coughing. This type of breathing pattern was originally developed to assist postpolio patients with severe muscle weakness. Today, if it is used at all because it is quite difficult to learn, it is most frequently taught to patients with high spinal cord injuries who can easily develop respiratory complications.[34,48,69]

Procedure. The patient takes in several "gulps" of air. Then the mouth is closed, and the tongue pushes the air back and traps it in the pharynx. The air is then forced into the lungs when the glottis is opened. This increases the depth of the inspiration and the patient's vital capacity.[34]

Pursed-Lip Breathing

Whether it is appropriate to teach pursed-lip breathing to a patient is debatable. Most therapists feel that gentle pursed-lip breathing with controlled expiration is a useful procedure, if it is performed appropriately. It is thought to keep airways open by creating a backpressure in the airways. It is taught to help a patient with chronic obstructive pulmonary dis-

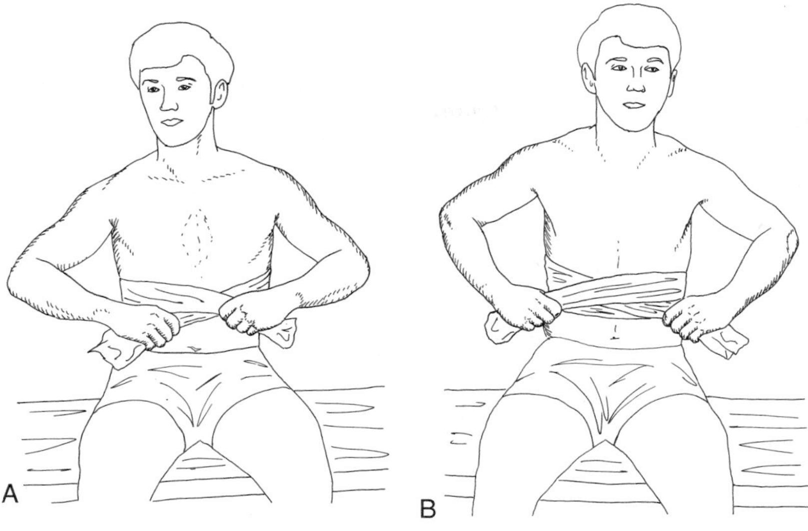

Figure 19–12 Belt exercises reinforce lateral costal breathing *(A)* by applying resistance during inspiration and *(B)* by assisting with pressure along the rib cage during expiration.

ease (COPD) deal with episodes of dyspnea.[7,44,52] Studies suggest that pursed-lip breathing decreases the respiratory rate, increases the tidal volume, and improves exercise tolerance.[14,44] Some patients spontaneously develop this pattern of breathing. If so, they should not be discouraged from using it.

Precaution: The use of *forced* expiration during pursed-lip breathing must be avoided. Forceful or prolonged expiration while the lips are pursed can increase the turbulence in the airways and cause further restriction of the small bronchioles. For this reason, some therapists have suggested that patients may perform pursed-lip breathing inappropriately and, therefore, should not be taught this form of breathing. Cognizant of this concern, it is the opinion of the authors of this textbook that pursed-lip breathing (with passive expiration) is a valuable means of dealing with episodes of dyspnea and *should* be taught to patients with COPD.

Procedure. Have the patient assume a comfortable position and relax as much as possible. Explain to the patient that expiration must be relaxed (passive) and that contraction of the abdominals must be avoided. Place your hand over the patient's abdominal muscles to detect any contraction of the abdominals. Instruct the patient to breathe in slowly and deeply. Then have the patient loosely purse the lips and exhale.

Preventing and Relieving Episodes of Dyspnea

Many patients with COPD (emphysema and asthma, for example) may suffer from periodic episodes of dyspnea (shortness of breath), particularly with physical exertion or when in contact with allergens. Whenever a patient's normal breathing pattern is interrupted, shortness of breath can occur. It is helpful to teach patients how to monitor their level of shortness of breath to *prevent* episodes of dyspnea with *controlled breathing,* by *pacing activities* and by becoming aware of what activity or situation causes dyspnea.

Pacing is the performance of functional activities, such as walking, stair climbing, or work-related tasks, within the limits of a patient's ventilatory capacity.[11] Although some patients may intuitively understand to what limits functional activities can be pushed, other patients must be taught to recognize

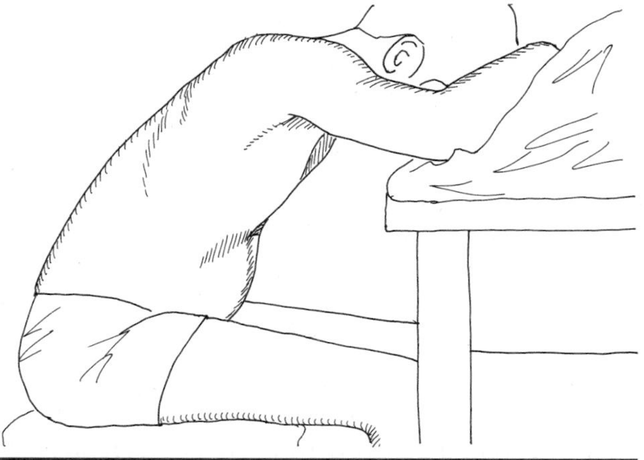

Figure 19–13 A patient can sit and lean forward on a pillow to relax and relieve an episode of dyspnea.

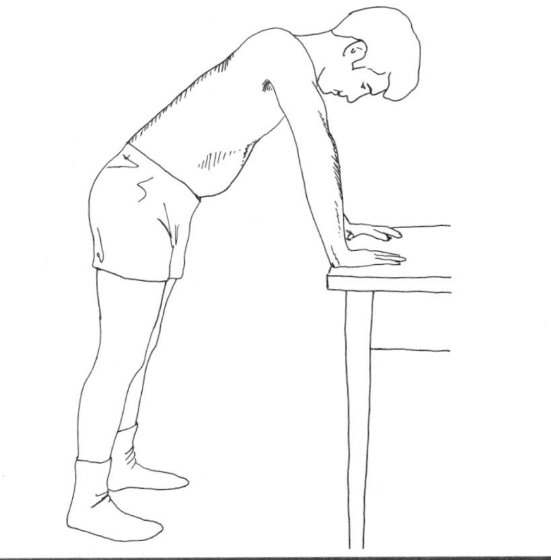

Figure 19–14 While standing, a patient can lean forward and place some weight on the hands to relieve dyspnea.

the early signs of dyspnea. If the patient becomes slightly short of breath, he or she must learn to stop an activity and use controlled, pursed-lip breathing until the dyspnea subsides.[5]

Procedure

- Have the patient assume a relaxed, forward-bent posture (Figs. 19–13 and 19–14; also see Fig. 19–5). This forward-bent position stimulates diaphragmatic breathing (the viscera drops forward and the diaphragm descends more easily). Use bronchodilators as prescribed.
- Have the patient gain control of his or her breathing and reduce the respiratory rate by using pursed-lip breathing during expiration. Have the patient emphasize the expiratory phase of breathing while being sure to avoid forceful expiration.
- After each pursed-lip expiration, have the patient breathe in diaphragmatically, avoiding the use of accessory muscles.
- Then have the patient remain in this posture and continue to breathe in as relaxed a manner as possible.

▶ Exercises to Mobilize the Chest

Chest mobilization exercises are any exercises that combine active movements of the trunk or extremities with deep breathing.[19,56] They are designed to maintain or improve mobility of the chest wall, trunk, and shoulder girdles when it affects ventilation or postural alignment. For example, a patient with hypomobility of the trunk muscles on one side of the body will not expand that part of the chest fully during inspiration. Exercises that combine stretching of these muscles with deep breathing improve ventilation on that side of the chest. Chest mobilization exercises are also used to reinforce or emphasize the depth of inspiration or controlled expiration. For example, a patient can improve expiration by leaning forward at the hips or flexing the spine as he or she breathes out. This pushes the viscera superiorly into the diaphragm and further reinforces expiration.

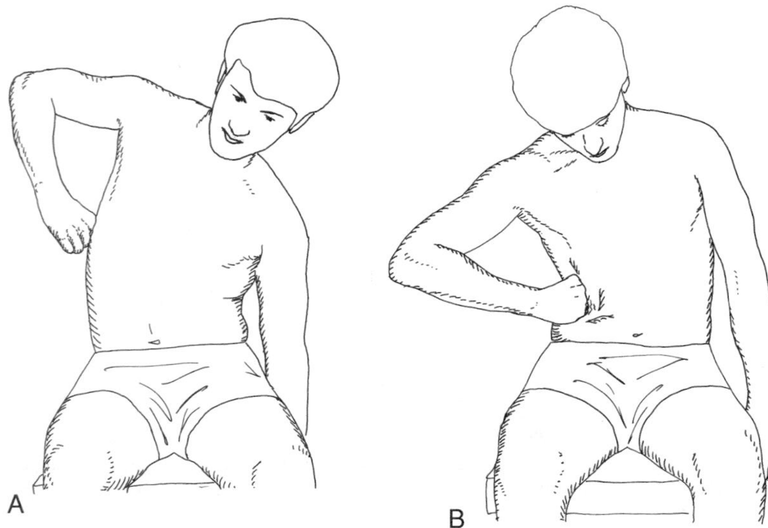

Figure 19–15 Chest mobilization during inspiration and expiration. To mobilize the lateral rib cage *(A)* have the patient bend away from the tight side during inspiration and *(B)* bend toward the tight side during expiration.

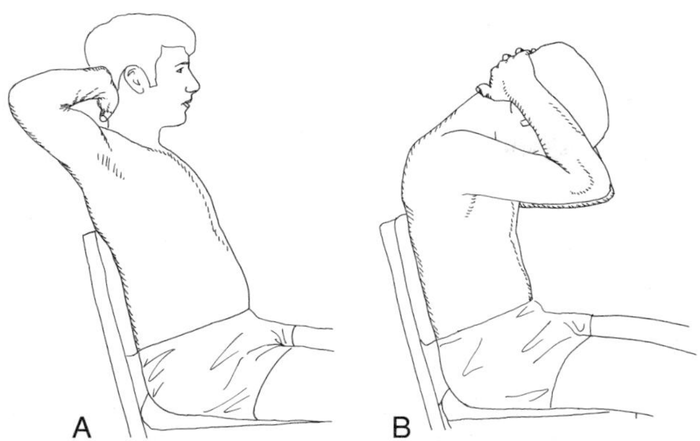

Figure 19–16 *(A)* A stretch is applied to the pectoralis muscles during inspiration, and *(B)* the patient brings the elbows together to facilitate expiration.

Specific Techniques

To Mobilize One Side of the Chest

- While sitting, have the patient bend away from the tight side to lengthen hypomobile structures and expand that side of the chest during inspiration (Fig. 19–15*A*).
- Then, have the patient push the fisted hand into the lateral aspect of the chest, as he or she bends toward the tight side and breathes out (Fig. 19–15*B*).
- Progress by having the patient raise the arm on the tight side of the chest over the head and side-bend away from the tight side. This will place an additional stretch on hypomobile tissues.

To Mobilize the Upper Chest and Stretch the Pectoralis Muscles

- While the patient is sitting in a chair with hands clasped behind the head, have him or her horizontally abduct the arms (elongating the pectoralis major) during a deep inspiration (Fig. 19–16*A*).
- Then, instruct the patient to bring the elbows together and bend forward during expiration (Fig. 19–16*B*).

To Mobilize the Upper Chest and Shoulders

With the patient sitting in a chair, have him or her reach with both arms overhead (180 degrees bilateral shoulder flexion and slight abduction) during inspiration (Fig. 19–17*A*). Then have the patient bend forward at the hips and reach for the floor during expiration (Fig. 19–17*B*).

Additional Activities

In addition to exercises specifically designed to mobilize the chest, the therapist may also instruct the patient in:

- Posture correction
- Manual stretching of the chest wall, trunk, and extremities

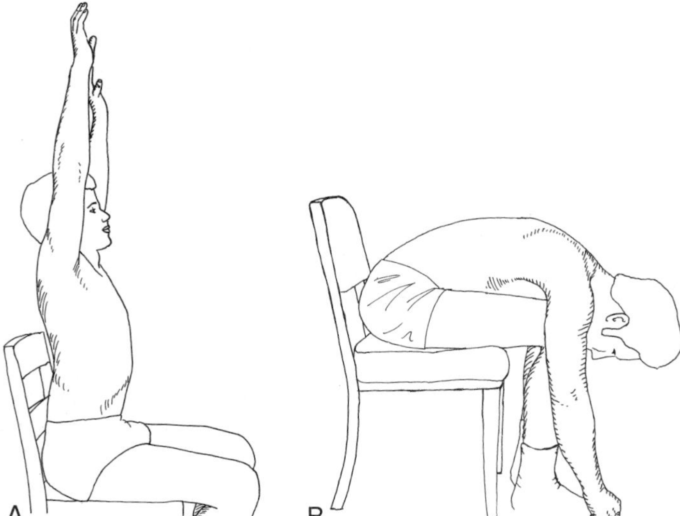

Figure 19–17 *(A)* Chest expansion is increased with bilateral movement of the arms overhead during inspiration. *(B)* Expiration is then reinforced by reaching the arms toward the floor.

Coughing

An effective cough is necessary to eliminate respiratory obstructions and keep the lungs clear. Airway clearance is an important part of management of patients with acute or chronic respiratory conditions.[23,42,47,56]

The Cough Mechanism

The following series of actions occur when a person coughs:[42]

- Deep inspiration occurs.
- Glottis closes and vocal cords tighten.
- Abdominal muscles contract and the diaphragm elevates, causing an increase in intrathoracic and intra-abdominal pressures.
- Glottis opens.
- Explosive expiration of air occurs.

The Normal Cough Pump

A cough may be reflexive or voluntary. In the normal individual, the cough pump is effective to the seventh generation of bronchi. (There are a total of 23 generations of bronchi in the tracheobronchial tree.) Ciliated epithelial cells are present up to the terminal bronchiole and raise secretions from the smaller to the larger airways in normal individuals.

Factors That Decrease the Effectiveness of the Cough Mechanism and Cough Pump

The effectiveness of the cough mechanism can be compromised for the following reasons:[23,34,47,56,69]

- ***Decreased inspiratory capacity because of***
  - Pain as a result of acute lung disease, rib fracture, trauma to the chest, or recent thoracic or abdominal surgery.
  - Specific muscle weakness that affects the diaphragm or accessory muscles of inspiration as a result of a high spinal cord injury or neuropathic or myopathic disease.
  - Depression of the respiratory center associated with general anesthesia or pain medication.
- ***Inability of the patient to forcibly expel air as the result of***
  - Spinal cord injury above T-12
  - Myopathic disease and weakness, such as muscular dystrophy
  - Tracheostomy
  - Critical illness that causes excessive fatigue
  - Chest wall or abdominal incision
- ***Decreased action of the cilia in the bronchial tree secondary to***
  - General anesthesia and intubation
  - COPD (chronic obstructive pulmonary disease), such as chronic bronchitis, which is associated with a decreased number of ciliated epithelial cells in the bronchi
  - Smoking
- ***Increase in the amount or thickness of mucus caused by***
  - Cystic fibrosis
  - Chronic bronchitis
  - Pulmonary infections, such as pneumonia
  - Dehydration
  - Intubation

Teaching an Effective Cough

Because an effective cough is an integral aspect of airway clearance, a patient must be taught the significance of an effective cough, how to produce an efficient and controlled voluntary cough, and when to cough. The following procedures are used when teaching an effective cough.[23,47,52,63]

1. Assess the patient's voluntary or reflexive cough.
2. Place the patient in a relaxed and comfortable position for deep breathing and coughing. Sitting or leaning forward is usually the best position for coughing. The patient's neck should be slightly flexed to make coughing more comfortable.
3. Teach the patient controlled diaphragmatic breathing, emphasizing deep inspirations.
4. Demonstrate a sharp, deep, double cough.
5. Demonstrate the proper muscle action of coughing (contraction of the abdominals). Have the patient place the hands on the abdomen and make three *huffs* with expiration to feel the contraction of the abdominals (see Fig. 19–8). Have the patient practice making a "K" sound to experience tightening the vocal cords, closing the glottis, and contracting the abdominals.
6. When the patient has put these actions together, instruct the patient to take a deep but relaxed inspiration, followed by a sharp double cough. The second cough during a single expiration is usually more productive.

7. Use an abdominal binder or glossopharyngeal breathing in selected patients with inspiratory or abdominal muscle weakness to enhance the cough, if necessary.

Precautions: When implementing coughing techniques:

- Never allow the patient to suck air in by gasping, because it increases the work (energy expenditure) of breathing and the patient fatigues more easily. It also tends to increase turbulence and resistance in the airways and may lead to increased bronchospasm (further constriction of airways). A gasping action may push mucus or a foreign object deep into air passages.
- Avoid uncontrolled coughing spasms *(paroxysmal coughing)*.
- Avoid forceful coughing with patients who have a history of a cerebrovascular accident or aneurysm. Have these patients *huff* several times to clear the airways, rather than cough.
- Be sure that the patient coughs while in a somewhat erect or, if necessary, a side-lying posture.

Additional Means of Facilitating a Cough

To maximize airway clearance, several techniques can be used to stimulate a stronger cough, make coughing more comfortable or improve the clearance of secretions.

Manual-Assisted Cough

If a patient has abdominal weakness (for instance, as the result of a midthoracic or cervical spinal cord injury), manual pressure on the abdominal area will assist in developing greater intra-abdominal pressure for a more forceful cough. Manual pressure for cough assistance can be applied by either the therapist or the patient.[3,23,34,47,63,69]

Therapist-Assisted Techniques

- With the patient in a supine or semi-reclining position, the therapist places the heel of one hand on the patient's abdomen at the epigastric area just distal to the xiphoid process. The other hand is placed on top of the first, either keeping the fingers open or interlocking them (Fig. 19–18). After the patient inhales as deeply as possible, the therapist manually assists the patient as he or she attempts to cough. The abdomen is compressed with an inward and upward force, which pushes the diaphragm upward to cause a more forceful and effective cough.

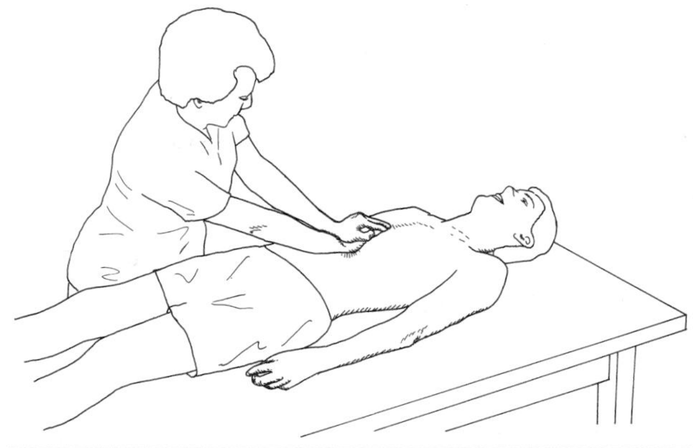

Figure 19–18 Therapist-assisted manual cough technique.

- This same maneuver can be performed with the patient in a chair (Fig. 19–19). The therapist or family member can stand in back of the patient and apply manual pressure during expiration.

Precaution: Avoid direct pressure on the xiphoid process during the maneuver.

Self-Assisted Technique (see Fig. 19–19)

- While the patient is in a sitting position, he or she crosses the arms across the abdomen or places the interlocked hands below the xiphoid process.

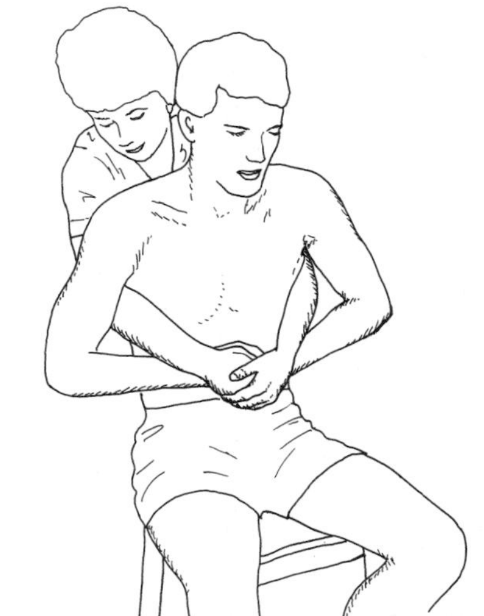

Figure 19–19 Therapist-assisted or self-assisted manual cough technique.

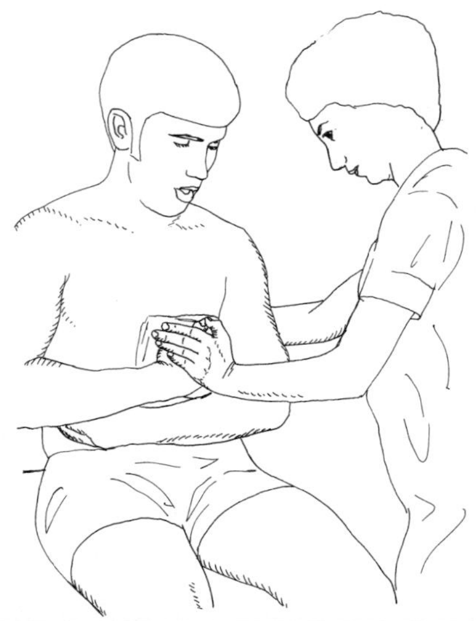

Figure 19–20 Splinting over an anterior surgical incision.

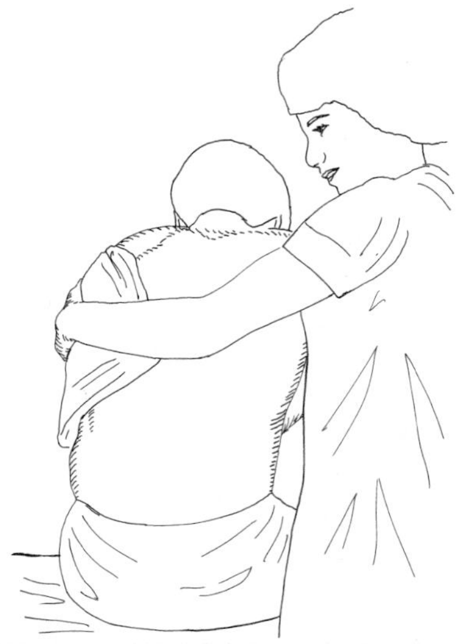

Figure 19–21 Splinting over a posterior lateral incision.

- After a deep inspiration, he or she pushes inward and upward on the abdomen with the wrists or forearms and simultaneously leans forward while attempting to cough.

Splinting

If chest wall pain from recent surgery or trauma is restricting the cough, teach the patient to splint over the painful area during coughing.[23,39,47] Have the patient press the hands or a pillow firmly over the incision to support the painful area as he or she coughs (Fig. 19–20). If the patient cannot reach the painful area, the therapist should assist (Fig. 19–21).

Humidification

If secretions are very thick, work with the patient after humidification therapy or ultrasonic nebulizer (USN) therapy, both of which enhance the mucociliary transport system and facilitate a productive cough.[63]

Tracheal Stimulation

Tracheal stimulation, sometimes called a *tracheal tickle,* may be used with infants or disoriented patients who cannot cooperate in the treatment.[63] This is a somewhat uncomfortable maneuver, performed to elicit a reflexive cough. The therapist places two fingers at the sternal notch and applies a circular motion with pressure downward into the trachea to facilitate a reflexive cough.

Suctioning: Alternative to Coughing

Endotracheal suctioning may be the only means of clearing the airways in patients who are unable to cough or huff voluntarily or after reflex stimulation of the cough mechanism.[56] Suctioning is indicated in all patients with artificial airways. The suctioning procedure clears only the trachea and the mainstem bronchi.

Precaution: Only individuals who have been instructed in proper suctioning technique should use this alternative means of clearing the airways. Suctioning, if performed incorrectly, can introduce an infection into the airways or damage the delicate mucosal lining of the trachea and bronchi. Improper suctioning can also cause hypoxemia, abnormal heart rates, and atelectasis. A complete description of proper endotracheal suctioning technique is described in another resource.[56]

▶ Postural Drainage

Postural drainage (bronchial drainage), another intervention for airway clearance, is a means of mobilizing secretions in one or more lung segments to the central airways by placing the patient in various positions so that gravity assists in the drainage process.[11,23,47,56] When secretions are moved to the larger airways, they are then cleared by coughing or endotracheal suctioning. *Postural drainage therapy* also includes the use of manual techniques, such as percussion, shaking, and vibration, as well as voluntary coughing. Box 19–5 lists the goals and indications for postual drainage.

Box 19–6 lists some relative contraindications to postural drainage. Despite the risks postural drainage still may be necessary in the unstable patient. Modified positioning to avoid a head-down or fully horizontal position is necessary for most high-risk patients.

Manual Techniques Used During Postural Drainage Therapy

In addition to the use of body positioning, deep breathing, and an effective cough to facilitate airway clearance, a variety of manual techniques are used in conjunction with postural drainage to maximize the effectiveness of the mucociliary transport system.[11,23,47,56,63,66] They include percussion, vibration, shaking, and rib springing. Findings from studies that have been implemented to evaluate the effectiveness of these manual techniques are inconsistent.[63]

Percussion

This airway clearance technique is used to further mobilize secretions by mechanically dislodging viscous or adherent mucus from the lungs. Percussion is performed with cupped hands (Fig. 19–22*A*) over the lung segment being drained. The therapist's cupped hands alternately strike the patient's chest wall in a rhythmic fashion (Fig. 19–22*B*). The therapist should try to keep shoulders, elbows, and wrists loose and mobile during the maneuver. Mechanical percussion is an alternative to manual percussion techniques. Percussion is continued for several minutes or until the patient needs to alter position to

Box 19–5 Goals of Postural Drainage

Prevent Accumulation of Secretions in Patients at Risk for Pulmonary Complications

- Patients with pulmonary diseases that are associated with increased production or viscosity of mucus, such as chronic bronchitis and cystic fibrosis
- Patients who are on prolonged bed rest
- Patients who have received general anesthesia and who may have painful incisions that restrict deep breathing and coughing postoperatively
- Any patient who is on a ventilator if he or she is stable enough to tolerate the treatment

Remove Accumulated Secretions from the Lungs

- Patients with acute or chronic lung disease, such as pneumonia, atelectasis, acute lung infections, and COPD
- Patients who are generally very weak or are elderly
- Patients with artificial airways

Box 19–6 Relative Contrandications to Postural Drainage

Severe Hemoptysis

Untreated Acute Conditions

- Severe pulmonary edema
- Congestive heart failure
- Large pleural effusion
- Pulmonary embolism
- Pneumothorax

Cardiovascular Instability

- Cardiac arrhythmia
- Severe hypertension or hypotension
- Recent myocardial infarction
- Unstable angina

Recent Neurosurgery

- Head-down positioning may cause increased intracranial pressure; if PD is required, modified positions can be used.

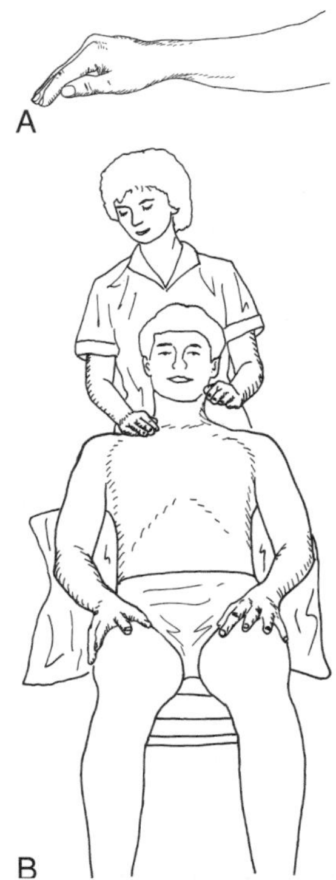

Figure 19–22 *(A)* Hand position for applying percussion. *(B)* The therapist alternately percusses over the lung segment being drained.

cough. This procedure should not be painful or uncomfortable. To prevent irritation to sensitive skin, have the patient wear a lightweight gown or shirt. Avoid percussion over breast tissue in women and over bony prominences.

Relative Contraindications to Percussion

Prior to implementing percussion in a postural drainage program, the therapist must compare the potential benefits with the possible risks to the patient. In most instances, avoid the use of percussion:

- Over fractures, spinal fusion, or osteoporotic bone
- Over tumor area
- If a patient has a pulmonary embolus
- If a patient has a condition in which hemorrhage could easily occur, such as in the presence of a low platelet count, or if a patient is receiving anticoagulation therapy
- If a patient has unstable angina
- If a patient has chest wall pain, for example, after thoracic surgery or trauma

Vibration

This airway clearance technique is used in conjunction with percussion in postural drainage. It is applied *only during expiration* as the patient is deep breathing to move the secretions to the larger airways.[23,47,66] Vibration is applied by placing both hands directly on the skin and over the chest wall (or one hand on top of the other) and gently compressing and rapidly vibrating the chest wall as the patient breathes out (Fig. 19–23). Pressure is applied in the same direction as that in which the chest is moving. The vibrating action is achieved by the therapist isometrically contracting (tensing) the muscles of the upper extremities from shoulders to hands.

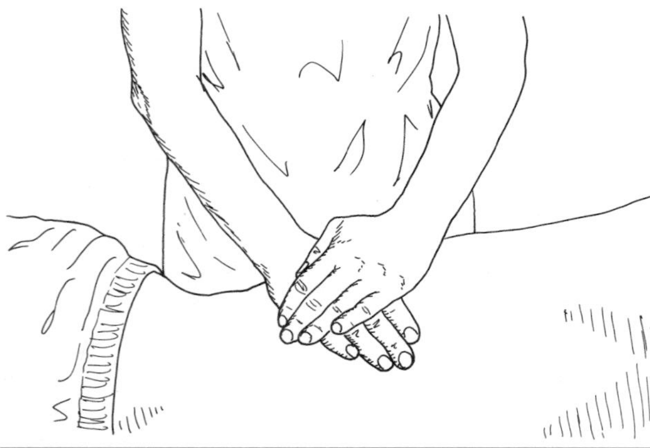

Figure 19–23 Hand placement for vibration during postural drainage.

Shaking

Shaking is a more vigorous form of vibration applied during exhalation using an intermittent bouncing maneuver coupled with wide movements of the therapist's hands. The therapist's thumbs are locked together, the open hands are placed directly on the patient's skin, and fingers are wrapped around the chest wall. The therapist simultaneously compresses and shakes the chest wall.[23,47,66]

Postural Drainage Positions

Positions are based on the anatomy of the lungs and the tracheobronchial tree (see Figs. 19–1 and 19–3). Each segment of each lobe is drained using the positions depicted in Figures 19–24 to 19–35. The shaded area in each illustration indicates the area of the chest wall where percussion or vibration is applied.

The patient may be positioned on a postural drainage table that can be elevated at one end, a tilt table, a reinforced padded table with a lift, or a hospital bed. A small child can be positioned on a therapist's or parent's lap.

Guidelines for Implementation of Postural Drainage

General Considerations

Time of day. Consider the following when scheduling postural drainage into a patient's day:

- Never administer postural drainage directly after a meal.
- Coordinate treatment with aerosol therapy. Some therapists feel that aerosol therapy combined with humidification prior to postural drainage will help loosen secretions and increase the likelihood of productivity. Others believe that aerosol therapy is best after postural drainage when the patient's lungs are clearer and maximal benefit can be gained from medication administered through aerosol therapy.
- Choose a time (or times) of day that will be of most benefit to the patient. A patient's cough

RIGHT AND LEFT UPPER LOBES

Anterior apical segments

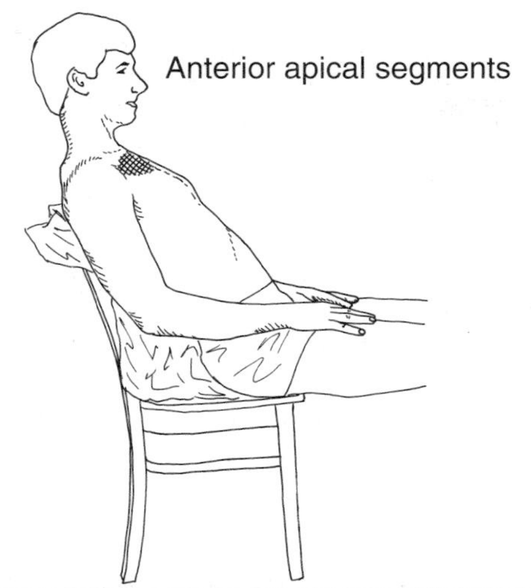

Figure 19–24 Percussion is applied directly under the clavicle.

Posterior apical segments

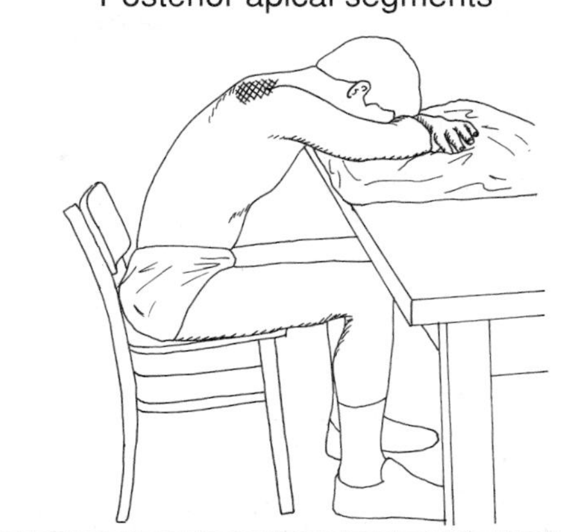

Figure 19–25 Percussion is applied above the scapulae. Your fingers curve over the top of the shoulders.

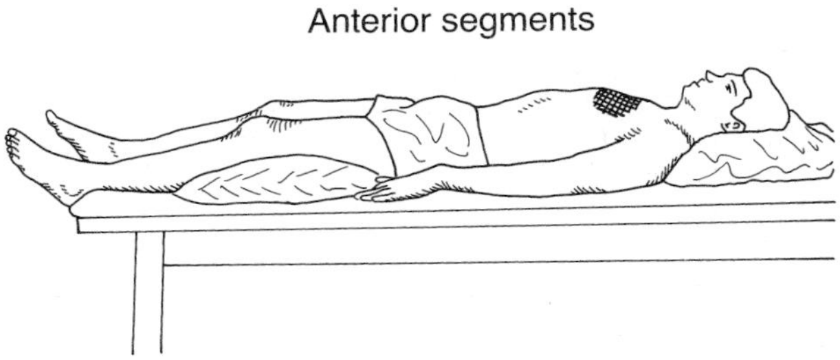

Anterior segments

Figure 19–26 Percussion is applied bilaterally, directly over the nipple or just above the breast.

Posterior segment
(left)
30° - 45°

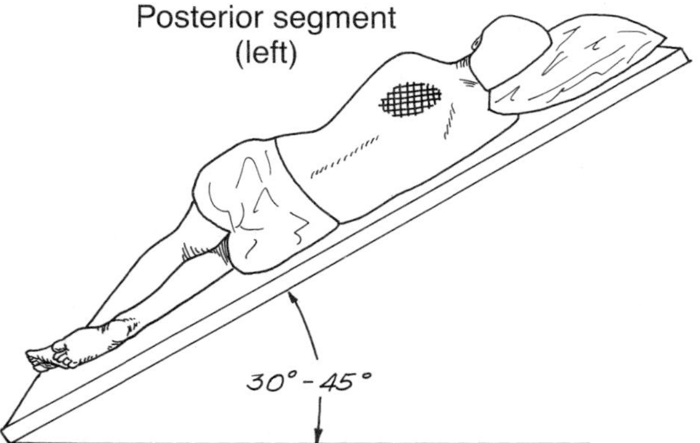

Figure 19–27 Patient lies one-quarter turn from prone and rests on the right side. Head and shoulders are elevated 45 degrees or approximately 18 inches if pillows are used. Percussion is applied directly over the left scapula.

Posterior segment
(right)

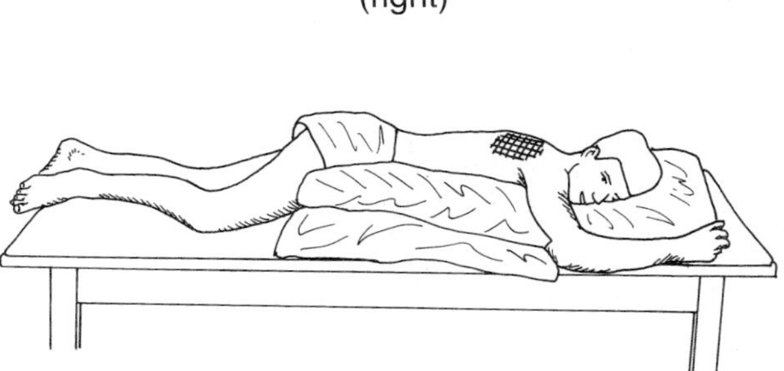

Figure 19–28 Patient lies flat and one-quarter turn from prone on the left side. Percussion is applied directly over the right scapula.

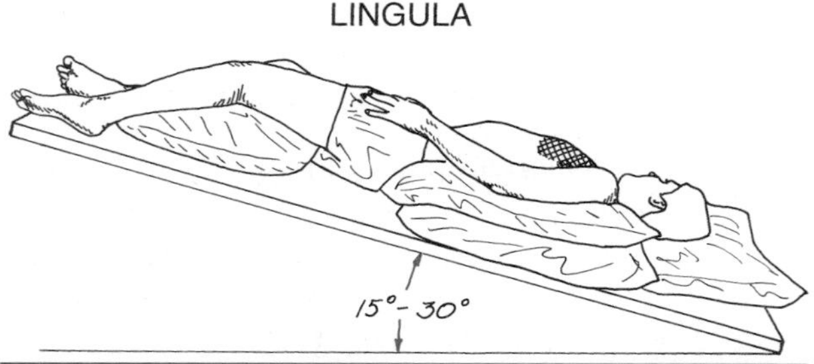

Figure 19–29 Patient lies one-quarter turn from supine on the right side, supported with pillows and in a 30-degree head-down position. Percussion is applied just under the left breast.

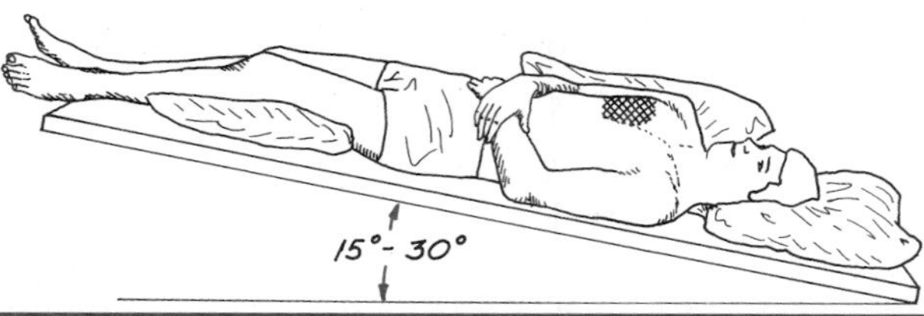

Figure 19–30 Patient lies one-quarter turn from supine on left side, supported with pillows behind the back, and in a 30-degree head-down position. Percussion is applied under the right breast.

RIGHT AND LEFT LOWER LOBES

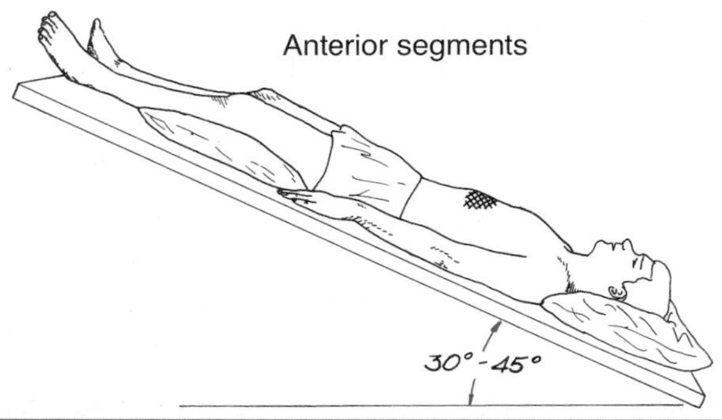

Figure 19–31 Patient lies supine, pillows under knees, in a 45-degree head-down position. Percussion is applied bilaterally over the lower portion of the ribs.

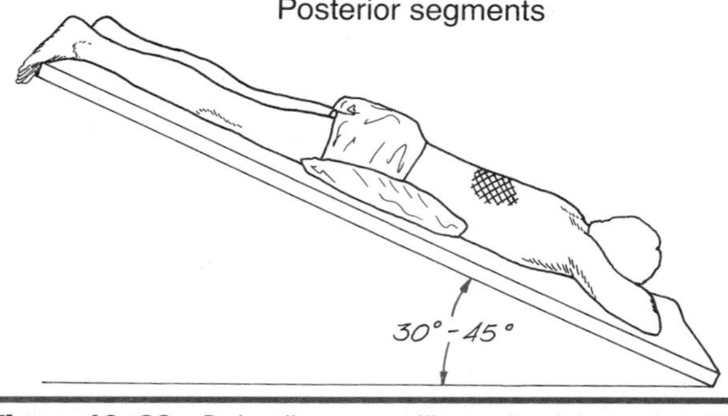

Figure 19–32 Patient lies prone, pillow under abdomen in a 45-degree head-down position. Percussion is applied bilaterally over the lower portion of the ribs.

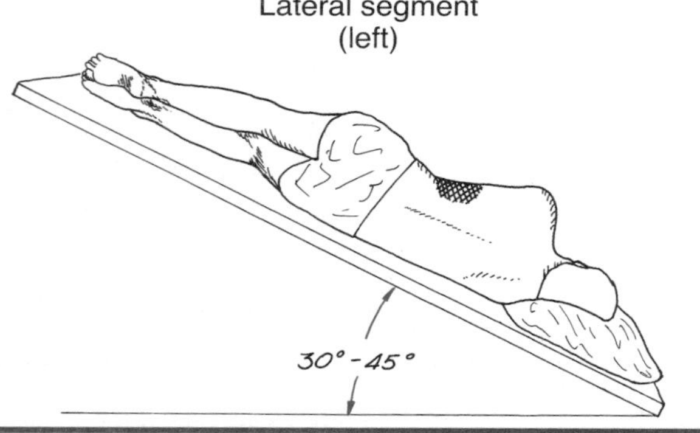

Figure 19–33 Patient lies on the right side in a 45-degree head-down position. Percussion is applied over the lower lateral aspect of the left rib cage.

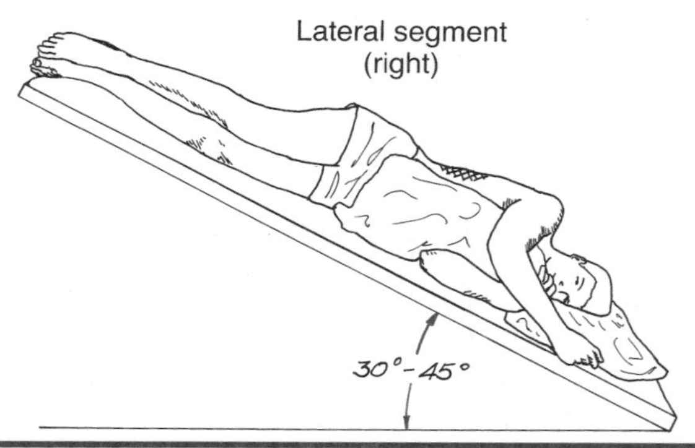

Figure 19–34 Patient lies on the left side in a 45-degree head-down position. Percussion is applied over the lower lateral aspect of the right rib cage.

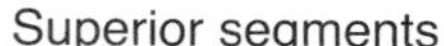

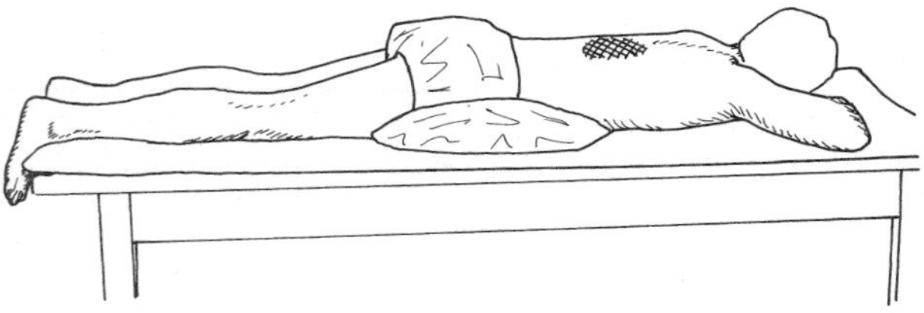

Figure 19–35 Patient lies prone, pillow under the abdomen to flatten the back. Percussion is applied bilaterally, directly below the scapulae.

tends to be very productive in the early morning because of accumulation of secretions from the night before. Postural drainage in the early evening will clear the lungs prior to sleeping and help the patient rest more easily.

Frequency of treatments. Frequency on a daily or weekly basis depends upon the pathology of the patient's condition. If secretions are thick and copious, two to four times per day is usually necessary until lungs are clear. If the patient is on a maintenance program, the frequency may be decreased.

Prepare the Patient

- Loosen tight or bulky clothing. It is not necessary to expose the skin. The patient may wear a lightweight shirt or gown.
- Have a sputum cup or tissues available.
- Have sufficient pillows for positioning and comfort.
- Explain the treatment procedure to the patient.
- Teach the patient deep breathing and an effective cough prior to beginning postural drainage.
- If the patient is producing copious amounts of sputum, instruct the patient to cough a few times or have the patient suctioned prior to positioning.
- Make any adjustments of tubes and wires, such as chest tubes, ECG wires, or catheters, so they remain clear during positioning.

Treatment Sequence

- Determine which segments of the lungs should be drained. Some patients with chronic lung diseases, such as cystic fibrosis, need to be drained in all positions. Other patients may require drainage of only a few segments in which secretions have accumulated.
- Check the patient's vital signs and breath sounds.
- Position the patient in the correct position for drainage. See that he or she is as comfortable and relaxed as possible.
- Stand in front of the patient, whenever possible, to observe his or her color.
- Maintain each position for 5 to 10 minutes if the patient can tolerate it, or as long as the position is productive.
- Have the patient breathe deeply in a relaxed manner during drainage, but do not allow the patient to hyperventilate or become short of breath.
- Apply percussion over the segment being drained while the patient is in the correct position.
- Encourage the patient to take a deep, sharp, double cough whenever necessary. It may be more comfortable for the patient to momentarily assume a semiupright position (resting on one elbow) and then cough.
- If the patient does not cough spontaneously during positioning with percussion, instruct the patient to take several deep breaths or huff several times in succession as you apply vibration during expiration. This may help elicit a cough.
- If the patient's cough is not productive after 5 to 10 minutes of positioning, go on to the next position. Secretions that have been mobilized during a treatment may not be coughed up by the patient until 30 minutes to 1 hour after treatment.
- The duration of any one treatment should not exceed 45 to 60 minutes, as the procedure is quite fatiguing for the patient.

Concluding the Treatment

- Have the patient sit up slowly and rest for a short while after the treatment. Watch for signs of postural hypotension when the patient rises from a supine position or from a head-down position to sitting.
- Advise the patient that, even if the cough was not productive during treatment, it may be productive a short while after treatment.
- Assess the effectiveness of the treatment by reassessing breath sounds.
- Note the type, color, consistency, and amount of secretions produced.
- Check the patient's vital signs after treatment, and note how the patient tolerated the treatment.

Criteria for Discontinuing Postural Drainage

- If chest x-ray is relatively clear
- If the patient is afebrile for 24 to 48 hours
- If normal or near-normal breath sounds are heard with auscultation
- If the patient is on a regular home program

Modified Postural Drainage

Some patients who require postural drainage cannot assume or cannot tolerate the positions that are optimal for treatment. For example, the patient with congestive heart failure may develop orthopnea (shortness of breath caused by lying flat). After neurosurgery a patient may not be allowed to assume a head-down (Trendelenburg) position because this position causes increased intracranial pressure. After thoracic surgery a patient may have chest tubes and monitoring wires that may limit positioning. Under these circumstances, as well as many others, positioning during postural drainage must be modified.[23,47,56,63] The positions in which postural drainage is undertaken are modified consistent with the patient's medical or surgical problems. This compromise, although not ideal, is better than not administering postural drainage at all.

Home Program of Postural Drainage

Postural drainage may have to be carried out on a regular basis at home for patients with chronic lung disease. Patients need to be shown how to position themselves using inexpensive aids. An adult may place pillows over a hard wedge or stacks of newspapers to achieve the desired head-down positions in bed. A patient may also lean the chest over the edge of the bed, resting with the arms on a chair or stool. A child may be positioned on an ironing board propped up against a couch. A family member should be instructed in positioning and percussion to assist the patient when needed. Guidelines and precautions, previously discussed, should be followed.

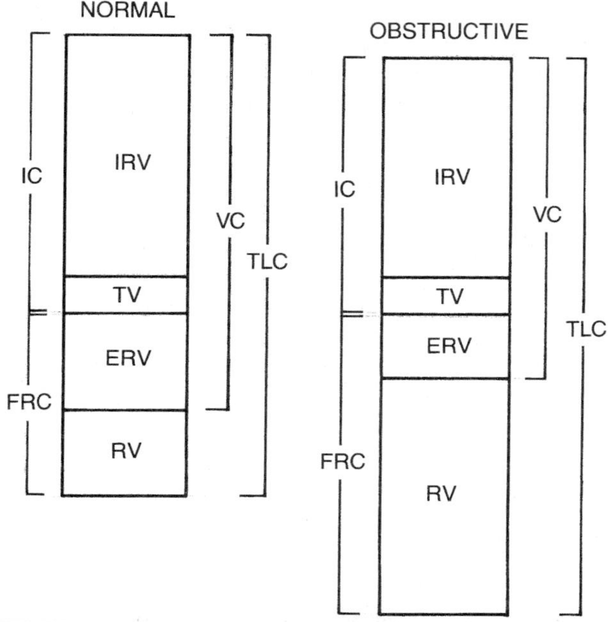

Figure 19–36 Normal lung volumes and capacities compared with abnormal lung volumes and capacities found in patients with obstructive pulmonary disease. (From Rothstein, J, Roy, A, and Wolf, SL: The Rehabilitation Specialist's Handbook. FA Davis, Philadelphia, 1991, p 604, with permission.)

▶ Management of Patients with Chronic Obstructive Pulmonary Disease

Chronic obstructive pulmonary disease (COPD) is a broad term that applies to a number of chronic conditions, all of which obstruct the flow of air in the conducting airways of the lower respiratory tract and alter ventilation and gas exchange.[6,25] A number of specific diseases can be classified as obstructive in nature. Each disease has its unique features and clinical manifestations and is distinguished by the cause of the obstruction of airflow, the onset of the disease, the location of the obstruction, and the reversibility of the obstruction.

Types of Obstructive Pulmonary Disorders

Typically, *peripheral airway disease, chronic bronchitis,* and *emphysema* are classified as COPD, but other obstructive pulmonary diseases that are chronic in nature, such as *asthma, bronchiectasis, cystic fibrosis,* and *bronchopulmonary dysplasia,* may also be included under this descriptor. The focus of discussion and management guidelines in this chapter is on chronic bronchitis and emphysema as patients with these diseases are commonly seen in pulmonary rehabilitation programs.[7]

The pathological changes that occur over time in COPD (specifically, chronic bronchitis and emphysema) are: inflammation of the mucus membranes of the airways; increased production and retention of mucus; narrowing and destruction of airways; and destruction of alveolar and bronchial walls.[6,25] These structural changes are reflected in pulmonary function tests depicted schematically in Figure 19–36. These changes in the patient's pulmonary status predispose the patient to frequent acute respiratory infections.

Impairments and Impact on Function

As a result of the pathophysiology of COPD, many physical impairments develop over time. Patients typically have a chronic, productive cough and are often short of breath. The characteristic impact of COPD on the pulmonary system is the inability to effectively remove air from the lungs, which, in turn, affects the ability of the respiratory system to transport oxygen into the lungs.

Box 19–7 Management Guidelines—Chronic Obstructive Pulmonary Disease (COPD)

Impairments:

An increase in the amount and viscosity of mucus production
A chronic, often productive cough
Frequent episodes of dyspnea
A labored breathing pattern that results in:

- Increased respiratory rate (tachypnea)
- Use of accessory muscles of inspiration and decreased diaphragmatic excursion
- Upper chest breathing

Inadequate exchange of air in the lower lobes
Most difficulty during expiration; use of pursed-lip breathing
Changes in pulmonary function

- Increased residual volume
- Decreased vital capacity
- Decreased expiratory flow rates

Decreased mobility of the chest wall; a barrel chest deformity develops
Abnormal posture: forward-head and rounded and elevated shoulders
Decreased general endurance during functional activities

Plan of Care	Interventions
1. Decrease the amount and viscosity of secretions and prevent respiratory infections.	1. Administration of bronchodialators, antibiotics, and humidification therapy. If patient smokes, he or she should be strongly encouraged to stop.
2. Remove or prevent the accumulation of secretions. (This is important if emphysema is associated with chronic bronchitis or if there is an acute respiratory infection.)	2. Deep and effective cough. Postural drainage to areas where secretions are identified. *Note:* Drainage positions may need to be modified if the patient is dyspneic in the head-down position.
3. Promote relaxation of the accessory muscles of inspiration to decrease reliance on upper chest breathing and to decrease muscle tension associated with dyspnea.	3. Positioning for relaxation. • Relaxed head-up position in bed: trunk, arms, and head are well supported. • Sitting: leaning forward, resting forearms on thighs or on a table. • Standing: leaning forward on an object, with hands on the thighs or leaning backwards against a wall. Relaxation exercises for shoulder musculature: active shoulder shrugging followed by relaxation; shoulder and arm circles; horizontal abduction and adduction of the shoulders.
4. Improve the patient's breathing pattern and ventilation. Emphasize diaphragmatic and lateral costal breathing and *relaxed* expiration; decrease the work of breathing, rate of respiration, and use of accessory muscles. Carry over controlled breathing exercises to functional activities.	4. Breathing exercises: controlled diaphragmatic breathing with minimal upper chest movement; lateral costal breathing; pursed-lip breathing (careful to *avoid forced* expiration); practice controlled breathing during standing, walking, climbing stairs, and other functional activities.
5. Minimize or prevent episodes of dyspnea.	5. Have a patient assume a comfortable position so the upper chest is relaxed and the lower chest is as mobile as possible. Emphasize controlled diaphragmatic breathing. Have the patient breathe out as rapidly as possible *without forcing* expiration. *Note:* Initially, the rate of ventilation will be rapid and shallow. As the patient gets control of breathing, he or she will slow down the rate. Administer supplemental oxygen in a severe episode, if needed.
6. Improve the mobility of the lower thorax.	6. Exercises for chest mobility, emphasizing movement of the lower rib cage during deep breathing.
7. Improve posture.	7. Exercises and postural training to decrease forward-head and rounded shoulders.
8. Increase exercise tolerance.	8. Graded endurance and conditioning exercises (see Chapter 4).

Consequently, functional limitations and eventually disability occur consistent with the disablement process.[37] Impairments such as decreased vital capacity and forced expiatory volume are associated with decreased tolerance to exercise, frequent episodes of dyspnea, decreased walking speed and distance, and eventual inability to perform activities of daily living at home or in the workplace or to remain an active participant in the community.

Management of COPD

Lifelong management includes appropriate medical management to lessen disabling symptoms and prevent infection, smoking cessation, and participation in a comprehensive pulmonary rehabilitation program.[7,11] Important aspects of management include ongoing airway clearance and participation in an individually designed exercise graded program.[7,11] Common impairments and guidelines for management are described in Box 19–7.

▶ Management of Patients with Restrictive Pulmonary Disorders

Restrictive pulmonary disorders are characterized by the inability of the lungs to fully expand as a result of extrapulmonary and/or pulmonary disease or restriction.[11,16] In other words, the patient has difficulty taking in a deep breath.

Acute and Chronic Causes of Restrictive Pulmonary Disorders

Pulmonary causes of restrictive disorders include:

- Diseases of the lung parenchyma such as *tumor, interstitial pulmonary fibrosis* (such as pneumonia, tuberculosis, and asbestosis) or *atelectasis*
- Disorders of cardiovascular/pulmonary origin, such as *pulmonary edema* or *pulmonary embolism*
- Inadequate or abnormal pulmonary development (hyaline membrane disease)
- Normal aging

Extrapulmonary sources of restrictive disorders include:

- Chest wall pain secondary to trauma or surgery
- Chest wall stiffness associated with extrapulmonary disease (such as scleraderma or ankylosing spondylitis)
- Postural deformities (scoliosis, kyphosis)
- Ventilatory muscle weakness of neuropathic or myopathic origin (such as spinal cord injury, cerebral palsy, Parkinson's disease, or muscular dystrophy)
- Pleural disease
- Insufficient diaphragmatic excursion because of ascites or obesity

Pathologic Changes in the Pulmonary System

As a result of these pulmonary or extrapulmonary conditions, a number of changes are reflected in pulmonary function tests. These alterations in lung volumes and capacities are depicted in Figure 19–37. Factors within the cardiopulmonary system that contribute to these changes are: decreased pulmonary compliance caused by inflammation or fibrosis (thickening of the alveoli, bronchioles, or pleura), pulmonary congestion, and decreased arterial blood gases (hypoxemia).

Management: Post-Thoracic Surgery

Although any number of acute or chronic disorders can be the underlying cause(s) of restrictive lung dysfunction, only one will be discussed in this section. Patients with cardiac or pulmonary conditions that require surgical interventions are at high risk for restrictive pulmonary complications after surgery. A

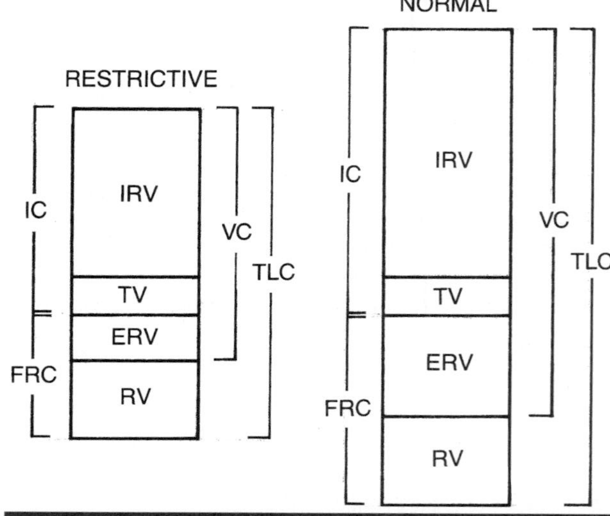

Figure 19–37 Normal lung volumes and capacities compared with abnormal lung volumes and capacities found in patients with restrictive pulmonary disorders. (From Rothstein, J, Roy, A, and Wolf, SL: The Rehabilitation Specialist's Handbook. FA Davis, Philadelphia, 1991, p 604, with permission)

thoracotomy, an incision into the chest wall, is necessary in many types of pulmonary surgery including *lobectomy* (removal of a lobe of a lung), *pneumonectomy* (removal of a lung), or *segmental resection* (removal of a segment of a lobe of a lung).[16,21,31,35]

Cardiac surgeries, such as coronary artery bypass graft surgery, replacement of one or more valves of the heart, repair of septal defects, or heart transplantation also require a thoracotomy.[16,21,31,35]

Note: Patients who undergo upper abdominal surgery also have a high risk of developing postoperative pulmonary complications. Postoperative pain is often greater after upper abdominal surgery than after thoracic surgery.[67] This results in hypoventilation (vital capacity is decreased 55% for the first 24 or 48 hours after surgery) and an ineffective cough, which place the patient at risk for developing pneumonia or atelectasis.[16,35] A postoperative program of cardiopulmonary physical therapy has been shown to be beneficial for these patients.[67]

Factors That Increase the Risk of Pulmonary Complications and Restrictive Lung Dysfunction After Pulmonary or Cardiac Surgery

The patient post-thoracotomy experiences considerable chest pain, which leads to chest wall immobility, poor lung expansion, and an ineffective cough. Pulmonary secretions also tend to be greater than normal postoperatively. Therefore, the patient is more likely to accumulate pulmonary secretions and develop secondary pneumonia or atelectasis. The factors that increase the risk of postoperative pulmonary complications are:[16,35]

General Anesthesia

- Decreases the normal ciliary action of the tracheobronchial tree
- Depresses the respiratory center of the central nervous system, which causes a shallow respiratory pattern (decreased tidal volume and vital capacity)
- Depresses the cough reflex

Intubation (Insertion of an Endotracheal Tube)

- Causes muscle spasm and immobility of the chest
- Irritates the mucosal lining of the tracheobronchial tree, which causes an increase in production of mucus
- Decreases the normal action of the cilia in the tracheobronchial tree, which leads to pooling of secretions

Incisional Pain

- Causes muscle splinting and decreases chest wall compliance, which, in turn, causes a shallow breathing pattern. Consequently, lung expansion is restricted and secretions are not adequately mobilized.
- Restricts a deep and effective cough. The patient usually has a weak, shallow cough that does not effectively mobilize and clear secretions.

Pain Medication

Although pain medication administered postoperatively tends to diminish incisional pain, it also:

- Depresses the respiratory center of the central nervous system
- Decreases the normal ciliary action in the bronchial tree

General Inactivity Postoperatively

- Causes secretions to pool, particularly in the posterior basilar segments of the lower lobes.

General Weakness and Fatigue

- Decreases the effectiveness of the cough pump
- Decreases postoperative functional mobility

Other Risk Factors Not Directly Related to the Surgery

- The patient's age (over age 50)
- History of smoking
- History of COPD or restrictive pulmonary disorder because of neuromuscular weakness

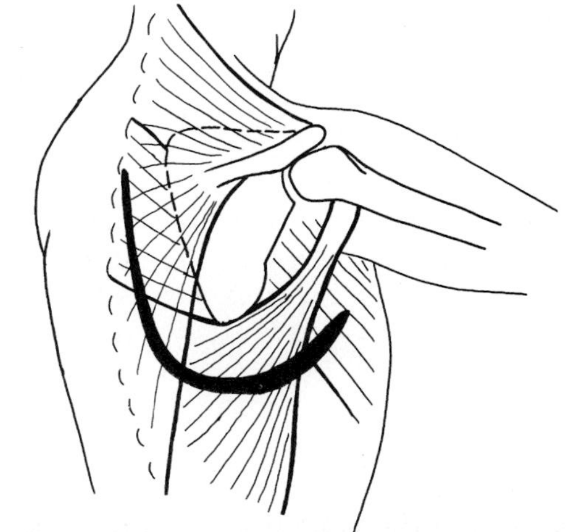

Figure 19–38 A posterolateral approach commonly used in thoracic surgery incises and divides the trapezius, rhomboids, latissimus dorsi, serratus anterior, and internal and external intercostal muscles.

Box 19–8 Management Guidelines: Post-Thoracic Surgery

Impairments:

Reduced lung expansion or an inability to take a deep inspiration because of incisional pain
Decreased effectiveness of the cough because of incisional pain and irritation of the throat from intubation
Possible accumulation of pulmonary secretions either preoperatively or postoperatively
Decreased chest wall and upper extremity mobility
Poor postural alignment because of incisional pain or chest tubes
Increased risk of deep vein thrombosis and pulmonary embolism
General weakness, fatigue, and disorientation

Plan of Care	Interventions
1. Ascertain the status of the patient before each treatment.	1. Evaluate orientation, color, respiratory rate, heart rate, breath sounds, sputum drainage into chest tubes.
2. Promote relaxation and reduce postoperative pain.	2. Position the patient in a semi-Fowler's position (head of bed elevated to 30 degrees and hips and knees slightly flexed). This position reduces traction on the thoracic incision. Coordinate treatment with administration of pain medication.
3. Optimize ventilation and re-expand lung tissue to prevent atelectasis and pneumonia.	3. Begin deep-breathing exercises on the day of surgery as soon as patient is conscious; diaphragmatic breathing; segmental expansion. Add incentive spirometry or inspiratory resistance exercises to improve inspiratory capacity. Emphasize a deep inhalation followed by a 3- to 5-second hold and then a relaxed exhalation. Continue deep-breathing exercises postoperatively, with six to ten consecutive deep breaths per hour until the patient is ambulatory.
4. Assist in the removal of secretions.	4. Begin deep, effective coughing as soon as the patient is alert and can cooperate. Implement early functional mobility (getting up to a chair, early ambulation). Institute modified postural drainage only if secretions accumulate.
5. Maintain adequate circulation in the lower extremities to prevent deep vein thrombosis and pulmonary embolism.	5. Begin active exercises of the lower extremities, with emphasis on ankle pumping exercises on the first day after surgery. Continue leg exercises until the patient is allowed out of bed and is ambulatory.
6. Regain ROM in the shoulders.	6. Begin relaxation exercises for the shoulder area on the first postoperative day. These can include shoulder shrugging or shoulder circles. Initiate active-assistive ROM of the shoulders, being careful not to cause pain. Reassure the patient that gentle movements will not disturb the incision. Progress to active shoulder exercises on the succeeding postoperative days to the patient's tolerance until full active ROM has been achieved.
7. Prevent postural impairments.	7. Reinforce symmetric alignment and positioning of the trunk on the first postoperative day when the patient is in bed *Note:* The patient will tend to lean toward the side of the incision. Instruct the patient in symmetric sitting posture when he or she is allowed to sit up in a chair or at the side of the bed.
8. Increase exercise tolerance.	8. Begin a progressive and graded ambulation or stationary cycling program as soon as the chest tubes are removed and the patient is allowed to be out of bed.

Precautions:

- Monitor vital signs throughout treatment.
- Be certain to show the patient how to splint over the incision to minimize incisional pain during coughing.
- Avoid placing traction on chest tubes when moving the patient.
- To prevent dislodging a chest tube for the patient who has a lateral incision, limit shoulder flexion to 90 degrees on the operated side for several days until the chest tube is removed.
- If postural drainage must be implemented, modify positioning to avoid a head-down position.
- Do not use percussion over the incision.
- When turning a patient, use a logroll technique to minimize traction on the incision.

- Obesity
- Poor mentation and orientation

Thoracic Surgery: Postoperative Considerations

Many factors contribute to a patient's postoperative impairments, any one of which has an impact on postoperative management.[16,21] The patient who has undergone a thoracotomy for a pulmonary or cardiac condition is hospitalized for approximately 1 week or less. In addition to the primary pulmonary or cardiac pathology, such as a malignant tumor, lung abscess, or coronary artery disease, the patient may also have related cardiopulmonary problems such as angina, congestive heart disease, chronic bronchitis, or emphysema. The patient with a long history of cardiac disease may also have preoperative pulmonary conditions such as hypoxemia, dyspnea on exertion, orthopnea, or pulmonary congestion. If this is the case, postoperative rehabilitation may be longer and more complicated.

Most patients undergoing pulmonary surgery will have a large posterolateral, lateral, or anterolateral chest incision. A standard posterolateral approach (Fig. 19–38), for example, is performed by incising the chest wall along the intercostal space that corresponds to the location of the lung lesion. The incision divides the trapezius and rhomboid muscles posteriorly and the serratus anterior, latissimus dorsi, and external and internal intercostals laterally.

Postoperatively the incision is painful, and the potential for pulmonary complications is significant. Many patients, quite understandably, complain of a great deal of shoulder soreness on the operated side. Loss of range of shoulder motion and postural deviations are possible because of the disturbance of the large arm and trunk musculature during surgery.

The most common incision used with cardiac surgery is a *median sternotomy.* A large incision extends along the anterior chest from the sternal notch to just below the xiphoid. The sternum is then split and retracted so that the chest cavity can be exposed. After completion of the surgical procedure, the sternum is closed with stainless steel sutures. Postoperatively there is actually less incisional pain after a median sternotomy than after a posterolateral thoracotomy, but deep breathing and coughing are still painful. After a median sternotomy, a patient tends to exhibit rounded shoulders and is at risk for developing shortened pectoralis muscles bilaterally.

After a thoracotomy or median sternotomy, one or two chest drainage tubes are put in place at the time of the surgery to prevent a *pneumothorax* or a *hemothorax*. While these tubes are in place, crimping, clamping, or traction on the tubes must be avoided during postoperative interventions.

The patient will fatigue easily in the first few postoperative days, so treatment sessions should be short but frequent. The duration and intensity of treatment should be slowly and gradually increased during the patient's hospital stay.

Check the patient's chart regularly to note any day-to-day changes in vital signs and laboratory test results. Always monitor vital signs such as heart rate and rhythm, respiratory rate, and blood pressure, prior to, during, and after every treatment session.

Typical postoperative impairments and guidelines for management of the patient who has undergone thoracic surgery are summarized in Box 19–8.[15,16,20,35,36,65]

Independent Learning Activities

CRITICAL THINKING AND DISCUSSION

1. Describe the structure of the lower respiratory tract from trachea to the alveoli, and discuss the impact of pulmonary diseases on those structures and their functions.
2. Describe the thorax and its movements during ventilation and the actions of the primary and accessory muscles of ventilation.
3. Organize a presentation that compares and contrasts the characteristics and management of obstructive and restrictive pulmonary disorders.
4. What factors contribute to placing the post-thoracic surgery patient at risk for the development of postoperative complications?
5. Under what circumstances (types of impairment or pathology) would it be appropriate to try to change a patient's breathing pattern? For what purpose?
6. Analyze how ventilation and coughing are affected by a spinal cord injury at a midthoracic level, a C-6 level, and a C-3 to C-4 level.

LABORATORY PRACTICE

1. Perform a systematic physical examination of a patient with a 5-year history of chronic bronchitis who has been referred to your outpatient facility to begin a graded conditioning program.

2. How would you alter or change the focus of your examination of a patient with a traumatic brain injury who is on a ventilator or a patient who is 1 day post-coronary artery bypass graft surgery?
3. Practice auscultation of breath sounds.
4. Practice a complete postural drainage sequence on your laboratory partner. Include manual techniques and cough instruction. Perform the activity for a minimum of 1 to 2 minutes per position to begin to appreciate the endurance needed by the therapist. Then have your partner perform the same sequence with you as the patient to appreciate how it feels from the patient's perspective to undergo postural drainage.
5. What methods of measurement should be used to document improvement in a pulmonary patient's condition as the result of a pulmonary rehabilitation program? Practice those techniques.

CASE STUDY

Case 1

TM is a 62-year-old man who underwent thoracic surgery (a RLL lobectomy) yesterday for bronchogenic carcinoma. He has a posterolateral incision. Although his cough is currently nonproductive, he has had a chronic cough for years. He has also smoked more than a pack a day for 35 years. He is currently febrile with a 99.8 degree temperature.

- What current and potential postoperative impairments might you find in your examination?
- Design a comprehensive management program that includes airway clearance, exercise, and functional mobility. How would you progress the program while the patient is hospitalized? What precautions should be built into his plan of care?
- Design a program that the patient can follow when he returns home.

Case 2

BA is a 21-year-old student with a 15-year history of asthma. Her chief complaint is episodes of dyspnea when she is physically active. She wheezes frequently, particularly with physical activity but sometimes at rest. Wheezing also is worse when in contact with household pets at friends' apartments. She is small for her age and underweight, but wants to participate in some form of regular physical activity for general health and fitness. What additional signs or symptoms would you expect to find in an examination of this young woman? How would you manage her problems and needs?

REFERENCES

1. Aldrich, T: The application of muscle endurance training to the respiratory muscles in COPD. Lung 163:15, 1985.
2. Aldrich, T, and Karpel, J: Inspiratory muscle resistive training in respiratory failure. Am Rev Respir Dis 131:461, 1985.
3. Alvarez, SE, Peterson, M, and Lunsford, BA: Respiratory treatment of the adult patient with spinal cord injury. Phys Ther 61:1737, 1981.
4. American Association of Respiratory Care: AARC clinical practice guidelines: Postural drainage therapy. Respir Care 36:1418, 1991.
5. American College of Chest Physicians and the American Thoracic Society Joint Committee on Pulmonary Nomenclature: Pulmonary terms and symbols. Chest 67:583, 1975.
6. American Thoracic Society: Standards for the diagnosis and care of patients with chronic obstructive pulmonary disease (COPD) and asthma. Am Rev Respir Dis 136:225, 1987.
7. Barr, RN: Pulmonary rehabilitation. In Hillegass, EA, and Sadowsky, HS (eds): Essentials of Cardiopulmonary Physical Therapy, ed 2. WB Saunders, Philadelphia, 2001, p 727.
8. Baskin, MW: Respiratory care practice overview. In Frownfelter, D, and Dean, E (eds): Principles and Practice of Cardiopulmonary Physical Therapy, ed 3. CV Mosby, St. Louis, 1996, p 749.
9. Basmajian, JV, and DeLuca, CJ: Muscles Alive, ed 5. Williams & Wilkins, Baltimore, 1985.
10. Berger, AJ: Control of breathing. In Murray, JF, and Nadel, JA (eds): Textbook of Respiratory Medicine, Vol 1, ed 2. WB Saunders, Philadelphia, 1994, p 199.
11. Brannon, FJ, et al: Cardiopulmonary Rehabilitation: Basic Theory and Application, ed 2. FA Davis, Philadelphia, 1993.
12. Butler, SM: Clinical assessment of the cardiopulmonary system. In Frownfelter, D, and Dean, E (eds): Principles and Practices of Cardiopulmonary Physical Therapy, ed 3. CV Mosby, St Louis, 1996, p 209.
13. Cahalin, LP, Semigran, MJ, and Dec, GW: Inspiratory muscle training in patients with chronic heart failure awaiting cardiac transplantation: Results of a pilot clinical trial. Phys Ther 77:830, 1997.
14. Casiari, RJ, et al: Effects of breathing retraining in patients with chronic obstructive pulmonary disease. Chest 79:393, 1981.
15. Ciesla, ND: Chest physical therapy for patients in the intensive care unit. Phys Ther 76:609, 1996.
16. Clough, P: Restrictive lung dysfuntion. In Hillegass, EA, and Sadowsky, HS (eds): Essentials of Cardiopulmonary Physical Therapy, ed 3. WB Saunders, Philadelphia, 2001, p 183.

17. Crane, LD: The chest examination. Phys Ther Health Care 1:11, 1987.
18. Crowe, JM, and Bradley, CA: The effectiveness of incentive spirometry with physical therapy for high-risk patients after coronary artery bypass surgery. Phys Ther 77:260, 1997.
19. Dean, E: Mobilization and exercise. In Frownfelter, D, and Dean, E (eds): Principles and Practice of Cardiopulmonary Physical Therapy, ed 3. CV Mosby, St Louis, 1996, p 265.
20. Dean, E, and Hobson, L: Cardiopulmonary physiology. In Frownfelter, D, and Dean, E (eds): Principles and Practice of Cardiopulmonary Physical Therapy, ed 3. CV Mosby, St Louis, 1996, p 53.
21. Dean, E, and Mathews, M: Acute surgical conditions. In Frownfelter, D, and Dean, E (eds): Principles and Practice of Cardiopulmonary Physical Therapy, ed 3. CV Mosby, St Louis, 1996, p 495.
22. Derrickson, J, et al: A comparison of two breathing exercise programs for patients with quadriplegia. Phys Ther 72: 763–769, 1992.
23. Downs, AM: Clinical application of airway clearance techniques. In Frownfelter, D, and Dean, E (eds): Principles and Practice of Cardiopulmonary Physical Therapy, ed 3. CV Mosby, St Louis, 1996, p 339.
24. Frownfelter, D: Pulmonary function tests. In Frownfelter, D, and Dean, E (eds): Principles and Practice of Cardiopulmonary Physical Therapy, ed 3. CV Mosby, St Louis, 1996, p 145.
25. Goodman, CC: The respiratory system. In Goodman, CC, and Boissonnault, WG (eds): Pathology: Implications for the Physical Therapist. WB Saunders, Philadelphia, 1998, p 399.
26. Goodman, CC, and Snyder, TEK: Differential Diagnosis in Physical Therapy, ed 3. WB Saunders, Philadelphia, 2000.
27. Gosselink, R, et al: Respiratory muscle weakness and respiratory muscle training in severly disabled multiple sclerosis patients. Arch Phys Med Rehabil 81:747, 2000.
28. Gross, D: The effect of training on strength and endurance of the diaphragm in quadriplegia. Am J Med 68:27, 1980.
29. Guyton, A, and Hall, JE: Human Physiology and Mechanisms of Disease, ed 6. WB Saunders, Philadelphia, 1997.
30. Hillegass, EA: Assessment procedures. In Hillegass, EA, and Sadowsky, HS (eds): Essentials of Cardiopulmonary Physical Therapy, ed 2. WB Saunders, Philadelphia, 2001, p 610.
31. Hillegass, EA, and Sadowsky, HS: Cardiovascular and thoracic interventions. In Hillegass, EA, and Sadowski, HS (eds): Essentials of Cardiopulmonary Physical Therapy, ed 2. WB Saunders, Philadelphia, 2001, p 452.
32. Hughes, RC: Does abdominal breathing affect regional gas exchange? Chest 76:258, 1979.
33. Humberstone, N, and Tecklin, JS: Respiratory evaluation: Respiratory assessment and respiratory treatment. In Irwin, S, and Tecklin, J: Cardiopulmonary Physical Therapy, ed 3. Mosby-Year Book, St Louis, 1995, p 334.
34. Imle, PC: Physical therapy and respiratory care for the patient with acute spinal cord injury. Phys Ther Health Care 1:45, 1987.
35. Imle, PC: Physical therapy for patients with cardiac, thoracic or abdominal conditions following surgery or trauma. In Irwin, S, and Tecklin, JS (eds): Cardiopulmonary Physical Therapy, ed 3. CV Mosby, St Louis, 1995, p 375.
36. Jenkins, SC, et al: Physiotherapy after coronary artery surgery. Are breathing exercises necessary? Thorax 44:634, 1989.
37. Jette, DU, et al: The disablement process in patients with pulmonary disease. Phys Ther 77:385, 1997.
38. Kigin, CM: Breathing exercises for the medical patient: The art and the science. Phys Ther 70:700, 1990.
39. Kigin, CM: Chest physical therapy for the postoperative or traumatic injury patient. Phys Ther 61:1724, 1981.
40. Lane, C: Inspiratory muscle weight training and its effect on vital capacity of patients with quadriplegia. Cardiopulmonary Quarterly 2:13, 1982.
41. Leith, D, and Bradley, M: Ventilatory muscle strength and endurance training. J Appl Physiol 41:508, 1976.
42. Leith, DE: Cough. Phys Ther 48:439, 1968.
43. Levangie, PK, and Norkin, CC: Joint Structure and Function: A Comprehensive Analysis, ed 3. FA Davis, Philadelphia, 2001.
44. Levenson, CR: Breathing exercises. In Zadai, CC (ed): Pulmonary Management in Physical Therapy. Churchill Livingstone, New York, 1992.
45. Liaw, MY, et al: Resistive inspiratory training: Its effectiveness in patients with acute complete cervical cord injury. Arch Phys Med Rehabil 81:752, 2000.
46. Martin, D, and Yountsey, J: Respiratory Anatomy and Physiology. CV Mosby, St Louis, 1988.
47. Massery, M, and Frownfelter, D: Facilitating airway clearance with coughing techniques. In Frownfelter, D, and Dean, E (eds): Principles and Practice of Cardiopulmonary Physical Therapy, ed 3. CV Mosby, St Louis, 1996, p 367.
48. Massery, M, and Frownfelter, D: Facilitating ventilatory patterns and breathing strategies. In Frownfelter, D, and Dean, E (eds): Principles and Practice of Cardiopulmonary Physical Therapy, ed 3. CV Mosby, St Louis, 1996, p 383.
49. Merrick, J, and Axen, K: Inspiratory muscle function following abdominal weight exercise in healthy subjects. Phys Ther 61:651, 1981.
50. Metcalf, VA: Vital capacity and glossopharyngeal breathing in traumatic quadriplegia. Phys Ther 46:835, 1966.
51. Reid, WD, and Dechman, G: Considerations when testing and training the respiratory muscles. Phys Ther 75:971, 1995.
52. Reinisch, E: Functional approach to chest physical therapy. Phys Ther 58:972, 1978.
53. Rutchnik, A, et al: Resistive inspiratory muscle training in subjects with chronic cervical spinal cord injury. Arch Phys Med Rehabil 79:293, 1998.
54. Sackner, MA, et al: Distribution of ventilation during diaphragmatic breathing in obstructive lung disease. Am Rev Respir Dis 109:331, 1974.
55. Sadowsky, HS: Cardiovascular and respiratory physiology. In Hillegass, EA, and Sadowsky, HS (eds): Essentials of Cardiopulmonary Physical Therapy, ed 2. WB Saunders, Philadelphia, 2001, p 48.
56. Sciaky, A, Stockford, J, and Nixon, E: Treatment of acute cardiopulmonary conditions. In Hillegass, EA, and Sadowsky, HS (eds): Essentials of Cardiopulmonary Physical Therapy, ed 2. WB Saunders, Phildelphia, 2001, p 647.
57. Shaffer, TH, Wolfson, MR, and Gault, JH: Respiratory physiology. In Irwin, S, and Tecklin, JS (eds): Cardiopulmonary Physical Therapy, ed 3. CV Mosby, St Louis, 1995, p 237.
58. Shearer, MC, et al: Lung ventilation during diaphragmatic breathing. Phys Ther 52:139, 1972.
59. Sheckleton, M, Berry, JK, and Covey, MK: Respiratory muscle weakness and training. In Frownfelter, D, and Dean, E (eds):

Principles and Practice of Cardiopulmonary Physical Therapy, ed 3. CV Mosby, St Louis, 1996, p 443.

60. Smakowski, PS: Ventilatory muscle training. Part I: The effectiveness of endurance training on rodent diaphragm. A scientific review of the literature from 1972–1991. Cardiopulmonary Physical Therapy Journal 4:2, 1993.
61. Sobush, DC: Breathing exercises: Laying a foundation for a clinical practice guideline. Cardiopulmonary Physical Therapy Journal 3:8, 1992.
62. Sonne, L, and Davis, J: Increased exercise performance in patients with severe: COPD following inspiratory resistive training. Chest 81:436, 1982.
63. Starr, JA: Manual techniques of chest physical therapy and airway clearance techniques. In: Zadai, CC (ed): Pulmonary Management in Physical Therapy. Churchill-Livingstone, New York, 1992.
64. Staub, NC, and Albertine, KH: Anatomy of the lungs. In Murray, JF, and Nabel, JA (eds): Textbook of Respiratory Medicine, Vol 1, ed 2. WB Saunders, Philadelphia, 1994, p 3.
65. Stiller, K, et al: Efficacy of breathing and coughing exercises in the prevention of pulmonary complications after coronary artery surgery. Chest 105:741, 1994.
66. Sutton, P, et al: Assessment of percussion vibratory shaking and breathing exercises in chest physiotherapy. Eur J Respir Dis 66:147, 1985.
67. Thomas, JA, and McIntosh, JM: Are incentive spirometry, intermittent positive pressure breathing and deep breathing exercises effective in the prevention of postoperative pulmonary complicaitons after upper abdominal surgery? A systematic overview and meta-analysis. Phys Ther 74:3, 1994.
68. Uijl, S, et al: Training of the respiratory muscles in individuals with tetraplegia. Spinal Cord 37:575, 1999.
69. Wetzel, J, et al: Respiratory rehabilitation of the patient with spinal cord injury. In Irwin, S, and Tecklin, J (eds): Cardiopulmonary Physical Therapy, ed 3. Mosby-Year Book, St Louis, 1995, p 579.
70. Wilkins, RL, et al: Lung sound nomenclature survey. Chest 98: 886, 1990.
71. Zadai, CC: Comprehensive physical therapy evaluation: Identifying potential pulmonary complications. In Zadai, CC (ed): Pulmonary Management in Physical Therapy. Churchill Livingstone, New York, 1992.
72. Zadai, CC: Physical therapy for the acutely ill medical patient. Phys Ther 61:1716, 1981.

Appendix A

Systematic Musculoskeletal Examination Guidelines

An examination consists of three primary parts: history, systems review, and tests and measures.[1] Details of the history and systems review are described in Chapter 1. Once the history and systems review are complete and determination is made to continue with a musculoskeletal examination, tests are systematically administered in order to define the impairments in terms of which tissues may be interfering with function, identify the resulting functional limitations, and establish a baseline of objective measurements from which progress can be measured.

Note: The following information is a suggested sequence for examining a patient with impairments in the musculoskeletal system, along with an explanation of various testing procedures that may be used to establish a diagnosis related to impairments. Specific tests are not described; they are determined by the area being examined and are beyond the scope of this text. All appropriate tests are performed with the patient in one position before moving him or her to another position. Common sequencing of the examination begins with the patient standing, then sitting, then lying down (supine, side-lying on one side, prone, and then side-lying on the other side).

▶ History

For a discussion on the history, see Chapter 1 and Box 1–8. Information generated from the initial history is summarized in Box A–1 at the end of this appendix.

▶ Systems Review

For a discussion on the systems review, see Chapter 1 and Table 1–1. An outline of the content of a systems review is summarized in Box A–2 at the end of this appendix.

▶ Tests and Measures

The following outline of the sequence of tests and measures is summarized in Box A–3 at the end of this appendix.

Note: Any tests that were conducted in the systems review are not repeated unless additional clarification is necessary.

Inspection

Observe appearance and basic abilities. Suggestions include the following.

Adaptive or Supportive Aids

Note use of braces, splints, or assistive devices.

Posture

Observe general posture and specific posture or shape of involved body parts such as contour changes, swelling, atrophy, hypertrophy, and asymmetry.

Transitional Activities (Supine-Sit-Stand) and Gait Patterns

Look at general ease of movement, coordination, balance, and ability to maneuver in preparation for the examination. From these observations and the results of the diagnostic testing, more detailed tests can be chosen for documentation of functional limitations, disabilities.

Tests of Provocation (Selective Tension)

Use the principle of selective tension by administering specific tests in a systematic manner to provoke or re-create the symptoms and to minimize or alleviate the symptoms described by the patient during the history. Systematically perform the tests in order to determine whether the lesion is within an inert structure (joint capsules, ligaments, bursae, fasciae, dura mater, and dural sheaths around nerve roots) or a contractile unit (muscle with its tendons and attachments).[2] Include joint integrity tests to verify problems within the joint.[3] From these tests, it is possible to identify the forces or stresses that cause or alleviate the patient's symptoms, the stage of healing, and in many cases, the tissue or tissues causing the symptoms; that is, identify the impairments(s).

From this information as well as the results of other special tests[5] and functional tests (described later) attempt to identify a relationship between the tissue impairments and the patient's functional losses. Minimizing and controlling the identified stresses on the involved tissues along with developing or modifying functional activities that can be performed safely form the foundation in designing an appropriate therapeutic exercise program.

1. **Active range of motion (ROM).** Ask the patient to move the body parts related to the symptoms through their ROM. From the way the patient moves and the amount of motion exhibited, determine if the patient is able and willing to move the part. Because both contractile and inert structures are influenced by active motion, specific impairments are not isolated. Note anything abnormal in the movement pattern, any experience of pain, or any changes in sensation.

2. **Passive ROM.** Repeat the same movements passively; when the end of the available range is reached, apply pressure to get a feel of the resistance of the tissues; the pressure is called **overpressure,** and the feel is called **end-feel.** With the muscles relaxed, only inert structures are being stressed. Note whether any of the tests provoke or alleviate the patient's symptoms.
   - Measure the ROM and compare it with the active ROM. Determine whether the limitation follows a pattern of restriction typical for that joint when joint problems exist. These are called **capsular patterns**[2,5] and are described for each peripheral joint under the respective sections on joint problems in Chapters 9 through 14.
   - Describe the **end-feel,** the feel that is experienced at the end of the range when overpressure is applied. Decide whether the feel is:
     - *Soft*—related to compressing or stretching soft tissues.
     - *Firm*—related to stretching joint capsules and ligaments.
     - *Hard*—related to a bony block.
     - *Empty*—no end-feel is detected because the patient will not allow movement to the end of the available range—related to an acutely painful condition in which the patient inhibits motion.
   - Decide if the end-feel is normal or abnormal for that joint. Abnormal end-feels include:
     - *Springy*—intra-articular block such as a torn meniscus or articular cartilage.
     - *Muscle guarding*—involuntary muscle contraction in response to acute pain.
     - *Muscle spasm*—prolonged muscle contraction in response to circulatory and metabolic changes.
     - *Muscle spasticity*—increased tone and contraction in muscle in response to central nervous system influences.
     - Any end-feel that is *different from normal* for that joint or at *a different part of the range* from normal for the joint being tested.
   - Determine the **stage of pathology** by observing when pain is experienced relative to the ROM. Is the pain or muscle guarding experienced before the end-feel *(acute),* concurrent with the end-feel *(subacute),* or after application of overpressure *(chronic)?*
   - Note whether there is a **painful arc,** which is pain experienced with either active or passive motion somewhere within the ROM. It indicates that some sensitive structure is being pinched during that part of the range. Sometimes pain-sensitive structures are pinched at the end of the range. This is not a painful arc, although such pain should be noted.

3. **Special joint tests**
   - Apply ligament stress tests and special tests for labral and meniscus tears based on joint anatomy.

- Apply joint play (accessory motion) tests to confirm or rule out joint involvement. Glide, distract and compress the joint surfaces together to see if there is reproduction of symptoms, alleviation of symptoms, or restricted or excessive motion. Note quality and quantity of joint play. These tests are passive tests used to rule out or confirm articular or capsular impairments. They are performed prior to testing for muscle lesions[3] since muscle contraction causes compression and shear forces on the joints,[4] and therefore pain with muscle contraction could give a false positive for contractile lesions.
- Determine the state of hypo- versus hyper mobility.

4. **Resisted tests.** Resist the related muscles so that they contract isometrically in midrange to determine whether there is pain or decreased strength in the contractile units. Midrange isometric contractions are used so that there is minimal movement or stress to the noncontractile structures around the joint. Initially perform the tests on groups of muscles; then, if pain or weakness is noted, isolate and test each muscle that is potentially involved. Decide if there is a problem in the neuromuscular system. Possible choices include:

- A *strong, yet painful* contraction indicates a contractile unit problem (assuming joint problems have been ruled out). Palpate along the entire musculotendinous unit to identify the site of injury.
- A *weak and painless* contraction may suggest a complete muscle tear, a disused muscle, or a neurologic problem.
  - A muscle tear will have a history of trauma or forceful muscle contraction in the region.
  - A disused muscle will usually demonstrate some atrophy and probably not be localized in only one muscle.
  - A neurologic problem will usually have a pattern of sensory loss, as well as weakness in related muscles following a pattern consistent with a nerve root, plexus, or peripheral nerve innervation.
- A *weak and painful* contraction usually suggests something serious, such as an active lesion, fracture, or inflammation. Relate this finding to information from the history.
- Document strength with a manual muscle test, tensiometer or dynamometer test grade. Relate strength to functional limitations.

5. **Other tests of muscle performance.** Look at other factors influencing muscle function such as endurance, coordination, stabilizing function, and flexibility (including flexibility of two-joint or multi-joint muscles).

Palpation

Palpate, if possible, the structures that are incriminated as the source of the impairments. Usually palpation is best done after the tests of provocation in order not to increase the irritability of the structures prior to testing, but some therapists prefer to palpate earlier in the sequence of testing or in conjunction with the tests of provocation. Palpation can be a confirming test in identifying anatomic structures involved if the tissue that was symptomatic under the selective tension stresses is also symptomatic when palpated. Include:

Skin and Subcutaneous Tissue

Note temperature, edema, texture, and mobility.

Muscles, Tendons, and Attachments

Note tone, tenderness, trigger points, tension, and swelling.

Tendon Sheaths and Bursae

Note tenderness, texture, crepitus, and mobility.

Joints and Ligaments

Note effusion, tenderness, changes in position or shape, synovial hypertrophy.

Nerves and Blood Vessels

Note tenderness, change in sensation, neuroma, and pulse.

Neurologic Tests

If there are any signs of muscle weakness or change in sensation, perform specific tests to determine nerve, nerve root, or central nervous system involvement. Examine:

Key Muscles

Determine strength and reflexes of muscles related to specific spinal levels and peripheral nerve patterns. Strength tests will have already been performed in the provocation tests; interpretation of the results based on nerve patterns is considered here for organizational purposes.

Motor Ability

Identify any control, balance, or coordination deficits. Identify abnormal associated reactions, synergies, synkinesis, or postural righting and protective reflexes if indicated.

Sensory Perception

Identify changes in perception of temperature, light touch, deep pressure, two-point discrimination, stereognosis, and proprioception. Relate loss to peripheral nerve or spinal cord patterns or to central nervous system control. If there is central nervous system impairments, test for body awareness of limbs and trunk, spatial awareness, and perception of vertical alignment.

Nerve Mobility

Determine whether there are symptoms with stretching or when applying pressure on the peripheral nerves, nerve trunks, or nerve roots.

Cranial Nerve Integrity

Test the cranial nerves if indicated.

Functional Performance Tests

Use standardized and consistently measured tests that focus on the patient's impairments and described limitations. In addition to information gained from self-reports from the patient or from functional limitations described in the history include examination of the patient's abilities when performing specific functional activities. Suggestions include:

Gait Performance

Observe ability to walk on even and uneven surfaces, change directions, speed, distance, and need for assistive devices.

Functional Mobility Performance

Observe ability to climb and descend steps, step over objects, rise up from a chair and sit down, move in and out of a motor vehicle, or other needed activities.

Body Mechanics and Related Abilities

Observe ability to lunge, squat, kneel, and bend over. Observe ability to lift objects of various sizes and weights from various heights and with various techniques.

Upper Extremity Functional Performance

Observe ability to reach, push, pull, grip, and carry objects of various sizes and weights.

Agility and Skill

Observe ability to hop, jump, catch, and throw. Observe eye-hand coordination and ability to manipulate objects with various prehension patterns.

Additional Tests

Cardiovascular/Pulmonary Endurance

Determine level of fitness.

Special Tests

Administer tests unique to specific tissues or functions that have not yet been described.

Adaptability to Environment

Identify barriers, safety, ability for self care and mobility in the home, job, school, and recreational facilities.

Tests by Other Professionals

Determine if additional medical or other health professional testing should be done to clarify the patient's condition, to receive care beyond the scope of physical therapy, or to receive care by a therapist in an area of specialty other than yours.

Box A–1 Information Generated from the Initial History

Demographic Data
- Age, sex, race, ethnicity
- Primary language
- Education

Social History
- Family and caregiver resources
- Cultural background
- Social interactions/support systems

Occupation/Leisure
- Current and previous employment Job/school-related activities
- Recreational, community activities/tasks

Growth and Development
- Developmental history
- Hand and foot dominance

Living Environment
- Current living environment
- Expected destination after discharge
- Community accessibility

General Health Status & Lifestyle Habits and Behaviors: Past/Present (based on self or family report)
- Perception of health/disability
- Lifestyle health risks (smoking, substance abuse, diet, exercise, sleep habits)

Medical/Surgical/Psychological History

Medications: current and past

Family History
- Health risk factors
- Family illnesses

Cognitive/Social/Emotional Status
- Orientation, memory
- Communication
- Social/emotional interactions

Current Conditions/Chief Complaints/Concerns
- Conditions, reasons PT services sought
- Patient's perceived level of disability
- Patient's needs, goals
- History, onset (date and course), mechanism of injury, pattern and behavior of symptoms
- Family or caregiver needs, goals, perception of patient's problems
- Current or past therapeutic interventions
- Previous outcome of chief complaint(s)

Functional Status and Activity Level
- Current/prior functional status: basic ADL, IADL related to self-care and home
- Current/prior functional status in work, school, community-related IADL

Other Laboratory and Diagnostic Tests

Box A–2 Areas of Screening for the Systems Review

Cardiovascular/Pulmonary
- Heart rate, respiratory rate and blood pressure
- Pain or heaviness in the chest or pulsating pain
- Light headedness; peripheral edema

Integumentary
- Skin temperature, color, texture
- Skin integrity
- Scars, lumps, growths

Musculoskeletal
- Height, weight
- Symmetry
- Gross ROM and strength

Neuromuscular
- General aspects of motor control (balance, locomotion, coordination)
- Sensation, changes in hearing or vision; severe headaches

Gastrointestinal/Genitourinary
- Heartburn, diarrhea, vomiting, severe abdominal pain
- Problems with swallowing
- Problems with bladder function
- Unusual menstrual cycles, pregnancy

Cognitive and Social/Emotional
- Communication abilities (expressive and receptive)
- Cognition, affect
- Level of arousal, orientation, ability to follow directions or learn
- Behavioral/emotional stressors and responses

General/Miscellaneous
- Persistent fatigue, malaise
- Unexplained weight gain or loss
- Fever, chills, sweats

Box A–3 Systematic Musculoskeletal Examination

1. History (see Box A–1)
2. Systems review (see Box A–2)
3. Tests and Measures

Inspection
- Use of adaptive or supportive aids
- Posture
- Transitional activities and gait

Tests of Provocation (Selective Tension)
- Active ROM
- Passive ROM
- Special joint tests
- Resisted tests
- Other tests of muscle performance

Palpation
- Skin and subcutaneous tissue
- Muscles, tendons, and attachments
- Tendon sheaths and bursae
- Joints and ligaments
- Nerves and blood vessels

Neurologic Tests
- Key muscles
- Motor ability
- Sensory perception
- Nerve mobility
- Cranial nerve integrity

Functional Performance Tests
- Gait performance
- Functional mobility performance
- Body mechanics and related abilities
- Upper extremity functional performance
- Agility and skill

Additional Tests
- Cardiovascular endurance
- Special tests
- Adaptability to environment
- Tests by other professionals

REFERENCES

1. American Physical Therapy Association: A Description of patient/client management in: Guide to Physical Therapist Practice, ed 2. Phys Ther 81 (1):39, 2001.
2. Cyriax, J: Textbook of Orthopaedic Medicine, Vol 1. Diagnosis of Soft Tissue Lesions, ed 8. Bailliere and Tindall, London, 1982.
3. Kaltenborn, FM: Manual Mobilization of the Joints: The Kaltenborn Method of Joint Examination and Treatment, Vol 1. The Extremities, ed 5. Olaf Norlis Bokhandel, Oslo, Norway, 1999.
4. Levangie, PK and Norkin, CC: Muscle structure and function, in: Joint Structure and Function A Comprehensive Analysis, ed 3. FA Davis, Philadelphia, 2001, pp 84-112.
5. Magee, DJ: Orthopedic Physical Assessment, ed 3. WB Saunders, Philadelphia, 1997.

Appendix B

Management Guidelines

The development and progression of therapeutic interventions using therapeutic exercise are the main focuses of this text. To lay a foundation, general management guidelines for various stages of tissue repair and pathologic conditions were described in several chapters of this text. The boxes that summarize the guidelines are reproduced in this appendix for easy reference.

In Chapter 4, principles of aerobic training programs are described. Guidelines are summarized in the following boxes.

Box 4–11 General Guidelines for an Aerobic Training Program

- Establish the target heart rate and maximum heart rate.
- Warm up gradually for 5 to 10 minutes. Include stretching and repetitive motions at slow speeds, gradually increasing the effort.
- Increase the pace of the activity so that the target heart rate can be maintained for 20 to 30 minutes. Examples include fast walking, running, bicycling, swimming, cross-country skiing, and aerobic dancing.
- Cool down for 5 to 10 minutes with slow, total body repetitive motions and stretching activities.
- The aerobic activity should be three to five times per week.
- To avoid injuries from stress, use appropriate equipment, such as correct footwear, for proper biomechanical support. Avoid running, jogging, or aerobic dancing on hard surfaces such as asphalt and concrete.
- To avoid overuse syndromes to structures of the musculoskeletal system, proper warm-up and stretching of muscles to be used should be performed. Progression of activities should be within the tolerance of the individual. Overuse commonly occurs when there is an increase in time or effort without adequate rest (recovery) time between sessions. Increase repetitions or time by no more than 10% per week. If pain begins while exercising, or lasts longer than 4 hours after exercising, heed the warning and reduce the stress.
- Individualize the program of exercise. All people are not at the same fitness level and therefore cannot perform the same exercises. Any one exercise has the potential to be detrimental if attempted by someone not able to execute it properly. During recovery following an injury or surgery choose an exercise that will not stress the vulnerable tissue. Begin at a safe level for the individual and progress as the individual meets the desired goals.

Box 4–13 Guidelines for Initiating an Aerobic Exercise Program for the Deconditioned Individual and Patient with Chronic Illness

- Determine the exercise heart rate response that can be safely reached using the Karvonen formula as a guide, accounting for medical conditions, medications and the individuals perceived exertion.
- Initiate a program of activities for the patient that will not elicit a cardiovascular response over the exercise heart rate (e.g., walking, repetitive activities, easy calisthenics).
- Provide the patient with clearly written instructions about any activity they perform on their own.
- Initiate an educational program that provides the patient with information about effort symptoms and exercise precautions, monitoring of heart rate, and modification when indicated.

Box 4–14 Guidelines for Progression of an Aerobic Training Program

- Determine the maximum heart rate or symptom-limited heart rate by multistage testing with ECG monitoring.
- Decide on the threshold stimulus (percentage of maximum or symptom-limited heart rate) that will elicit a conditioning response for the individual tested and that will be used as the exercise heart rate.
- Determine the intensity, duration, and frequency of exercise that will result in attainment of the exercise heart rate and a conditioning response.
- Determine the mode of exercise to be used based on the individual's physical capabilities and interest.
- Initiate an exercise program with the patient and provide clearly written instructions regarding the details of the program.
- Educate the patient about:
  - Effort symptoms and the need to cease or modify exercise when these symptoms appear and to communicate with the physical therapist and/or physician about these problems.
  - Monitoring heart rate at rest as well as during and following exercise.
  - The importance of exercising within the guidelines provided by the physical therapist.
  - The importance of consistent long-term follow-up about the exercise program so that it can be progressed within safe limits.
  - The importance of modifying risk factors related to cardiac problems.

Chapter 8 is the key chapter in which principles for treating various conditions is discussed. Management guidelines are summarized in the following boxes. Treatment interventions described in Chapters 9 through 14 make reference to these boxes.

Box 8–1 Management Guidelines—Acute Stage/Protection Phase

Impairments:

Inflammation, pain, edema, muscle spasm
Impaired movement
Joint effusion (if the joint is injured or if there is arthritis)
Decreased use of associated areas

Plan of Care	Intervention (up to 1 week postinjury)
1. Educate the patient.	1. Inform patient of anticipated recovery time and how to protect the part while maintaining appropriate functional activities.
2. Control pain, edema, spasm.	2. Cold, compression, elevation, massage (48 hours). Immobilize the part (rest, splint, tape, cast). Avoid positions of stress to the part. Gentle (grade I) joint oscillations with joint in pain-free position.
3. Maintain soft tissue and joint integrity and mobility.	3. Appropriate dosage of passive movements within limit of pain, specific to structure involved. Appropriate dosage of intermittent muscle setting or electrical stimulation.
4. Reduce joint swelling if symptoms are present.	4. May require medical intervention if swelling is rapid (blood). Provide protection (splint, cast).
5. Maintain integrity and function of associated areas.	5. Active-assistive, free, resistive, and/or modified aerobic exercises, depending on proximity to associated areas and effect on the primary lesion. Adaptive or assistive devices as needed to protect the part during functional activities.

Precautions: The proper dosage of rest and movement must be used during the inflammatory stage. Signs of too much movement are increased pain or increased inflammation.

Contraindications: Stretching and resistance exercises should not be performed at the site of the inflamed tissue.[71]

Box 8–2 Management Guidelines—Subacute Stage/Controlled Motion Phase

Impairments:

- Pain when end of available ROM is reached
- Decreasing soft tissue edema
- Decreasing joint effusion (if joints are involved)
- Developing soft tissue, muscle, and/or joint contractures
- Developing muscle weakness from reduced usage
- Decreased functional use of the part and associated areas

Plan of Care	Intervention (up to 3 weeks postinjury)
1. Educate the patient.	1. Inform patient of anticipated healing time and importance of following guidelines. Teach home exercises and encourage functional activities consistent with plan; monitor and modify as patient progresses.
2. Promote healing of injured tissues.	2. Monitor response of tissue to exercise progression; decrease intensity if inflammation increases. Protect healing tissue with assistive devices, splints, tape, or wrap; progressively increase amount of time the joint is free to move each day and decrease use of assistive device as strength in supporting muscles increases.
3. Restore soft tissue, muscle, and/or joint mobility.	3. Progress from passive to active-assistive to active ROM within limits of pain. Gradually increase mobility of scar, specific to structure involved. Progressively increase mobility of related structures if they are tight; use techniques specific to tight structure.
4. Develop neuromuscular control, muscle endurance, and strength in involved and related muscles.	4. Initially, progress multiple-angle isometric exercises within patient's tolerance; begin cautiously with mild resistance. Initiate AROM and protected closed-chain stabilization exercises. As ROM, joint play, and healing improve, progress isotonic exercises with increased repetitions. Emphasize control and proper mechanics. Progress resistance later in this stage.
5. Maintain integrity and function of associated areas.	5. Apply progressive strengthening and stabilizing exercises, monitoring effect on the primary lesion. Resume low-intensity functional activities involving the healing tissue that do not exacerbate the symptoms.

Precautions: The signs of inflammation or joint swelling normally decrease early in this stage. Some discomfort will occur as the activity level is progressed, but it should not last longer than a couple of hours. Signs of too much motion or activity are resting pain, fatigue, increased weakness, and spasm.[71]

Box 8–4 Management Guidelines—Chronic Stage/Return to Function Phase

Impairments:

Soft-tissue and/or joint contractures and adhesions that limit normal ROM or joint play
Decreased muscle performance: weakness, poor endurance, poor neuromuscular control
Decreased functional usage of the involved part
Inability to function normally in an expected activity

Plan of Care	Interventions (>3 weeks postinjury)
1. Educate the patient.	1. Instruct patient in safe progressions of exercises and stretching. Monitor understanding and compliance. Teach ways to avoid reinjuring the part. Teach safe body mechanics. Provide ergonomic counseling.
2. Increase soft tissue, muscle and/or joint mobility.	2. Stretching techniques specific to tight tissue: • Joint and selected ligaments (joint mobilization). • Ligaments, tendons and soft tissue adhesions (cross-fiber massage). • Muscles (neuromuscular inhibition, passive stretch, massage, and flexibility exercises).
3. Improve neuromuscular control, strength, muscle endurance.	3. Progress exercises: • Submaximal to maximal resistance. • Specificity of exercise using resisted concentric and eccentric, open- and closed-chain. • Single plane to multiplane motions. • Simple to complex motions, emphasizing movements that simulate functional activities. • Controlled proximal stability, superimpose distal motion. • Safe biomechanics. • Increase time at slow speed; progress complexity and time; progress speed and time.
4. Improve cardiovascular endurance.	4. Progress aerobic exercises using safe activities.
5. Progress functional activities.	5. Continue using supportive and/or assistive devices until the ROM is functional with joint play, and strength in supporting musclesis adequate. Progress functional training with simulated activities from protected and controlled to unprotected and variable. Continue progressive strengthening exercises and advanced training activities until the muscles are strong enough and able to respond to the required functional demands.

Precautions: There should be no signs of inflammation. Some discomfort will occur as the activity level is progressed, but it should not last longer than a couple of hours. Signs that activities are progressing too quickly or with too great a dosage are joint swelling, pain that lasts longer than 4 hours or that requires medication for relief, a decrease in strength, or fatiguing more easily.[71]

Box 8–5 Management Guidelines—Chronic Inflammation/Cumulative Trauma Syndromes

Impairments:

Pain in the involved tissue of varying degrees:[53]

- Only after doing repetitive activities
- When doing repetitive activities as well as after
- When attempting to do activities; completion of demands prevented
- Continued and unremitting

Soft-tissue, muscle, and/or joint contractures or adhesions that limit normal ROM or joint play

Muscle weakness and poor muscular endurance in postural or stabilizing muscles as well as primary muscle at fault

Imbalance in length and strength between antagonistic muscles; biomechanical dysfunction

Decreased functional use of the region

Faulty position or movement pattern perpetuating the problem

Plan of Care	Interventions During Chronic Inflammation
1. Educate the patient.	1. Counsel as to cause of chronic irritation and need to avoid stressing the part while inflamed. Adapt the environment to decrease tissue stress. Home exercise program to reinforce therapeutic interventions.
2. Promote healing; decrease pain and inflammation.	2. Cold, compression, massage. Rest to the part (stop mechanical stress, splint, tape, cast).
3. Maintain integrity and mobility of involved tissue.	3. Nonstressful passive movement, massage, and muscle setting within limits of pain.
4. Develop support in related regions.	4. Posture training. Stabilization exercises.

Plan of Care	Interventions—Controlled Motion and Return to Function Phases
1. Educate the patient.	1. Ergonomic counseling in ways to prevent recurrence. Home instruction in safe progression of stretching and strengthening exercises. Instruction on signs of too much stress (see Box 8–3).
2. Develop strong, mobile scar.	2. Friction massage. Soft-tissue mobilization.
3. Develop a balance in length and strength of the muscles.	3. Correct cause of faulty muscle and joint mechanics with appropriately graded stretching and strengthening exercises.
4. Progress functional independence.	4. Train muscles to function according to demand; provide alternatives or support if it cannot. Train coordination and timing. Develop endurance.
5. Analyze job/activity.	5. Adapt home, work, sport environment/tools.

Precaution: If there is progressive loss of range of motion as the result of stretching, do not continue to stretch. Re-evaluate the condition and determine if there is still a chronic inflammation with contracting scar or if there is protective muscle guarding. Emphasize stabilizing the part and training in safe adaptive patterns of motion.

Box 8–7 Management Guidelines—Rheumatoid Arthritis/Active Disease Period

Impairments:

Tenderness and warmth over the involved joints with joint swelling
Muscle guarding and pain on motion
Joint stiffness and limited motion
Muscle weakness and atrophy
Potential deformity and ankylosis from the degenerative process and asymmetric muscle pull
Fatigue, malaise, sleep disorders
Restricted ADLs and IADLs

Plan of Care	Interventions
1. Educate the patient.	1. Inform the patient on importance of rest, joint protection, energy conservation, and performance of ROM. Teach home exercise program and activity modifications that conserve energy and minimize stress to vulnerable joints.
2. Relieve pain and muscle guarding and promote relaxation.	2. Modalities. Gentle massage. Immobilize in splint. Relaxation techniques.
3. Minimize joint stiffness and maintain available motion.	3. Passive or active-assistive ROM within limits of pain, gradual progression as tolerated. Gentle joint techniques using grade I or II oscillations.
4. Minimize muscle atrophy.	4. Gentle isometrics in pain-free positions, progression to ROM when tolerated.
5. Prevent deformity and protect the joint structures.	5. Use of supportive and assistive equipment for all pathologically active joints. Good bed positioning while resting. Avoidance of activities that stress the joints.

Precautions: Respect fatigue and increased pain; do not overstress osteoporotic bone or lax ligaments.

Contraindications: Do not stretch swollen joints or apply heavy resistance exercise that cause joint stress.

Box 8–8 Management Guidelines: Osteoarthritis

Impairments:

- Pain with mechanical stress or excessive activity
- Pain at rest in the advanced stages
- Stiffness after inactivity
- Limitation of motion
- Muscle weakness
- Decreased proprioception and balance
- Functional limitations in ADLs and IADLs

Plan of Care	Intervention
1. Educate the patient.	1. Teach about deforming forces and prevention. Teach home exercise program to reinforce interventions and minimize symptoms.
2. Decrease effects of stiffness.	2. Active ROM. Joint-play mobilization techniques.
3. Decrease pain from mechanical stress and prevent deforming forces.	3. Splinting and/or assistive equipment to minimize stress or to correct faulty biomechanics. Strengthen supporting muscles. Alternate activity with periods of rest.
4. Increase ROM.	4. Stretch muscle, joint, or soft-tissue restrictions with specific techniques.
5. Improve neuromuscular control, strength, and muscle endurance.	5. Low-intensity resistance exercises and muscle repetitions.
6. Improve balance.	6. Balance training activities.
7. Improve physical conditioning.	7. Nonimpact or low-impact aerobic exercise.

Precautions: When strengthening supporting muscles, increased pain in the joint during or following resistive exercises probably means that too great a weight is being used or stress is being placed at an inappropriate part of the ROM. Analyze the joint mechanics and at what point during the range the greatest compressive forces are occurring. Maximum resistance exercise should not be performed through that ROM.

Box 8–9 Management Guidelines—Postfracture/Period of Immobilization

Impairments:

- Initially, inflammation and swelling
- In the immobilized area, progressive muscle atrophy, contracture formation, cartilage degeneration, and decreased circulation
- Potential overall body weakening if confined to bed
- Functional limitations imposed by the fracture site and method of immobilization used

Plan of Care	Intervention
1. Educate the patient.	1. Teach functional adaptations. Teach safe ambulation, bed mobility.
2. Decrease effects of inflammation during acute period.	2. Ice, elevation.
3. Decrease effects of immobilization.	3. Intermittent muscle setting. Active ROM to joints above and below immobilized region.
4. If patient is confined to bed, maintain strength and ROM in major muscle groups.	4. Resistive exercises to major muscle groups not immobilized, especially in preparation for future ambulation.

Box 8–10 Management Guidelines—Postfracture/Postimmobilization

Impairments:

- Pain with movement, which progressively decreases
- Decreased ROM
- Decreased joint play
- Scar tissue adhesions
- Decreased strength and endurance

Plan of Care	Interventions
1. Educate the patient.	1. Inform patient of limitations until fracture site is radiologically healed. Teach home exercises that reinforce interventions.
2. Provide protection until radiologically healed.	2. Use partial weight bearing in lower extremity and nonstressful activities in the upper extremity.
3. Initiate active exercises.	3. Active ROM, gentle multiangle isometrics.
4. Increase joint and soft-tissue mobility.	4. Initiate joint play stretching techniques (using grades III and IV) with the force applied proximal to the healing fracture site. For muscle stretching, apply the force proximal to the healing fracture site until radiologically healed.
5. Increase strength and muscle endurance.	5. As the ROM increases and the bone heals, initiate resistive and repetitive exercises.
6. Improve cardiorespiratory fitness.	6. Initiate safe aerobic exercises that do not stress the fracture site until it is healed.

Precautions: No stretch or resistive forces distal to the fracture site until the bone is radiologically healed. No excessive joint compression or shear for several weeks after the period of immobilization. Use protected weight bearing until the site is radiologically healed.

Box 8–14 Management Guidelines—Postoperative Rehabilitation

Impairments:

- Postoperative pain because of disruption of soft tissue
- Postoperative swelling
- Potential circulatory and pulmonary complications
- Joint stiffness or limitation of motion because of injury to soft tissue and necessary postoperative immobilization
- Muscle atrophy because of immobilization
- Loss of strength for functional activities
- Limitation of weight bearing
- Potential loss of strength and mobility in unoperated joints

Maximum Protection Phase

Plan of Care	Interventions
1. Educate the patient in preparation for self-management.	1. Instruction in safe positioning and limb movements and special postoperative precautions or contraindications.
2. Decrease postoperative pain, muscle guarding, or spasm.	2. Relaxation exercises. Use of modalities such as transcutaneous nerve stimulation (TNS), cold, or heat. Continuous passive motion (CPM) during the early postoperative period.
3. Prevent wound infection.	3. Instruction or review of proper cleaning and dressing the incision.
4. Minimize postoperative swelling.	4. Elevation of the operated extremity. Active muscle pumping exercises at the distal joints. Use of compression garment. Gentle distal-to-proximal massage.[69]
5. Prevent circulatory and pulmonary complications such as deep vein thrombosis, pulmonary embolus, or pneumonia.	5. Active exercises to distal musculature. Deep-breathing and coughing exercises.
6. Prevent unnecessary, residual joint stiffness, or soft tissue contractures.	6. CPM or passive or active-assistive ROM initiated in the immediate postoperative period.
7. Minimize muscle atrophy across immobilized joints.	7. Muscle-setting exercises.
8. Maintain motion and strength in areas above and below the operative site.	8. Active and resistive ROM exercises to unoperated areas.
9. Maintain functional mobility while protecting the operative site.	9. Adaptive equipment and assistive devices.

Moderate Protection/Controlled Motion Phase

Plan of Care	Interventions
1. Educate the patient.	1. Teach the patient to monitor the effects of the exercise program and make adjustments if swelling or pain increases.
2. Gradually restore soft-tissue and joint mobility.	2. Active-assistive or active ROM within limits of pain. Joint mobilization procedures.
3. Establish a mobile scar.	3. Gentle massage across and around the maturing scar.
4. Strengthen involved muscles and improve joint stability.	4. Multiple-angle isometrics against increasing resistance. Alternating isometrics and rhythmic stabilization procedures. Dynamic exercise against light resistance in open- and closed-chain positions. Light functional activities with operated limb.

cont'd on page 790

Box 8–14 Management Guidelines—Postoperative Rehabilitation *(continued)*

Minimum Protection/Return to Function Phase

Plan of Care	Interventions
1. Continue patient education.	1. Emphasize gradual but progressive incorporation of improved muscle performance, mobility, and balance into functional activities.
2. Prevent reinjury or postoperative complications.	2. Reinforce self-monitoring and review the signs and symptoms of excessive use; identify unsafe activities.
3. Restore full joint and soft-tissue mobility, if possible.	3. Joint stretching (mobilization) and self-stretching techniques.
4. Maximize muscle performance, dynamic stability, and neuromuscular control.	4. Progressive strengthening exercises using higher loads and speeds and combined movement patterns. Integrate movements and positions into exercises that simulate functional activities.
5. Restore balance and coordinated movement.	5. Progressive balance and coordination training.
6. Acquire or relearn specific motor skills.	6. Apply principles of motor learning (appropriate practice and feedback during task-specific training).

Precautions: In addition to the precautions already addressed that relate to the stages of tissue repair and healing, there are several additional precautions that are of particular importance to the postsurgical patient.

- Avoid positions, movements, or weight bearing that could compromise the integrity of the surgical repair.
- Keep the wound clean to avoid postoperative infection. Monitor for wound drainage and signs of systemic or local infection, such as elevated temperature.
- Avoid vigorous/high-intensity stretching or resistance exercises with soft tissues, such as muscles, tendons, or joint capsules that have been repaired or reattached for at least 6 weeks to ensure adequate healing and stability.
- Modify level and selection of physical activities, if necessary, to prevent premature wear and tear of repaired or reconstructed soft tissues and joints.

Chapter 15 describes principles of interventions for spinal and postural conditions. Management guidelines are summarized as follows.

Box 15–5 Management Guidelines—Acute Spinal Problems/Protection Phase

Impairments and Functional Limitations:
- Pain and/or neurological symptoms
- Inflammation
- Inability to perform ADLs and IADLs
- Guarded posture (prefers flexion, extension, or nonweight-bearing)

Plan of Care	Intervention
1. Learn self-management.	1. Engage patient in all activities.
2. Decrease acute symptoms.	2. Modalities, massage, traction as needed. Rest only for first couple days if needed.
3. Demonstrate awareness of neck and pelvic position and movement.	3. Kinesthetic training: cervical and scapular motions, pelvic tilts, neutral spine.
4. Demonstrate safe postures.	4. Practice positions and movement and experience effect on spine. Provide passive support/bracing if needed.
5. Initiate neuromuscular control of stabilizing muscles.	5. Core Technique: drawing-in maneuver. Basic stabilization: with arm and leg motions (passive support, progress to active control).
6. Safely perform basic ADLs and progress to IADLs.	6. Roll, sit, stand, and walk with safe postures. Progress tolerance to sitting >30 min., standing >15 min., and walking >1 mile.

Box 15–6 Management Guidelines—Subacute Spinal Problems/Controlled Motion Phase

Impairments and Functional Limitations:
- Pain: only when excessive stress is placed on vulnerable tissues
- Poor neuromuscular control of stabilizing muscles
- Flexibility postural awareness
- Generalized deconditioning
- Inability to perform IADLs for extended periods of time
- Poor body mechanics

Plan of Care	Intervention
1. Learn self-management and decrease episodes of pain.	1. Engage patient in all activities emphasizing safe movement and postures. Ergonomic adaptation of work or home environment.
2. Progress awareness and control of spinal alignment.	2. Practice active spinal control in pain free positions and with all exercises and activities. Practice posture correction.
3. Increase mobility in tight muscles/joint/fascia.	3. Joint mobilization/manipulation, muscle inhibition, self-stretching.
4. Develop neuromuscular control, strength and endurance in stabilizing muscles.	4. Progress stabilization exercises; increase repetitions and challenge.
5. Increase dynamic trunk and extremity strength.	5. Initiate dynamic trunk and extremity resistance exercises.
6. Develop general aerobic endurance.	6. Low to moderate intensity aerobic exercises; emphasize spinal bias.
7. Learn techniques of stress relief/relaxation.	7. Relaxation exercises and postural stress relief.
8. Learn safe body mechanics.	8. Functional exercises to prepare for safe mechanics. Practice stable spine lifts, push/pull activities.
9. Develop functional skills.	9. Functional exercises specific to desired outcome emphasizing spinal control, endurance, and timing.

Box 15–7 Management Guidelines—Chronic Spinal Problems/Return to Function Phase

Impairments and Functional Limitations:

Pain: only when excessive stress is placed on vulnerable tissues in repetitive or sustained nature for prolonged periods
Poor neuromuscular control and endurance in high intensity or destabilized situations
Flexibility and strength imbalances
Generalized deconditioning
Inability to perform high intensity physical demands for extended periods of time

Plan of Care	Intervention
1. Learn spinal control in high intensity and repetitive activities.	1. Practice active spinal control in various transitional and disturbed balance activities.
2. Increase mobility in tight muscles/joints/fascia.	2. Joint mobilization/manipulation, muscle inhibition, self-stretching.
3. Increase dynamic trunk and extremity strength.	3. Progress dynamic trunk and extremity resistance exercises emphasizing functional goals.
4. Develop general cardiovascular endurance.	4. Progress intensity of aerobic exercises.
5. Habitually use techniques of stress relief/relaxation and posture correction.	5. Reinforce motions and postures to relieve stress and any ergonomic changes needed.
6. Return to high level/high intensity activities for prolonged periods of time without exacerbating symptoms.	6. Progressive practice using activity-specific training consistent with desired functional outcome, emphasizing spinal control, endurance, timing, and speed.
7. Develop healthy exercise habits for self-maintenance.	7. Engage patient in all activities and educate as to benefits of maintaining fitness level and safe body mechanics.

Chapter 17 describes principles of exercise for the obstetric patient. Management guidelines are summarized in the following boxes.

Box 17–2 Management Guidelines—Pregnancy and Postpartum

Potential Impairments and Functional Limitations:

Stress, pain, and muscle imbalances from faulty postures
Poor body mechanics; related to changing body size and caring for growing child
Changing body image
Lower extremity edema and discomfort from altered circulation, varicose veins
Pelvic floor dysfunction, urinary incontinence from pelvic floor stress, or trauma superimposed on poor proprioceptive awareness
Abdominal muscle stretch, trauma, and diastasis recti
Potential decrease in cardiovascular fitness
Lack of knowledge of body changes and safe exercises to use during pregnancy and after childbirth
Lack of physical preparation (strength, endurance, relaxation) necessary for labor and delivery
Lack of knowledge of appropriate positioning for optimal comfort in labor and delivery
Lack of adequate postpartum rehabilitation

Plan of Care	Interventions
1. Develop awareness and control of posture during and after pregnancy.	1. Stretch, train, and strengthen postural muscle. Posture awareness training.
2. Learn safe body mechanics.	2. Body mechanics in sitting, standing, lifting, and lying as well as transitions from one position to another. Body mechanics with baby equipment and childcare activities. Positioning options for labor and delivery.
3. Develop upper extremity strength for the demands of infant care.	3. Resistive exercises to appropriate muscles.
4. Promote increased body awareness and a positive body image.	4. Body awareness and proprioception activities. Posture reinforcement
5. Prepare the lower extremities for the demands of increased weight bearing and circulatory compromise.	5. Use of elastic support stockings. Stretching exercises. Resistive exercises to appropriate muscles.
6. Develop awareness and control of the pelvic floor musculature.	6. Awareness of pelvic floor muscle contraction and relaxation. Train and strengthen for muscle control.
7. Maintain abdominal function and prevent or correct diastasis recti pathology.	7. Monitor diastasis recti. Diastasis recti exercises. Safe abdominal-strengthening exercises with diastasis recti protection.
8. Promote or maintain safe cardiovascular fitness.	8. Safe progression of aerobic exercises.[16]
9. Learn about the changes of pregnancy and birth.	9. Client/family instruction. Refer to other disciplines as indicated.
10. Learn relaxation skills.	10. Relaxation techniques.
11. Prevent impairments associated with pregnancy (i.e., low back pain, pelvic floor weakness, decreased circulation).	11. Education about potential problems of pregnancy. Teach prevention techniques and appropriate exercises.
12. Prepare physically for labor, delivery, and postpartum activities.	12. Strengthen muscles needed in labor and delivery, and train responses. Teach comfort measures for labor and delivery.
13. Provide education on safe postpartum exercise progression.	13. Postpartum exercise instruction.
14. Develop awareness of treatment options for pelvic floor dysfunction.	14. Comprehensive approach for prolapse, incontinence, or hypertonus.

Box 17–4 Management Guidelines—Postcesarean Section

Impairments and Functional Limitations:

- Risk of pulmonary complications
- Postsurgical pain and discomfort
- Risk of vascular complications
- Development of adhesions at incisional site
- Faulty posture
- Pelvic floor dysfunction
- Abdominal weakness; diastasis recti
- General functional restrictions of postdelivery

Plan of Care	Interventions
1. Improve pulmonary function and decrease the risk of pneumonia.	1. Breathing instruction; coughing and/or huffing[24,32]
2. Decrease incisional pain associated with coughing, movement, or breast-feeding.	2. Postoperative TENS; support incision with pillow when coughing or breast-feeding. Incisional support with pillow or hands when exercising. Education regarding incisional care and risk of injury.
3. Prevent postsurgical vascular complications.	3. Active leg exercises. Early ambulation.
4. Enhance incisional circulation and healing; prevent adhesion formation.	4. Gentle abdominal exercise with incisional support. Scar mobilization and friction massage.
5. Decrease postsurgical discomfort from flatulence, itching, or catheter.	5. Positioning instruction, massage, and supportive exercises.
6. Correct posture.	6. Posture instruction.
7. Prevent injury and reduce low back pain.	7. Instruction in incisional splinting and positioning for ADL Body mechanics instruction.
8. Prevent pelvic floor dysfunction.	8. Pelvic floor exercises; education regarding risk factors and types of pelvic floor dysfunction.
9. Develop abdominal strength.	9. Abdominal exercises including corrective exercises for diastasis recti.

Box 17–5 Management Guidelines—High-Risk Pregnancy

Impairments and Functional Limitations[37,46]:

- Primary functional limitation is inability to be out of bed and prolonged static positioning with the potential of the following impairments.
- Joint stiffness and muscle aches
- Muscle weakness and atrophy
- Vascular complications including risk of thrombosis and decreased uterine blood flow
- Decreased proprioception in distal body parts
- Constipation caused by lack of exercise
- Postural changes
- Boredom
- Emotional stress; patient may be at risk of losing the baby
- Guilt from the belief that some activity caused the problem or that the patient did not take good enough care of herself
- Anxiety about her home situation or the impending birth

Plan of Care	Interventions
1. Decrease stiffness.	1. Positioning instructions; assess for supports. Facilitation of joint motion in available range.
2. Maintain muscle length and bulk.	2. Stretching and strengthening exercises within limits imposed by the physician.
3. Maximize circulation; prevent deep-vein thrombosis.	3. Ankle pumping; ROM.
4. Improve proprioception.	4. Movement activities for as many body parts as possible.
5. Improve posture within available limits.	5. Posture instruction, modified as necessary based on allowed activity level. Bed mobility and transfer techniques if able (avoid Valsalva).
6. Relieve boredom.	6. Vary activities and positioning for exercises.
7. Enhance relaxation.	7. Relaxation techniques/stress management.
8. Prepare for delivery.	8. Childbirth education, breathing training, and exercises to assist and prepare for labor.
9. Enhance postpartum recovery.	9. Exercise instruction and home program for postpartum period. Body mechanics instruction.

Chapter 18 describes principles of exercise for the patient with vascular disorders of the extremities. Management guidelines are summarized in the following boxes.

Box 18–2 Management Guidelines—Acute Arterial Occlusion

Impairments:

Severe ischemia
Severe pain
Potential for tissue necrosis and amputation
Risk of local or systemic infection

Plan of Care	Interventions
1. Decrease ischemia by restoration or improvement of blood flow.	1. Medical: bed rest; complete systemic anticoagulation therapy. Physical: reflex heating of the torso or opposite extremity.[29,50] Positioning the patient in bed, with the head slightly raised, increases the blood flow to the distal portion of the extremity. Note: Thromboembolectomy and reconstructive arterial or bypass graft surgery are alternatives to nonoperative treatment.
2. Protect the limb.	2. The limb must be protected from any trauma. Pressure on skin must be minimized by a special mattress, implementation of a turning schedule, and periodic repositioning of the patient.[29,49,59]

Precautions/Contraindications: With an acute arterial occlusion any form of exercise is *contraindicated.* Local, direct heating of the involved extremity is *contraindicated* because it could easily cause a burn to ischemic tissue. Use of support hose is also *contraindicated* as they may increase peripheral resistance to blood flow. In addition, avoid wearing restrictive clothing that could compromise blood flow.

Box 18–3 Management Guidelines—Chronic Arterial Insufficiency

Impairments:

Decreased endurance and increased frequency of muscular fatigue with functional activities such as walking
Pain with exercise or at rest
Skin breakdown and ulcerations
Limitation of passive and active motion
Weakness and disuse atrophy

Plan of Care	Interventions
1. Teach the patient how to minimize or prevent potential impairments and correct impairments or functional limitations currently affecting functional capabilities.	1. Self-management of current or potential impairments through patient education.
2. Communicate with health professionals from other disciplines appropriate for consultation with the patient.	2. Medical or surgical management including medications; nutritional counseling for weight control and to decrease salt, sucrose, cholesterol and caffeine intake; smoking cessation.
3. Improve exercise tolerance for ADL and decrease the incidence of intermittent claudication.	3. Regular, graded aerobic conditioning program of walking or bicycling[31,50,59,69,70,81] (see Chapter 4).
4. Relieve pain at rest.	4. Sleep with the legs in a dependent but supported position over the edge of the bed or with the head of the bed slightly elevated.
5. Prevent skin ulcerations.	5. Proper care and protection of the skin, particularly the feet[14] or hands. Proper nail care.[14] Proper shoe selection and fit.[14] Avoid use of support hose and restrictive clothing. Avoid exposure to extremes of temperature, both hot and cold.
6. Improve vasodilation in affected arteries.	6. Vasodilation by iontophoresis.[2] Vasodilation by reflex heating.[2] ***Note:*** Although these physical measures have been advocated, their effectiveness is questionable.
7. Prevent or minimize joint contractures and muscle atrophy, particularly if the patient is confined to bed.	7. Repetitive, active ROM against low loads and/or gentle stretching exercises; proper positioning in bed to maintain joint and muscle extensibility.
8. Promote healing of any skin ulcerations that develop.	8. Wound management procedures for treating ischemic ulcers, including electrical stimulation and oxygen therapy.[29,60,61]

Box 18–6 Management Guidelines—Acute Thrombophlebitis

Impairments:

Dull ache or pain usually in the calf
Tenderness, warmth, and swelling with palpation

Plan of Care	Interventions
1. Relieve pain during the acute inflammatory period.	1. Bed rest, pharmacologic management (systemic anticoagulant therapy); elevation of the affected lower extremity, keeping the knee slightly flexed.
2. In later stages, as the acute symptoms subside, regain functional mobility.	2. Graded ambulation with legs wrapped in elastic bandages or when pressure-gradient support stockings are worn.
3. Prevent recurrence of the acute disorder.	3. Continuation of appropriate medical and pharmacologic management. Use of strategies to prevent DVTs.

Contraindications: Passive or active motion or application of moist heat; use of a sequential pneumatic compression pump.

Box 18–7 Management Guidelines—Chronic Venous Insufficiency and Varicose Veins

Impairments:

Edema
Increased risk of skin ulcerations and infections
Aching of involved limb
Decreased functional mobility, strength, and endurance

Plan of Care	Interventions
1. Teach the patient how to prevent or minimize impairments.	1. Patient education and self-management skills for skin care, self-massage for lymphedema, and a home exercise program.
2. Prevent lymphedema; minimize venous stasis.	2. Use of individually tailored pressure-gradient support stockings donned before getting out of bed in the morning and worn every day. Support garment worn during exercise and ambulation. Light active exercise, such as walking, on a regular basis. Elevate the lower extremities after graded ambulation until the heart rate returns to normal. Avoid prolonged periods of standing still and sitting with legs dependent. Elevate involved limb(s) above the level of the heart (about 30–45 degrees) when resting or sleeping (see Box 18–9 for additional methods to prevent lymphedema).
3. Increase venous return and reduce lymphedema if already present.	3. Use intermittent mechanical compression pump and sleeve with involved limb elevated for several hours a day. Manual massage to drain edema. Stroke in a distal-to-proximal direction clearing the proximal nodes and areas of lymphedema first, then the middle, and finally the distal areas. Relaxation and active ROM (pumping exercises) of the distal muscles while involved limb is elevated.
4. Prevent skin abrasions, ulcerations, and wound infections.	4. Proper skin care (see Box 18–9).

Box 18–12 Management Guidelines after Surgery for Breast Cancer

Potential Postoperative Impairments:

Pulmonary and circulatory complications
Lymphedema
Restricted mobility of the upper extremity
Postural malalignment
Weakness and decreased functional use of the upper extremity
Fatigue and decreased endurance for functional activities
Emotional and social adjustments

Plan of Care	Interventions
1. Prepare the patient for postoperative self-management.	1. Interdisciplinary patient education involving all aspects of potential impairments and functional limitations. Self-management activities and preparation for participation in a home program on the first postoperative day.
2. Prevent postoperative pulmonary complications and thromboemboli.	2. Pre- or postoperative instruction in deep breathing, emphasizing maximal inspirations and effective coughing (see Chapter 19). Active ankle exercises (calf pumping exercises).
3. Prevent or minimize postoperative lymphedema.	3. Elevation of the involved upper extremity on pillows (about 30 degrees) while the patient is in bed or sitting in a chair. Wrapping the involved upper extremity with bandages or wearing an elastic pressure gradient sleeve. Pumping exercises of the arm on the side of the surgery. Early ROM exercises. ***Precaution:*** Avoid static, dependent positioning of the arm.
4. Decrease lymphedema if or when it develops.	4. Daily use of a sequential pneumatic compression pump followed by wrapping. Continued elevation of the involved upper extremity while at rest. Compressive bandaging with nonelastic or low-stretch wraps worn continually (during activity and at rest). Manual lymphatic drainage massage. Daily regimen of exercises to reduce lymphedema. Use of custom-fit elastic compression garment when lymphedema is stabilized. Adherence to precautions for skin care (see Box 18–9).
5. Prevent postural deformities.	5. Instruction in proper bed positioning preoperatively or on the first postoperative day, emphasizing midline and symmetric positioning of the shoulders and trunk. Posture awareness training; encourage the patient to assume an erect posture when sitting or standing to minimize a rounded shoulder posture. Posture exercises with an emphasis on scapular retraction exercises.
6. Prevent muscle tension and guarding in cervical musculature.	6. Active ROM of the cervical spine to promote relaxation. Shoulder shrugging and shoulder circle exercises. Gentle massage to cervical musculature.

cont'd on page 799

Box 18–12 Management Guidelines after Surgery for Breast Cancer *(continued)*

7. Prevent restricted mobility of the upper extremity.	7. Active-assistive and active ROM exercises of the shoulder, elbow, and hand initiated as soon as possible but cautiously usually on the first postoperative day. *Note:* Exercise may be initiated even when the drainage tubes and sutures are still in place. After the incision has healed, self-stretching to the shoulder.
8. Regain strength and functional use of the involved upper extremity.	8. Low-intensity isometric exercises of shoulder musculature initiated on the first or second postoperative day. Resistance exercises with a light handheld weight or a light grade of elastic resistance material, emphasizing scapular and glenohumeral musculature. Scapular and glenohumeral stabilization exercises in standing with hands against a table or wall. Upper extremity ergometry initially against minimal and, later, moderate resistance. Use of the involved extremity for light functional activities.
9. Improve exercise tolerance and sense of well-being, and reduce fatigue.	9. Graded, low-intensity aerobic exercise such as walking or cycling.
10. Provide information about resources for patient and family support and ongoing patient education.	10. Resources include: American Cancer Society family support and ongoing patient education (www.cancer.org), National Breast Cancer Coalition; National Lymphedema Network.

Precautions: Shoulder exercise should be performed within a *protected* ROM usually no more than 90 degrees of elevation of the arm until after removal of drains. Observe the incision and sutures carefully during exercises. Avoid any undue tension on the incision or blanching of the scar during shoulder exercises. Avoid exercises with the involved arm in a dependent position. Progress graded exercise program very slowly, particularly if the patient is receiving adjuvant therapy.

Chapter 19 describes principles of exercise for the patient with pulmonary disorders. Management guidelines are summarized in the following boxes.

Box 19–7 Management Guidelines—Chronic Obstructive Pulmonary Disease (COPD)

Impairments:

An increase in the amount and viscosity of mucus production
A chronic, often productive cough
Frequent episodes of dyspnea
A labored breathing pattern that results in:

- Increased respiratory rate (tachypnea)
- Use of accessory muscles of inspiration and decreased diaphragmatic excursion
- Upper chest breathing

Inadequate exchange of air in the lower lobes
Most difficulty during expiration; use of pursed-lip breathing
Changes in pulmonary function

- Increased residual volume
- Decreased vital capacity
- Decreased expiratory flow rates

Decreased mobility of the chest wall; a barrel chest deformity develops
Abnormal posture: forward-head and rounded and elevated shoulders
Decreased general endurance during functional activities

Plan of Care	Interventions
1. Decrease the amount and viscosity of secretions and prevent respiratory infections.	1. Administration of bronchodialators, antibiotics, and humidification therapy. If patient smokes, he or she should be strongly encouraged to stop.
2. Remove or prevent the accumulation of secretions. (This is important if emphysema is associated with chronic bronchitis or if there is an acute respiratory infection.)	2. Deep and effective cough. Postural drainage to areas where secretions are identified. *Note:* Drainage positions may need to be modified if the patient is dyspneic in the head-down position.
3. Promote relaxation of the accessory muscles of inspiration to decrease reliance on upper chest breathing and to decrease muscle tension associated with dyspnea.	3. Positioning for relaxation. • Relaxed head-up position in bed: trunk, arms, and head are well supported. • Sitting: leaning forward, resting forearms on thighs or on a table. • Standing: leaning forward on an object, with hands on the thighs or leaning backwards against a wall. Relaxation exercises for shoulder musculature: active shoulder shrugging followed by relaxation; shoulder and arm circles; horizontal abduction and adduction of the shoulders.
4. Improve the patient's breathing pattern and ventilation. Emphasize diaphragmatic and lateral costal breathing and *relaxed* expiration; decrease the work of breathing, rate of respiration, and use of accessory muscles. Carry over controlled breathing exercises to functional activities.	4. Breathing exercises: controlled diaphragmatic breathing with minimal upper chest movement; lateral costal breathing; pursed-lip breathing (careful to *avoid forced* expiration); practice controlled breathing during standing, walking, climbing stairs, and other functional activities.
5. Minimize or prevent episodes of dyspnea.	5. Have a patient assume a comfortable position so the upper chest is relaxed and the lower chest is as mobile as possible. Emphasize controlled diaphragmatic breathing. Have the patient breathe out as rapidly as possible *without forcing* expiration. *Note:* Initially, the rate of ventilation will be rapid and shallow. As the patient gets control of breathing, he or she will slow down the rate. Administer supplemental oxygen in a severe episode, if needed.
6. Improve the mobility of the lower thorax.	6. Exercises for chest mobility, emphasizing movement of the lower rib cage during deep breathing.
7. Improve posture.	7. Exercises and postural training to decrease forward-head and rounded shoulders.
8. Increase exercise tolerance.	8. Graded endurance and conditioning exercises (see Chapter 4).

Box 19–8 Management Guidelines: Post-Thoracic Surgery

Impairments:

- Reduced lung expansion or an inability to take a deep inspiration because of incisional pain
- Decreased effectiveness of the cough because of incisional pain and irritation of the throat from intubation
- Possible accumulation of pulmonary secretions either preoperatively or postoperatively
- Decreased chest wall and upper extremity mobility
- Poor postural alignment because of incisional pain or chest tubes
- Increased risk of deep vein thrombosis and pulmonary embolism
- General weakness, fatigue, and disorientation

Plan of Care	Interventions
1. Ascertain the status of the patient before each treatment.	1. Evaluate orientation, color, respiratory rate, heart rate, breath sounds, sputum drainage into chest tubes.
2. Promote relaxation and reduce postoperative pain.	2. Position the patient in a semi-Fowler's position (head of bed elevated to 30 degrees and hips and knees slightly flexed). This position reduces traction on the thoracic incision. Coordinate treatment with administration of pain medication.
3. Optimize ventilation and re-expand lung tissue to prevent atelectasis and pneumonia.	3. Begin deep-breathing exercises on the day of surgery as soon as patient is conscious; diaphragmatic breathing; segmental expansion. Add incentive spirometry or inspiratory resistance exercises to improve inspiratory capacity. Emphasize a deep inhalation followed by a 3- to 5-second hold and then a relaxed exhalation. Continue deep-breathing exercises postoperatively, with six to ten consecutive deep breaths per hour until the patient is ambulatory.
4. Assist in the removal of secretions.	4. Begin deep, effective coughing as soon as the patient is alert and can cooperate. Implement early functional mobility (getting up to a chair, early ambulation). Institute modified postural drainage only if secretions accumulate.
5. Maintain adequate circulation in the lower extremities to prevent deep vein thrombosis and pulmonary embolism.	5. Begin active exercises of the lower extremities, with emphasis on ankle pumping exercises on the first day after surgery. Continue leg exercises until the patient is allowed out of bed and is ambulatory.
6. Regain ROM in the shoulders.	6. Begin relaxation exercises for the shoulder area on the first postoperative day. These can include shoulder shrugging or shoulder circles. Initiate active-assistive ROM of the shoulders, being careful not to cause pain. Reassure the patient that gentle movements will not disturb the incision. Progress to active shoulder exercises on the succeeding postoperative days to the patient's tolerance until full active ROM has been achieved.
7. Prevent postural impairments.	7. Reinforce symmetric alignment and positioning of the trunk on the first postoperative day when the patient is in bed *Note:* The patient will tend to lean toward the side of the incision. Instruct the patient in symmetric sitting posture when he or she is allowed to sit up in a chair or at the side of the bed.
8. Increase exercise tolerance.	8. Begin a progressive and graded ambulation or stationary cycling program as soon as the chest tubes are removed and the patient is allowed to be out of bed.

Precautions:

- Monitor vital signs throughout treatment.
- Be certain to show the patient how to splint over the incision to minimize incisional pain during coughing.
- Avoid placing traction on chest tubes when moving the patient.
- To prevent dislodging a chest tube for the patient who has a lateral incision, limit shoulder flexion to 90 degrees on the operated side for several days until the chest tube is removed.
- If postural drainage must be implemented, modify positioning to avoid a head-down position.
- Do not use percussion over the incision.
- When turning a patient, use a logroll technique to minimize traction on the incision.

Glossary

A

abruptio placentae Premature detachment of the placenta from the uterus

accessory movement Movement within a joint and surrounding soft tissues that is necessary for normal range of motion but cannot be voluntarily performed

accommodating resistance exercise A term used synonymously with **isokinetic exercise**

active inhibition A type of stretching exercise in which there is reflex inhibition and subsequent elongation of the contractile elements of muscles

adaptation The ability of an organism to change over time in response to a stimulus

adenosine triphosphate (ATP) A high-energy compound from which the body derives energy

adhesions Abnormal adherence of collagen fibers to surrounding structures during immobilization, following trauma, or as a complication of surgery, which restricts normal elasticity of the structures involved

aerobic exercise Submaximal, rhythmic, repetitive exercise of large muscle groups, during which the needed energy is supplied by inspired oxygen

aerobic system An aerobic energy system in which ATP is manufactured when food is broken down

airway clearance techniques Therapeutic procedures to improve mucociliary transport; includes coughing, postural drainage, manual techniques (percussion, vibration, shaking) and deep breathing exercise

airway resistance The resistance to the flow of air in the lungs offered by the bronchioles

amniotic fluid The liquid contained in the amniotic sac. The fetus floats in the fluid, which serves as a cushion against injury and helps maintain a constant fetal body temperature

anaerobic exercise Exercise that occurs without the presence of inspired oxygen

anaerobic glycolytic system (lactic acid system) An anaerobic energy system in which ATP is manufactured when glucose is broken down to lactic acid

apnea Cessation of breathing

apneusis The cessation of breathing during the inspiratory phase of respiration

arteriosclerosis obliterans (ASO) See **arteriosclerotic vascular disease**

arteriosclerotic vascular disease (ASVD) Progressive narrowing, loss of elasticity, fibrosis, and eventual occlusion of the large and middle-sized arteries, usually in the lower extremities

arteriovenous oxygen difference (a-$\bar{v}O_2$ difference) The difference between the oxygen content of arterial and venous blood

arthritis Inflammation of the structures of a joint

arthrodesis Surgical fusion of bony surfaces of a joint with internal fixation such as pins, nails, plates, and bone grafts; usually done in cases of severe joint pain and instability in which mobility of the joint is a lesser concern

arthroplasty Any reconstructive joint procedure, with or without a joint implant, designed to relieve pain and/or restore joint motion

arthroscopy Examination of the internal structures of a joint by means of an endoscopic viewing apparatus inserted into the joint

arthrotomy Surgical incision into a joint

asthma An obstructive lung disease seen in young patients, associated with a hypersensitivity to specific allergens and resulting in bronchospasm and difficulty in breathing

atelectasis Collapse or incomplete expansion of the lung

ATP-PC system An anaerobic energy system in which adenosine triphosphate (ATP) is manufactured when phosphocreatine (PC) is broken down

atrophy The wasting or reduction of size of cells, tissues, organs, or body parts

auscultation Listening to heart or lung sounds within the body, usually with a stethoscope

B

balance The ability to maintain the body's center of gravity over the base of support

bradypnea Slow rate of respiration; depth either shallow or normal

bronchiectasis A chronic obstructive lung disease characterized by dilation and repeated infection of medium-sized bronchioles

bursitis Inflammation of a bursa

C

capsular pattern A pattern of limitation, characteristic for a given joint, that indicates that a problem exists with that joint

cardiac output The volume of blood pumped from a ventricle of the heart per unit of time; the product of heart rate and stroke volume

cardiopulmonary endurance The ability of the lungs and heart to take in and transport adequate amounts of oxygen to the working muscle, allowing activities that involve large muscle masses to be performed over long periods of time

chondromalacia patellae Deterioration of the articular cartilage at the posterior aspect of the patella

chondroplasty A débridement procedure to repair joint cartilage, usually at the patellofemoral joint; also called abrasion arthroplasty

chronic bronchitis An inflammation of the bronchi that causes an irritating, productive cough that lasts up to 3 months and recurs over at least 2 consecutive years

chronic obstructive pulmonary disease (COPD) A term used to describe a variety of chronic lung conditions such as chronic bronchitis, emphysema, and peripheral airway disease

chronic pain syndrome Used to describe patients with long-standing low back pain who have developed illness behavior and hopelessness. There is no longer a direct relationship between the pain and the apparent disability, and treatment of the painful symptoms usually does not change the condition. The patient may require psychological and sociological intervention and behavior modification techniques

circuit training A training program that uses selected exercises or activities performed in sequence

closed-chain exercise Exercise in which the distal end of the segment is fixed to a supporting surface as the trunk and proximal segments move over the fixed part. This includes functional exercises, especially for the lower extremities, in which the foot is stabilized on the ground and the muscles control the hips, knees, and ankles in activities such as squatting, climbing steps, and getting in and out of a chair

clubbing, digital Broadening or thickening of the soft tissues of the terminal phalanges of the fingers and toes; often seen in persons with chronic pulmonary disease

co-contraction Simultaneous contraction of muscles on opposite sides of a joint; source of dynamic stability of a joint

comparable sign A test procedure that can be repeated following a therapeutic maneuver to determine the effectiveness of the maneuver

compression dressing A sterile bandage applied around or over a new surgical incision to compress the wound site and control swelling

concentric exercise An overall shortening of the muscle occurs as it generates tension and contracts against resistance

conditioning An augmentation of the energy capacity of the muscle through an exercise program

continuous training A training program that uses exercise over a given duration without rest periods

contracture Shortening or hypomobility of the

skin, fascia, muscle, or joint capsule that prevents normal mobility or flexibility of that structure

contusion Bruising from a direct blow, resulting in capillary rupture

coordination Using the right muscles at the right time with correct intensity. Coordination is the basis of smooth and efficient movement, which often occurs automatically

crackles Fine or coarse lung sounds heard with a stethoscope primarily during inspiration and caused by movement of secretions in the small airways of the lungs; formerly referred to as **rales**

cumulative trauma disorder Musculoskeletal symptoms from excessive or repetitive motion causing connective tissue or bony breakdown. Initially, the inflammatory response from the microtrauma is subthreshold but eventually builds to the point of perceived pain and resulting dysfunction. Syndromes include shin splints, carpal tunnel, bursitis, tendinitis, cervical tension, thoracic outlet, tennis elbow, and marching fracture. Also known as cumulative trauma syndrome, repetitive strain injury, and **overuse syndrome**

cyanosis A bluish appearance of skin and mucous membranes due to insufficient oxygenation of the blood

cystic fibrosis A genetically-based disease that involves malfunction of the exocrine glands and leads to chronic lung infections and pancreatic dysfunction

D

deconditioning A change that takes place in cardiovascular, neuromuscular, and metabolic functions as a result of prolonged bed rest or inactivity

decongestive lymphatic therapy A comprehensive approach to management of lymphedema that combines elevation, compression, exercise, massage, and skin care

degenerative joint disease (DJD) See **osteoarthritis**

delayed-onset muscle soreness (DOMS) Exercise-induced muscle tenderness or stiffness that occurs 24 to 48 hours after vigorous exercise

derangement (disk protrusion) Any change in the shape of the nucleus pulposus of the intervertebral disk that causes it to protrude beyond its normal limits

disability The inability to undertake normal activities of daily living (ADL) as a result of physical, mental, social, or emotional impairments

diagnosis The recognition or the determination of the cause and nature of a pathologic condition

diastasis recti Separation of the rectus abdominis muscle in the midline at the linea alba; continuity of the abdominal wall is disrupted

dislocation Displacement of a part, usually the bony partners within a joint

distensibility The ability of an organ or tissue to be stretched out or enlarged

distraction A pulling apart or separation of joint surfaces

dorsal clearance Surgical removal of diseased synovium from the extensor tendons of the fingers and wrist

dynamic stabilization An isometric or stabilizing contraction of trunk or proximal girdle muscles to maintain control of the functional position in response to imposed fluctuating forces through the moving extremities

dynamometer A device that quantitatively measures muscle strength

dysfunction A loss of function as a result of adaptive shortening of soft tissues and loss of mobility

dyspnea Shortness of breath; labored, distressed breathing

E

eccentric exercise Overall lengthening of the muscle occurs as it develops tension and contracts to control motion against the resistance of an outside force; negative work is done

efficiency The ratio of work output to work input

elasticity The ability of soft tissue to return to its original length after a stretch force has been released

embolus A thrombus or clot of material that has been dislodged and transported in the bloodstream from a larger to a smaller vessel, resulting in occlusion of the vessel

emphysema A chronic obstructive pulmonary disease that is characterized by inflammation, thickening, and deterioration of the respiratory bronchioles and alveoli

end-feel The quality of feel the evaluator experiences when passively applying pressure at the end of the available range of motion

endurance The ability to resist fatigue

endurance, general (total body) The ability of an individual to sustain low-intensity exercises, such as walking, jogging, or climbing, over an extended period

endurance, muscular The ability of a muscle to perform repeated contractions over a prolonged period

energy systems Metabolic systems involving a series of chemical reactions resulting in the formation of waste products and the manufacture of adenosine triphosphate (ATP). The systems include the ATP-PC (adenosine triphosphate-phosphocreatine) system, the anaerobic glycolytic system, and the aerobic system

ergometer An apparatus, such as a stationary bicycle or treadmill, used to quantitatively measure the physiologic effects of exercise

exercise bouts The number of sets of a repetition maximum performed during each exercise session

exercise duration The total number of days, weeks, or months during which an exercise program is performed

exercise frequency The number of times exercise is performed within a day or within a week

exercise load The amount of weight used as resistance during an exercise

exercise prescription Individualized exercise program involving the duration, frequency, intensity, and mode of exercise

expiratory flow rate The volume of air exhaled per unit of time

expiratory reserve volume (ERV) The maximum amount of air an individual can exhale after a normal, relaxed expiration

extension bias Describes the preferred position of spinal extension (lordosis) in which the patient's symptoms are decreased. Usually the symptoms increase in spinal flexion

extensor lag The range of active extension is less than the range of passive extension of a joint; in the knee, usually the result of inhibition or dysfunction of the quadriceps mechanism; synonymous with **quadriceps lag;** in the fingers, usually the result of adhesions restricting mobility of the extensor tendons

extrapment A tissue trapped on the outside of a structure unable to assume its normal relationship. When a meniscoid tissue becomes trapped outside a zygapophyseal joint as the surfaces slide together, the motion is blocked and tension is placed on the capsular tissue

extrusion A protrusion of the nucleus pulposus of the intervertebral disk in which the nuclear material ruptures through the outer annulus and lies under the posterior longitudinal ligament

F

fast-twitch (FT) fiber A skeletal muscle fiber with a fast reaction time that has a high anaerobic capacity and is suited for phasic muscle activity

fatigue, general (total body) The diminished response of a person during prolonged physical activity, such as walking or jogging, that may be due to a decrease in blood sugar (glucose) levels, a decrease in glycogen stores in muscle and liver, or a depletion of potassium, especially in the elderly

fatigue, local (muscle) A diminished response of the muscle due to a decrease in energy stores, insufficient oxygen, and a buildup of lactic acid; protective influences from the central nervous system; or a decrease in the conduction of impulses at the myoneural junction

fetus The developing embryo in the uterus from 7 to 8 weeks after fertilization until birth

fitness A general term indicating a level of cardiovascular functioning that results in heightened energy reserves for optimum performance and well-being

flat low-back posture A posture characterized by decreased lumbosacral angle, decreased lumbar lordosis, and posterior tilting of the pelvis

flexibility The ability of muscle and other soft tissue to yield to a stretch force

flexibility exercise A general term used to describe exercises performed by a person to passively or actively elongate soft tissues without the assistance of a therapist

flexion bias Describes the position of spinal flexion in which the patient's symptoms are lessened. Usually the symptoms are provoked in spinal extension

forward head posture A posture characterized by increased flexion of the lower cervical and upper thoracic regions, increased extension of the occiput on the first cervical vertebra, and increased extension of the upper cervical vertebrae

fremitus, vocal or tactile The vibration that can be felt on the chest wall as a person speaks

functional excursion The distance a muscle can shorten after it has been stretched to its maximum length

functional exercise Exercise that mimics functional activities but is performed in a controlled manner or environment

functional limitation A limitation from an impairment that is not disabling yet interferes with normal function

functional position The position or range of motion in which the patient experiences the greatest comfort or least amount of stress on the tissues in the region. It may also be referred to as the **resting position** or neutral position. The position is not static and may change as the patient's condition changes

functional residual capacity The amount of air remaining in the lungs after a resting expiration

functional skills Motor skills that are necessary to independently perform activities or tasks of daily living; refined movements requiring coordination, agility, balance, and timing

G

ganglion (pl., ganglia) A ballooning of the wall of a joint capsule or tendon sheath

gestation The period of development from the time of fertilization to birth (pregnancy)

glossopharyngeal breathing A type of breathing exercise used to increase a patient's inspiratory capacity by gulping in air

glycogen The storage form of carbohydrates in the body, found predominantly in the muscles and the liver

H

handicap The social disadvantage resulting from an impairment or disability that prevents or limits persons in their occupation, environment, or social setting

hemarthrosis Bleeding into a joint, usually from severe trauma

hemoptysis The expectoration of blood or blood-streaked sputum from the bronchial tree and lungs

hemothorax A collection or effusion of blood in the pleural cavity

herniation Abnormal protrusion of an organ or other body structure through a defect or natural opening in a covering membrane, muscle, or bone

hyperplasia An increase in the number of fibers or cells

hypertrophy An increase in the cross-sectional size of a fiber or cell

hyperventilation An increase in the rate and depth of respiration above a level necessary for normal ventilatory function

I

impairment Any loss or abnormality of psychological, physiologic, or anatomic structure or function that limits or changes an individual's ability to perform a task or activity

incentive spirometry A form of inspiratory muscle training in which the patient inhales maximally and sustains the inspiration

incontinence, urinary or fecal Involuntary loss of bladder or bowel contents; often a result of both neuromuscular and musculoskeletal impairments; may occur in combination with prolapse of the uterus

inspiratory capacity The amount of air a person can inhale after a resting expiration

inspiratory reserve volume (IRV) The maximum amount of air a person can inhale after a relaxed inspiration

inspiratory resistance training A method of strengthening the muscles of inspiration

intermittent claudication The cramping of muscles after short periods of exercise; often seen in patients with occlusive arterial disorders

intermittent traction A traction force that is alternately applied and released at frequent intervals, usually in a rhythmic pattern

interval training A training program that alternates bouts of heavy work with periods of rest or light work

intrinsic muscle spasm The prolonged contraction of a muscle in response to the local circulatory and metabolic changes that occur when a muscle is in a continued state of contraction

intubation Insertion of a tube, such as an endotracheal or nasogastric tube, into the body

involution The progressive contraction of the uterus following childbirth, returning the organ to near its prepregnant size

isokinetic exercise A form of active-resistive exercise in which the speed of movement of the limb is controlled by a preset rate-limiting device

isometric (static) exercise A form of exercise in which tension develops in the muscle but no mechanical work is performed. There is no appreciable joint movement, and the overall length of the muscle remains the same

J

joint mobilization/manipulation Passive traction and/or gliding movements applied to joint surfaces that maintain or restore the joint play normally allowed by the capsule, so that the normal roll-slide joint mechanics can occur as a person moves

joint play Capsular laxity or elasticity that allows movements of the joint surfaces. The movements include distraction, sliding, compression, rolling, and spinning

K

kypholordotic posture A posture characterized by an exaggerated thoracic kyphosis and lumbar lordosis and usually forward head

kyphosis A posterior convexity in the spinal column. A posterior curve is primary because it is present at birth and remains in the thoracic and sacral regions of the spine

kyphotic posture A posture characterized by an exaggerated posterior curvature of the thoracic spine; syn: **humpback, round back**

L

labor The physiologic process by which the uterus contracts and expels the products of conception after 20 or more weeks of gestation

load-resisting exercise Any exercise in which a load or a weight producing an external force resists the internal force generated by a muscle as it contracts

lobectomy Surgical removal of a lobe of a lung

lordosis An anterior convexity in the spinal column. An anterior curve is secondary or compensatory and occurs in the cervical and lumbar spinal regions as the spine of a young child adapts to the upright position

lordotic posture A posture characterized by an increase in the lumbosacral angle, causing an increased lumbar lordosis, anterior pelvic tilt, and hip flexion

lung compliance Refers to the distensibility or elastic recoil of lung tissue

lymphedema Excessive accumulation of extravascular and extracellular fluid in tissue spaces

M

manipulation/mobilization Passive, skilled manual therapy techniques applied to joints and related soft tissues at varying speeds and amplitudes using physiologic or accessory motions, for therapeutic purposes

mastectomy Removal of a breast

maximal aerobic power (max $\dot{V}O_2$) The maximum volume of oxygen consumed per unit of time

maximal heart rate reserve (HRR) The difference between the resting heart rate and the maximum heart rate

mediastinal shift Asymmetric positioning of the trachea, palpable at the suprasternal notch

meniscectomy An intra-articular procedure at the knee by which the meniscus (fibrocartilage) is removed surgically

metabolic equivalent (MET) The amount of oxygen required per minute under quiet resting conditions; equal to 3.5 milliliters of oxygen consumed per kilogram of body weight per minute

mobilization See **manipulation**

multiple-angle isometrics The application of resistance at multiple points in the ROM to isometric muscle contractions

muscle-setting exercise A form of isometric exercise but one not performed against any appreciable resistance; gentle static muscle contractions used to maintain mobility between muscle fibers and to decrease muscle spasm and pain

muscle soreness, acute Pain or tenderness in muscle that occurs during strenuous exercise as the muscle fatigues

muscle soreness, delayed-onset See **delayed-onset muscle soreness**

muscle spasm See **intrinsic muscle spasm**

N

nonweight-bearing bias Describes the preferred position in which the patient's symptoms are lessened when in nonweight-bearing positions such as lying down or in traction or when reducing spinal pressure by leaning on the upper extremities (using arm rests to unweight the trunk), by leaning the trunk against a support, or while in a pool. The condition is considered gravity sensitive because the symptoms are worsened during standing, walking, running, coughing, or similar activities that increase spinal pressure

O

occlusion Closure or obstruction of a vessel such as an artery or vein

open-chain exercise Exercise in which a distal segment of the body moves freely in space

orthopnea Difficulty breathing while lying supine

osteoarthritis (degenerative joint disease) A chronic degenerative disorder primarily affecting the articular cartilage with eventual bony overgrowth at the margins of the joints

osteoporosis (bone atrophy) A condition of bone that leads to a loss of bone mass, a narrowing of the bone shaft, and widening of the medullary canal

osteotomy The surgical cutting and realignment of bone to correct deformity and reduce pain

outcome measure An activity that is objectively documented and is part of the goal for therapeutic intervention

overload Stressing the body or parts of the body to levels above that normally experienced

overpressure A stretch force applied to soft tissues at the end of the ROM

overstretch A stretch beyond the normal range of motion of a joint and the surrounding soft tissues

overtraining A term synonymous with **overwork**

overuse syndromes See **cumulative trauma disorders**

overwork A phenomenon that causes temporary or permanent deterioration of strength as a result of exercise, most often observed clinically in patients with nonprogressive lower motor neuron diseases who participate in excessively vigorous resistance exercise programs. Also known as overwork weakness or **overtraining**

oxygen deficit The time period during exercise in which the level of oxygen consumption is below that necessary to supply all the ATP required for the exercise

oxygen transport system Composed of stroke volume, heart rate, and arterial-mixed venous oxygen difference

P

pacing The performance of functional activities within the available cardiopulmonary capacity

pallor Chalky white appearance or blanching of the skin

paresthesia Abnormal sensation perceived as burning, tingling, or prickling

pathologic fracture A fracture that occurs as the result of minor stresses to bone already weakened by disease (osteoporosis)

pendulum (Codman's) exercises Self-mobilization techniques that use the effects of gravity to distract the humerus from the glenoid fossa and gentle pendulum motions to move the joint surfaces

percussion A technique used with postural drainage to mobilize secretions by mechanically dislodging viscous or adherent secretions in the lungs

percussion, mediate A technique used to assess the air-to-solid ratio in the lungs

peripheral airway disease An early form of obstructive lung disease characterized by inflammation, fibrosis, and narrowing of the small airways

perturbation Displacement or disturbance of the body. Anterior/posterior and medial/lateral movement of a person, or the supporting surface under the person, is used to test and develop balance and postural reactions

phlebitis Inflammation of a vein

phosphocreatine (PC) Creatine phosphate; an energy-rich compound that plays a critical role in providing energy for muscular contraction

physiologic movement Movement that a person normally can carry out, such as flexion, extension, rotation, abduction, and adduction

plasticity The quality of soft tissue that allows it to maintain a lengthened state after a stretch force has been removed

pleural effusion The presence of fluid in the pleural cavity

pleurectomy An incision into the pleura

plyometric training High-intensity, high-velocity resistance exercise characterized by a resisted eccentric muscle contraction followed by a rapid concentric contraction and designed to increase muscular power and coordination, also known as **stretch-shortening drills**

pneumonectomy Surgical excision of lung tissue. In some instances, the term denotes removal of an entire lung

pneumonia An inflammation of the lungs characterized by consolidation and exudation; often caused by a bacterial or viral infection

pneumothorax The presence or accumulation of air in the pleural cavity

postural drainage A means of clearing the airways of secretions by placing the patient in various positions so that gravity will assist in the flow of mucus

postural dysfunction A faulty posture in which adaptive shortening of soft tissues and muscle weakness has occurred

postural fault (postural pain syndrome) A posture that deviates from normal alignment but has no structural limitations

posture A position or attitude of the body, the relative arrangement of body parts for a specific activity, or a characteristic manner of bearing one's body

power Work per unit of time (force × distance/time) or force times velocity

progressive resistance exercise (PRE) An approach to exercise whereby the load or resistance to the muscle is applied by some mechanical means and is quantitatively and progressively increased over time

pulmonary edema An infiltration of fluid (serum) in the lungs

pumping exercises Active repetitive exercises, usually of the ankles or wrists, performed to maintain or improve circulation in the extremities

Q

Q angle The angle formed by intersecting lines drawn from the anterior-superior iliac spine through the midportion of the patella and from the anterior tibial tuberosity through the midpatella. The norm is 15 degrees

quadriceps lag A term synonymous with **extensor lag** of the knee

R

rales A term used synonymously with **crackles**

range of motion (ROM) The amount of angular motion allowed at the joint between any two bony levers

range of motion, active (AROM) Movement within the unrestricted ROM for a segment that is produced by an active contraction of the muscles crossing that joint

range of motion, active-assistive (A-AROM) A type of active ROM in which assistance is provided by an outside force, either manually or mechanically, because the prime-mover muscles need assistance to complete the motion

range of motion, passive (PROM) Movement within the unrestricted ROM for a segment that is produced entirely by an external force. There is no voluntary muscle contraction

Raynaud's disease A functional vasospasm of the small arteries, particularly in the hands, caused by an abnormality of the sympathetic nervous system

reflex muscle guarding The prolonged contraction of a muscle in response to a painful stimulus. Guarding ceases when the pain is relieved but may progress to muscle spasm

reflux A backward or return flow of urine back toward the kidneys from the bladder

relaxation A conscious effort to relieve tension in muscles

relaxed (slouched) posture Also called **sway back posture.** A posture characterized by a shifting of the pelvic segment anteriorly, resulting in hip extension, and shifting of the thoracic segment posteriorly, resulting in flexion of the thorax on the upper lumbar spine. An increased lordosis in the lower lumbar region, an increased kyphosis in the thoracic region, and a forward head are usually observed with relaxed posture

repetition maximum (RM) The greatest amount of weight a muscle can move through the range of motion a specific number of times in a load-resisting exercise routine

residual volume (RV) The amount of air that is left in the lungs after a maximum expiration

resistance exercise Any form of active exercise in which a dynamic or static muscular contraction is resisted by an outside force

resistance exercise, manual A type of active exercise in which resistance is provided by a therapist or other health professional to either a dynamic or static muscular contraction

resistance exercise, mechanical A type of active exercise in which resistance is applied through the use of equipment or mechanical apparatus

resistance exercise, variable A form of dynamic exercise carried out using equipment that varies the resistance to the contracting muscle throughout the ROM

respiration, external The exchange of gas at the alveolar capillary membrane and the pulmonary capillaries

respiration, internal The exchange of gas between the pulmonary capillaries and the cells of the surrounding tissues

respiratory resistance training The use of resistance to improve the strength or endurance of the muscles of ventilation; used interchangeably with ventilatory muscle training and inspiratory or expiratory resistance training.

resting position The position of the joint in which there is maximum laxity in the capsule and surrounding structures

rheumatoid arthritis A chronic connective tissue disease that is often systemic; characterized by inflammation of synovial joints with periods of exacerbation and remission

rhonchi The former term used to describe **wheezes**

rhythmic stabilization A form of isometric exercise in which manual resistance is applied to one side of a proximal joint, then to the other; no movement occurs as the individual stabilizes against the antagonistic forces

round-back posture A posture characterized by an increased thoracic curve, protracted scapulae, and a forward head

rubor Redness of the skin associated with inflammation

S

scaption Elevation of the humerus in the plane of the scapula that is 30 to 45 degrees anterior to the frontal plane; also called scapular plane abduction

scoliosis An abnormal lateral curvature of the vertebral column

scoliosis, functional A nonstructural reversible lateral curvature of the spine, also called nonstructural or postural scoliosis

scoliosis, structural An irreversible lateral curvature of the spine with fixed rotation of the vertebrae

selective tension The administration of specific tests in a systematic manner to determine whether the site of a lesion is in an inert structure (joint capsule, ligament, bursa, fascia, dura mater, or dural sheath around nerve roots) or in a contractile unit (muscle with its tendons and attachments)

self-mobilizing Techniques whereby the patient is taught to apply joint mobilization techniques to restricted joints using proper gliding techniques

self-stretching Techniques whereby the patient is taught to stretch a joint or soft tissue passively by using another part of the body for applying the stretch force

setting exercise See **muscle-setting exercise**

short-arc extension (terminal extension) exercise Active or active-resisted extension of a joint through the final degrees of its range of motion; most often applied to the knee from 35 degrees flexion to full extension

slow-twitch (ST) fiber A skeletal muscle fiber with a slow reaction time and a high aerobic capacity, suitable for tonic muscle activity

specificity of training The principle underlying the development of a training program for a specific activity or skill and the primary energy systems involved during performance

sprain Severe stress, stretch, or tear of soft tissues such as joint capsule, ligament, tendon, or muscle

stability The synergistic coordination of muscle contractions around a joint that provides a stable base for movement

stabilization exercise A form of exercise designed to develop control of proximal areas of the body in a stable, symptom-free position in response to fluctuating resistance loads. Exercises begin very easy so that control is maintained, and they progress in duration, intensity, speed, and variety. Often called **dynamic stabilization** exercise

static traction A steady traction force applied and maintained for an extended time interval. It may be continuous (prolonged) or sustained

steady state Pertaining to the time period during which a physiologic function remains at a constant value

strain Overstretching, overexertion, overuse of soft tissue; tends to be less severe than a sprain; occurs from slight trauma or unaccustomed repeated trauma of a minor degree. This term also refers to the amount of deformation that occurs in tissues when a stress is applied

strength The force output of a contracting muscle. It is directly related to the amount of tension a contracting muscle can produce

stress A load or force applied to tissues per unit area

stress testing A multistage test that determines the cardiovascular functional capacity of the individual

stretch-shortening drills A term synonymous with **plyometric training**

stretch weakness The weakening of muscles that are habitually kept in a stretched position beyond their physiologic resting length

stretching Any therapeutic maneuver designed to lengthen (elongate) pathologically shortened soft tissue structures and thereby to increase range of motion

stretching, cyclic A repeated passive stretch usually applied by a mechanical device

stretching, passive A type of mobility exercise in which manual, mechanical, or positional stretch is applied to soft tissues and in which the force is applied opposite to the direction of shortening

stretching, selective The process of stretching some muscle groups while selectively allowing others to adaptively shorten to improve function in a patient with paralysis

stretching, self See **self-stretching**

stroke volume The amount of blood pumped out of the ventricles with each contraction (systole)

subluxation An incomplete or partial dislocation that often involves secondary trauma to surrounding soft tissue

sway-back posture See **relaxed (slouched) posture**

synovectomy Surgical removal of the synovium (lining of the joint) in patients with chronic joint swelling

synovitis Inflammation of a synovial membrane; an excess of normal synovial tissue and fluid within a joint or tendon sheath

T

target heart rate A predetermined heart rate to be obtained during exercise

tendinitis Scarring or calcium deposits in a tendon

tendinosis Degeneration of a tendon from repetitive microtrauma; collagen degeneration without inflammation

tendon-gliding exercises Exercises designed to maintain or develop mobility between the multijoint-musculotendinous units and other connective tissue structures in the wrist and hand; also used to develop neuromuscular control and coordinated movement

tenosynovectomy Surgical removal of proliferated synovium from tendon sheaths

tenosynovitis An inflammation of the synovial sheath covering a tendon

tenovaginitis A thickening of a tendon sheath

terminal extension See **short-arc extension**

thoracotomy Any surgical cutting of the chest wall

thromboangiitis obliterans (Buerger's disease) An inflammatory reaction and subsequent vasospasm of the arteries as a result of exposure to nicotine

thrombophlebitis An inflammatory occlusion of a deep or superficial vein with a thrombus

thrombosis The formation of a clot in a blood vessel

thrombus A blood clot

tidal volume (TV) The amount of air that a person breathes in and breathes out during a relaxed inspiration and expiration

total lung capacity (TLC) The total amount of air in the lungs; the vital capacity plus the residual volume

traction The process of drawing or pulling

transfer of training Carryover of the effects of an exercise program from one mode of exercise or performance to another. Also known as cross-training

transitional stabilization A stabilization technique whereby the functional position of the spine is stabilized by the trunk muscles while the body moves from one position to another. This requires graded contractions and adjustments between the trunk flexor and extensor muscles

V

Valsalva maneuver An expiratory effort against a closed glottis

vasoconstriction Narrowing of a blood vessel because of contraction of smooth muscle in the walls of the vessels, resulting in a decrease in blood flow

velocity spectrum rehabilitation Isokinetic exercises performed over a wide range of exercise speeds

ventilation The movement or mass exchange of air in and out of the body

ventilatory muscle training (VMT) The process of improving the strength or endurance of the muscles of ventilation, usually the inspiratory muscles

vibration A technique of rapid shaking with small amplitude used with postural drainage to mobilize secretions

vital capacity (VC) The greatest amount of air that a person can inspire and expire

W

wheezes Abnormal breath sounds heard during exhalation characterized by high- or low-pitched sounds or musical tones; formerly called **rhonchi**

Index

A

B

I

J

M

S

T

U